PATHOLOGY
for the PHYSICAL THERAPIST ASSISTANT

Second Edition

CATHERINE CAVALLARO GOODMAN, PT, MBA, CBT
Private Practice
Missoula, Montana

KENDA S. FULLER, PT, NCS
ABPTS Board Certified Specialist in Neurologic Physical Therapy
Co-owner South Valley Physical Therapy, PC
Denver, Colorado
Invited Lecturer, Physical Therapy Program
University of Colorado Health Sciences Center
Denver, Colorado

ASSOCIATE EDITOR **CHARLENE MARSHALL**, BS, PTA
Formerly Physical Therapist Assistant Program Faculty
Great Falls College
Montana State University
Great Falls, Montana

ELSEVIER

ELSEVIER

3251 Riverport Lane
St. Louis, Missouri 63043

Content Strategy Director: Penny Rudolph
Content Development Manager: Jolynn Gower
Senior Content Development Specialist: Courtney Sprehe
Publishing Services Manager: Julie Eddy
Senior Project Manager: David Stein
Design Direction: Ashley Miner

Printed in China

Last digit is the print number: 9 8 7 6 5 4 3 2

Working together
to grow libraries in
developing countries

www.elsevier.com • www.bookaid.org

Charlene Marshall, BS, PTA
Formerly Physical Therapist Assistant
  Program Faculty
Great Falls College
Montana State University
Great Falls, Montana

Sue Queen, PT, PhD
Associate Professor Emeritus
Division of Physical Therapy
University of New Mexico
Albuquerque, New Mexico

Carolyn Heather Senn, BSPH, PTA, CHES
Health Educator
Las Vegas, Nevada

CONTRIBUTORS TO THE FIRST EDITION

Stefanie L. Cozad, PT, NCS CCCE
Out Patient Staff Physical Therapist
Frye Regional Medical Center
Hickory, North Carolina
*Introduction to Central Nervous System
Disorders; Degenerative Diseases of the
Central Nervous System*

David J. Diers, EdD, PT, MHS, ATC
Professor
Governors State University
College of Health Professions
Department of Physical Therapy
University Park, Illinois
*Introduction to Pathology of the Musculoskel-
etal System*

Kenda S. Fuller, PT, NCS
ABPTS Board Certified Specialist in Neuro-
logic Physical Therapy
Co-owner South Valley Physical Therapy, PC
Denver, Colorado
Invited Lecturer, Physical Therapy Program
University of Colorado Health Sciences
Center
Denver, Colorado
*Introduction to Central Nervous System
Disorders; Infectious Disorders of the
Central Nervous System; Degenerative
Diseases of the Central Nervous System;
Stroke; Traumatic Brain Injury; Traumatic
Spinal Cord Injury; Epilepsy; Headache;
Vestibular Disorders*

Allan M. Glanzman, PT, DPT, PCS
Co-Chair, Research and Scientific Review
Committees
Physical Therapy Department
The Children's Hospital of Philadelphia
Philadelphia, Pennsylvania
*Genetic and Developmental Disorders;
Cerebral Palsy*

Catherine C. Goodman, PT, MBA, CBP
Private Practice
Missoula, Montana
*Introduction to the Concepts of Pathology;
Problems Affecting Multiple Systems;
Injury and Inflammation; The Immune
System; Infectious Disease; Oncology; The
Integumentary System; The Endocrine and
Metabolic Systems; The Cardiovascular
System; The Hematologic System; The
Respiratory System; The Hepatic, Pancre-
atic, and Biliary Systems; Introduction to
Pathology of the Musculoskeletal System;
Infectious Diseases of the Musculoskeletal
System; Musculoskeletal Neoplasms; Bone,
Joint, and Soft Tissue Diseases and Disor-
ders; Behavioral, Social, and Environmen-
tal Factors Contributing to Disease and
Dysfunction; The Psychosocial-Spiritual
Impact on Health Care; Environmental
and Occupational Medicine; The Gastro-
intestinal System; The Renal and Urologic
Systems; The Male Genital or Reproductive
System; The Female Genital or Reproduc-
tive System; Laboratory Tests and Values*

Ira Gorman, PT, MSPH
Assistant Dean/Associate Professor
Department of Physical Therapy
Rueckert-Hartman College for Health
Professions
Regis University
Denver, Colorado
*Behavioral, Social, and Environmental Factors
Contributing to Disease and Dysfunction*

Donna S. Hurley, PT, DPT
Research Assistant Professor
Department of Physical Therapy and Human
Movement Sciences
Northwestern University
Chicago, Illinois
*The Integumentary System: The Renal and
Urologic Systems; The Male Genital or
Reproductive System; The Female Genital
or Reproductive System*

**Elizabeth (Beth) Ikeda, PT, DPT, MTC,
OCS**
Professor Emeritus of Physical Therapy and
Rehabilitation Sciences
University of Montana
Missoula, Montana
The Respiratory System

Glenn L. Irion, PhD, PT, CWS
Professor
Department of Physical Therapy
Emory & Henry College
Emory, Virginia
Laboratory Tests and Values

Zoher F. Kapasi, PT, PhD, MBA
Director and Associate Professor
Division of Physical Therapy
Department of Rehabilitation Medicine
Emory University School of Medicine
Atlanta, Georgia
The Immune System

Laura Kelley, PT
Rehabilitation Manager
Adventist La Grange Hospital
La Grange, Illinois
*The Hepatic, Pancreatic, and Biliary Systems;
The Gastrointestinal System*

Michele Komp, PT, PTA, MPT, DPT
Dove Healthcare
Eleva, Wisconsin
*Problems Affecting Multiple Systems; The
Immune System; Infectious Disease;
Oncology; The Endocrine and Metabolic
Systems; The Cardiovascular System;
Cerebral Palsy: The Peripheral Nervous
System; Behavioral, Social, and
Environmental Factors Contributing to
Disease and Dysfunction; Environmental
and Occupational Medicine; Headache;
Vestibular Disorders; Laboratory Tests and
Values*

Sharon M. Konecne, MHS, PT
National Oncology Rehabilitation Consultant and Lecturer
Clinician Denver Visiting Nurses Association
Affiliate Faculty Physical Therapy Program
Regis University
Denver, Colorado;
Lecturer Physical Therapy Program
University of Colorado
Denver, Colorado
Central Nervous System Neoplasms

Harriett B. Loehne, PT, DPT, CWS, FCCWS
Harriett B. Loehne & Associates
WISE: Wound & Integumentary Specialty Education
President, Academy of Clinical Electrophysiology and Wound Management
American Physical Therapy Association
Thomasville, Georgia
The Integumentary System

Nicole Marquardt, MS, PT
Physical Therapist
Mayo Clinic Health System
Eau Claire, Wisconsin
Infectious Diseases of the Musculoskeletal System; Musculoskeletal Neoplasms

Jane Morse, PT, DPT, GCS
Adjunct Professor
Physical Therapy Assistant Program
South College
Asheville, North Carolina
Central Nervous System Neoplasms

Roberta Kuchler O'Shea, PT, PhD
Professor
Physical Therapy Department
Governors State University
University Park, Illinois
Introduction to the Concepts of Pathology; Genetic and Developmental Disorders

Celeste Peterson, MD
Medical Consultant
Missoula, Montana
Problems Affecting Multiple Systems; Infectious Disease; The Hematologic System; The Hepatic, Pancreatic, and Biliary Systems; The Renal and Urologic Systems

Tim Rylander, PT, MPT
Adjunct Professor
Program in Physical Therapy
Governors State University
University Park, Illinois
The Hematologic System

Susan A. Scherer, PT, PhD
Associate Dean/Professor
Department of Physical Therapy
Rueckert-Hartman College for Health Professions
Regis University
Denver, Colorado
Behavioral, Social, and Environmental Factors Contributing to Disease and Dysfunction

Donnalee Milette Shain, PT, MS, DPT
Physical Therapist
Braintree Rehabilitation
Milford, Massachusetts
Infectious Disorders of the Central Nervous System; Stroke: Traumatic Brain Injury; Traumatic Spinal Cord Injury; The Psychosocial-Spiritual Impact on Health Care: Epilepsy

Irina V. Smirnova, PhD
Director, PhD in Rehabilitation Science Program
Associate Professor
Department of Physical Therapy and Rehabilitation Science
University of Kansas Medical Center
Kansas City, Kansas
The Cardiovascular System

Marcia B. Smith, DPT, PhD, FAPTA
Professor
Department of Physical Therapy
Rueckert-Hartman College for Health Professions
Regis University
Denver, Colorado
The Peripheral Nervous System

Dawn M. Stackowicz, PT, MS, CCS
Physical Therapist
Stroger Hospital of Cook County
Chicago, Illinois
The Respiratory System

Ann M. Vendrely, PT, EdD, DPT
Associate Provost/Professor of Physical Therapy
Office of the Provost
Governors State University
University Park, Illinois
Bone, Joint, and Soft Tissue Diseases and Disorders

Patricia A. Winkler, PT, DSc, NCS
Assistant Professor (retired) and Affiliate
Department of Physical Therapy
Regis University
Denver, Colorado
Degenerative Diseases of the Central Nervous System

Bonnie Yost, PT, LCCE
Physical Therapist
Centennial, Colorado
The Psychosocial-Spiritual Impact on Health Care

Martha Y. Zimmerman, PT, MA
PTA Program Director/ACCE
Physical Therapist Assistant Program
Caldwell Community College and Technical Institute
Hudson, North Carolina
Injury and Inflammation

PREFACE

The second edition of *Pathology for the Physical Therapist Assistant* is possible because of the tremendous support from physical therapist assistant (PTA) educators and the PTA community.

The foundation of this book remains the same, providing concise information regarding disease processes and systemic disorders. While the demand continues to grow for the PTA to be educated in making sound clinical decisions, the role of the PTA also continues to progress and change according to the needs of today's health care environment. This demand places stress on the educators to fit more information into an already packed curriculum while leaving the PTA students hungry for more physical therapy treatment ideas specific to the expectations placed on them in a clinical setting.

I believe that the updated material in this text builds on the vision that Robbie O'Shea and her team of experts had to create a special text that would provide the PTA with the essential tools required to assist the physical therapist in treating patients effectively and competently. Each chapter has a new look, with **vocab builders** and **chapter objectives** added to help streamline the classroom experience for both students and instructors. More emphasis has been placed on presenting the information in practical terms, with a focus on the role of the PTA. The **Special Implications for the PTA** boxes continue to be a strength of the text, offering practical information in an easy-to-read format.

The new addition on Evolve of clinical scenarios and critical thinking questions for each chapter provides further learning opportunities for the reader to build critical knowledge of pathology. As Catherine Goodman stated in the previous edition, "The PTA who has a good background in the underlying pathology of diseases will be able to ask appropriate questions, recognize patients' responses and tolerance, and more readily see the need to change or progress therapeutic exercise programs. All of these advanced competencies improve the contribution PTAs make to health care in general and, more specifically, to the physical therapist and individual patient care."

Charlene M. Marshall

Special Implications for the PTA

4.5 Special Implications for the PTA: Hypersensitivity Disorders

Type IV reactions may occur in response to lanolin added to lotions, ultrasound gels, or other preparations used in massage or soft tissue mobilization, necessitating careful observation of all people for delayed skin reactions to any of these substances.

With the first exposure, no reaction necessarily occurs but antigens are formed, and on subsequent exposures, hypersensitivity reactions are triggered. Anyone with known hypersensitivity should have a small area of skin tested before use of large amounts of topical agents in the therapy setting. Careful observation throughout treatment is recommended.

Beginning in the 1980s, the use of latex gloves to protect health care workers against exposure to blood and body fluids increased. Since then, the number of reported cases of latex sensitivity also has increased. Reactions to latex range from contact dermatitis (type IV hypersensitivity) to anaphylactic shock (type I hypersensitivity).

PTAs who are allergic to latex should avoid contact with latex gloves and other products that contain latex. Use of low-powder, powder-free, and nonlatex gloves provides PTAs with a strategy for preventing exposure to latex allergens.[86]

Incorporated throughout the text, the **Special Implications for the PTA** boxes give you a starting point when addressing a particular condition for the first time. In addition, you can easily reference these sections when working with patients.

Medical Management

Medical Management

Differentiating an ADE from underlying disease requires a thorough history, especially when a symptom appears 1 to 2 months after a medication regimen has been started. Monitoring blood cell counts, liver enzymes, electrolytes, blood urea nitrogen (BUN), and creatinine is indicated for certain drugs. Digoxin and other cardiotropic drugs cause arrhythmias that require electrocardiographic monitoring. With dose-related ADEs, dose modification is usually all that is required, whereas with non–dose-related ADEs, the drug therapy is usually stopped and reexposure avoided.

The **Medical Management** sections, set off for easy recognition within the text, address diagnosis, treatment, and prognosis for each condition discussed.

Question Icon

Question Icons are included throughout the text to indicate when there is an accompanying critical thinking question and/or case scenario on Evolve.

Pedagogy

CHAPTER OBJECTIVES

1. Understand the role of the study of pathology in the field of physical therapy.
2. Introduce health and disease as concepts, variables that affect human health, and theories of health.
3. Understand the differences between incidence and prevalence, acute and chronic.
4. Understand the relevance of enablement/disablement for the field of physical therapy.
5. Understand the relevance of health promotion and disease prevention in the field of physical therapy.

OUTLINE

Chapter Objectives, Outlines, and **Vocab Builders** set the stage by framing the information to be presented in the chapter. They also serve as "checkpoints" to which you can refer to ensure content comprehension and study for examinations.

VOCAB BUILDERS

Complex problem solving	Functional symptoms	Narcissistic
Compliance	Immunotics	Noncompliance
Disability	Information processing	Organic symptoms
DNA	Learning disability	RNA
Executive function	Memory deficit	Stoic

ACKNOWLEDGMENTS

I have to begin by saying that the first person that I would like to acknowledge is Catherine Goodman for your support and belief in me to take on this project. You are always there for me with words of encouragement and wisdom. I have learned so much from you and look forward to learning more. Thank you for being such a wonderful mentor and friend.

To the editorial staff at Elsevier: Kathy Falk, Courtney Sprehe, David Stein, and Suzi Epstein. Thank you for all your hard work, for your detail-oriented "eagle eyes," and most importantly for teaching me so much along the way.

A special thank you to Heather Senn for all your hard work and terrific ideas on the Evolve materials and chapter objectives. You helped make this book even better than it already was.

And finally, a very special thank you to Robbie O'Shea and the contributors to the first edition; without all of you this second edition would not be possible. Thank you for all your countless hours of hard work to develop an awesome text that will forever benefit the PTA. I hope that you find the updates in this edition useful and worthy of your efforts.

Charlene M. Marshall

CONTENTS

Introduction to Concepts of Pathology

CHAPTER OBJECTIVES

1. Understand the role of the study of pathology in the field of physical therapy.
2. Introduce health and disease as concepts, variables that affect human health, and theories of health.
3. Understand the differences between incidence and prevalence, acute and chronic.
4. Understand the relevance of enablement/disablement for the field of physical therapy.
5. Understand the relevance of health promotion and disease prevention in the field of physical therapy.

OUTLINE

VOCAB BUILDERS

Complex problem solving
Compliance
Disability
DNA
Executive function

Functional symptoms
Immunotics
Information processing
Learning disability
Memory deficit

Narcissistic
Noncompliance
Organic symptoms
RNA
Stoic

PATHOGENESIS OF DISEASE

Pathology is defined as the branch of medicine that investigates the essential nature of disease, especially changes in body tissues and organs that cause or are caused by disease.[23] *Clinical pathology* in medicine refers to pathology applied to the solution of clinical problems, especially the use of laboratory methods in clinical diagnosis. *Pathogenesis* is the development of unhealthy conditions or disease or more specifically, the cellular events and reactions and other pathological mechanisms that occur in the development of disease.

This text examines the pathogenesis of each disease or condition—that is, the progression of each pathological condition both at its cellular level and with regard to its clinical presentation whenever signs and symptoms are manifested. For the physical therapist assistant (PTA), *clinical pathology* has a different meaning with regard to the effects of pathological processes (i.e., disease) on the individual's functional abilities and limitations. The relationship between impairment and functional limitation is the key focus in therapy.

In addition, how the person with the pathological condition is able to participate in his or her family and community is paramount. Current clinical practice should include an emphasis on the person's activity level, participation, level of supports, and environment. Thus despite the disease process and related loss of function, the whole person must be considered.

Advances in medicine have resulted in a population with greater longevity but also with a more complex pathological picture. Orthopedic and neurological conditions are no longer present as singular phenomena; they often occur in a person with other medical pathology. As health care professionals, we must be knowledgeable about the impact other conditions and diseases have on the individual's neuromusculoskeletal system and the necessary steps that must be taken to provide safe, effective treatment.

Recently the profession has moved toward using the World Health Organization (WHO) International Classification of Functioning, Disability, and Health (ICF) to describe the impact of a pathology on a person's lifestyle and plan of care. This model expands on the previous disablement model by also considering the individual's participation and environmental constraints or supports. Throughout the book, we will describe certain scenarios using the WHO ICF model.

CONCEPTS OF HEALTH, ILLNESS, AND DISABILITY

Health

Many people and organizations have attempted to define the concept of health, but no universally accepted definition has been adopted. A dictionary definition describes health in terms of an individual's ability to function normally in society. Some definitions characterize health as a disease-free state or condition. WHO[33] has defined *health* as a state of complete physical, mental, and social well-being and not merely as the absence of disease or infirmity. All of these definitions present health as an either–or circumstance, meaning an individual is either healthy or ill.

Health is more accurately viewed as a continuum; wellness, on one end, is the optimal level of function and illness, on the other, may be so unfavorable as to result in death. Health is a dynamic process that varies with changes in interactions between an individual and the internal and external environments. This type of definition recognizes health as an individual's level of wellness.

Health reflects a person's biologic, psychologic, spiritual, and sociologic state. The *biologic* or *physical state* refers to the overall structure of the individual's body tissues and organs and to the biochemical interactions and functions within the body. The *psychologic* state includes the individual's mood, emotions, and personality.

The *spiritual* aspect of health addresses the individual's religious needs, which may be affected by illness or injury. The spiritual dimension in health care focuses on the integration of mind, body, and spirit, with the goal of promoting whole-person healing. The *sociologic* or *social state* refers to the interaction between the individual and the social environment. A high level of wellness or holistic health is achieved when the biopsychosocial–spiritual needs of a person are met.

Illness

Definition

Illness is often defined as sickness or deviation from a healthy state, and the term has a broader meaning than disease. *Webster's Dictionary* defines illness as "an unhealthy condition of mind or body." *Disease* refers to a biologic or psychologic alteration that results in a malfunction of a body organ or system. The term *disease* usually describes a biomedical condition that is substantiated by objective data such as elevated temperature or the presence of infection (as demonstrated by positive blood cultures). *Webster's* describes disease as: "an impairment of the normal state of the living animal or plant body or one of its parts that interrupts or modifies the performance of the vital functions, is typically manifested by distinguishing signs and symptoms, and is a response to environmental factors (e.g., malnutrition, industrial hazards, or climate), to specific infective agents (as worms, bacteria, or viruses), to inherent defects of the organism (as genetic anomalies), or to combinations of these factors."

Illness is the perception and response of the person to not being well. Illness includes disturbances in normal human biological function and personal, interpersonal, and cultural reactions to disease. Disease can occur in an individual without that person being aware of illness and without others perceiving illness, and a person can feel very ill even though no obvious pathological processes can be identified.

Incidence and Prevalence

When various diseases, disorders, and conditions are discussed, incidence and prevalence may be reported. *Incidence* is the number of new cases of a condition in a specific period of time (e.g., 6 months or 1 year) in relation to the total number of people in the population who are "at risk" at the beginning of the period. *Prevalence* measures all cases of a condition (new and old) among those at risk for developing the condition. Measures of prevalence are made at one point in time (e.g., on a specific day).

Natural History

The natural history of a condition, disorder, or disease describes how it progresses over time. The natural history of some conditions, such as cancer, can be judged based on the stage of the tumor at the diagnosis and the response to treatment. Scientists are actively engaged in identifying *predictive factors* that help tell what the patient/client's prognosis and outcome might be. In medicine, predictive factors (both negative and positive) are the closest thing we have to a crystal ball.

Even with known predictive factors, the natural history is not always clear; predicting what is going to happen and when it is going to happen can have wide or narrow margins, depending on the condition. For example, individuals with some forms of muscular dystrophy have a more predictive natural history, whereas individuals with cerebral palsy may not be so easy to gauge, especially during the early years of growth and development.

The PTA must maintain a plan of care keeping in mind the natural history of the condition and where the individual is in the lifespan or life stage. Some thought should be given to dovetailing our view of impairments, dysfunctions, and disabilities with the natural history of the disease, condition, or illness. This is particularly important when working with individuals who have degenerative, progressive, or chronic neurological conditions.

Improvements in treatment for neurological and other conditions that previously were considered fatal (e.g., cancer, cystic fibrosis) are now extending the life expectancy for many individuals. Improved interventions bring new areas of focus, such as quality-of-life issues. With some conditions (e.g., muscular dystrophy, cerebral palsy), the artificial dichotomy of pediatric versus adult care is gradually being replaced by a lifestyle approach that takes into consideration what is known about the natural history of the condition.

Many individuals with childhood-onset diseases now live well into adulthood. For them, their original pathology or disease process has given way to secondary impairments. These secondary impairments create further limitation and issues as the person ages. For instance, a 30-year-old with cerebral palsy may experience chronic pain, changes or limitations in ambulation and endurance, and increased fatigue. These symptoms result from the atypical movement patterns and musculoskeletal strains caused by chronic increase in tone and muscle imbalances that were caused by cerebral palsy originally. In this case the therapy would not be focused on decreasing the primary signs and symptoms of cerebral palsy but instead would focus on the issues that have developed as a result of the cerebral palsy.

Acute Illness

Acute illness usually refers to an illness or disease that has a relatively rapid onset and short duration; it is not synonymous with "severe." The condition often responds to a specific treatment and is usually self-limiting, although exceptions to this definition are numerous. If no complications occur, most acute illnesses end in a full recovery and the individual returns to the previous level of functioning.

Subacute refers to how long a disease has been present, but there is no set time that divides subacute from the other time descriptions (i.e., acute and chronic). Subacute describes a time course that is between acute and chronic. A symptom that is subacute has been present for longer than a few days but less than several months. Chronic conditions sometimes flare up and may be referred to as subacute.

Acute illnesses usually follow a specific sequence, or stages of illness, from onset through recovery. The first stage involves the development of physical symptoms (e.g., pain, shortness of breath, fever), cognitive awareness (i.e., the symptoms are interpreted to have meaning), and an emotional response, usually one of denial, fear, or anxiety.

Subsequent stages of an acute illness may include assumption of a sick role as the person recognizes the problem as being sufficient to require contact with a health care professional. If the illness is confirmed, the individual continues in the sick role; if it is not confirmed, a return to normalcy may occur, or the person may continue to seek health care to identify the illness.

A stage of dependency occurs when the person receives and accepts a diagnosis and treatment plan. This type of dependency in the psychologically and emotionally balanced person represents awareness, acceptance, reliance on diagnosis, and care beyond self-help. This definition of dependency differs from dependency associated with dependent personality disorder, in which the affected person lacks self-confidence or the ability to function independently and allows others to assume responsibility for his or her care. Depending on the severity of the illness, the individual may give up independence and control and assume a more dependent sick role. During this stage, sick people often become more passive and concerned about themselves.

Most people move from acute or subacute to the final stage of recovery or rehabilitation. During this stage the individual gives up the sick role and resumes more normal activities and responsibilities. Individuals with long-term or chronic illnesses may require a longer period to adjust to new lifestyles.

Chronic Illness

Chronic illness describes illnesses that include one or more of the following characteristics: permanent impairment or *disability*, residual physical or cognitive disability, and the need for special rehabilitation and/or long-term medical management. Chronic illnesses and conditions may fluctuate in intensity as acute exacerbations occur that cause physiologic instability and necessitate additional medical management (e.g., diabetes mellitus, fibromyalgia, rheumatoid arthritis). A person who has exacerbations of chronic illness may progress through the stages of illness described in the previous section. Often in rehabilitation the person must adjust to not "getting better" but "getting different," especially after a life-changing illness.

Psychologic Aspects

One of the most important factors influencing psychologic reactions to illness is the premorbid (before illness) psychologic profile of the affected person. For example, a person with a dependent-type personality may become very dependent, perhaps seeking unusually large amounts of advice or reassurance from the health care specialist or expecting attention beyond that required for the degree of illness present. A *narcissistic* (self-centered) person may be particularly concerned about the need to take medication or the loss of the ability to work. The *stoic* person (indifferent to or unaffected by pain) may have difficulty admitting to being sick at all.

Other factors that affect a person's psychologic reaction include the extent of the illness and the particular symptoms that develop. Extremely mild disease may have little effect, whereas completely unexpected and debilitating illness may be very distressing. A common reaction to any illness is fear or anxiety related to the loss of control over one's own body. Denial is an unconscious defense mechanism that allows a person to avoid painful reality for as long as possible. Denial can be a natural part of the process of dealing with illness, which culminates in acceptance.

Noncompliance with treatment may have a psychologic basis (e.g., denial: "There is nothing wrong with me, so I do not need medical treatment"), but it may also occur as a result of previous experience. For example, noncompliance with prescribed corticosteroid therapy may be based on an aversion to side effects experienced during use of this drug in a previous disease flare-up. With chronic autoimmune diseases (e.g., connective tissue diseases), denial may continue for years as a coping mechanism for individuals who continue to decline in physical functional capacity.

It is important to recognize that psychologic or psychiatric symptoms—such as impairment of memory, personality changes (e.g., paranoia), loss of impulse control, or mood disorders (e.g., persistent depression or elation)—can have a functional or organic basis. *Functional symptoms* occur without significant physical dysfunction of brain cells, whereas *organic symptoms* can be caused by abnormal physiologic changes in brain tissue. An example of a functional symptom is depression that is considered to be the psychologic consequence of a general medical condition (e.g., myocardial infarction).

Organic symptoms occur as a direct physiological consequence of a medication or medical condition. For example, onset of corticosteroid-induced psychologic symptoms is often dose related, and symptoms subside as the corticosteroids are tapered. Another example of an organic basis for symptomatology is someone with systemic lupus erythematosus who experiences symptoms of organic mental disorders secondary to systemic lupus erythematosus–mediated vasculitis, called *lupus cerebritis,* or someone with end-stage liver disease who develops hepatic encephalopathy when toxic substances in the blood, such as ammonia, reach the brain.

Disability

Disability is a large public health problem in the United States. According to the 2000 U.S. Census, 50 million people report experiencing a disabling condition. This figure illustrates that nearly 20% of the U.S. population currently lives with a disability. Prevalence of disability is higher in men than in women under age 65 and higher in women than in men over age 65. People 65 years of age and older report the highest incidence of disability (40% to 43% of the age group). One of the national health goals for 2020 is to eliminate health disparities among different segments of the population, including among people with disabilities. National estimates of disability range from 15% to 20% for adults over the age of 18 years, but these figures are most likely underestimated and do not account for severity or duration of disability.[8]

Disability can be viewed from a biopsychosocial model, which incorporates and integrates the traditional medical model with the less stringent and more flexible social model of disability. The medical model confines disability as a descriptor of the affected individual. In this context, disability requires intervention by others (usually health care providers) to correct the problem. The social model of disability is more likely to see an unaccommodating environment and lack of social response to individuals with disabilities as the problem, which requires a social or political response.[19]

Classification Models

Many contemporary models have been proposed to describe disability classifications and give us a framework for identifying the consequences of diseases, disorders, and injuries.[18]

Individually, none of these models focuses on what or how the person with a disability experiences his or her problems. The American Physical Therapy Association's (APTA) adoption of the ICF helps physical therapists avoid some of the pitfalls associated with other models of disability. The ICF can be used to more accurately identify and address the multiple factors that affect and contribute to an individual's recovery. The model briefly summarized here has been incorporated into this text whenever possible.

International Classification of Functioning, Disability, and Health. The WHO framework to classify and code information about health and provide standardized language is the *International Classification of Functioning, Disability, and Health,* established in 2001. The ICF is presented as the international standard to describe and measure health, function, and ability (rather than disability) from a biopsychosocial perspective by all health care professionals. The ICF Health and Disability Model is a good framework for research from a global perspective.

Whereas traditional health indicators are based on the mortality (i.e., death) rates of populations, the ICF shifts focus to "life" (i.e., how people live with their health conditions and how these can be improved to achieve a productive and fulfilling life). The ICF model is an interactive, integrative, and universal model focused on human functioning, not disability. Most notable in the current structure is the inclusion of "host factors" that affect the behavior of the individual, such as demographic background, physical and social environments, and psychologic status. The full description of this model can be found at http://www.who.int/classifications/icf/. The ICF Health and Disability Model includes the following five components (Fig. 1.1):

- Body functions
- Body structures
- Activities and participation
- Environmental factors
- Personal factors

The ICF describes how people live with their health conditions. The ICF uses these health-related domains to describe body functions and structures and activities and participation from body, individual, and societal perspectives. Because an individual's functioning and disability occur in a context, the ICF also includes a list of environmental factors.[35]

The ICF changes our understanding of disability, no longer presenting disability as a problem of a minority group or only people who have a visible impairment or are in a wheelchair. For example, a person living with human immunodeficiency virus (HIV) infection or acquired immunodeficiency syndrome (AIDS) could be disabled in terms of his or her ability to participate actively in a profession. In that case, the ICF provides different perspectives as to how measures can be targeted to optimize that person's ability to remain in the workforce and live a full life in the community.[37]

ICF—language. The ICF introduces new "enablement" language to replace older disablement terminology that implied distinctions between individuals who are healthy and those who have disabilities. The new language defines *body functions and structures* as physiologic or psychologic functions of body systems or anatomical parts (e.g., organs, limbs). *Impairments* are defined as problems in body function or structure.

Activity is defined as the execution of specific tasks or actions by an individual. *Activity limitations* are the difficulties that an individual might have in executing activities, and *participation*

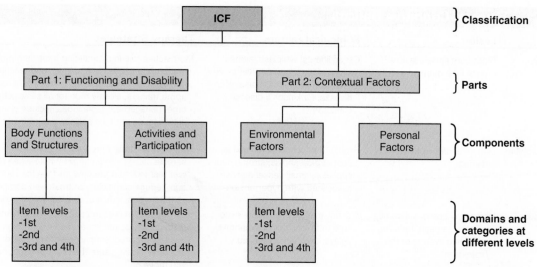

FIG. 1.1 Structure of the International Classification of Functioning, Disability, and Health (ICF). (From World Health Organization [WHO]: Principles and process for including classifications in the Family of International Classifications, Geneva, Revised 2004, WHO.)

is the individual's involvement in life situations. *Participation restrictions* are problems the individual might have in real-life situations.[18,35]

Secondary conditions or impairments of body structures can result from limitation of activity and participation. Joint contractures, disuse atrophy, and heart disease are examples of changes from inactivity. If not prevented, these changes can lead to further limitation of activity but are not part of the underlying health condition. It is important to remember that the same impairments may not result in the same extent of activity limitation—or that activity limitation may not limit the participation in a life role in the same way in two different individuals.

An example of this continuum could be described this way: A person has survived a stroke in the left side of the brain and has the impairments of hemiparesis and aphasia. This person may not be able to walk or talk but can participate in work with the assistance of a walker and communication board. On the other hand, a person who survived a stroke on the right side of the brain may be able to walk but not be able to participate in work because of loss of executive function and poor judgment.

If the first individual does not have access to a walker and communication board because of lack of funding, he or she may not be able to return to work. In many cultures, it is tradition that if a person is injured or has a medical condition, it is the responsibility of the family to provide passive or palliative care; that person may never have the opportunity to rehabilitate to full potential.

The ICF framework takes a broad biopsychosocial view that looks beyond mortality and disease to focus on how people live with their conditions.[18,19] The ICF framework promotes international exchange using a common and consistent framework and universal language to discuss disability and related phenomena.[19] The APTA has joined the WHO, the World Confederation for Physical Therapy, the American Therapeutic Recreation Association, and other organizations in endorsing the ICF model.

Cognitive Disability[32]

Although responsible for only about 1% of deaths, problems such as mental illness (including depression, alcoholism, schizophrenia, and cognitive impairments) are seriously underestimated sources of disabilities, accounting for 11% of the world's disease burden.[34] These conditions are often undiagnosed, and although therapists cannot diagnose these impairments, recognizing the deficits is important. Only cognitive disability is discussed in this section. Five types of cognitive deficit most commonly encountered by the PTA are presented here. Each one is associated with a specific area of brain damage and linked to possible causes that may be barriers to successful treatment (Table 1.1).

Executive functions may be described as cortical functions involved in formulating goals and in planning, initiating, monitoring, and maintaining behavior.[20] *Behavior* is defined here in its broadest terms to include not only overt motor behavior but also affective and social behavior. A person with executive function deficits typically appears inert or apathetic. Clinically, these clients typically have a right hemisphere lesion and apraxia, unilateral neglect, or both. When frontal lobe damage occurs, the effects of impaired executive functions may be attributed to depression. Although the two may occur simultaneously, depression is usually characterized by a lack of energy, whereas impaired executive functions are demonstrated by a lack of involvement.

Complex problem solving may be described as the effective handling of new information. Impaired problem solving results in concrete thinking, inability to distinguish the relevant from the irrelevant, erroneous application of rules, and difficulty generalizing from one situation to another. For example, when a client learns how to accomplish wheelchair transfers and then generalizes that information to various settings (bed to chair, chair to toilet, chair to car, in hospital, at home), he or she is using new information in complex problem solving.

Information processing involves the speed with which information travels from one part of the brain to another and the amount of information assimilated at that speed.[20] Whereas

TABLE 1.1   Types of Cognitive Deficits

Type	Lesion	Etiological Factors	Therapy Strategies
Decreased executive functions	Right hemisphere lesion Frontal lobe damage	Car accidents, whiplash injuries, exposure to organic solvents, HIV/AIDS complications, Korsakoff's disease, Parkinson's disease, craniotomy	More active role in maintaining treatment program, educating family and client's employer, and teaching self-monitoring skills; include pacing in treatment regimen; use home trainers; closely monitor all clinic activities; teach time-management techniques; include client in group activities; do not take socially inappropriate behavior personally
Poor complex problem solving	Diffuse and/or global cortical damage	Exposure to occupational toxins, postsurgical anoxia, stroke, hydrocephalus, small-vessel disease associated with hypertension	Fragment treatment program into small pieces and reassemble pieces into coherent whole when each has been well learned; turn the new into the familiar through repetition; reduce complexity of treatment components; avoid abstract visual aids and abstract verbal explanations
Slowed information processing	Diffuse cortical or subcortical system damage, reticular activating system of the brainstem	Alcohol abuse, drug abuse, exposure to toxins, developmental delays, traumatic brain injury	Slow the rate of presentation; remove environmental distractions; do not speak loudly as though client were hearing impaired; simply present one type of information at a time, making sure the client understands you before you move on
Memory deficits	Temporal lobe damage	Alcohol abuse, temporal lobe injuries, seizures, traumatic brain injury, exposure to toxins, age-related deterioration	Make certain that no learning or emotional disorder is involved; use external aids and multichannel approaches to improve retention of information; determine which aid or approach works best for each individual
Learning disabilities	Unclear	Unknown, possibly traumatic birth or genetic predisposition, early acquired brain damage, metabolic abnormalities	Avoid written material unless it is appropriate to the person's reading level; use nonverbal modes of communication

AIDS, Acquired immunodeficiency syndrome; *HIV,* human immunodeficiency virus.
Modified from Woltersdorf MA: Beyond the sensorimotor strip, Clin Manage 12:63–69, 1992.

complex problem solving has to do with the orchestration of information, information processing involves the efficient transfer of information.

Some people are more proficient processors than others, a result of genetic, environmental, and educational factors. As a result of trauma, some people may lose processing ability and speed. Noise levels, external sensory stimulation (e.g., presence of other people and other activities), and presentation of more than one kind of information at a time (e.g., providing a written home program then discussing the time of the next appointment) are examples of distractions to people with reduced information-processing abilities.

Memory deficits result from a failure to store or retrieve information. Before it can be determined that the person is experiencing a memory lapse, it must be established that the material was learned in the first place. Memory problems typically are acquired, not developmental. Depression may masquerade as memory loss, but the depressed person is usually less attentive or interactive with the environment and therefore registers (or learns) less. For example, a client may appear to have a memory dysfunction when in fact the decreased attention span is a result of depression that has reduced learning.

Learning disability occurs in a person with normal or near-normal intelligence as difficulty acquiring information in specific domains such as spelling, arithmetic, reading, and visual–spatial relationships. Therapists most commonly encounter learning disabilities manifested as noncompliance with written treatment programs, repeated tardiness or absence for treatment sessions, and an overly anxious approach to the physical symptoms that have brought the client to the therapist in the first place.

1.1 Special Implications for the PTA: Disability Classifications The medical model and the ICF Health and Disability Model are reflected in this text. Diagnosis and treatment of disease are presented after the medical model, along with the ICF Model's assessment of the impact of acute and chronic conditions on the functioning of specific body systems (impairments) and basic human performance (functional limitations). The ICF Model extends the scope of the medical model of disease by placing the focus on the functional consequences of disease. Thus the reader will see terminology reflecting these two models such as *etiology, pathogenesis, diagnosis,* and *prognosis* from the traditional medical model and *impairments, interventions, desired outcomes, functional and activity limitations, participation, personal support,* and *environmental influences* from the ICF Model.

Using these tools and the definition of clinical pathology, we ask the following: How does this particular disease or condition affect this person's functional abilities and functional outcome? What precautions should be taken when someone with this condition is exercising? Should vital signs be monitored during therapy for this disease? How will that information affect the plan of care or intervention? How does the disease affect the person's ability to participate in his or her chosen livelihood? How do the person's support systems and environment affect his or her ability to complete relevant activities and participate to the person's fullest ability?

Physical Disability

Each individual client must be evaluated and treated on the basis of the clinical presentation in conjunction with the underlying pathology. For example, the person with osteoporosis may require joint mobilization, but this technique must be modified for the presence of osteoporosis. The individual with cardiac valvular disease may need a different exercise program from that prescribed for a healthy athlete. The adult with musculoskeletal symptoms of thoracic spine pain, muscle spasm, and loss of thoracic motion who has a primary medical diagnosis (e.g., posterior penetrating ulcer) will be unaffected by therapy techniques aimed at the human movement system.

Cognitive Disability

Although therapists cannot diagnose cognitive deficits, the PTA's clinical observations may help identify cognitive deficits that might interfere with treatment. Appropriate referral is always recommended when problems beyond our expertise are suspected.

There is a new prevalence of executive function impairments as a result of new information regarding the impact of multiple concussions on cognitive performance. Soldiers serving in combat zones or training to serve have a large incidence of blast injuries and concussions. In addition, athletes are being monitored for the effects of single concussion versus multiple concussions. These topics will be discussed in more depth in subsequent chapters related to neurological pathologies.

Overall, a person with cognitive impairments requires adapted intervention and follow-up strategies. The treatment area may have to be modified to reduce noise, lighting, and the amount of activity so that the person can concentrate and improve. Home programs may need to be in an altered format (and not exclusively written). Multisensory formatting such as audio recording, video recording, or many repetitions may need to be implemented to assist the client in succeeding with the home program.

HEALTH PROMOTION AND DISEASE PREVENTION

The topic of health promotion and disease prevention has moved front and center in many arenas within the health care industry. There has been a change in health care focus from intervention for cure and healing to healing, health, wellness, and prevention. Traditional health promotion has not been to take care of the sick and disabled but rather to prevent disease and disability in the healthy.[15] Today's concepts of health place all health on a continuum. The focus is on practicing healthy behaviors, even in the presence of disease and disability. Although disability can increase a person's risk of—or susceptibility to—secondary health conditions, the primary disability does not mean that the individual is "unhealthy."

Research has proved beyond a shadow of a doubt that many of today's illnesses, disorders, and conditions can be prevented altogether. Diseases related to longevity, lifestyle, and health behaviors are prevalent, and more people are living longer with chronic diseases, all of which drive up the cost of health care. The health care industry as a whole (and especially third-party payers) has been slow to respond with ways to change our approach to this information.

The first set of national health targets was published in 1979 in *Healthy People: The Surgeon General's Report on Health Promotion and Disease Prevention. Healthy People 2000* was released in 1990 as a management tool with goals to reduce mortality, increase independence among older adults, reduce disparities in health among different population groups, and achieve access to preventive health services.

This program has become an ongoing comprehensive program of public health planning now called *Healthy People 2020. Healthy People* provides science-based, 10-year national objectives for promoting health and preventing disease. *Healthy People 2020* is a tremendously valuable asset to all who work to improve health. *Healthy People 2020* (available

at http://health.gov/healthypeople) has a series of objectives to bring better health to all people in this country and eliminate disparities among different segments of the population, including people of either gender or any race or ethnicity, education or income level, disability, residence in rural localities, and sexual orientation. This program has a built-in means to measure progress toward achieving 10-year targets across a broad range of health behaviors and outcomes. The program has now been expanded to look toward *Healthy People 2020.* There are new initiatives and objectives that reflect assessments of major risks to health and wellness, changing public health priorities, and emerging issues related to our nation's health preparedness and prevention.

Health Promotion

Health promotion as a concept and as an active process is built on the principles of self-responsibility, nutritional awareness, stress reduction and management, and physical fitness. Health promotion is not limited to any particular age or level of ability but extends throughout the lifespan from before birth (e.g., prenatal care) through old age, including anyone with a disability of any kind.

Health promotion programs that encompass the entire lifespan are applicable to people of both genders and all socioeconomic and cultural backgrounds, to those who have no health problems, and to those with chronic illnesses and disabilities. Many types of health promotion programs are in existence, such as health screening; wellness, safety, and stress management programs; and support groups for specific diseases.

Disease Prevention

In recent times disease prevention has gained momentum and today sits at the forefront of the health care industry. Greater numbers of health care professionals now recognize that preventing disease is more cost effective than treating disease. Many new areas of study have developed as a result of this paradigm shift in focus from treatment to prevention. Scientists are revolutionizing the way we fight infection, manage chronic illness, and stay well. For example, one group has coined the term *immunotics* to describe this new approach to preventing and treating disease.[9]

Immunotics is to the 21st century what antibiotics were to the 20th—but perhaps even better. Whereas antibiotics are used to treat illness after it occurs, immunotics is designed to prevent illness in the first place. Unlike antibiotics, which can have serious side effects, immunotics has no side effects; at the very least it adopts the Hippocratic philosophy of *do no harm.*[9] Immunotics represents the group of immunity boosters that fend off infection and keep the immune system working by using natural and organic substances.

In another area, strategies to reduce the incidence of cancer occurrence and recurrence have commanded the attention of oncology researchers. Chemoprevention—the use of agents to inhibit and reverse cancer—has focused on diet-derived agents. Another discipline, *preventive oncology,* is a relatively new branch of medicine that includes both primary and secondary prevention.

Preventive medicine as a branch of medicine is categorized as primary, secondary, or tertiary. *Primary* prevention is geared toward removing or reducing disease risk factors. Examples include maintaining adequate levels of calcium intake and regular exercise as a means of preventing osteoporosis and subsequent bone fractures or giving up or not starting smoking to reduce multiple causes of morbidity. Use of seat belts, use of helmets by motorcyclists and bicyclists, and immunizations are other examples of primary prevention strategies.

Secondary prevention techniques are designed to promote early detection of disease and to employ preventive measures to avoid further complications. Examples of secondary prevention include skin tests for tuberculosis or screening procedures such as mammography, colonoscopy, or routine cervical Papanicolaou smear.

Tertiary prevention measures are aimed at limiting the impact of established disease (e.g., radiation or chemotherapy to control localized cancer). Tertiary prevention involves rehabilitation and may end when no further healing is expected. The goal of tertiary prevention is to return the person to the highest possible level of functioning and to prevent severe disabilities.

Although specific preventive interventions are not the focus of this text, whenever possible, risk-factor reduction strategies are offered because risk factors are a part of the discussion surrounding each disease and therapists play an important role in disease prevention and health promotion.

1.2 Special Implications for the PTA: Health Promotion and Disease Prevention The practice of physical and occupational therapies is becoming increasingly complex. Rapid changes in the health care system are placing increased pressure for effective and efficient management of clients amid fast client turnover and high productivity quotas. Intervention and client–family education must be done quickly and accurately.

In many hospitals, decreased acute care length of stay means that physical and occupational therapy staff are being called on to treat clients earlier in the course of the hospitalization to help prevent secondary complications of immobility. Understanding the diseases, surgeries, and medications frequently encountered in practice is necessary for safe and appropriate interventions and for establishing a reasonable prognosis.

Physical and occupational professionals play major roles in secondary and tertiary care. Clients with musculoskeletal, neuromuscular, cardiopulmonary, or integumentary conditions are often treated initially by another health care practitioner and then referred to therapy for secondary care. PTAs provide secondary care in a wide range of settings from hospitals to preschools.

Role in Prevention and Wellness[2]

Physical and occupational therapy professionals are involved in prevention and wellness activities, screening programs, and the promotion of positive health behavior. These initiatives decrease costs by helping clients achieve and restore optimal functional capacity; minimize impairments, functional limitations, and disabilities related to congenital and acquired conditions; maintain health and thereby prevent further deterioration or future illness; and create appropriate environmental adaptations to enhance independent function.

Prevention is not confined to a single form of presentation but instead takes one of three forms: primary, secondary, or tertiary. All individuals are included—even those who already have one or more primary disabilities.

Primary prevention involves preventing disease in a susceptible or potentially susceptible population through general health promotion. Secondary prevention involves decreasing duration of illness, severity of disease, and sequelae through early diagnosis and prompt intervention. Tertiary prevention includes limiting the degree of disability and promoting rehabilitation and restoration of function in clients with chronic and irreversible diseases.

The beneficial role of prescriptive exercise for health and disease has been documented many times and in many ways. When prescribed appropriately, exercise—including cardiovascular training, endurance training, and strength training—is effective for developing fitness and health, for increasing life expectancy, for preventing injury and disease, and in undergoing rehabilitation because of impairments and disabilities (Box 1.1).

Prescriptive exercise programs to develop and maintain a significant amount of muscle mass, endurance, and strength contribute to overall fitness and health. Exercise plays a vital role in reducing risk factors associated with disease states (e.g., osteoporosis, diabetes mellitus, heart disease), the risk of falls and associated injuries, and the morbidity associated with chronic disease.[13]

Although not as abundant, there is also evidence that suggests that involvement in regular exercise can provide a number of psychologic benefits related to preserved cognitive function, alleviation of depression symptoms and behavior, and an improved concept of personal control and self-direction. It is important to note that although participation in physical activity may not always elicit increases in the traditional markers of physiologic performance and fitness in older adults (e.g., VO_{2max}, body composition, blood pressure changes), it does improve health as measured by a reduction in disease risk factors and improved functional capacity and quality of life in the aging population.[1]

As always, when planning treatment interventions, including client education, the therapy staff must take into consideration the comorbidities and pathologic processes present. This requires identification of lifestyle factors (e.g., amount of exercise, stress, weight) that lead to increased risk for serious health problems and identification of risk factors for disease or injury. As a final reminder, the study and understanding of basic mechanisms of disease physiology and pathokinesiology along with the identification of lifestyle or risk factors are necessary but insufficient guides for clinical practice. Many variables affect the relationships among pathology, impairments, and disability. Attention must be paid to the psychosocial, spiritual, educational, and environmental variables that can modify client outcomes.[11]

BOX 1.1   Benefits of Exercise

- Increased cardiovascular functional capacity, decreased myocardial oxygen demand
- Reduced mortality in people with coronary artery disease
- Favorable change in metabolism of carbohydrates and lipids, including an increase in level of high-density lipoproteins
- Improved hemodynamic, hormonal, metabolic, neurological, and respiratory function
- Improved immune function (stressful or excessive exercise can have the opposite effect)
- Facilitation of biorhythms and thermoregulation; prevention of insomnia
- Favorable effect on fibrinogen levels in older men
- Increased sensitivity to insulin
- Increased bone density; prevention of osteoporosis
- Greater strength and flexibility; maintenance of muscle mass
- Improved postural stability; reduction in falls
- Improved psychologic functioning, self-confidence, and self-esteem
- Reduction in some type A behaviors

Modified from American Heart Association: Recommendations: benefits of exercise, and guidelines for becoming—and remaining—active, J Musculoskelet Med 14:60–65, 1997; and Mayo Clinic Staff: You know exercise is good for you—but do you know how good? Available from http://www.mayoclinic.org/healthy-lifestyle/fitness/in-depth/exercise/art-20048389.

GENETIC ASPECTS OF DISEASE

Advances in immunology and molecular genetics have accelerated our understanding of the genetic and cellular basis of many diseases. Remarkable progress has been made in recombinant deoxyribonucleic acid (DNA) technology, making it possible to offer molecular and cellular treatments for infectious diseases, inherited disorders, and cancer. The monoclonal antibody technique is finding ever-increasing uses in the treatment of diseases such as rheumatoid arthritis, cancer, and AIDS.[24]

At the same time, innovations in gene therapy have advanced the field of vaccine development, especially recombinant vaccine technology. Although the field of vaccination has historically focused on the prevention of infectious diseases, this technology provides a broader base for immune modulation of pathological responses underlying other conditions.[24]

Technological advances and the completion of the Human Genome Project just 50 years after the discovery of the structure of DNA have enabled researchers to begin identifying the actual genes that encode particular disorders.[26] It may be possible in the near future to treat altered gene structure (gene therapy) in an attempt to cure or control previously incurable diseases. Laboratory studies and advances in the collection of immune cells made it possible to begin clinical trials of gene therapy in the early 1990s. The recent explosion in biotechnology has advanced the field of genetic testing, which is a necessary component in the genetic treatment of diseases and disorders.

The Human Genome Project

The Human Genome Project, an international project led in the United States by the National Human Genome Research Institute and the Department of Energy, was completed in April 2003 and provides a reference DNA sequence of the human genome. Researchers identified all 30,000 genes existing in 23 pairs of chromosomes and deciphered the genetic code by sequencing the 3.1 billion base pairs of human DNA and mapping their location in the chromosomes.

The goals of this project have been to identify all human genes, map the genes' locations on chromosomes, and ultimately provide detailed information from the genetic coding about how the genes function. Because virtually every human illness and even many lifestyle-related conditions have a hereditary component, the Human Genome Project may hold the key to the prevention or cure of many, if not all, diseases and disorders.[27]

The Human Genome Project dispelled the idea that race- or ethnicity-based biologic differences existed when they discovered that 99.99% of the genome is the same across the human population, regardless of race or ethnic origin. Individual variations can increase the risk of disease, as some people can become more vulnerable to bacteria, viruses, toxins, and chemicals, but the Human Genome Project disproved many previously held beliefs about biologically based racial differences.

Knowing the order in which these chemical units are arranged on each strand of DNA does not tell where the genes are located within the genome, the specific function of each gene in the sequence, or which genes make which proteins. The study of genomes has been labeled *genomics,* which includes the investigation of an organism's entire hereditary information encoded in the DNA. The term comes from the words *gene* and *chromosome.*

The genome of any organism (including humans) is a complete DNA sequence of one set of chromosomes. Genomics is different from genetics, which is generally the study of single genes or groups of genes. Genomics, with its unfolding of the complete DNA sequences, will provide a basis for the study of susceptibility to disease, the pathogenesis of disease, and the development of new preventive and therapeutic approaches.

In addition, the completion of the Human Genome Project has enhanced the widespread use of prenatal diagnosis and DNA chip technology and will make it possible to analyze a sample of DNA collected from saliva. The design and prescription of drugs to accommodate individual differences in metabolism may be possible from the data derived from this project. All of these areas of interest will be the substance of future studies.

Information about the genes is made available immediately on the Internet to scientists, clinicians, librarians, educators, and the general public. The cataloging and filing of this information are under the auspices of the Cancer Genome Anatomy Project (CGAP). The Human Cancer Genome Project is another program that is attempting to develop a comprehensive description of the genetic basis of human cancer and specifically the complete identification and characterization of genetic alterations present in a large number of major types of cancer (Fig. 1.2).

Gene Therapy

Genes are the chemical messengers of heredity; 30,000 human genes—composed of DNA molecules along a double helix and

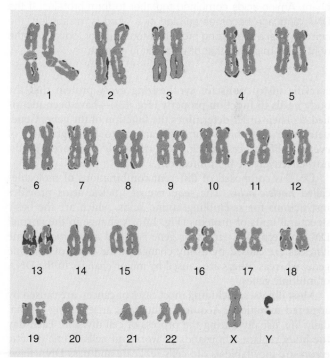

FIG. 1.2 Example of genetic basis for cancer found in early cervical carcinoma. The gain of chromosome 3q (tumor deoxyribonucleic acid [DNA] seen as green) that occurs with HPV16 infection defines the transition from severe dysplasia or carcinoma in situ to invasive carcinoma of the uterine cervix. Genetic testing can help identify chromosomal aberrations such as this that occur during carcinogenesis. (From Heselmeyer K, Schrock E, du Manoir S, et al.: Gain of chromosome 3q defines the transition from severe dysplasia to invasive carcinoma of the uterine cervix, Proc Natl Acad Sci U S A 93:479–484, 1996.)

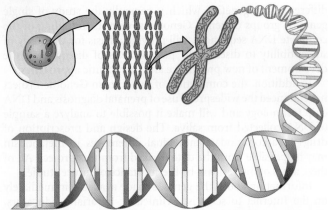

FIG. 1.3 Schematic diagram of the chemical called *deoxyribonucleic acid* (DNA). Inside the nucleus of nearly every cell in the body, a complex set of genetic instructions known as the *human genome* is contained on 23 pairs of chromosomes. Chromosomes are made of long chains of DNA packaged into short segments called *genes*. Every cell of every human body contains a copy of the same DNA. Genes contain instructions to direct all body functions written in a molecular language. This molecular language is made up of four letters; each letter represents a molecule on the DNA: *a*denine, *c*ytosine, *g*uanine, *t*hymine. The As, Cs, Gs, and Ts form in triplets, constituting a code; each triplet of letters instructs the cell to attach to a particular amino acid (e.g., TGG attaches to amino acid tryptophan). Amino acids combined together to form proteins. If the DNA language becomes garbled or a word is misspelled, the cell may make the wrong protein or too much or too little of the right one—mistakes that often result in disease.

carrying instructions for synthesizing every protein that the body needs to function properly (Fig. 1.3)—have been identified.[30a] Their order determines the function of the gene. Genes determine everything from appearance to the regulation of everyday life processes (e.g., how efficiently we process foods, how effectively we fight infection).

DNA is composed of different combinations of molecules called *nucleic acids*. The sequence of nucleic acids provides instructions for assembling amino acids, which are the basic structural units of proteins (Fig. 1.4). A change in the normal DNA pattern of a particular gene is called a *mutation*. Some illnesses are caused by a tiny change in the DNA of just one gene, whereas others are caused by major changes in the DNA of multiple genes.

Most illnesses, including most cases of cancer, are caused by acquired mutations. Acquired mutations arise during normal daily life, usually during the process of cell division. Each day the body replaces thousands of worn-out cells. Some genetic errors are inevitable as old cells replicate and pass DNA flaws along to replacement (daughter) cells. When all goes well, daughter cells recognize these mutations and repair them, but the repair mechanism can fail or be disabled by environmental toxins and diet. Although acquired mutations can be passed on to daughter cells, they cannot be inherited.

More specifically, gene therapy (also known as *human genetic engineering*) is the process by which specific malfunctioning cells are targeted and repaired or replaced with corrected genes (Fig. 1.5). A gene can be delivered to a cell using a carrier known as a *vector*. The most common types of vectors used in gene

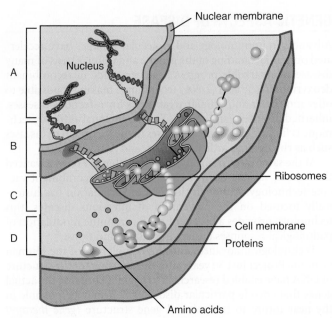

FIG. 1.4 The chain of events from deoxyribonucleic acid (DNA); this is how the DNA directs the cell. (A) Ribonucleic acid *(RNA)* receives instructions from the DNA code in the chromosomes. (B) The RNA travels from the nucleus to link up with ribosomes (protein-making units). (C) Instructions from the code contained within the DNA are used by the RNA-ribosome complex to assemble amino acids. (D) Cellular function is now directed by proteins containing the amino acids.

therapy are genetically altered viruses, but nonviral vectors are being developed as potential gene delivery vehicles as well. Essentially, DNA is used like a drug, allowing it to replace or repair defective genes. It is hoped that the altered cells will yield daughter cells with healthy genes and that these offspring cells will help eliminate the diseased cells. Alternately, cells can be genetically altered to contain a toxin-producing suicide gene to treat some cancers.[22]

Uses for Gene Therapy

Research is ongoing into such cures for a wide variety of hereditary disorders and diseases caused by aging (Box 1.2); some diseases, such as hemophilia, are being studied as a good model for gene therapy. Gene therapy for the treatment of diseases in children before birth is being actively pursued at many medical centers using animal models. In utero gene therapy (IUGT) could be beneficial for those with genetic diseases if gene therapy is performed before symptoms are manifested.[25,31]

Gene therapy is being investigated as a means of helping injuries heal, replacing worn-out tissue, reducing scar tissue, or fusing spinal segments together. The gene for bone growth has been injected into the disk space and shown to signal enough bone growth to bridge the bone on either side of the space. Investigational studies using animals may find an injectable method to fuse bone to replace the costly and complicated spinal fusion surgery.[28]

Gene insertion has been used to successfully treat humans with inoperable coronary artery disease. Researchers injected a gene that makes a protein called *vascular endothelial growth factor* (VEGF) into the hearts of candidates with severe chest

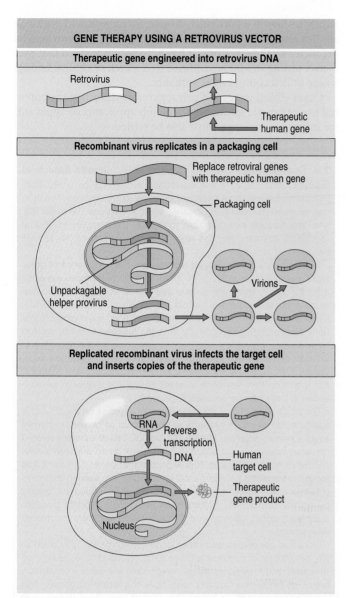

GENE THERAPY USING A RETROVIRUS VECTOR

Therapeutic gene engineered into retrovirus DNA

Retrovirus

Therapeutic human gene

Recombinant virus replicates in a packaging cell

Replace retroviral genes with therapeutic human gene

Packaging cell

Unpackagable helper provirus

Virions

Replicated recombinant virus infects the target cell and inserts copies of the therapeutic gene

RNA

Reverse transcription

DNA

Human target cell

Therapeutic gene product

Nucleus

FIG. 1.5 Gene therapy. A therapeutic gene is engineered genetically into the retrovirus deoxyribonucleic acid (DNA) and replaces most of the viral DNA sequences. The recombinant virus that carries the therapeutic gene is allowed to replicate in a special "packaging cell," which also contains normal virus that carries the genes required for viral replication. The replicated recombinant virus is allowed to infect the human diseased tissue, or "target cell." The recombinant virus may invade the diseased tissue but cannot replicate or destroy the cell. The recombinant virus inserts copies of the normal therapeutic gene into the host genome and produces the normal protein product. (From Yanoff M, Duker JS: Ophthalmology, ed 4, Edinburgh, 2009, Mosby.)

pain caused by ischemia that could not be corrected with bypass surgery or angioplasty.

Tests suggest that once installed, the gene produces blood vessel–promoting proteins for 2 or 3 weeks (enough to grow a permanent new blood supply) before ceasing to work. The heart actually sprouts tiny new blood vessels (therapeutic angiogenesis) too small to be seen but with improved blood flow to the heart readily demonstrated.[17,29] Investigations continue to

BOX 1.2   Potential Uses of Gene Therapy[a]

- Adenosine deaminase (ADA) deficiency
- Acquired immunodeficiency syndrome (AIDS)
- Alzheimer's disease
- Arthritis
- Cancer (not all forms)
- Chronic pain
- Congenital heart defects
- Cystic fibrosis
- Diabetes mellitus
- Familial hypercholesterolemia
- Heart disease
- Hemophilia
- Hepatitis
- Hepatocellular carcinoma (liver cancer)
- Huntington's disease
- Liver failure
- Marfan syndrome
- Mesothelioma
- Muscular dystrophy (Duchenne's)
- Neurofibromatosis
- Peripheral vascular disease
- Schizophrenia
- Severe combined immunodeficiency (SCID)
- Sickle cell anemia

[a]This is only a partial list of diseases or disorders being studied and compiled from research reported but should give the reader an idea of the broad and varied applications of genetic manipulation.

examine gene therapy strategies to deliver genes that code for the angiogens.

Approaches to Gene Therapy

Gene therapy may take a number of different approaches. The original design was to inject one or more genes into the person to replace genes that are absent or not functioning properly. A second approach called *small-molecule therapy* injects a small molecule (i.e., a drug) to modify the function of one or more genes in the body that is making a normal product but too much or too little of it.

Other approaches include transferring a gene into cancer cells to sensitize them to drugs[12] or restoring immune function in people with HIV infection by transferring a therapeutic gene into target cells, rendering them resistant to HIV replication. Infusion of protected cells may limit virus spread and delay AIDS disease progression. Efforts are underway to deliver antiviral genes to hematopoietic stem cells to ensure a renewable supply of HIV-protected cells for the life of the individual.[6,7,21]

Germ-line gene therapy is an approach that delivers genes to sperm or eggs (or to the cells that produce them). It might prevent defective genes from being transmitted to subsequent generations by repairing the original genetic defect in germ cells. Gene modification at an early stage of embryonic development might also be a way of correcting gene defects in both the germ-line and body cells. This therapy is highly controversial because it carries an unknown level of risk (interference with another gene, specificity of the insertion). As a consequence, germ-line gene therapy is not being considered for application in humans at this time. The safety of germ-line gene therapy procedures might be dramatically increased in the future if scientists determine ways to make sure that a transferred gene goes into the cell's genome at the same position as the already mutated gene.

Obstacles to Gene Therapy

Some obstacles to gene therapy must be overcome before this procedure is considered a viable treatment option. Examples include finding appropriate harmless viral vectors to carry the normal gene to the target cells that do not provoke an immune response against them as foreign invaders or cause toxic side effects, engineering the transplanted genes to be efficient and effective, and finding ways to modify retrovirus vectors so they can carry the genes into nondividing cells (presently, genes can be delivered only to actively dividing cells when delivered by retrovirus vectors).

Ethical concerns have also been raised about the use of human genetic engineering for purposes other than therapy (e.g., eugenics). These include the use of genes to improve ourselves cosmetically, improve memory, increase intelligence, accomplish ethnic cleansing ("designer babies" genetically engineered before birth), or cause permanent changes in the gene pool. Some researchers are advocating the use of human genetic engineering for the treatment of serious diseases only.[3]

Gene doping. Gene therapy in athletes, called *gene doping*, involves transferring genes directly into human cells to blend with an athlete's own DNA, enhancing muscle growth and increasing strength or endurance. Gene doping is banned in sports, and although there has been no direct evidence yet to prove it, there is some concern that gene doping has already begun.

Concerns have been raised about long-term effects such as leukemia, other forms of cancer, and unknown effects, including the potential harm in passing changes on to the athlete's children. Although gene doping is not currently in use, its potential to enhance performance has been discussed in the literature.[16,30]

Gene Testing

The rapidly expanding field of genetic testing holds great promise for detecting many devastating illnesses long before their symptoms become apparent. Such testing identifies people who have inherited a faulty gene that may (or may not) lead to a particular disorder. In the last 15 years, such predictive tests have been developed for more than 200 of the 4000 diseases thought to be caused by inherited gene mutations. The result has been earlier monitoring, preventive treatments, and in some cases, planning for long-term care.

Gene testing is not without its difficulties, however. For example, the presence of a particular mutation does not mean that illness is inevitable, which makes the interpretation of test results a highly complex task. The psychologic implications of predictive testing must be considered. Identifying who is a candidate for testing remains to be determined. Inheritance accounts for a limited number of diseases, suggesting that genetic testing should be reserved for people with a strong family history of a particular disease. Safeguards and protocols are not always in place before testing finds its way into general practice. For these reasons, it has been recommended that predictive testing should be confined to research or clinical settings where skilled counseling is available.

Other ethical issues and privacy concerns, such as the potential use of genetic testing to screen job applicants or applicants for insurance coverage, must also be settled.

1.3 Special Implications for the PTA: Genetic Aspects of Disease Understanding the interaction and influence of environmental factors (such as exercise) on gene expression and function has taken on increasing importance as scientists use the molecular and genetic tools now available to unravel the complex etiological factors of diseases such as obesity, diabetes, and cardiovascular disease.

The Human Genome Project emphasizes the importance of other factors in disease susceptibility when genetic differences are eliminated. For example, regular exercise has been shown to improve glucose tolerance, control of lipid abnormalities, diabetes mellitus, hypertension, bone density, immune function, psychologic function, sleep patterns, and obesity, with the greatest benefits realized by sedentary individuals who begin to exercise for the first time or after an extended period of inactivity. Responses to exercise interventions are often highly variable among individuals, and research has indicated that response to exercise may be mediated or influenced in large part by variation in genes.[5]

The study of acute and chronic effects of exercise on the structure and function of organ systems is now a field of research referred to as *exercise science*. During the last 30 years, exercise-related research has rapidly transitioned from focus on an organ to a subcellular or molecular focus. It is expected that genetic research will focus on translating fundamental knowledge into solving the complexities of a number of degenerative diseases influenced heavily by activity or inactivity factors such as cardiopulmonary disease, diabetes mellitus, obesity, and the debilitating disorders associated with aging.[4]

Individual genotypes and other genetic information may eventually help therapists assess a client's risk for conditions, enable us to understand why some people respond to the same intervention faster or better than others who have the same diagnosis, and develop and execute an appropriate plan of care. Gene therapy and the elimination of some diseases and conditions may contribute to the continuing trend for physical therapists to focus on health and fitness in the future.[27]

REFERENCES/SUGGESTED READINGS

To enhance this text and add value for the reader, references and suggested readings are included on the companion Evolve site that accompanies this textbook. The reader can view the source and access it online whenever possible.

Problems Affecting Multiple Systems

CHAPTER OBJECTIVES

1. Understand the interconnected nature of human physiology and the connection between primary and secondary pathology.
2. Recognize the secondary effects of primary treatments.
3. Recognize pharmacokinetic effects and the symptoms of adverse drug reactions.
4. Become familiar with primary conditions affecting multiple systems.

OUTLINE

VOCAB BUILDERS

Alopecia	Malaise	Purpura
Cachexia	Necrosis	Somnolence
Concomitant	Neuroleptic	Striae
Ecchymoses	Paresis	Tachycardia
Fluid shift	Petechiae	Tardive dyskinesia
Hepatotoxicity	Pharmacodynamics	Urticaria
Leukocytosis	Pharmacokinetic	
Lymphocytosis	Plexopathy	

Many conditions and diseases seen in the rehabilitation setting can affect multiple organs or systems (Box 2.1). Given the kinds of multiple comorbidities and system impairments encountered in the health care arena, the physical therapist assistant (PTA) must go beyond a systems approach and use a biopsychosocial–spiritual approach to client management. Chronic diseases and multiple system impairments require such an approach because risk factors correlate with health outcomes; early intervention and intervention results are correlated with improved outcomes.

Individual modifying (risk) factors (IMFs) such as lifestyle variables and environment affect pathology and modify how a person responds to health, illness, and disease. For example, adverse drug reactions (ADRs) are correlated with increasing age and obesity, whereas fitness level has a profound impact on recovery from injury, anesthesia, and illness.

In addition, a single injury, disease, or pathologic condition can predispose a person to associated secondary illnesses. For example, the victim of a motor vehicle accident sustained a traumatic brain injury (TBI) and *concomitant* pelvic fracture then developed pneumonia and pulmonary compromise, subsequently experiencing a myocardial infarction.

Although medical conditions encountered in the clinic or home health care setting are discussed individually in the appropriate chapter, the health care provider must understand the systemic and local effects of such disorders. This chapter provides a brief listing of the systemic effects of commonly encountered pathologic conditions and a basic presentation of acid–base and fluid and electrolyte imbalances.

SYSTEMIC EFFECTS OF PATHOLOGY

Systemic Effects of Acute Inflammation

Acute inflammation can be described as the initial response of tissue to injury—particularly bacterial infections and *necrosis*—involving vascular and cellular responses. Local signs of inflammation are commonly observed in the therapy setting. Local inflammation can lead to abscesses when excessive formation of pus occurs.

Systemic effects of acute inflammation include fever, *tachycardia,* and a hypermetabolic state. These effects produce characteristic changes in the blood, such as elevated serum protein levels.

Systemic Effects of Chronic Inflammation

Chronic inflammation is the result of persistent injury, repeated episodes of acute inflammation, infection, cell-mediated immune responses, and foreign body reactions. The tissue response to injury is characterized by accumulation of lymphocytes, plasma cells, and macrophages and production of fibrous connective tissue. Grossly, fibrotic tissue is light gray and has a dense, firm texture that causes contraction of the normal tissue.

The associated fibrosis may cause progressive tissue damage and loss of function. Systemic effects of chronic inflammation may include low-grade fever, *malaise,* weight loss, anemia, fatigue, *leukocytosis,* and *lymphocytosis.*[22] Inflammation is reflected by an increased erythrocyte sedimentation rate (ESR). In general, as the disease improves, the ESR decreases.

Systemic Factors Influencing Healing

In addition to local factors that affect healing, a variety of systemic factors influence healing as well. Systemic factors may include general nutritional status; psychologic well-being; presence of cardiovascular disease, cancer, hematologic disorders, systemic infections, and diabetes mellitus; and whether the person is undergoing corticosteroid or immunosuppressive therapy.[70]

BOX 2.1   Conditions that Affect Multiple Systems

- Autoimmune disorders
- Burns
- Cancer
- Cystic fibrosis
- Congestive heart failure (CHF)
- Connective tissue diseases:
  - Rheumatoid arthritis
  - Progressive systemic sclerosis (scleroderma)
  - Polymyositis
  - Sjögren's syndrome
  - Systemic lupus erythematosus
  - Polyarteritis nodosa
- Endocrine disorders (e.g., diabetes, thyroid disorders)
- Environmental and occupational diseases
- Genetic diseases
- Infections (e.g., tuberculosis, human immunodeficiency virus [HIV])
- Malnutrition or other nutritional imbalance
- Metabolic disorders
- Multiple organ dysfunction syndrome (MODS)
- Renal failure (chronic)
- Sarcoidosis
- Shock
- Trauma
- Vasculitis

Consequences of Immunodeficiency

Immunodeficiency diseases are caused by congenital (primary) or acquired (secondary) failure of one or more functions of the immune system, predisposing the affected individual to infections that a noncompromised immune system could resist. The PTA is more likely to encounter individuals with acquired (rather than congenital) immunodeficiency from nonspecific causes, such as those that occur with viral and other infections; malnutrition; alcoholism; aging; autoimmune diseases; diabetes mellitus; cancer, particularly myeloma, lymphoma, and leukemia; chronic diseases; steroid therapy; cancer chemotherapy; and radiation therapy.[46]

The primary consequence of immunodeficiency is predisposition to opportunistic infections that results in clinical manifestations of those infections. Selective B-cell deficiencies predispose an individual to bacterial infections. T-cell deficiencies predispose to viral and fungal infections. Combined deficiencies, including acquired immunodeficiency syndrome (AIDS), are particularly severe because they predispose to many kinds of viral, bacterial, and fungal infections.

Systemic Effects of Neoplasm

Malignant tumors, by their destructive nature of uncontrolled cell proliferation and spread, produce many local and systemic effects. Locally, the rapid growth of the tumor encroaches on healthy tissue, causing destruction, necrosis, ulceration, compression, obstruction, and hemorrhage.

Pain may or may not occur, depending on the proximity of tumor cells, swelling, or hemorrhage to the nerve cells. Pain may occur as a late symptom as a result of infiltration, compression, or destruction of nerve tissue. Secondary infections often occur as a result of the host's decreased immunity and can lead to death.[137]

The person with a malignant neoplasm often manifests systemic symptoms such as gradual or rapid weight loss, muscular weakness, anorexia, anemia, and coagulation disorders. Continued spread of the cancer may lead to bone erosion or liver, gastrointestinal (GI), pulmonary, or vascular obstruction. Other vital organs may be affected, and tumor cells can increase intracranial pressure in the brain and cause partial paralysis and eventual coma. Hemorrhage caused by direct invasion or necrosis in any body part leads to further anemia—or even death if the necrosis is severe.

Advanced cancers produce *cachexia* (wasting) as a result of tissue destruction and the body's nutrients being used by the malignant cells for further growth.

2.1 Special Implications for the PTA: Systemic Effects of Pathology[26,27] Medical advances, the aging of America, the increasing number of people with multisystem problems, and the expanding scope of practice require that the PTA anticipate, reassess, and manage the manifestations of disease and pathology in consultation with the physical therapist.

Interventions to maximize oxygen transport should be an important focus even in people who are acutely and critically ill. Enhancing oxygen transport centrally and peripherally improves the body's ability to respond to stress. At the same time, many therapy interventions elicit an exercise stimulus that stresses an already strained oxygen transport system. Exercise is now recognized as a prescriptive intervention in pathology that has indications,

---

contraindications, and side effects. These factors necessitate careful and close monitoring of cardiopulmonary status, especially in the person with multisystem involvement.

Blood abnormalities require that the results of the client's blood analysis and clotting factors be monitored so that therapy intervention can be modified to minimize risks. Individualized treatment programs are developed for each person, addressing the special needs of that client and the family and responding to physical, psychologic, emotional, and spiritual needs.

ADVERSE DRUG EVENTS

Drugs were once developed through a hit-or-miss process in which researchers would identify a compound and test it in cells and animals to determine its effect on disease. When a compound appeared to be successful, it was often tested in humans with little knowledge of how it worked or what side effects it might have. Today biochemists know much more about disease processes and work at the molecular level designing drugs to interact with specific molecules.

Definition and Overview

Adverse drug events (ADEs) are unwanted and potentially harmful effects produced by medications or prescription drugs. The term usually excludes nontherapeutic overdosage such as accidental exposure or attempted suicide. Most ADEs are medication reactions or side effects. A *drug–drug* interaction occurs when medications interact unfavorably, possibly adding to the pharmacologic effects. A *drug–disease* interaction occurs when a medication causes an existing disease to worsen. *Side effects* are usually defined as predictable pharmacologic effects that occur within therapeutic dose ranges and are undesirable in the given therapeutic situation. Overdosage toxicity is the predictable toxic effect that occurs with dosages in excess of the therapeutic range for a particular person.[43]

ADEs are classified as *mild* (no antidote, therapy, or prolongation of hospitalization necessary), *moderate* (change in drug therapy required, although not necessarily a cessation of therapy; may prolong hospitalization or require special treatment), *severe* (potentially life-threatening, requires discontinuation of the drug and specific treatment of the adverse reaction), and *lethal* (directly or indirectly leads to the death of the person).

Incidence

ADEs have been declared a national public health problem, with more than 700,000 emergency department visits and 120,000 hospitalizations required for further treatment after the emergency visit.[116] The annual incidence of death caused by ADEs is estimated to be between 0.08/100,000 and 0.12/100,000 people.[116] According to one study of primary care (outpatients), ADEs were common (25%) and often preventable.[59] Adults older than age 65 years are twice as likely to go to an emergency department because of an ADE and are almost seven times more likely to experience an ADE requiring hospitalization than a younger person.[16] Death rates secondary to an ADE are also highest in people older than age 55 years, with the greatest risk in those older than 75 years.[116] The Centers for Disease Control and Prevention (CDC) reports that inappropriate medications are prescribed to older adults in about 1 out of every 12 visits (8%).[58]

Etiologic and Risk Factors

Definite risk factors for experiencing a serious ADE can include age, gender, ethnicity, concomitant alcohol consumption, new drugs, number of drugs, dosages, concomitant use of herbal compounds,[24] duration of treatment, noncompliance (e.g., unintentional repeated dosage), small stature, and presence of underlying conditions.[19,20,98]

Of all the risk factors, age has the most prevalent effect in the aging American population. Factors that contribute to ADEs in older people include age-related physiologic changes, a greater degree of frailty, an increased number of underlying diseases, and the presence of polypharmacy.[41,77] Age-related physiologic changes affect the distribution of drugs. A decrease in lean body mass and an increase in the proportion of body fat result in a decrease in body water. As a result, water-soluble drugs have a lower volume of distribution, which speeds up onset of action and raises peak concentration. High peak concentrations are associated with increased toxicity.

On the other hand, lipid-soluble drugs are distributed more widely, have a delayed onset of action, and accumulate with repeated dosing. Aging adults are also at risk for drug accumulation because of changes in both metabolism and elimination. Functional liver tissue diminishes and hepatic blood flow decreases with advanced age. Consequently, the capacity of the liver to break down and convert drugs and their metabolites declines. This may be exacerbated by other changes, such as age-related reduction in renal mass and blood flow, cancer, heart failure, and cirrhosis.

The drugs most commonly associated with ADRs in the aging are listed in Box 2.2. ADRs may be dose-related or non–dose-related. Dose-related effects include drug toxicity from overdose, variations in pharmaceutical preparations, preexisting liver disease, presence of comorbidities such as renal or heart failure, and drug interactions. Non–dose-related effects may occur as a result of hypersensitivity.

Cardiac or pulmonary toxicity may occur as a result of irradiation and immunosuppressive drugs given to prepare recipients for organ transplantation or for treatment of cancer.

Clinical Manifestations

Rashes, fever, and jaundice are common signs of drug toxicity. Adverse skin reactions include erythema, discoloration, itching, burning, *urticaria*, eczema, acne, alopecia, blisters, and *purpura* (Fig. 2.1). Onset may be within minutes to hours to days. Signs and symptoms suggestive of a mild reaction include anxiety, dizziness, headache, nasal congestion, shakiness, and brief vomiting. Persons with a moderate drug reaction may present with abdominal cramps, dyspnea, hypertension or hypotension, palpitations, tachycardia, and persistent vomiting. Severe reactions can include arrhythmia, seizures, laryngeal edema, profound hypotension,

pulmonary edema, and cardiopulmonary arrest. Arthralgias and myalgias can be part of the mild or moderate reactions.

Older adults may develop ADEs that are clearly different from those seen in younger persons (Box 2.3).[105] The PTA may observe motor tics called *tardive dyskinesia,* which is a neurologic syndrome caused by the long-term use of neuroleptic drugs. *Neuroleptic* drugs are usually prescribed for psychiatric disorders but may be used for some GI and neurologic disorders. Tardive dyskinesia is characterized by repetitive, involuntary, and purposeless movements. The client may demonstrate

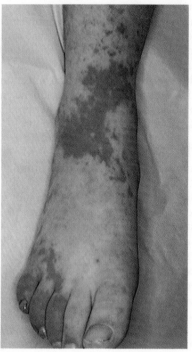

FIG. 2.1 Purpura. Hemorrhaging into the tissues, particularly beneath the skin or mucous membranes, producing raised or flat ecchymoses or petechiae. Seen most often in a physical therapy practice as a result of thrombocytopenia (e.g., drug reaction or medication induced, especially with nonsteroidal antiinflammatory drugs [NSAIDs], methotrexate, Coumadin or warfarin; radiation or chemotherapy induced); also occurs in older adults as blood leaks from capillaries in response to minor trauma. (From Hurwitz S: Clinical pediatric dermatology: a textbook of skin disorders of childhood and adolescence, ed 2, Philadelphia, 1993, Saunders.)

BOX 2.2   Drugs that Most Commonly Cause Adverse Drug Reactions in the Aging

- Corticosteroids
- Digoxin
- Aminoglycoside antibiotic
- Anticoagulants (heparin and warfarin)
- Insulin overdose
- Aspirin
- Tranquilizers (phenothiazines)
- Sedative-hypnotics
- Antacids
- Oral hypoglycemics

BOX 2.3   Common Signs and Symptoms of Adverse Drug Reactions in the Aging

- Dry mouth (xerostomia)
- Restlessness
- Orthostatic hypotension (dizziness, weakness, decreased blood pressure, falls)
- Depression
- Confusion, delirium
- Impaired memory or concentration
- Nausea
- Constipation
- Incontinence
- Extrapyramidal syndromes (e.g., parkinsonism, tardive dyskinesia)
- Fatigue

repetitive grimacing; tongue protrusion; lip smacking, puckering, and pursing; and rapid eye blinking. Rapid movements of the arms, legs, and trunk may also occur. Involuntary movements of the fingers may give the person the appearance of playing an invisible guitar or piano.

Medical Management

Differentiating an ADE from underlying disease requires a thorough history, especially when a symptom appears 1 to 2 months after a medication regimen has been started. Monitoring blood cell counts, liver enzymes, electrolytes, blood urea nitrogen (BUN), and creatinine is indicated for certain drugs. Digoxin and other cardiotropic drugs cause arrhythmias that require electrocardiographic monitoring. With dose-related ADEs, dose modification is usually all that is required, whereas with non–dose-related ADEs, the drug therapy is usually stopped and reexposure avoided.

2.2 Special Implications for the PTA: Adverse Drug Events Many people treated by the PTA today have a pharmacologic profile. It is not unusual to find out during the client interview that the person is taking many different prescription or nonprescription medications. Often there is an equally long list of nutritional aids, supplements, herbs, or vitamins. Adults aged 65 years or older commonly have complicated medication regimens that may result in ADEs. Age-related physiologic changes result in altered pharmacokinetic and *pharmacodynamic* responses to medications that contribute to ADRs.[51]

Knowing when a person is having an ADE to medication or supplements versus experiencing symptoms of disease or illness is not always easy. Knowing about potential drug effects and using a drug guide to look up potential side effects are good places to start.

Client/patient education is important. The PTA can remind his or her clients to take their medication as prescribed and to report any unusual signs and symptoms to their doctor, physician's assistant, or nurse practitioner. Encourage your clients to keep follow-up appointments with the health care professional who prescribed the drug and to make sure that person knows all drugs and supplements currently being taken.

If the PTA suspects drug- or nutraceutical-related signs or symptoms, several observations can be made and reported to the physician, such as correlation between the time medication is taken and length of time before signs and symptoms appear (or increase). In addition, family members can be asked to observe whether the signs or symptoms increase after each dose. Documentation of observed or reported behavior or signs and symptoms and the date first observed is important. Make note of the client's clinical condition and your interventions. Follow your facility's policies for notification of suspected ADE.

Any signs of tardive dyskinesia should be reported to the physician. There is no standard treatment for tardive dyskinesia. The first step is generally to stop or minimize the use of the neuroleptic drug. This may not be possible for anyone with a severe underlying condition. Replacing the neuroleptic drug with substitute drugs may help some people. Other drugs, such as benzodiazepines, adrenergic antagonists, and dopamine agonists, may also be beneficial.

Symptoms of tardive dyskinesia may continue even after the person has stopped taking the drugs. Some symptoms may improve and/or disappear over time with proper medical management.

Exercise and Drugs

Exercise can produce dramatic changes in the way drugs are absorbed, distributed, localized, metabolized, and excreted in the body *(pharmacokinetics)*. The magnitude of these changes is dependent on the characteristics of each drug (e.g., route of administration, chemical properties) and exercise-related factors (e.g., exercise intensity, mode, and duration).

A single exercise session can cause sudden changes in pharmacokinetics that may have an immediate impact on people who exercise during therapy. Exercise training can also produce changes in pharmacokinetics, but these tend to occur over a longer period and cause a slower and fairly predictable change in a person's response to certain medications. Drugs that are administered locally by transdermal techniques or by subcutaneous or intramuscular injection may have altered or increased absorption in the presence of exercise, local heat, or massage of the administration site.

In addition, allergic and potentially fatal anaphylactic drug reactions are mediated by exercise. The therapist should always consider the possibility that anyone in therapy taking drugs may have an altered response to those drugs as a result of interventions used in therapy.[115] The possibility of drug–exercise interactions requires careful and consistent monitoring of vital signs.

SPECIFIC DRUG CATEGORIES

Nonsteroidal Antiinflammatory Drugs

Nonsteroidal antiinflammatory drugs (NSAIDs) are a heterogeneous group of drugs that reduce inflammation, provide pain relief, and reduce fever. NSAIDs are commonly used postoperatively for discomfort; for painful musculoskeletal conditions, especially among the older adult population; and in the treatment of inflammatory rheumatic diseases.

Although the incidence of serious side effects from using NSAIDs is rather low, the widespread use of readily available nonprescription NSAIDs results in a substantial number of people being adversely affected. Risk factors associated with increased toxicities include older age, higher doses, volume depletion, concurrent use of corticosteroids or anticoagulants, previous history of GI bleeding or ulcer, and serious comorbidities.[18,135] The use of NSAIDs is associated with a wide spectrum of potential clinical toxicities (Table 2.1), but serious side effects are most often seen with the GI tract, kidneys, and cardiovascular system.

NSAIDs may cause GI symptoms ranging from mild dyspepsia to more serious complications such as GI bleeding, ulceration, and perforation. These serious side effects may occur without previous symptoms (e.g., dyspepsia) and are particularly more likely to occur in persons taking higher doses, in older adults, and with chronic use.

NSAIDs have multiple mechanisms of action that affect the body both locally and systemically.

One of these mechanisms is to inhibit the enzymes cyclooxygenase (COX)-1 and COX-2. COX-1 is involved in synthesizing prostaglandins and is felt to be a "housekeeping" enzyme. When COX-1 is inhibited, there is a decrease in the protective mucosal barrier of the GI tract.

COX-2 is thought to be produced during states of inflammation. For this reason, NSAIDs were created that selectively inhibit COX-2 but not COX-1 (Vioxx, Celebrex, and Bextra), with the hope of reducing GI side effects. Yet further scrutiny and clinical trials[14,15] noted that users of Vioxx exhibited an increase in myocardial infarctions and stroke. Also, to varying degrees, all NSAIDs can cause sodium retention and edema in susceptible people. NSAIDs are also known to interact with hypertension medications, particularly angiotensin-converting enzyme (ACE) inhibitors and β-blockers, thereby modestly increasing blood pressure in persons with hypertension.[103] Kidney dysfunction may also occur. Careful monitoring is required in older adults taking NSAIDs for both short- and long-term treatment.[94]

NSAIDs are also reversible platelet inhibitors that result in antiplatelet activity. Aspirin is the most powerful agent because

TABLE 2.1   Possible Systemic Effects of Nonsteroidal Antiinflammatory Drugs

Site	Signs and Symptoms
Gastrointestinal	Indigestion, abdominal pain Gastroesophageal reflux Peptic ulcers GI hemorrhage and perforation Nausea, vomiting, diarrhea, constipation
Hepatic	Jaundice Transaminase elevation
Renal	Edema (exacerbation of CHF) Hypertension (particularly in clients with hypertension) Hyperkalemia Renal insufficiency Papillary necrosis Nephrotic syndrome Interstitial nephritis Renal dysgenesis (infants of mothers given NSAIDs during third trimester)
Hematologic	Thrombocytopenia, ASA-related anemia Prolonged bleeding time
Cardiovascular	Blunt action of cardiovascular drugs (e.g., diuretics, ACE inhibitors, β-blockers) Increase in blood pressure CHF (for those on diuretics or otherwise volume depleted)
Musculoskeletal	Suppression of cartilage repair and synthesis
Cutaneous	Skin reactions and rashes Pruritus Urticaria (hives), angioedema Sweating
Respiratory	Bronchospasm, ASA-sensitive asthma Rhinitis
Central nervous system	Headache Dizziness, lightheadedness Drowsiness Aseptic meningitis, rarely seen with ibuprofen therapy Tinnitus Confusion (elderly treated with ASA, indomethacin, ibuprofen)
Ophthalmologic	Blurred vision, decreased acuity Scotomata
Other	Anaphylaxis

ACE, Angiotensin-converting enzyme; *ASA*, aspirin; *CHF*, congestive heart failure; *GI*, gastrointestinal; *NSAIDs*, nonsteroidal antiinflammatory drugs.

it irreversibly binds to platelets. A single dose of aspirin impairs clot formation for 5 to 7 days, and two aspirin tablets can double bleeding time. These characteristics of aspirin also make it an important drug in the treatment of coronary artery disease, myocardial infarctions, and stroke.

2.3 Special Implications for the PTA: Nonsteroidal Antiinflammatory Drugs The PTA is advised to observe for any side effects or adverse reactions to nonsteroidal antiinflammatory drugs (NSAIDs), especially among older adults; those taking high doses of NSAIDs for long periods (e.g., for rheumatoid arthritis [RA]); those with peptic ulcers or renal or hepatic disease, congestive heart failure (CHF), or hypertension; and those treated with anticoagulants. NSAIDs have antiplatelet effects that can be synergistic with the anticoagulant effects of drugs such as warfarin (Coumadin). Easy bruising and bleeding under the skin may be early signs of hemorrhage.

Ulcer presentation without pain occurs more often in older adults and in those taking NSAIDs. People who take prescription NSAIDs often take Advil or aspirin also. Combining these medications or combining these medications with drinking alcohol increases the risk for development of peptic ulcer disease.[98] Any client with gastrointestinal (GI) symptoms should report these to the physician.

Musculoskeletal symptoms may recur after discontinuation of NSAIDs because of the pain-relieving effects of antiinflammatory agents and the fact that they do not prevent tissue injury or affect the underlying disease process.[81]

Depending on the therapy intervention planned, the PTA may schedule the client according to the timing of the medication dosage. For example, with a chronic condition such as adhesive capsulitis, the goal may be to increase joint accessory motion, which requires more vigorous joint mobilization techniques. Relieving local painful symptoms may help the client remain relaxed during mobilization procedures.

When pain can be predicted, the drug's peak effect should be timed to coincide with the painful event. For nonopioids, such as NSAIDs, the peak effect occurs approximately 2 hours after oral administration. NSAIDs produce modest increases in blood pressure, averaging 5 mm Hg, and should be avoided in people with borderline blood pressures or who are hypertensive.[103] All NSAIDs are renal vasoconstrictors with the potential for increasing blood pressure, resulting in increased fluid retention, especially lower-extremity edema.

Immunosuppressive Agents

Immunosuppressive agents have been used traditionally and most frequently in organ and bone marrow transplantation. These medications have also been found to be helpful in treating a few other diseases, but because of their significant toxicities are indicated only for serious, debilitating, and nonresponding diseases (e.g., RA and psoriasis that have not responded to any other medication).

Intravenous immune globulins (IVIGs) are used for graft-versus-host disease.[9] These medications are often used at different times of transplantation, during the first few days after transplant, during maintenance, or with acute rejection.

Drugs are administered at the lowest possible doses while still maintaining adequate immunosuppression. Individual medical factors often determine the choice of immunosuppressive agent. Intensive immunosuppression is usually only required during the first few weeks after organ transplantation or during rejection crises. Subsequently the immune system accommodates the graft, which can be maintained with relatively small doses of immunosuppressive drugs with fewer adverse effects.

Complications of immunosuppressive medications are many and can be serious. Most agents exhibit three effects: the desired immunosuppressive effect, nonimmune toxicities, and adverse effects related to immunosuppression.[60] Nonimmune toxicities vary depending on the drug.

Serious adverse reactions include anaphylactic reactions, renal failure, *hepatotoxicity*, cytokine-release syndrome, and neurotoxicities.[102] Careful drug monitoring is required. Adverse effects related to immunosuppression are often the most serious consequences of transplantation. Almost all immunosuppressive agents render transplant recipients prone to infection, particularly cytomegalovirus. There is also an increased risk of developing fungal and bacterial infections. Viruses, such as herpes simplex and varicella zoster, may disseminate or reactivate.

An increase in certain kinds of malignancy occurs with long-term use of immunosuppressants, including lymphoma and other lymphoproliferative malignancies and nonmelanoma skin cancers.[99] Host and graft survival are improving, making infection and cancer more relevant complications. Newer protocols are being developed to reduce the risk of infection and cancer.[60]

2.4 Special Implications for the PTA: Immunosuppressants
Careful handwashing is essential before contact with any client who is immunosuppressed. If the PTA has a known infectious or contagious condition, he or she should *not* work with the immunosuppressed client. Both client and PTA can wear a mask in the presence of an upper respiratory infection.

Corticosteroids

Corticosteroids are naturally occurring hormones produced by the adrenal cortex and gonadal tissue. These hormones are steroid based with similar chemical structures but quite different physiologic effects. Generally, they are divided into *glucocorticoids* (cortisol), which mainly affect carbohydrate and protein metabolism; *mineralocorticoids* (aldosterone), which regulate electrolyte and water metabolism; and *androgens* (testosterone), which cause masculinization. Many steroid hormones can be synthesized for clinical use.

Glucocorticoids are used to decrease inflammation in a broad range of local or systemic conditions for immunosuppression. Therapists most often see people who have received prolonged, systemic glucocorticoid therapy in the treatment of cancer, transplantation, autoimmune disorders, and respiratory diseases. Mineralocorticoids are given for adrenal insufficiency, whereas androgens are given for deficiency states.

Generally, glucocorticoids cause fluid imbalances, and mineralocorticoids cause electrolyte imbalances, but mineralocorticoids are used minimally. Most adverse effects seen by the clinical therapist will be related to glucocorticosteroids. Adverse effects of anabolic steroids primarily occur in an athletic or sports-training setting.

Adverse Effects of Glucocorticoids

Glucocorticoids are effective antiinflammatory agents. They reduce inflammation by interacting with cell membrane receptors and activating antiinflammatory proteins. They also turn off genes involved with producing inflammatory agents while turning on genes that produce antiinflammatory proteins.[121] But long-term use to sustain the benefits of these drugs is accompanied by an increased risk of side effects and adrenal suppression.[133]

Glucocorticoids affect many functions of the body, especially in persons taking long-term steroids. PTAs should be familiar with common adverse effects such as change in sleep and mood, GI irritation, hyperglycemia, and fluid retention (Table 2.2); side effects are related to dose and duration of treatment. The most serious side effect of steroid use is increased susceptibility to infection and the masking of inflammatory symptoms from infection or intraabdominal complications.

Most clients taking glucocorticoids notice a change in mood, behavior, or sleep. Individuals often describe a nervous or "jittery" feeling. Symptoms may range from mild anxiety to confusion or psychosis. Changes are typically noted 5 to 14 days after glucocorticoid therapy begins; improvement is seen with withdrawal of the medication.

Effects on skin and connective tissue. Effects on the skin and connective tissue include thinning of the subcutaneous tissue accompanied by splitting of elastic fibers with resultant red or purple *striae* (stretch marks). *Ecchymoses* (bruising) and *petechiae* (small reddish blood-containing spots) are caused by decreased vascular strength.[13] Clients who are taking steroids experience delayed wound healing with decreased wound strength, inhibited tissue contraction for wound closure, and impeded epithelization.

TABLE 2.2 Possible Adverse Effects of Prolonged Systemic Corticosteroids

System	Symptom
Metabolic system	Increased glucose and protein metabolism Stimulation of appetite, weight gain Fluid retention, edema Potassium loss (hypokalemia)
Endocrine system	Delayed puberty Glucose intolerance, insulin resistance Hirsutism (hair growth) Cushing's syndrome (hypercortisolism)
Cardiovascular system	Dyslipidemia Increased blood pressure
Immune system	Increased risk of opportunistic infections Activation of latent viruses Masking of infection
Musculoskeletal system	Increased muscle catabolism (degenerative myopathy, muscle wasting) Retardation of bone growth Tendon rupture Other musculoskeletal injuries Osteoporosis Osteonecrosis, avascular necrosis of femoral head Bone fractures
Gastrointestinal system	Peptic ulcer disease Gastrointestinal bleeding, nausea, increased appetite
Nervous system	*Central nervous system:* Change in behavior (insomnia, euphoria, nervousness) Psychosis, depression Changes in cognition, mood, and memory Cerebral atrophy Pseudotumor cerebri *Autonomic nervous system (ANS):* ANS dysfunction *Peripheral nervous system:* Peripheral neuropathy
Ophthalmologic structures	Cataracts, glaucoma
Integument	Acne Striae (stretch marks) Bruising, petechiae Skin atrophy, delayed wound healing Hirsutism

---

Steroid-induced myopathy. At high doses, glucocorticoids can cause muscle weakness and atrophy called *steroid-induced myopathy.* There is a breakdown of muscle protein, resulting in muscle wasting and atrophy severe enough to interfere with daily function and activities. There is an increased variation in size and atrophy of muscles fibers, particularly type IIb.

Steroid-induced myopathy is often insidious, appearing as painless weakness weeks to months after the initiation of treatment. Clients manifest bilateral atrophy and weakness of proximal muscles; the pelvis, hips, and thighs are typically affected first.[69] Upper limb muscles can be affected, and occasionally distal limb muscles are involved. The diaphragm may also be involved, which results in difficulty breathing, especially in people with underlying pulmonary disease.

Recovery from chronic myopathy is possible with reduction or discontinuation of the drug but may take from 1 to 4 months up to 1 to 2 years. Prognosis depends on the underlying diagnosis before treatment with corticosteroids.

Effect of steroids on growth. Long-term use of glucocorticoids in children leads to growth retardation. Although there is an increase in bone synthesis once the drug has been discontinued, full height may not be achieved.[125] In adults, prolonged use of glucocorticoids inhibits bone mineralization, destroys osteoblasts, and encourages osteoclastic activity. Decreased GI calcium absorption and increased calcium excretion by the kidney also occur. These combined changes result in osteoporosis.[110] Strategies should be in place before extended therapy with glucocorticoids (greater than 3 months) to avoid bone loss.

Long-term exposure to corticosteroids increases the risk of avascular necrosis, which often requires orthopedic intervention. Glucocorticosteroids are also associated with an increase in the prevalence of vertebral fracture compared with individuals who are not treated with corticosteroids.[112]

Individuals already requiring oral diabetic agents or insulin frequently need an increase in their dosage. Persons at risk for diabetes may require a diabetic agent. Glucose monitoring is essential. Long-term treatment with inhaled glucocorticoids is common for clients with asthma. Glucocorticoids decrease inflammation and aid in counteracting the vasodilatation. Animal studies suggest that glucocorticoids may play a role in the development of diaphragm dysfunction in anyone with pulmonary impairment. Consistent with the previous discussion of glucocorticoids causing muscle weakness and atrophy, these drugs can cause a decrease in the force generation of the diaphragm. Physical therapy intervention may be helpful in counteracting this glucocorticoid-induced muscle dysfunction.[39]

The GI effects of steroids are fewer than those of NSAIDs, yet steroids are known to cause gastritis, esophageal irritation, GI bleeding, and less commonly, peptic ulcers. Many clients take both glucocorticoids and NSAIDs, increasing their risk for adverse GI events. Glucocorticoids are also known to cause cataracts. Cataract formation is dependent on dose and duration of use. They typically develop bilaterally but slowly. Clients with a history of glaucoma and taking glucocorticoids long term may have an increase in pressure while taking glucocorticoids, making pressure checks advisable.

Because glucocorticoids cause the adrenal gland to stop working, withdrawal must be slow and tapered. Severe adrenal problems may follow sudden withdrawal of the medication, particularly in the presence of infection or other stress. The person may experience vomiting, orthostatic hypotension, hypoglycemia, restlessness, arthralgia, anorexia, malaise, and fatigue. These symptoms should be reported to the physician.

Designer glucocorticoids. New glucocorticoids are in development that would selectively enhance the antiinflammatory aspects of the drug while selectively decreasing or avoiding the adverse side effects, although there are many overlapping factors.

Anabolic–androgenic steroids. Anabolic–androgenic steroids (AASs), anabolic steroids, or "roids" are synthetic derivatives of the hormone testosterone. They are most commonly used in a nonmedical setting to develop secondary male characteristics and to build muscle tissue.[10–12] The use of anabolic steroids to enhance physical performance by athletes has been declared illegal by all national and international athletic committees. Even so, an estimated 3 million individuals in the United States alone are current or past nonmedical users of AASs.[30] These compounds can be administered orally, intramuscularly, or by injection.

Studies indicate that adolescent AAS users are significantly more likely to be males and to use other illicit drugs, alcohol, and tobacco.[5] Previously, more athletes were found to use AASs than nonathletes, to enhance sports performance.[7] However, questions are being raised as to the percentage who now use AASs for cosmetic reasons alone.[96] The goal is to advance to a more mature body build and enhance the masculine appearance.

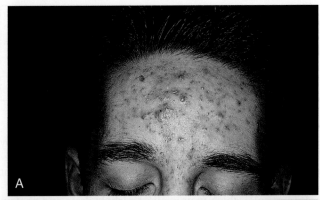
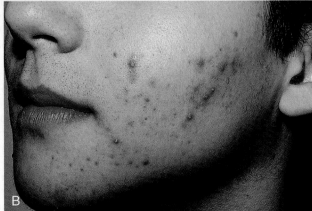

FIG. 2.2 Acne vulgaris on the forehead (A) and lower face (B) associated with the use of anabolic steroids. It is considered an abnormal response to normal levels of the male hormone testosterone. The face, chest, back, shoulders, and upper arms are especially affected. There are many other causes of this form of acne; its presence does not necessarily mean the individual is using anabolic steroids.

Athletes tend to take doses that are 10, 100, or even 1000 times larger than the doses prescribed for medical purposes. They cycle the drugs before competition, a technique known as *stacking*, alternately tapering the dosage upward and downward before a competitive event. Human growth hormone has been used alone and in combination with anabolic steroids to further enhance athletic performance.

Nearly all users of AASs report side effects. The most common include an increase in sexual drive, acne vulgaris (Fig. 2.2), increased body hair, and an increase in aggressive behavior.[89] Individuals may also exhibit an increase in low-density lipoproteins and a decrease in high-density lipoproteins, complicating atherosclerosis and coronary artery disease.[4] The development of thrombosis (i.e., venous thromboembolism, stroke, retinal vein occlusion) is also seen in persons taking AAS.[71]

Misuse of supraphysiologic doses of AASs for nonmedical reasons has been linked with serious side effects such as hypertension, left ventricular hypertrophy, myocardial ischemia, liver dysfunction, and sudden and premature death.

Users of anabolic steroids may experience an increased susceptibility to tendon strains and injuries, especially biceps and patellar tendons, because muscle size and strength increase at a rate far greater than tendon and connective tissue strength. Steroid use by adolescents may lead to accelerated maturation and premature epiphyseal closure.[120]

Homicides, suicides, poisonings, and other accidental deaths associated with AAS use have been attributed to impulsive, disinhibited behavior characterized by violent rages, mood swings, and/or uncontrolled drug intake.[101,122] Shared use of multi-dose vials, dividing drugs using syringes, and increased sexual risk-taking behavior are risk factors associated with AAS use and are potential routes for human immunodeficiency virus (HIV) and hepatitis infection.[79]

There are, however, legitimate medical uses for anabolic steroids that have come about as a result of physiologic evidence that anabolic steroids prevent loss of lean body mass. Oxandrolone, a synthetically derived testosterone, is approved as an adjuvant therapy to promote weight gain after weight loss secondary to chronic infections, severe trauma (severe burns), and extensive surgery to relieve bone pain associated with osteoporosis.[29–31,44]

Other areas of testosterone use include in premenopausal women with a loss of libido and in aging men to prevent loss in muscle mass and strength.[11,45,57] The adverse effects of these steroids, however, make long-term use inadvisable, particularly in the doses often required for efficacy.

2.5 Special Implications for the PTA: Corticosteroids

Inflammation and Infection

In the rehabilitation setting, large doses of steroids are administered early in the treatment of TBI and in some clients with spinal cord injury (SCI) to control cerebral or spinal cord edema. Suppression of the inflammatory reaction in people who are given large doses of steroids may be so complete as to mask the clinical signs and symptoms of major diseases, intraabdominal complications, or spread of infection. In the orthopedic population, local symptoms of pain or discomfort are also masked, so the therapist must exercise caution during treatment to avoid exacerbating the underlying inflammatory process.

Increased susceptibility to the infections associated with impaired cellular immunity and the decreased rate of recovery from infection associated with corticosteroid use necessitate careful infection control. Special care should be taken to avoid exposing immunosuppressed clients to infection, and everyone in contact with that person should follow strict handwashing policies.

If back pain occurs in a person who is receiving corticosteroids, diagnostic measures should be undertaken to rule out osteoporosis or compression fracture.

Intensive Care Setting

Although clients in the intensive care unit (ICU) are often treated with steroids for various serious illnesses, the use of these medications may increase the risk for complications such as infection, impaired wound healing, ICU-acquired *paresis*, muscle weakness,[28] or death.

Intraarticular Injections

Intraarticular injections of corticosteroids are occasionally necessary to control acute pain in a joint that is not responding to oral analgesics, particularly if an effusion is present. Such injections can provide short-term relief and improve the client's mobility and function.[67] The rationale for use in the joint is to suppress the synovitis because no evidence currently indicates that intraarticular injections retard the progression of erosive disease. Intraarticular injections must be carefully selected, and no single joint should have more than three or four injections before other procedures are pursued.[87]

Most steroid injections are accompanied by an anesthetizing agent, such as lidocaine or bupivacaine, which usually provides immediate pain relief, although the antiinflammatory effect may

require 2 to 3 days. During this time, the client should be advised to continue using proper supportive positioning and avoid movements that would otherwise aggravate the previous symptoms.

Some controversy remains as to whether the person can bear weight on the joint for several days after the injection; a less conservative approach permits nonstrenuous activity. Vigorous exercise may speed resorption of the steroid from the joint and reduce the intended effect. Intraarticular injection of corticosteroids may also result in pigment changes that are most noticeable among dark-skinned people.

Exercise and Steroids

The harmful side effects of glucocorticoids can be delayed or reduced in their severity by physical activity, regular exercise (aerobic or fitness), strength training, and proper nutrition. Unfortunately, these clients are often too sick to engage in exercise at all, much less at a level of intensity that would reverse myopathy. When possible, the PTA can help emphasize the importance of exercise, especially activities that produce significant stress on the weight-bearing joints.

Strength training or stair exercise is one way to maintain the large muscle groups of the legs, which are most affected by the muscle-wasting properties of corticosteroids. The treatment plan should also include closed-chained exercises to prevent shearing forces across joint lines and to allow for normal joint loading, prevention of vertebral compression fractures, and education about proper body mechanics during functional activities.

Client education on the importance of proper footwear and choice of exercise surfaces is important for the individual receiving long-term corticosteroid therapy. For the person at risk for avascular necrosis of the femoral head, exercising the surrounding joint musculature in a non–weight-bearing position may be required.

Monitoring Vital Signs

Long-term use of corticosteroids may result in electrolyte imbalances, which necessitate monitoring of vital signs during aerobic activity because of the demand placed on the cardiovascular system in conjunction with these adverse effects.

Many glucocorticoids have mineralocorticoid activity as well. This causes sodium and fluid retention, leading to hypertension. Careful monitoring of blood pressure should be performed in clients with previously existing high blood pressure.

Steroids, Nutrition, and Stress

People taking steroids may be advised to increase their dietary intake of calcium and vitamin D to counteract the loss of calcium in the urine.[97] Clients may also require a medication to decrease the loss of bone.[109] Protein intake is recommended for muscle growth. Individuals may also require potassium supplementation because of increased potassium loss in the urine.

Corticosteroids interfere with the action of insulin, which may result in glucose intolerance or diabetes mellitus or may aggravate existing conditions in diabetes. Regular blood glucose monitoring is recommended to detect steroid-induced diabetes mellitus.

Psychologic Considerations

Corticosteroid use can result in a range of mood changes from irritability, euphoria, and nervousness to more serious depression and psychosis. Insomnia is often also a reported problem during corticosteroid therapy. The intensity of changes in mood may depend on the dosage administered, the sensitivity of the individual, and the underlying personality. When intense changes are observed, the physician should be notified so that an adjustment in dosage can be made.

Chronic corticosteroid use may alter a person's body image because of changes in adipose tissue distribution, thinning of skin, and development of stretch marks. Some people may be extremely self-conscious about these cosmetic changes, and others may be emotionally devastated by them; caution is required in discussing assessment findings with the client. These cosmetic changes do reverse when the drug is discontinued slowly.

Anabolic Steroids

Athletes, especially adolescent athletes, may display signs and symptoms of (nonmedical, illegal) anabolic steroid use, including rapid weight gain (10 to 15 lb in 3 weeks); elevated blood pressure and associated peripheral edema; acne on the face, upper back, and chest; alterations in body composition, with marked muscular hypertrophy; and disproportionate development of the upper torso along with stretch marks around the back and chest. Jaundice may develop after prolonged anabolic steroid use.

PTAs working with adolescents may see cases of recurrent tendon or muscle strain. Soft tissues working under the strain of added muscle bulk and body mass take longer than expected for physiologic healing to occur. Reinjury is not uncommon under these conditions.

Other signs of steroid use include needle marks in the large muscle groups, development of male pattern baldness, and gynecomastia (breast enlargement). Abscesses from injection use may also develop. Among females, secondary male characteristics may develop, such as a deeper voice, breast atrophy, and abnormal facial and body hair. Irreversible sterility can occur (females being affected more than males), and menstrual irregularities may develop in women.

Changes in personality may occur; the user may become more aggressive or experience mood swings and psychologic delusions (e.g., believe he or she is indestructible). "Roid rage," sometimes referred to as *steroid psychosis* and characterized by sudden outbursts of uncontrolled emotion, may be observed. Severe depression is one of the signs of withdrawal from steroids. Withdrawal from AASs is a risk factor for suicide.

RADIATION INJURIES

Definition and Overview

Radiation therapy, or radiotherapy, is the treatment of disease (usually cancer) by delivery of radiation to a particular area of the body. Radiation therapy is one of the major treatment modalities for cancer and is used in approximately 60% of all cases of cancer. Radiotherapy is used in the local control phase of treatment but has both direct and indirect toxicities associated with its use. Radiation reactions and injuries to body tissues are the harmful effects (acute, delayed, or chronic) of exposure to ionizing radiation.

Today, a pencil-thin beam of radiation can be targeted to deliver extremely high doses of radiation to within a millimeter of a cancer site. Advanced computer technology creates a three-dimensional model of the tumor to allow target mapping. Careful preplanning and delivery of targeted, modulated radiation doses have contributed to a reduced number of radiation side effects.

Etiologic and Risk Factors

Risk factors for developing radiation toxicities arising from therapeutic radiation are often multifactorial, depending on the organ irradiated, individual variations and tolerance, tumor type, volume irradiated, and fraction size.

People may also be exposed to radiation found in the environment, such as radon in their homes, or when rare nuclear events release large amounts of radioactivity, exposing people to total body irradiation. According to the seventh report on the Biological Effects of Ionizing Radiation (BEIR VII) issued by the National Academy of Science, exposure to even low-dose imaging radiology (including computed tomography [CT] scans) can result in the development of malignancy. Exposure to medical x-rays is linked with leukemia, thyroid cancer, and breast cancer. There is a 1 in 1000 chance of developing cancer from a single CT scan of the chest, abdomen, or pelvis. The latency period for leukemias is 2 to 5 years, and 10 to 30 years for solid tumors.[84]

Pathogenesis

Radiation therapy uses high-energy ionizing radiation to kill cancer cells. Irradiation is an effective treatment for cancer because it directly destroys hydrogen bonds between deoxyribonucleic acid (DNA) strands within cancer cells. This prevents cellular replication.

Ionizing radiation also causes the production of free radicals, which leads to membrane damage and the breakdown of proteins, resulting in cell death. Arterioles supplying oxygenated blood are often damaged, resulting in inadequate nutritional supply and leading to ischemia and death of the irradiated tissues.

Clinical Manifestations and Medical Management

Similar to risk factors associated with radiation therapy, the clinical manifestations of radiation depend on individual variations, location and type of tumor, radiation volume and fraction dose, and organ system involved. Although newer techniques allow for organ shielding and lower volumes and fraction doses, radiation therapy continues to cause symptoms and injuries.

Each organ has its own tolerance to radiation, therefore injuries vary among organ systems—yet there are some general principles that encompass radiation therapy injuries. Most organ systems exhibit both acute injuries that occur within 30 days of irradiation and delayed injuries that occur more than 30 days later (Table 2.3). Acute injuries are frequently self-limiting, whereas delayed effects are often irreversible and difficult to treat. Acute symptoms may delay further radiation treatments because of damage to GI mucosa, bone marrow, and other vital tissues.

Acute injuries are often treated symptomatically with red blood cells (RBCs) and platelet transfusions, antibiotics, fluid and electrolyte maintenance, and other supportive medical measures as needed. More effort is being placed on prevention because of poor prognosis in many cases of delayed radiation complications. Clinicians have been attempting to optimize total dose, fractionation size, and total volume being radiated.[40,73]

Modifications are made when chemotherapy is used in conjunction with radiation, and prophylactic medications to prevent damage or complications are under investigation.[64,108,124,139] Because there are unique or specific injuries to different organ systems, the following sections specify clinical manifestations, treatment, and research pertaining to different organ systems.

Radiation Esophagitis and Enterocolitis

The esophagus is often involved in the radiation fields under treatment for lung cancer. An acute reaction may occur within 2 to 3 weeks after the initiation of radiation therapy, manifested by abnormal peristalsis activity, odynophagia (pain with swallowing), and dysphagia (difficulty swallowing).

Resolution of symptoms typically occurs 1 to 3 weeks after completion of radiotherapy. Late esophagitis is a result of inflammation and fibrosis of tissue, causing stricture and fistula formation. Dilation and surgical repair may be necessary.[132]

TABLE 2.3 Immediate and Delayed Effects of Ionizing Radiation[a]

System Affected	Immediate Effect	Delayed Effect
Musculoskeletal		Soft tissue (collagen) fibrosis, contracture, atrophy Orthopedic deformity
Neuromuscular	Fatigue Decreased appetite Subtle changes in behavior and cognition Short-term memory loss Ataxia (subacute)	Myelopathy (spinal cord dysfunction) Cerebral injury, neurocognitive deficits Radionecrosis (headaches, changes in personality, seizures) Plexopathy (brachial, lumbosacral, or pelvic plexus) Gait abnormalities
Cardiovascular and pulmonary	Fatigue, decreased endurance Radiation pneumonitis	Radiation fibrosis (lung) Cardiotoxicity • Coronary artery disease • Myocardial ischemia or infarction • Pericarditis Lymphedema
Integumentary	Erythema Edema Dryness, itching Epilation or hair loss (alopecia) Destruction of nails Epidermolysis (loose skin) Delayed wound healing	Skin scarring, delayed wound healing, contracture Telangiectasia (vascular lesion) Malignancy (basal cell, squamous cell, melanoma)
Other	Gastrointestinal: anorexia, nausea, dysphagia, vomiting, diarrhea, xerostomia (dry mouth), stomatitis (inflammation of mouth mucosa), esophagitis, intestinal stenosis Renal and urologic: urinary dysfunction	Bone marrow suppression (anemia, infection, bleeding) Cataracts Endocrine dysfunction (cranial radiation) including amenorrhea, menopause, infertility, decreased libido Hepatitis Nephritis, renal insufficiency Malignancy • Skin cancer • Leukemia • Lung cancer • Thyroid cancer • Breast cancer

[a]Some of the delayed effects of radiation (e.g., cranial injury, pericarditis, pulmonary fibrosis, hepatitis, nephritis, gastrointestinal disturbances) may be signs of recurring cancer. The physician should be notified of any new symptoms, change in symptoms, or increase in symptoms.

As in other organs receiving radiation, the intestines exhibit both acute and chronic symptoms of radiation treatment. This increased rate of stem cell loss contributes to acute radiation enteritis, reducing the surface area required for nutrient absorption and leading to dehydration and malnutrition.

Intestinal motility also changes, causing diarrhea, abdominal cramping, and nausea. Abnormal intestinal motility can occur after the first treatment, but symptoms become most pronounced at around the third week of treatment.

Radiation frequently causes fibrosis of tissues that may lead to strictures in the intestines, bowel obstruction, fistulas with abscess formation, ulceration with bleeding, and malabsorption.

Radiation Heart Disease

Radiation to the chest can cause pericarditis, coronary heart disease, and myocardial disease.

Radiation Lung Disease

The lung is a radiosensitive organ that can be affected by radiation therapy. Pulmonary toxicity is fairly uncommon and is determined by the volume of lung irradiated and the dose and fraction rate of therapy, along with risk factors such as concurrent chemotherapy, older age, lower baseline pulmonary function, and lower performance status.[74]

The two syndromes of pulmonary response to radiation are an acute phase (radiation pneumonitis) and a chronic phase (radiation fibrosis). *Radiation pneumonitis* is caused by significant interstitial inflammation creating a reduction of gas exchange. It usually occurs 2 to 3 months (range of 1 to 6 months) after completion of radiotherapy and typically resolves within 6 to 12 months.

Symptoms range from a dry cough with dyspnea on exertion to severe cough and dyspnea at rest.[74] Rarely, clients may develop acute respiratory distress requiring intubation and ventilation.

Diagnosis of radiation pneumonitis can prove difficult if underlying disease, such as chronic obstructive pulmonary disease (COPD), is present. Clients with grade 1 or 2 radiation pneumonitis respond well to corticosteroids, although their use can increase the risk for serious infection. Grades 3 and 4 radiation pneumonitis typically have a poor outcome.

Pulmonary radiation fibrosis may occur months after radiation therapy. Radiation fibrosis is progressive, and symptoms may develop slowly. Only supportive therapy is available, such as oxygen supplementation, bronchodilators, and treatment of infection.

Radiation Dermatitis

Damage to the skin is one of the more common side effects of radiation because it is involved in most therapies, despite tumor location. Although most injury to the skin is reversible, severe reactions can cause delay in therapy or a change in administration. The cutaneous effects of radiation can be separated into acute, consequential-late, and chronic.

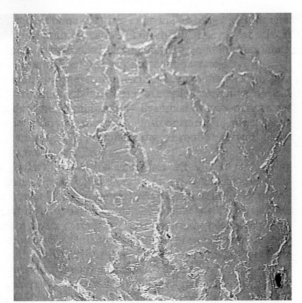

FIG. 2.3 Dry desquamation with scaling associated with radiation. (From Habif TP: Clinical dermatology: a color guide to diagnosis and therapy, ed 6, St. Louis, 2016, Mosby.)

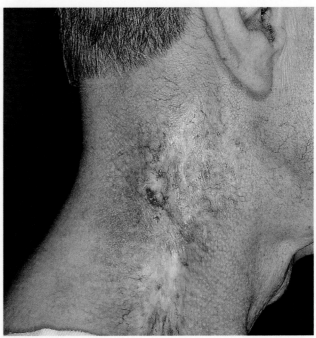

FIG. 2.4 Radiation dermatitis. Acute or chronic inflammation of the skin caused by exposure to ionizing radiation (radiation therapy for cancer). Symptoms may include redness, blistering, and sloughing of the skin. The condition can progress to scarring, fibrosis, and atrophy as shown here.

The National Cancer Institute has provided guidelines for grading acute cutaneous damage to the skin after radiation. Grade 1 reactions resemble sunburn and are accompanied by hair loss, dry desquamation, pruritus, dyspigmentation, and scaling (Fig. 2.3). These changes are secondary to damage of the hair follicles and sebaceous glands. Grade 2 reactions produce persistent erythema or patchy moist desquamation in the folds and creases of the skin, often associated with pain and edema. Bullae may form, rupture, and become superinfected. These changes manifest 4 to 5 weeks into therapy and peak 1 to 2 weeks after treatment completion. Complete healing requires 1 to 3 months.[65]

Moist desquamation of the skin with pitting edema characterizes grade 3 reactions. Compared with grade 2 reactions, the edematous erythema of grade 3 is not confined to the skin folds. Grade 4 reactions (rare) are severe, with skin necrosis or ulceration of full-dermis thickness associated with bleeding.

Sebaceous glands, hair follicles, and nails may be permanently affected. Fibrosis of the dermis accompanied by absorption of collagen creates contracted, atrophic skin, which is susceptible to tearing and ulceration (Fig. 2.4). An abnormal proliferation of arteriole cells may occur, causing thrombosis of the vessels, which, combined with fibrosis, inhibits healing and predisposes ulcers to infection. These complex ulcers are painful and difficult to heal.

Treatment of acute cutaneous injury is typically symptomatic. For grade 1 and 2 reactions, washing with water or a gentle, low pH agent is sufficient to keep the skin clean and reduce bacterial load. Antiperspirants and talcum powders should be avoided in the radiation field. Ointments and creams can often benefit irritated and dry skin after radiotherapy.

Treatment of ulcers and erosions from radiation does not require specific therapy, but the same general principles of wound care apply. Other modalities that have been used include biosynthetic, artificial, and bioengineered skin; lasers;[113] and recombinant platelet-derived growth factor (PDGF).[136] Diligence is required to keep fibrotic tissue intact. Active and

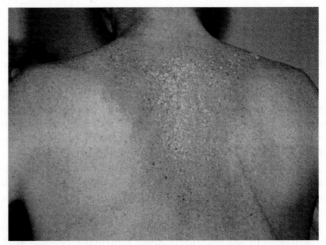

FIG. 2.5 Radiation recall. This person had small cell cancer of the lung treated with radiation. Cytoxan treatment some months later elicited erythema and desquamation within the portal of radiation. This lesion is in the healing phase.

passive range-of-motion exercises are important for retention of mobility and reduction of contractures.

Another type of radiation-induced reaction is *radiation recall*. Radiation recall reactions (Fig. 2.5) are inflammatory reactions that occur in a previously irradiated site after the administration of certain chemotherapeutic drugs or antibiotics.[68]

Recall may occur in the skin, mucous membranes, lungs, central nervous system (CNS), esophagus, and GI tract, although the skin is most frequently involved.[111] Months and even years may pass from the time of the initial radiation therapy to the onset of this reaction. A more immediate reaction (within 2 to

3 days) often occurs after the initiation of chemotherapy and is usually characterized by a mild, sunburned appearance. The skin may itch or burn; the reaction can last hours to days.

Effects of Radiation on Connective Tissue

Radiation therapy is well known to cause significant long-term or chronic effects on the connective tissue. Acute irradiation toxicity is less likely because connective tissue has a slower turnover or reproductive rate and striated muscle tolerates relatively high doses of radiation.

Late changes—such as fibrosis, atrophy, and contraction of tissue—can occur to any area irradiated but especially to collagen tissue. Irradiation can cause profound and irreversible changes in growing bones and limbs, resulting in limb-length discrepancies and scoliosis requiring orthopedic surgical correction. Weakness of the bone may lead to pathologic fractures.

Fibrosis of connective tissue can result in edema, decreased range of motion, and functional impairment. The fibrotic effect of radiation on the circulatory and lymphatic system is typically seen in a loss of elasticity and contractility of the irradiated vessels that are required to transport the blood, lymph, and waste products from the area of the body being exposed.[6]

Although lymphatic vessels maintain their structural integrity after being irradiated, fibrosis occurs in the surrounding tissue. This effect can inhibit normal growth of lymphatic vessels into healing tissues and delay lymphatic proliferation in response to inflammation.[78]

Currently, physical therapy and supportive measures are the mainstay of therapy, although newer modalities and medications are under investigation.[92]

Effects of Radiation on the Nervous System

As radiation therapy is used more frequently and aggressively in treating malignancies, toxicities to the nervous system increase. The incidence of nervous system toxicity related to radiation increases as the volume of nervous tissue being irradiated, the total dose, and the fraction size increase.[23]

Clinical manifestations of nervous system radiation toxicity can be separated into three categories: acute, subacute, and delayed. Neurologic symptoms relating to acute and subacute complications are most often self-limiting, requiring only supportive measures. The chronic or delayed complications are more often severe and progressive. Therapies for these complications are often palliative at best, although hyperbaric oxygen and anticoagulation have demonstrated questionable improvement.[56,72,106,140]

Acute symptoms. Acute symptoms generally occur during the period of treatment. The most common symptom is progressive and sometimes debilitating fatigue. Other clinical manifestations of cranial irradiation may include lethargy, short-term memory difficulties, and subtle changes in behavior and cognition. General symptoms that may occur during brain irradiation include decreased appetite, dry skin, hearing loss, hair loss, and decreased salivation.

Acute radiation encephalopathy, probably related to edema, is an uncommon reaction secondary to brain irradiation, causing headache, nausea and vomiting, lethargy, seizures, new focal deficits, and mental status changes. Because of careful planning and use of the drug dexamethasone, the incidence has significantly decreased, although it can be life threatening in clients who do develop this complication.

Subacute symptoms. Subacute symptoms (early delayed), noted 1 to 4 months after the completion of therapy, are fairly uncommon. If treatment included the cervical spine (and to a lesser degree the thoracic), clients may experience subacute myelopathy, a tingling, shocklike sensation passing down the arm or trunk when the neck is flexed (Lhermitte's sign).

Symptoms are usually self-limiting and peak 4 to 6 months after treatment. Irradiation of the brainstem may cause ataxia, nystagmus, and dysarthria.

Delayed complications. Late or delayed complications (late delayed) can be more serious and do not appear for months to years after therapy. For example, cerebral vasculature and other arteries, such as the carotid and coronary arteries, may be damaged when exposed to radiation, leading to coronary artery disease, transient ischemic attacks, stroke, or myocardial infarction. Other late effects are described as follows and in Table 2.3.

Radionecrosis. One of the best-described complications of whole-brain radiotherapy is delayed cerebral radionecrosis. Symptoms include headache, changes in cognition and personality, focal neurologic deficits, and seizures. Another serious long-term complication of radiotherapy of the brain is the development of tumors, including meningiomas, gliomas, lymphomas, fibrosarcomas, and malignant schwannomas. These tumors are often aggressive and difficult to cure.

Myelopathy. Radiotherapy of the spinal cord may cause a radiation-induced myelopathy. This can manifest as the Brown-Séquard syndrome or as a motor neuron syndrome. The Brown-Séquard syndrome is loss of the lateral hemisection of the spinal cord, resulting in muscle weakness that ultimately leads to paraparesis on the same side as the lesion and loss of sensation on the opposite side of the lesion.

Plexopathy. The brachial and lumbar plexuses may also be damaged after treatment. Clinical manifestations of radiation-induced brachial *plexopathy* include paresthesias with progressive motor deficits, lymphedema, and pain. Many clients lose hand function or develop arm paralysis[8,42] with associated loss of sensation.

The incidence of brachial plexopathy after radiation therapy has been reduced significantly with improved treatment, but women who were treated in the axillary, supraclavicular, and parasternal lymph node regions years ago have shown a progression of both prevalence and severity of the late effects many years later, including arm paralysis.[66]

Today, with improved irradiation techniques, the overall incidence is approximately 0.5% of all cases of irradiated breast cancer. Lumbar plexopathy is also possible when the pelvic area is irradiated. Clinical manifestations of radiation-induced plexopathy appear to be a result of fibrosis around the nerve trunks and include paresthesias, hypesthesia, progressive weakness, decreased reflexes, and pain.

Currently no curative treatment is available for either brachial or lumbar plexopathies, although therapeutic interventions can achieve significant pain control and improve strength and function in the affected limb.[59]

Pregnancy

The fetus is very sensitive to radiation. Pregnant women or those who suspect they may be pregnant must avoid all possible exposure to sources of radiation. Congenital anomalies that develop after intrauterine exposure, especially if it occurs during early pregnancy or 2 to 12 weeks after conception during organ development, may include microcephaly, growth and mental retardation, hydrocephalus, spina bifida, blindness, cleft palate, and clubfoot. Later development of cancer, especially leukemia and thyroid cancer, is most often reported when the fetus was exposed to a source of radiation.[126]

2.6 Special Implications for the PTA: Radiation

Radiation Hazard for Health Care Professionals

People who receive external radiation do not give off radiation to those who come in contact with them. Internal implants can present some hazards to others as long as the implant is in place. Pregnant staff members should avoid all contact with the internally radiated client.

When administering direct care, staff members should plan interventions so that each task can be accomplished as quickly as possible. Distance provides some protection; therefore it is advisable to use positions that place the staff person as far away from the radioactive implant as possible. For example, if the implant is in the pelvis, the caregiver might stand at the head or foot, not the side, of the bed.

The use of protective lead aprons or portable shields may be recommended according to the hospital protocol. Each staff member is encouraged to know and follow the recommended policies and procedures for the given institution. A film badge or ring badge worn on the outside of any protective devices or clothing of the caregiver records the cumulative dose of radiation received and is used to monitor exposure over a period. When removed, this badge should be stored in a location where no additional radiation exists.

Careful removal and disposal of any personal protective equipment worn by the PTA must be done according to radiation safety instructions posted. Thorough handwashing after glove removal is essential.[138]

Postradiation Therapy

Handwashing before treating the client who is in the process of receiving external radiation therapy is essential to protect him or her from infection. Skin care precautions include the following:

- Avoid topical use of alcohol or other drying agents, lotions, gels, oils, or salves; creams and gels on the skin can potentiate the received skin dosage and lead to increased adverse effects; do not wash away markings for the target area.
- Avoid positions in which the client is lying on the target area.
- Avoid exposure to direct sunlight, heat lamps, or other sources of heat, including thermal modalities.

Delayed wound healing associated with radiotherapy requires assessment early on of other factors that impair wound healing such as smoking or tobacco use, poor nutrition, weight loss before the start of treatment, and infection.

Radiation to the low back may cause nausea, vomiting, or diarrhea because the lower digestive tract is exposed to the radiation.[85] Radiation of the pelvic cavity often causes dense pelvic adhesions that can result in painful motion restrictions. The PTA's role in the postradiation treatment of these clients is to increase range of motion and provide stretching exercises.

Anyone with neurologic signs or symptoms of unknown cause must be questioned about medical history (e.g., cancer, heart disease) and the possibility of prior radiation treatment, keeping in mind that progressive disease or a vascular event can also cause an acute or subacute neurologic event. The physician must rule out cancer recurrence in anyone with a previous history of cancer and evaluate for the presence of some other cause of new onset neurologic signs and symptoms.

Postradiation Infection

Signs and symptoms of infection are often absent because the immunosuppressed person cannot mount an adequate inflammatory response. Fever may be the first and only sign of infection. Swelling, redness, and pus may be absent in infected tissue.

Radiation Therapy and Exercise

Radiation and chemotherapy can cause permanent scar formation in the lungs and heart tissues, whereas drug-induced cardiomyopathies can contribute to limitations in cardiovascular function.

Both of these variables necessitate monitoring of vital signs when working with people who are recovering or in remission from cancer treatments. Clients should be taught to monitor their own vital signs—including pulse rate, respiratory rate, and perceived exertion rate (PER), which is not to exceed 15 to 17 for moderate intensity training or submaximal testing—and observe for early signs of cardiopulmonary complications of cancer treatments such as dyspnea, pallor, excessive perspiration, or fatigue during exercise.

Low- to moderate-intensity aerobic exercise (e.g., self-paced walking) during the weeks of radiation treatment can help manage treatment-related symptoms by improving physical function and lowering reported levels of fatigue, anxiety, depression, and sleep disturbance.[80,114]

A successful aerobic training protocol for a client with cancer should include client education, an exercise evaluation, and an individualized exercise prescription. Ideally, these components of cancer treatment should begin when the person receives the diagnosis. Current guidelines recommend that clients should be advised not to exercise within 2 hours of chemotherapy or radiation therapy because increases in circulation may increase the effects of the treatments.[54] In addition, it is very important that the client carry out careful, daily stretching during and after radiation treatment. Postradiated tissue can tear when stretching. Therapy staff and client must observe for blanching of the skin and avoid stretching beyond that point. Stretching must be continued for 18 to 24 months postradiation, as the fibrotic process continues for that amount of time.

CHEMOTHERAPY[82]

Systemic chemotherapy plays a major role in the management of the 60% of malignancies that are not curable by regional modalities. As with radiation therapy, chemotherapy acts by interfering with cellular function and division.

In contrast to most cells in the body, tumor cells undergo frequent cell division, leading to an accumulation of cells that are cytologically and histologically defective. Cellular processes needed to support this increased cell division, such as DNA synthesis, DNA repair, DNA replication, and ribonucleic acid (RNA) transcription, are themselves accelerated. The principal goal of chemotherapy is to destroy malignant cells with the least harm to normal cells or the host. However, most chemotherapeutic agents are nonspecific and therefore affect both malignant and normal cells.[110]

Researchers first used these unique characteristics of tumor cells as targets for antitumor drugs in the mid-1940s. This discovery led to the development of many new drugs, commonly referred to as *chemotherapeutic drugs*, that specifically target those processes needed to support mitotic activity and cell division. Although such drugs have been successful in treating a wide variety of cancers, they are unable to distinguish cancerous from noncancerous cells (i.e., they lack specificity), often attacking normal, as well as cancerous, cells.

Characteristics and Categories of Chemotherapeutic Drugs

Chemotherapeutic drugs are *systemic drugs,* meaning that they travel throughout the body rather than remain confined to a specific area. They are able to reach cells in the primary tumor and cancerous cells that may have escaped from the primary tumor.

Normal cells most at risk for damage by chemotherapeutic agents are those that normally have high mitotic rates such as hepatic cells, cells that make up epithelial layers, bone marrow cells, and hair cells. However, virtually every organ in the body can be affected by these drugs; for this reason, chemotherapy is often accompanied by multisystem problems and disease.

Adverse Effects of Chemotherapy

Many chemotherapy agents have unique, dose-limiting toxicities. Chemotherapy drugs are used in combination for their specific actions on cells, and care is taken not to use agents with significant overlapping toxicities.

Most chemotherapeutic agents have the propensity to cause nausea and vomiting with the administration of the drug, and mucositis, diarrhea, myelosuppression, and alopecia often occur after treatment. Many cause sterility and are toxic to a fetus.[100]

Cognitive deficits referred to as *chemotherapy-related cognitive dysfunction* (CRCD) can have a dramatic effect on a person's quality of life. These deficits can be subtle or dramatic, transient or permanent, and stable or progressive.[52]

Alopecia

Alopecia (hair loss) is the most noticeable cutaneous side effect of chemotherapy and often the most distressing because it has a profound social and psychologic impact on the individual. Actively growing hair is the most rapidly proliferating cell population in the human body and therefore is very susceptible to the effects of systemic chemotherapeutic agents. Depending on which drugs and doses are used, clients may experience varying amounts of hair loss, ranging from thinning of hair to complete loss of hair, including eyelashes, eyebrows, and body hair.

Hair loss typically occurs within 1 to 3 weeks after the onset of chemotherapy. Hair loss is not restricted to the scalp, but because this area has the greatest amount of hair, the greatest losses occur here. Hair loss is temporary, with regrowth typically occurring 2 to 3 months after termination of treatment. Full hair restoration may require 1 to 2 years and may be accompanied by changes in hair color, texture, and type.[62]

Gastrointestinal Toxicity

Chemotherapy drugs have a varying ability to cause nausea/vomiting, known as emetogenic potential. High-dose platinum-based agents are among the most strongly emetogenic drugs. Chemotherapy-induced nausea and vomiting (CINV) can be acute or delayed. Acute CINV typically occurs 1 to 2 hours after the administration of the agent, with the effects peaking at 4 to 10 hours after administration and lasting approximately 12 to 24 hours.

The mechanisms responsible for nausea and vomiting are varied and not completely understood, and different drugs may cause nausea by using different pathways. Chemotherapy drugs affect cells that normally divide quickly, such as cells of the oral cavity and GI tract. Damage to the cells lining the GI tract results in the diarrhea so often seen after treatment. The cytotoxic effects of many chemotherapy drugs cause an inflammation of the mucosal epithelium in the GI tract. The resulting mucositis occurs when these injured cells are unable to replace themselves. This effect can occur anywhere in the GI tract and manifests differently depending on where the damage occurs.[55] Like nausea and vomiting, mucositis and diarrhea lead to dehydration and malnutrition.

Myelosuppression

Myelosuppression, a frequent side effect of cancer treatments, is defined as the inhibition of bone marrow cells resulting in fewer red cells, white cells, and platelets. Myelosuppression often results in anemia, infections, and bleeding as a result of a reduced number of cells. A reduction of white cells, referred to as leukopenia, or more specifically, neutropenia (reduced number of neutrophils), is a major dose-limiting toxicity of cancer treatment and often delays further treatment, possibly compromising outcomes. It is also one of the most serious adverse effects of chemotherapy, resulting in significant morbidity, mortality and cost.[74] Prolonged neutropenia can result in severe, life-threatening infections requiring prolonged hospital stays and aggressive antibiotic therapy.

Fatigue

It has been estimated that 70% to 100% of all individuals with cancer will experience cancer-related fatigue.[49] Symptoms of cancer related fatigue may include persistent sense of tiredness that is not relieved by rest, shortness of breath, decreased ability to focus or concentrate, and decreased ability to perform daily tasks.[93] Although most people will experience fatigue during treatment, upwards of 35% still experience fatigue 24 months after completing therapy.[86]

Fatigue often peaks within a few days after receiving cyclic chemotherapy then declines until the next treatment cycle. Fatigue significantly reduces quality of life. It is generally agreed that fatigue has multiple cancer-related or treatment-induced causes that can be described as being either physiologic or psychologic. Physiologic causes of fatigue include underlying disease; cancer treatment; anemia; infection; accompanying pulmonary, hepatic, cardiac, and renal disorders; sleep disorders; poorly controlled pain; and malnutrition. Psychologic causes of fatigue include anxiety disorders, depressive disorders, and cognitive losses that include decreased attention span and concentration.[104]

Cardiotoxicity

Therapies for cancer have improved over the last 20 years, and more people are surviving. However, the aggressive therapies have led to more toxicities with resulting long-term effects, including toxicities of the heart.

Chemotherapy drugs known as antimetabolites can produce ischemia and sequelae. High-dose regimens and a high total dose per course increase the likelihood of developing cardiac disease. Cessation of the drug will often decrease symptoms.[141]

The earliest signs of drug-induced cardiomyopathy include tachycardia and inability to return to baseline heart rate after exertion.

Renal Toxicity

Many chemotherapy agents, antibiotics, and other drugs used in cancer treatment are metabolized and excreted by the kidneys, making the renal system prone to injury or exacerbating underlying disease. Renal abnormalities are one of the most commonly encountered problems associated with cancer therapy, which may alter dosing or require a change in therapy. Renal impairment can be manifested as a range of abnormalities spanning from an asymptomatic increase in BUN and creatinine on laboratory tests, to more serious disorders such as acute renal failure.

A serious complication of chemotherapy that has critical adverse effects on the kidneys is tumor lysis syndrome. Tumor lysis syndrome occurs when cytotoxic drugs destroy malignant cells, releasing large amounts of metabolic byproducts and intracellular ions into the bloodstream (e.g., potassium, phosphate, and uric acid). The kidneys are unable to tolerate the sudden load, leading to hyperkalemia, hyperuricemia, hypocalcemia, and uremia. This can be life threatening, leading to cardiac dysrhythmias and renal failure. Clients who have renal insufficiency before treatment, large tumors, or rapidly dividing tumors that are sensitive to chemotherapy are at highest risk for this syndrome.

Neuropathies

Many chemotherapeutic agents adversely affect the nervous system, either peripherally or systemically, depending on the pharmacologic properties of the class of chemotherapy drug.

Chemotherapy-induced peripheral neuropathy symptoms can develop within hours after an infusion or may not appear for several days to weeks after treatment has stopped. Although most symptoms will improve or resolve, some clients report their symptoms persist for years after completing treatment.[107] Clients will often describe numbness, tingling (paresthesias/dysesthesias), or burning of their hands or feet that will progress in a distal to proximal pattern as the neuropathy becomes more severe.

Other common impairments include diminished or absent deep tendon reflexes, increased vibration and touch thresholds, hyperalgesia, allodynia, and reduced sural and peroneal nerve conduction amplitudes. In cases where motor neuropathy occurs, clients will present with weakness and/or cramping of distal muscles in the hands and feet. Orthostatic hypotension, constipation, and dysfunction of sexual organs and urinary bladder may be reported in the rare case of autonomic neuropathy.

The severity of neuropathy is related to several factors, including cumulative-dose coexisting peripheral neuropathy and combination therapy of several neurotoxic chemotherapy agents.

2.7 Special Implications for the PTA: Chemotherapy Anyone receiving chemotherapeutic drugs is at increased risk for acquiring an infection because these drugs often reduce white blood cell (WBC) numbers.

The importance of strict handwashing technique with an antiseptic solution cannot be overemphasized.

The PTA should be alert to any sign of infection and report any potential site of infection such as mucosal ulceration or a skin abrasion or tear. Check skin for petechiae, ecchymoses, cellulitis, and secondary infection.

Myelosuppression or bone marrow suppression is the most frequent side effect of many chemotherapeutic drugs. These drugs can cause the circulating numbers of mature RBCs to fall to dangerous levels. Significantly decreased hemoglobin, hematocrit, and

---

RBC numbers can compromise an individual's ability to engage in physical activity.

Drug-induced mood changes ranging from feelings of well-being and euphoria to depression and irritability may occur; depression and irritability may also be associated with the cancer. Knowing these and other potential side effects of medications used in the treatment of cancer can help the therapist better understand client reactions during rehabilitation or therapy intervention.

As part of the cancer care team, the therapy staff should keep abreast of reliable up-to-date information about treatment. The American Cancer Society (ACS) publishes many patient education materials such as *Understanding Chemotherapy: A Guide for Patients and Families*. These types of introductory materials may help the PTA come to a better understanding of the patient's own early experiences and questions. Patient education materials are usually provided free. Contact the local ACS office; if there is no local or district office, then contact the national organization (http://www.cancer.org/ or 1-800-ACS-2345).

Late Effects of Chemotherapy

It is important for the PTA to realize that the adverse effects of many chemotherapeutic agents may not appear for many years after treatment has been completed.

Survivors face an increased risk of morbidity, mortality, and diminished quality of life associated with cancer treatment. Risk is further modified by the survivor's genetics, lifestyle habits, and comorbid health conditions. Because a therapist is less likely to see individuals receiving these drugs acutely, the greater concern is for the cardiac and other organ damage, which manifests itself months to years after the cancer treatment has ended. Survivors of childhood and adolescent cancer are one of the higher risk populations seen. The curative therapy administered for the cancer also affects growing and developing tissues.[90]

Neuropathy

Neuropathy can occur as a result of the neurotoxic effects of chemotherapy, causing sensory, motor, and/or autonomic deficits. The PTA should pay attention to any reports of pain, burning pain, numbness, and/or the sensation of pins and needles in the hands and/or feet, as well as motor deficits in lower extremity muscles.

Sensory or motor loss in the lower extremities can lead to gait abnormalities, loss of balance, and increased risk of falls. Careful attention should be paid to lower extremity peripheral sensation and manual muscle testing during the history taking and physical assessment of anyone currently on these drugs or who has recently discontinued their use.

For the immobile client, prevention of pressure ulcers through client and family education and positioning with appropriate protection are also important. For the mobile client, safety standards must be followed during ambulation because of weakness and numbness of the extremities.

Chemotherapy and Exercise[33]

Fatigue is a common and severe problem for many individuals undergoing chemotherapy or chemoradiotherapy to the extent that some people are unable to carry out usual daily activities both during treatment and for months afterward. The PTA can identify cancer-related fatigue (CRF) as a potential problem by asking individuals undergoing cancer treatment to quantify their fatigue level from zero (no fatigue) to 10 (extreme fatigue) using the visual analog scale (VAS).

Before beginning or advancing an exercise program, the PTA should screen for possible energy-draining conditions such as dehydration, malnutrition, anorexia, and sleep disturbances.

In addition, other effects of treatment, such as anemia and cardiotoxicity, can severely affect a person's functional ability. Research has shown that people recovering from high-dose chemotherapy should not be instructed to rest but should increase physical activity to reduce fatigue and improve physical performance.[38] Prolonged rest and decreased activity coupled with sleep disturbances or too much sleep can contribute to CRF. An optimal balance of rest and physical exercise is essential to the successful treatment of these symptoms.[2,3,33,35,134]

Results indicate that 6 weeks of endurance training consisting of low to moderate levels of aerobic exercise (walking for 30 minutes daily on a treadmill after an interval-training program) yield a significant improvement of physical performance and a reduction of fatigue, along with an improved mood and reduced mental stress, in patients undergoing chemotherapy.[34] In addition, no reported increases in chemotherapy-related complications were associated with an endurance-training program.

Clearly, low to moderate physical levels of aerobic activity yield a reduction in fatigue and an improvement in quality of life,[33–36,93] so the challenge to the therapy staff is to keep the client active in the context of the fatigue. The PTA can monitor the presence and extent of fatigue in these individuals and schedule treatment times that coincide with periods when they have the most energy. Activities and activity demands need to be tailored to match the energy levels of the client. Teaching the use of energy conservation techniques can increase the energy available for activities of daily living (ADLs) and participation in therapy sessions.

Winningham suggests that exercise should be restricted when hemoglobin levels fall below 10 g/dL; however, clients can experience fatigue with values of 10 to 13 g/dL. Chemotherapeutic drugs often cause thrombocytopenia or depress the number of platelets. Because platelets are essential for clot formation, symptoms of this condition include easy or excessive bruising, nosebleeds or gum bleeds, skin rashes, or petechiae. Platelet counts of less than 50,000 per µL have been suggested as a contraindication to physical activity, but people with platelet counts of 10,000 per µL have been successfully treated.

SPECIFIC DISORDERS AFFECTING MULTIPLE SYSTEMS

Vasculitic Syndromes

Vasculitis is a term that applies to a diverse group of diseases characterized by inflammation in blood vessel walls. The pathogenesis of most forms of vasculitis remains poorly understood, and cases of vasculitis show great variability; it may not be possible to apply a specific disease label to such cases. Such instances of vasculitis may be diagnosed as *systemic vasculitis.*

Blood vessels of different sizes in various parts of the body may be affected by vasculitis, causing a wide spectrum of clinical manifestations. The inflammation often causes narrowing or occlusion of the vessel lumen and produces ischemia of the tissues that are supplied by the involved vessels. The inflammation may weaken the vessel wall, resulting in aneurysm or rupture. Large-vessel disease often produces limb claudication, aortic dilation, and bruits. Vasculitis of the medium vessels causes cutaneous nodules (Fig. 2.6), gangrene of the digits, mononeuritis multiplex, and microaneurysms.

Most clients with vasculitis will exhibit constitutional symptoms such as fever, arthralgias, arthritis, weight loss, and malaise.[119] Vasculitis may occur as a primary disease; as a secondary manifestation of other illnesses such as RA, infection, malignancy, or serum sickness; or as a drug-induced illness.

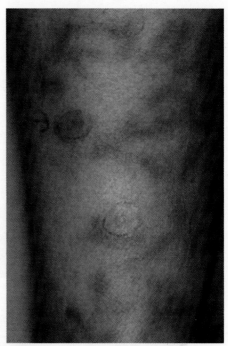

FIG. 2.6 Nodular vasculitis caused by inflammation of the medium blood vessels. (From Mahr A, Battistella M, Bouaziz J, et al.: Single-organ vasculitis: conceptual and practical considerations. La Presse Médicale 42:628-634, 2013.)

Rheumatoid Arthritis

RA is best known as a progressive autoimmune disease affecting the synovial tissue and joints. Yet RA has many extraarticular manifestations involving bone, muscle, eyes, lung, heart, and the skin. The most frequent skin manifestation is the rheumatoid nodule. These are most commonly found subcutaneously on extensor surfaces such as the forearm, but have been noted on the heart, lung, sacrum, and larynx (Fig. 2.7).

Rheumatoid vasculitis has become much less frequent over the last decade, probably because of disease-modifying agents, yet it remains the most feared complication of RA, with considerable morbidity and mortality. Vasculitis is more common in men and usually develops in persons with the most significant active disease. Clinical features of systemic rheumatoid vasculitis are diverse because the disease affects both medium and small vessels throughout the body. The most common findings are cutaneous lesions such as nail-edge infarctions, purpura (see Fig. 2.1), and skin ulcers. Skin ulcers usually develop suddenly as deep, punched-out lesions at sites that are unusual for venous ulceration, such as the dorsum of the foot or the upper calf.

Neurologic manifestations of RA vasculitis most commonly involve either a mild distal sensory neuropathy (paresthesia or numbness) or a severe sensorimotor neuropathy such as wrist or foot drop (mononeuritis multiplex). These may be the only extraarticular manifestations of RA.

Systemic manifestations of rheumatoid vasculitis may include unexplained weight loss, anorexia, and malaise. Individuals with severe RA who experience any of these symptoms should be referred to the physician for further evaluation. Clients with multiple manifestations of vasculitis have a poor prognosis and require aggressive treatment.

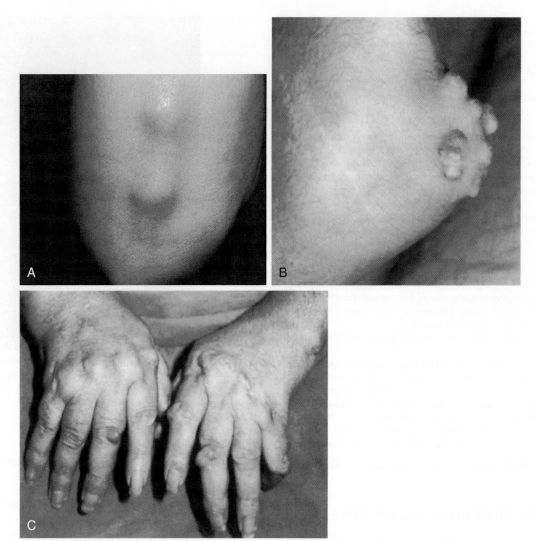

FIG. 2.7 (A) Rheumatoid nodules may be firm, raised, nontender bumps over which the skin slides easily. Common sites are in the olecranon bursa (elbow), along the extensor surface of the forearm, and behind the heel (calcaneus). (B) These nodules are also associated with rheumatoid arthritis and are firm, nontender, and freely movable. These are most common in people with severe arthritis, high-titer rheumatoid factor, or rheumatoid vasculitis. (C) Multiple rheumatoid nodules of the digits with typical ulnar deviation deformity from long-standing rheumatoid arthritis. Histologically identical lesions have been found in the sclera (eye), larynx, heart, lungs, and abdominal wall. The lesions develop insidiously and may regress spontaneously but usually persist.

Systemic Lupus Erythematosus

Lupus erythematosus is an autoimmune disease that appears in two forms: discoid lupus erythematosus (DLE), which affects only the skin, and systemic lupus erythematosus (SLE), which affects both multiple organ systems and the skin and can be fatal. SLE most commonly causes rashes of the skin, polyarthritis, and myalgias. The most serious complications affect the heart, kidneys, and CNS. Like RA, SLE is characterized by recurring remissions and exacerbations, although complete remission is rare.

Systemic Sclerosis

Systemic sclerosis, also known as *progressive systemic sclerosis* (PSS) or *scleroderma*, is a generalized connective tissue disorder of unknown cause characterized by thickening and fibrosis of the skin. It may also affect internal organs, namely the heart, lungs, GI tract, and kidneys.

Although there are many subgroups termed *scleroderma*, it is often categorized into two main subgroups: diffuse cutaneous scleroderma (skin involvement of the trunk, face, and proximal and distal extremities) and limited cutaneous scleroderma (involvement of the skin of the face and neck but distal to the elbow and knee). There is significant variability of symptoms and organ involvement among clients. It affects women more than men and occurs most frequently at 35 to 50 years of age. Although scleroderma has no current significant disease-modifying treatments, there has been a significant improvement in survival. This is most likely a result of better management of the specific organ disease.

Tuberculosis

Tuberculosis (TB) is an acute or chronic infection caused by *Myco-bacterium tuberculosis*. Although the primary infection site is the lung, mycobacteria commonly exist in other parts of the body; this is referred to as *extrapulmonary tuberculosis*. The extrapulmonary sites may include the renal system and skeletal system.

Sarcoidosis

Sarcoidosis is a multisystem disorder characterized by the formation of noncaseating granulomas, which are inflammatory cells usually surrounded by a rim of lymphocytes. These granulomas may develop in any organ but often are noted in multiple organs at once, including the lungs, lymph nodes, liver, bones, or eyes and may be accompanied by skin lesions. Presenting symptoms of sarcoidosis can often be confused with other inflammatory or infectious processes, making the diagnosis difficult. In the United States sarcoidosis occurs predominantly among African Americans and affects twice as many women as men.

Sarcoidosis is often referred to as either *acute* or *chronic*. Acute sarcoidosis is abrupt in onset, frequently involving the eyes and skin. Bell's palsy may also be seen. Acute sarcoidosis is transient, often with a good prognosis and complete resolution of symptoms. Chronic sarcoidosis typically is more insidious in onset and occurs in older individuals. Fibrosis formation is prevalent, involving the heart, lung, kidneys, and bone. Significant morbidity and mortality are associated with chronic sarcoidosis, with recurrence of the disease despite treatment.

Multiple Organ Dysfunction Syndrome
Overview

Care of critically ill people has progressed significantly during the last 50 years. Substantial advances have been made in the care of shock, acute renal failure, acute brain injury, and acute respiratory failure, with more people surviving these conditions.

However, despite these advances, progressive deterioration of organ function may occur in people who are critically ill or injured. People often die of complications of disease, rather than from the disease itself. Multiple organ dysfunction syndrome (MODS) is often the final complication of a critical illness; it is one of the most common causes of death in the ICU.[47]

Definition and Etiologic and Risk Factors

MODS, also called *multiple organ failure syndrome* (MOFS), is the progressive failure (more than 24 hours) of two or more organ systems after a severe illness or injury. Sepsis and septic shock are the most common causes.[142] MODS carries a high mortality rate that increases with each organ that fails.

Systemic inflammatory response syndrome (SIRS) characterizes the clinical manifestations of hypermetabolism (e.g., increased temperature, heart rate, and respirations) present in many clients with MODS. Because it is a response to tissue insult or injury, SIRS is present in many individuals admitted to an ICU.

Pathogenesis

Although MODS may be a final common pathway in critical illnesses, actual causes and cellular changes leading to MODS are not completely understood. Most likely multiple mechanisms and factors are responsible or contribute to the development of MODS. In response to illness or traumatic injury, the neuroendocrine system activates stress hormones to be released into the circulation, whereas the sympathetic nervous system is stimulated to compensate for complications such as fluid loss and hypotension.

Because of the initial insult, proinflammatory cells and enzymes are released, with the overall effect of massive uncontrolled systemic immune and inflammatory responses. This hyperinflammation and hypercoagulation perpetuates edema formation, cardiovascular instability, endothelial damage, and clotting abnormalities.

At the same time, initial oxygen consumption demand increases because the oxygen requirements at the cellular level increase. Flow and oxygen consumption are mismatched because of a decrease in oxygen delivery to the cells caused by maldistribution of blood flow, myocardial depression, and a hypermetabolic state. The outcome is abnormal cellular respiration and function, resulting in the multiple organ dysfunction characteristic of MODS.[95]

Clinical Manifestations

A clinical pattern has been well established in the development of MODS. After the precipitating event, low-grade fever, tachycardia, dyspnea, SIRS, and altered mental status develop. The lung is the first organ to fail.

At 7 to 10 days, the hypermetabolic state intensifies, GI dysfunction is common, and signs of liver and kidney failure develop. During days 14 to 21, renal and liver failures progress to a severe status and the GI and immune systems fail, with eventual cardiovascular collapse. Ischemia and inflammation are responsible for the CNS manifestations. Protein metabolism is also affected, and amino acids derived from skeletal muscle, connective tissue, and intestinal viscera become an important energy source. The result is a significant loss of lean body mass.

Medical Management

Prevention, early detection, and supportive therapy are essential for MODS, as no specific medical treatment exists for this condition. A way to halt the process once it has begun has not yet been discovered. Pharmacologic treatment may include antibiotics to treat infection and supplemental oxygen and ventilation to keep oxygen saturation levels at or above 90%.

Fluid replacement and nutritional support are also provided. MODS is the major cause of death (usually occurring at days 21 to 28) after septic, traumatic, and burn injuries. If the affected individual's condition has not improved by the end of the third week, survival is unlikely. The mortality rate of MODS is 60% to 90% and approaches 100% if three or more organs are involved, sepsis is present, and the individual is older than 65 years of age.

FLUID AND ELECTROLYTE IMBALANCES

Observing clinical manifestations of fluid or electrolyte imbalances may be an important aspect of client care, especially in the acute care and home health care settings. Identifying clients at risk for such imbalances is the first step toward early detection.

The causes of fluid and electrolyte imbalance are many and varied and include disease processes, injury, medications, medical treatment, dietary restrictions, and imbalance of fluid intake with fluid output.[123] The most common causes of fluid and electrolyte imbalances in a therapy practice include burns, surgery, diabetes mellitus, malignancy, alcoholism, and the various factors affecting the aging adult population (Box 2.4).

BOX 2.4   Factors Affecting Fluid and Electrolyte Balance in the Aging

- Acute illness (fever, diarrhea, vomiting)
- Bowel cleansing for gastrointestinal (GI) diagnostic testing
- Change in mental status
- Constipation
- Decreased thirst mechanism
- Difficulty swallowing
- Excessive sodium intake:
  - Diet
  - Sodium bicarbonate antacids (e.g., Alka-Seltzer)
  - Water supply or water softener
  - Decreased taste sensation (increased salt intake)
- Excessive calcium intake:
  - Alkaline antacids
- Immobility
- Laxatives (habitual use for constipation)
- Medications:
  - Antiparkinsonian drugs
  - Diuretics
  - Propranolol
  - Tamoxifen (breast cancer therapy)
- Sodium-restricted diet
- Urinary incontinence (voluntary fluid restriction)

BOX 2.5   Clinical Manifestations of Dehydration

- Absent perspiration, tearing, and salivation
- Body temperature (subnormal or elevated)
- Confusion
- Disorientation; coma; seizures
- Dizziness when standing
- Dry, brittle hair
- Dry mucous membranes, furrowed tongue
- Headache
- Incoordination
- Irritability
- Lethargy
- Postural hypotension
- Rapid pulse
- Rapid respirations
- Skin changes:
  - Color: gray
  - Temperature: cold
  - Turgor: poor
  - Feel: warm, dry if mild; cool, clammy if severe
- Sunken eye
- Sunken fontanel (children)

Aging and Fluid and Electrolyte Balance

The volume and distribution of body fluids composed of water, electrolytes, and nonelectrolytes vary with age, gender, body weight, and amount of adipose tissue. Throughout life, a slow decline occurs in lean body or fat-free mass, with a corresponding decline in the volume of body fluids. Only 45% to 50% of the body weight of aging adults is water, compared with 55% to 60% in younger adults. This decrease represents a net loss of muscle mass, and it places older people at greater risk for water-deficit states.

There are also changes in the kidney that further potentiate the risk for fluid and electrolyte disturbances. With increasing age, there is a decrease in renal mass and glomerular filtration rate (GFR). This in turn may lead to the inability of the aging kidney to excrete free water in the face of fluid excess, causing hyponatremia (decreased levels of sodium in the blood).

Yet hypernatremia (increased levels of sodium in the blood) can also be problematic in the aging adult secondary to a defect in the ability of the kidney to concentrate urine combined with a decreased thirst despite dehydration, which is often seen with age. Although these changes are seen in normal aging, factors that depress the sensation of thirst will complicate hypernatremia further.

Fluid Imbalances
Overview

Approximately 45% to 60% of the adult human body is composed of water, which contains the electrolytes that are essential to human life. This life-sustaining fluid is found within various body compartments, including the intracellular, interstitial, intravascular, and transcellular compartments.

Fluid in the transcellular compartment is present in the body but is separated from body tissues by a layer of epithelial cells. This fluid includes digestive juices, water, and solutes in the renal tubules and bladder, intraocular fluid, joint-space fluid, and cerebrospinal fluid. The fluid in the interstitial and intravascular compartments comprises approximately one third of the total body fluid, called the *extracellular fluid* (ECF). Fluid found inside the cells accounts for the remaining two thirds of the total body fluid, called the *intracellular fluid* (ICF).

The cell membrane is water permeable, with equal concentrations of dissolved particles on each side of the membrane maintaining equal volumes of ECF and ICF and preventing passive shifts of water. Passive shifts occur only if an inequality occurs between the sides of the membrane in the concentration of solutes that cannot permeate the membrane. For example, water will move from one compartment to another if there is a change in sodium ion concentration.

Increased intravascular fluid results in CHF and increased pulse and respiration. *Decreased intravascular fluid* results in decreased blood pressure and increased pulse and respirations. However, *increased extravascular fluid* may cause edema, ascites, or pleural effusion. *Decreased extravascular fluid* results in decreased skin turgor and fatigue.

Etiologic Factors and Pathogenesis

Maintaining constant internal conditions (homeostasis) requires the proper balance in volume and distribution of ECF and ICF to provide nutrition to the cells, allow excretion of waste products, and promote production of energy and other cell functions. Maintenance of this balance depends on the differences in the concentrations of ICF and ECF fluids, the permeability of the membranes, and the effect of the electrolytes in the fluids.

A fluid imbalance occurs when either the ICF or the ECF gains or loses body fluids or electrolytes, causing a fluid deficit or a fluid excess. Sodium is the major ion that influences water retention and water loss. A deficit of body fluids occurs with either an excessive loss of body water or an inadequate compensatory intake. The result is an insufficient fluid volume to meet the needs of the cells. It is manifested by dehydration (Box 2.5), blood or plasma loss, or both. Severe *fluid volume deficit* (FVD) can cause vascular collapse and shock.

An *excess* of water occurs when an overabundance of water is in the interstitial fluid spaces or body cavities (edema) or within the blood vessels (hypervolemia). A *fluid shift* occurs when vascular fluid moves to interstitial or intracellular spaces or interstitial fluid or ICF moves to vascular fluid space.

Clinical Manifestations

FVD is most often accompanied by symptoms related to a decrease in cardiac output, such as decreased blood pressure, increased pulse, and orthostatic hypotension. FVD can occur from loss of blood (loss of plasma) or loss of body fluids resulting in dehydration.

Hypernatremia occurs if the body fluid loss is a loss of body water without solute components. Most often, however, body fluid losses contain both body water and its solute components. The affected individual experiences symptoms of thirst, weakness, dizziness, decreased urine output, weight loss, and altered levels of consciousness. Significant decreases in systolic blood pressure (less than 70 mm Hg) result in symptoms of shock and require immediate medical treatment and possibly life-sustaining emergency management.

Fluid volume excess (FVE) is primarily characterized by weight gain, edema of the extremities, dyspnea, engorged neck veins, and a bounding pulse. The person may not exhibit any of these symptoms in the early stages.

Fluid shift from the vascular to the extravascular (interstitial) spaces (e.g., in burns or peritonitis) is manifested by signs and symptoms similar to FVD and shock, including skin pallor, cool extremities, weak and rapid pulse, hypotension, oliguria, and decreased levels of consciousness. When the fluid returns to the blood vessels, the clinical manifestations are similar to those of fluid overload, such as bounding pulse and engorgement of peripheral and jugular veins.

Medical Management

The ECF is the only fluid compartment that can be readily monitored; clinically, the status of ICF is inferred from analysis of plasma and the condition of the person. A fluid balance record is kept on any individual who is susceptible or already experiencing a disturbance in the balance of body fluids. In addition, medical evaluation of clinical signs and laboratory tests are helpful in the assessment of a person's hydration status.

Serum osmolality measures the concentration of particles in the plasma portion of the blood. Osmolality increases with dehydration and decreases with overhydration. Serum sodium is an index of water deficit or excess; an elevated level of sodium in the blood (hypernatremia) would indicate that the loss of water from the body has exceeded the loss of sodium, such as occurs in the administration of osmotic diuretics, uncontrolled diabetes insipidus, and extensive burns. Hematocrit increases with dehydration and decreases with excess fluid. BUN serves as an index of kidney excretory function; BUN increases with dehydration and decreases with overhydration.

Treatment is directed to the underlying cause; in the case of FVD, the aim is to improve hydration status. This may be accomplished through replacement of fluids and/or electrolytes by oral, nasogastric, or intravenous means.

2.8 Special Implications for the PTA: Fluid Imbalances

Monitoring Fluid Balance

Fluid balance is so critical to physical well-being and cardiopulmonary sufficiency that fluid input and output records are often maintained at bedside. Body weight may increase by several pounds before edema is apparent. The dependent areas manifest the first signs of fluid excess. Individuals on bed rest show sacral swelling; people who can sit on the edge of the bed or in a chair for prolonged periods tend to show swelling of the feet and hands.[25]

Water and fluids should be offered often to older adults and clients with debilitating diseases to prevent body fluid loss and hypernatremia. However, increasing fluid intake in clients with CHF or severe renal disease is usually contraindicated.

Caffeinated fluids and alcohol can increase water loss; these beverages should be avoided to prevent fluid loss caused by this diuretic effect. Water is the preferred fluid for hydration except in athletic or marathon race situations, which necessitate replacement of electrolytes.[48]

Thirst is not always a reliable signal for fluid intake or even dehydration. A person may not feel "thirsty" until the body reaches a dangerous point of fluid loss. Therapists and clients should both be encouraged to keep water and clear fluids on hand and drink on a schedule rather than wait until they feel thirsty. Many people confuse thirst for hunger and eat instead of drinking when the thirst mechanism does kick in.

Urine is good gauge of adequate hydration. A low volume of dark or highly concentrated urine is a yellow flag. When accompanied by other signs of dehydration, it becomes a red flag.

Dehydration

Healthy older adults can become at risk for dehydration for many physiologic and psychosocial reasons. Older individuals have an impaired thirst response to dehydration, abnormal circadian rhythm, and increased fluid loss. Other contributing medical factors include diabetes, urinary tract infections, renal failure, and medications such as diuretics.[83]

Psychosocial factors also play a key role in the development of dehydration in the older age group. Isolation, depression, and confusion are associated with reduced oral intake and impaired fluid status and can make dehydration worse.[83]

Dehydration degrades endurance exercise performance, and physical work capacity is diminished even at marginal levels of dehydration. Alterations in VO_{2max} occur with a 2% or more deficit in body water. Greater body water deficits are associated with progressively larger reductions in physical work capacity.

For individuals in any age group, dehydration results in larger reductions in physical work capacity in a hot environment (e.g., aquatic or outdoor setting) compared with a thermally neutral environment. Prolonged exercise that places large demands on aerobic metabolism is more likely to be adversely affected by dehydration than is short-term exercise.[21]

Core body temperature increases predictably as the percentage of dehydration increases. The heart rate increases about 6 beats/minute for each 1% increase in dehydration. This is not true for older adults, who may have limited rate changes with increased activity.

Older individuals are especially at risk for negative sequelae associated with dehydration. Hospitalization for dehydration is common, and mortality is high. Almost 50% of Medicare patients who are hospitalized with dehydration die within a year of admission.[83,128,129]

Individuals exercising in the heat, including aquatic exercise, should be encouraged to drink water in excess of normally desired amounts. When exercise is expected to cause an increase of more than 2% in dehydration, target heart rate modifications are necessary.[76]

Dehydration may contribute to underlying disabilities caused by orthostatic hypotension and dizziness. It may result in symptoms, such as confusion and weakness, that can interfere with rehabilitation outcomes, especially after orthopedic surgery.[83]

Skin Care
Careful handling of edematous tissue is essential to maintaining the integrity of the skin, which is stretched beyond its normal limits and has a limited blood supply. Turning and repositioning the client must be done gently to avoid friction. A break in or abrasion of edematous skin can readily develop into a pressure ulcer.

Client education may be necessary in the proper application and use of antiembolism stockings, lower-extremity elevation, and the need for regular exercise. Clients should be cautioned to avoid crossing the legs, putting pillows under the knees, or otherwise creating pressure against the blood vessels.[37,88]

Electrolyte Imbalances

Overview
Electrolytes are chemical substances that separate into electrically charged particles, called *ions,* in solution. The electrolytes that consist of positively charged ions, or *cations,* are sodium (Na^+), potassium (K^+), calcium (Ca^{2+}), and magnesium (Mg^{2+}). Those that consist of negatively charged ions, or *anions,* are chloride (Cl^-); bicarbonate (HCO_3^-); and phosphate (PO_4^{3-}).

Concentration gradients of sodium and potassium across the cell membrane produce the membrane potential and provide the means by which electrochemical impulses are transmitted in nerve and muscle fibers. *Sodium* affects the osmolality of blood and therefore influences blood volume and pressure and the retention or loss of interstitial fluid.

Adequate *potassium* is necessary to maintain function of sodium–potassium membrane pumps, which are essential for the normal muscle contraction–relaxation sequence. Imbalances in potassium affect muscular activities—notably those of the heart, intestines, and respiratory tract—and neural stimulation of the skeletal muscles.

Calcium influences the permeability of cell membranes and thereby regulates neuromuscular activity. Calcium plays a role in the electrical excitation of cardiac cells and in the mechanical contraction of the myocardial and vascular smooth muscle cells. An imbalance in calcium concentrations affects skeletal muscle, bones, kidneys, and the GI tract. *Magnesium,* an important intracellular enzyme activator, exerts physiologic effects on the nervous system that resemble the effects of calcium. Magnesium plays a role in maintaining the correct level of electrical excitability in the nerves and muscle cells by acting directly on the myoneural junction. Magnesium depresses acetylcholine release at synaptic junctions; neuromuscular irritability results from hypomagnesemia, and magnesium excess causes neuromuscular depression, affecting the musculoskeletal and cardiac systems.[91]

Etiologic and Risk Factors
An electrolyte imbalance exists when the serum concentration of an electrolyte is either too high or too low. Stability of the electrolyte balance depends on adequate intake of water and the electrolytes and on homeostatic mechanisms within the body that regulate the absorption, distribution, and excretion of water and its dissolved particles.

Bodily fluid loss associated with weight loss, excessive perspiration, or chronic vomiting and diarrhea are the most common causes of electrolyte imbalance. Many other conditions can interfere with these processes and result in an imbalance (Table 2.4).

Ischemia is accompanied by electrolyte disturbances, particularly the release of potassium, calcium, and magnesium from cells when cellular death ensues. Myocardial cells deprived of necessary oxygen and nutrients lose contractility, thereby diminishing the pumping ability of the heart. Diuretics also can produce mild to severe electrolyte imbalances. These factors explain the careful observation of specific electrolyte levels in the cardiac client.

TABLE 2.4 **Causes of Electrolyte Imbalances**	
	Risk Factors for Imbalance
Potassium	
Hypokalemia	Dietary deficiency (rare)
	Intestinal or urinary losses as a result of diarrhea or vomiting (anorexia, dehydration), drainage from fistulas, overuse of gastric suction
	Trauma (injury, burns, surgery): damaged cells release potassium, are excreted in urine
	Medications such as potassium-wasting diuretics, steroids, insulin, penicillin derivatives, amphotericin B
	Metabolic alkalosis
	Cushing's syndrome, severe magnesium deficiency
	Hyperaldosteronism
	Integumentary loss (sweating)
	Type 2 renal tubular acidosis
	Diabetic ketoacidosis
Hyperkalemia	Conditions that alter kidney function or decrease its ability to excrete potassium (chronic renal disease or renal failure)
	Intestinal obstruction that prevents elimination of potassium in the feces
	Addison's disease
	Chronic heparin therapy, lead poisoning, insulin deficit, NSAIDs, ACE inhibitors, cyclosporine
	Trauma: crush injuries, burns
	Metabolic acidosis
	Rhabdomyolysis
	Tumor lysis syndrome
	Hyperglycemia
	Digitalis toxicity
	Hypoaldosteronism

TABLE 2.4   Causes of Electrolyte Imbalances—cont'd

Risk Factors for Imbalance

Sodium

Hyponatremia
Inadequate sodium intake (low-sodium diets)
Excessive intake or retention of water (kidney failure and heart failure)
Excessive water loss and electrolytes (vomiting, excessive perspiration, tap water enemas, suctioning, use of diuretics, diarrhea)
Loss of bile (high in sodium) as a result of fistulas, drainage, GI surgery, and suction
Trauma (loss of sodium through burn wounds, wound drainage from surgery)
IV fluids that do not contain electrolytes
Adrenal gland insufficiency (Addison's disease) or hypoaldosteronism
Cirrhosis of the liver with ascites
SIADH: brain tumor, cerebrovascular accident, pulmonary disease, neoplasm with ADH production, medications, pain, nausea
Hypothyroidism
Nephrotic syndrome

Hypernatremia
Decreased water intake (comatose, mentally confused, or debilitated client)
Water loss (excessive sweating, osmotic diarrhea), fever, heat exposure, burns
Hyperglycemia
Excess adrenocortical hormones (Cushing's syndrome)
IV administration of high-protein, hyperosmotic tube feedings and diuretics
Diabetes insipidus
Central: loss of neurohypophysis from trauma, surgery, neoplasm, CVA, infection
Nephrogenic: renal resistance to ADH drugs (lithium), hypercalcemia papillary necrosis, pregnancy

Calcium

Hypocalcemia
Inadequate dietary intake of calcium and inadequate exposure to sunlight (vitamin D) necessary for calcium use (especially older adults)
Impaired absorption of calcium and vitamin D from intestinal tract (severe diarrhea, overuse of laxatives, and enemas containing phosphates; phosphorous tends to be more readily absorbed from the intestinal tract than calcium and suppresses calcium retention in the body)
Hypoparathyroidism (injury, disease, surgery)
Severe infections or burns
Overcorrection of acidosis
Pancreatic insufficiency
Renal failure
Hypomagnesemia (especially with alcoholism)
Medications (anticonvulsive medications)

Hypercalcemia
Hyperparathyroidism, hyperthyroidism, adrenal insufficiency
Multiple fractures
Excess intake of calcium (excessive antacids), excess intake of vitamin D, milk-alkali syndrome
Osteoporosis, immobility, multiple myeloma
Thiazide diuretics
Sarcoidosis
Tumors that secrete PTH (bone, lung, stomach, and kidney)
Multiple endocrine neoplasia (MEN) tumors (types I and II)

Magnesium

Hypomagnesemia
Decreased magnesium intake or absorption (chronic malnutrition, chronic diarrhea, bowel resection with ileostomy or colostomy, chronic alcoholism, prolonged gastric suction, acute pancreatitis, biliary or intestinal fistula)
Excessive loss of magnesium (diabetic ketoacidosis, severe dehydration, hyperaldosteronism, and hypoparathyroidism)
Vitamin D deficiency
Impaired renal absorption
Acute tubular necrosis (ATN)
Medications: diuretics, cisplatin, foscarnet, cyclosporine, amphotericin B
Hyperthyroidism
Metabolic acidosis
SIADH
Pregnancy

Hypermagnesemia
Chronic renal and adrenal insufficiency
Overuse of antacids and laxatives containing magnesium
Severe dehydration (resulting oliguria can cause magnesium retention)
Overcorrection of hypomagnesemia
Near-drowning (aspiration of sea water)
Intestinal obstruction
Trauma, burns
Hypothyroidism
Addison's disease
Shock, sepsis

ACE, Angiotensin-converting enzyme; *ADH,* antidiuretic hormone; *CVA,* cerebrovascular accident; *GI,* gastrointestinal; *IV,* intravenous; NSAIDs, nonsteroidal antiinflammatory drugs; *PTH,* parathyroid hormone; *SIADH,* syndrome of inappropriate antidiuretic hormone.
Modified from Horne M, Bond E: Fluid, electrolyte, and acid–base imbalances. In Lewis S, Heitkemper M, Dirksen S, editors: Medical-surgical nursing: assessment and management of clinical problems, ed 5, St. Louis, 2000, Mosby.

Clinical Manifestations

In a therapy practice, paresthesias, muscle weakness, muscle wasting, muscle tetany, and bone pain are the most likely symptoms first observed with electrolyte imbalances (Table 2.5).

Medical Management

As with fluid imbalances, the underlying cause of electrolyte imbalances must be determined and corrected. Electrolyte supplementation, when needed, can be given orally or intravenously.

2.9 Special Implications for the PTA: Electrolyte Imbalances

Encourage adherence to a sodium-restricted diet prescribed for clients. The use of over-the-counter (OTC) medications for people on a sodium-restricted diet should be approved by the physician. Encourage activity and alternate with rest periods. Monitor for worsening of the underlying cause of fluid or electrolyte imbalance, and report significant findings to the nurse or physician.

Frequent position changes are important in the presence of edema; edematous tissue is more prone to skin breakdown than normal tissue.

TABLE 2.5 Clinical Features of Various Electrolyte Imbalances

SYSTEM DYSFUNCTION		
Potassium Imbalance		
	Hypokalemia	**Hyperkalemia**
Cardiovascular	Dizziness, hypotension, arrhythmias, ECG changes, cardiac arrest (with serum potassium levels 2.5 mEq/L)	Tachycardia and later bradycardia, ECG changes, cardiac arrest (with levels >7.0 mEq/L)
GI	Nausea and vomiting, anorexia, constipation, abdominal distention, paralytic ileus or decreased peristalsis	Nausea, diarrhea, abdominal cramps
Musculoskeletal	Muscle weakness and fatigue, leg cramps	Muscle weakness, flaccid paralysis
Genitourinary	Polyuria	Oliguria, anuria
CNS	Malaise, irritability, confusion, mental depression, speech changes, decreased reflexes, pulmonary hyperventilation	Areflexia progressing to weakness, numbness, tingling, and flaccid paralysis
Acid–base balance	Metabolic alkalosis	Metabolic acidosis
Calcium Imbalance		
	Hypocalcemia	**Hypercalcemia**
CNS	Anxiety, irritability, twitching around mouth, laryngospasm, seizures, apathy, irritability, confusion, Chvostek's sign (facial muscle spasms induced by tapping the branches of the facial nerve)	Drowsiness, lethargy, headaches, depression, or Trousseau's sign
Musculoskeletal	Paresthesia (tingling and numbness of the fingers), tetany or painful tonic muscle spasms, facial spasms, abdominal cramps, muscle cramps, spasmodic contractions	Weakness, muscle flaccidity, bone pain, pathologic fractures
Cardiovascular	Arrhythmias, hypotension	Signs of heart block, cardiac arrest in systole, hypertension
GI	Increased GI motility, diarrhea from dehydration	Anorexia, nausea, vomiting, constipation, dehydration, polyuria, prerenal azotemia
Sodium Imbalance		
	Hyponatremia	**Hypernatremia**
CNS	Anxiety, headaches, muscle twitching and weakness, confusion, seizures	Agitation, restlessness, seizures, ataxia, confusion
Cardiovascular	Hypotension; tachycardia; with severe deficit, vasomotor collapse, thready pulse	Hypertension, tachycardia, pitting edema, excessive weight gain
GI	Nausea, vomiting, abdominal cramps	Rough, dry tongue; intense thirst
Genitourinary	Oliguria or anuria	Oliguria
Respiratory	Cyanosis with severe deficiency	Dyspnea, respiratory arrest, and death (from dramatic rise in osmotic pressure)
Cutaneous	Cold clammy skin, decreased skin turgor	Flushed skin; dry, sticky mucous membranes
Magnesium Imbalance		
	Hypomagnesemia	**Hypermagnesemia**
Neuromuscular	Hyperirritability, tetany, leg and foot cramps, Chvostek's sign	Diminished reflexes, muscle weakness, flaccid paralysis, respiratory muscle paralysis that may cause respiratory impairment
CNS	Confusion, delusions, hallucinations, seizures	Drowsiness, flushing, lethargy, confusion, diminished sensorium
Cardiovascular	Arrhythmias, vasomotor changes (vasodilation and hypotension), occasionally hypertension	Bradycardia, weak pulse, hypotension, heart block, cardiac arrest

CNS, Central nervous system; *ECG*, electrocardiogram; *GI*, gastrointestinal.

Older adults have frequent problems with *hypokalemia* (severe potassium loss) most often associated with the use of diuretics. Decreased potassium levels can result in fatigue, muscle cramping, and cardiac dysrhythmias, usually manifested by an irregular pulse rate or complaints of dizziness and/or palpitations. Fatigue and muscle cramping increase the chance of musculoskeletal injury. Observing for accompanying signs and symptoms of fluid and electrolyte imbalances will help promote safe and effective exercise for anyone with the potential for these disorders.

With appropriate medical therapy, cardiac, muscular, and neurologic manifestations associated with electrolyte imbalances can be corrected. Delayed medical treatment may result in irreversible damage or death.

Common Causes of Fluid and Electrolyte Imbalances
Overview

The exact mechanisms of fluid and electrolyte imbalances are outside the scope of this text. A brief description of the common causes and overall clinical picture encountered in a therapy practice is included here. Burns, surgery, and trauma may result in a fluid volume shift from the vascular spaces to the interstitial spaces. Tissue injury causes the release of histamine and bradykinin, which increases capillary permeability, allowing fluid, protein, and other solutes to shift into the interstitial spaces.

In the case of burns, the fluid shifts out of the vessels into the injured tissue spaces, as well as into the normal (unburned) tissue. This causes severe swelling of these tissues and a significant loss of fluid volume from the vascular space, which results in hypovolemia. Severe hypovolemia can result in shock, vascular collapse, and death. In the case of major tissue damage, potassium is also released from the damaged tissue cells and can enter the vascular fluids, causing hyperkalemia.

In an attempt to treat shock, large quantities of fluid are administered intravenously to maintain blood pressure, cardiac output, and renal function. After 24 to 72 hours, capillary permeability is usually restored and fluid begins to leave the tissue spaces and shift back into the vascular space. If renal function is not adequate, the accumulation of fluid used for treatment and fluid returning from the tissue spaces into the vascular space can cause fluid volume overload. Fluid overload can then lead to CHF or pulmonary edema.

Diabetes mellitus (type 1) may result in a condition called *diabetic ketoacidosis,* which is caused by a lack of insulin. This leads to hyperglycemia, polyuria, and an overproduction of ketones that results in metabolic acidosis. Movement of hydrogen into the cells promotes the movement of potassium out of the cells and into the ECF. As the potassium enters the vascular space, the plasma potassium levels increase. Significant diuresis occurs, and the excess accumulated potassium is quickly excreted in the urine. Hypokalemia occurs as a result, which causes life-threatening cardiac dysrhythmias unless treated immediately.

Tumors often produce peptides that can affect fluid and electrolyte balance. These peptides cause neurologic, hormonal, dermatologic, and hematologic symptoms or syndromes. An ectopic hormone arises at or is produced at an abnormal site or in a tissue where it is not normally found, often causing serious electrolyte imbalances. A more local effect of malignancy occurs when metastases to the skeletal system produce hypercalcemia from the osteolysis of bone. The treatment of malignancies also can create fluid and electrolyte imbalances, as occurs with hormonal treatment for breast cancer. Hyponatremia and hypokalemia may also result from nausea and vomiting caused by chemotherapy. Hyponatremia is also the most common electrolyte imbalance affecting hospitalized patients. Causes of hyponatremia in this population group include sodium loss from diuretics, vomiting, or wound draining and water gain if the person receives too much of a hypotonic intravenous fluid.

Clinical Manifestations

The effects of a fluid or electrolyte imbalance are not isolated to a particular organ or system (Box 2.6). Symptoms most commonly observed may include skin changes, neuromuscular irritability, CNS involvement, edema, and changes in vital signs, especially tachycardia and postural hypotension.

Skin changes include changes in skin turgor and alterations in skin temperature. In a healthy individual, pinched skin will immediately fall back to its normal position when released, a measure of skin turgor. In a person with dehydration, the skin flattens more slowly after the pinch is released and may even remain elevated for several seconds, referred to as *tenting* of tissue (Fig. 2.8).

Neuromuscular irritability can occur as a result of imbalances in calcium, magnesium, potassium, and sodium. Specific signs of neuromuscular involvement associated with these imbalances occur because of increased neural excitability, specifically increased acetylcholine action at the nerve ending, resulting in lowering of the threshold of the muscle membrane.

Tetany is the most characteristic manifestation of hypocalcemia. The affected person may report a sensation of tingling around the mouth and in the hands and feet, and spasms of the muscles of the extremities and face. *Nervous system* involvement may occur in the peripheral system or the CNS. CNS

BOX 2.6 Clinical Manifestations of Fluid and Electrolyte Imbalance[a]

Skin Changes
- Poor skin turgor
- Changes in skin temperature

Neuromuscular Irritability
- Muscle fatigue
- Muscle twitching
- Muscle cramping
- Tetany

Central Nervous System Involvement
- Changes in deep tendon reflexes
- Seizures
- Depression
- Memory impairment
- Delusions
- Hallucinations

Edema
- Changes in vital signs
  - Tachycardia
  - Postural hypotension
  - Altered respirations

[a]Only signs and symptoms most likely to be seen in a therapy practice are included here.

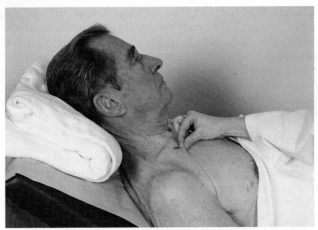

FIG. 2.8 Testing skin turgor (normal resiliency of a pinched fold of skin). Turgor is measured by the time it takes for the skin and underlying tissue to return to the original contour after being pinched up. If the skin remains elevated (i.e., tented) for more than 3 seconds, turgor is decreased. Normal turgor is indicated by a return to baseline contour within 3 seconds when the skin is mobile and elastic. Turgor decreases with age as the skin loses elasticity; testing turgor on the forearm (the standard site for testing) of some older persons is less valid because of decreased skin elasticity in this area. (From Jarvis C: Physical examination and health assessment, ed 7, St. Louis, 2016, Elsevier.)

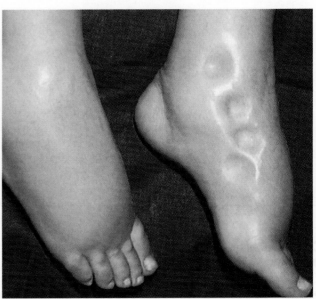

FIG. 2.9 Severe, dependent, pitting edema occurs with some systemic diseases, such as congestive heart failure and hepatic cirrhosis. Note the finger-shaped depressions that do not refill after pressure has been exerted by the examiner. (From Thidodeau GA, Patton KT: The human body in health and disease, ed 6, St. Louis, 2014, Mosby.)

manifestations of hypocalcemia may include seizures, irritability, depression, memory impairment, delusions, and hallucinations. In chronic hypocalcemia, the skin may be dry and scaling, the nails become brittle, and the hair is dry and falls out easily.

Signs and symptoms of hyponatremia occur when a drop in the serum sodium level pulls water into cells. When this happens, the client may experience headaches, confusion, lethargy, muscle weakness, and nausea. These symptoms are easily mistaken for complications from anesthesia or analgesia.

Hypokalemia seen in a therapy practice can be associated with diuretic therapy; excessive sweating, vomiting, or diarrhea; diabetic acidosis; trauma; or burns. It is accompanied by muscular weakness that can progress to flaccid quadriparesis. The weakness is initially most prominent in the legs, especially the quadriceps; it extends to the arms, with involvement of the respiratory muscles soon after.[91] Severe hypokalemia can cause paralysis, respiratory failure, cardiac arrhythmias, and hypotension. Finally, a condition called *rhabdomyolysis*, disintegration of striated muscle fibers, can occur with potassium or phosphorus depletion.

Edema, defined as an excessive accumulation of interstitial fluid, may be either localized or generalized. Generalized edema may be characterized by shortness of breath, ankle swelling, nocturia, and orthopnea. Other manifestations of generalized edema may include decreased urinary output; weight gain; labored, shallow, and increased respiratory rate; changes in blood pressure; and abnormal laboratory findings.

Pulmonary edema results from excessive shifting of fluid from the vascular space into the pulmonary interstitium and air spaces. When edema forms secondary to fluid retention, the clinical picture is usually one of pitting edema (Fig. 2.9).

Vital sign changes, including changes in pulse, respirations, and blood pressure, may signal early development of fluid volume changes. Decreased blood pressure and tachycardia are usually the first signs of the decreased vascular volume as the

heart pumps faster to compensate for the decreased plasma volume. Irregular pulse rates and dysrhythmias may also be associated with magnesium, potassium, or calcium imbalances.

Orthostatic hypotension is another sign of volume depletion. Moving from a supine to standing position causes an abrupt drop in venous return.

In contrast, for the person with FVD, systolic pressure may fall 20 mm Hg or more, accompanied by an increase in the pulse rate greater than 15 beats/minute.[63] The decreased volume results in compensatory increases in pulse rate as the heart attempts to increase output in the face of decreased stroke volume.

As fluid volume depletion worsens, blood pressure becomes low in all positions because of loss of compensatory mechanisms and autonomic insufficiency.

> **2.10 Special Implications for the PTA: Assessment of Fluid and Electrolyte Imbalance** Ongoing assessment of fluid and electrolyte balance is based on both subjective and objective findings (Table 2.6). At the bedside or in the home health care setting, the PTA must be alert to complaints of headache, thirst, and nausea and changes in dyspnea, skin turgor, and muscle strength. More objective assessment of fluid and electrolyte balance is based on fluid intake and output and body weight.

ACID–BASE IMBALANCES

Overview

Normal function of body cells depends on regulation of hydrogen ion concentration (H^+) so that H^+ levels remain within very narrow limits. Acid–base imbalances occur when these limits are exceeded and are recognized clinically as abnormalities of serum pH. Normal serum pH is 7.35 to 7.45. Cell function is seriously impaired when pH falls to 7.2 or lower or rises to 7.55 or higher.

TABLE 2.6 Assessment of Fluid and Electrolyte Imbalance

Area	Fluid Excess and Electrolyte Imbalance	Fluid Loss and Electrolyte Imbalance
Head and neck	Distended neck veins, facial edema	Thirst, dry mucous membranes
Extremities	Dependent pitting edema, discomfort from weight of bed covers	Muscle weakness, tingling, tetany
Skin	Warm, moist; taut, cool feeling when edematous	Dry, decreased turgor
Respiration	Dyspnea, orthopnea, productive cough, moist breath	Changes in rate and depth of breathing sounds
Circulation	Hypertension, distended neck veins, atrial arrhythmias	Pulse rate irregularities, arrhythmia, postural hypotension, tachycardia
Abdomen	Increased girth, fluid wave	Abdominal cramps

Modified from Briggs J, Drabek C: Fluid and electrolyte imbalance. In Phipps WJ, Sands J, Marek J, editors: Medical-surgical nursing: concepts and clinical practice, ed 5, St Louis, 1999, Mosby.

Three physiologic systems act interdependently to maintain normal pH: immediate buffering of excess acid or base by the *blood buffer systems*, excretion of acid by the *lungs* (occurs within hours), and excretion of acid or reclamation of base by the *kidneys* (occurs within days). *Acidosis* refers to any pathologic process causing a relative excess of acid in the body. This can occur as a result of accumulation of acid or depletion of the alkaline reserve in the blood and body tissues.

Acidemia refers to excess acid in the blood and does not necessarily confirm an underlying pathologic process. The same distinction may be made between the terms *alkalosis* and *alkalemia*; alkalosis indicates a primary condition resulting in excess base in the body. Although efforts have been made to standardize acid–base terminology, these terms are often used interchangeably.

Incidence

The incidence of acid–base imbalances in hospital settings is high. Acid–base imbalances are often related to respiratory and/or metabolic problems typical of the critically ill or injured individual. Some people have more than one acid–base imbalance at the same time.

Clinical Manifestations

A guide to the clinical presentation of acid–base imbalances is shown in Table 2.7.

Medical Management

Diagnosis

Pulse oximetry is used most often to measure oxygen saturation, yet it does not provide needed information regarding the effectiveness of ventilation or the pH of the blood. A more comprehensive procedure is the arterial blood gas (ABG) test.

This measurement is important in the diagnosis and treatment of ventilation, oxygen transport, and acid–base problems. The test measures the amount of dissolved oxygen and carbon dioxide in arterial blood and indicates acid–bases status by measurement of the arterial blood pH. As the hydrogen ion concentration (H+) increases (acidosis), the pH decreases; as the hydrogen ion concentration (H+) decreases (alkalosis), the pH increases.

The Pco_2 is a measure of the *partial pressure of carbon dioxide* in the blood. Pco_2 is termed the *respiratory component* in acid–base measurement because the carbon dioxide level is primarily controlled by the lungs. As the carbon dioxide level increases, the pH decreases (respiratory acidosis); as the carbon dioxide level decreases, the pH increases (respiratory alkalosis).

Treatment

Treatment in acid–base imbalances is directed toward the underlying cause and correction of any coexisting electrolyte imbalance.

Respiratory Acidosis

Respiratory acidosis is nearly always the result of hypoventilation and subsequent retention of carbon dioxide (CO_2). In a therapy setting, respiratory acidosis is most commonly observed in people with COPD, asthma, or depressed CNS or whenever the diaphragm is impaired (secondary to burns and as a result of lesions of the CNS).

The respiratory system plays an important role in maintaining acid–base equilibrium. The respiratory rate increases in response to an increase in the hydrogen ion concentration in body fluids, causing more CO_2 to be released from the lung.

Anything that impairs this CO_2 exhalation causes the CO_2 to accumulate in the blood, where it unites with water to form carbonic acid (H_2CO_3), decreasing the blood pH. In addition, the kidneys begin to excrete more acid and retain more bicarbonate to further correct the acid imbalance.

Respiratory acidosis can be acute, because of a sudden failure in ventilation, or chronic, as with long-term pulmonary disease (e.g., COPD). In the *acute* episode, the blood buffer systems cannot compensate to restore the acid–base balance because normal blood circulation and tissue perfusion are impaired. The lungs may not be functioning properly, and the kidneys require more time to compensate than the acute condition permits.

Chronic respiratory acidosis results from gradual and irreversible loss of ventilatory function. Although there is increased retention of CO_2, the kidneys have time to compensate by retaining bicarbonate and thereby maintaining a pH within tolerable limits. If even a minor respiratory infection develops, however, the person is subjected to a rapidly developing state of acute acidosis because the lungs remove only a limited amount of carbon dioxide.

Clinical manifestations. Acute respiratory acidosis produces CNS disturbances. Effects range from restlessness, confusion, and apprehension to *somnolence* (sleepiness), with a fine or flapping tremor or coma. The person may report headaches and shortness of breath with retraction and use of accessory muscles. On examination, deep tendon reflexes (DTRs) may be depressed. This disorder may also cause cardiovascular abnormalities such as tachycardia, hypertension, atrial and ventricular arrhythmias, and, in severe acidosis, hypotension with vasodilation.

Respiratory Alkalosis

Respiratory alkalosis, the opposite of respiratory acidosis, occurs as a result of a loss of acid without compensation and

TABLE 2.7   Overview of Acid–Base Imbalances

Mechanism	Etiologic Factors	Clinical Manifestations	Treatment
Respiratory Acidosis			
Hypoventilation	Acute respiratory failure COPD Neuromuscular disease Guillain-Barré syndrome Myasthenia gravis Respiratory center depression Drugs • Barbiturates • Sedatives • Narcotics • Anesthetics CNS lesions Tumor Stroke Inadequate mechanical ventilation	Hypercapnia, restlessness, disorientation, confusion, sleepiness, visual disturbances, headache, flushing, dyspnea, cyanosis, decreased deep tendon reflexes, hyperkalemia, palpitation, pH <7.35, $Paco_2$ >45 mm Hg	Treat underlying cause; support ventilation; correct electrolyte imbalance
Excess carbon dioxide production	Hypermetabolism Sepsis Burns		
Respiratory Alkalosis			
Hyperventilation	Hypoxemia Pulmonary embolus High altitude Impaired lung expansion Pulmonary fibrosis Ascites Scoliosis Pregnancy[a] Congestive heart failure Stimulation of respiratory center Anxiety hyperventilation Encephalitis or meningitis (hepatic failure) Salicylates (aspirin overdose) Theophylline CNS trauma CNS tumor Excessive exercise Extreme stress Severe pain Mechanical overventilation	Tachypnea, hypocapnia, dizziness, difficulty concentrating, numbness and tingling, blurred vision, diaphoresis, dry mouth, muscle cramps, carpopedal spasm, muscle twitching and weakness, hyperreflexia, arrhythmias, pH >7.45, $Paco_2$ <35 mm Hg, hypokalemia, hypocalcemia	Treat underlying cause; increase carbon dioxide retention (rebreathing, sedation)
Metabolic Acidosis			
Acid excess	Renal failure (acid retention) Diabetic or alcoholic ketoacidosis Lactic acidosis Starvation Ingested toxins Aspirin Antifreeze	Hyperventilation (compensatory), muscular twitching, weakness, malaise, nausea, vomiting, diarrhea, headache, hyperkalemia (cardiac arrhythmias), pH <7.35, HCO_3^- <22 mm Hg, $Paco_2$ normal or slightly decreased, coma (death)	Treat underlying cause, correct electrolyte imbalance; $NaCO_3$ for severe acidosis (pH <7.2)
Base deficit	Severe diarrhea (HCO_3^- loss) Renal failure (inability to reabsorb HCO_3^-)		
Metabolic Alkalosis			
Fixed acid loss (with base excess)	Hypokalemia Diuresis Steroids Vomiting Nasogastric suctioning	Hypoventilation (compensatory): dysrhythmias, nausea, prolonged vomiting, diarrhea, confusion, irritability, agitation, restlessness, muscle twitching, cramping, hypotonia, weakness, Trousseau's sign, paresthesias, seizures, coma, hypokalemia, pH >7.45, $Paco_2$ normal or slightly increased	Treat underlying cause; administer potassium chloride
Excessive HCO_3^- intake	Peptic ulcer Milk-alkali syndrome Excessive intake of antacids Overcorrection of acidosis Massive blood transfusion	Hypochloremia	
Excessive HCO_3^- resorption	Hyperaldosteronism Cushing's disease		

CNS, Central nervous system; *COPD,* chronic obstructive pulmonary disease; *HCO₃⁻,* bicarbonate; *NaCO₃,* sodium bicarbonate; *Paco₂,* partial pressure of carbon dioxide (arterial).
[a]In the third trimester of pregnancy, the hormone progesterone also stimulates respiration.

most commonly when the lungs excrete excessive amounts of carbon dioxide (hyperventilation).

Conditions associated with respiratory alkalosis fall into the following two categories:

1. *Pulmonary,* caused by hypoxemia in early stage pulmonary problems and by overuse of a mechanical ventilator
2. *Nonpulmonary,* which includes anxiety, hysteria, pain, fever, high environmental temperature, pregnancy, drug toxicities, CNS conditions, and hyperthyroidism (see Table 2.7)

Clinical manifestations. The cardinal sign of respiratory alkalosis is deep, rapid breathing, possibly exceeding 40 breaths/minute. Such hyperventilation usually leads to CNS and neuromuscular disturbances such as dizziness or light-headedness; inability to concentrate; tingling and numbness of the extremities and around the mouth; blurred vision; diaphoresis; dry mouth; muscle cramps; carpopedal (wrist and foot) spasms; twitching (possibly progressing to tetany); and muscle weakness. Severe respiratory alkalosis may cause cardiac arrhythmias, seizures, and syncope.

Metabolic Acidosis

Metabolic acidosis is an accumulation of acids or a deficit of bases in the blood. This type of acidosis can occur with an acid gain or bicarbonate loss, as may occur in someone with diarrhea.

Ketoacidosis occurs when insufficient insulin for the proper use of glucose results in increased breakdown of fat. This accelerated fat breakdown produces ketones and other acids. Although the body attempts to neutralize these increased acids, the plasma bicarbonate (HCO_3^-) is depleted.

In the case of *renal failure,* the failing kidney cannot rid the body of excess acids and cannot produce the necessary bicarbonate to buffer the acid load that is accumulating in the body. *Lactic acidosis* occurs as excess lactic acid is produced during strenuous exercise or when oxygen is insufficient (hypoxemia).

Clinical manifestations. The symptoms of metabolic acidosis can include muscular twitching, weakness, malaise, nausea, vomiting, diarrhea, and headache (see Table 2.7). If the acidosis is severe, myocardial depression and hypotension can occur. Compensatory hyperventilation may occur as a result of stimulation of the hypothalamus as the body attempts to rid itself of excess CO_2. As the acid level goes up, these symptoms progress to stupor, unconsciousness, coma, and death. The breath may have a fruity odor in the presence of acetone associated with ketoacidosis.

Metabolic Alkalosis

Metabolic alkalosis occurs when either an abnormal loss of acid or excess accumulation of bicarbonate occurs. Postoperative loss of acids through vomiting or gastric suctioning may also result in metabolic alkalosis. In the outpatient setting, diarrhea, excessive use of laxatives, diuretics, antacids, and milk also lead to metabolic alkalosis. Other causes are listed in Table 2.7.

Clinical manifestations. Signs and symptoms occur as the body attempts to correct the acid–base imbalance, primarily through hypoventilation. Respirations are shallow and slow as the lungs attempt to compensate by building up carbonic acid stores. Clinical manifestations may be mild at first, with muscle weakness, irritability, confusion, and muscle twitching. If untreated, the condition progresses and the person may become comatose, with possible seizures, cardiac arrhythmias, and respiratory paralysis.

Aging and Acid–Base Regulation

The normal aging process results in decreased ventilatory capacity and loss of alveolar surface area for gas exchange; thus older adults are prone to respiratory acidosis caused by hypoventilation and to respiratory alkalosis caused by hypoxemia and subsequent hyperventilation. Older adults are often taking multiple medications for hypertension or cardiovascular disease that may contribute to hypokalemia and metabolic alkalosis. Respiratory compensation in these conditions can be compromised because of the structural and functional changes mentioned.

Older adults who are unable to excrete an acid load may develop a chronic metabolic acidosis. While the bicarbonate level and pH of the blood remain normal, mild metabolic acidosis may contribute to muscle wasting and bone loss.

2.11 Special Implications for the PTA: Acid–Base Imbalances The PTA must observe clients at risk for acid–base imbalance for any early symptoms. This is especially true for people with known pulmonary, cardiovascular, or renal disease; clients in a hypermetabolic state, such as occurs in fever, sepsis, or burns; clients receiving total parenteral nutrition or enteral tube feedings that are high in carbohydrates; mechanically ventilated clients; clients with insulin-dependent diabetes; older clients whose age-related decreases in respiratory and renal function may limit their ability to compensate for acid–base disturbances; and clients with vomiting, diarrhea, or enteric drainage.[105]

Client and family education is essential in the prevention of acute episodes of metabolic acidosis, particularly diabetic ketoacidosis. A fruity breath odor from rising acid levels (acetone) may be detected by the therapy staff treating someone who has uncontrolled diabetes.

The PTA should not hesitate to ask the client about this breath odor because immediate medical intervention is required for diabetic ketoacidosis. Dehydration occurs rapidly as a result of severe hyperglycemia. A rising pulse rate and a drop in blood pressure are critical (and often late), indicators of a FVD caused by dehydration.

Safety measures to avoid injury during involuntary muscular contractions are the same as for convulsions or epileptic seizures. Vigorous restraint can cause orthopedic injuries as the muscles contract strongly against resistance. Placing padding to protect the person is a key to prevention of injury.

Measures that facilitate breathing are essential to client care during respiratory acidosis. Frequent turning, coughing, and deep breathing exercises to encourage oxygen–carbon dioxide exchange are beneficial. Postural drainage, unless contraindicated by the client's condition, may be effective in promoting adequate ventilation.

In the case of respiratory hyperventilation, rebreathing CO_2 in a paper sack is helpful, as is holding the breath. Oxygen may be given to reduce respiratory effort and the resultant blowing off of CO_2. Individuals with COPD may retain CO_2; the use of oxygen is contraindicated in these clients because it can further depress the respiratory drive, causing death.

Any client receiving diuretic therapy must be monitored for signs of potassium depletion. Decreased respiratory rate may be an indication of compensation by the lungs, but the physician must make this assessment.

REFERENCES/SUGGESTED READINGS

To enhance this text and add value for the reader, references and suggested readings are included on the companion Evolve site that accompanies this textbook. The reader can view the source and access it online whenever possible.

3

Injury, Inflammation, and Healing

CHAPTER OBJECTIVES

1. Understand the process of tissue healing from cellular level.
2. Introduce the types of agents and factors that cause and contribute to cellular injury.
3. Understand the phases of normal and abnormal tissue healing.
4. Discuss differences between acute and chronic tissue injury.
5. Understand when it is appropriate for the physical therapist assistant (PTA) to begin mechanical stress stimulation in the healing process for musculoskeletal tissue.

OUTLINE

VOCAB BUILDERS

Anaphylaxis	Exogenous	Karyolysis
Blebs	Exudate	Karyorrhexis
Caseous	Free radical	Keloid
Comorbidities	Granuloma	Kwashiorkor
Contracture	Hemostasis	Marasmus
Cytokines	Hepatocytes	Metaplasia
Diapedesis	Hydroxyl radicals	Oxidative stress
Dysplasia	Hyperplasia	Psychoneuroimmunology
Effusion	Hypertrophy	Senescence
Endogenous	Ionizing radiation	Sepsis

Pathology is defined as the structural and functional changes in the body caused by disease or trauma. Understanding the normal structure and function of the tissues is required before the discussion of pathology. The organization of the material presented in this chapter parallels the processes underlying pathology, that is, cell injury and the factors causing this injury; inflammation as a secondary response to cell injury; and tissue healing, which is the third step of the process toward homeostasis.

The role of nerve–immune interactions in regulation and tissue healing is just beginning to be revealed and will continue to enhance our understanding of and intervention in injury, inflammation, and recovery. A new area of science called *psychoneuroimmunology* describes the influences of the nervous system on immune and inflammatory responses and how these contribute to the healing and repair process. For example, it is now clear that mast cells, T cells, neutrophils, and monocytes can directly alter tissue physiology through the release of mediators and cytokines. In addition, aging, age-related changes, and various other factors can influence homeostasis and the recovery process and are the major focus of the next two sections.

CELLULAR AGING

Various components of cells (e.g., mitochondria, ribosomes, cell membrane) are subject to changes caused by aging. The mitochondrial deoxyribonucleic acid (DNA) is a prime target for age-related changes. Preserving genetic messages, DNA replicates and maintains itself. This division can result in alterations of the genetic code by anything that can damage DNA (e.g., physical, chemical, or biologic factors; spontaneous mutations of genes; exposure to radiation). Anything that can alter the information content of the cell can cause changes in function and affect the ability of the cell to maintain homeostasis.

The ability of a cell to resist disease-causing microorganisms or to recover from injury or inflammation is dependent in part on the underlying state or health of the cells. Although researchers are working to find cellular age-related biomarkers, age-related changes at the cellular level are present but remain difficult to measure or quantify. Age-associated deterioration in cells leads to tissue or organ deficiencies and ultimately to the expression of aging or disease. The best described age-associated change in the component of lysosomes of mature cells, especially neurons and cardiac muscle cells, is the presence of a component called *lipofuscin,* an aging-pigment granule found in high concentrations in old cells. The increase, and effects on

function, of lipofuscin with age remain under investigation, but it is suspected that pressure on the cell nucleus may interfere with cellular function.[123,145]

Theories of Cellular Aging

The aging process is often associated with impaired wound healing, but the cellular and molecular mechanisms implicated are not completely understood.[38,78] More than 300 theories exist to explain the aging phenomenon on a cellular level. Many of these theories originate from the study of changes that accumulate with time. In organs composed of cells that cannot regenerate, such as those of the heart and brain, the *wear-and-tear theory* may account for the decline in function of these organs. Other factors may also play a role, such as the influence of genetics, suggested by the genetic hypothesis that aging is a genetically predetermined process.

The *free radical theory* of aging is the most popular and widely tested and is based on the chemical nature and wide presence of free radicals causing DNA damage and cellular oxidative stress as it relates to the aging process (see the Chemical Factors section under Mechanisms of Cell (Tissue) Injury).

The discovery of the telomeres, the structures at the end of chromosomes, has added the *telomere aging clock theory* for the molecular mechanisms that lead to *senescence,* or *growing old.* This theory suggests that the telomere acts as a molecular clock signaling the onset of cell senescence. Normal human cells will not divide forever but eventually enter a viable nondividing state (senescence). The progressive accumulation of senescent cells contributes to but does not exclusively cause the aging process. Cell senescence acts as an anticancer mechanism to control the potential for cellular proliferation.[72,148] Because of the close association between telomere dysfunction and malignancy or the uncontrolled cell division of cancer, both pathologists and clinicians expect this molecule to be a useful malignancy marker.

Pathologic changes associated with aging vary from individual to individual but usually consist of reduced functional reserve caused by atrophy of tissues or organs. Resistance to infection declines with age, and pathologic processes such as atherosclerosis result in increased cardiovascular and cerebrovascular injuries or death.

Studies have shown that considerable potential exists for improving aerobic capacity by training. This observation has cellular implications. For example, mitochondria of cardiac and skeletal[78] muscle cells improve function under appropriate training conditions. If changes in diet and exercise or treatment with hormones or compounds, such as antioxidants, are able to modify damage by reactive oxygen species (ROS) and the body can reestablish cellular norms, then this information has great implications for the various cellular and molecular theories on aging and our approach to the aging process.

CELL INJURY

Understanding cell injury, inflammation, and tissue healing serves as a solid foundation for clinical decision making. We begin by acknowledging that the structural and functional changes produced by pathology start with injury to the cells that make up the tissues. Mild injury produced by stressors leads to sublethal alterations of the affected cells, whereas moderate or severe injury leads to lethal alterations. After cell injury, the body reacts by initiating the process of inflammation. The amount, type, and severity of the inflammatory reaction are dependent on the amount, type, and severity of the injury. As part of the healing process, the inflammatory process is responsible for the removal of the injurious agent, removal of cellular debris, and the initiation of the healing process. The healing process occurs to allow restoration of structure and function whenever possible.

To achieve complete restoration of function, regeneration of the damaged tissue must occur. Often, regeneration of the tissue is not possible, and the body must settle for tissue repair by nonfunctional connective tissue (fibrosis or scar tissue). This connective tissue helps maintain structural integrity but has none of the functional properties of the original cells and tissues.

Mechanisms of Cell (Tissue) Injury

Cells may be damaged by a variety of mechanisms. The most important mechanisms are listed in Box 3.1. Each of these mechanisms leads to either a reversible (sublethal) or irreversible (lethal) injury. Whether the injury is reversible is dependent on the cell's ability to withstand the derangement of homeostatic mechanisms and its adaptability (i.e., ability to return to a state of homeostasis). Reversing the injury and achieving homeostasis (a balanced state) are determined by a combination of factors including the mechanism of injury, length of time the injury is present without intervention, and the severity of the injury.

Ischemia

At the tissue or organ level, *ischemia* occurs when the blood flow is insufficient to maintain cell homeostasis and metabolic function. This can be caused by a reduction in flow or an increase in metabolism of the tissue beyond the capability of the arterial vascular system. Insufficient blood flow results in a critical reduction in oxygen delivery to the tissue that is partial (hypoxia) or total (anoxia), decreased delivery of nutrients, and decreased removal of waste products from the tissue. The

---

BOX 3.1   Mechanisms of Cell Injury

- Ischemia (lack of blood supply)
- Infectious agents
- Immune reactions
- Genetic factors
- Nutritional factors
- Physical factors
- Chemical factors

---

lack of oxygen leads to loss of aerobic metabolism. The resulting reduction in adenosine triphosphate (ATP) synthesis leads to accumulation of ions and fluid inside the cell, and this cell swelling compromises function. This concept is discussed further in the section Reversible Cell Injury.

Hypoxia or anoxia may occur under many circumstances, including obstruction of the respiratory tree (e.g., suffocation secondary to drowning), inadequate transport of oxygen across the respiratory surfaces of the lung (e.g., pneumonia), inadequate transport of oxygen in the blood (e.g., anemia), or an inability of the cell to use oxygen for cellular respiration (e.g., carbon monoxide poisoning).[26]

Ischemia is usually the result of arterial lumen obstruction and narrowing caused by atherosclerosis and/or an intravascular clot called a *thrombus*. Ischemia, resulting in myocardial infarction (MI) and stroke (lack of blood flow to the heart or brain, respectively), can cause death of tissue (necrosis) and accounts for two of the three leading causes of death or mortality in industrialized nations.

Infectious Agents

Infectious agents, such as bacteria, viruses, mycoplasmas, fungi, rickettsiae, protozoa, prions, and helminths, may also cause cell injury or death. Bacterial and viral agents are responsible for the vast majority of infections. Bacterial infections cause cell injury primarily by invading tissue and releasing exotoxins and endotoxins that can cause cell lysis or death and degradation of extracellular matrix and aid in the spread of the infection. Injury can also result from the inflammatory or immunologic reactions induced by bacteria in the host. For example, exotoxins may be released by clostridial organisms that cause gas gangrene, tetanus, and botulism.

Clostridium tetani, for example, releases an exotoxin that is preferentially absorbed by the alpha motor neurons and delivered into the central nervous system (CNS). Once inside the CNS, the exotoxin crosses the synapse of the anterior horn cell and interferes with release of inhibitory neurotransmitters. This disruption of homeostasis eventually causes the activation of motor neurons that in turn cause involuntary muscular contractions (tetanus).[131]

When microorganisms or their toxins are present in the blood, thus throughout the entire body, a condition called *sepsis* can occur. Endotoxins released from gram-negative bacteria induce the synthesis of cytokines (extracts of normal leukocytes such as tumor necrosis factor [TNF] and interleukins [ILs]) that are responsible for many of the systemic manifestations of sepsis (see Box 3.5).

In sepsis, endothelial cell damage, loss of plasma volume, and maldistribution of blood flow result in hypovolemia. Cardiovascular collapse may ensue and lead to a condition called *septic shock.* The detection of an infectious agent initiates an inflammatory reaction designed to contain and inactivate the pathogen, but the magnitude of this defensive response by the host may also cause cellular or tissue destruction in the infected area.

Viruses kill cells by one of two mechanisms (Fig. 3.1) and are the consequence of complete redirection of the cell's biosynthesis toward viral replication. The first is a direct cytopathic effect usually found with ribonucleic acid (RNA) viruses. These viruses kill from within by disturbing various cellular processes or by disrupting the integrity of the nucleus and/or plasma membrane.

Virally encoded proteins become inserted into the plasma membrane of the host cell (forming a channel) and alter the permeability of the cell membrane to ions. The resulting loss of the ionic barrier leads to cell swelling and death. DNA-type viruses also kill cells through an indirect cytopathic effect by integrating themselves into the cellular genome. These viruses encode the production of foreign proteins, which are exposed on the cell surface and recognized by the body's immune cells.

Immunocompetent cells, such as the T lymphocyte, recognize these virally encoded proteins inserted into the plasma membrane of host cells and attack and destroy the infected cells. When the immune system is compromised or if the number

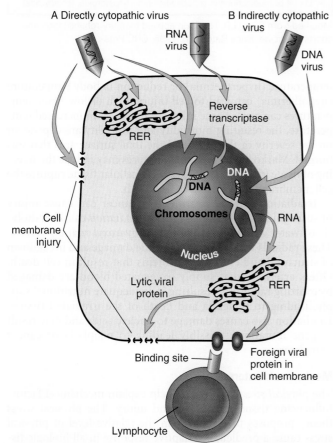

FIG. 3.1 Mechanisms of cell destruction by viruses. (A) Direct cytopathic effect: RNA virus inserts itself into a receptor on the cell membrane and is brought into the cell. The RNA virus is altered into DNA by reverse transcriptase. The DNA within the nucleus of the cell forms various types of RNA that allow for protein synthesis in the rough endoplasmic reticulum (RER). The protein formed inserts itself into the cell membrane, forming a channel that allows ions and extracellular fluid to enter, leading to cell lysis (directly killing the cell). (B) Indirect cytopathic effect mediated by immune mechanisms: DNA virus inserts itself into a receptor on the cell membrane and is brought into the cell. The DNA virus within the nucleus of the cell forms various types of RNA that allow for protein synthesis in the RER. This foreign viral protein inserts into the cell membrane and becomes a neoantigen. This neoantigen will be recognized by the T lymphocytes that will react to and kill (indirectly) the infected cell. (From Damjanov I: Pathology for the health-related professions, ed 4, St Louis, 2012, Saunders.)

of invading microorganisms overwhelms the immune system, then disease (and the symptoms of illness) occurs.

Immune Reactions

Although the immune system normally functions in defense against foreign antigens, sometimes the system becomes overzealous in its activity, leading to hypersensitivities ranging from a mild allergy to life-threatening anaphylactic reactions or autoimmune disorders (attacking oneself). The mechanisms by which the immune system can lead to cell injury or death include antibody attachment, complement activation, and activation of the inflammatory cells.

Cell injury and disease can be caused by the immune system in numerous ways. For example, allergies are caused by the presence of high numbers of a specific antibody, immunoglobulin E (IgE), on the surface of specialized cells (mast cells and basophils, which release histamine), resulting in mild, moderate, or severe allergic reactions. Examples of mild reactions include the runny nose and watery eyes caused by a mild allergic response.

Moderate reactions include severe hypoxia caused by asthmatic bronchoconstriction. Severe reactions can result in a potentially life-threatening circulatory collapse seen in *anaphylaxis* (a whole-body allergic reaction). The presence of what would normally be considered optimal ratios of antigen to antibody in the circulation may lead to damage of filtration in the kidney because of excess deposition of antigen–antibody complexes in the glomeruli.

Cross-reactivity between foreign and host antigens is another immune mechanism that can compromise the body. For example, cross-reaction between streptococcal and myocardial antigens can occur in rheumatic fever and result in injury of cardiac valves. Alternately, the chronic persistence of a foreign antigen by a foreign body or microorganism that cannot be cleared by the body may lead to a specific type of chronic inflammatory reaction called a *granuloma* (e.g., tuberculosis). Finally, sensitization to endogenous antigens can lead to type 1 diabetes mellitus caused by destruction of islet cells by T lymphocytes sensitized by islet antigens released during an antecedent viral infection.

Genetic Factors

Genetic alterations lead to cellular injury or death by three primary means: (1) alterations in the structure or number of chromosomes that induce multiple abnormalities, (2) single mutations of genes that cause changes in the amount or functions of proteins, and (3) multiple gene mutations that interact with environmental factors to cause multifactorial disorders. These genetic alterations can be severe enough to cause fetal death in utero, resulting in spontaneous abortion. Some may cause congenital malformations, whereas others do not manifest pathologic alterations, such as Huntington's disease, until midlife. Down syndrome is an example of an alteration in the number of chromosomes that results in multiple abnormalities. This condition, caused by the abnormal presence of a third chromosome in the 21st pair, includes cardiac malformations, increased susceptibility to severe infections, cognitive and developmental delays, and increased risk of leukemia and Alzheimer's dementia.

Sickle cell anemia, low-density lipoprotein (LDL) receptor deficiency, and α-antitrypsin deficiency are examples of single gene mutations. In α-antitrypsin deficiency, the deficiency in a protease inhibitor causes enhanced degradation of elastic

---

BOX 3.2   Connective Tissue Symptoms Associated with Vitamin C Deficiency

- Reduced collagen tensile strength (scurvy)
- Altered capillary structure (petechiae and hemorrhage)
- Osteopenia (bone pain and pathologic fractures)
- Skin and gum lesions
- Impaired skin and wound healing (decreased collagen formation, lack of scar formation, and impaired vascularization)
- Bilateral femoral neuropathy
- Muscle weakness
- Joint pain and effusions
- Edema

Modified from Bucci LR: Nutrition applied to injury rehabilitation and sports medicine, Boca Raton, FL, 1995, CRC Press.

BOX 3.3   Risk Factors for Vitamin C Deficiency

- Inadequate food intake (anorexia, chronic dieters, older adults, and bedridden individuals)
- Malabsorption syndromes
- Moderate to severe physical injury or emotional stress
- Pregnancy and lactation
- Use of tobacco products (smoking or chewing)
- Obesity
- Alcoholism
- Rheumatoid arthritis
- Kidney dialysis (hemodialysis or peritoneal dialysis)
- Diabetes mellitus
- Oral contraceptives
- Drugs or medications (e.g., salicylates, corticosteroids, tetracycline)

Modified from Bucci LR: Nutrition applied to injury rehabilitation and sports medicine, Boca Raton, FL, 1995, CRC Press.

tissue surrounding the alveoli of the lungs, which in turn leads to emphysema. Examples of multiple gene mutations that can cause disease include hypertension and type 2 diabetes mellitus. In type 2 diabetes mellitus, obesity and other environmental factors induce the expression of the diabetic genetic trait.

Nutritional Factors

Imbalances in essential nutrients can lead to cell injury or cell death. For example, deficiencies of essential amino acids interfere with protein synthesis. Synthesis of proteins is required to replace cell proteins lost through normal catabolism, through growth, and in preparation for cell replication. Cell replication is essential for the healing processes after cell injury and the replacement of cells lost through normal turnover.

The consequence of protein malnutrition is a condition called *kwashiorkor; marasmus,* another form of malnutrition, is a consequence of generalized dietary deficiency. These two diseases are still leading causes of death in impoverished countries. In many industrialized countries, excessive nutrient intake leads to obesity and its many complications.

Nutritional imbalance can also occur as a result of abnormal levels of either vitamins or minerals. These nutrients function as cofactors for biosynthetic reactions or are essential components of proteins or membranes; their deficiency usually affects selected cells or tissues. For example, a deficiency of iron leads to anemia, and the presence of excessive amounts of iron in the tissues can cause damage by the formation of free radicals.

Vitamin C (ascorbic acid) deficiency can be associated with a wide range of connective tissue symptoms (Box 3.2). Frank deficiencies of ascorbate are uncommon in the United States, although certain population groups may be at increased risk for deficient intake sometimes referred to as *biochemical scurvy* (Box 3.3).

Physical Factors

Trauma and physical agents can lead to cell injury and/or death. Blunt trauma caused by motor vehicle accidents is a leading killer in the United States. Massive brain contusions, injury to internal organs and soft tissues, and blood loss may lead to immediate mortality. Survivors may succumb to infections and multiple organ failure. Repair of injuries to soft tissue, skeletal and muscular systems, and internal organs often requires prolonged periods of rehabilitation. Penetrating trauma inflicted by a variety of weapons can result in multiple complications.

Extremes of physical agents, such as temperature, radiation, and electricity, may damage cells. Generalized increases in body temperature (hyperthermia) or reduction in body temperature (hypothermia) can lead to cell injury; high or low tissue temperatures can cause tissue injury or death. With increased temperature, the resulting morbidity and mortality are dependent on the severity of the burn and the total surface area that was burned. Markedly reduced temperatures may induce the freezing of tissue (frostbite). Ice crystals in cellular tissue rupture the cell membrane, which leads to cell death.

Irradiation for the treatment of cancer can cause injury of susceptible normal cells. *Ionizing radiation* causes radiolysis of water and the production of *hydroxyl radicals* (OH^-). These radicals will lead to membrane damage and breakdown of structural and enzymatic proteins that result in cell death. Often, arterioles that supply oxygenated blood are damaged by ionizing radiation, resulting in inadequate nutritional supply, leading to ischemia and death of the irradiated tissues. Irradiation also causes damage to nucleic acids and may result in gene mutations, possibly leading to neoplasia or cancer years later.

Mechanical Factors

The *physical stress theory* may help explain mechanical factors influencing tissue adaptation and injury. The physical stress theory proposes that changes in the relative level of physical stress cause a predictable adaptive response in all biologic tissue. Typical tissue response to physical stress includes decreased stress tolerance (e.g., atrophy), maintenance, increased stress tolerance (e.g., hypertrophy), injury, and death.[100]

Failure of a tissue occurs when the applied load exceeds the failure tolerance of the tissue. Soft tissues are influenced by the history of recent physical stresses, so that the accumulation of individual stresses can cause injury. Characteristics of the load, such as rate, compression, and forces (e.g., torsion, shear), along with the properties of the affected tissue, determine the type and extent of tissue damage. The time elapsed since injury and the extent of tissue damage determine the inflammatory response.[8,90]

With repetitive and/or forceful tasks, the initiating stimuli for inflammatory responses include repeated overstretch, compression, friction, and anoxia. These insults lead to mechanical injury of cellular membranes and intracellular structures and a localized release of proteins such as collagen, fibronectin, and cytokines.[8]

A single high load or stress from a traumatic fall, car accident, or other traumatic event can cause significant injury. Bones can fracture from one episode of high-magnitude force, and workers lifting heavy boxes repeatedly can incur a slow degradation of the tissue tolerance. Decreasing tissue tolerance may explain why there are no active acute inflammatory indicators in tendons associated with tendinitis. Instead, antiinflammatory mediators and fibrotic proliferation are observed, suggesting the acute inflammatory phase has resolved. Tennis elbow or golfer's elbow is recognized in many cases as a noninflammatory condition after an inflammatory episode,[8] and research is ongoing to find ways to reinitiate the inflammatory cascade and promote healing in an otherwise degenerative process.[36] Low loads sustained over a long period of time, such as in workers who remain in a fixed, flexed posture for prolonged periods of time, can also result in tissue injury because of decreased tissue tolerance.[100]

Some soft tissues, such as ligaments, can rupture with a single high-magnitude force but can also fail from repeated bouts of moderate-magnitude stress. Likewise, as mentioned previously, bone can fracture from high-magnitude force but can also develop stress fractures or stress reactions from repeated episodes of moderate-magnitude force.[71] Altering mechanical stress (either increasing or decreasing forces) can be used to benefit individuals under varying circumstances. For example, reducing mechanical stress by offloading or pressure reduction is a concept used for healing ulcers and preventing their recurrence.

Controlled increase in physical stress is the underlying principle of progressive resistive exercise used to cause muscle fibers to hypertrophy and able to withstand and generate greater force. Higher than normal levels of physical stress can promote remodeling in bone. Musculoskeletal tissues subjected to higher than normal levels of stress become more tolerant to subsequent physical stresses and are more resistant to injury.[100]

Chemical Factors

Toxic substances cause chemical injury. These substances can be divided into two categories: those that can injure cells directly and those that require metabolic transformation into the toxic agent. Examples of chemicals that injure cells directly are heavy metals, such as mercury, that bind to and disrupt critical membrane proteins and a number of toxins and drugs, such as alkylating agents, used in chemotherapy.

Alkylating agents, such as nitrogen mustards, induce cross-linking of DNA and inactivation of other essential cellular constituents. Carbon tetrachloride and acetaminophen are examples of inert substances that must be metabolized to reactive intermediates to cause cell injury. Taken in large amounts, most medications can be toxic, and many are even lethal. Suicide by drug overdose is a common example of drug-induced chemical toxicity.

Free radical formation. An important mechanism of cell injury and disease is the production of ROS, sometimes referred to as the formation of *free radicals*. Free radicals are an integral part of metabolism and are formed continuously in the body. They can exert positive effects (e.g., on the immune system) or negative effects (e.g., lipid, protein, DNA oxidation). A variety of normal and pathological reactions can lead to the activation of oxygen by the sequential addition or subtraction, respectively, of one electron at a time (Fig. 3.2).

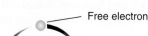
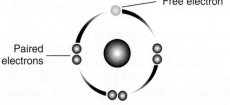
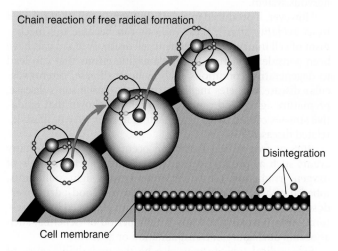
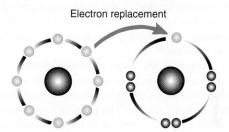

FIG. 3.2 The oxidative process and formation of free radicals. Normal metabolic processes and a variety of other extrinsic factors, such as pollution, poor nutrition, and exposure to toxic chemicals, can result in the formation of free radicals when normal oxygen atoms lose one of their four paired electrons. The resulting unstable atom attempts to replace the missing electron by "stealing" an electron from a healthy cell, creating another unstable atom (free radical) and setting off a chain reaction referred to as *oxidation*. Oxidation as a by-product of metabolism damages cell membranes, leading to intrinsic cellular damage, a part of the normal aging process. Free radical damage (oxidation) is believed to alter the way cells encode genetic information in the DNA and may contribute to a variety of diseases and disorders. Antioxidant molecules freely give up an electron to stabilize the oxygen atom without becoming unstable and without initiating a chain reaction.

For example, the body's natural process of using oxygen and food to produce energy can create free radicals as a by-product of these functions. These unpaired electrons are reactive and commonly bind to oxygen for stabilization. The oxygen then binds to hydrogen for stabilization. This series of reactions generated by normal cellular metabolism results in a phenomenon referred to as *oxygen toxicity* and yields superoxide (O_2^-), hydrogen peroxide (H_2O_2), and hydroxyl radical (OH^-). These forms of reactive oxygen are referred to as *oxygen radicals,* which are toxic to cells.

The cellular enzymes always scavenging the body to protect cells from this type of injury normally inactivate these radicals and convert the radical back to usable oxygen. Some unstable oxygen molecules (i.e., free radicals) enable the body to fight inflammation, kill bacteria, and help regulate the autonomic nervous system.

However, if produced in excess amounts (a situation referred to as *oxidative stress*), these radicals can become the mechanism of cell injury and subsequent cell death. Free radicals have been considered central to the damaging effects that can lead to degenerative conditions such as heart disease, cerebrovascular disease, diabetes mellitus, cataracts, Parkinson's disease, premature aging, and cancer. Research has shown that oxidative stresses caused by ROS are factors in over 90% of lifestyle-related diseases.[98]

ROS or free radical formation occurs as a result of many events such as prolonged exercise; exposure to high levels of oxygen, irradiation, ultraviolet or fluorescent light, pollutants, tobacco smoke, and pesticides (airborne or in food); drug overdose; heat stress; and the reperfusion injury induced by the restoration of normal blood flow after a period of ischemia, such as occurs during organ transplantation or after MI.

Free radical toxicity may also be the underlying cause of degeneration of neurons located in the *substantia nigra* of the brain, leading to the loss of dopamine necessary for the normal control of movements that produces the abnormal movements seen in Parkinson's disease.[24]

Antioxidants. Oxygen is the most common form of free radical in the human body, but the use of oxygen as a life-supporting mechanism means oxidative stress is an inescapable part of the human biologic system. The simultaneous presence of antioxidants is an adaptive response to help the body ward off the potentially harmful effects of oxygen and its derivatives, including free radicals.[156]

Antioxidants neutralize the extra free radicals and keep them from taking electrons from other molecules, resulting in cellular and DNA damage. A variety of enzymatic and non-enzymatic defense mechanisms are present within cells to perform the function of antioxidants, detoxifying ROS and protecting the cells from this type of injury. These are called *endogenous antioxidants.* Researchers are finding a variety of uses for natural antioxidants in combating the effects of aging and disease.

There are also *exogenous antioxidants* that can be taken from outside the body through our diet. Vitamin C, vitamin E, and β-carotene are three important exogenous antioxidants. Over 200 antioxidants have been identified in food or plant substances. For example, vitamin E effectively scavenges several types of free radicals and other reactive species in lipid membranes and other lipid concentrations, making it a potentially effective antioxidant (able to neutralize the free radical before damage occurs) in preventing LDL cholesterol from adhering to the walls of arteries. In the case of the prostate, lycopene (the compound that makes tomatoes red) is a potent antioxidant potentially effective in promoting prostate health.[52,79]

Adequate intake of folate, a B vitamin, has been shown to reduce the risk of breast cancer associated with alcohol consumption by providing bioactive compounds to counteract the formation of oxidative compounds.[49,157]

Multiple trials are ongoing to investigate oxidation and its effect on cellular injury, aging, and disease (e.g., cancer, heart disease, cataracts) and the use of antioxidants found naturally in food and plants to combat oxidative stress, preventing or possibly modifying diseases at the cellular level. Animal and human studies have confirmed that regular, moderate physical activity and exercise strengthen the antioxidant defense system, whereas intense or prolonged, strenuous exercise (especially in a person who has a sedentary lifestyle) constitutes an oxidative stress.[39,116,119]

Nitric oxide. The nitric oxide (NO) molecule is composed of one nitrogen atom and one oxygen atom. It is present in all mammals including humans and is one of the few gaseous signaling molecules known. It should not be confused with nitrous oxide (N_2O), a general anesthetic, or with nitrogen dioxide (NO_2), which is a poisonous air pollutant.

The nitric oxide molecule is a free radical, which is relevant to understanding its high reactivity. NO is recognized as an important modulator of an enormous number of physiologic responses. Reduced NO bioavailability that is a result of oxidative stress seems to be the common molecular disorder causing many pathologic effects within the body.

NO assists in long-term memory. It also influences neuronal transmission by increasing the permeability of nerve endings, making acetylcholine transfer across the synapses easier. It alters the ability of the gastrointestinal (GI) mucosa to resist injury induced by toxins, influencing the immune system. NO inhibits virally induced cytokine and chemokine production, possibly combating the common cold.[120] It also stimulates collagen synthesis for wound healing, modulates fracture healing, and is useful in the treatment of tendinopathy.[108,109]

NO is an antilipid that provides a nonstick coating to the lining of blood vessels, much like Teflon. These two effects have helped explain how NO might prevent heart attacks and strokes and why nitroglycerin works. Nitroglycerin is converted to NO inside vascular tissue, where it relaxes smooth muscle in arteries and causes blood vessels to dilate. It also controls platelet function by preventing platelets from clumping together, preventing the formation of blood clots.

Researchers are studying the effect of NO on free radicals that cannot be stabilized or removed. Studies show that NO appears to play a role in exercise-induced dilation of blood vessels supplying cardiac and skeletal muscle. Exercise training enhances NO-mediated vasodilation. The exact mechanism is not clear yet, but a growing number of studies suggest that exercise training, perhaps via increased capacity for NO formation, retards atherosclerosis.[85] There is also accumulating evidence that NO is involved in skeletal muscle glucose uptake during exercise.[86]

Exercise and free radicals. Physical activity and exercise can have positive or negative effects on oxidative stress depending on training load, training specificity, and basal level of training. Oxidative stress seems to be involved in muscular fatigue and overtraining.[44] Excessive exercise has been shown to induce DNA damage in peripheral leukocytes. Exhaustion of the leukocyte ROS may reduce the body's ability to combat microbial invasions (i.e., infections) before the system has been restored.[105] On the other hand, moderate stress in the form of regular exercise training may have protective effects against exercise-induced DNA damage.

Evidence is emerging to support a role for improved NO bioavailability with exercise training.[128] Upregulation of endogenous antioxidant defense systems and complex regulation of repair systems are seen in response to training and exercise. Upregulation of antioxidants and modulation of the repair response may be mechanisms by which exercise can influence our health in a positive way.[42]

Regular, long-term aerobic exercise has been shown to reduce migraine pain severity, frequency, and duration, which is possibly a result of increased NO production.[104]

If you are going to introduce NO, it is essential to recognize the position of the U.S. Food and Drug Administration (FDA) on infrared treatments to stimulate NO for peripheral vascular disease (PVD). The FDA recognizes that NO is increased during the episode of infrared treatments, but if the patient does not develop normal exercise habits to produce his or her own NO, when infrared interventions are stopped the tissue damage is exponentially increased, resulting in severe distal tissue necrosis. Therefore Medicare is not reimbursing for infrared interventions for PVD.

Psychosocial Factors

Psychosocial factors can impact tissue adaptation, especially as related to tissue injury.[89] Psychosocial factors (e.g., fear, tension, anxiety) may influence individual threshold values for tissue adaptation and injury. Many studies have investigated the role of mechanical and psychosocial factors in the onset of musculoskeletal (and other regional) acute and chronic pain.[121] For example, people who are only occasionally or never satisfied in their work settings or who describe their work as "monotonous" have a higher risk of injury than those who are satisfied or completely satisfied with support from supervisors and colleagues.[11,58,59,102]

Reversible Cell Injury

Alteration in a cell's functional environment, either acute or chronic, produces a stress to the cell's ability to attain or maintain homeostasis. The extent to which the cell is able to alter mechanisms and regain homeostasis in the altered environment is considered an adaptation by the cells or tissues. When the cell is unable to adapt, injury can occur. A sublethal or reversible injury occurs if the stress is sufficiently small in magnitude or short enough in duration that the cell is able to recover homeostasis after removal of the stress.

Cells react to injurious stimuli by changing their steady state to continue to function in a hazardous environment. Reversible (sublethal) injury caused by any of the mechanisms of cell injury listed in Box 3.1 is a transient impairment in the cell's normal structure or function. Normal cell structure and function can return after removal of the stressor or injurious stimulus (Fig. 3.3).

Acute reversible injury causes an impairment of ion homeostasis within the cell and leads to increased intracellular levels of sodium and calcium. An influx of interstitial fluid into the cell accompanies these ionic shifts and causes increased cell volume (swelling). Swelling occurs within the cytosol (liquid medium of the cytoplasm) and within organelles such as mitochondria and the endoplasmic reticulum (ER). Swollen mitochondria generate less energy. Thus instead of oxidative ATP production, the cell reverts to less efficient anaerobic glycolysis, which results in excessive production of lactic acid. The pH of the cell becomes acidic, which slows down the cell metabolism,

resulting in further cellular damage. The injured cell forms plasma membrane *blebs* that can seal off and detach from the cell surface. In severely injured cells, ribosomes detach from the rough ER (RER), and a decrease in the number of polysomes occurs. These changes lead to reduced protein synthesis by the affected cells, and the cycle of damage continues. However, if the cell nucleus remains undamaged and the energy source is restored or the toxic injury is neutralized, the cell is able to recover and pump the ions and excess fluid back out. The swelling disappears, and the cell is returned to the original steady state, constituting a reversible cell injury.

Cellular Adaptations in Chronic Cell Injury

When a sublethal stress remains present over a period of time, stable alterations (adaptations) take place within the affected cells, tissues, and organs. Adaptation enables the cells to function in an altered environment, avoiding injury. Characteristics of cell adaptation, such as change in size, number, or function, increase the cell's ability to survive; these changes are also potentially reversible. In many but not all cases, these changes benefit the function of the parent organ or structure within which the cell resides. Common cellular adaptations include atrophy, hypertrophy, hyperplasia, *metaplasia*, and dysplasia (Fig. 3.4).

Atrophy is a reduction in cell and organ size. It can occur with vascular insufficiency, reduction in hormone levels, malnutrition, immobilization, pain that limits function, and chronic inflammation. Bone loss, muscle wasting, and brain cell loss are examples of either tissue or organ atrophy associated with aging. Pathologic atrophy occurs as a consequence of cell injury caused by ischemia, inadequate nutrition, or physical factors (see Box 3.1). For example, ischemia of the viscera results in atrophied organs; cancer or malnutrition can result in cachexia, a general wasting of the body; and spinal cord injury results in atrophy of the affected muscles.

Hypertrophy is an increase in the size of the cell and organ and can occur when increased functional demands are placed on the cells, tissues, or organs and with increased hormonal input (e.g., exercise stress can induce skeletal muscle hypertrophy). Pure hypertrophy occurs only in the heart and striated muscles because these organs consist of cells that cannot divide. Hypertrophy of the heart is a common pathologic finding that occurs as an adaptation of heart muscle to an increased workload. Specifically, hypertrophy of the left ventricle is a typical complication of hypertension. Increased blood pressure requires that the heart produce more force to eject the blood. The additional force is produced by hypertrophy of muscle fibers in the left ventricle.

Hyperplasia is an increase in the number of cells leading to increased organ size. In tissues consisting of cells that are capable of dividing, the presence of excessive functional demands can cause a consequent increase in cell number. Pure hyperplasia typically occurs because of hormonal stimulation (e.g., prolonged estrogen exposure causes the endometrium of the uterus to become thick) or chronic stimulation (e.g., persistent pressure on the skin induces hyperplasia and the formation of a callus). Some hyperplasia has no discernible cause and may represent early neoplasia. Hypertrophy and hyperplasia often occur together, such as in prostate enlargement and obstruction of the urethra and bladder. The result is an increase in size and number of smooth muscle cells in the wall of the urinary bladder.

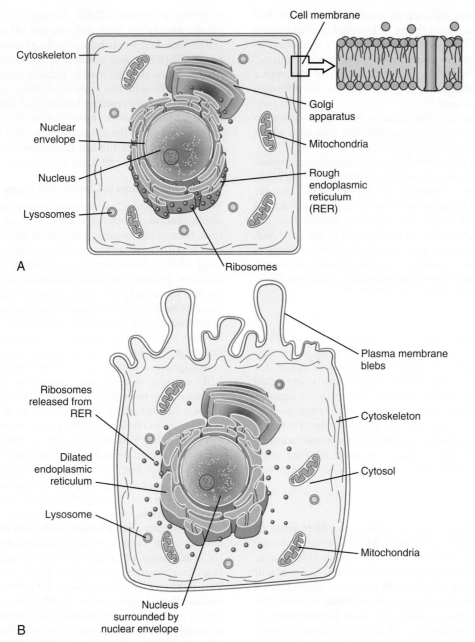

FIG. 3.3 (A) A normal cell with its organelles. (B) Reversible cell injury with cellular swelling, accumulation of fluid in endoplasmic reticulum, and the release of ribosomes and formation of membrane blebs. (Courtesy Steven H. Tepper, PT, PhD, FAPTA, Rehab Essentials, Inc.)

Metaplasia is a change in a cell's makeup or morphology and function resulting from the conversion of one adult cell type into another. For example, in smokers, portions of the respiratory tract change from ciliated pseudostratified columnar epithelium into stratified squamous epithelium, leading to a thickening of the respiratory epithelium and loss of the functional clearance of mucus and debris along the respiratory tree.

Dysplasia is an increase in cell numbers accompanied by altered cell morphology and loss of histologic or cell organization. Considered to be a preneoplastic alteration, dysplasia can be found in areas that are chronically injured and undergoing hyperplasia or metaplasia.

Intracellular Accumulations or Storage

Intracellular accumulations are increases in the storage of lipids, proteins, carbohydrates, or pigments within the cell that occur as a result of an overload of various metabolites or exogenous material. These accumulations can also be caused by metabolic disturbances altering cell function. For example, when the liver is sublethally injured, lipid (triglyceride) accumulates within the liver cells (*hepatocytes*). This lipid accumulation occurs when a reduction in protein synthesis occurs as a result of disaggregation of the ribosomes from the RER, as previously discussed. Hepatocytes normally produce our endogenous lipoproteins.

With sublethal damage to hepatocytes (e.g., alcohol abuse), a lack of protein shell formation occurs so that lipoproteins

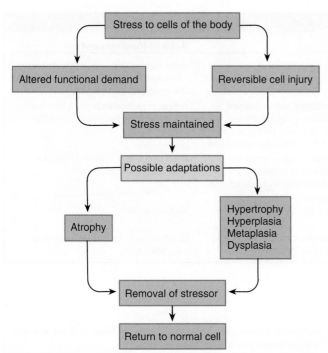

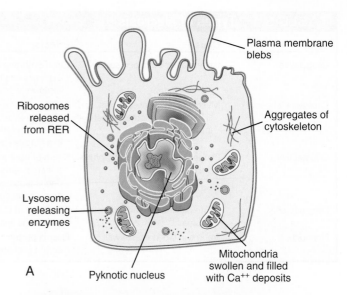

FIG. 3.4 Cellular adaptations and reversible cell injury in response to stress. When the body is under persistent stress leading to either reversible cell injury or altered functional demand, the tissues adapt. Adaptations could include atrophy, hypertrophy, hyperplasia, metaplasia, or dysplasia. All of these changes are reversible with removal of the stressor. (Courtesy Steven H. Tepper, PT, PhD, FAPTA, Rehab Essentials, Inc.)

cannot be packaged and transported to the plasma. As a result, lipids remain within the hepatocyte, causing the characteristic "fatty liver" found in alcoholics.

Irreversible Cell Injury

If the injurious or stressful stimulus is of sufficient magnitude or duration or if the cell is unable to adapt, the cell will be irreversibly injured. Irreversible cell injury is synonymous with cell death. Hallmarks of lethally injured cells include alterations in the cell nucleus, mitochondria, and lysosomes and rupture of the cell membrane.

Damage to the nucleus can occur in three forms: pyknosis, karyorrhexis, and karyolysis. Nuclei undergo clumping or pyknosis, which is a degeneration of the cell as the nucleus shrinks in size and the chromatin condenses to a solid mass. The pyknotic nuclei can fragment, a process termed *karyorrhexis,* or it can undergo dissolution *(karyolysis).*

Mitochondria lose their membrane potential and become unable to synthesize ATP, leaving the cell without the necessary energy production for cell function. Morphologically, irreversibly injured mitochondria appear swollen, contain large lipid-protein aggregates called *flocculent densities,* and may also contain dense crystalline deposits of calcium (Fig. 3.5).

After cell death, lysosomes release their digestive enzymes within the cytoplasm of the cell, initiating enzymatic degradation of all cellular constituents, a process that may be aided by enzymes released from inflammatory cells. The active process of degradation of dead cells is called *necrosis.* Enzymes help dissolve the dead tissue, making it easier for phagocytic cells to remove the dead tissue in preparation for healing by repair (laying

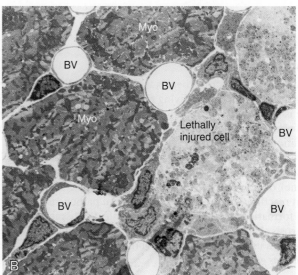

FIG. 3.5 Irreversible cell injury: ultrastructural alterations in an irreversibly killed cell. (A) Mitochondria are nonfunctional and filled with flocculent densities. Lysosomes are releasing their digestive enzymes. The nucleus is condensing on itself (pyknosis). Membrane breakdown allows intracellular enzymes to be released into the interstitial area. (B) Electron micrograph of lethally injured cardiomyocytes next to healthy viable cardiomyocytes *(Myo).* Note lethally injured cells to the right of the Myo are swollen, mitochondria are filled with flocculent densities, there is a loss of myofilaments, and mononuclear phagocytic cells are beginning to remove these dead cells. *BV,* Blood vessel. Original magnification ×1500. (A, Courtesy Steven H. Tepper, PT, PhD, FAPTA, Rehab Essentials, Inc.; B, From Tepper SH, Anderson PA, Mergner WJ: Recovery of the heart following focal injury induced by dietary restriction of potassium, Pathol Res Prac 186:265–285, 1990.)

down of a collagenous tissue scar) or regeneration (regrowth of parenchymal tissue). Dead cells release their contents into the extracellular fluid, eventually making their way into the circulation, in which they can be measured as clinically useful signs of cell injury. For example, levels of aspartate aminotransferase (AST), creatine kinase (CK), and lactate dehydrogenase (LDH)

TABLE 3.1   Types of Necrosis

Type	Cause	Effects	Area of Involvement
Coagulative	Ischemia (lack of blood supply	Cell membrane is preserved; nucleus undergoes pyknosis and karyolysis (dissolution); organelles dissolve	Solid internal organs (e.g., heart, liver, kidneys)
			Dry gangrene (extremities)
Caseous ("cheesy")	Mycobacterium tuberculosis (TB); seen with other fungal infections	Cell membrane is destroyed; debris appears cheeselike and does not disappear by lysis but persists indefinitely; damaged area is walled off in a fibrous calcified area, forming a granuloma	Lungs, bronchopulmonary lymph nodes, skeletal bone (extrapulmonary TB)
Liquefactive	Pyogenic bacteria (e.g., *Staphylococcus aureus*)	Death of neurons releases lysosomes that liquefy the area, leaving pockets of liquid and cellular debris (abscess of fluid-filled cavity); shapeless, amorphous debris remains	Brain tissue (e.g., brain infarct); skin, wound, joint infections
Fatty necrosis	Acute pancreatitis, abdominal trauma	Formation of calcium soaps by the release of pancreatic lipases	Abdominal area
Fibrinoid	Trauma in blood vessel wall	Plasma proteins accumulate; cellular debris and serum proteins form pink deposits	Blood vessels (tunica media, smooth muscle cells)

are typically elevated in the serum of people with myocardial infarct or viral hepatitis.

Types of Necrosis

The process of necrosis begins with the dissolution of irreversibly injured cells within living tissue. Removal of this dead tissue is essential for healing to take place. Histologically, several different types of necrosis are recognized (Table 3.1), with some additional subcategories.

Gangrene caused by bacterial infection and associated with tissue ischemia (PVD) may form coagulative necrosis (dry gangrene) or liquefactive necrosis (wet gangrene). The fermentation reactions caused by certain bacterial pathogens may cause the formation of gas bubbles in the infected tissue. In muscle necrosis, one of the causative agents is *Clostridium perfringens*. The term used to describe this condition is *clostridial myonecrosis* or *gas gangrene*.

3.1 Special Implications for the PTA: **Cell Injury: Multiple Cell Injuries** The concepts discussed in the section Mechanisms of Cell (Tissue) Injury are essential for understanding the pathogenesis of a variety of acute illnesses and injuries the physical therapist assistant (PTA) may see in any clinical setting. Often, multiple episodes of care with complex cases involving simultaneous multiple diseases or comorbidities occur in clinical practice. For example, the victim of a motor vehicle accident experiencing a traumatic brain injury (TBI) and pelvic fracture may develop pneumonia and pulmonary compromise and subsequently experience myocardial infarction (MI). The therapy staff following this client throughout the entire continuum of care—from the intensive care unit through rehabilitation to a home health service setting and possibly on an outpatient basis—can better meet the needs of such an individual during the healing process by understanding these concepts of injury and recovery.

TBI could occur during motor vehicle accidents. With direct trauma to the head, primary and secondary injury can lethally damage the brain tissue. Primary injury to the brain may occur in the following areas: (1) local brain damage occurs at the site in which the brain impacts the skull (coup injury) and the site opposite the impact (contrecoup injury); (2) polar brain damage occurs at the tips (poles) of the frontal, temporal, and occipital lobes and the undersurface of the frontal and temporal lobes when the brain moves inside the skull; or (3) diffuse axonal injury occurs throughout the subcortical white

matter (and brainstem if the magnitude of force is great enough) with sufficient shear force to injure axons.

Secondary injury is usually the result of hypoxic-ischemic injury caused by cerebral edema. Because the soft and pliable brain is enclosed within the rigid skull, abnormal brain fluid dynamics caused by cerebral edema result in increased intracranial pressure (ICP). Signs and symptoms of increased ICP include headache, loss of sense of smell, and altered level of consciousness. Even a mild increase in ICP is sufficient to cause death of neural tissue from inadequate perfusion. Moderate and severe increases in ICP can cause brain tissue to shift position or herniate from one chamber into another, and may also cause compression on neural structures. Intracranial bleeds or hematomas (epidural, subdural, and intracerebral) are another source of secondary brain damage.

Passive imaging techniques (e.g., computed tomography and magnetic resonance imaging) are useful to visualize the structural changes that occur with TBI, whereas active imaging techniques (e.g., electroencephalography, positron emission tomography, evoked potentials) are useful to visualize physiologic changes that occur with TBI.

Open wounds and fractures are common sequelae associated with motor vehicle accidents. In this case a fracture resulted from the mechanical force distributed during a motor vehicle accident. Fractures are often diagnosed by radiograph. When a bone is fractured, its normal blood supply is disrupted. Osteocytes (bone cells) die of the trauma and the resulting ischemia. Bone macrophages remove the dead bone cells and damaged bone.

A precursor fibrocartilaginous growth of tissue occurs before the laying down of primary bone, eventually followed by the laying down and remodeling of normal adult bone. This process, from fracture to full restoration of the bone, will take weeks to months, depending on the type of fracture, location, vascular supply, health, and age of the individual.

In this example, if the myocardium is subjected to ischemia for a sufficient duration, the myocytes become irreversibly injured. A cascade of physiologic and anatomic changes leads to the death of myocardial cells. Coagulative necrosis ensues, followed by acute inflammation, and finally repair by scar tissue formation (Fig. 3.6).

Coagulative necrosis begins with the release of lysosomal enzymes that cause dissolution of the normal structural relationships found within myocytes. The dead cells attract acute inflammatory cells that phagocytize the necrotic debris and release growth factors. The growth factors initiate the proliferation of blood vessels (angiogenesis) and fibroblasts, resulting in the eventual production of a collagenous scar.

Signs and symptoms correlate with the different stages of lethal cell injury and differ according to the organ or structure(s) involved. During acute MI, the individual often experiences angina, shortness of breath, sweating, and nausea. These symptoms of physiologic stress are caused by the release of histamines, bradykinins, and prostaglandins such as substance P from the lethally injured myocytes.

An electrocardiogram reveals ST segment elevation and Q waves over the affected area. The person is also at an increased risk for life-threatening dysrhythmias because of the loss of electrical conductivity of lethally injured myocytes and disrupted conductivity (irritability) of the adjacent cells. If a significant percentage of the myocardium is infarcted, cardiogenic shock or congestive heart failure may ensue.

Cytoplasmic enzymes or proteins (e.g., CK-MB) are released from the dead cells. Normally, the plasmalemma is impermeable to these large molecules and contains them within the confines of the cytoplasm. After lethal injury the plasmalemma is broken down by the actions of phospholipases, and these molecules are released from inside the cell. A number of cytoplasmic proteins are released into the interstitial area and are taken up by adjacent lymphatic vessels and finally enter the bloodstream. Lactate dehydrogenase, CK-MB, and troponin are clinically relevant for diagnosis and assessment of the severity of an MI.

The PTA must understand the process of injury to and repair of the brain, bones, and myocardium (or other involved organs and/or structures), as appropriate client care is determined by the different stages of this process. For example, recovery from TBI tends to follow the progression outlined by the Rancho Los Amigos Levels of Cognitive Function (LOCF).

Generally, intervention is directed by the current LOCF level. During LOCF levels I to III, primary goals involve increasing tolerance of activities, including intervention, tolerating upright posture, and increasing interaction with the environment. During levels IV to VI the emphasis shifts to increasing physical and cognitive endurance. During levels VII and VIII, intervention focuses on the skills necessary to reenter the community.

After fracture of bone, a period of immobilization usually occurs to remove longitudinal stress. This period allows for the phagocytic removal of necrotic bone tissue and the initial deposition of the fibrocartilaginous callus. As the fracture heals, as revealed by radiograph, gradual progression of stress is applied. Mobilization of this individual will occur depending on the type of fixation used on the bone. For example, if external fixation is applied for fracture stabilization, mobilization can occur almost immediately within tolerance of the symptoms.

The highest risk of death during the first hours after MI stems from dysrhythmias. Rupture of the myocardium is possible during days 3 to 10 after a transmural MI (from outside epicardium to inside endocardium). The risk of these events dictates that exercise during this time must not subject damaged cells to excessive stress. Proper mobilization soon after infarction may decrease the likelihood of succumbing to the negative effects of bed rest but may be complicated by variables such as fracture, pneumonia, and the TBI in this case.

TISSUE HEALING

The process of tissue healing begins soon after tissue injury or death and occurs either by regeneration (regrowth of original tissue) or by repair (formation of a connective tissue scar). The inflammatory cells recruited from the blood circulation begin the healing process by breaking down and removing the necrotic tissue. This is accomplished primarily by phagocytes that secrete degradative enzymes and also phagocytose the cellular debris, connective tissue fragments, and plasma proteins present in the dead tissue.

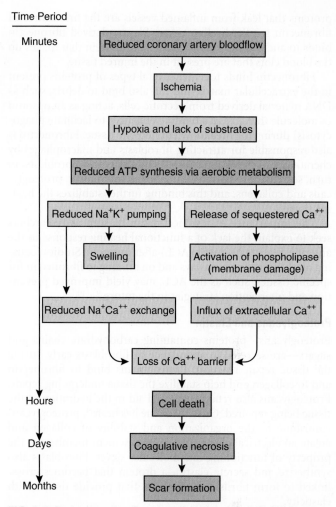

FIG. 3.6 Pathogenesis of myocardial infarction (MI). With reduction in coronary artery blood flow caused by a thrombus formation, ischemia results in a reduction of aerobic metabolism. Irreversible cell injury occurs, followed by necrosis of the heart tissue. Intracellular enzymes (creatine kinase [CK]-MB, troponin) released from the dead heart tissue serve as biochemical markers in the early diagnosis of MI. In the following weeks, healing occurs by repair, and there is the formation of a connective tissue scar. (Courtesy Steven H. Tepper, PT, PhD, FAPTA, Rehab Essentials, Inc.)

The healing process is complex and influenced by many components such as fibronectin, proteoglycans and elastin, collagen, and parenchymal (organ) and endothelial (skin) cells. In addition, there is a wide range of factors that affect tissue healing and must be taken into account during recovery and rehabilitation. Both the components and the factors that affect tissue healing are presented in this section followed by a discussion of the multiphasic process of tissue healing and recovery.

Components of Tissue Healing
Fibronectin
Fibronectin has numerous functions in wound healing, the most important of which are the formation of scaffold, the provision of tensile strength, and the ability to "glue" other substances and cells together. It is one of the earliest proteins to provide the structural support that stabilizes the healing tissue. Plasma

proteins that leak from inflamed vessels are the first source of fibronectin for the healing tissue. Plasma-derived fibronectin binds to and stabilizes fibrin, which is a protein that makes up the blood clots that are present in the injured tissue.

Fibronectin binds together several types of proteins present in the extracellular matrix and can also bind to debris, such as DNA material derived from necrotic cells, acting as an opsonin (a molecule that acts as a binding enhancer to facilitate phagocytosis) during the breakdown of necrotic tissue. Fibronectin is also responsible for attracting fibroblasts and macrophages by chemotaxis to the healing tissue. The stimulated fibroblasts, in turn, secrete more fibronectin. Fibronectin binds to proteoglycans and collagens, and this binding further stabilizes the healing tissue.

The importance of fibronectin can be seen as researchers seek to explain the lack of a functional healing response in the anterior cruciate ligament (ACL) after injury.[156] Studies focusing on the signaling pathways and on binding to fibronectin for specific tissues, such as the ACL, may yield improved prevention and intervention strategies in the future.[92,140,155]

Proteoglycans and Elastin

Proteoglycans—proteins containing carbohydrate chains and sugars—are secreted in abundance by fibroblasts early during the tissue repair reaction. Proteoglycans bind to fibronectin and to collagen and help stabilize the tissue undergoing repair. Proteoglycans also retain water and aid in the hydration of the tissue being repaired. Once the tissue has healed, proteoglycans contribute to the organization and stability of collagen and create an electrical charge that gives basement membranes the property of functioning like molecular sieves. Fibroblasts also synthesize and secrete elastin, a protein that becomes cross-linked to form fibrils or long sheets that provide tissues with elasticity.

Collagen

Collagen most importantly provides structural support and tensile strength for almost all tissues and organs of the body. The different types of collagen give stability to healing tissue; the word *collagen* is derived from Greek and means *glue producer*. Collagen is a fibrous protein molecule consisting of three chains of amino acid coiled around one another in a triple helix (Fig. 3.7). Improved technology has made it possible to identify collagen types and measure protein turnover. It is the most abundant protein in the body; at least 27 collagen types have been identified.

We know that exercise is a potent stimulus for protein synthesis in skeletal muscle. Collagen in the extracellular matrix of muscle and tendon is also sensitive to mechanical stimuli. Collagen does not appear to be nutritionally sensitive, which may contribute to the loss of muscle during aging. It is possible that the tissue is unable to respond adequately to the increased availability of nutrients.[152]

Organization of collagen. Each collagen type has a specialized function (Table 3.2). The amino acid makeup of the collagen molecule and the manner in which the molecules are assembled together vary for each collagen type. The differences in organization and composition account for the structural properties of each collagen type; for example, collagen organized in unidirectional or parallel bundles contributes to the strength of tendons. Collagen is the principal extracellular component of a normal tendon.

Collagen in random arrangement provides flexibility of the skin and rigidity of bone. When organized at right angles, collagen allows transmission of light in the cornea and vitreous. Collagen laid down in a tubular fashion contributes to the elasticity of the blood vessels.

Some collagen molecules are assembled into progressively thicker and stronger filamentous structures, allowing the molecules to become cross-linked. These cross-links impart tensile strength to collagen fibers and prevent slippage of molecules past one another when under tension. The structural stability of the extracellular matrix is primarily a consequence of collagen and the extent of cross-linking.[23]

Types of collagen. Type I collagen, the most common form, is assembled as a thick bundle that is structurally very strong and can be found in all body tissues, in which it forms bundles together with other collagen types. It is the main component of mature scars and is predominant in strong tissues such as tendons and bones.

Type II collagen is assembled into thin supporting filaments and is the predominant collagen type found in cartilaginous tissue. Type II fibers have a half-life of about 3 months. This allows maintenance of the nutritive exchanges between degenerative external annulus and any healthy remaining tissue, possibly delaying or avoiding further degeneration.[49]

Type III collagen is assembled into thin filaments that make tissues strong but supple and elastic. It contains interchain disulfide bonds or bridges not found in type I or II collagen and is the collagen type first deposited in wound healing (i.e., fresh scars). This type of highly soluble collagen accounts in part for the plasticity of skin and blood vessels. Overexposure to the sun speeds up the breakdown of collagen and elastin, two proteins that give skin its strength and resilience, thus contributing to the development of skin wrinkling.

Type III collagen is more prevalent in newborns; with each passing decade, collagen-producing cells make less soluble collagen and progressively convert to synthesizing an insoluble, more stable type I collagen. The changing ratio of collagen types I and III throughout the body is so reliable that chronologic age can be determined by analyzing the collagen type III content of a skin sample.[7]

During the initial stages of tissue repair, fibroblasts secrete large amounts of type III collagen, which provides support for the developing capillaries. Within a few days after the tissue injury, type III collagen is degraded by enzymes secreted by fibroblasts and other cells and is replaced by newly synthesized type I collagen. Type I collagen enhances wound tensile strength and is the main component of the scar tissue that remains after repair is completed. Type IV collagen is not assembled into fibers. Together with other proteins, it forms the basement membrane to which epithelial, endothelial, and certain mesenchymal cells are anchored.

Mutations in the genes for collagen cause a wide spectrum of diseases of bone, cartilage, and blood vessels, including osteogenesis imperfecta, a variety of chondrodysplasias, Alport syndrome, Ehlers–Danlos syndrome, and more rarely, some forms of osteoporosis, osteoarthritis, and familial aneurysms. Scientists are finding that extremely unusual or aberrant collagen cross-linking and increased collagen synthesis are present in some malignancies,[12] whereas the presence of free radical scavengers inhibits the rate of collagen formation.[94]

When either collagen or elastin becomes resorbed, elements are released into blood and concentrate in urine. Determining

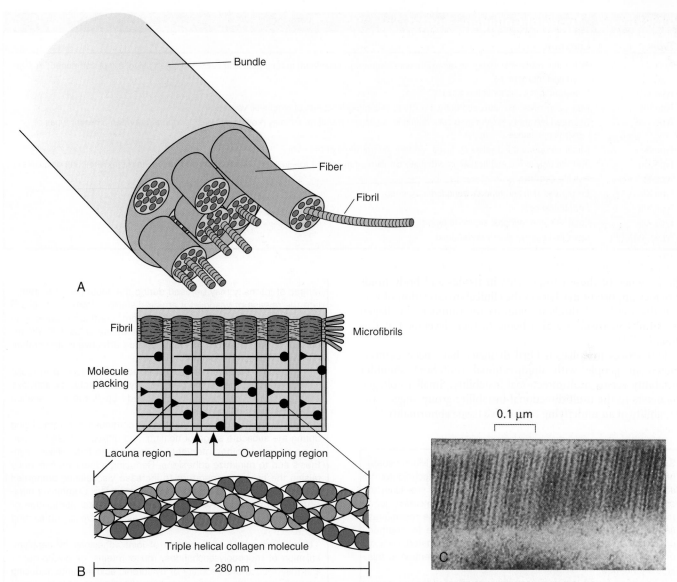

FIG. 3.7 Structure of collagen. (A) The collagen fiber is composed of fibrils, each of which is composed of microfibrils. (B) The molecule itself consists of three polypeptide chains called *alpha chains* that wrap around one another in a triple helix. The helix is made possible because each third amino acid in the polypeptide chain is glycine. The molecules are quarter-staggered one to another, which ensures that no weak points occur across the fibril to prevent overload and slippage. (C) Visualized by transmission electron microscopy, the individual collagen fibrils are seen to have two orders of banding. The larger bands result from the gaps between the individual molecules of collagen, which then overlap the adjacent molecules to form a strong bond. (From Bullough PG: Bullough and Vigorita's orthopaedic pathology, ed 3, St Louis, 1997, Mosby.)

TABLE 3.2	**Types of Collagen**
Type	**Location**
Type I	Predominant structural collagen of the body; constitutes 80%-85% of dermal collagen; prominent in mature scars, tendon, bone, and dentin; joints
Type II	Predominant component of hyaline cartilage (e.g., outer ear, end of nose, joint); not present in skin; found in nucleus pulposus external annulus
Type III	Prominent in vascular and visceral structures (e.g., blood vessels, gastrointestinal tract, liver, uterus) but absent in bone and tendon; constitutes 15%-20% of dermal collagen; abundant in embryonic tissues; first collagen deposited in wound healing (granulation tissue)
Type IV	Found in basement membranes (base of epithelial, endothelial, and mesenchymal cells found in developing fetus), glomeruli of kidney nephron

Continued

TABLE 3.2	Types of Collagen—cont'd
Type	**Location**
Type V	Present in most tissues but never as a major component; prominent in fetal membrane, cornea, heart valve; minor component of skin; synovial membranes
Type VI	Prevalent in most connective tissues
Type VII	May be involved in matrix and bone disorders; anchoring filaments of lymphatic vessels
Type VIII	Secreted by rapidly proliferating cells; found in basement membranes; may provide a molecular bridge between different types of matrix molecules
Type IX	Minor component in hyaline cartilage; vitreous humor (fluid of the eye)
Type X	Formed only in the epiphyseal growth plate cartilage; may have a role in angiogenesis; may be involved in matrix and bone disorders
Type XI	Hyaline cartilage
Type XII	Embryonic skin and tendon, periodontal ligament
Type XIII	Endothelial cells
Type XIV	Fetal skin and tendons; similar to type I
Types XV-XXVII	Identified but not clearly understood

the presence of these components in tissues and body fluids provides important markers in the clinical investigation of various diseases.[135] Methods to quantify the number of collagen cross-links in tissue are also being further developed at this time.[113,132,149]

Differences in collagen fibril diameter have been demonstrated in people with unidirectional (anterior) shoulder instability versus multidirectional instability. Smaller collagen diameters in the multidirectional instability group suggest the possibility of an underlying connective tissue abnormality.[127]

3.2 Special Implications for the PTA: Collagen Much debate has been directed toward the ability of myofascial techniques or soft tissue mobilization techniques (including friction massage) to change collagen structures and improve mobility, increase joint range of motion, or alter scar tissue. Whether these techniques can break the collagen cross-links and allow slippage to lengthen or realign the collagen fibers continues to be investigated. Clinical research and determination of evidence-based intervention in this area are needed.

It has been found that regular mobility of affected tissues helps maintain lubrication and critical fiber distance.[1,45,154] Immobilization is associated with excessive deposition of connective tissue in associated areas. This is accompanied by a loss of water and subsequent dehydration. The result is an increase in intermolecular cross-linking, which further restricts normal connective tissue flexibility and extensibility.

Therapeutic Ultrasound

The use of ultrasound to increase collagen tissue extensibility, increase enzymatic activity at the site of wound healing, absorb joint adhesions, and reduce fibrous tissue volume and density in scar tissue has been widely accepted, although some of these effects remain to be definitively proved. Ultrasound has been shown to facilitate the development of stronger and better aligned scar tissue[19]; findings of the first study to examine the ability of ultrasound to heat human tendon have been published.[20] Ultrasound as a therapeutic intervention in the treatment of human tendinopathy remains under investigation.[35,50,153]

In the physiologic response to injury or wound healing, the key to growth or replacement tissue at sites of injury is stimulation of protein synthesis in fibroblasts. Exposure of injured tissue to ultrasound at clinically practical doses seems to provide this stimulation.[87] Continuous ultrasound during the first week of wound healing may hinder repair, but pulsed ultrasound at the lower ranges of intensity may be used during the acute phase to stimulate the release of vasodilator amine histamine from mast cells.[46] Other research has shown that 0.1-W/cm² continuous ultrasound provides the same total amount of ultrasound as 0.5 W/cm² pulsed, but the pulsed ultrasound is more effective in its nonthermal wound healing effects.[34]

It is thought that the nonthermal effects of ultrasound increase cellular diffusion, membrane permeability, and fibroblastic activities such as protein synthesis, which speeds up tissue regeneration during the proliferative phase.[20,122]

After 3 weeks, collagen synthesis continues for remodeling during the subacute stage of healing, and ultrasound can be used as an adjunct to other interventions to promote this collagen synthesis and to minimize adhesions. Reducing adhesions occurs by raising the tissue temperature to increase viscoelastic properties during the proliferation to remodeling stage.[39,40] Combining ultrasound with other interventions, such as electrical stimulation or laser photo stimulation, may not be as effective as ultrasound alone.[56]

Ultrasound aids in reabsorption of joint adhesions by depolymerization of mucopolysaccharides, mucoproteins, or glycoproteins and may reduce the viscosity of hyaluronic acid in joints, reducing joint adhesions. Slow, static stretching after ultrasound is important in increasing viscoelastic properties and maintaining length of the structure.[55,124]

Tight capsular tissue, tendon, and mature scar tissue can also achieve increased extensibility when ultrasound is properly applied and followed immediately by slow, static stretching. This increased extensibility occurs as the mechanical effects of ultrasound disrupt the glucoside bonds forming scar tissue, and the thermal effects increase the viscoelastic properties of the connective tissue.

Again, ultrasound must be accompanied or immediately followed by a slow, controlled stretching and then active motion through the full available range of motion to assist in restoring mobility in tissue and between the tissue interfaces.[20,65] The stretch must be held until the collagen reaches a deformation phase. Without these follow-up techniques, the bond will reform in its original position.[55,77]

The therapy professional is advised to make careful assessment of the phase of injury and clinical results in the use of ultrasound and discontinue its use if there are increases in pain or edema or decreases in range of motion or function. Continuous ultrasound at low intensities may be used for nonthermal or thermal effects during the subacute and proliferative phase (fibroblastic infiltration and collagen formation) and early into the remodeling phase.

Factors That Affect Tissue Healing

Many variables regulate or affect the healing process and facilitate, inhibit, or delay wound healing (Box 3.4). Because local blood supply is vital to the delivery of the materials necessary for wound healing, factors that impede local circulation or deplete the necessary materials could delay rehabilitation. Certain tissues (e.g., tendons, ligaments, cartilage, disk) have a decreased blood supply; thus the healing process may require additional time.

Growth Factors

The cells involved in the tissue repair response produce proteins called *growth factors,* which regulate a number of cellular reactions involved in healing. Growth factors regulate cell proliferation, differentiation, and migration; biosynthesis and degradation of proteins; and angiogenesis. Through all of these varying functions, growth factors integrate the inflammatory events with the reparative processes. When these complex mechanisms are disturbed, the result can be delayed healing and an inferior (hypotrophic) scar or elevated levels of growth factor, resulting in hypertrophic scarring such as occurs after a burn injury or in the formation of keloids.[117,147]

Growth factors act by binding to receptors on the plasma membranes of specific cells and have a stimulatory or inhibitory effect on these cells. This binding initiates a process of transmembrane signaling that results in the phosphorylation of proteins (the process of attaching a phosphate group to the protein). These steps lead to the activation of gene expression and DNA synthesis in the cell.

The signals that turn on proliferation of normal cells and cause tissue healing are also responsible for turning on proliferation of cancer cells. With continued growth of neoplastic cells, a neoplasm or tumor may occur. The significant difference between the healing process and cancer is that the growth of the cancer cells goes on unchecked. These analogies have led to the designation of cancers as wounds that do not heal.

Platelets, endothelial cells, fibroblasts, macrophages, and cytokines are important sources of growth factors. Two important growth factors are platelet-derived growth factor (PDGF), which activates fibroblasts and macrophages, and fibroblast growth factor (FGF), which stimulates endothelial cells to form new blood vessels. An example of a growth factor that inhibits cell growth and inactivates macrophages is transforming growth factor-β (TGF-β).

Several growth factors (e.g., recombinant human PDGF-BB, granulocyte colony-stimulating factor) are being tested clinically to establish whether these can boost the healing process in people who have deficiencies in wound healing (e.g., diabetic lower extremity ulcers).[37,101]

PDGF-BB has been approved by the FDA for the treatment of neuropathic ulcers when there is adequate blood supply.[111] Wound dressings of the future may include several growth factors, each with a specific function. The application of topically active growth factors to chronic ulcers remains in the experimental phase.[31,151] Efforts to improve methods of delivering growth factors are also under investigation.[111]

Finally, it should be mentioned that cytokines, such as IL-1, IL-2, IL-15, and TNF, can also regulate some aspects of the healing response. Some ILs have been identified as T-cell growth factors with proinflammatory properties or TGF, associated with hypertrophic scarring. Further studies are necessary to clarify the mechanism of cytokine release in normal postoperative wounds before therapeutic use can be developed.[68]

Nutrition

Nutrition is an important factor influencing healing. Adequate nutritional intake is necessary to support the active metabolism of cells involved in repair. Trauma, including surgery, infections, or large draining wounds, often increases the systemic rate of protein catabolism (loss). This has adverse effects on the synthesis of proteins required for healing. Inadequate intake of specific nutritional factors can specifically affect collagen production and remodeling. Examples are vitamin C deficiency, which causes defective collagen molecules to form, and deficiency of zinc.

Zinc is essential for the activity of enzymes that degrade collagen and of enzymes that are responsible ultimately for the induction of protein synthesis; therefore zinc deficiency impairs healing. People with cancer often manifest delayed healing because of poor nutritional status often associated with the cancer process or the medical treatment (e.g., chemotherapy). Particularly notable is the poor healing in tissues that have been subjected to radiation therapy. For an excellent source of information related to nutrition and healing in the therapist's practice, see the book *Nutrition Applied to Injury Rehabilitation and Sports Medicine.*[16]

Other Factors

Other factors that influence healing include vascular supply, presence of infection, immune reaction, client's age, and the presence of other medical conditions, which are referred to as *comorbidities.* Healing is often adversely affected in people who smoke, who are immunosuppressed, or who have other compromising medical conditions. For example, incontinence, PVD, confusion associated with dementia or Alzheimer's disease, or other neurologic impairment can contribute to delayed wound healing.

Diseases associated with decreased oxygen (tissue) perfusion (e.g., anemia, congestive heart failure, chronic obstructive pulmonary disease, diabetes mellitus) can also delay healing. Diabetes mellitus is associated with poor healing; one of the causes appears to be impaired function of phagocytic cells, and another is a defect in granulation tissue formation.[27]

Medications can directly affect healing, especially the prolonged use of corticosteroids, as can chemotherapy or radiation treatment. Anyone taking prednisone or other corticosteroids may be at risk because steroids are well known to impair the healing process by inhibiting the inflammatory response necessary for tissue regeneration or repair.

An adequate vascular supply is critical to provide oxygen and nutrients to support healing. Vascular insufficiency, particularly in the lower limbs, is an important cause of slow-healing or nonhealing wounds. When blood return is not normal, a buildup of fluid can occur, reducing the body's ability to supply nutrients and oxygen to the wound site.

Infection interferes with healing by inciting a severe and prolonged inflammatory reaction that can increase tissue damage. Certain microorganisms can also release toxins that directly cause tissue necrosis and lysis. Foreign bodies may retard healing by inducing a chronic inflammatory reaction by interfering with closure of a tissue defect and by providing a site protected from leukocytes and antibiotics in which bacteria can multiply.

It may be necessary to off-load weight-bearing surfaces to relieve pressure on the wound and surrounding area. Immobility, lack of desire to exercise or follow a plan of care, and refusal to change dietary or other lifestyle behaviors contributing to poor wound healing must also be considered.

Healing may be delayed or inhibited for individuals who are in a constant state of survival or sympathetic nervous system (SNS) stimulation. When the SNS is locked in hyperactive mode, exaggerated responses to relatively minor stimuli cause the body to work against itself for healing and recovery.

3.3 Special Implications for the PTA: Tissue Healing

Tissue Injury

The physical therapist assistant (PTA) is often involved with individuals who have chronic tissue injury, often caused by stresses of moderate magnitude that are repeated many times a day. Injuries from this mechanism range from cervical and back pain to patellofemoral dysfunction, tendinitis, impingement syndromes, stress fractures, and carpal tunnel syndrome.[100] The therapy team must identify and modify all factors that may contribute to excessive stress on injured tissues. This includes movement and alignment (e.g., motor control, posture, muscle length), extrinsic factors (e.g., footwear, gravity, ergonomic environment), psychosocial factors, medications, age, obesity, or other comorbidities.[100]

After sources of excessive stress have been addressed, injured tissues are still less tolerant of stress than before the injury. Once pain and inflammation have subsided, previously injured tissue must be exposed gradually to higher levels of physical stress. This progression will help restore the tissues' ability to tolerate greater levels of stress. Once healing has occurred and tissue integrity has been restored, activity tolerance can be increased.[100]

Mueller and Maluf offer a good example of how to think about our clients in this way. An older adult has asked the PTA to help her stand independently from a sitting position. The examining therapist identifies the primary modifiable factors limiting this activity as being lower extremity muscle atrophy resulting in poor force production, decreased ankle dorsiflexion, poor motor control (movement and alignment factors), and a low seat surface (extrinsic factor).[100]

A plan of care that considers her age as an important physiologic factor includes a progressive resistive exercise program for lower extremity extensor muscles with at least 70% of maximum effort, two to three times a week, to increase muscle force production. At the same time, the client is instructed in stretching exercises to increase ankle range of motion and appropriate movement

---

strategies with good alignment to practice going from a seated to a standing position. Finally, the client is advised to use a higher chair to lower muscle force needed to meet her goal of independently standing from a seated position.[100]

Delayed Wound Healing

Understanding the interaction of the wound, wound microorganisms, and the immune response is central to developing successful therapeutic interventions for wound care and management. This chapter has carefully explained how wounding of normal tissue initiates an inflammatory response that ordinarily contributes to the healing process orchestrated by specific and nonspecific immune responses. Inflammatory cells provide growth factors and stimulate the deposition of matrix proteins and phagocytose debris. However, the maturation and resolution of a wound may be complicated by the presence of microorganisms. The effects of microorganisms on oxygen consumption and pH or toxin production may interrupt the natural course of wound healing.

Also, ineffective medications and numerous other factors may delay or inhibit wound healing. Box 3.4 lists factors that could delay recovery from an injury. Because local blood supply is vital to the delivery of the materials necessary for wound healing, factors that impede local circulation or deplete the necessary materials could delay rehabilitation. Certain tissues (e.g., tendons, cartilage, disks) have a decreased blood supply; thus the healing process may require additional time.

PTAs should screen a client's medical history for the presence of conditions, such as diabetes, chemical dependency (alcoholism), cigarette smoking, and so on, to identify factors that could delay recovery and report any findings to the supervising physical therapist.

Finally, local infection delays healing. If an abscess is present, the expected fever, chills, and sweats associated with infection may not be present in someone who is taking steroid medications. A sudden worsening of symptoms; the presence of a hot, acutely inflamed joint; or the onset of fever should warn the PTA that something more serious may exist. Generally, the more compromised the host, the greater the chance of a slow or incomplete recovery.

The wound may not progress from the acute phase but may become a nonhealing chronic wound as long as the antigens from microorganisms or underlying pathology remain, leading to wound infection. Even so, most chronic wounds progress toward healing, depending on the wound-care strategy used.[146] For example, a venous leg ulcer will heal once the proper compression and support have been provided to counteract the underlying venous hypertension and once appropriate wound care has been provided. Similarly, diabetic neuropathic foot ulcers do not heal until the disordered glucose metabolism is controlled, adequacy of the vascular supply is ensured, and causative pressure on the foot is off-loaded.

Successful healing of chronic wounds involves intervention to address the underlying causes and clinical wound management that provides an environment to tip the balance in favor of healing. The therapy team is more likely to select appropriate intervention measures if the evaluation and assessment process takes into consideration the physiology of tissue repair along with the many factors that can affect wound healing. Investigating the status of these other factors (e.g., nutritional status; mobility status; turning schedule for the immobile; continence status; use of substances such as tobacco, alcohol, caffeine; medication schedule) requires collaboration with other health care specialists and with the family.[141]

Laboratory values, such as prealbumin levels, indicating nutritional status 48 hours before may be helpful. Glucose levels, hemoglobin, and hematocrit provide the PTA with necessary information to monitor wound healing when performing an appropriate intervention plan.

Specific techniques for wound management are beyond the scope of this text. The reader is referred to other texts for this information.

❓ PHASES OF HEALING

Acute wounds caused by trauma or surgery usually heal according to a well-defined process with the following four phases that overlap and can take months to years to complete[6]:
- Hemostasis and degeneration
- Inflammation
- Proliferation and migration
- Remodeling and maturation

Hemostasis and Degeneration

When tissue injury occurs, hemostasis is the first step. It occurs immediately after an acute injury as the body tries to stop the bleeding by initiating coagulation. Blood fills the gap, and the coagulation cascade commences immediately, clumping platelets together to form a loose clot. Platelets release chemical messengers, including growth factors that summon inflammatory cells to the wounded tissue. Growth factors stimulate proliferation and migration of epithelial cells, fibroblasts, and vascular endothelial cells. They also regulate the differentiation of cells such as expression of extracellular matrix proteins.[6]

The inflammatory process described in detail in the next section begins right away, bringing fluid to the area to dilute harmful substances and support infection-fighting and scavenger cells (neutrophils and macrophages). Some sources describe this first phase as degeneration and inflammation.

The degeneration phase is characterized by the formation of a hematoma, necrosis of dead cells, and, as mentioned, the start of the inflammatory cell response. After the removal of the dead tissue, the healing process undertakes the repair of the tissue defect that remains. Tissue repair begins within 24 hours of the injury with the migration of fibroblasts from the margins of the viable tissue into the defect caused by the injury. The fibroblasts proliferate and synthesize and secrete proteins such as fibronectin, various proteoglycans and elastin, and several types of collagen. The function of these proteins is to reconstitute the extracellular matrix and provide a scaffolding-like framework for the developing endothelial and parenchymal cells.

At this point proliferation and migration occur as epidermal skin cells in the top layer move down the sides of the wound to help fill in the gap. Fibroblasts move in from the dermis, and new blood vessels form to create granulation tissue, which later becomes scar tissue. The next phase of remodeling eventually progresses into the final maturation phase as the regenerated tissue reorganizes into healthy scar tissue.

We have just jumped ahead to tell you the "rest of the story" by discussing proliferation and migration before describing the inflammatory process. Because the phases of tissue healing overlap, it is difficult to describe the process from start to finish without interrupting the discussion.

Inflammation
Overview and Definition

Inflammation serves a vital role in the healing process, and it has both protective and curative features. Every step serves a specific purpose and is necessary as the body responds to tissue injury or damage. The ultimate goal of the inflammatory process is to replace injured tissue with healthy regenerated tissue, a fibrous scar, or both.[8]

The inflammatory phase begins once the blood clot has formed. Vasodilation and increased capillary permeability activate the movement of various cells, such as polymorphonuclear leukocytes and macrophages, to the wound site. These cells destroy bacteria; release proteases, such as elastase and collagenase; and secrete additional growth factors.

Growth factors, cytokines, and chemokines are the key molecular bioregulators of the inflammatory phase of tissue healing. The functions of these three bioregulators overlap considerably. About 5 days after injury, fibroblasts, epithelial cells, and vascular endothelial cells move into the wound to form granulation tissue. This newly developing tissue is not strong, so there is a higher risk of wound reopening or dehiscence during this time.[6]

In contrast to cell injury, which occurs at the level of single cells, inflammation is the coordinated reaction of body tissues to cell injury and cell death that involves vascular, humoral, neurologic, and cellular responses. Regardless of the type of cell injury or death, the inflammatory response follows a basically similar pattern. As a result of all of these factors, inflammation occurs only in living organisms.

The functions of the inflammatory reaction are to inactivate the injurious agent, to break down and remove the dead cells, and to initiate the healing of tissue. The key components of the inflammatory reaction are as follows:
- Blood vessels
- Circulating blood cells
- Connective or interstitial tissue cells (fibroblasts, mast cells, and resident macrophages)
- Chemical mediators derived from inflammatory cells or plasma cells
- Specific extracellular matrix constituents, primarily collagen, and basement membranes

Basement membranes are thin, sheetlike structures deposited by endothelial cells (cells that line the heart, blood vessels, lymph vessels, and serous body cavities) and epithelial cells (cells that cover the body and viscera) but are also found surrounding nerve and muscle cells. They provide mechanical support for resident cells and function as a scaffold for accurate regeneration of preexisting structures of tissue. Basement membrane tissue also serves as a semipermeable filtration barrier for macromolecules in organs such as the kidney and the placenta and act as regulators of cell attachment, migration, and differentiation. The major constituents are collagen type IV and proteoglycans.

Inflammation of sudden onset and short duration is referred to as *acute inflammation*, whereas inflammation that does not resolve but persists over time is called *chronic inflammation*. Although inflammation has been linked with many other conditions (e.g., Alzheimer's disease, cardiovascular disease, cancer, diabetes, insulin resistance syndrome, obesity), the focus of this chapter is inflammation and the musculoskeletal system.

Acute Inflammation

Normally, inflammation has a protective role and is generally beneficial to the body. However, inflammation, whether in the acute or chronic stage (and with all of its components), can be detrimental, causing damage and even death to adjacent healthy tissue.

In the acute stage the inflammatory stimulus acts on blood cells and plasma constituents. Chemical mediators are produced that alter vascular tone and permeability. These mediators also cause the accumulation of plasma proteins, fluid (edema), and blood cells in the injured site (Fig. 3.8).

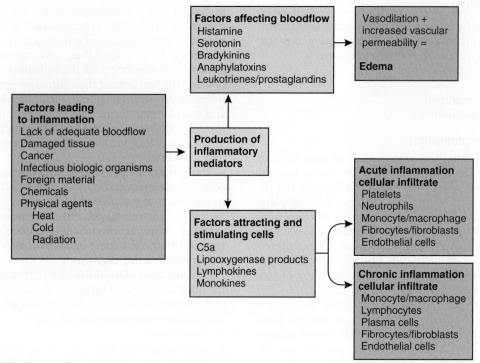

FIG. 3.8 Contributing factors and components of inflammation. Note the vascular alterations associated with factors affecting blood flow (vasoactive mediators), leading to edema, and the factors attracting and stimulating cellular alterations (chemotactic factors), resulting in acute (and sometimes) chronic inflammation. (Courtesy Steven H. Tepper, PT, PhD, FAPTA, Rehab Essentials, Inc.)

TABLE 3.3   Four Cardinal Signs and Symptoms of Inflammation

Sign or Symptom	Precipitating Events
Erythema	Vasodilation and increased blood flow
Heat	Vasodilation and increased blood flow
Edema	Fluid and cells leaking from local blood vessels into the extravascular spaces
Pain	Direct trauma; chemical mediation by bradykinins, histamines, serotonin; internal pressure secondary to edema; swelling of the nerve endings

The clinical manifestations of this inflammatory reaction are redness, swelling, increased temperature, pain, and decreased function of the affected site (Table 3.3). Arteriolar constriction followed by vasodilation gives rise to the redness and heat. The *exudation* or the emigration of cells and leukocyte infiltration give rise to the swelling. Pain and loss of function occur as a result of the increased pressure from the edema on the peripheral nerves.[8]

Accompanying clinical findings include increased muscle tone or spasm and loss of motion or function. Cyriax describes two components of passive movement testing that also suggest acute inflammation: a spasm end feel and pain reported before resistance is noted by the practitioner as the limb is moved passively.[25] If movement testing suggestive of acute inflammation persists, inflammation can become chronic, with proliferation of blood vessels and connective tissue components.

In the normal, healthy individual, symptoms may be more intense because the body is vital and capable of healing quickly. Conversely, immunocompromised individuals and especially older adults with multiple comorbidities often require a much longer time to heal. The symptoms may be less intense, but healing and repair are often delayed, and chronic inflammation may occur.

There are three primary outcomes of acute inflammation: (1) complete resolution with restoration of normal tissue structure, (2) healing with scar formation, and (3) chronic fibrosis. There is usually complete resolution after mild trauma and minimal tissue damage. Healing with scar formation occurs after substantial tissue destruction in tissues with little capacity for regeneration or after prolonged edema. The soft tissue structures of the musculoskeletal system are often characterized by this result.

Chronic Inflammation

As previously described, acute inflammation follows injury. Once the injurious agent has been removed, acute inflammation subsides. If little necrosis is present and replacement of lost parenchymal cells is possible, restitution of normal structure and function of the tissue occurs. In the presence of extensive necrosis or if regeneration of parenchymal cells is not possible (e.g., heart, CNS, peripheral nervous system cells), the inflammatory reaction can become chronic. Chronic inflammation also develops if the underlying cause is not addressed and the injurious agent persists for a prolonged period. Repeated episodes of acute inflammation in the same tissue over time or low-grade, persistent immune reactions can also result in a chronic inflammatory response (Fig. 3.9).

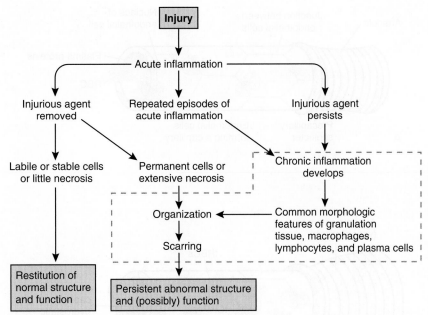

FIG. 3.9 Overview after tissue injury: acute inflammation, chronic inflammation, and the likely healing process. (Courtesy Steven H. Tepper, PT, PhD, FAPTA, Rehab Essentials, Inc.)

The hallmark of chronic inflammation in a tissue is the accumulation of macrophages, lymphocytes, and plasma cells (see Fig. 3.8). The macrophage accumulation is the result of chemotaxis of monocytes (precursors to macrophages) to the area of injury. Macrophages modulate lymphocyte functions and promote growth of endothelial cells and fibroblasts by the release of growth factors. Eosinophils may also be present, particularly if allergic reactions or parasite invasions are involved.

Granulation tissue made up of proliferating endothelial cells and fibroblasts is also seen in areas of chronic inflammation. Granulation tissue can be seen in well-healing, open wounds. Inspection of the wound site reveals red "beefy" tissue with pinpoint red dots (new capillaries) and a granular surface composed of newly formed collagen.

Certain diseases cause the formation of a specific type of chronic inflammation called a *granuloma*, which is a microscopic (less than 2 mm in diameter) aggregate of macrophages often surrounded by lymphocytes. Most of the macrophages are flattened and "epithelioid" in appearance, and some may fuse together, giving rise to large cells with multiple nuclei (Langerhans and foreign body giant cells).

The presence of granulomatous inflammation is clinically important because it aids in the diagnosis of the injurious stimulus. Tuberculosis, a disease caused by *Mycobacterium tuberculosis,* classically causes granulomas or tubercles in this condition with a central focus of *caseous* necrosis. The presence of a foreign body (e.g., a suture) is another common cause of granulomatous inflammation.

Chronic inflammation can contribute to the healing of injured tissue but usually without a full return of function. The proliferation of endothelial cells reconstitutes the vasculature in the injured tissue, whereas proliferation of fibroblasts and the production of collagens and proteoglycans (polymers that form the gel between collagen fibrils) reconstitute the extracellular matrix. These constituents make up the granulation tissue and

lead to the formation of a connective tissue scar. This process is regulated by growth factors derived from macrophages, platelets, and plasma.

Components of the Inflammatory Reaction

Vascular alterations. Acute inflammation can last from a few minutes (e.g., redness and swelling from scratching your skin) to a few days (e.g., after an open cut on the finger), during which time a series of vascular events occurs. After an injury that disrupts the integrity of a vessel wall, the small arteries supplying blood to the area undergo vasoconstriction. This is mediated by a neural reflex and results in a slowing down of blood flow to the affected area.

At the same time, the blood flowing into the surrounding tissue exerts pressure on the damaged vessels, compressing them from outside. The slowdown of the blood flow promotes aggregation of platelets, which leads to the formation of a blood clot, resulting in a reduction in the amount of blood loss.

In the case of an injury that does not disrupt the integrity of the blood vessel wall but does cause tissue injury, the temporary neurally mediated constriction of arterioles is followed by a more sustained and overriding vasodilation, resulting in increased blood flow to the affected area. The increased blood volume raises hydrostatic pressure, and an increased loss of protein-poor fluid occurs from the vasculature into the injured tissue.

At this stage, clinical manifestations include redness (erythema) and warmth of the injured area caused by the increased blood flow. The leakage of protein-poor fluid (transudate) from the vasculature into the interstitial spaces is called *transudation* and causes the affected area to appear swollen (Fig. 3.10).

Transudation, the passage of fluid through a membrane or tissue surface, occurs as a result of a difference in hydrostatic pressure, primarily in conditions in which there is protein loss

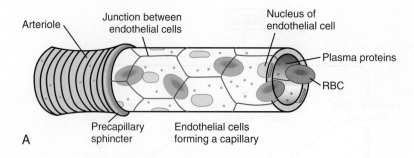

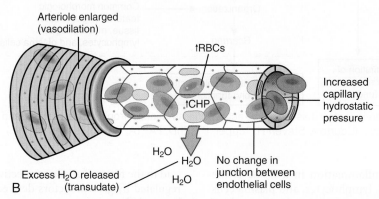

FIG. 3.10 Normal capillary (A) reveals endothelial cells connected by tight junctions limiting flow of plasma proteins into the interstitium. With mild injury (B) vasodilation results in increased capillary hydrostatic pressure pushing more water into the interstitial area (transudate). (Courtesy Steven H. Tepper, PT, PhD, FAPTA, Rehab Essentials, Inc.)

and low protein content (e.g., left ventricular failure, cirrhosis, nephrosis). Typically, transudate is thin and watery, containing few blood vessels or other large proteins. The terms *transudate, exudate, effusion,* and *edema* are often used interchangeably, although each of these has its own clinical significance. When fluid transudates or leaks from blood vessels and accumulates inside an anatomic space, such as the pleural, pericardial, or peritoneal cavities or the joint space, these accumulations are called effusions.

Effusion is a more general term referring to the escape of a fluid and is often used to describe fluid escaping into a compartment such as into a joint capsule; such fluid can be either a transudate or an exudate. Exudates occur when an increase in capillary permeability allows proteinaceous fluid and/or cells to leak out primarily through openings created between adjacent endothelial cells in the capillaries or venules (Fig. 3.11).

Exudate contains much more protein than transudate. It may also contain inflammatory phagocytic cells that occur in response to necrotic tissue and/or an infection. Protein-rich fibrinous (stringy) material found within some blisters or pus is sometimes identified as exudate. Various types of exudate are evident, depending on the stage of inflammation and its cause (Table 3.4).

Removal of the fluid for analysis is required when differentiating between transudates and exudates and helps establish a specific diagnosis. Sometimes exudates are described by visual appearance (e.g., serosanguineous exudate, a fluid containing erythrocytes or red blood cells [RBCs]).

The time of onset of the vascular reaction to injury varies. Mild injuries may induce an increase in vascular permeability that occurs very soon after injury and resolves in a few minutes. In this case the anatomic site responsible for the leak is the capillary or venule.[88] The leak occurs because endothelial cells lining the lumen of the capillaries or venules actively contract and open up their intercellular junctions. This increase in vascular permeability allows proteins to shift from the plasma into the interstitium, causing a greater attraction and retention of fluid in this area.

The increase in vascular permeability caused by the injury may be delayed for some time and may persist for days; for example, in the delayed reaction seen in tissue injury caused by ultraviolet light (sunburn) or irradiation (radiation therapy); typically, the vascular leak begins a few hours after exposure to the sun. In severely injured tissues (e.g., trauma, extensive burns), all vascular structures may be directly injured and become leaky instantly.

Leukocyte accumulations. An important consequence of the exudation of protein and fluid from the vasculature is the engorgement of vessels with blood cells. This causes a slowing or cessation of blood flow in the affected vessels, which is a phenomenon called *stasis.* During stasis, the leukocytes (white blood cells [WBCs]) accumulate and adhere to the endothelial cells of blood vessel walls at the site of injury in a process called *margination.* Inflammatory mediators cause an increased expression of specific glycoproteins called *adhesion molecules* on the surface membrane of leukocytes and endothelial cells. These

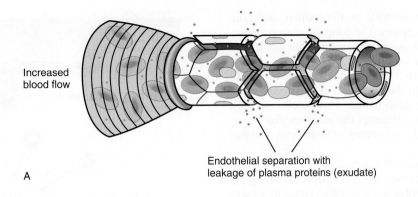

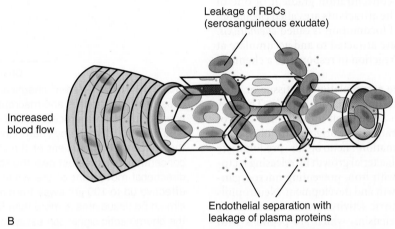

FIG. 3.11 (A) With a more severe inflammatory response, endothelial cells separate, causing leakage of plasma proteins into the interstitium (exudate). This accentuates the edema. (B) With damage to the endothelial cells, the separation between the damaged cells may allow even erythrocytes to extravasate (serosanguineous exudate). (Courtesy Steven H. Tepper, PT, PhD, FAPTA, Rehab Essentials, Inc.)

TABLE 3.4 Inflammatory Exudates

Type	Appearance	Significance
Hemorrhagic; sanguineous	Bright red or bloody; presence of red blood cells (RBCs)	Small amounts expected after surgery or trauma; large amounts may indicate hemorrhage; sudden large amounts of dark, red blood may indicate a draining hematoma
Serosanguineous	Blood-tinged yellow or pink; presence of RBCs	Expected for 48-72 hours after injury or trauma to the microvasculature; a sudden increase may precede wound dehiscence (rupture or separation)
Serous	Thin, clear yellow, or straw colored; contains albumin and immunoglobulins	Occurs in the early stages of most inflammations; common with blisters, joint effusion with rheumatoid arthritis, viral infections (e.g., skin vesicles caused by herpesvirus); expected for up to 1 week after trauma or surgery; a sudden increase may indicate a draining seroma (pocket of serum within tissue or organ)
Purulent	Viscous, cloudy, pus; cellular debris from necrotic cells and dying neutrophils (polymorphonuclear neutrophils)	Usually caused by pus-forming bacteria (streptococci and staphylococci) and indicates infection; may drain suddenly from an abscess (boil)
Catarrhal	Thin, clear mucus	Seen with inflammatory process within mucous membranes (e.g., upper respiratory infection)
Fibrinous	Thin, usually clear; may be yellow or pink, tinged, or cloudy	Occurs with severe inflammation or bacterial infections (e.g., strep throat, pneumonia); does not resolve easily; can cause fibrous scarring and restriction (e.g., constrictive pericarditis)

Modified from Black JM, Hawks JH, editors: Medical-surgical nursing: clinical management for positive outcomes, ed 8, St. Louis, 2009, Saunders.

adhesion glycoproteins, by adhering to one another, function as receptors and counterreceptors. The adhesion glycoproteins are the glue that binds the leukocytes to one another and to the endothelium of venules and capillaries.

The binding of leukocytes to receptors on endothelial cells of venules is the first step in the migration of leukocytes from the vasculature to the interstitial tissues. This process initiates the circulation of leukocytes through the extravascular space in normal conditions and the infiltration of leukocytes into the site of inflammation.

In the next stage, the leukocytes actively migrate out of the vessels, passing through the vascular walls without damaging the blood vessels and entering the interstitial space in a process called *diapedesis,* or oozing (Fig. 3.12). The continued migration of leukocytes in interstitial space is directed by a chemical trail created by a concentration gradient of one of many possible attractants. The attractants are called *chemotactic agents,* and the process of locomotion is called *chemotaxis.* In other words, leukocytes are attracted to and accumulate at the site of an inflammatory reaction in response to a chemical stimulus.

The presence of leukocyte accumulations in tissue or fluid specimens is diagnostic of an inflammatory process. The predominant cell type found in a specimen identifies the type of inflammation and/or its duration and original stimulus. Typically during acute inflammation, neutrophils predominate (neutrophilia). They inhibit bacterial growth by releasing lactoferrin, a protein that binds with iron, preventing microorganisms from using iron for growth and development. Neutrophils also demonstrate direct cytotoxic activity toward viruses, fungi, and bacteria by releasing defensins, which are peptides with natural antibiotic activity.

If the inflammatory stimulus subsides, the neutrophils rapidly die out because their life span (after extrusion from the circulation) is approximately 24 hours; they are replaced by monocytic or macrophage cells responsible for cleaning up the cellular debris left after neutrophils have done their job. Certain inflammatory stimuli can induce a sustained neutrophil response (e.g., first defense against pyogenic bacteria), a predominantly lymphocytic response (e.g., fight tumor cells or respond to viruses), or an eosinophilic response (e.g., plays a role in asthma and allergies or attacks parasites).

In addition to the types of WBCs present, the total and differential counts of the leukocytes in the circulating blood are also very important diagnostic tools. An increased number of circulating leukocytes (leukocytosis) is often an indication of an active inflammatory reaction (typically to an infection or tissue injury). A decreased WBC count (leukopenia) can, for example, be seen in certain types of infections and is an indicator of grave prognosis in severe systemic infections (sepsis).

The main function of the leukocytes recruited to the affected tissue is to remove or eliminate the injurious stimulus. Leukocytes achieve this function by releasing enzymes and toxic substances that kill, inactivate, and degrade microbial agents, foreign antigens, or necrotic tissue. Leukocytes also take up these materials by phagocytosis and release growth factors necessary for healing or regeneration (see Fig. 3.17).

In addition to the role played by blood vessels in inflammation, a contribution is made from a system of thin-walled channels formed by endothelial cells with loose junctions. These channels are called the *lymphatics* and ultimately drain into the subclavian vein via the thoracic duct. These channels

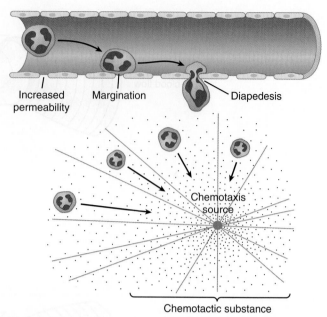

FIG. 3.12 Many different chemical substances in the tissues cause both neutrophils and macrophages to move through the capillary pores in a process called diapedesis and toward the area of tissue damage by chemotaxis. Chemotaxis depends on the concentration gradient of the chemotactic substance. The concentration is greatest near the source, which directs the unidirectional movement of the white blood cells. Chemotaxis is effective up to 100 μm away from an inflamed tissue. Because almost no tissue area is more than 50 μm away from a capillary, the chemotactic signal can easily move vast numbers of white blood cells from the capillaries into the inflamed area. (From Hall JE: Guyton and Hall textbook of medical physiology, ed 13, Philadelphia, 2016, Elsevier.)

in physiologic conditions help drain fluid and protein from the interstitium, reducing edema. They also serve as a conduit for the removal of certain leukocytes and inflammatory stimuli.[144]

The movement of the phagocytic cells into the lymphatic vessels allows presentation of the engulfed material to immunocompetent cells located in the lymph nodes. Hyperplasia of immunocompetent cells (T and B lymphocytes) in the lymph nodes leads to an enlargement of the nodes called *lymphadenopathy.* During the process of removing infectious agents, lymphatics and their lymph nodes may become actively inflamed. Clinically, the inflamed lymphatics may appear as red streaks under the epidermis and may be painful to palpation; this condition is called *lymphangitis.*

Chemical mediators of inflammation. A large number of chemical mediators are responsible for the vascular and leukocytic responses generated by the cells involved in an acute inflammatory response. These mediators are either released from inflammatory cells (cell derived) or are generated by the action of plasma protease (plasma derived). Mediators of inflammation are multifunctional and have numerous effects on blood vessels, inflammatory cells, and other cells in the body. Some of their primary effects in the inflammatory response include vasodilation or vasoconstriction, modulation of vascular permeability, activation of inflammatory cells, chemotaxis, cytotoxicity, degradation of tissue, pain, and fever.

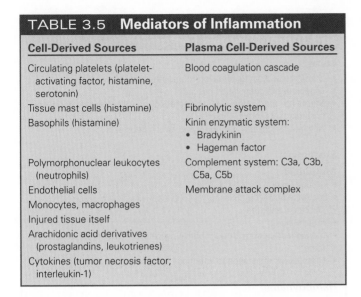

TABLE 3.5	Mediators of Inflammation
Cell-Derived Sources	**Plasma Cell-Derived Sources**
Circulating platelets (platelet-activating factor, histamine, serotonin)	Blood coagulation cascade
Tissue mast cells (histamine)	Fibrinolytic system
Basophils (histamine)	Kinin enzymatic system:
	• Bradykinin
	• Hageman factor
Polymorphonuclear leukocytes (neutrophils)	Complement system: C3a, C3b, C5a, C5b
Endothelial cells	Membrane attack complex
Monocytes, macrophages	
Injured tissue itself	
Arachidonic acid derivatives (prostaglandins, leukotrienes)	
Cytokines (tumor necrosis factor; interleukin-1)	

These mediators include histamine, serotonin, bradykinin, the complement system, platelet-activating factor (PAF), arachidonic acid derivatives (e.g., prostaglandins, leukotrienes), and cytokines (Table 3.5).

Histamine. Histamine is synthesized and stored in granules (for quick availability and release) of mast cells, basophils, and platelets. Histamine causes endothelial contraction leading to the formation of gaps, which increase blood vessel permeability and allow fluids and blood cells to exit into the interstitial spaces (vascular leak). Histamine's effect occurs quickly but is short-lived because it is inactivated in less than 30 minutes. Histamine is also a potent vasodilator and bronchoconstrictor. Serotonin is another mediator released from platelets; it induces vasoconstriction, but its effect is usually overridden by the vasodilator action of histamine.

Platelet-activating factor. Leukocytes and other cells on stimulation also synthesize three classes of inflammatory mediators that are derived from phospholipids (the major lipids present in cell membranes). The first of these mediators is an acetylated lysophospholipid named *platelet-activating factor*. The other two classes of mediators are derived from a fatty acid (arachidonic acid) of membrane phospholipids and are called *prostaglandins* and *leukotrienes*. All three of these lipid mediators have potent and wide-ranging inflammatory activities. In addition, these mediators have hormone-like functions that modulate physiologic responses and induce pathology in a variety of organ systems.

PAF was so named because it was first found to induce platelet activation and secretion. It is now known to be a potent activator of cells, such as smooth muscle cells, endothelial cells, and leukocytes, by receptor binding and intracellular signaling mechanisms. Consequently, PAF can induce the aggregation of leukocytes and leukocyte infiltration in tissues and can profoundly affect vasomotor tone and permeability.[137] PAF can potentiate (increase or strengthen) the activity of other inflammatory mediators.

Arachidonic acid derivatives. The synthesis of prostaglandins and leukotrienes begins with the cleavage (splitting) of arachidonic acid from membrane phospholipids by the action of the phospholipase (Fig. 3.13). Once this step is completed, either a cyclooxygenase (COX) enzyme or a

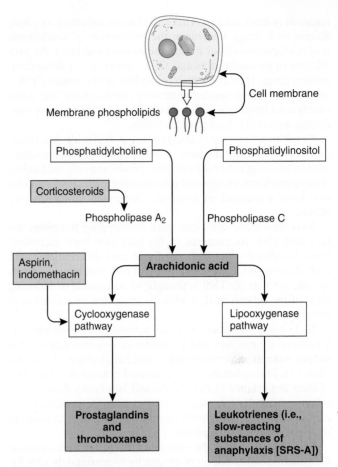

FIG. 3.13 Production of prostaglandins and leukotrienes from damaged cell membranes. Note sites for pharmacologic (aspirin and prednisone) interventions. (Courtesy Steven H. Tepper, PT, PhD, FAPTA, Rehab Essentials, Inc.)

lipoxygenase enzyme further metabolizes the arachidonic acid. The COX pathway leads to the production of several types of prostaglandins that modulate vasomotor tone and platelet aggregation (e.g., thromboxane is a strong platelet aggregator and vasoconstrictor, whereas prostacyclin [PGI2] is a strong platelet inhibitor and vasodilator). Clinically, prostaglandins are also important because they are mediators of the fever and pain responses associated with inflammation.[24]

The lipoxygenase pathway leads to the production of leukotrienes, which occur naturally in leukocytes and produce allergic and inflammatory reactions similar to those of histamine. They are extremely potent mediators of immediate hypersensitivity reactions and inflammation, producing smooth muscle contraction, especially bronchoconstriction; increased vascular permeability; and migration of leukocytes to areas of inflammation. They are thought to play a role in the development of allergic and autoimmune disease such as asthma and rheumatoid arthritis. Certain leukotrienes (C4, D4, and E4) are collectively known as a *slow-reacting substance of anaphylaxis* (SRS-A), which is the name given when their potent bronchoconstrictor activity was discovered; they also cause leakage of fluid and proteins from the microvasculature.

The importance of the arachidonic acid metabolites in the inflammatory process is made evident by the excellent clinical response to treatment of acute and chronic inflammatory conditions with drugs that block the production of arachidonic acid (corticosteroids) or inhibit the enzyme and block the production of prostaglandins and COX (nonsteroidal antiinflammatory drugs [NSAIDs] such as aspirin or the newer COX-2 inhibitors). These antiinflammatory medications are commonly used by people with somatic pain or inflammatory conditions, especially rheumatoid arthritis.

Cytokines. Leukocytes also produce polypeptide substances called *cytokines,* which have a wide range of inflammatory actions affecting either the cytokine-producing cells themselves (autocrine effects) or adjacent cells (paracrine effects). Cytokines also have a number of systemic "hormonal" inflammatory effects.

Two important cytokines with overlapping functions are IL-1 and TNF. As many as 15 ILs have now been identified. Most ILs direct other cells to divide and differentiate, with each IL acting on a particular group of cells that have receptors specific for that IL. TNF is thought to be capable of inducing most of the actions of IL-1 with the exception of activation of lymphocytes.

IL-1 has a number of local actions that promote the inflammatory reaction and a number of systemic actions that induce metabolic, hemodynamic, and hematologic alterations (Box 3.5). These alterations are discussed in some detail because of their importance in the clinical and laboratory diagnosis of inflammation. IL-1 causes fever by raising the production of prostaglandins in the hypothalamus, resetting the threshold of temperature-sensitive neurons.

Fever in turn raises the systemic metabolism and increases the systemic consumption of oxygen by approximately 10% for each degree Celsius of body temperature elevation. As a result, a decrease in systemic vascular resistance occurs, producing hypotension and an increase in cardiac output to increase the flow of blood and the delivery of oxygen to various organs. These hemodynamic changes are characteristic of severe systemic infections and a febrile condition. The situation is very interesting and has huge implications for acute care.

IL-1 also causes characteristic changes in blood chemistry. Albumin and transferrin levels are decreased, whereas levels of coagulation factors, complement components, C-reactive protein, and serum amyloid A increase. These changes occur because IL-1 alters the rate of synthesis of these proteins by the liver. IL-1 also increases the number of neutrophils and decreases the number of lymphocytes in the circulation.

Blood coagulation, fibrinolytic, and complement systems. Plasma proteins produce chemical inflammatory mediators by the enzymatic activity of proteases on plasma proteins. Plasma proteases are enzymes that act as a catalyst in the breakdown of proteins. These plasma protein systems are the blood coagulation and fibrinolytic, kinin enzymatic, and complement systems.

All of these systems can become activated by contact with by-products of cell injury or foreign materials. Examples include contact with components of denuded vascular endothelial cells, revealing their underlying basement membrane, which occurs with trauma to the vessel wall and contact with bacterial endotoxins. The key plasma protein in the activation sequence of these systems is clotting factor XII, also known as *Hageman factor.*

The blood coagulation system (Fig. 3.14) is formed in part by plasma proteins. The design is to bandage injuries with clots

---

BOX 3.5   Actions of Cytokines: Interleukin-1 and Tumor Necrosis Factor

Local
- Stimulate leukocyte adhesion to endothelium
- Modulate the coagulation cascade
- Stimulate production and/or secretion of inflammatory mediators (including interleukin-1 itself)
- Activate fibroblasts, chondrocytes, and osteoclasts

Systemic
Metabolic
- Induce fever
- Increase body metabolism
- Decrease appetite
- Induce sleep
- Induce adrenocorticotropic hormone release to secrete corticosteroids
- Nonspecific resistance to infection

Hemodynamic
- Cause hypotension
- Cause hypovolemia (sepsis)

Hematologic
- Cause changes in blood chemistry (see text)
- Activate endothelial, macrophage, and resting T cells
- Increase neutrophils in circulation
- Decrease lymphocytes in circulation
- Stimulate synthesis of collagen and collagenases

(coagulation) and then disassemble (lyse) the clots when the job is done. The system protects against both hemorrhage and catastrophic clotting. To maintain homeostasis, these two processes must remain in balance.

Platelets circulating throughout the bloodstream are always ready to seal any damage to blood vessels with a hemostatic plug. When there is no need for the platelets, the smooth vascular walls prevent platelets from adhering and aggregating. At the same time, endothelial cells in the walls of the blood vessels make tissue plasminogen activator to prevent fibrin deposits from forming and for breaking down existing clots.

More specifically, when injury or bleeding occurs, a series of enzymes are activated sequentially to generate the enzyme thrombin, which converts the plasma protein fibrinogen to fibrin, the essential component of a blood clot. Fibrin forms a meshwork at bleeding sites to stop the bleeding and trap exudate, microorganisms, and foreign materials and keep this content contained in an area where eventually the greatest number of phagocytes will be found. This localizing effect prevents the spread of infection to other sites and begins the process of healing and tissue repair.

The fibrinolytic system (designed to dissolve these clots) is activated by the conversion of plasminogen to the enzyme plasmin (also known as *fibrinolysin,* which means "to loosen"). Plasmin splits or divides fibrin and lyses the blood clots. Both the coagulation and the fibrinolytic systems are activated in inflammation and function together in a system of checks and balances to preserve vascular function.

The products of fibrin degradation are chemotactic for leukocytes and increase vascular permeability. The kinin enzymatic system is also activated by Hageman factor and functions

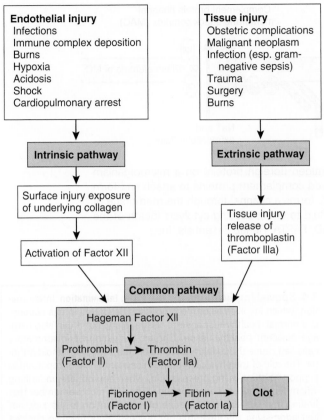

FIG. 3.14 Clinical causes of the activation of a clotting cascade, intrinsic and extrinsic pathways of activation, and the mechanism by which both pathways lead to the formation of fibrin threads, or clot. In the chain reaction, inactive proenzymes (represented by Roman numerals) are converted into active enzymes (represented by Roman numerals followed by the letter "a"). The clotting cascade can follow two pathways: intrinsic and extrinsic. The intrinsic pathway is activated within the vascular compartment. The extrinsic pathway is activated outside the vascular compartment, when blood comes in contact with any tissue other than blood vessels. In the case of internal bleeding, both pathways are activated. (Courtesy Steven H. Tepper, PT, PhD, FAPTA, Rehab Essentials, Inc.)

to produce bradykinin. Bradykinin is a mediator that causes dilatation and leakage of blood vessels and induces pain.

The complement system is composed of a group of plasma proteins that normally lie dormant in the blood, interstitial fluid, and mucosal surfaces. Then, through a series of enzymatic reactions, several plasma protein fragments (C3a, C3b, C5a, and C5b) are formed that are potent inflammatory mediators. These components are also active in immunologic processes. In the nomenclature used for the complement system, each complement component (C) is designated by a number (1 to 9). The individual subunits that make up each component are designated by a letter. For example, the first component of a complement is designated C1, which is made up of three subunits designated as C1q, C1r, and C1s. The protein fragments that are generated from the proteolytic degradation of complement components are also identified by a letter (a, b).

The complement system is activated by microorganisms or antigen–antibody complexes causing four events to occur that promote inflammation: (1) vasodilation of the capillaries, which increases blood flow to the area; (2) facilitation of the movement of leukocytes into the area by chemotaxis; (3) coating of the surfaces of microbes to make them vulnerable to phagocytosis; and (4) formation of a membrane attack complex (MAC).

Complement activation can follow one of two pathways, the classic or the alternate pathway, and each pathway produces the same active complement components. The products of the complement system bind to particles of foreign material, microorganisms, or other antigens, coating them to make them vulnerable to phagocytosis by leukocytes, a process called *opsonization.* Activation of the complement cascade by either pathway also results in the formation of the MAC. The MAC is inserted in cell membranes of the microorganism, where it creates an opening (pore or channel) in the cell membrane. This leads to an influx of sodium and extracellular fluid, eventually leading to its lysis (Fig. 3.15). For example, in hemolytic anemia, the MAC bores holes in the cell membrane of RBCs, causing their destruction.

The plasma protease systems (blood coagulation, fibrinolytic, kinin enzymatic, and complement systems) are interconnected at several steps. This arrangement serves to amplify the stimulus for the inflammatory reaction as a balance mechanism. For example, the activation of the plasma protein Hageman factor can initiate both the coagulation system (blood clotting) and the kinin system (produces bradykinin, causing dilation and vascular leakage).

The kinin system can in turn activate the fibrinolytic system by producing plasmin (splits or divides fibrin and lyses blood clots). Plasmin then can activate the complement system and further amplify these protease loops by activating the Hageman factor, once again starting the cycle (Fig. 3.16).

Phagocytosis. One of the most important functions of the inflammatory reaction is to inactivate and remove the inflammatory stimulus to begin the process of healing. The process of ingestion (phagocytosis) of microorganisms, other foreign substances, necrotic cells, and connective tissue constituents by specialized cells (phagocytes) is important in achieving this goal.

Although phagocytosis could be considered the next step in the process of acute inflammation, it is included here as part of the section on chemical mediators because the chemical mediators are what attract phagocytic cells to the area for removal of the dead tissue or microorganisms. After ingestion by phagocytic cells, microorganisms are killed or inactivated, and necrotic debris is removed to allow tissue healing to proceed.

The most important phagocytes involved in the inflammatory and healing reactions are neutrophils, monocytes, or, when found in tissues of the body, macrophages. Macrophages have different names depending on their location (e.g., histiocytes in the skin, osteoclasts in bone, microglial cells in the CNS).

The mechanism of phagocytosis is well understood. Phagocytosis is facilitated by the coating (opsonization) of particles to be ingested by IgG antibody or by the C3b component of complement. These opsonins bind to specific receptor sites located on the cell surfaces of neutrophils and macrophages. This receptor binding initiates a process of transmembrane

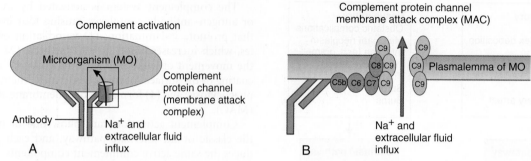

Complement activation

Complement protein channel
membrane attack complex (MAC)

FIG. 3.15 (A) When an antibody attaches to an antigen (foreign protein) on a microorganism (MO), the antibody–antigen stimulates plasma-derived complement proteins to attach and form the membrane attack complex (MAC). (B) This MAC forms a channel through the membrane of the invading cell and allows ions and extracellular fluid to enter, causing cytolysis (death of the microorganism). (Courtesy Steven H. Tepper, PT, PhD, FAPTA, Rehab Essentials, Inc.)

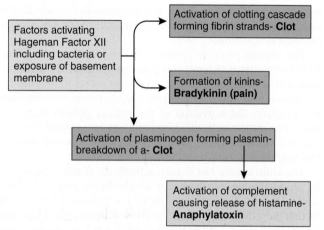

FIG. 3.16 Clot formation. Revealed in this figure are the mechanisms for activating both the intrinsic and the extrinsic pathways for clot formation. Either of these pathways leads to activation of the Hageman factor XII, which results in the formation of a fibrin clot. (Courtesy Steven H. Tepper, PT, PhD, FAPTA, Rehab Essentials, Inc.)

signaling, allowing calcium influx, which activates cytoskeletal proteins within the cell. These cytoskeletal structures allow the movement of cell membranes that is necessary for phagocytosis.

The internalization of the opsonized particle begins by the enfolding of the cell surface membrane (Figs. 3.17 and 3.18). The membrane folds surround the particle to be ingested and seal it within a pouch that separates it from the cell surface and becomes an intracellular vacuole called the *phagosome*. The phagosomes fuse with lysosomes (containing digestive materials and bactericidal components) and acquire enzymes and other substances that allow the killing and degradation of microorganisms and other ingested materials. Many neutrophils (e.g., polymorphonuclear neutrophils [PMNs]) die in their battle with bacteria. Dead and dying leukocytes, mixed with tissue debris and lytic enzymes, form a viscous yellow fluid known as *pus*. Inflammations identified by their pus formations are called *purulent* or *suppurative* (see Table 3.4).

3.4 Special Implications for the PTA: Inflammation Inflammation, which involves all of the processes described in this section, is a normal, healthy response to tissue injury, but it can also damage adjacent healthy tissue. Chronic activation of inflammatory cells can cause tissue injury such as occurs with rheumatoid arthritis. The role of the physical therapist assistant (PTA) is important in supporting the healing process and, when appropriate, in limiting inflammation and its consequences. The PTA must remember that finding and correcting the cause of inflammation is the key, not just addressing the inflammatory process. Poor lifestyle choices including poor nutrition, improper posture and body mechanics, and poor breathing habits can contribute to the chronicity of this condition.

Rheumatoid arthritis illustrates how the inflammatory mediators discussed are activated and how this process leads to clinical manifestations observed in a therapy practice. Inflammatory activity can be detected by the erythrocyte sedimentation rate (ESR). The PTA can review laboratory values to assess systemic factors; generally, as the inflammation improves, the ESR decreases.

Clinical Example
The majority of people with rheumatoid arthritis produce rheumatoid factor, an antibody that is made against the person's own antibodies of the immunoglobulin G (IgG) class. In this case the IgG antibody actually functions as an antigen (Ag) capable of inducing an immune response.

This antibody-to-antibody attachment can occur in the joint space in which it leads to the formation of large antibody–antigen (Ig–Ag) aggregates. Ig–Ag complexes stimulate complement activation by the classic pathway and to the formation of the strongly chemotactic cleavage products C3a and C5a. These products attract neutrophils, which then release free radicals (see Fig. 3.2) and enzymes that degrade the joint cartilage, prostaglandins, and leukotrienes that amplify the inflammatory reaction. The Ig–Ag complex is phagocytosed by synovial-lining cells that are stimulated to release collagen-degrading enzymes, prostaglandins, and interleukin (IL)-1.

Lymphocytes contribute to the acute reaction by the production of rheumatoid factor and are responsible for the evolution of a chronic inflammatory reaction by producing cytokines that attract and activate macrophages. The macrophages produce cytokines, such as IL-1, that further amplify the inflammatory reaction by attracting more neutrophils and lymphocytes and by stimulating the synthesis and release from fibroblasts, chondrocytes, and osteoclasts of enzymes that degrade cartilage and bone.

Clinically, the joints affected by the inflammatory process appear red and swollen and are painful; a low-grade fever may also be present. A prominent symptom is joint stiffness that is relieved by activity. With disease progression, damage to the joints occurs; with loss of cartilage, narrowing of the joint space occurs, and resorption of bone is evident on radiograph. These changes are associated with a decrease in the range of motion of the affected joints. In later stages, obvious joint deformities develop that are accompanied by muscle wasting. Antiinflammatory agents, such as aspirin and corticosteroids, are effective in providing symptomatic relief and in slowing the progression of the disease.

The inflammatory process associated with rheumatoid arthritis may also affect other organ systems. Foci of chronic inflammation can develop in muscles, tendons, blood vessels, nerves, and various organs of the body (e.g., heart and lungs). In the skin, these foci cause the deposition of connective tissue called *subcutaneous nodules*.

Proliferation and Migration

Within 2 days after a skin wound or injury, endothelial cells from viable blood vessels near the edge of the necrotic tissue begin to proliferate. The purpose of the endothelial cell proliferation is to establish a vascular network that can transport oxygen and nutrients and support the metabolism of the healing tissue. The endothelial cells bud out from the vessels and form new capillary channels that merge with one another as they develop and grow toward the tissue defect caused by the injury. This process of formation of new blood vessels is called *neovascularization* or *angiogenesis*.

The rich network of developing blood vessels with its connective tissue matrix can be seen with the naked eye in healing wounds. As described previously, the appearance of a reddish granular layer of tissue was therefore given the name "granulation tissue." Histologically, the main cellular components of granulation tissue are the endothelial cells and the fibroblasts, although some inflammatory cells are also commonly present.

Initially, the newly formed vessels are leaky, and this leak contributes to the edematous appearance of tissue undergoing repair. As tissue healing is completed, blood flow to the newly formed vasculature shuts down, and the nonfunctional vessels are degraded, leaving few blood vessels in mature scar tissue.

Tissue gaps are replaced during the proliferation phase when the number of inflammatory cells decreases and fibroblasts, endothelial cells, and keratinocytes take over synthesis of growth factors. The result is the continued promotion of cell migration, proliferation, and formation of new capillaries and synthesis of extracellular matrix components.[6] The next step is the removal of damaged matrix as new matrix builds up to fill the wound. The wound initially fills with provisional wound matrix, which consists primarily of fibrin and fibronectin. As fibroblasts are drawn into the matrix, they synthesize new collagen, elastin, and proteoglycan molecules, which cross-link the collagen of the matrix and produce the initial scar.[6]

Damaged proteins in the matrix have to be removed before the newly synthesized matrix components can be properly integrated. This process is facilitated by proteases secreted by neutrophils, macrophages, fibroblasts, epithelial cells, and endothelial cells. Epithelial cells are at the front of the wound

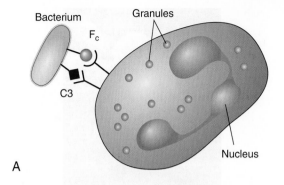

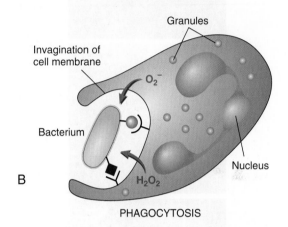

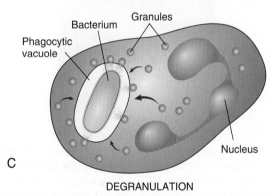

FIG. 3.17 Phagocytosis of bacteria. (A) The bacterium that was opsonized (coated with IgG and complement [C3]) binds to the Fc and complement receptors on the surface of the leukocytes. (B) Engulfment of the bacterium into an invagination of surface membrane is associated with an oxygen burst and formation of oxygen radicals that are bactericidal and thus kill the bacterium. (C) Inclusion of the bacterium into a phagocytic vacuole is associated with the fusion of the vacuole with lysosomes and specific granules of the leukocyte. The contents of the lysosomes and specific granules are bactericidal and contribute to final inactivation and degradation of the bacterium. The cytoplasm of the leukocyte becomes devoid of granules in a process referred to as *degranulation of leukocytes*. (From Damjanov I: Pathology for the health-related professions, ed 4, St Louis, 2012, Saunders.)

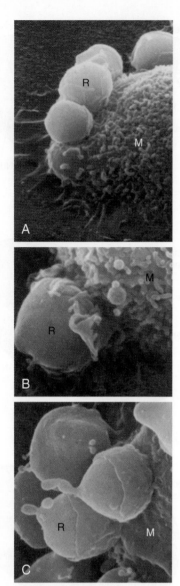

FIG. 3.18 Phagocytosis. This series of scanning electron micrographs shows the progressive steps in phagocytosis of damaged red blood cells (RBCs) by a macrophage. (A) RBCs *(R)* attach to the macrophage *(M)*. (B) Plasma membrane of the macrophage begins to enclose the RBC. (C) The RBCs are almost totally ingested by the macrophage. (From Patton KT, Thibodeau GA: The human body in health and disease, ed 6, St Louis, 2014, Mosby. Courtesy Emma Shelton.)

edge, traveling across the highly vascularized extracellular matrix, forming granulation tissue to reform the epidermal layer. This process can take several weeks.[6]

Remodeling and Maturation

In the maturation phase of healing, the scar tissue is reduced and remodeled, leaving tissue smoother, stronger, less dense, and less red in color (in Caucasians) as the concentration of blood vessels in the area decreases. In all skin colors, the scar tissue becomes more like the natural skin tones of the person. The density of fibroblasts and capillaries needed in the early phase of healing but no longer needed now declines, primarily through apoptosis or programmed cell death.[6] The remodeling

phase can take years, as the skin produces collagen fibers that are broken down and rearranged to withstand stress. Over time, scar tissue grows stronger, relaxes, and then lightens.

Tissue Contraction and Contracture

As the healing process proceeds, the newly formed extracellular matrix draws together, causing a shrinkage (contraction) of the healing tissue. In this manner the size of the tissue defect caused by the injury is diminished. Some fibroblasts within the healing tissue differentiate and acquire some of the morphologic and functional characteristics of smooth muscle cells (myocytes). These specialized fibroblasts are called *myofibroblasts.* Myofibroblasts contain abundant contractile proteins and apparently contract and contribute to the shrinkage of the healing tissue.

Tissue contraction is a normal process that contributes to tissue repair by approximating the margins of the healing tissue and speeding up the closure of wounds. In some cases, excessive shrinkage of the healing tissue occurs. This condition is called *contracture.* Contracture is an undesirable outcome of healing because it can be disfiguring and can impair movement or organ function. For example, people with severe burns often develop skin contractures because of the process of "hypertrophic scarring," which can result in significant movement impairments and subsequent disability.

Contracted tissue with excessive arthrofibrosis can occur in the joints (most often the shoulder and knee) after either injury or surgery. Postoperative or posttraumatic arthrofibrosis is characterized by local or global periarticular scarring that can be restrictive, and in some cases a thickened, fibrotic capsule inhibits motion. Arthrofibrosis can be caused by a variety of factors including prolonged immobilization, infection, or graft malposition after ligament reconstruction (e.g., ACL reconstruction).[95]

Studies have not been done to identify when scar tissue can be broken up by manual therapy techniques, but anecdotal evidence indicates that immature scar tissue can be successfully treated conservatively (e.g., analgesia and antiinflammatory medications, early motion, bracing, strengthening, electrical stimulation, manual therapy techniques).

Exactly when scar tissue becomes mature is variable and remains a topic of debate. Some estimate an open window of 3 to 4 months, after which time surgical (arthroscopic) manipulation is required. Forceful manipulation of the stiff joint is never advised because this can create excessive joint compression leading to articular cartilage damage and even fracture.[96]

Tissue Regeneration

Within a few hours after lethal injury to skin, epithelial cells, the viable cells that surround the necrotic tissue, detach from their extracellular matrix anchorage sites and separate from the other epithelial cells. The remaining epithelial cells flatten out to cover the area left bare by the necrotic cells. These epithelial cells also divide and migrate into the tissue, using the extracellular matrix support provided by the proteins secreted by the fibroblasts. This process of replacement of dead parenchymal cells by new cells is called *regeneration,* which is a very desirable healing process because it restores normal tissue structure and function. In most cases, healing of tissue is achieved by both cell regeneration and replacement by connective tissue (scarring) called *repair.* In the case of skin, for example, this type of healing occurs after wounds that involve both the epidermis and dermis. In some instances, tissue healing occurs almost exclusively by the progress of regeneration (regrowth of original tissue).

Regeneration can occur only if the parenchymal cells can undergo mitosis. Cells are classified as *permanent, stable,* and *labile* based on their ability to divide. Regeneration does not occur in permanent tissues that cannot divide (e.g., cardiac myocytes, central or peripheral neurons); they are long-lived and irreplaceable. It can also occur only in labile or stable tissues and only if the inflammatory reaction that follows injury is short-lived and does not disrupt the basement membranes, other extracellular components, and vascular structures of labile or stable parenchymal cells. Labile cells, such as epithelial cells of the skin and GI system, and bone marrow divide continuously. Hematopoietic (blood cell–forming) stem cells continuously divide, giving rise to specialized cells, such as erythrocytes and neutrophils, with finite life spans.

Under these conditions the regenerating parenchymal cells can use the existing connective tissue scaffolding to reconstitute the normal structure and function of the organ. This type of tissue healing can be seen after superficial mechanical injury to epithelia. An example is a superficial abrasion of the skin that causes only necrosis of the epidermis. In this case regeneration occurs with little or no scarring.

Stable cells, such as hepatocytes, skeletal muscle fibers, and kidney cells, normally do not divide but can be induced to undergo mitosis by an appropriate stimulus. For example, if a portion of the liver is removed by surgery or if liver cells are killed by a viral infection (hepatitis), the remaining hepatocytes divide and sometimes can fully replace the missing liver tissue.

Studies have revealed some capability of neurons to regenerate (neurogenesis), but only in certain areas of the brain (e.g., hippocampus, olfactory bulb).[10] The reasons for the restriction of neurogenesis to a few regions of the brain in mammals compared with a more widespread neurogenesis in other vertebrates remain unknown.[106] It may be that neuronal stem cells persist in these areas throughout the life span, but why they do not persist in all areas is still a mystery.[3] What we do know is that neural stem cells residing in specific niches are able to proliferate and differentiate, giving rise to migrating neuroblasts, which in turn mature into functional neurons. These new neurons integrate into the existing circuits and contribute to the structural plasticity of certain brain areas.[112] Scientific evidence suggests that the process could become more general under pathologic conditions. For example, adult neurogenesis increases under acute and chronic brain diseases. Neuronal precursors are directed to the lesions where they contribute to tissue repair. Investigations are underway to find ways to manipulate and direct the neurogenic process toward the amelioration of neurodegenerative diseases.[112,140]

Tissue Repair (Formation of Scar Tissue)

Skin has the remarkable ability to heal, often without scarring. Growth factors, blood components, and epithelial (skin) cells mobilize to seal off wounds and protect the body. Scarring does not occur unless the cut, incision, damage, or trauma extends beneath the surface layer (epidermis).

Tissue repair, including the formation of a connective tissue scar, requires removal of the connective tissue matrix. Without this matrix, labile cells do not regenerate, or they regenerate in an incomplete fashion. Therefore the structural integrity of the parenchymal tissue depends on the formation of this connective tissue scar (dense, irregular laying down of collagen).

In many cases, however, healing of tissue is achieved by both cell regeneration and replacement by connective tissue (which is what constitutes scarring). In the case of skin, for example, both types of healing occur in wounds that involve both the epidermis and dermis.

Minimizing tissue scarring is important not only for cosmetic reasons, as is the case in skin, but also because excessive scarring can interfere with organ function. Very large tissue defects may require the use of grafts or flaps of tissue to achieve optimal healing. It is possible to minimize scarring by surgical obliteration of the tissue defect caused by injury and cell necrosis. For example, treatment of skin wounds begins with careful cleansing of the wound to remove foreign materials and bacterial contamination, which interfere with healing. This is followed by debridement to remove nonviable tissue that normally would be broken down by the inflammatory reaction.

Careful attention to hemostasis minimizes the deposition of blood into the wound. During closure, the wound margins are closely apposed under the right amount of tension by surgical sutures. A clean, closed wound is free of infectious and other foreign material, fibrin, and necrotic debris. As a result, the duration and intensity of the inflammatory reaction are minimized. Little granulation tissue forms, and the epithelial cell surface is readily reconstituted.

The healing that occurs in the type of wound described is called *primary union* or *healing by first intention* and results in a small scar (Fig. 3.19). In the presence of large tissue defects or infections, and in other conditions in which surgical closure is not possible or desirable, healing occurs by secondary union. In this situation the time required for healing is longer and the amount of scarring is greater. There is a distinction between closure and healing; the wound or skin may close but healing takes much longer, as much as 2 years in some situations.

Even after wound closure is complete, degradation and resynthesis of collagen continue. This is a response at least in part to shifts in the stress forces to which the tissue is subjected. Cross-linking of collagen fibers continues for a period of several weeks, providing progressive strengthening of scar tissue. However, even under optimal conditions, the repaired tissue never fully regains its original stability. In the case of skin, a fully mature fibrous scar requires 12 to 18 months and is about 20% to 30% weaker than normal skin.

In some people, especially people of African or Asian descent, there is an inherited tendency to produce excessive amounts of collagen during the healing process, causing large amounts of collagen arranged in thick bundles to accumulate in the tissue. These collagenous masses are called *keloids* and can be seen protruding from the skin surface (Fig. 3.20). Keloids are more than just raised, hypertrophic scar tissue. Both keloid and hypertrophic scar tissue result from excess collagen formation, but hypertrophic scars generally calm down in 12 to 24 months, whereas keloids tend to grow larger and appear worse, often invading surrounding tissue.

Several methods are used to treat keloids, although none of them are 100% successful. Surgical keloid excision followed by high dose–rate brachytherapy, form-pressure garments, and pulsed dye lasers have some reported success.[14,30]

Necrosis of heart tissue (myocardial infarct) results in a fibrous scar because cardiac myocytes do not replicate to any great extent. Outcomes that can result from tissue repair in various tissue and conditions are summarized in Fig. 3.9. The CNS

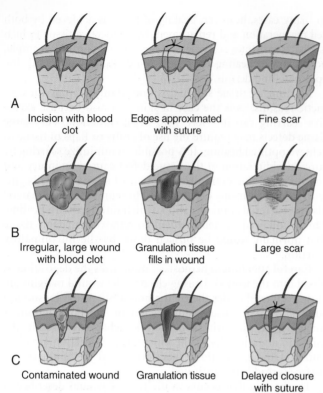

A Incision with blood clot   Edges approximated with suture   Fine scar

B Irregular, large wound with blood clot   Granulation tissue fills in wound   Large scar

C Contaminated wound   Granulation tissue   Delayed closure with suture

FIG. 3.19 (A) Healing by primary intention is the initial union of the edges of a wound, progressing to complete healing without granulation. (B) Healing by secondary intention is wound closure in which the edges are separated, granulation tissue develops to fill the gap, and epithelium grows in over the granulations, producing a scar. (C) Healing by tertiary intention is wound closure in which granulation tissue fills the gap between the edges of the wound, with epithelium growing over the granulation at a slower rate and producing a larger scar than results from healing from second intention. Suppuration is also usually found in tertiary wound closure. (From Lewis SL, Dirksen SR, Heitkemper MM et al (eds): Medical-surgical nursing: assessment and management of clinical problems, ed 9, St Louis, 2014, Mosby.)

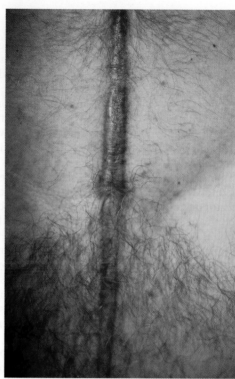

FIG. 3.20 Keloid (hypertrophic) scar composed predominantly of type III collagen, rather than type I collagen. Keloids result from defective remodeling of scar tissue and the persistence of type III collagen, which is typical of immature scar. The epidermis is elevated by excess scar tissue, which may continue to increase long after healing occurs. The tissue looks smooth, rubbery, and "clawlike." Young women, and people of Mediterranean and African descent are particularly susceptible to keloid formation. (From Rakel RE: Textbook of family medicine, ed 7, Philadelphia, 2007, Saunders.)

differs in its healing process because neurons are permanent cells and do not replicate.

After tissue necrosis neither regeneration nor tissue scarring occurs. No fibroblasts are present in the brain parenchyma, and no collagen is produced. After a brain infarct (stroke), the inflammatory cells arrive from the blood circulation and clear away the necrotic tissue, leaving behind an empty cavity (cyst). Specialized CNS cells called *astrocytes (glial cells)* proliferate, forming dense aggregates around the necrotic area called *glial scars* or *gliosis*.

Chronic wounds. When a wound fails to heal normally, reepithelialization and closure do not occur. Chronic wounds can occur when the wrong biochemicals are present in the wrong amounts at the wrong times and fail to function effectively. There may be a deficiency in endogenous growth factors, which have the primary role of stimulating cell migration, proliferation, and extracellular matrix deposition. Chronic wounds remain in the inflammatory and proliferative phases.[6] Understanding the normal repair process and factors that affect tissue healing can help guide the PTA in removing barriers to healing. Preparing

the wound bed appropriately changes the wound's biochemical environment back to an acute state, thus reinitiating the healing cascade.

3.5 Special Implications for the PTA: Scar Tissue The clinical implications of tissue repair can be seen in two examples presented earlier in this chapter (see 3.1 Special Implications for the PTA: Cell Injury: Multiple Cell Injuries and 3.2 Special Implications for the PTA: Collagen). In this example, after a transmural myocardial infarction (MI), a symptom-limited stress test will usually be given after phase II of cardiac rehabilitation, which is around 8 to 12 weeks after MI. With understanding of the material presented in this chapter, one can see the logical explanation.

Heart healing, which occurs primarily through the process of tissue repair, requires 8 to 12 weeks for the formation of a dense connective tissue scar. This dense scar allows for structural integrity and force transduction of the viable myocardium, leading to a complete heart contraction. Because the connective tissue scar is not contractile, this area of the heart will never return to full function. Of great importance is the fact that after an MI (heart attack), a person's aerobic fitness can improve to (or exceed) the level present before his or her premorbid state with proper exercise.

SPECIFIC TISSUE OR ORGAN REPAIR

Throughout this chapter, examples of cell types and healing processes within various organs and systems of the body have been discussed. Some organs are composed of cells that cannot regenerate (e.g., heart, CNS, peripheral nervous system cells), whereas other organs such as the liver and epithelial cells of the integumentary and GI systems can replace missing tissue through cell division (mitosis). Some cells, such as skeletal muscle cells and renal cells, do not divide but can be induced to undergo mitosis. The extent to which cells can regenerate depends on the type of cell (e.g., permanent, stable, labile), the cell's ability to divide, the type of damage incurred (e.g., lethal, sublethal), and other factors discussed (e.g., nutrition, age, immunocompetency, vascular supply, presence of microorganisms leading to infection). The proliferation and migration of cells, including parenchymal cells, have been discussed; regeneration only occur can if the parenchymal cells can undergo mitosis. When regeneration of parenchymal cells is not possible, the inflammatory reaction can become chronic.

Using an example of a person with traumatic brain injury (TBI) who also experiences MI (see 3.1 Special Implications for the PTA: Cell Injury: Multiple Cell Injuries), healing of brain and myocardial tissue was discussed earlier in this chapter. In this final section, only those tissues not specifically included in the main body of this chapter are discussed further.

Lung

After lethal injury to alveolar cells (type I and II pneumocytes), regeneration can occur only when the basement membrane remains intact. After the phagocytic removal of the necrotic cells, adjacent living epithelial cells migrate onto the remaining basement membrane and differentiate into type II pneumocytes (cells that primarily produce surfactant).

Eventually, some of these cells differentiate into type I pneumocytes (cells that permit gas exchange), and full lung function is restored. If the damage to the lung disrupts the basement membrane, healing must be achieved by repair that is characterized by fibrosis and scar formation. Also, certain injurious agents induce lung healing by the formation of scar tissue, leading to restrictive lung disease. An example of this would include inhalation of asbestos.

Digestive Tract

The healthy gut is lined with multiple rows of villi structures. These finger-like projections are responsible for nutrient absorption and the production of digestive enzymes. Gut cells grow single file from the base of the villi up toward the top. They slough off into the intestinal tract and pass out of the body every 5 days or so. Damaged or injured cells are constantly leaving, whereas healthy cells renew the GI environment. It takes about 3 to 4 weeks for a complete turnover of all gut cells throughout the digestive tract. A mildly to moderately impaired gut takes 3 to 6 months to heal, and 12 to 18 months are required for healing of a more severe intestinal injury.[29]

Because two-thirds of all immune system function and 90% of serotonin function take place in the gut, healing the gut can assist in bringing both of these functions back into balance. Serotonin is needed to produce melatonin, which is an essential component for good, restful sleep; the proper amount of circulating and functioning serotonin is also needed to stabilize mood.[29]

Peripheral Nerves

When a nerve is cut, the peripheral portion rapidly undergoes a myelin degeneration and axonal fragmentation. The lipid debris is removed by macrophages mobilized from the surrounding tissues in a process referred to as *Wallerian degeneration.* Within 24 hours of section, new axonal sprouts from the central stump are observed with proliferation of Schwann cells from both the central and peripheral stumps.

Careful microsurgical approximation of the nerve may result in reinnervation. The most important factor in achieving successful nerve regeneration after repair is the maintenance of the neurotubules (basement membrane and connective tissue endoneurium), along which the new axonal sprouts can pass.[17]

Skeletal Muscle

Skeletal muscle is composed of contractile and connective tissue elements. Actin and myosin myofilaments make up the sarcomere units of muscle fibers. Each individual myofiber is surrounded by a delicate sheath called the *endomysium* (basement membrane) and then arranged in bundles. Satellite cells surround the muscle fibers and are important for tissue regeneration after injury. The greater the degree of muscle injury, the larger the amount of connective tissue that is disrupted.[15]

Muscle Injury

Muscle injuries, including contusion, strain, or laceration, are common injuries, occurring particularly in sports; about 90% of all muscle injuries are either contusions or strains. A muscle *contusion* occurs when the muscle is subject to a sudden, heavy compressive force such as a direct blow to the muscle. Muscle *strains* occur when excessive tensile force leads to overstraining of the myofibers.[76] This is more likely to occur during eccentric contraction when the muscle is lengthening because tension is greater than the muscle's resistance to stretch; the resultant forces are large. Muscles that cross two joints (e.g., hamstrings, gastrocnemius) are especially vulnerable to stretch injury because they are simultaneously affected by angular positions and velocities of the adjacent joints.[15]

The most common site of strain injury is the myotendinous junction, a region of highly folded basement membranes between the end of the muscle fiber and the tendon. These involutions maximize surface area for force transmission. The transition from compliant muscle fibers to relatively noncompliant tendon may account for the vulnerability of the myotendinous junction.

If the force of stretch on a muscle is too great to be resisted by the contractile unit, resistance shifts from the contractile unit to the connective tissues. Pathogenic stretch (passive or active) that is beyond the threshold length of the entire musculotendinous unit can result in disruption at the myotendinous junction. Complete tears do occur but less often than muscle strains.[15]

Muscle Regeneration or Repair

Contrary to widespread belief, muscle tissue can regenerate, but the restoration of normal structure and function is strongly dependent on the type of injury sustained. In *severe infections* the muscle fibers may be extensively destroyed. However, the sarcolemmal sheaths (basement membrane and connective tissue endomysium) usually remain intact, and rapid regeneration of muscle cells within the sheaths occurs so that the function of the muscle may be completely restored.

After *transection* of a muscle, muscle fibers may regenerate either by growth from undamaged stumps or by growth of new, independent fibers.[17] Once again, this type of regeneration after lethal cell injury to skeletal muscle fibers is possible when the basement membrane remains intact through mitotic division of "satellite cells." Satellite cells play an integral role in normal development of skeletal muscle and are essential to the repair of injured muscle by serving as a source of myoblasts for fiber regeneration. These proliferating satellite cells support the process of regeneration by either combining with other myogenic cells causing the development of new fibers, or by fusing with remaining muscle fibers.[9]

A muscle that is *contused* or *strained,* has the capability to repair itself, but the period of recovery is markedly prolonged, and results in loss of strength. At the conclusion of the healing process, the repaired site shows a high rate of reinjury.[70] Recovery is largely dependent on the severity of the injury but follows the same phases of degeneration, inflammation, regeneration, and fibrosis described in this chapter.

As with all healing, muscle fiber injury is regenerated or repaired through a consistent sequence of events that goes into motion as soon as an injury occurs. Hemostasis with hematoma formation and inflammation overlap in the first phase, starting in the first 24 to 48 hours after injury. This phase is followed by phagocytosis with the removal of detritus, activation of satellite cells, and subsequent myofiber regeneration. This second phase can last 6 to 8 weeks after injury. The final phase involves tissue remodeling. This phase is characterized by complete reorganization and maturation of the regenerated muscle.[70,82]

With death of the muscle cell and ensuing necrosis, chemotactic agents attract macrophages within the basement membrane confines to engulf the remnants of the dead cell. Macrophages release growth factors, stimulating the division of the satellite cells. These cells migrate to the central region and begin to differentiate into expressing the usual characteristics of a skeletal muscle fiber. This healing process can occur after lethal cell injury (e.g., muscular dystrophy) when the connective tissue matrix (primarily basement membrane) is disrupted and regeneration is attempted, but disruption of basement membrane leaves the satellite cells no place to set up and multiply.

The end result is that the muscle tissue heals by forming a connective tissue scar (i.e., repair). This at least maintains the structural integrity of the tissue but not the complete functional capability. This type of healing of muscle (repair versus regeneration) could occur after the trauma of a motor vehicle accident or a knife wound.

The formed scar tissue that replaces the damaged muscle fibers is disorganized and therefore has decreased ability to withstand tensile forces. The result is that these repaired muscles have a higher risk of injury.[82,143]Many reports indicate that the overproduction of TGF-β in response to injury is a major cause of tissue fibrosis. Scientists have been able to use antagonists to block the profibrotic effects of TGF-β, improving both muscle structure and function, enabling nearly complete recovery of muscle strength.[45,83]

Muscle Stiffness

Muscle deficiency (weakness and stiffness) is a common problem as we age. Humans lose about 1% of muscle mass every year beginning in their late twenties, which is a process known as *sarcopenia.* Without regular exercise, we can lose up to 30% in midlife. By age 40, the elasticity of muscle also decreases.

Connective tissue changes involving the musculotendinous unit also occur with age as small amounts of fibrinogen (produced in the liver and normally converted to fibrin to serve as a clotting factor) leak from the vasculature into the intracellular spaces, adhering to cellular structures.

The resulting microfibrinous adhesions among the cells of muscle and fascia cause increased muscular stiffness. Activity and movement normally break these adhesions; however, with the aging process, production of fewer and less efficient macrophages combined with immobility for any reason results in reduced lysis of these adhesions.[133] Other possible causes of aggravated stiffness include increased collagen fibers from reduced collagen turnover, increased cross-links of aged collagen fibers, changes in the mechanical properties of connective tissues, and structural and functional changes in the collagen protein. Tendons and ligaments also have less water content, resulting in increased stiffness.[118]

In the athlete, prolonged exercise can result in fatigue or damage as a result of muscle membrane leakage lasting several days after the exercise event. Research studies suggest that initiation of degenerative processes in muscles after severe exercise may be the result of changes in sodium, potassium, and calcium ion content.[53,107]

Release of muscle enzymes, such as LDH and CK, has also been reported as an indicator of muscle damage associated with intense exercise. These enzymes are found within 6 to 24 hours of muscle injury, and their levels remain elevated up to 4 days postinjury.[21,22]

Motor Control and Muscle Inhibition

Neurophysiologic adaptation to chronic pain appears to result in changes in motor control and muscle recruitment strategies. Three important motor control issues seem to be part of musculoskeletal dysfunction and human movement impairment observed: feedforward mechanisms, cortical plasticity, and task specificity.[32,150] For example, studies of low back pain are reporting muscle inhibition after injury, a state in which there is no activation seen in the muscle on electromyography even when the particular muscle under surveillance is expected to serve as the prime mover. Inhibition can be task specific (i.e., related only to one task) or global (i.e., as if the brain has forgotten that muscle altogether).[61]

Task-specific inhibition shows a muscle recruitment pattern that is perfectly normal in one motion or direction but absent in another. With global inhibition, the muscle is inactive throughout most (but not all) motions and tasks involving that muscle. The presence of global inhibition signals that a different approach is required in intervention. Pain management and muscle strengthening must be done in conjunction with treatment to restore normal motor recruitment patterns.[61,62]

New information in the areas of motor control and muscle inhibition as these topics relate to muscle injury and repair is being reported. We may expect to see more information in the near future. Greater knowledge and understanding in these areas may help direct treatment interventions in the future.

Bone

Bone is composed of two types of tissue: cortical and cancellous (trabecular). Cortical bone accounts for approximately 80% of skeletal tissue. It is the tough outer layer of bone, densely packed, and surrounds trabecular or cancellous bone. The remaining 20% is cancellous bone, which consists of spongy, intermeshing thin plates (trabeculae) that are in contact with the bone marrow. Bone has two surfaces referred to as *periosteal* (external) and *endosteal* (internal).

Loss of bone occurs when there is an imbalance between destruction and production of bone cells or when there is a defective mineralization of bone matrix. An increase in osteoclasts or failure of osteoblasts to assemble can result in bone resorption faster than bone is being built up.

A variety of conditions can affect bone and require a reparative process, including fracture, infection, inflammation (e.g., tuberculosis, sarcoidosis), metabolic disturbances (e.g., Paget disease, osteoporosis, osteogenesis imperfecta), tumors, response to implanted prostheses, bone infarction, and any other systemic diseases that have skeletal manifestations (e.g., sickle cell disease, amyloidosis, hemochromatosis). For a discussion of these specific conditions and their impact on bone, the reader is referred to each individual chapter that includes those diseases. Only the bone response to injury and the reparative process (specifically fracture) are discussed in this chapter.

Fracture Healing

Fracture repair is a process of healing by regeneration and remodeling (i.e., without a scar) and with the potential for a return of optimal function in many cases. After an uncomplicated fracture, bone heals in similar overlapping phases previously discussed in this chapter (Fig. 3.21). At the moment of fracture, tiny blood vessels through the haversian systems are torn at the fracture site. A brief period of local internal bleeding occurs, resulting in a hematoma around the fracture site called a *fracture hematoma*. Bleeding from the fracture site delivers fibroblasts, platelets, and osteoprogenitor cells, which secrete numerous growth factors and cytokines. They stimulate transformation of the initial hematoma into a more organized granulation tissue, eventually promoting callus formation.

The inflammatory phase occurs as inflammatory cells arrive at the injured site, accompanied by the vascular response and cellular proliferation. Clinical evidence of this phase includes pain, swelling, and heat.

Clotting factors from the blood initiate the formation of a fibrin meshwork, which is the scaffolding for the ingrowth of fibroblasts and capillary buds around and between the bony ends. By the end of the first week, phagocytic cells have removed a majority of the hematoma, and neovascularization and initial fibrosis are occurring.

The *reparative phase* begins during the next few weeks and includes the formation of the soft callus seen on radiographs around 2 weeks after the injury, which is eventually replaced by a hard callus. During this phase, osteoclasts (bone macrophages) clear away the necrotic bone while the periosteum and endosteum regenerate and begin to differentiate into hyaline cartilage (soft callus) and primary bony spicules (hard callus). Bone growth factors, including bone morphogenetic proteins, FGF, insulin-like growth factors, PDGF, TGF-β, and vascular endothelial growth factor, are major components of the fracture healing (reparative) phase.[33]

Once the callus is sufficient to immobilize the fracture site, repair occurs between the fractured cortical and medullary bones when the fibrocartilaginous union (soft callus) is replaced by a fibroosseous union (hard callus). The process is called *endochondral ossification*. Delayed union and nonunion fractures result from errors in this phase of bone healing. The completion of the reparative phase (usually occurring at 6 to 12

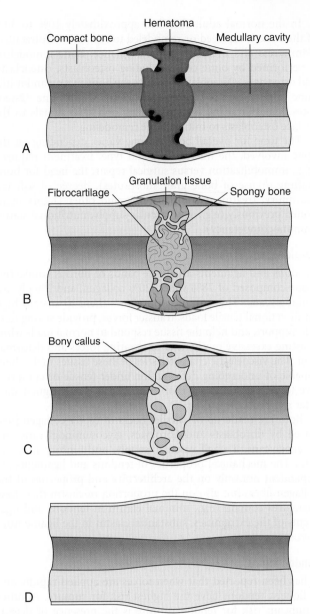

FIG. 3.21 Fracture healing occurs in overlapping stages or phases. (A) Immediate vascular response with hematoma formation and inflammatory response. (B) Granulation tissue and fibrocartilage formation during early reparative phase. (C) Fibrocartilaginous union (soft callus) is replaced by a fibroosseous union (bony callus). (D) Remodeling phase with complete restoration of the medullary canal. (From Damjanov I: Pathology for the health-related professions, ed 4, St Louis, 2012, Saunders.)

weeks) is indicated by fracture stability. Radiographically, the fracture line begins to disappear.[69]

The *remodeling phase* begins with clinical and roentgenographic union (no movement occurs at the fracture site) and persists until the bone is returned to normal, including restoration of the medullary canal. During this phase, which may take months to years, the immature, disorganized woven bone is replaced with a mature organized lamellar bone that adds further stability to the fracture site. The excessive bony callus is resorbed, and the bone remodels in response to the mechanical stresses placed on it.

In the normal adult skeleton, approximately 10% to 30% of the bone is replaced or remodeled to replace microfractures from stress and maintain mineral balance. Bone remodeling is performed by bone cells, including osteoblasts, osteoclasts, and osteocytes. Osteoblasts produce the bone matrix and initial bone mineralization, whereas osteoclasts resorb bone. Osteocytes detect local mechanical loading and send signals to the surface osteoblasts to initiate bone remodeling.[2]

The time for overall bone healing varies depending on the bone involved, the fracture site and type, treatment required (e.g., immobilization versus surgical repair, the need for bone grafting or use of bone graft substitutes), degree of soft tissue injury, treatment complications, and other factors mentioned previously (e.g., age, vascular supply, nutritional status, immunocompetency).

Tendons and Ligaments

Tendons and ligaments are dense bands of fibrous connective tissue composed of 78% water, 20% collagen, and 2% glycosaminoglycans. This composition allows them to sustain high unidirectional tensile loads, transfer forces, provide strong flexible support, and help the tissue respond to normal loads while resisting excessive mechanical or shearing forces and deformation. The viscoelastic characteristics of these tissues make them capable of undergoing deformation under tensile or compressive force, yet still capable of returning to their original state after removal of the force.

Both are made up of parallel fibers of type I collagen produced by fibroblasts and fibrocytes, glycosaminoglycans and proteoglycans, a small vascular supply, and sensory innervation. The mechanical properties of tendons and ligaments are dependent not only on the architecture and properties of the collagen fibers but also on the proportion of elastin that these structures contain (e.g., minimal elastin in tendons and ligaments of the extremities, substantial elastin in the ligamentum flavum).

Tendon Injury

It has been reported that when forces are applied rapidly and obliquely, tendons have the highest risk for rupture. Another significant risk for tendon rupture is the presence of degenerative changes in the tendon itself because tensile strength is decreased under degenerative conditions.[158]

In the case of acute injury and tendon rupture, tendons may heal either as a result of proliferation of the tenoblasts from the cut ends of the tendon or more likely as a result of vascular ingrowth and proliferation of fibroblasts derived from the surrounding tissues that were injured at the time of the tendon injury. Because the surrounding tissues contribute so much to the healing of a tendon, adhesions are very common. With rupture of the Achilles tendon, rotator cuff tendons, or cruciate ligament(s), functional restoration requires surgical repair to appose and suture the cut ends.[17] Tendon healing progresses through the same overlapping phases as other tissues: hemostasis and inflammation, cellular proliferation and matrix deposition, and long-term remodeling. Hemostasis begins immediately and is followed by the inflammatory process, which begins during the first 72 hours (3 to 5 days) after injury and/or surgical intervention.

Hemostasis occurs as platelets from blood plasma enter the tear to initiate clot formation. Fibrin and fibronectin form cross-links with collagen fibers to form a fragile bond, which helps reduce hemorrhage. The activity of phagocytic cells clears away the debris in the area from damaged and devitalized tissue. Chemotactic mediators attract inflammatory WBCs to the area, including polymorphonuclear leukocytes and monocytes. The *inflammatory phase* overlaps and transforms into the *proliferative phase*, which usually occurs 2 to 3 weeks after tendon injury or repair but can begin as early as 48 hours after injury.[18] Granulation tissue is formed by the migration and proliferation of fibroblasts and vascular buds from the surrounding connective tissue. Capillary sprouts grow out of blood vessels around the edges of the wound-forming loops by joining with one another or with capillaries already carrying blood. The new blood vessels enhance delivery of nutrients to the healing tissue.

While this is occurring, the fibroblasts are secreting soluble type III collagen molecules, which form fibrils. A new extracellular matrix is formed. In this step, the original fibrin clot and scaffolding are replaced with more permanent repair tissue.

Approximately 2 weeks into the healing process, the collagen fibrils are oriented and rearranged into thick bundles, providing the tissue with greater strength. During this period the affected area remains immobilized to relieve stress from the healing tissue and prevent rupture recurrence. The lack of stress causes the newly forming collagen to be deposited in random alignment without the formation of cross-links. The immature collagen is randomly oriented and has limited strength.

Now the transition from the proliferative phase to the *maturation phase* takes place. The maturation and remodeling phase begins around week 3 after the initial injury. The immature type III collagen is replaced by mature type I collagen; the latter aligns along tensile forces. The collagen is continually remodeled until permanent repair tissue is formed that is oriented along the lines of stress and organized to provide increasing resistance to stretch and tearing.[80] On the basis of animal models, we know that tendon healing takes at least 12 to 16 weeks to reach a level at which the tendon can be stressed.[96,147]

Aggressive early motion that stresses the repair and exceeds the mechanical strength of the repair should be avoided. During the early weeks of the remodeling phase, the force required to rupture a lacerated and repaired tendon can be less than the force generated by a maximum muscle contraction. These findings suggest that maximum muscle contraction forces should be avoided for at least 8 weeks after tendon repair; the PTA can expect to see significant tendon weakness for a considerable period afterward.[18,67]

When the healing tissue has achieved adequate integrity, motion is permitted once again. The remodeling collagen then aligns to the lines of stress produced by the motion, permitting the healed tendons and ligaments to provide support in line with the stress. Realignment of collagen to its usual parallel arrangement also permits the restoration of full, normal range of motion after repair. In animal studies, at 24 weeks after surgery, the tensile strength of lacerated and repaired tendons was only 50% that of healthy intact tendon.[67] Human tendons and ligaments regain normal strength in 40 to 50 weeks postoperatively; this means that even as long as a year after injury, the tendon or ligament may not have achieved premorbid tensile strength.

Although the process of healing is by repair (formation of a connective tissue scar), this constitutes regeneration because tendons and ligaments are originally composed of connective tissue. However, the scar tissue is weaker and larger and has compromised biomechanical integrity, with increased minor collagens (types III, V, and VI), decreased collagen cross-links, and increased glycosaminoglycans.[66]

These changes lead to impaired function, increased risk of reinjury, and increased risk of osteoarthritis. Research on ligament healing includes studies on low-load and failure-load properties, alterations in the expression of matrix molecules, cytokine modulation of healing, and gene therapy as a method to alter matrix protein and cytokine production.[84,103]

Ligament Injury

Sprains and tears of the tendinous or ligamentous structures around a joint can be caused by abnormal or excessive joint motion. These injuries can be classified as first, second, or third degree, depending on the changes in structural or biomechanical integrity (ranging from injury of a few fibers without loss of integrity to a complete tear).

Common sites for this type of injury include the ankle, knee, and fingers, with clinical manifestations of local pain, edema, increased local tissue temperature, ecchymosis, hypermobility or instability, and loss of motion and/or function. If after injury the PTA notes quick onset of joint effusion, and the joint feels hot to the touch with extremely painful and limited movement, the joint needs to be examined by a physician to rule out hemarthrosis.

In many extraarticular ligaments (e.g., medial collateral ligament [MCL]), healing occurs by the same basic phases described in the previous section. However, there is variation in the manner in which ligaments heal; some intraarticular ligaments (e.g., ACL) have a poor healing response. After the ligament ruptures, the thin synovial sheath is disrupted and blood dissipates, preventing clot and hematoma formation. Healing cannot take place without a foundation for repair or localization of chemotactic cytokines and growth factors.[115]

Recent studies have revealed that after injuries, ligament tissues such as the ACL release large amounts of matrix metalloproteinases (MMPs). These enzymes have a devastating effect on the healing process of the injured ligaments. MMPs are critically involved in the extracellular matrix turnover, which may help explain one of the reasons why the injured ACL repairs minimally. The higher levels of active MMP-2 seen in ACL injuries may disrupt the delicate balance of extracellular matrix remodeling. MMP activity is less in the MCL, which may account for the difference in healing capacities between the MCL and the ACL.[158]

Cartilage

Several forms of cartilage are recognized, including articular cartilage, found at the ends of the bones; fibrocartilage, found in the menisci of the knee, at the annulus fibrosus, at the insertions of the ligaments and tendons into the bone, and on the inner side of tendons as they angle around pulleys (e.g., at the malleoli); and elastic cartilage, found in the ligamentum flavum, external ear, and epiglottis (Table 3.6).

Articular cartilage has many individual zones that make up the whole (Fig. 3.22). It is composed of hyaline cartilage, made up of water (75%), chondrocytes, type II collagen (20%), and glycosaminoglycans or proteoglycans (5%). It is aneural, avascular, and alymphatic and does not appear to regenerate well after adolescence, most likely because of its

TABLE 3.6	**Types of Cartilage**
Types of Cartilage	**Location**
Articular (hyaline)	Joint surfaces, bone apophyses, epiphyseal plates, costal cartilage (ribs), fetal skeleton
Fibrocartilage	Tendon and ligament insertion, meniscus, and disk
Elastic	Trachea (epiglottis), earlobe, and ligamentum flavum
Fibroelastic	Meniscus

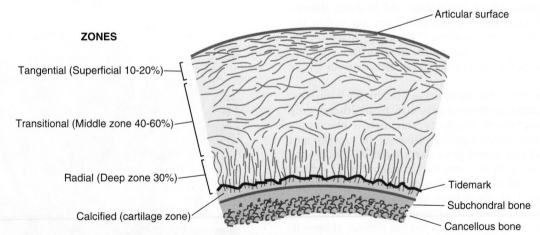

FIG. 3.22 Zones of cellular distribution in adult articular cartilage. Superficial tangential zone: type II collagen fibers are oriented tangentially to the surface, providing the greatest ability to resist shear stresses. Transitional (middle) zone: composed primarily of proteoglycans, but collagen fibers present are arranged obliquely to provide a transition between the shearing forces of the surface layer and the compression forces in the cartilage layer. Radial (deep) zone: collagen fibers are attached vertically (radial) into the tidemark; distributes loads and resists compression. Tidemark layer is located in the calcified zone. The tidemark is the line that straddles the boundary between calcified and uncalcified cartilage; it separates hyaline cartilage from subchondral bone. Calcified zone: layer just above the subchondral bone containing type X collagen. Subchondral bone. Cancellous bone.

ZONES

Tangential (Superficial 10-20%)
Transitional (Middle zone 40-60%)
Radial (Deep zone 30%)
Calcified (cartilage zone)

Articular surface
Tidemark
Subchondral bone
Cancellous bone

avascularity and low cell-to-matrix ratio. Proteoglycan, produced by the chondrocytes and secreted into the matrix, is responsible for the compressive strength of cartilage. It binds growth factors and traps and holds water used to regulate matrix hydration.

Cartilage Healing

Ideal conditions for healing of articular cartilage require a source of cells, provision of matrix, removal of stress concentration, and intact subchondral bone plate with some mechanical stimulation.

Following cartilage injury, the normal inflammatory process that involves the migration of repair cells to the site is impeded because the articular cartilage lacks the vascularization to bring these cells to the area.[98] Therefore, in adults without intervention, the healing of articular cartilage occurs by fibrous scar tissue, or the cartilage fails to heal at all. This replacement tissue does not function as well as the original, and the adjacent joint surface can be affected. Fibrous scarring of the articular cartilage leads to local degenerative arthritis (Fig. 3.23).

In people with rheumatoid arthritis, stiffness and pain are common. Researchers are still investigating the underlying mechanisms contributing to mechanical stiffness. One hypothesis is that chronic pain leads to CNS plasticity. Chronic pain may elicit joint, ligament, and capsule mechanoreceptor sensitivity alterations at the spinal level, impairing proprioceptive joint responses and ultimately resulting in perceived joint stiffness.[57,63]

Menisci (Knee)

The menisci are fibrocartilaginous structures consisting of cartilage bundles composed mainly of collagen, although some proteoglycan is also present. The amount of proteoglycan increases dramatically in the injured, degenerate meniscus. The cells of the meniscus sometimes are called *fibrochondrocytes* because of their appearance and the fact that they synthesize a fibrocartilaginous matrix.[54] The principal orientation of collagen fibers in the menisci is circumferential, designed to disperse compressive load, resist shear, aid in shock absorption, and withstand the circumferential tension within the meniscus during normal loading (Fig. 3.24). A few small, radially oriented fibers present on the tibial surface probably act as ties to resist lateral splitting of the menisci from undue compression.

At birth, the entire meniscus is vascular; by age 9 months, the inner one-third has become avascular. By adulthood, only the outer 10% to 30% of vascularity remains, with blood supplied via the perimeniscal capillary plexus off the superior and inferior medial and lateral genicular arteries.[129] Blood supply to the meniscus flows from the peripheral to the central meniscus principally through diffusion or mechanical pumping (movement).[4] Meniscal tears heal by migration of cells from the synovial membrane adjacent to the meniscus. The remodeling events of the healing process remain unknown. Healing of meniscal tears may be inhibited based on the location of the tear; less vascular locations have less vigorous healing capability.

Water accounts for 70% of meniscal composition, contributing to the meniscal function of joint lubrication. Water in the menisci also provides resistance to compressive loads. Collagen makes up 60% to 70% of the dry weight; 90% of it is type I collagen fibers, with types II, III, V, and VI present in much smaller amounts.[54] In the young individual, the menisci are

usually white, translucent, and supple on palpation. In the older individual, the menisci lose their translucency, become more opaque and yellow in color, and become less supple.

Injury and degeneration leading to laceration are the two most common causes of symptoms that require surgical intervention.[17] The presence of clinical symptoms of pain, swelling, locking and catching, and loss of motion often necessitates surgical intervention. Proper management depends on the type of tear and its location (Fig. 3.25).[54]

Synovial Membrane

The synovial membrane lines the inner surface of the joint capsule and all other intraarticular structures (e.g., subcutaneous and subtendinous bursae sacs, tendon sheaths), with

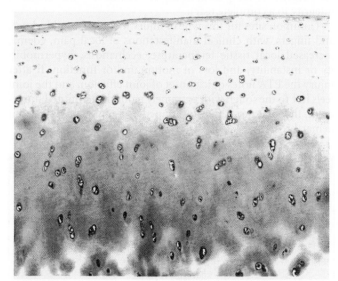

A   Normal

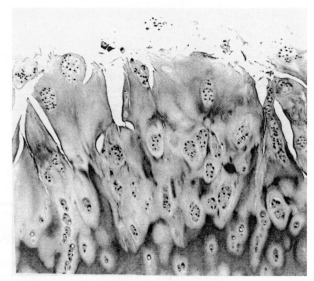

B   Osteoarthritis

FIG. 3.23 Histologic sections of normal (A) and osteoarthritic (B) articular cartilage obtained from the femoral head. The osteoarthritic cartilage demonstrates surface irregularities, with clefts to the radial zone and cloning of chondrocytes. (From Firestein GS, Budd RC, Bariel SE et al (eds): Kelley's textbook of rheumatology, ed 9, Philadelphia, 2013, Saunders.)

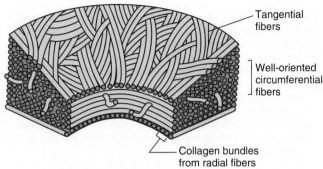

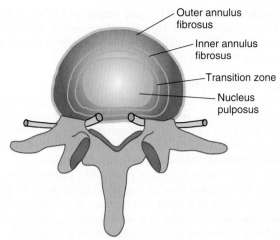

FIG. 3.24 Diagrammatic representation of the distribution of collagen fibers in the meniscus of a knee. Collagen is oriented throughout the connective tissues in such a way as to maximally resist the forces placed on these tissues. The majority of the fibers in the meniscus are circumferentially arranged, with a few fibers on or near the tibial surface placed in a radial pattern. This structural arrangement enables the meniscus to resist the lateral spread that occurs during high loads generated during weight bearing. Longitudinally arranged collagen fibers facilitate shock absorption and sustain the tension generated between the anterior and posterior attachments. (From Bullough PG: Bullough and Vigorita's orthopaedic pathology, ed 3, St Louis, 1997, Mosby.)

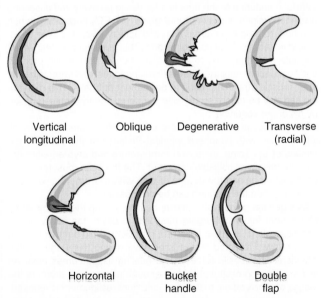

FIG. 3.25 Classification of most common meniscal tears.

the exception of articular cartilage and the meniscus. Synovial membrane consists of two components: the intimal (cellular layer or synoviocytes) layer next to the joint space, and the subintimal or supportive layer, made of fibrous and adipose tissue.

The synovial membrane has three principal functions: secretion of synovial fluid hyaluronate, phagocytosis of waste material, and regulation of the movement of solutes, electrolytes, and proteins from the capillaries into the synovial fluid. This last function provides a regulatory mechanism for maintenance of the matrix through various chemical mediators such as ILs.

Injury to any of the joint structures affects the synovium and results in hemorrhage, hypertrophy, and hyperplasia of the synovial lining cells and mild chronic inflammation.[17] In the

FIG. 3.26 Zones of the adult human lumbar intervertebral disk.

case of prolonged, chronic synovitis, such as occurs in hemophilia, abnormal synovial fluid, joint immobilization, and fibrous adhesions, a progressive destructive condition in the joint can result.

Any type of immobilization leads to contraction of the capsule. Loss of glycosaminoglycans with the associated water loss further increases capsule stiffness and results in decreased joint motion. The synovial membrane lining the inside of the capsule hypertrophies and forms adhesions between itself and the adjacent articular cartilage.[99]

Disk

The intervertebral disk sits between each pair of vertebrae and is made of connective tissue (collagen fibers) that helps the disk withstand tension and pressure (Fig. 3.26). The disk is made of three zones: (1) the outer annulus fibrosus, a lamellated ring of alternately obliquely oriented, densely packed type I collagen fibers that insert onto the vertebral bodies; (2) the fibrocartilaginous inner annulus fibrosus, consisting of a type II collagen fibrous matrix; and (3) the viscoelastic central nucleus pulposus with type II collagen fibers along with various mucopolysaccharides and a high concentration of proteoglycans.[5] This composition supports the high water content of the nucleus, which behaves biomechanically as a fluid cushion that transmits loading forces to the outer annulus fibrosus, as well as to the vertebral endplate.[139]

The nucleus is held in place by the *annulus,* a series of strong ligament rings surrounding it. The annulus is primarily composed of type I collagen arranged in multiple concentric layers. This fiber arrangement allows the annulus to resist tensile, radial, and torsional forces. With acute trauma or degenerative changes and microtrauma over time, the fibers of the annulus may be disrupted.[139] The normal disk's blood supply is restricted to the peripheral outer annulus. The vertebral body's blood vessels lie directly against the endplates but do not enter the disk itself. The nutrition of the more centrally located disk cells is derived from diffusional and convection transport of nutrients and wastes through the porous solid matrix.[5] The metabolism of the avascular disk is so slow that the turnover of proteoglycans takes 20 years.[142]

Although the nucleus has no nerve supply, the outer third of the annulus is innervated, receiving supply from both the sinuvertebral nerve, which innervates the posterior and posterolateral regions, and the gray ramus, which is distributed primarily anteriorly and laterally. More recent studies have confirmed that the annulus is a source of pain in people with chronic low back pain.[139]

Aging and Disk Degeneration

Our intervertebral disks change with age and demonstrate degenerative changes relatively early in life. Cell senescence in the disk has been linked with degenerative disease, with more senescence of cells in the nucleus pulposus compared with the annulus fibrosus in individuals with herniated disks.[125]

Disk degeneration follows a predictable pattern. First, the nucleus in the center of the disk begins to lose its ability to absorb water. This occurs as a result of a decrease in cell density in the disk accompanied by a reduction in synthesis of cartilage-specific extracellular matrix components such as type II collagen.[48]

As the proteoglycan content of the disk decreases, a loss of water-binding capacity by the disk matrix occurs, and the disk becomes dehydrated. Then the nucleus becomes thick and fibrous, so that it looks much the same as the annulus. As a result, the nucleus is not able to absorb shock as well. Routine stress and strain begin to take a toll on the structures of the spine. Tears called *fissures* form around the annulus. In addition to these, continued compressive forces to the spine caused by inactivity, weight gain, poor posture, and poor tone of the muscles supporting the spine further slow the ability of the disk to heal.[139]

Along with the pathology of degeneration, changes in the extracellular matrix content affecting collagen fibers can reduce the disk's load-bearing capacity. Calcification of the vertebral endplates is another factor thought to contribute to disk degeneration. Alterations in permeability adversely affect chondrocyte metabolism. The passage of nutrients and waste products across the endplate depends on fluid flowing into the disk during the night while an individual rests and flowing out during the day when he or she moves about.[48]

Injury to the disk (herniation) is more likely in the morning soon after waking, when the nucleus pulposus is maximally hydrated after a prolonged period of rest. Vigorous early morning activities increase the vertical load beyond the strength of the collagen in the annulus. Other proposed risk factors for lumbar disk herniation include lifting heavy loads, torsional stress, strenuous physical activity, and occupational driving of motor vehicles.[5]

Conditions such as a major back injury or fracture can affect how the spine works, making the changes happen even faster. Daily wear and tear and certain types of vibration can also speed up degeneration in the spine. In addition, strong evidence suggests that smoking speeds up degeneration of the spine. Scientists have also found links among family members, showing that genetics plays a role in how fast these changes occur.

3.6 Special Implications for the PTA: **Specific Tissue or Organ Repair** Physical therapist assistants (PTAs) have an important role in the rehabilitation of acute injuries. Certain components of the inflammatory process must be controlled quickly for recovery to proceed. For example, if edema is a component of a joint injury, it must be controlled as quickly as possible. Studies have demonstrated that joint edema can inhibit or hinder local muscle activity, which could result in altered joint mechanics and further irritation.[28,136] The anticipated goals are to facilitate wound healing and maintain the normal

---

function of noninjured tissue and body regions. The overall goal of the rehabilitation program is to return the person to normal activity as soon as possible, yet not so fast that irritation and further inflammation of the injured area occur. A fine line exists between maximizing activity and overdoing the activity to the point of injury aggravation.

Client education is essential regarding the injured individual's role in facilitating tissue healing is essential. Adherence to weight-bearing guidelines, avoiding aggravating movements, applying ice appropriately, and performing the prescribed exercises are key to the recovery process.

Prevention

Appropriate rehabilitation is necessary for soft tissue injuries, especially severe muscle strains and frank rupture of any tendon or muscle. Return to full activity, especially high-impact sports, can (and often does) result in recurrence of injury. Injury prevention should include addressing issues such as muscle fatigue, weakness, and lack of flexibility. Stronger muscles are better able to absorb energy, limiting the magnitude of tissue stretch. In other words, muscle strengthening is an important way to avoid muscle strain. The value of stretching before activity continues to be a topic of controversy. Although some studies have shown that a warm-up program that includes stretching may reduce strain. More studies are needed to confirm this relationship.[91]

Rehabilitation of Repaired Soft Tissues

Careful monitoring of the time line for tissue recovery and observing presenting signs and symptoms guide the PTA in deciding when and how to progress intervention and activity level. The type of tissue involved also makes a difference, because tendon tear repair requires prolonged rest to avoid disruption of the healing process and subsequent reinjury, whereas prolonged rest and immobilization after muscle strain can result in permanent stiffness. This monitoring can also be taught so the client understands the limits imposed by his or her condition.

The process is somewhat more difficult with acute back or neck injuries than with peripheral injuries. Because of the depth of the tissues of the spine, increased temperature and erythema are not always present or palpable if present. The therapist must rely more on muscle tone and the degree of pain with movement changes in deciding when the program can be progressed.

As a general guideline for tissue healing, during the inflammatory phase after injury or surgery (first 3 to 5 days), the ability of the soft tissue (e.g., tendon, ligament, muscle) to hold sutures is at an all-time low. Protected rest is imperative during this stage. Gradually increasing tensile force on the healing tissue comes next. An incremental approach that is slow enough to allow and promote the stages of proliferation, maturation, and fiber realignment is required.

Tendon or Muscle Rupture

During the proliferative phase (usually 5 to 28 days after tendon injury or repair), controlled passive movement is allowed. The repaired tissue is kept protected to avoid excessive force. Passive range of motion is continued as healing progresses and until the tissue moves into the remodeling phase of healing (around 4 to 8 weeks after injury or repair). Active range of motion is then initiated with controlled movements (e.g., gravity-eliminated positions). The idea is to prevent excessive resistance from the weight of the limb while still working on gradually increasing the force of the muscle contraction. As the repair strengthens, the PTA can allow increased muscle force through increased antigravity movements.[18]

Resistance with weights, rubber tubing, elastic bands, and so on is not started until at least 8 weeks after the repair. Once again, resistance is increased progressively (8 to 12 weeks). At the end of 12 weeks, if there have been no complications (e.g., infection, wound dehiscence) and there are no comorbidities to delay healing (e.g., tobacco use, diabetes, peripheral vascular disease), then full-force muscle contraction can be tolerated.

Muscle Strain

Recovery from severe muscle strain may begin with a short period of immobilization to provide pain relief and protect the tissue during the initial phase of healing. Immobilization followed by mobilization of muscle may help muscle fiber regeneration and fiber orientation with reduced scar formation.[75] As soon as pain and swelling subside, a program can be initiated to recover range of motion, strength, and endurance. Return to sports is considered safe when there is 80% return of strength compared with the noninvolved side. Surgical repair of a complete muscle tear has its own protocol. Repair is difficult, as the muscle fibers do not hold sutures well.[15]

Modalities

Physical therapy modalities, such as transcutaneous electrical nerve stimulation, iontophoresis, and ultrasound, may be used to manage pain and achieve limited motion, but their impact on the underlying tear and healing tissue is not known. Use of high-voltage electrical stimulation and cryotherapy with compression helps control postoperative pain, decreases swelling and muscle spasm, suppresses inflammation, and decreases metabolism. Transverse friction massage in the treatment of tendinitis or tendinosis is based on the soft tissue work of Cyriax.[25] However, there are no scientific data to support the use of this technique.

Guidelines for nonsurgical and postoperative rehabilitation for ligament, tendon, and muscle tear and repair vary based on geographic regions and physician preferences and protocols and are reported widely in the literature. The plan of care should always be based on an understanding of the healing stages of injured tissue. The goal is to restore motion and strength without subjecting the healing tissue to excessive forces that may hinder healing or rupture the repair.

Medications

A significant percentage of those coming to outpatient therapy clinics are taking salicylates or nonsteroidal antiinflammatory drugs (NSAIDs).[13] These medications can play a key role in recovery from an acute injury, facilitating therapy and clinical decision making. The common clinical practice to administer NSAIDs should be limited to early symptom control during the early phases of tissue healing. Prolonged NSAID use may be counterproductive for the biologic healing process because complete tissue recovery involves delicate and finely coordinated elements of cellular and metabolic inflammatory reactions, which can be interrupted by NSAIDs.[93,110]

Considering the widespread use of salicylates and NSAIDs, PTAs must also be aware of potential side effects that would warrant communication with a physician. Irritation of the gastrointestinal (GI) system is the most common potential side effect. The risk of developing peptic ulcer disease increases significantly if someone is taking more than one of these types of drugs. With new topical NSAIDs, the GI system can be avoided; phonophoresis or iontophoresis can aid in the delivery of these newer drugs. A pattern of drug use exists in the therapy population, in which significant numbers of subjects are taking one or more over-the-counter antiinflammatory agents along with a prescribed NSAID.[13]

Tissue Response to Immobilization

In addition to having an important role in the rehabilitation of acute injuries, PTAs often deal with clinical problems secondary to the effects of immobilization. Although not traumatic in the classic sense, immobilization of a limb or joint can result in significant impairment and functional limitations.

Immobilization takes a variety of forms, including bed rest, casting or splinting of a body part, or non–weight-bearing status of a lower extremity. On a tissue level, significant changes can occur with immobilization (Table 3.7). Along with the inert joint structures, changes also occur in muscle, particularly a loss of strength. Such changes can occur without injury, which magnifies the importance of maintaining function in uninjured tissue and body areas. A rehabilitation program should be designed to address the needs of each of the tissues.

Deep Venous Thrombosis

While initiating rehabilitation after immobilization, the PTA must remain vigilant for the possible presence of deep vein thrombosis (DVT). A potential complication of DVT is pulmonary embolus, which represents one of the leading causes of morbidity and mortality after orthopedic surgical procedures.[43] Although a large percentage of clients with DVT are asymptomatic, severe local pain and edema, fever, chills, and malaise are all possible manifestations. The types of immobilization that carry the risk of DVT include bed rest, a limb being placed in a cast or splint, and non–weight-bearing status after a lower extremity injury, a surgical procedure, or a long car or plane ride.

Stiffness

Joint or muscular stiffness is not uncommon after immobilization and in conjunction with conditions such as arthritis that are accompanied by pain and stiffness contributing to movement dysfunction and causing mobility impairments. Affected individuals often use the term *stiffness* to generally describe various joint sensations that may be unrelated to mechanical stiffness (increased resistance to motion). It may be necessary for the PTA to concentrate on disrupting the pain cycle to relieve "stiffness" when pain sensations are misinterpreted or poorly described as stiffness.[57,64]

When muscular stiffness occurs as a result of aging, increased physical activity and movement can reduce associated muscular pain. As part of the diagnostic evaluation, consider a general conditioning program for the older adult reporting generalized muscle pain. Even 10 minutes a day on a stationary bike or treadmill or in an aquatics program can bring dramatic and fast relief of painful symptoms when caused by muscle deficiency.

Cartilage

Immobility or immobilization causes marked changes in articular cartilage. The collagen content remains unchanged, but there is a loss of glycosaminoglycans and water from the matrix, which leads to weakening and deterioration of the cartilage. Damage to the cartilage results in impairment of cartilage nutrition.[99] Normally, synovial fluid accumulates in the peripheral part of the joint where the cartilage is not in contact with its opposing cartilage, and nutrition from the synovial fluid takes place there. Proliferation of the synovial membrane from immobilization causes a loss to this space and thus a reduction in cartilage nutrition. These types of alteration in the structure, quality, and nutrition of cartilage can lead to changes similar to those seen with osteoarthritis.[99]

Cartilage degeneration results from both loss of normal loading and loss of motion. The adverse effects of immobilization are seen in both the internal and external surfaces of cartilage. Lack of normal use also leads to loss of smoothness and the presence of fibrillation of the outer surface, potentially leading to arthritic joint changes.[99]

Current research is examining the effects of replacing damaged cartilage with cartilage harvested from the individual, grown in culture, and reinjected into the area of damaged cartilage to avoid this postoperative or postinjury sequela. This technology may allow the individual to regenerate a smooth, weight-bearing surface and avoid the rough, degenerative fibrocartilage formation that leads to osteoarthritis.

Advances in the fields of biotechnology and biomaterials are providing new techniques for regeneration or repair of tissue lost to injury, disease, or aging. Bioengineered tissues, including skin, bone, articular cartilage, ligaments, and tendons, are under investigation for clinical use.[73,74]

TABLE 3.7	**Effects of Prolonged Immobilization**
Tissue	**Results of Immobilization**
Muscle	Atrophy, decreased strength, contracture, reduced capillary-to-muscle fiber ratio, reduced mitochondrial density, reduced endurance
Bone	Generalized osteopenia of cancellous and cortical bone
Tendons and ligaments	Disorganization of parallel arrays of fibrils and cells; increased deformation with a standard load or compressive force
Ligament insertion site	Destruction of ligament fibers attaching to bone, reduced load to failure
Cartilage	Adherence of fibrofatty connective tissue to cartilage surfaces; loss of cartilage thickness; pressure necrosis at points of contact where compression has been applied
Synovium	Proliferation of fibrofatty connective tissue into joint space
Menisci	Adhesions of synovium villi; decreased synovial intima length; decreased synovial fluid hyaluronan concentrations; decreased synovial intima macrophages
Joint	*0-12 weeks:* Impaired range of motion; increased intraarticular pressure during movements; decreased filling volume of joint cavity
	After 12 weeks: Force required for the first flexion–extension cycle is increased more than 12-fold
Heart	Reduced strength of contraction (SV), reduced maximal cardiac output, reduced endurance, increased work of the heart for a submaximal load
Lung	Reduced airway clearance of mucus, increased likelihood of pneumonia, reduced maximal ventilatory volume
Blood	Reduced hematocrit and plasma volume, reduced endurance and temperature regulation

REFERENCES/SUGGESTED READINGS

To enhance this text and add value for the reader, references and suggested readings are included on the companion Evolve site that accompanies this textbook. The reader can view the source and access it online whenever possible.

The Immune System

Immunology is the study of the physiologic mechanisms that allow the body to recognize materials as foreign and to neutralize or eliminate them. When the immune system is working properly, it protects the organism from infection and disease; when it is not, the failure of the immune system can result in localized or systemic infection or disease. In fact, the significance of a healthy immune system is apparent in states or diseases characterized by immunodeficiency, such as occurs in human immunodeficiency virus (HIV) infection or in people on immunosuppressive medication.

Without an effective immune system, an individual is at risk for the development of overwhelming infection, malignant disease, or both. Not all immune system responses are helpful, as in the case of organ or tissue transplant rejection.

In addition, excessive or inappropriate activity of the immune system can result in hypersensitivity states, immune complex disease, or autoimmune disease. For a complete understanding of the immune system as it relates to injury, inflammation, and healing, the reader is encouraged to read this chapter along with, Chapter 3.

TYPES OF IMMUNITY

Innate and Acquired Immunity

Two types of immunity are recognized: innate immunity (natural or native immunity) and acquired immunity (adaptive or specific immunity). *Innate immunity* acts as the body's first line of defense to prevent the entry of pathogens.

Two nonspecific, nonadaptive lines of defense are involved in innate immunity. *Nonspecific* refers to the fact that this part of the immune system does not distinguish among different types of invaders (e.g., bacteria, fungus, virus) and is nonadaptive—that is, it does not remember the encounter with specific invaders for future encounters. Each time that potential pathogen is introduced, the innate immune system reacts in the same predictable manner.

The first line of defense is the skin and its mucosal barriers, and the second is a nonspecific inflammatory response to all forms of cellular injury or death. Innate responses occur to the same extent no matter how many times the infectious agent is encountered (Fig. 4.1).

Acquired immunity is characterized by specificity and memory. The primary role of the immune system as a more specific line of defense (acquired immunity) is to recognize and destroy foreign substances such as bacteria, viruses, fungi, and parasites and to prevent the proliferation of mutant cells such as those involved in malignant transformation.

This type of immunity results when a pathogen gains entry to the body and the body produces a specific response to the invader. Acquired immunity has a memory, so that when the same organism is encountered again, the body can respond even more rapidly to it and with a stronger reaction. The two components to acquired immunity (humoral immunity and cell-mediated immunity) are discussed in greater detail later in the following section.

Acquired Immunity: Active or Passive Immunity

Acquired immune responses can occur as a result of active or passive immunity. Active immunity includes natural immunity and artificial immunity, which is intended or deliberate.

Active acquired immunity refers to protection acquired by introduction (either naturally from environmental exposure

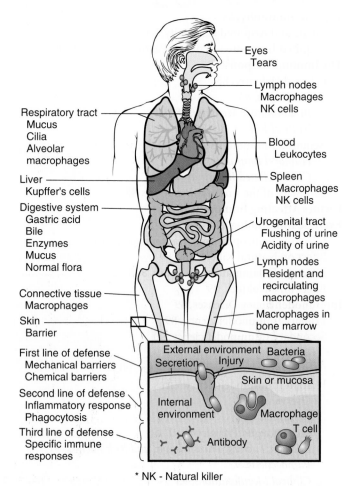

* NK - Natural killer

FIG. 4.1 Natural protective mechanisms of the human body. (From Damjanov I: Pathology for the health-related professions, ed 4, St. Louis, 2012, Saunders.)

or artificially by vaccination) of an antigen (microscopic component of a pathogen that causes an immune response) into a responsive host.

The concept of vaccination is based on the fact that exposure to a harmless version of a pathogen generates memory cells but not the disease the pathogen causes. The immune system becomes primed with strong and immediate protection if the pathogen or microorganism is encountered in the future.[33] Some of the most promising prophylactic and therapeutic vaccine strategies are currently being investigated for malaria, cancer, HIV, asthma, influenza, diabetes, hepatitis C, and many other diseases.

For example, the transplacental transfer of antibodies from mother to fetus, the transfer of antibodies to an infant through breast milk, or the administration of immune serum globulin (γ-globulin) provides immediate protection but does not result in the formation of memory cells and therefore provides only temporary immunity. This type of immunity (passively acquired) lasts only until the antibodies are degraded, which may be only a few weeks to months.

THE IMMUNE RESPONSE

External Defenses

As a covering for the entire body (with the exception of any openings), the skin offers the first and best line of protection (see Fig. 4.1), which is clearly demonstrated in cases of significant burns when infection becomes a major problem. The body openings also offer their own unique protection such as *lysozyme* in tears to kill bacteria, waxy secretions in the ear canal to prevent bacteria from advancing inside, nasal hair, stomach acid and unfavorable rapid pH change at the gastroduodenal junction to protect against ingested organisms, protective low pH vaginal secretions, acidic urine, and so on.

When organisms enter the body by penetrating the epithelial surface of the respiratory, gastrointestinal (GI), or genitourinary tract, biochemical defenses offer additional protection in the form of mediators, phagocytes that engulf and destroy foreign particles, and NK cells that attack and destroy virus-infected cells and tumor cells.

Phagocytes

Phagocytes are involved in nonspecific or innate immunity. These cells readily eat (ingest) microorganisms such as bacteria or fungi and kill them as a means of protecting the body against infection.

The two principal phagocytes are neutrophils and monocytes, which are white blood cells (WBCs), or leukocytes. The five types of leukocytes are neutrophils, eosinophils, basophils, monocytes, and lymphocytes. Because of their granular appearance, neutrophils, eosinophils, and basophils are collectively referred to as *granulocytes*. Granulocytes are short-lived (2 to 3 days) compared with monocytes and macrophages, which may live for months or years.

Phagocytes emigrate out of the blood and into the tissues in which an infection has developed, and each of these cell types has a specific phagocytic function in the immune system. Neutrophils, eosinophils, basophils, and monocytes are classified as phagocytic leukocytes that function in nonspecific or innate immunity. A severe decrease in the blood level of these cells is the principal cause of susceptibility to infection in people treated with intensive radiotherapy or chemotherapy. These treatments suppress blood cell production in the marrow, resulting in deficiencies of these phagocytic cells.

Neutrophils, also referred to as polymorphonuclear cells (PMNs), derive from bone marrow and increase dramatically in number in response to infection and inflammation. Neutrophils can directly kill invading organisms but may also damage host tissues. In the process of *phagocytosis,* bacteria or debris is engulfed and then digested by enzymes contained within the neutrophils. Neutrophils die after phagocytosis; the accumulation of dead neutrophils and phagocytosed bacteria contributes to the formation of pus.

Monocytes circulate in the blood, but when they migrate to tissues they mature into *macrophages,* which means "large eaters." The engulfment of a pathogen by a macrophage is an essential first step leading to a specific immune response. After neutrophils kill the invading organism and the process of phagocytosis has begun, macrophages appear to clear up the debris produced by the neutrophils and to kill any damaged-but-not-dead bacteria or bacteria that are too large for neutrophils. After phagocytes—in this case macrophages—digest the pathogens, antigenic material appears on their surface to identify them as foreign invaders. In this process, macrophages introduce the pathogen to lymphocytes.

Microscopically, T lymphocytes appear identical, but they can be distinguished by means of distinctive molecules called *cluster designations (CDs)* located on their cell surface. For example, all mature T cells carry markers known as T2, T3, T5, and T7 (or CD2, CD3, CD5, and CD7). T4 (CD4) lymphocytes are the helper T cells, and T8 (CD8) lymphocytes are cytotoxic T cells. Other T lymphocytes are identified as NK cells for their ability to kill certain tumor cells and virus-infected cells. Macrophages release a chemical messenger, interleukin-1 (IL-1), to prompt T4 lymphocytes to recognize that they have ingested a pathogen. Once the lymphocytes are aware of the pathogen, they will trigger a specific immune response.

ILs are one type of *cytokine,* a protein released by macrophages to trigger the immune response (see the discussion of cytokines later in this section). Some of the multiple functions of IL-1 include increasing the temperature set point in the hypothalamus; increasing serotonin in the brainstem and duodenum, causing sleep and nausea, respectively; stimulating the production of prostaglandins, leading to a decrease in the pain threshold, resulting in myalgias and arthralgias; increasing the synthesis of collagenases, resulting in the destruction of cartilage; and, most important, kicking the T4 cells into action.

Macrophages also participate in the defense against tumor cells and secrete numerous molecules that assist in the immune and inflammatory response. Stimulation of macrophages can boost the immune response.

Eosinophils are the next group of leukocytes that participate in the innate immunity process. Eosinophils are derived from bone marrow and multiply in both allergic disorders and parasitic infestations. When organisms are too large for neutrophils and macrophages, eosinophils get within close proximity of the invading organisms and release the contents of their granules to kill them.

Basophils and *mast cells* are WBCs (leukocytes) that circulate in peripheral blood and function similarly to mast cells in allergic disorders. Basophils and mast cells are located close to blood vessels throughout the body and have similar functional characteristics; *mast cells* contain histamine, which dilates blood vessels when released.

Mast cells are derived from stem cells and travel in the blood in such small numbers that they are not recognized as blood cells. Basophils and mast cells cause an increase in blood supply in the area where the bacteria or viral antigen is located. This increase in circulation brings more phagocytes to the area.

Inflammatory Mediators

The complement system and *interferons* act as mediators of inflammation. Along with phagocytes, they destroy organisms that breach the first line of defense. The complement system consists of 20 proteins that are key components in the acute inflammatory response designed to enhance immune function.

When activated, these proteins interact in a cascade-like process to assist immune cells by coating microorganisms so they can be more easily phagocytosed. They also participate in bacterial lysis. In some cases the invading organisms are eliminated from the body. Sometimes the inflammation produced by the complement cascade (immune response) walls off the microorganism by forming, for example, a cyst or tubercle that protects the rest of the body from infection.

The second group of mediators is the cytokines, especially interferons. They act as messengers, both within the immune system and between the immune system and other systems of the body, forming an integrated network that is highly involved in the regulation of immune responses.[99]

Once a cell becomes infected by a virus, certain genes in the cell that produce interferons are turned on. Interferons coat the surrounding, uninfected cells, making them viral resistant.

Natural Killer Cells

Natural killer (NK) cells are large granular lymphocytes that function to kill viruses, other intracellular microbe-infected cells, and tumor cells. NK cells respond by releasing cytotoxic granules and by secreting cytokines.[81]

Acquired Immunity

To establish an infection, the pathogen must first overcome numerous surface barriers and the innate immune responses (see Fig. 4.1). In these cases, acquired immunity is tailored to recognize each different type of organism and kill it.

The two types of acquired immune responses that occur are *humoral immunity* and *cell-mediated immunity*. Although these two responses are often discussed separately, they are two arms of the immune system and work together; failure in one can alter the effectiveness of the other. These two types of responses overlap and interact considerably, but the distinction is useful in understanding how the immune system is activated.

Humoral Immunity

The humoral immune response is mediated by antibodies present in different body fluids, such as saliva, blood, or vaginal secretions, such as those produced by B lymphocytes. *B lymphocytes,* or *B cells,* are called such because they originate in the bone marrow and then circulate throughout the extracellular fluid. Antibodies produced by B lymphocytes are very effective against organisms that are free floating in the body that can be easily reached and neutralized.

The surface of B lymphocytes is coated with *immunoglobulin* (Ig), and each B cell has a receptor (an antibody) that can recognize a specific foreign substance or antigen. When this happens, B cells change into protein-synthesizing cells known as *plasma cells* and *memory B cells.*

The plasma cell produces and secretes into body fluids a specific antibody to that antigen. Memory cells produced in connection with humoral immunity circulate among the blood, lymphoid system, and tissues for about 1 year or even longer. They are responsible for the more rapid and sustained (stronger) immune response that occurs with repeated exposure to the same antigen. This humoral response is particularly useful in fighting bacterial infections.

The type of antibody produced depends on genetic variability, the specific antigenic stimulus, and whether it is a first or subsequent exposure to that antigen. The humoral immune response is more rapid than the cell-mediated response and is more often a factor in resistance to acute bacterial infections. Humoral immunity can be transmitted to another person, either by inoculation or by maternal transfer via placenta or breast milk. This transfer is called *passive immunity.*

Cell-Mediated Immunity

Some organisms (all viruses and some bacteria) actually hide inside cells, where antibodies cannot reach them. A second arm of the immune system, called *cell-mediated immunity,* uses T lymphocytes, which can recognize hidden organisms, search them out, and destroy them on a cell-to-cell basis.

Lymphocytes originate from stem cells in the bone marrow and differentiate or mature into either B or T cells. T lymphocytes, or T cells, are called such because the precursors of these cells start from the bone marrow but then mature in the thymus, located right behind the sternum, where they learn to discriminate self from nonself (Fig. 4.2). Both T and B lymphocytes continuously circulate through blood, lymph, and lymph nodes.

After interaction with a specific antigen, the activated lymphocyte produces numerous additional lymphocytes called *sensitized T cells.* This T-cell subpopulation has several functions, including (1) helping B cells enhance the production of antibodies, (2) activating macrophages and helping them destroy large bacteria, (3) helping other T lymphocytes recognize and destroy virally infected cells, and (4) helping NK cells kill infected cells (Fig. 4.3).

The immune system also consists of regulatory and suppressor T cells (CD4+, CD25+), which suppress activation of the immune system and prevent pathologic self-reactivity, or autoimmune disease. Cell-mediated immunity is responsible for the rejection of transplanted tissue, delayed hypersensitivity reactions (e.g., contact dermatitis), and some autoimmune diseases. Cell-mediated immunity is the basis for many skin tests (e.g., tuberculin test, allergy testing). Cellular immunity cannot be transferred passively to another person.

Conditions known to affect T-cell number or responsiveness include HIV infection, acquired immunodeficiency syndrome (AIDS), stress, malignancy, general anesthesia, thermal injury, surgery, diabetes, and immunosuppressive drugs (including corticosteroids). Older adults (aged 65 years and older) show reduced numbers of circulating lymphocytes, and malnourished people show defects in most tests of T-cell function.

Summary of the Immune Response

The immune system has evolved to protect multicellular organisms from a vast array of threats. Immunology is the study of how the immune system works and the consequences of its dysfunction. Through past and present research on various immune response mechanisms, ways in which the immune

Major lymphoid organs

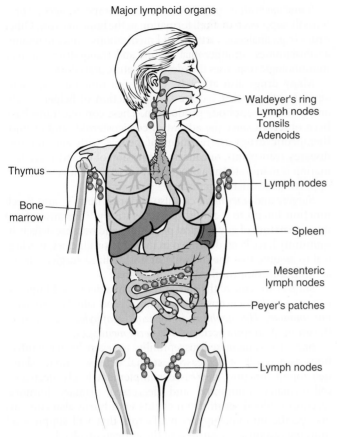

FIG. 4.2 Immune system. Organs of the immune system are referred to as *lymphoid tissues*. The bone marrow and thymus are referred to as primary lymphoid organs, because these organs are the central sites of all cells of the immune system and B- and T-cell differentiation, respectively. Immature lymphocytes migrate through the central lymphoid tissues and later reside as mature lymphocytes in the peripheral or secondary lymphoid tissues (e.g., lymph nodes, Peyer's patches, tonsils, spleen, mucosa-associated lymphoid tissue [MALT] from the mouth to the rectum). (From Damjanov I: Pathology for the health-related professions, ed 4, St. Louis, 2012, Saunders.)

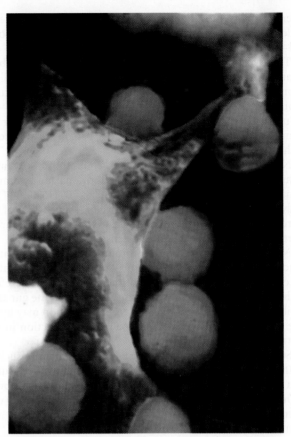

FIG. 4.3 T cells. The *purple spheres* seen in this scanning electron microscope view are T cells attacking a much larger cancer cell. T cells are a significant part of our defense against cancer and other types of foreign cells. (From Patton KT, Thibodeau GA: The human body in health and disease, ed 6, St. Louis, 2014, Mosby.)

system can be manipulated to benefit the host are being discovered. The principal function of the immune system is to eliminate infectious agents and abnormal "self" components (e.g., cancer cells) without attacking the body's own tissues. The immune system must maintain a state of balance such that when an external or internal threat is encountered, an appropriate response is generated to control the invader, and then the system returns to equilibrium. This encounter with a particular insult educates the immune system to produce memory so that upon reencountering a foreign invader, it reacts more rapidly and with a stronger response.

Most pathogens and antigens are encountered after they have been inhaled or ingested (see Fig. 4.2).[34]

Keeping in mind that innate immunity and acquired immunity function in tandem—and that within the acquired immune system humoral immunity and cellular immunity are also working simultaneously—a variety of immune responses can occur when an extracellular pathogen attempts to invade the body.

If the pathogenic organism gets past the first line of defense (innate immunity) and is presented to the body, the following can happen: (1) a B lymphocyte recognizes it as a bacterium and produces antibodies that bind to it and neutralize it (humoral response), (2) a T lymphocyte recognizes it as a bacterium and produces cytokines to help the macrophages lyse and phagocytose the bacteria (cell-mediated response), (3) in the case of a virus, a cytotoxic T lymphocyte can recognize the cell and destroy it (cell-mediated response), and (4) the complement system can recognize the invading organism and destroy it (innate immunity).

Dysfunction of the immune system can contribute to diseases. Two types of genetic alterations could lead to abnormalities: (1) mutations that inactivate the receptors or signaling molecules involved in innate immune recognition, and (2) mutations that render them active all the time. The first type of mutation would result in immunodeficiencies. The second type of mutation triggers antiinflammatory reactions and thereby contributes to a variety of conditions with an inflammatory component (e.g., asthma, allergy, arthritis, autoimmune diseases).[96]

FACTORS AFFECTING IMMUNITY

In addition to the effects of aging, other factors can affect the immune system. These factors may include nutrition; environmental pollution and exposure to chemicals that influence the host defense; prior or ongoing trauma or illnesses; medications;

splenectomy (removal of the spleen); influences of the enteric, endocrine, and neurochemical systems; stress; and psychosocial–spiritual well-being and socioeconomic status.

These factors, as well as clinical conditions that contribute to an immunocompromised state, are listed in Box 4.1. Sleep deprivation has also been shown to have important effects—similar to the effects of stress on the immune system—by reducing cellular immunity.[11,119] Some factors do not alter the immune system directly but increase a person's exposure to pathogens.

New information is being discovered about the sensory functions of the intestine and how neural, hormonal, and immune signals interact. The gut immune system has 70% to 80% of the body's immune cells, and the protective blocking action of the secretory response in the gut is crucial to the integrity of the GI tract immune function and host defense.[13]

Nutritional status can have a profound effect on immune function. Nutrients have fundamental and regulatory influences on the immune response of the GI tract and therefore on host defense. Reduction of normal bacteria in the gut after antibiotic treatment or in the presence of infection may interfere with the nutrients available for immune function in the GI tract.

Severe deficits in calories, protein intake, or vitamins such as vitamin A or vitamin E can lead to deficiencies in T-cell function and numbers. Deficient zinc intake can profoundly depress both T- and B-cell function. Zinc is required for at least 70 different enzymes, some of which are found in lymphocytes and are necessary for their function.

Dietary changes may alter aspects of immunity, although research in this area is ongoing. In addition, morbid obesity may alter the immune system by creating a vulnerability to certain diseases, including cancer.

BOX 4.1   Factors Affecting Immunity

Factors That Alter the Immune System
- Aging
- Sex and hormonal influences
- Nutrition and malnutrition
- Environmental pollution
- Exposure to toxic chemicals
- Trauma
- Burns
- Sleep disturbance
- Presence of concurrent illnesses and diseases
  - Malignancy
  - Diabetes mellitus
  - Chronic renal failure
  - Human immunodeficiency virus (HIV) infection
- Medications, immunosuppressive drugs
- Hospitalization, surgery, general anesthesia
- Splenectomy
- Stress, psychosocial–spiritual well-being, socioeconomic status

Factors That Increase Exposure to Pathogens
- Iatrogenic factors
  - Urinary catheters
  - Nasogastric tubes
  - Endotracheal tubes
  - Chest tubes
  - Intracranial pressure monitor
  - External fixation devices
  - Implanted prostheses
  - Sexual practices

Some *medications* (e.g., cancer chemotherapeutic agents) profoundly suppress blood cell formation in the bone marrow. Other drugs (e.g., analgesics, antithyroid medications, anticonvulsants, antihistamines, antimicrobial agents, and tranquilizers) induce immunologic responses that destroy mature granulocytes.

Many drugs also affect B- and T-cell function, especially against antigens that require the interaction of helper T cells and B cells for antibody production. These complications have been observed since the advent of corticosteroids and chemotherapeutic drugs as treatment of people with autoimmune diseases, transplants, or cancer. Depression of B- and T-cell formation is manifested as a progressive increase in infections with opportunistic microorganisms.

Surgery and *anesthesia* can also suppress both T- and B-cell function for up to 1 month postoperatively.[91] Because of the invasive nature of any surgical procedure and because defects in immunity have been described in most major illnesses, it is logical to assume that the majority of hospitalized surgical clients are immunocompromised to some degree.

Surgery to remove the spleen results in a depressed humoral response against encapsulated bacteria, especially *Streptococcus pneumoniae, Haemophilus influenzae, Staphylococcus aureus,* the group A streptococci, and *Neisseria meningitidis.*

Burns cause increased susceptibility to severe bacterial infections as a result of decreased external defenses (intact skin), neutrophil function, decreased complement levels, decreased cell-mediated immunity, and decreased primary humoral responses. Blood serum from clients with burns also contains nonspecific immunosuppressive factors that will suppress all immune responses, regardless of the antigen involved.

The relationship among *stress, psychosocial–spiritual well-being,* and *socioeconomic status* and susceptibility to disease through depressed immune function has become an area of intense research interest. In the past there were anecdotal reports of increased incidence of infection, diseases, and malignancy associated with periods of both intense and relatively minor stress.

EXERCISE IMMUNOLOGY

The effect of physical activity and exercise (aerobic, endurance, and resistance) on the immune and neuroimmune systems has been an area of research interest. A brief summary of the results is presented here, but a more detailed accounting of exercise and the immune system and future direction for studies is available.[5,105]

Depending on the intensity, activity or exercise can enhance or suppress immune function. In essence, the immune system is enhanced during moderate exercise. Moreover, regular, moderate physical activity can prevent the neuroendocrine and detrimental immunologic effects of stress.[43]

In contrast to the beneficial effects of moderate exercise on the immune system, strenuous or intense exercise or long-duration exercise such as marathon running is followed by impairment of the immune system. Intense exercise can suppress the concentration of lymphocytes, suppress NK cell activity, and leave the host open to microbial agents, especially viruses, which can invade during this open window of opportunity and may lead to infections.

Extreme and long-duration strenuous exercise appears to lead to deleterious oxidation of cellular macromolecules. The oxidation of DNA is important because the oxidative modifications of DNA bases are mutagenic and have been implicated in a variety of diseases, including aging and cancer.[112]

Effect on Neutrophils and Macrophages

Exercise triggers a rise in blood levels of neutrophils (PMNs) and stimulates phagocytic activity of neutrophils and macrophages. The exercise-evoked increase in the PMN count is greater if the exercise has an eccentric component, such as downhill running. If the exercise goes beyond 30 minutes, a second—or delayed—rise in PMNs occurs over the next 2 to 4 hours while the exerciser is at rest.

This delayed rise in PMNs is probably the result of cortisol, which spurs release of PMNs from the bone marrow and hinders the exit of PMNs from the bloodstream.[95] After brief, gentle exercise, the PMN count soon returns to baseline, but after prolonged, strenuous exercise, this return to normal may take 24 hours or longer.[40]

Effect on Natural Killer Cells

Most researchers agree that the number of NK cells and the function or activity of these cells in the blood increase during and immediately after exercise of various types, duration, and intensity.[5]

This phenomenon, referred to as *NK enhancement,* is temporary and seems to be the result of a surge in epinephrine levels and from cytokines released during exercise. NK enhancement by exercise occurs in everyone regardless of sex, age, or level of fitness training. Once a person is accustomed to a given exercise level, however, the NK enhancement falls off, suggesting it is a response not to exercise per se, but to physiologic stress.

After intense exercise of long duration the concentration of NK cells and NK cytolytic activity declines below preexercise values. Maximal reduction in NK cell concentrations and lower NK cell activity occurs 2 to 4 hours after exercise.[5] Although this depression in NK cell count seems too brief to have major practical importance for health, there may be a cumulative adverse effect in athletes who induce these changes several times per week. Further study is warranted before specific exercise guidelines are determined.[134]

Effect on Inflammatory Response

Regular moderate exercise as well as resistance training and long-lasting endurance exercise is known to induce proinflammatory cytokines.[53] Brisk exercise (even brief, heavy exertion such as maximal bicycle ergometry for 30 or 60 seconds) increases the WBC count in proportion to the effort.[44,103] This exercise-induced increase in WBCs (including lymphocytes and NK cells) is largely the result of the mechanical effects of an increased cardiac output and the physiologic effects of a surge in serum epinephrine concentration. The number of cells that enter the circulation is determined by the intensity of the stimulus.[5]

The number of lymphocytes in circulation increases during exercise but decreases below the normal levels for several hours after intense exercise. Decreased numbers of lymphocytes are associated with decreased lymphocyte responsiveness and antibody response to several antigens after intense exercise.[73]

Effect on Cytokines

Strenuous exercise, defined as exercising at a minimum of 80% of maximal oxygen consumption ($\dot{V}O_{2max}$), can suppress immune function.

Regular exercise protects against diseases associated with chronic low-grade systemic inflammation, however. This long-term effect of exercise may be ascribed to the antiinflammatory response elicited by a short-term bout of exercise.[109]

4.1 Special Implications for the PTA: Exercise Immunology

PTAs use exercise in the treatment of patients of all ages with a variety of clinical problems, thereby influencing immune function. Exercise as a means of preventing illness and attaining a healthy lifestyle and as an intervention tool in immunodeficiency states is becoming a larger part of preventive services. Research in the area of exercise immunology is growing. Keeping abreast of research results is the first step to examining the clinical implications in this area.

Aged adults constitute a growing and important consumer group of therapy services. Because immune function declines with advancing age, it is important that we understand the effects of exercise on immune function. Very few absolute guidelines have been developed; it seems that intense or strenuous exercise may be detrimental to the immune system, whereas a lifetime of moderate exercise and physical activity enhances immune function. Further research is needed to clarify or modify this guideline.

It takes 6 to 24 hours for the immune system to recover from the acute effects of severe exercise. Each individual client must be evaluated after exercise to determine the perceived intensity of the exercise or intervention session. For example, in the deconditioned older adult with compromised cardiopulmonary function, reduced oxygen transport, and impaired mobility, ambulating from the bed to the bathroom may be perceived by his or her body as strenuous exercise.

Although intense exercise causes suppression of immune parameters in young subjects, data from aged animals[73,74] and human beings[75] show that intense exercise has no detrimental effect on immune function or rate of infections in older adults. Thus relatively intense exercise programs may be prescribed that could maximize cardiopulmonary and musculoskeletal function without impairing immune function in frail elderly people.

Nevertheless, intense exercise during an infectious episode should be avoided. A "neck check" should be conducted for anyone—especially a competitive athlete—who wonders whether to exercise in the presence of an acute viral or bacterial infection.

If the symptoms are located above the neck—such as a stuffy or runny nose, sneezing, or a scratchy throat—exercise should be performed cautiously through the scheduled workout at half-speed. If after 10 minutes the symptoms are alleviated, the workout can be finished with the usual amount of frequency, intensity, and duration. If instead the symptoms are worse and the head is pounding or throbbing with every footstep, the exercise program should be stopped and the person should rest. If a fever or symptoms below the neck are evident, such as aching muscles, a hacking cough, diarrhea, or vomiting, exercise should not be initiated.[40]

IMMUNODEFICIENCY DISEASES

In immunodeficiency the immune response is absent or depressed as a result of a primary or secondary disorder. Primary immunodeficiency reflects a defect involving T cells, B cells, or lymphoid tissues. Secondary immunodeficiency results from an underlying disease or factor that depresses or blocks the immune response.

Primary Immunodeficiency

The recognition of impaired immunity in children 50 years ago has resulted in a tremendous increase in knowledge of the functions of the immune system. More than 95 inherited immunodeficiency disorders have now been identified. Genetically determined immunodeficiency can cause increased susceptibility to infection, autoimmunity, and increased risk of cancer.

The defects may affect one or more components of the immune system, including T cells, B cells, NK cells, phagocytic cells, and complement proteins. No further discussion of these conditions is included in this book because the PTA rarely encounters these congenital conditions. A review of the pathophysiology of primary immunodeficiency is available.[16]

Secondary Immunodeficiency

Secondary immunodeficiency disorders, such as leukemia and Hodgkin's disease, follow and result from an earlier disease or event. Defects in the immune defenses occur in viral infections, other infections, malnutrition, alcoholism, aging, autoimmune disease, diabetes mellitus, cancer, chronic disease, steroid therapy, cancer chemotherapy, and radiation. More specific causes such as AIDS also contribute to secondary immunodeficiency.

Iatrogenic Immunodeficiency

Iatrogenic immunodeficiency refers to immunodeficiency caused by a physician, such as occurs with immunosuppressive drugs, radiation therapy, or splenectomy. Immunosuppressive drugs include cytotoxic drugs, corticosteroids, cyclosporine, and antilymphocyte serum or antithymocyte globulin.

Cytotoxic drugs kill cells while they are replicating, but because most cytotoxic drugs are not selective, all rapidly dividing cells are affected. Not only are lymphocytes and phagocytes eliminated, but these drugs also interfere with lymphocyte synthesis.

Other effects of this nonselectivity of cytotoxic drugs may include bone marrow suppression with neutropenia, anemia, and cytopenia; gonadal suppression with sterility; alopecia; hemorrhagic cystitis; and vomiting, nausea, and stomatitis. The risk of lymphoproliferative malignancy is also increased.

Corticosteroids are used to treat immune-mediated disorders because of their potent antiinflammatory and immunosuppressive effects. Corticosteroids stabilize the vascular membrane, blocking tissue infiltration by neutrophils and monocytes, thus inhibiting inflammation. They also kidnap T cells in the bone marrow, causing lymphopenia.

Cyclosporine (immunosuppressive drug) selectively suppresses the proliferation and development of helper T cells, resulting in depressed cell-mediated immunity. This drug is used primarily to prevent rejection of organ transplants but is also being investigated for use in several other disorders.

Radiation therapy is cytotoxic to most lymphocytes, inducing profound lymphopenia, which results in immunosuppression. Irradiation of all major lymph node areas—a procedure known as *total nodal irradiation*—is used to treat disorders such as Hodgkin's lymphoma. It is being investigated for its effectiveness in severe rheumatoid arthritis and lupus nephritis and the prevention of kidney transplant rejection.

Splenectomy increases a person's susceptibility to infection, especially with pyogenic bacteria such as *S. pneumoniae*.

Consequences of Immunodeficiency

People who are immunocompromised from any of the immunodeficiency disorders are at increased risk for developing infection because their impaired immune system does not provide adequate protection against invading microorganisms. Normal mechanical defense mechanisms may be affected (respiratory, GI systems). Body flora that are normally harmless, such as *Candida,* may become pathogenic and a source of infection.

Additional risk factors for people who are already immunocompromised include poor physiologic and psychologic health status, old age, coexistence of other diseases or conditions, invasive procedures (e.g., surgery, invasive lines), and treatments (e.g., chemotherapy, radiation therapy, bone marrow transplantation).

The weakened immune system can cause the person to become susceptible to common everyday infectious agents, such as influenza viruses.

4.2 Special Implications for the PTA: Infection Control in Immunodeficiency Disorders Although infection control strategies such as handwashing, standard precautions, and disinfection are important for all people treated in the health care system, they are especially critical for individuals whose immune systems are altered by primary immunodeficiency disorders, secondary immunodeficiency disorders, and HIV infection.

It is important that health care providers stop to think about altered defense mechanisms, infectious agents, reservoirs, modes of transmission, and infection control strategies to prevent infection in this population (Fig. 4.4).

Pulmonary complications are common among the immunocompromised, accompanied by poor cough reflexes, an inability to cough effectively, and susceptibility to pulmonary and other opportunistic infections. In addition, these individuals are often debilitated and easily fatigued. Frequent mobilization and body positioning enhance gas exchange and promote comfort while maintaining strength.[31]

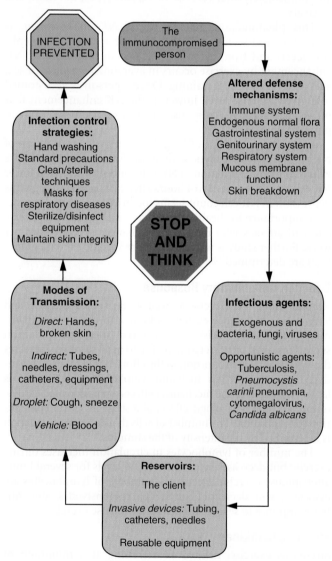

FIG. 4.4 Factors affecting the immunocompromised person, leading to the selection of the correct infection control strategies to prevent infectious complications. (From Schaffer SD, Garzon LS, Heroux DL, et al.: Pocket guide to infection prevention and safe practice, St. Louis, 1996, Mosby.)

Human Immunodeficiency Virus

Overview

HIV is an infection of the immune system. If untreated, it results in progressive and ultimately profound immune suppression. AIDS was first recognized in homosexual men in 1981 (the earliest sample of HIV-infected blood dates back to 1959,[64] but computer analysis suggests an emergence date of 1930[78]).

AIDS is characterized by progressive destruction of cell-mediated (T-cell) immunity and changes in humoral immunity and even elements of autoimmunity.

The resultant immunodeficiency leaves the affected person susceptible to opportunistic infections, including unusual cancers, tuberculosis (TB), and other abnormalities that characterize this syndrome. For example, HIV-positive individuals are nearly 2.5 times more likely than HIV-negative persons to have a recurrence of TB[137] and 8 to 10 times more likely to develop Hodgkin's disease compared with the general population.[84]

In addition, 25% to 40% of Americans with HIV are believed to be infected with the hepatitis C virus (HCV), primarily among injection drug users (IDUs) and those with hemophilia as a result of blood products used to treat the hemophilia.[6] Mortality rates are higher and life expectancy is lower in people with hemophilia who are HIV positive.[110]

Definition

The term *HIV infection* includes the entire spectrum of illness from initial diagnosis to full-blown expression of AIDS. Three distinct points identify this continuum: (1) asymptomatic HIV seropositive, (2) early symptomatic HIV, and (3) HIV advanced disease (AIDS).

Not everyone who is exposed to HIV becomes infected, and not everyone who is infected develops AIDS. The explanation for this phenomenon remains unknown, but researchers have shown that infection with HIV and progression to AIDS are controlled by both host genetic factors and viral factors.

Incidence and Prevalence

Since the first AIDS cases were reported in the United States in 1981, the number of cases and deaths among people with AIDS increased rapidly during the 1980s, followed by substantial declines in new cases and deaths in the late 1990s.

New infections in the United States have declined to an estimated 40,000 per year (down from a peak of 150,000 per year in the mid-1980s). The number of people living with AIDS in the United States is the highest ever reported, at more than 1 million.[145] Deaths from AIDS declined 63% from approximately 52,000 to 19,000 in the late 1990s.[58]

In the United States the greatest impact of the epidemic is among IDUs, sex workers, and men who have sex with men (MSM), with an 8% increase in this last group[54,130,144] and among racial and ethnic minorities.[21] Increases have been observed in the number of cases attributed to heterosexual transmission among minority women and women older than 50 years of age. The total number of people living with AIDS has increased as deaths have declined (Fig. 4.5).[101,144]

Most people diagnosed with AIDS in the United States are aged 20 to 49 years; however, the number of adolescents with HIV in the United States doubles every year. Teens account for one quarter of the cases of new STDs reported

each year, and AIDS in older adults accounts for 11% of all AIDS cases.[101]

Etiologic Factors, Transmission, and Risk Factors

The primary cause of AIDS is the type 1 retrovirus (HIV). Transmission of HIV occurs by exchange of body fluids (notably blood and semen) and is associated with high-risk behaviors.

High-risk behaviors include unprotected anal and oral sex, having six or more sexual partners in the past year, sexual activity with someone known to carry HIV, exchanging sex for money or drugs, or injecting drugs. HIV is not transmitted by fomites (e.g., coffee cups, drinking fountains, or telephone receivers) or casual household or social contact.

As mentioned, injection drug use also continues to play a key role in the HIV epidemic. In some large drug-using communities, HIV seroincidence and seroprevalence among IDUs have declined in recent years.[37] This decline has been attributed to several factors, including increased use of sterile injection equipment, declines in needle sharing, shifts from injection to noninjection methods of using drugs, and cessation of drug use.[2]

Ethnicity is not directly related to increased AIDS risk, but it is associated with other determinants of health status such as poverty, illegal drug use, access to health care, and living in communities with a high prevalence of AIDS. Adolescents are one of the groups at greatest risk for HIV infection, particularly minority inner-city youth. Runaway and homeless youth are especially likely to engage in high-risk

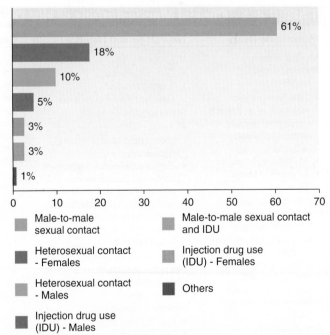

Diagnoses of HIV infection among adults and adolescents, by transmission category, 2010–46 States and 5 U.S. dependent areas, N = 48,079

Male-to-male sexual contact — 61%
Male-to-male sexual contact and IDU — 18%
Heterosexual contact - Females — 10%
Heterosexual contact - Males — 5%
Injection drug use (IDU) - Males — 3%
Injection drug use (IDU) - Females — 3%
Others — 1%

FIG. 4.5 Proportion of acquired immunodeficiency syndrome (AIDS) cases and population by race and ethnicity, reported in 2010 (50 states and Washington, DC). (Reprinted from Centers for Disease Control and Prevention: HIV/AIDS surveillance by race/ethnicity (through 2010).http://www.cdc.gov/hiv/topics/surveillance/resources/slides/race-ethnicity/.)

sexual activity. The use of amphetamines, ecstasy, and amyl nitrate is associated with increased frequency of unprotected anal sex, especially among homosexual and bisexual individuals younger than 23 years of age.[38]

Pathogenesis

The rapid convergence of information from diverse areas of AIDS research makes it impossible to present the most up-to-date information. Scientists are reporting new discoveries daily about the pathogenesis of HIV disease.

The natural history of AIDS begins with infection by the HIV retrovirus detectable only by laboratory tests. This retrovirus predominantly infects human T4 (helper) lymphocytes (also known as *CD4 cells*), the major regulators of the immune response, and destroys or inactivates them. Macrophages and B cells are also infected.

Replication of the virus can cause cell death, although the person remains asymptomatic. Seroconversion (becoming positive for HIV) usually takes place during the first 3 to 6 weeks of this replication process but can take longer. After a few months, very little virus is found in the blood; only HIV antibodies remain in the serum.

During the asymptomatic period (also called the *early stage*), the virus migrates from the serum into the tissues to infect CD4 cells in lymph tissue. The virus continues to kill the CD4 cells in the lymph nodes.

Once all the cells are depleted, the virus again enters the blood to infect any remaining lymphocytes, and clinically apparent disease occurs. By the time this happens, the immune system has been compromised and is ineffective and unable to mount a specific immune response. The immune system dysfunction is even more exaggerated if the host has become further immunocompromised by opportunistic diseases.

The decline in CD4 cells results in progressive loss of immune system function and the development of a wide variety of clinical signs and symptoms (Table 4.1). This describes the middle stage or symptomatic phase of AIDS.

HIV has an extremely high mutation rate even within a single individual, producing competing strains of the same virus that fight for survival against the weapons produced by the immune system. Researchers are studying how different strains of HIV use cell surface molecules, in addition to the CD4 molecule, to bind to and enter target cells.

Clinical Manifestations

HIV infection manifests itself in many different ways (see Table 4.1) and differs between adult and pediatric populations. Great variation exists among individuals as to the amount of time that passes between acute HIV infection, the appearance of symptoms, the diagnosis of AIDS, and death.

Asymptomatic stage (CD4 count of 500 cells/mm³ or more). During the early stage the person demonstrates laboratory evidence of seroconversion (positive for HIV) but remains asymptomatic. Some individuals develop an acute, self-limiting infectious mononucleosis-like illness or a subtle, viral-like syndrome, followed by a period of clinical latency that may last a decade or more.

During the asymptomatic period, the infected person is clinically healthy and capable of normal daily activities, normal work habits, and unrestricted level and duration of exercise. Fatigue and generalized lymphadenopathy with swollen and firm lymph glands may be reported during this stage.

TABLE 4.1 Clinical Manifestations of HIV Disease

Musculoskeletal	Neurologic and Neuromuscular	Cardiopulmonary	Integumentary	Other
Myalgia, arthralgia Rheumatologic manifestations: • Inflammatory joint disorders (e.g., Reiter's syndrome, reactive arthritis, psoriatic arthritis) • Myositis, pyomyositis • Connective tissue disease Avascular necrosis (osteonecrosis) Musculoskeletal pain syndrome, HIV wasting syndrome Myopathy (disease- or drug-induced) Pelvic pain (e.g., pelvic inflammatory disease [PID]) Extrapulmonary tuberculosis Delayed healing (can lead to sepsis and death) Myositis ossificans	HIV encephalitis: • Gait disturbance • Intention tremor • Delayed release of reflexes HIV-associated dementia: • *Behavioral:* Apathy, lethargy, social withdrawal, irritability, depression • *Cognitive:* Memory impairment, confusion, disorientation • *Motor:* Ataxia, leg weakness with gait disturbances, loss of fine motor coordination, incontinence, paraplegia (advanced stage) Guillain–Barré syndrome Headache, seizures (toxoplasmosis) HIV myelitis (osteomyelitis) Radiculopathy Peripheral neuropathy: • Pain (burning tingling • Sensory loss • Secondary motor deficits, gait disturbances • Brachial neuropathy Vacuolar spinal myelopathy	Dyspnea, especially on exertion Nonproductive cough Hypoxia Symptoms associated with opportunistic infections of the pulmonary system Pericardial effusion Cardiomyopathy Endocarditis Vasculitis	Alopecia (hair loss) Basal cell carcinoma Kaposi's sarcoma Mucocutaneous ulcers Rash Urticaria (diffuse skin reaction, wheals) Delayed wound healing	Constitutional symptoms: • Flulike symptoms • Fever, sore throat • Generalized adenopathy • Weight loss • Lethargy, fatigue • Night sweats, fevers Opportunistic infections: • Cytomegalovirus • Bacterial pneumonia • Tuberculosis • Toxoplasmosis • *Pneumocystis carinii* Sinusitis Vaginal infection Malignancy (most common): • Non-Hodgkin's lymphoma • Kaposi's sarcoma • Cervical cancer Gastrointestinal disturbance, including wasting syndrome Lymphedema Lipodystrophy Renal (kidney) failure Hepatic (liver) failure Oral thrush Gingivitis Visual disturbance (DMV) HIV-related psychiatric disorders

Early symptomatic stage (CD4 count of 200 to 500 cells/mm³). As the infection progresses and the immune system becomes increasingly more compromised, a variety of symptoms may develop, including persistent generalized adenopathy; nonspecific symptoms such as diarrhea, weight loss, fatigue, night sweats, and fevers; neurologic symptoms resulting from HIV encephalopathy; or an opportunistic infection.

More than half the adults with HIV in this stage report fatigue that limits physical and recreational activities. Half the adults who report fatigue are unable to attend school or work.[131]

HIV advanced disease (AIDS; CD4 count of 200 cells/mm³ or less). The neurologic manifestations of more advanced HIV disease are numerous and can involve the central nervous system (CNS), the peripheral nervous system (PNS), and the autonomic nervous system (ANS). The CNS appears to be more commonly attacked by HIV than the PNS.

HIV or AIDS encephalopathy, also referred to as *HIV-associated dementia* (HAD), formerly called *AIDS dementia complex,* is a primary infection of the brain by HIV. Symptoms can vary and are listed in Table 4.1. In the most advanced stages of the disease, severe dementia, mutism, incontinence, and paraplegia may occur. A detailed summary of nervous system disorders associated with HIV, including treatment, is available.[48,131,146]

Dermatologic conditions are common and can be extensive, including malignancies; bacterial, viral, and fungal infections (Fig. 4.6); and reactions to drug treatment. Cutaneous manifestations of HIV can include dry flaking skin, telangiectasias, and thinning of the skin (and hair).

The prevalence of conditions such as seborrheic dermatitis, psoriasis, Reiter syndrome, acquired ichthyosis, Kaposi's sarcoma, and scabies is on the rise. Kaposi's sarcoma (purple nodular skin lesions) predominantly affects homosexual men (Fig. 4.7). HIV-associated nutritional disorders may also contribute to nail and hair changes. HIV-associated wounds may occur as a result of Kaposi's sarcoma, herpes simplex virus, syphilis, injection drug use, *Candida* and fungal infections, postoperative infections, and herpes zoster.[61]

Pain syndromes. Pain syndromes seen in HIV-infected individuals are divided into three groups: pain directly related to HIV infection or immunosuppression, pain caused by HIV diagnostic procedures and treatment, and pain unrelated to AIDS or its treatment.

Painful sensory peripheral neuropathy is the most commonly reported pain syndrome, followed by pain associated with extensive Kaposi's sarcoma and other dermatologic conditions, headache, abdominal pain, chest pain, and arthralgias and myalgias. Women infected with HIV experience pain more often and with greater intensity than men; women also have unique gynecologic syndromes related to opportunistic infections and cancers of the pelvis and genitourinary tract.[141]

Peripheral neuropathy, disease- or drug-induced myopathy, and musculoskeletal pain syndromes occur most often in advanced stages of HIV disease but can occur at any stage of HIV infection and may be the presenting manifestation.

Peripheral neuropathies affect a large portion of people with AIDS and are usually distal, symmetric, and predominantly sensory, but other parts of the body may be affected, such as the face or trunk. Peripheral neuropathies generally manifest in a stocking-glove distribution, with the feet and legs most commonly affected. Involvement of the upper extremities is less common and often occurs much later in the disease process.

AIDS is associated with *neuromusculoskeletal diseases* such as osteomyelitis, bacterial myositis, and infectious (reactive) arthritis. Osteonecrosis, osteopenia, and osteoporosis are increasingly observed in clients with HIV disease. Avascular necrosis (osteonecrosis) of the femoral head(s) has been reported.

Musculoskeletal pain syndromes are associated with the wasting process in AIDS, referred to as *HIV wasting syndrome.* HIV wasting is characterized by a disproportionate loss of metabolically active tissue, specifically body cell mass. These conditions occur secondary to low food intake, altered metabolism, and poor nutrient absorption, with manifestations such as extreme weight loss, chronic diarrhea, unexplained weakness, fever, and malnutrition.

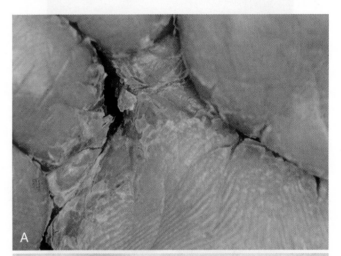

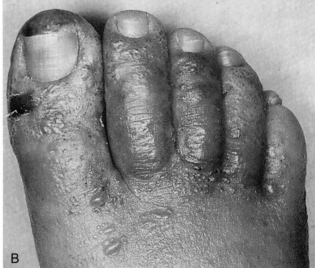

FIG. 4.6 Tinea pedis. (A) Fungal infections such as tinea pedis (also known as athlete's foot) often begin between the toes and extend to the surface of the toes and foot. Red, itching skin may begin to peel or cause foot odor. (B) The condition can progress, as shown here. Skin changes can become even more severe, with complete destruction of the nail beds (not shown). (A, From Lemmi FO, Lemmi CAE: Physical assessment findings CD-ROM, Philadelphia, 2000, Saunders. B, From Cohen J, Powderly WG: Infectious diseases, ed 2, St. Louis, 2004, Mosby.)

Rheumatologic manifestations are transient or subtle and appear more often as HIV disease progresses. The arthritis can be severe and does not necessarily respond to conventional medications. Polymyositis involves bilaterally symmetric proximal muscle weakness, and arthritis may precede or accompany seroconversion.

HIV-associated myopathy manifests as a progressive painless weakness in the proximal limb muscles. The weakness is symmetric and often involves the muscles of the face and neck. This type of myopathy may occur in individuals with HIV at every stage of illness.

Lipodystrophy or *lipodystrophic syndrome* (LDS), a syndrome of defective fat metabolism, dyslipidemia, and insulin resistance, manifests as central fat accumulation (Fig. 4.8)

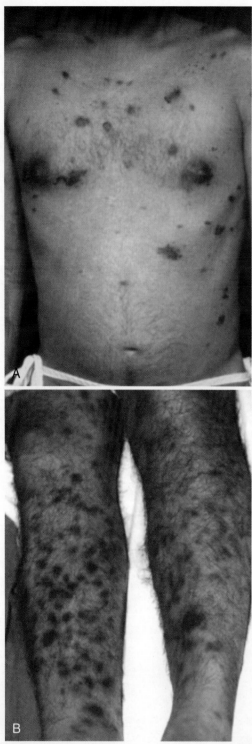

FIG. 4.7 (A) Kaposi's sarcoma. There is a reduced incidence of Kaposi's sarcoma in the human immunodeficiency virus (HIV)–infected population because of better treatment, so fewer people progress this far in the disease. With better treatment have come fewer complications. Kaposi's sarcoma appears primarily in the upper body, sometimes starting as a bulbous lesion on the end of the nose but also involving the face, chest, and lymph nodes. (B) Kaposi's sarcoma is not limited to the upper body and can also appear in the lower quadrant. (Courtesy Julie Hobbs, Kingwood MEDICAL Center, Clingwood, TX.)

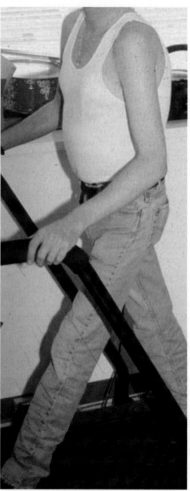

FIG. 4.8 Lipodystrophic syndrome (LDS) in clients with human immunodeficiency virus (HIV) and acquired immunodeficiency syndrome (AIDS) has become more prevalent as a result of highly active antiretroviral therapy (HAART) treatment. LDS with cardiac complications from hyperlipidemia affects men and women, with fat deposits in the upper body and breasts contributing to body image problems, emotional trauma, and cardiac involvement. Additional fat deposits in the upper thoracic area and abdomen with loss in the extremities are seen in this client with AIDS. (Courtesy Julie Hobbs, Kingwood Medical Center, Kingwood, TX.)

with visceral fat deposition documented by computed tomographic scans. It is a common problem that occurs soon after starting highly active antiretroviral therapy (HAART). Loss of fat occurs in the arms, legs, or face, with concomitant fat deposits in the abdomen, breasts (men and women), and back of the neck.

AIDS-related lymphomas (ARLs), including Burkitt's lymphoma, non-Hodgkin's lymphoma, Hodgkin's lymphoma, and other more uncommon types (e.g., primary effusion lymphoma), are more likely to occur in HIV-infected people than in the general population. ARLs are now the second most common cancer associated with HIV after Kaposi's sarcoma and increase with time after infection. The incidence of non-Hodgkin's lymphoma appears to be declining with the use of HAART, whereas the incidence of Hodgkin's lymphoma may actually have increased in the HIV-infected population.[84]

Cardiopulmonary diseases continue to be an important cause of illness and death in people with HIV infection. Bacterial pneumonia, bronchitis, TB (pulmonary and extrapulmonary), and cytomegalovirus (CMV) infection are common opportunistic diseases in the HIV/AIDS population. Emphysema, asthma, and pulmonary hypertension are also observed in this population.

Cardiac involvement (heart and blood vessels) occurs as a result of a combination of the HIV infection, medical management, and secondary opportunistic infections.

Cardiovascular diseases have become a major cause of mortality among HIV-infected people who respond well to antiretroviral therapy. Myocardial infarction, cardiomyopathy, pericardial effusion, and pericarditis are some other cardiovascular conditions that occur as a result of HIV and/or its treatment. There is increasing evidence to suggest that cardiovascular disease appears earlier and more often among HIV-infected adults than in the general public.[66,97]

Medical Management

Prevention

HIV prevention in the United States has placed the primary focus on persons who are not HIV infected to help them avoid becoming infected. Reducing sexual and drug-using risk behavior has been the main emphasis of public health prevention programs. The overarching HIV prevention goals of the Centers for Disease Control and Prevention (CDC) are to reduce the number of new HIV infections and to eliminate racial and ethnic disparities by promoting HIV counseling, testing, and referral and by encouraging HIV prevention among persons living with HIV and those at high risk for contracting the virus.[145]

However, further reduction of HIV transmission will require new strategies, including increased emphasis on appropriate routine screening, identification of new cases, partner notification, increased availability of sustained treatment, and prevention services for those infected. The addition of a simple, rapid HIV test may help overcome some of the traditional barriers to early diagnosis and treatment of infected persons. The CDC also recommends routine HIV testing of all pregnant women and routine screening of any infant whose mother was not screened.[15,69]

Diagnosis

Early diagnosis is important so that early and preventive therapies may be initiated and sex partners can be notified of their risk of HIV and the subsequent need for HIV testing. To establish uniformity in reporting AIDS cases, the CDC has established diagnostic criteria for the confirmation of AIDS.

The most commonly performed screening test is the HIV-1 antibody enzyme immunoassay test, an antibody test to indicate HIV infection indirectly by revealing HIV antibodies (indicating exposure to the virus). However, antibody testing is not always reliable because the body takes a variable amount of time to produce a detectable level of antibodies. Consequently, a person with HIV could test negative for HIV antibodies. Antibody tests are also unreliable in neonates because transferred maternal antibodies persist for 6 to 10 months. The Western blot test is a more expensive test that may be used when there is a concern about false-positive results.

Treatment

No cure has been found for AIDS, but advances in treatment have successfully transformed AIDS into a manageable chronic condition. The national HIV Vaccine Trials Network has been established to develop and test possible vaccine compounds, but an effective vaccine is not imminent. Until a vaccine is available, the goals of intervention are to stop HIV from replicating, increase the number of CD4 cells, and delay HIV disease progression.

Current efforts are focused on (1) simplifying the drug regimens to improve adherence (once-daily dosing), (2) developing alternatives for those in whom the current medications have failed, (3) preventing viral rebound (return of high levels of the virus when drugs are discontinued), and (4) managing the wide range of pharmacologic side effects.

Development of drug resistance is the inevitable consequence of incomplete suppression of virus plasma levels in individuals with HIV treated with HAART. Noncompliance with the drug regimen, which involves taking multiple drugs throughout the day, can lead to mutation of the virus and resistance to the treatment. Drug resistance is one of the most significant threats to effective therapy.

Potential toxicities from drug treatment include metabolic disorders (e.g., LDS), avascular necrosis of the femoral head(s), and lactic acidosis. There is no known treatment to stop treatment-induced osteonecrosis.

Palliative treatment may include nonsteroidal antiinflammatory drugs (NSAIDs) and pain medications. Surgical procedures to improve blood flow to the affected area or joint replacement to improve function may be considered. When present, dyslipidemia may be associated with accelerated atherosclerosis and insulin resistance, contributing to increased cardiovascular morbidity and mortality rates in the population with HIV.[53,80]

Nonpharmacologic intervention includes nutritional therapy, exercise, mental health support, and alternative or complementary interventions. AIDS-associated weight loss, nutritional deficiencies, loss of muscle mass (wasting syndrome), and other effects contribute to immune dysfunction, faster disease progression in some people, and a variety of complications that can be ameliorated with proper nutrition. The use of alternative and complementary intervention techniques remains an area of controversy and investigation.

Prognosis

AIDS has changed from an acute to a subacute chronic illness. The development of combination therapies is extending the lives of AIDS clients, keeping many healthy enough to avoid hospitalization and/or return to their baseline after illness, extending survival, and even resulting in return to work status for some people. People with AIDS are living longer with lower CD4 levels because of prophylaxis, improved supportive care, and treatment.

Changes in treatment rather than changes in human behavior account for the decline in AIDS-related deaths.[111]

4.3 Special Implications for the PTA: Acquired Immune Deficiency Syndrome With advances in treatment, improved care, and longer survival, PTAs can expect to see increasing numbers of people in their practices who may have HIV infection. Maximal effectiveness from physical therapy requires a PTA who is knowledgeable about HIV disease and the unique rehabilitation issues surrounding individuals with HIV or AIDS.[128]

It is possible for individuals with HIV infection or AIDS to come to a therapy practice undiagnosed or unwilling to provide this information. Women who have been attacked or are the victims of domestic violence have an increased risk of HIV transmission and do not always report this information.

It is important to include questions in the history that consider the possibility of sexual violence and HIV-related disease and correlate this information with objective evaluation results. For example, anyone with musculoskeletal or neuromuscular symptoms of unknown origin (with or without constitutional symptoms) should be interviewed more specifically about the presence of past or current HIV risk behaviors. This may potentially lead to early medical referral, early diagnosis, and early appropriate therapy. Early treatment choices will also determine future therapies because of viral resistance and other factors.

Health care providers who routinely assess the HIV and sexually transmitted disease (STD) risks of their clients can encourage at-risk MSM to be tested annually for HIV, syphilis, gonorrhea, and chlamydia and to accept or seek vaccination against hepatitis A and hepatitis B virus (HBV).[153] Providing a discreet and nonjudgmental environment with the assurance of confidentiality while emphasizing the importance of disclosing accurate risk information may help facilitate risk disclosure from young MSM.

Clients at all stages of HIV infection need psychosocial support to deal with depression, anxiety, and other emotional problems that can develop as the person's condition changes. Screening for depression and anxiety is essential; referral for further treatment may be indicated. PTAs also may have a role in osteoporosis education, prevention, and screening. Risk factor assessment is advised for anyone with HIV infection. Anyone at high risk for osteopenia or osteoporosis should be referred for dual x-ray absorptiometry measurement of bone mineral density. Clients should be encouraged to minimize risk for developing osteoporosis with dietary calcium and vitamin D intake, maintaining a normal body mass index, avoiding tobacco and alcohol abuse, and maintaining a long-term weight-bearing exercise program.[117]

Prevention of Transmission

Health care workers may be concerned about potential contact in the workplace with clients who have AIDS; however, the risk of transmission of the virus from client to health care worker is exceedingly small.

Sources of HIV that may pose a risk of transmission through these routes include blood and visibly bloody fluids, tissues, and other body fluids, including semen, vaginal secretions, and cerebrospinal, synovial, pleural, peritoneal, pericardial, and amniotic fluids. In addition, any direct cutaneous or mucosal contact—without barrier protection—with concentrated HIV in a research laboratory or production facility is considered to be an exposure.[92]

In the absence of visible blood in the saliva, exposure to saliva from a person with HIV is not thought to pose a risk for HIV transmission. Exposure to tears, sweat, or nonbloody urine or feces from individuals with the virus does not constitute exposure to HIV. Occupational exposure to breast milk does not constitute an exposure unless ingested directly.[92]

Health care considerations are primarily directed at preventing the transmission of the virus when caring for someone with AIDS by avoiding occupational blood exposure. Recommendations for preventing the spread of the virus consist of the use of standard precautions.

Specific recommendations for health care professionals working with AIDS and HIV-positive clients are included in Box 4.2. Everyone with AIDS is immunodeficient, and every precaution must be taken to prevent infection in that person.

An individual with HIV does not need a private room unless he or she has a communicable disease that requires respiratory isolation. Hepatitis necessitates standard precautions but not isolation. The virus is not transmitted through casual, nonintimate contact or social encounters such as eating in restaurants or using public transportation or public bathroom facilities because the virus does not live long or replicate outside the body.

There are no documented cases of HIV being transmitted during participation in sports. The very low risk of transmission during sports participation would involve sports with direct body contact in which bleeding might be expected to occur. There is no risk of HIV transmission through sports activities in which bleeding does not occur. Athletes in contact and collision sports are at greater risk for HBV transmission and should be vaccinated against this virus.[79]

Postexposure Prophylaxis

HIV postexposure prophylaxis (PEP) is a form of secondary HIV prevention that may reduce the incidence of HIV infections.[107] The two types of PEP are occupational and nonoccupational. Occupational exposure should be considered an urgent medical concern requiring timely postexposure management.[23]

Occupational HIV PEP is an accepted form of therapy for health care workers exposed to HIV through their jobs.[24] Health care providers caring for persons with occupationally acquired HIV infection or who have acquired HIV themselves through occupational exposure should contact their state health department and follow guidelines.

Well-established U.S. national guidelines for occupational HIV PEP exist. No national guidelines are available for nonoccupational HIV PEP, after nonconsensual sexual intercourse (sexual abuse and assault), injection drug use, or needlestick and sharp injuries in non–health care providers.[98] Health care providers with occupational exposure to HIV should receive follow-up counseling, postexposure testing, and medical evaluation regardless of whether they receive PEP.

Follow-up care provided to exposed health care providers is important, including follow-up testing, monitoring, and counseling—especially psychologic counseling for those with needlestick exposure or exposure to blood or body fluid. Exposed health care providers are advised to use precautions to prevent secondary transmission, especially during the first 6 to 12 weeks postexposure (e.g., avoid blood or tissue donations, breastfeeding, or pregnancy). Other guidelines for HIV PEP are available.[23,98,107]

HIV and Rehabilitative Therapy

Over the past 20 years, the rehabilitation of the person with HIV or AIDS has changed significantly. In the middle of the 1980s, the person with AIDS often developed *Pneumocystis pneumonia* (PCP) and/or other opportunistic infections and quickly succumbed.

During this period, the PTA's role was primarily that of pain control, energy conservation, and instruction in the use of adaptive equipment to maximize functional ability. Today prophylactic medications are highly effective in the prevention of PCP and many other opportunistic infections and HIV-associated conditions.

Chronic conditions such as cardiovascular disease related to LDS and rheumatologic and musculoskeletal conditions are much more common in those living with HIV. Therefore PTAs are generally focused on assisting the individual with the management of physical dysfunctions related to this chronic disease.

From a rehabilitation point of view, HIV is considered a chronic illness on a continuum (i.e., from being asymptomatic to exhibiting mild to severe symptoms) rather than a terminal illness. The individual with HIV disease may demonstrate clinical manifestations of overlapping pathologic processes and HIV-related physical disabilities that necessitate appropriate rehabilitation intervention.

In addition to physical fitness and strength training, PTAs must look at quality-of-life issues; work simplification; activities of daily living (ADLs), including community management skills such as access to transportation, socialization opportunities, shopping, banking, and ability to negotiate health care and insurance systems[48]; and participation in church, synagogue, or other spiritual network. Home programs must be simple and easily incorporated into ADLs.

Often individuals with AIDS are overwhelmed by the disease process, the complicated treatment, the multiple health care appointments, and the scheduling to manage all of these tasks. Adding an exercise program may result in frustration and noncompliance unless the person can see a clear benefit and way to manage yet another aspect of the treatment program.

The PTA must be prepared for seizures, which may occur as a result of nervous system involvement, sometimes for the first time during a therapy session. Cognitive deficits in attention, concentration, and memory necessitate consistency, structure, and environmental cures to minimize confusion.[48]

Quickly progressive peripheral neuropathy is one of the most common types of pain experienced by people with HIV, sometimes as a result of drugs used to treat HIV or possibly related to HIV-induced immune complexes.[49]

Conventional transcutaneous electrical nerve stimulation may exacerbate peripheral pain in HIV-related peripheral neuropathies and should not be used. Joint and soft tissue mobilization, stretching, gait and balance training, and desensitization techniques can also be very effective. The alternate use of microcurrent electroacupuncture has been reported to reduce pain, improve functional status, and increase perceived strength. Discussion of the possible mechanisms for these effects is available.[49]

The body may begin to draw from its own stores of fat, affecting the myelin sheaths of nerves, which are protected by fat. Without proper nutrition, therapy involving balance training, extremity strengthening and stretching, and motor skills—although extremely important—may be limited in benefit.

Diminished sensory information associated with peripheral neuropathies of the lower extremities makes balance and gait control more difficult. Clients with AIDS may have balance deficits at lower movement speeds compared with healthy adults. Motor slowness is associated with both neuropathy and myopathy.[87] Formulating a rehabilitation approach must be based on the underlying neurophysiologic deficit(s) present.[50] Other guidelines for management of the lower extremity complications and balance and postural derangements associated with distal symmetric polyneuropathy are available.[51,132]

For individuals with painful myopathy in the large muscle groups, progressive resistance training with weights or elastic bands or tubing to strengthen specific muscles may be beneficial. Muscle spasms accompanying myopathy may respond well to gentle but consistent stretching exercises. Postexercise soreness is common in AIDS patients experiencing muscle pain. A longer rest period between exercises may be necessary.

Improper body mechanics, poor postural alignment and postural instability, balance and gait problems, and other biomechanical changes may occur in the person who has developed muscle weakness and fatigue from progression of the disease process, malnutrition, or the wasting syndrome. Again, postural awareness, stretching and strengthening of specific muscles, and attention to nutrition may be part of the treatment plan.

Cardiopulmonary complications (see Table 4.1) in advanced stages of AIDS contribute to morbidity and mortality. Oxygen transport mechanisms can be adversely affected. Muscle and joint mobilization techniques and breathing exercises are essential for the person who has been immobilized for any length of time as a result of respiratory or other disease involvement. The rib cage is one area where normal respiratory and accessory movements are essential for adequate lung ventilation, energy conservation, correct posture, and balance reactions.

Exercise and HIV/AIDS

Unlike other infections, HIV directly affects the immune system. Exercise has clinically significant effects on immune responsiveness; therefore a potential exists to alter the natural history of HIV infection in a beneficial manner through the use of exercise (see discussion in the section on exercise immunology in this chapter). A growing number of studies are now addressing the issue of the relationship between exercise and HIV infection.[39,77] The results are summarized here (Box 4.3).

Early Stage HIV Disease

Exercise is considered safe for people with HIV and an important way to increase the CD4 cells at earlier stages of the disease, possibly delaying symptoms while increasing muscle strength and size. During asymptomatic stages of HIV disease metabolic parameters are within normal limits, with no limitations placed on the individual. Individuals with asymptomatic HIV disease should be encouraged to exercise regularly, including both aerobic and resistance exercise components.[77]

The effect of HIV and its treatment with protease inhibitors on exercise and activity tolerance has been reported. Physical activity intolerance resulting in functional limitations may be caused by diminished aerobic capacity (decreased peak $\dot{V}O_2$) far below that occurring as a result of physiologic deconditioning alone. Individuals who receive HAART may have a reduced ability to extract and use oxygen from the muscle during exercise, limiting their ability to increase the intensity of activity.[18]

Symptomatic and Advanced Stages of HIV Disease

During symptomatic and advanced stages of HIV disease, functional capacity is reduced, requiring more individualized exercise prescription and lower intensities.[82] Neurologic dysfunction and deconditioning are common. Regular physical activity and exercise are just as important in this group but are more difficult and symptom limited. Among people with HIV who have known cardiovascular disease, pulmonary limitations, or muscle dysfunction, exercise prescription should address impairments and limitations. Collaboration with the physician to determine any contraindications for exercise is advised.

Strenuous exercise training is not recommended; aerobic exercise at moderate levels of intensity is suggested with medical clearance.[140] Constant or interval aerobic exercise for at least 20 minutes, at least three times per week for 4 weeks may lead to improved cardiopulmonary fitness and improved psychologic status with an accompanying maintenance of immunologic function.[106] Supervised aerobic exercise training safely decreases fatigue, weight, body mass index, fat, and central fat in HIV-1–infected individuals. It may not affect dyspnea.[136]

Clients with advanced disease may be at greater risk for exercise-related injuries caused by chronic myopathic and neuropathic tissue changes. Recovery periods after exercise may be prolonged compared with asymptomatic or early stage individuals. Response to exercise should be carefully monitored.[77]

Chronic Fatigue and Immune Dysfunction Syndrome
Overview

Chronic fatigue and immune dysfunction syndrome, chronic fatigue syndrome, chronic Epstein–Barr virus, myalgic encephalomyelitis, neuromyasthenia, and the "yuppie flu" all denote a highly publicized but not new illness.

The name *chronic fatigue syndrome* (CFS) indicates that this illness is not a single disease but the result of a combination of factors and is actually a subset of *chronic fatigue*, a broader category defined as unexplained fatigue of greater than or equal to 6 months' duration. This distinction is made to facilitate epidemiologic studies of populations with prolonged fatigue and chronic fatigue.

Incidence and Risk Factors

Two U.S. community-based CFS studies found prevalences among adults of 0.23% and 0.42%; the rates were higher in women, members of minority groups, and people with lower educational attainment and occupational status.[70,121]

People of every age, gender, ethnicity, and socioeconomic group can have CFS. Demographic data show that in most studies 75% or more of people with CFS are female. The mean age at onset of CFS is 29 to 35 years. The mean illness duration ranges from 3 years to 9 years.[19] Although CFS is much less common in children than in adults, children can develop the illness, particularly during the teen years.

Etiologic Factors and Pathogenesis

Many somatic and psychosocial hypotheses on the etiology of CFS have been explored. Explanations for CFS were sought in viral infections, immune dysfunction, neuroendocrine responses, dysfunction of the CNS, muscle structure, exercise capacity, sleep patterns, genetic constitution, personality, and (neuro)psychologic processes.

Abnormalities of the neuroendocrine system and CNS alone are not sufficient to explain the symptoms of CFS. More complex interactions between regulating systems are assumed to be at work and seem to involve the CNS, the immune system, and the hormonal regulation system. The etiology and pathogenesis are generally believed to be multifactorial.[26,30]

Personality and lifestyle are presumed to influence vulnerability to CFS. Personality characteristics of neuroticism and introversion have been reported as risk factors for the disorder.[116]

Inactivity in childhood and inactivity after infectious mononucleosis have been found to increase the risk of CFS in adults.[147,150] Also, acute physical or psychologic stress might trigger the onset of CFS.

Three quarters of the individuals with this disorder have reported an infection such as a cold, flulike illness, or infectious mononucleosis as the trigger,[32,129] and high rates of chronic fatigue after Q fever and Lyme disease have been found.[85] Finally, serious life events, such as the loss of a loved one or a job, and other stressful situations have been found to precipitate the disorder.[59,143]

Clinical Manifestations

The most commonly reported CFS symptoms at illness onset are sore throat, fever, muscle pain, and muscle weakness. As the illness progresses, muscle pain and forgetfulness increase, along with prolonged (lasting more than 6 months) and often overwhelming fatigue that is exacerbated by minimal physical activity.

BOX 4.2   Standard AIDS/HIV Precautions for Health Care Professionals

- Use protective barriers (gloves, eye shields, gowns) when handling blood, body fluids, and infectious fluids.
- Wash hands, skin, and mucous membranes immediately and thoroughly if contaminated by blood or other body fluids.
- Prevent needlesticks or scalpel sticks.
- Ventilation devices are available for resuscitation.
- Any health care professional (HCP) with open wounds or skin lesions should not treat clients or handle equipment until the lesion(s) heals.
- Pregnant health care professionals should take extra precautions.
- Occupational exposure to HIV should be followed immediately by evaluation of exposure source and postexposure prophylaxis.

From U.S. Public Health Service: Updated guidelines for the prevention of HIV and hepatitis virus transmission and the management of occupational exposures to HIV, BHV, and HCV, MMWR Recomm Rep 54:RR-9, 2005.

BOX 4.3   Exercise Recommendations for Athletes with HIV[a] Disease

- Before initiating any exercise program, the athlete must have a complete physical examination.
- A graded exercise test may be a necessary part of the evaluation to determine how much exercise the person can tolerate and what baseline of exercise should be established to start.
- Exercise is a safe and beneficial activity for the HIV-infected person.
- For healthy individuals who are asymptomatic of HIV, unrestricted exercise activity and competition are acceptable; overtraining should be avoided.
- For people with more advanced HIV infection who are experiencing mild to moderate symptoms, athletic competition is not considered advisable given the stress of competition and its effect on the immune system; training may continue without competition.

- Symptomatic people should avoid exhaustive exercise but may be able to continue exercise training under close supervision.
- Exercise training programs may need to be modified to include mild exercise and energy conservation techniques for anyone during the acute stage of an opportunistic infection.
- For the noncompetitive person, exercise should begin while healthy with strategies to help maintain an exercise program throughout the course of the illness.
- People with HIV, through the use of exercise, can play an important role in the management of their illness while improving quality of life.
- Exercise has the potential to offer subtle and effective behavioral therapeutic benefits regardless of ethnicity, exposure category, or gender.

Modified from Calabrese LH, LaPerriere A: Human immunodeficiency virus infection, exercise, and athletics, Sports Med 15:6, 1993.
[a]General principles included here apply to all individuals with HIV, including those who are not athletes or competitive in athletics or sports.

Neurally mediated hypotension (NMH) caused by disturbances in the autonomic regulation of blood pressure and pulse is common in people with CFS. This condition is characterized by lowered blood pressure and heart rate accompanied by lightheadedness, visual dimming, or slow response to verbal stimuli. Many people with NMH experience lightheadedness or worsening fatigue as they stand for prolonged periods or when in warm places (e.g., hot shower, sauna, indoor pool environment).

The severity of CFS varies from person to person, with some people able to maintain fairly active lives. By definition, however, CFS significantly limits work, school, and family activities.

Symptoms vary from person to person in number, type, and severity, but all individuals with CFS are functionally impaired to some degree. CDC studies show that CFS can be as disabling as multiple sclerosis (MS), lupus, rheumatoid arthritis, heart disease, end-stage renal disease, chronic obstructive pulmonary disease, and similar chronic conditions.

CFS often follows a cyclical course, alternating between periods of illness and relative well-being. Some people experience partial or complete remission of symptoms during the course of the illness, but symptoms often recur.

This pattern of remission and relapse makes CFS especially hard for clients and their health care professionals to manage. People who are in remission may be tempted to overdo activities when they are feeling better, which can exacerbate symptoms and fatigue and cause a relapse. In fact, postexertional malaise is a hallmark of the illness.[22]

Treatment. Because there is no known cure for CFS, treatment is aimed at symptom relief and improved function. A combination of drug and nondrug therapies is usually recommended.

Lifestyle changes, including prevention of overexertion, reduced stress, dietary restrictions, gentle stretching, and nutritional supplementation, are frequently recommended in addition to drug therapies used to treat sleep disturbances, pain, and other specific symptoms.

Carefully supervised physical therapy may also be part of treatment for CFS, but symptoms can be exacerbated by overly ambitious physical activity. A very moderate approach to exercise and activity management is recommended to avoid overactivity and to prevent deconditioning.[22] Systematic reviews have investigated the effectiveness of several CFS treatments, and cognitive behavior therapy and graded exercise therapy are the only interventions found to be beneficial.[115,120,151]

4.4 Special Implications for the PTA: Chronic Fatigue Syndrome The client with chronic fatigue syndrome (CFS) is treated according to guidelines and protocols for autoimmune disorders such as fibromyalgia. Pacing, energy conservation, stress management, and balancing life activities are extremely helpful in preventing worsening of fatigue and maintaining an even flow of energy from day to day. Support groups may be beneficial in providing emotional and psychologic support and in helping the individual keep up with the latest research results and progress in medical interventions.

Exercise and Chronic Fatigue Syndrome

Carefully controlled and graded exercise is the center of effective intervention for CFS.[46,47,108,113] Many affected individuals fear a relapse and avoid physical activity and exercise, but deconditioning and muscle atrophy increase fatigue and make other symptoms even worse.

The PTA can be very instrumental in providing a prescriptive program of regular, moderate exercise to avoid deconditioning while advising against overexertion during periods of remission. People with CFS are unable to sustain physical activity or exercise during acute onset or flare-ups. Beginning with low-level, intermittent physical activity throughout the day to accumulate 30 minutes of exercise has been shown to be effective without exacerbating symptoms.[28]

People with CFS may also have a significantly reduced exercise capacity. Always assess for conditioning before initiating even a simple exercise program with anyone who has had CFS longer than 6 months. Athletes and sports participants may require special help to develop a progressive exercise regimen. Impairments of peak aerobic power and muscle strength may occur with self-imposed or physician-imposed inactivity.[133]

The PTA must observe for altered breathing patterns, components of poor posture, and inefficient or biomechanically faulty movement patterns contributing to pain. Addressing these areas is an important part of the rehabilitation process.

Stretching, strengthening, and cardiovascular training are essential aspects of therapy. Like people with fibromyalgia, those diagnosed with CFS must progress slowly and avoid overexertion because they often do not have the internal mechanism to alert them to stop an activity.

Soft tissue and joint mobilization combined with stretching are important components of intervention, especially in the presence of postural components or faulty mechanics. Prolonged inactivity, rest in poorly supported positions for long periods, and assuming postures dictated by pain can contribute to muscle shortening.

Over time, some individuals can be progressed to graded aerobic exercise therapy. Continuous exercise must be started at a short duration appropriate to the client's baseline ability. A more specific description of how to deliver a graded exercise therapy program to people with CFS is available.[45] This has been shown to be significantly more effective than just stretching and relaxation exercises.[46,149]

Monitoring Vital Signs

Assessment of vital signs in adults with CFS may demonstrate very large fluctuations in pulse rate and blood pressure that are not consistent with the person's position or movement. Whereas the blood pressure and pulse rate normally show a slight increase as a physiologic response to a change in position from sitting to standing, orthostatic hypotension is marked in the CFS population. Vital signs may stay the same or even decrease, resulting in dizziness, lightheadedness, or loss of balance. The symptoms may result in decreased self-confidence in the ability to pursue activities.

During the initiation of an exercise program, it is advised to monitor blood pressure, rate of perceived exertion, heart rate, and respiratory rate for any signs of physiologic distress. Although the rate of perceived exertion may not change during the exercise session, the individual may perceive fatigue as worse after initiating exercise. However, if this increase in fatigue does not exceed 1 unit on a scale from 1 to 5 from the baseline level established before exercise, symptom exacerbation after exercise can potentially be avoided.[28]

TABLE 4.2	**Clinical Manifestations of Hypersensitivity Disorders**		
Type I	**Type II**	**Type III**	**Type IV**
Varies according to the allergies present Classic symptoms • Wheezing • Hypotension • Swelling • Urticaria • Rhinorrhea Anaphylaxis	*General:* malaise, weakness *Dermal:* hives, erythema *Respiratory:* sneezing, rhinorrhea, dyspnea *Upper airway:* hoarseness, stridor; tongue and pharyngeal edema *Lower airway:* dyspnea, bronchospasm, asthma (air trapping), chest tightness, wheezing *Gastrointestinal:* increased *peristalsis*, vomiting, dysphagia, nausea, abdominal cramps, diarrhea *Cardiovascular:* tachycardia, palpitations, hypotension, cardiac arrest *Central nervous system:* anxiety, seizures	Headache Back (flank) pain Chest pain similar to angina Nausea and vomiting Tachycardia Hypotension Hematuria Urticaria	Fever Arthralgias Lymphadenopathy Urticaria Anemia

HYPERSENSITIVITY DISORDERS

An exaggerated or inappropriate immune response may lead to various hypersensitivity disorders. Such disorders are classified as type I, II, III, or IV, although some overlap exists (Table 4.2).

Overreaction to a substance, or hypersensitivity, is often referred to as an *allergic response,* and although the term *allergy* is widely used, the term *hypersensitivity* is more appropriate. Hypersensitivity designates an increased immune response to the presence of an antigen (referred to as an *allergen*) that results in tissue destruction. The damage and suffering come predominantly from the immune response itself rather than from the substances that provoke it.

The several types of hypersensitivity reactions include immediate, late phase, and delayed, based on the rapidity of the immune response. *Immediate hypersensitivity reactions* usually occur within minutes of exposure to an allergen. If the skin is affected, blood vessels dilate and fluid accumulates, causing redness and swelling. In the eyes and nose, increased fluid and mucous secretions cause tearing and a runny nose.

Late-phase inflammation and symptoms persist for hours to days after the allergens have been removed and can cause cumulative damage (e.g., progressive lung disease) if they persist. *Delayed hypersensitivity reaction* occurs after sensitization to certain drugs or chemicals (e.g., penicillin, poison ivy). These reactions often take several days to cause symptoms.

Type I Hypersensitivity (Immediate Hypersensitivity, Allergic Disorders, Anaphylaxis)

Type I hypersensitivity reactions include hay fever, allergic rhinitis, urticaria, extrinsic asthma, and anaphylactic shock. Allergens are a special class of antigens that cause an allergic response. These normally harmless substances are inhaled (e.g., mold spores, animal dander, dust mites, grasses, weeds), eaten (e.g., nuts, fruits, shellfish, eggs), or injected (e.g., venom from fire ants, wasps, bees, hornets), or they come in contact with the skin or mucous membranes (e.g., plants, cosmetics, metals, drugs, dyes, latex).

Immunoglobulin E (IgE), one of the five types of antibodies produced in response to specific antigens, resides on mast cells in connective tissue, especially the upper respiratory tract, GI tract, and dermis. When IgE meets the pathogen again, an immediate response occurs with histamine release, along with other inflammatory mediators (e.g., chemotactic factors, prostaglandins, and leukotrienes) that enhance and prolong the response initiated by histamine.

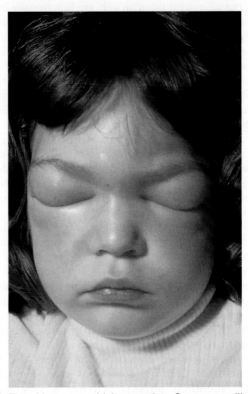

FIG. 4.9 Type I hypersensitivity reaction. Severe swelling of the eyelids in this child is the result of an allergic response to a bee sting. In some children and adults, difficulty breathing may be the first symptom of anaphylaxis. Intervention can be delayed until it is too late because there is no visible sign of narrowed airways. (From Fireman P: Atlas of allergies and clinical immunology, ed 3, Philadelphia, 2006, Mosby.)

If this response becomes systemic, widespread release of histamine (rather than just local tissue response) results in systemic vasodilation, bronchospasm, increased mucus secretion, and edema, referred to as *anaphylaxis.*

Classic associated signs and symptoms are wheezing, hypotension, swelling, urticaria, and rhinorrhea (clear, runny nose often accompanied by sneezing) (Fig. 4.9). Anaphylaxis is a life-threatening emergency and requires immediate intervention with injected epinephrine to restore blood pressure, strengthen the heartbeat, and open the airways. Bee stings remain the number one cause of anaphylaxis; other triggers include penicillin, foods, animal dander, children, semen, and latex.

Type II Hypersensitivity (Cytotoxic Reactions to Self-Antigens)

When the body's own tissue is recognized as foreign or nonself, the cellular membrane of normal tissues is disrupted and ultimately destroyed. Self-antigen disorders include blood transfusion reactions, hemolytic disease of the newborn, autoimmune hemolytic anemia, and myasthenia gravis.

Type III Hypersensitivity (Immune Complex Disease)

When circulating immune complexes (antigen–antibody complexes) successfully deposit in tissues around small blood vessels, they cause acute inflammation and local tissue injury.

The subsequent vasculitis most commonly affects the skin, causing urticaria (wheals); joints, causing synovitis, such as in rheumatoid arthritis; kidneys, causing nephritis; pleura, causing pleuritis; and pericardium, causing pericarditis.

Systemic lupus erythematosus (SLE) is the classic picture of vasculitis, occurring in various organ systems. The antigen is the individual's own nucleus of cells; antinuclear antibodies (ANAs) are made, which in turn form a complex with the antigen and are deposited in the skin, joints, and kidneys, causing acute immune injury.

Type IV Hypersensitivity (Cell-Mediated Immunity)

Type IV is a delayed hypersensitivity response such as the reaction that occurs in contact dermatitis after sensitization to an allergen (commonly a cosmetic, adhesive, topical medication, or plant toxin such as poison ivy), latex sensitivity, or the response to a TB skin test present 48 to 72 hours after the test.

4.5 Special Implications for the PTA: Hypersensitivity Disorders

Type IV reactions may occur in response to lanolin added to lotions, ultrasound gels, or other preparations used in massage or soft tissue mobilization, necessitating careful observation of all people for delayed skin reactions to any of these substances.

With the first exposure, no reaction necessarily occurs but antigens are formed, and on subsequent exposures, hypersensitivity reactions are triggered. Anyone with known hypersensitivity should have a small area of skin tested before use of large amounts of topical agents in the therapy setting. Careful observation throughout treatment is recommended.

Beginning in the 1980s, the use of latex gloves to protect health care workers against exposure to blood and body fluids increased. Since then, the number of reported cases of latex sensitivity also has increased. Reactions to latex range from contact dermatitis (type IV hypersensitivity) to anaphylactic shock (type I hypersensitivity).

PTAs who are allergic to latex should avoid contact with latex gloves and other products that contain latex. Use of low-powder, powder-free, and nonlatex gloves provides PTAs with a strategy for preventing exposure to latex allergens.[86]

 ## AUTOIMMUNE DISEASES

Definition and Overview

Autoimmune diseases fall into a category of conditions in which the cause involves immune mechanisms directed against self-antigens. More specifically, the body fails to distinguish self from nonself, causing the immune system to direct immune responses against normal (self) tissue and become self-destructive.

More than 56 autoimmune diseases have been identified, affecting everything from skin and joints to vital organs. Autoimmune diseases can be viewed as a spectrum of disorders, some of which are systemic and others of which involve a single

TABLE 4.3 Autoimmune Disorders

Organ-Specific Disorders	Systemic Disorders
Addison's disease	Amyloidosis
Crohn's disease	Ankylosing spondylitis
Chronic active hepatitis	Mixed connective tissue disease
Diabetes mellitus	Multiple sclerosis
Giant cell arteritis	Myasthenia gravis
Hemolytic anemia	Polymyalgia rheumatica
Idiopathic thrombocytopenic purpura	Progressive systemic sclerosis (scleroderma)
Polymyositis, dermatomyositis	Psoriasis (psoriatic arthritis)
Postviral encephalomyelitis	Reiter's syndrome
Primary biliary cirrhosis	Rheumatoid arthritis
Thyroiditis	Sarcoidosis
Graves' disease	Sjögren's syndrome
Hashimoto's disease	Systemic lupus erythematosus
Ulcerative colitis	

organ. Some the known diseases most likely to be seen in a rehabilitation setting are listed in Table 4.3.

At one end of the continuum are organ-specific diseases, in which localized tissue damage occurs that results from the presence of specific autoantibodies.

In the middle of the continuum are disorders in which the lesion tends to be localized in one organ, but the antibodies are not organ specific. An example is primary biliary cirrhosis, in which inflammatory cell infiltration of the small bile ductule occurs, but the serum antibodies are not specific to liver cells.

At the other end of the spectrum are non–organ-specific diseases, in which lesions and antibodies are widespread throughout the body and not limited to one target organ.

Etiologic and Risk Factors

Although the autoimmune disorders are regarded as acquired diseases, their causes often cannot be determined. Autoimmunity is believed to result from a combination of factors, including genetic, hormonal (women are affected more often than men by autoimmune diseases), and environmental influences (e.g., exposure to chemicals, other toxins, or sunlight and drugs that may destroy suppressor T cells).

Although no single gene has been identified as being responsible for autoimmune diseases, clusters of genes seem to increase susceptibility.

The influence of hormonal factors is confusing because some autoimmune diseases occur among women in their 20s and 30s, when estrogen is high, and others develop after menopause or before puberty, when estrogen levels are low. During pregnancy, many women with rheumatoid arthritis or MS experience complete remission, whereas pregnant women with SLE often experience exacerbations.

Other factors implicated in the development of immunologic abnormalities resulting in autoimmune disorders include viruses, stress, cross-reactive antibodies, and various autoimmune diseases occurring in women who have had silicone gel breast implants. This organ-specific autoimmune disease has been associated with musculoskeletal problems.

Pathogenesis

Autoimmune disorders involve disruption of the immunoregulatory mechanism, causing normal cell-mediated and humoral immune responses to turn self-destructive, resulting in tissue damage.

The exact pathologic mechanisms for this process remain unknown. It has been shown that the innate immune system plays an important role in determining whether T cells become activated and functional in autoimmune disorders.[96] Researchers suspect that more than one part of the immune system must be involved for autoimmune disease to develop.

Some autoimmune diseases affect a single organ (e.g., pancreas in type 1 diabetes), whereas others affect a large system or more than one system (e.g., MS). In some cases the autoimmune process overstimulates organ function, as in Graves' disease, in which excess thyroid hormone is produced.

Many autoimmune diseases are associated with characteristic autoantibodies. In other words, the body begins to manufacture antibodies directed against the body's own cellular components or specific organs. These antibodies are known as *autoantibodies*—in this case, producing autoimmune diseases.

Antibodies specific to hormone receptors on the surface of cells have been found and determined to be partially responsible for some conditions. Examples include myasthenia gravis, in which antiacetylcholine receptor antibodies are involved; Graves' disease, in which antibodies against components of thyroid cell membranes, including the receptors for thyroid-stimulating hormone, are responsible; and certain cases of insulin-resistant diabetes mellitus, in which the antibodies affect insulin receptors on cells.

Other diseases involving autoimmune mechanisms include rheumatic fever, rheumatoid arthritis, autoimmune hemolytic anemia, idiopathic thrombocytopenic purpura, and postviral encephalomyelitis.

Clinical Manifestations

Autoimmune disorders share certain clinical features, and differentiation among them is often difficult because of this. Common findings include synovitis, pleuritis, myocarditis, endocarditis, pericarditis, peritonitis, vasculitis, myositis, skin rash, alterations of connective tissues, and nephritis. Constitutional symptoms such as fatigue, malaise, myalgias, and arthralgias are also common.

Medical Management

Diagnosis
Diagnosis can be difficult because autoimmune diseases are poorly understood, mimic one another, and often consist of vague symptoms such as lethargy or migratory joint pain. Laboratory tests may reveal thrombocytopenia, leukopenia, Ig excesses or deficiencies, ANAs, rheumatoid factor, cryoglobulins, false-positive serologic test results, elevated muscle enzymes, and alterations in serum complement.

Treatment
Treatment of autoimmune diseases varies with the specific disease. Treatment must maintain a delicate balance between adequate suppression of the autoimmune reaction to avoid continued damage to the body tissues and maintenance of sufficient functioning of the immune mechanism to protect the person against foreign invaders. In general, autoimmune diseases are treated by the administration of corticosteroids to produce an antiinflammatory effect and salicylates to provide symptomatic relief.

The wealth of new information gleaned from research in the last decade has been used to improve immunization strategies and hopefully will lead to new approaches to the reinduction of immune tolerance. The development of an effective vaccine is under close scrutiny,[72] as is the use of intense immunosuppression (immunoablation) followed by stem cell transplantation for the treatment of autoimmune diseases.

Because autoimmune disease is the result of genetic dysregulation, gene therapy may become a viable alternative in the future. Scientists have been involved in developing new drugs aimed at the mechanism of autoimmunity rather than treating its effects.

Systemic Lupus Erythematosus
Definition and Overview
Lupus erythematosus, sometimes referred to as *lupus*, is a chronic inflammatory autoimmune disorder that appears in several forms, including *discoid lupus erythematosus* (DLE), which affects only the skin (usually face, neck, scalp), and *systemic lupus erythematosus*, which can affect any organ or system of the body.

The clinical picture of SLE reflects a continuum with different combinations of organ system involvement. The most common of these presentations are latent lupus, drug-induced lupus, antiphospholipid antibody syndrome, and late-stage lupus. *Latent lupus* describes a constellation of features suggestive of SLE but does not qualify as classic SLE. Many people with latent lupus persist with their clinical presentation of signs and symptoms over many years without ever developing classic SLE.

Drug-induced lupus may be diagnosed in people without prior history suggestive of SLE in whom the clinical and serologic manifestations of SLE develop while the person is taking a drug. The symptoms cease when the drug is stopped, with gradual resolution of serologic abnormalities.

Late-stage lupus is defined as chronic disease duration of greater than 5 years. In such cases, morbidity and mortality are affected by long-term complications of SLE that result either from the disease itself or as a consequence of its therapy. These late complications may include end-stage renal disease, atherosclerosis, pulmonary emboli, and avascular necrosis. In late-stage lupus, when no evidence of active disease exists and the client is on low-dose or no corticosteroids, cognitive disabilities are a common manifestation.

Incidence

SLE is primarily a disease of young women; it is rarely found in older people. It usually develops in young women of childbearing years, but many men and children also develop lupus. Lupus is three times more common in African American women than in Caucasian women and is also more common in women of Hispanic, Asian, and Native American descent.[41]

SLE also appears in the first-degree relatives of individuals with lupus more often than it does in the general population, which indicates a strong hereditary component. However, most cases of SLE occur sporadically, indicating that both genetic and environmental factors play a role in the development of the disease.

Etiologic and Risk Factors

The cause of SLE remains unknown, but evidence points to interrelated immunologic, environmental, hormonal, and genetic factors. Immune dysregulation in the form of autoimmunity is thought to be the prime causative mechanism. SLE shows a strong familial link, with a much higher frequency among first-degree relatives. Evidence for genetic susceptibility is present, and linkage studies in conjunction with genome scans may delineate this more specifically in the future.[155] As the human genome becomes more extensively mapped, a susceptibility gene may be found, although it remains possible that the differences in disease course among ethnic groups relate solely to their environment and other social factors.

Other factors predisposing to SLE may include physical or mental stress, which can provoke neuroendocrine changes affecting immune cell function; streptococcal or viral infections; exposure to sunlight or ultraviolet light, which can cause inflammation and tissue damage; immunization; pregnancy; and abnormal estrogen metabolism.

A higher incidence of SLE exacerbation occurs among women taking even low-dose estrogen contraceptives. Because an increased risk of thrombosis is possible in young women with SLE, estrogen-containing contraceptives are avoided or used at the lowest effective dose.

The role of the Epstein–Barr virus as a possible risk factor for SLE remains under investigation.[68] SLE may also be triggered or aggravated by treatment with certain drugs (e.g., hydralazine, anticonvulsants, penicillins, sulfa drugs, and oral contraceptives), which could modify both cellular responsiveness and immunogenicity of self-antigens.

Pathogenesis

The central immunologic disturbance in SLE is autoantibody production. The body produces antibodies (e.g., ANAs) against its own cells. Deposition of the formed antigen–antibody complexes at various tissue sites can suppress the body's normal immunity and damage tissues.

In fact, one significant feature of SLE is the ability to produce antibodies against many different tissue components such as red blood cells (RBCs), neutrophils, platelets, lymphocytes, or almost any organ or tissue in the body. This wide range of antigenic targets has resulted in SLE being classified as a disease of generalized autoimmunity. Given the clinical diversity of SLE, the disease may be mediated by more than one autoantibody system and several immunopathogenic mechanisms.

Skin lesions demonstrate inflammation and degeneration at the dermal–epidermal junction, with the basal layer being the primary site of injury. Other organ systems affected by SLE are usually studied only at autopsy. Although these tissues may show nonspecific inflammation or vessel abnormalities, pathologic findings are sometimes minimal, suggesting a mechanism other than inflammation as the cause of organ damage or dysfunction.

Clinical Manifestations

Generally, SLE is more severe than discoid lupus, and no two people with SLE will have identical symptoms. For some people, only the skin and joints will be involved. For others, joints, lungs, kidneys, blood, or other organs and/or tissues may be affected.

Musculoskeletal system. Arthralgias and arthritis constitute the most common presenting manifestations of SLE, but the onset of SLE may be acute or insidious and may produce no characteristic clinical pattern. Other early symptoms may include fever, weight loss, malaise, and fatigue.

Acute arthritis can involve any joint but typically affects the small joints of the hands, wrists, and knees. It may be migratory or chronic; most cases are symmetric, but asymmetric polyarthritis is not uncommon.

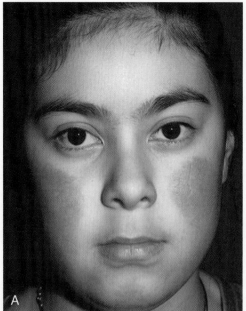

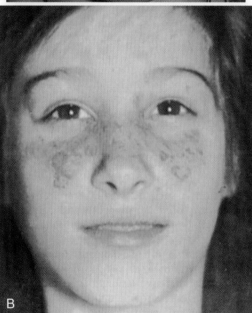

FIG. 4.10 The butterfly rash of systemic lupus erythematosus (SLE). The rash can vary from an erythematous blush (A) to thickened epidermis to scaly patches (B). (From Kliegman RM, Behrman RE, Jenson HB, et al.: Nelson textbook of pediatrics, ed 18, Philadelphia, 2007, Saunders.)

Unlike rheumatoid arthritis, the arthritis of SLE is not usually erosive or destructive of bone, and symptoms are not usually severe enough to cause joint deformities, but pain can cause temporary functional impairment. When deformities do occur, ulnar deviation, swan-neck deformity, or fixed subluxations of the fingers often occur as well. Tenosynovitis and tendon ruptures may occur.

Cutaneous and membranous lesions. The skin rash occurs most commonly in areas exposed to sunlight (ultraviolet rays) and may be exacerbated by the use of cosmetic products containing alpha hydroxy acids. The classic butterfly rash over the nose and cheeks is common (Fig. 4.10).

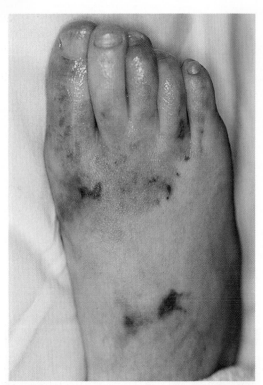

FIG. 4.11 A 12-year-old girl with systemic lupus erythematosus (SLE) and antiphospholipid antibodies with painful cutaneous vasculitis of the right foot. Arterial thrombosis documented by angiography resulted in cyanosis of the large toe. Symptoms resolved with treatment with heparin and corticosteroids. (From Kliegman RM, Behrman RE, Jenson HB, et al.: Nelson textbook of pediatrics, ed 18, Philadelphia, 2007, Saunders.)

Discoid lesions associated with DLE are raised, red, scaling plaques with follicular plugging and central atrophy. This raised edging and sunken center gives them a coinlike appearance.

Vasculitis (inflammation of cutaneous blood vessels) involving small and medium-sized vessels may cause other skin lesions, including infarctive lesions of the digits (Fig. 4.11), splinter hemorrhages, necrotic leg ulcers, or digital gangrene. Raynaud's phenomenon occurs in about 20% of people.

Diffuse or patchy alopecia (hair loss) may be temporary, with hair regrowth occurring once the disease is under control. However, permanent hair loss can occur from the extensive scarring of discoid lesions. Painless ulcers of the mucous membranes are common and involve the mouth, vagina, and nasal septum.

Cardiopulmonary system. Signs of cardiopulmonary abnormalities may develop, such as pleuritis, pericarditis, and dyspnea. Myocarditis, endocarditis, tachycardia, and pneumonitis (acute or chronic) may also occur. Pulmonary hypertension and congestive heart failure are less common and usually secondary to a combination of factors.

Central nervous system. A significant number of people with SLE will have CNS involvement at some point in their illness, sometimes referred to as *neuropsychiatric manifestations.* Clinical manifestations may be related to specific autoantibodies that react with nervous system antigens and/or cytokine-mediated brain inflammation and include headaches, irritability, and depression (most commonly).

Emotional instability, psychosis, seizures, cerebrovascular accidents, cranial neuropathy, peripheral neuropathy, and organic brain syndrome can also occur. Return to the previous level of intellectual function may follow remission of the neuropsychiatric flare, or permanent cognitive impairment may occur.

The pattern of cognitive dysfunction is diverse; intensity can vary within the same person and can be affected by mood.[35] The person may have difficulties with verbal memory, attention, language skills (verbal fluency, productivity), and psychomotor speed. Progressive cognitive impairment, sometimes subtle and sometimes obvious, may develop even in the absence of clinically diagnosed episodes of neuropsychiatric disease.[36] People with SLE may or may not have other signs of lupus when they experience neurologic symptoms.

Renal system. Pathologic changes may also occur in the kidneys, where the glomerulus is the usual site of destruction; other renal effects may include hematuria and proteinuria, progressing to kidney failure.

Other systems. Anemia from decreased erythrocytes is a common finding, with associated amenorrhea (cessation of menstrual flow) in women. Sometimes the spleen and cervical, axillary, and inguinal nodes are enlarged; hepatitis may also develop. Nausea, vomiting, diarrhea, and abdominal pain may occur with GI involvement. All symptoms mentioned in this section can occur at the onset or at any time during the course of lupus. Nearly all people with SLE experience fluctuations in disease activity with exacerbations and remissions.

4.6 Special Implications for the PTA: Systemic Lupus Erythematosus As in fibromyalgia, physical and occupational therapy intervention can be important components of the overall treatment plan. Recurrence of disease can be managed with carefully controlled and sometimes restricted activities. After an exacerbation, gradual resumption of activities must be balanced by maximum rest periods, usually 8 to 10 hours of sleep a night and several rest periods during the day.

Most of the principles and reference materials outlined in the section on fibromyalgia also apply to SLE. Management of joint involvement follows protocols for rheumatoid arthritis. Clients with skin lesions should be examined thoroughly at each visit by the physical therapist. The PTA can be instrumental in teaching and assisting with skin care and prevention of skin breakdown.

Functional limitations among people with SLE vary according to the type and degree of the disease. Generalized fatigue, defined as "the inclination to rest, even though pain and weakness are not limiting factors," is a common problem and can be very debilitating, especially for those individuals with both SLE and fibromyalgia.[3]

The PTA can instruct clients how to pace activities and conserve energy, follow a prescriptive exercise plan, avoid excessive bed rest, and protect joints. Excessive bed rest can worsen fatigue, promote muscle disuse and atrophy, and promote osteoporosis. Prescriptive exercise should strengthen the muscles and improve endurance while avoiding undue stress on inflamed joints.

Septic arthritis or osteonecrosis may develop as a complication of SLE or its treatment. Septic arthritis is uncommon in SLE, but it should be suspected when one joint is inflamed out of proportion to the others. People with SLE may develop a drug-related myopathy secondary to corticosteroids or as a complication of antimalarials. Anyone taking corticosteroids or immunosuppressants must be monitored carefully for signs of infection, especially people at heightened risk of infection such as those with renal failure, cardiac valvular abnormalities, or ulcerative skin lesions. The client should contact the physician if a fever or any other new symptoms develop. The PTA can provide osteoporosis prevention and intervention management.

High-dose oral corticosteroid treatment remains the major predisposing cause of avascular necrosis in SLE and other disorders. The most common site is the femoral head of the hip; less commonly, the femoral condyle of the knee is affected. Although the condition may be bilateral, it most often manifests as an insidious onset of unilateral hip or knee pain that is worse with ambulating but often present at rest. Symptoms are progressive over weeks to months.

Observe carefully for any sign of renal involvement such as weight gain, edema, or hypertension. Take seizure precautions if there are signs of neurologic involvement. The PTA may recognize signs of cognitive dysfunction or decline, either directly observed in the client or by family report. These manifestations should be reported to the physician for consideration in evaluating medications. If Raynaud's phenomenon is present, teach the client to warm and protect the hands and feet.

Fibromyalgia

Definition and Overview

Fibromyalgia or fibromyalgia syndrome (FMS) is a chronic muscle pain syndrome. It is considered a syndrome and not a disease and has now been defined by the American College of Rheumatology (ACR) as pain that is widespread in at least 11 of 18 tender points.

FMS currently falls under the auspices of rheumatology, having originally been determined to have no known organic basis. However, with the recent advances in understanding of FMS with documented objective biochemical, endocrine, and physiologic abnormalities, it may be best characterized as a biologic (organic) disorder associated with neurohormonal dysfunction of the ANS.

It is commonly associated with many other conditions (e.g., hypothyroidism, rheumatoid arthritis, connective tissue disease, SLE, CFS); the link between FMS and these disorders is under investigation.

Fibromyalgia has been differentiated from myofascial pain in that fibromyalgia is considered a systemic problem with widespread multiple tender points as one of the key symptoms.

Myofascial pain is a localized condition specific to a muscle and may involve as few as one or as many as several areas with characteristic trigger points that are painful and refer pain to other areas when pressure is applied. The person with FMS may have both tender points and trigger points, requiring specific treatment interventions for each.

The person with myofascial pain syndrome does not exhibit other associated constitutional or systemic signs or symptoms unless palpation elicits a painful enough response to elicit an ANS response with nausea and/or vomiting, increased blood pressure, and increased pulse.

It has been proposed that fibromyalgia and CFS are two names for the same syndrome, with CFS being an early form of FMS, but at present CFS is thought to differ by the greater degree of fatigue. People with fibromyalgia tend to experience more pain. In contrast to CFS, fibromyalgia is associated with a variety of initiating or perpetuating factors such as psychologically distressing events, primary sleep disorders, inflammatory rheumatic arthritis, and acute febrile illness.

Fibromyalgia and CFS have similar disordered sleep physiology, and evidence suggests a reciprocal relationship of the immune and sleep-wake systems. Interference with either system has effects on the other and will be accompanied by the symptoms of CFS.[100] A significant number of people with FMS meet the criteria for CFS and vice versa.

Incidence

Fibromyalgia occurs in more than 6 million Americans. It has now surpassed rheumatoid arthritis as the most common musculoskeletal disorder in the United States. Women are affected more often than men (90% are women), with symptoms appearing from ages 20 to 55 years, although it has been diagnosed in children as young as 6 years and adults as old as 85 years of age.

Risk Factors

Risk factors or triggering events for the onset of fibromyalgia may include prolonged anxiety and emotional stress, trauma (e.g., motor vehicle accident, work injury, surgery), rapid steroid withdrawal, hypothyroidism, and viral and nonviral infections.

Fibromyalgia may also develop with no obvious precipitating events or illnesses. It is more prevalent in minimally to moderately physically fit persons and is not usually found in highly trained athletes; a strong correlation exists between fibromyalgia and anxiety or depression (it remains unclear whether these factors are contributory or a result of this condition).

Etiologic Factors

Research is now ongoing to determine the cause of fibromyalgia; most likely the initiation of this condition is multifactorial. Debate continues over whether fibromyalgia is even an organic disease and, if so, whether it is caused by abnormal biochemical, metabolic, or immunologic pathology.

Possible etiologic theories include diet; viral origin; sleep disorder; occupational, seasonal, or environmental influences; psychologic distress; adverse childhood experiences, including sexual abuse[42,93]; and a familial or hereditary link.

Pathogenesis

Autonomic nervous system. The activity of the skeletal muscles, heart, stomach, intestines, blood vessels, and sweat glands during daily stress tends to be excessive in fibromyalgia. These organs overactivate, resulting in the heart beating faster, the stomach secreting excessive digestive juices and contracting erratically, the smooth muscles of the intestines and bowel contracting abnormally, breathing becoming rapid and shallow, and blood vessels constricting, which decreases blood flow to body parts. These and other ANS responses may occur in response to a relatively mild life stressor and linger even after cognitive memory of the event is gone.

In FMS the nervous system's ability to modulate and return to normal is fragile and lacks the subtle ability to respond quickly; responses are more exaggerated and the return to normal takes more time.[65,156]

The enteric system (autonomic nervous control of the digestive system) is often significantly disrupted in fibromyalgia. Digestion is often compromised, and the absorption of nutrients into the bloodstream where they can be used by the body for cell function is often inadequate for healthy daily function.

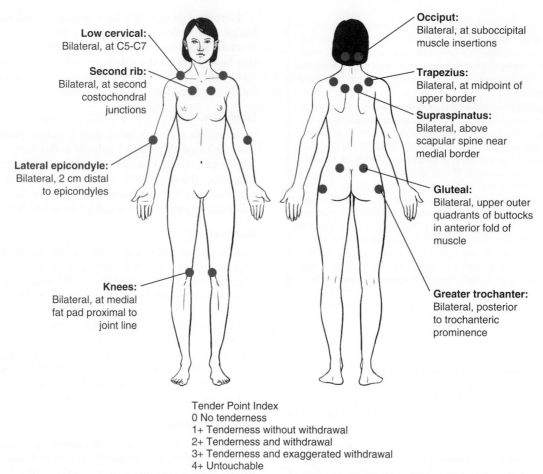

Low cervical:
Bilateral, at C5-C7

Second rib:
Bilateral, at second
costochondral
junctions

Lateral epicondyle:
Bilateral, 2 cm distal
to epicondyles

Knees:
Bilateral, at medial
fat pad proximal to
joint line

Occiput:
Bilateral, at suboccipital
muscle insertions

Trapezius:
Bilateral, at midpoint of
upper border

Supraspinatus:
Bilateral, above
scapular spine near
medial border

Gluteal:
Bilateral, upper outer
quadrants of buttocks
in anterior fold of
muscle

Greater trochanter:
Bilateral, posterior
to trochanteric
prominence

Tender Point Index
0 No tenderness
1+ Tenderness without withdrawal
2+ Tenderness and withdrawal
3+ Tenderness and exaggerated withdrawal
4+ Untouchable

FIG. 4.12 Anatomic locations of tender points associated with fibromyalgia. According to the literature, digital palpation should be performed with an approximate force of 4 kg (enough pressure to indent a tennis ball), but clinical practice suggests much less pressure is required to elicit pain. For a tender point to be considered positive, the subject must state that the palpation was "painful." A reply of "tender" is not considered a positive response. Counting the number of points as part of the clinical diagnosis of fibromyalgia syndrome (FMS) has been discounted,[152] but the presence of multiple tender points is still a key feature of FMS. (From Goodman CC, Snyder T: Differential diagnosis for physical therapists: screening for referral, ed 5, St. Louis, 2013, Saunders.)

Sleep disturbances may contribute to fibromyalgia symptoms; researchers are investigating alterations of the neuro-immunoendocrine systems that accompany disordered sleep physiology, resulting in the nonrestorative sleep, pain, fatigue, and cognitive and mood symptoms that people with fibromyalgia (and CFS) experience.

Immune system. Immune cells, activated in response to infection, inflammation, or trauma, release proinflammatory cytokines that signal the CNS to release glia within the brain and spinal cord. Pain has been classically viewed as being mediated solely by neurons, but the discovery that spinal cord glia (microglia and astrocytes) amplify pain has changed this view.

When glial cells become activated by sensory signals arriving from the periphery, they can release a variety of substances known to be involved in chronic pain.

Clinical Manifestations

Fibromyalgia is characterized by muscle pain as the major symptom, often described as aching or burning, a "migraine headache of the muscles." Diffuse pain or tender points are present on both sides of the body in many muscle groups, including the neck, back, arms, legs, jaw, feet, and hands (Fig. 4.12).

Sleep disturbances result in fatigue and exhaustion, even after a night's sleep. Men with fibromyalgia typically have fewer symptoms and milder tender points (less "hurt all over" reports), less fatigue, and fewer incidences of irritable bowel syndrome compared with women who have FMS.[1]

Other symptoms or associated problems occur with a high frequency (Table 4.4), sometimes more incapacitating than the pain and tender points. Symptoms are often exacerbated by stress; overloading physical activity, including overstretching; damp or chilly weather; heat exposure or humidity; sudden change in barometric pressure; trauma; or another illness.

People with fibromyalgia who are aerobically fit manifest fewer symptoms than those who remain physically deconditioned and aerobically unfit. Biofeedback specialists have shown that blood circulation to the affected areas is often significantly decreased while the individual is at rest, and a noticeable decrease in circulation occurs with changes in barometric pressure.

During exercise—when circulation should normally increase to muscles and the brain—in fibromyalgia just the opposite happens, and circulation is decreased considerably.[65]

The diaphragm is significantly affected in fibromyalgia to the point that it ceases to function as the major breathing muscle, and accessory muscles of the neck and upper chest take over.

This overwork results in tender points or tightness of the neck and chest muscles.

In general, the level of muscular activity in fibromyalgia is high, even when the body is sitting or reclining. The muscles used for daily activities such as cleaning, cooking, typing, and even socializing are at a higher level of activity than the muscles of a normal person doing the same tasks.

When the activity is over and the person with fibromyalgia is resting, those same muscles continue to repeat the activity over and over at a lower intensity so that no outward movement is apparent. This factor, combined with increased central pain processing, may lower tender point thresholds.[12]

TABLE 4.4 Clinical Manifestations of Fibromyalgia

Sign or Symptom	Incidence (%)[a]
Muscle pain (myalgia), tender points	99[b]
Visual problems (e.g., blurring, double vision, bouncing images)	95
Mental and physical fatigue	85
Sleep disturbance, morning fatigue	80
Morning stiffness (persists >30 min)	75
Mitral valve prolapse	75
Global anxiety	72
Cognitive (memory) problems (e.g., decreased attention span, impaired short-term memory, decreased concentration, increased distractibility)	71
Irritable bowel syndrome	70
Inflammatory bowel disease (Crohn's disease, ulcerative colitis)	50–60
Headaches	70
Hypersensitivity to noise, odors, heat, or cold (cold intolerance)	50–60
Paresthesias	50
Swollen feeling (joint or soft tissues)	50
Muscle spasms or nodules	50
Reactive hypoglycemia (e.g., weakness, irritability, disorientation)	45–50
Pelvic pain	43
Irritable bladder syndrome, female urethral syndrome	40
Hypotension (low blood pressure, elevated heart rate); neurally mediated hypotension or vasopressor syncope	40
Raynaud's phenomenon	38
Sicca syndrome (dry eyes, mouth)	33
Respiratory dysfunction (e.g., dyspnea, erratic breathing patterns during exertion)	33
Restless leg syndrome, nocturnal myoclonus, periodic leg movement disorder (PLMD)	30–60
Auditory problems	31
Temporomandibular dysfunction	25
Depression	20
Allergies	Unknown
Lack of libido	Unknown
Skin discoloration	Unknown
Sciatica	Unknown

[a]These figures were compiled from a variety of sources but represent a fairly accurate clinical perspective.
[b]Although the American College of Rheumatology requires the identification of at least 11 out of 18 tender points to qualify for a diagnosis of fibromyalgia syndrome (FMS), some clinicians report isolated individuals without pain but whose condition is characterized by the physiologic effects and manifestations of FMS or patients with fewer than 11 tender points.
Modified from Hulme J: Fibromyalgia: a handbook for self-care and treatment, ed 3, Missoula, MT, 2000, Phoenix Publishing Company.

4.7 Special Implications for the PTA: Fibromyalgia PTs and PTAs are often the first to recognize the history and clinical manifestations suggestive of fibromyalgia and then request medical diagnosis and intervention.

Rehabilitative therapy is an important component in managing fibromyalgia. Many people with FMS have undergone unnecessary exploratory or corrective surgery and have residual functional limitations. Chronic musculoskeletal conditions that are sources of noxious neural input to the CNS often involve the shoulder(s) and spine.

Therapy is helpful first in directing individuals to reach goals of lessening pain and fatigue and eliminating sleep disturbance. Outcomes can be measured in a variety of ways, not only by reduction in tender points but also by global scores of pain, fatigue, sleep, reduction of other distressing symptoms, improved quality of life, reduced visits to the physician, reduction or elimination of medications, increased sexual activity, improved work performance, and so on.

Many people with FMS have been told they must "learn to live with it." A more positive approach is to suggest working together to learn how to move forward with FMS, respecting limitations but not being controlled by them. The PTA can be very instrumental in guiding the client to understand how to manage this condition.

Strategies for work modification and applying ergonomic techniques to increase efficiency and decrease pain are important interventions. A chronic pain program may be appropriate. The reader is referred to more specific literature for treatment regimens, self-stabilizing techniques, and therapy protocols for this condition.[25,65,108,118]

Modalities and Fibromyalgia
Ultrasound can be an effective therapeutic modality for the treatment of pain in people with FMS when combined with connective tissue manipulation and high-voltage pulsed galvanic stimulation.[27] Also, pulsed ultrasound has been shown to be effective in treatment of pain in FMS as combined therapy with interferential current.[4]

There have been some reports on the use of ultrasound as an effective therapeutic modality for its thermal effects and for the treatment of myofascial trigger points often present in people with FMS. Continuous ultrasound is preferable to pulsed ultrasound and should be combined with a complete trigger point protocol.[142] The intensity must be reduced from standard settings to accommodate hypersensitivity in most people with FMS. Specific positions, tissue effects, intervention techniques, and treatment parameters are available.[62,63]

Given the proposed mechanism of muscle pain (hyperresponsive myofascial mechanoreceptors, impaired CNS pain-inhibiting system), soft tissue techniques must be applied gently and slowly to increase circulation while avoiding an increase in nociceptive signal transmission. With the typical FMS client, posttreatment discomfort can be avoided by keeping the discomfort level during treatment between 1 and 5 on a self-assessment scale of 1 to 10. Cross-friction massage is not advised.[90]

Exercise and Fibromyalgia

The primary nonpharmacologic modality in the management of FMS is prescriptive exercise. Improvement in both subjective pain and objective measurement has been demonstrated with cardiovascular fitness training or simple flexibility training.[94]

Aerobic exercise also contributes by increasing the metabolic rate of the lean tissues in those individuals with a thyroid component.[135] Resistance exercise contributes to the increase in metabolism by increasing lean tissue mass, which has a higher metabolic rate than fat tissue.[114] Well-managed prescriptive exercise regimens improve sleep and result in a decrease in pain and fatigue.[29]

Gentle stretching exercises performed routinely throughout the day may reduce fatigue. A cardiopulmonary fitness component should be included at whatever level is appropriate for the individual.

Sometimes the person's condition is so acute that exercise is not tolerated immediately. This is often the reason for using modalities in the early stage of therapy. Exercising too soon and committing to too much can set the person back considerably, but at the same time the PTA must keep in mind the long-term goal to increase strength and improve aerobic fitness.

Aquatic therapy is an ideal way to begin conditioning, especially for those individuals with FMS who have injuries, are overweight, or are sensitive to axial load. Aquatic therapy provides low-level progressive exercises, gradually increasing strength and endurance while improving overall cardiovascular fitness.[7,57] Ideal pool temperature is 84° to 90° F. As with all exercise programs with this population (whether aquatic or other therapy), people with fibromyalgia fatigue quickly and may have a low tolerance for exertion. The key is to avoid activating the peripheral sensory mechanisms in order to avoid increasing pain postexercise.

The person with FMS will respond to stimuli that would not ordinarily be perceived as painful (referred to as *allodynia*). This requires short exercise sessions—possibly even only 3 to 5 minutes at first—according to individual tolerance using the rate of perceived exertion.

The client is encouraged to increase exercise duration in small daily increments, sometimes only by seconds or minutes. Reaching a goal of 30 minutes of daily exercise may take weeks to months; some individuals are able to tolerate only one to three daily exercise cycles, each lasting only 5 to 10 minutes, but this will produce beneficial effects.

The individual with FMS must be taught to set aside the philosophy of "no pain, no gain" and to avoid "pushing through the pain." In the normal individual, growth hormone is increased with exercise, but this does not happen in the person with FMS.

Poor compliance is common when the use of muscle relaxants, sedatives, or other medications reduce desire or drive to exercise. Symptoms of pain and fatigue increase during exercise, resulting in limited compliance and limited long-term benefits. The PTA can explain that pain may result in part from muscle spasm and reduced blood flow to muscles, both of which can be aided by persistence in managing exercise.

People with fibromyalgia are also more vulnerable to overuse syndromes than are people with normal muscle histology, requiring a slower, longer rehabilitation process. This may not be activity induced as once thought, but rather may occur as a result of sarcolemmal abnormality.[71]

Other resources include the National Fibromyalgia Association (http://www.fmaware.org) and the American Fibromyalgia Syndrome Association (http://www.afsafund.org/).

REFERENCES/SUGGESTED READINGS

To enhance this text and add value for the reader, references and suggested readings are included on the companion Evolve site that accompanies this textbook. The reader can view the source and access it online whenever possible.

5

Infectious Disease

1. Understand the types of infectious microorganisms that cause disease.
2. Understand the chain of infection and infection control practices.
3. Recognize the common signs and symptoms of infectious disease.

OUTLINE

VOCAB BUILDERS

Amenable
Asymptomatic
Bullae
Coagulase
Delirium
Dysuria
Effusion
ELISA
Emesis
Exotoxin
Extrinsic
Fomites

Friable
Incubation
Inoculated
Intrinsic
Latent
Maculopapular
Morbidity
Mortality
Neutropenia
Nosocomial
Oliguria
Opportunistic

Petechial
Prophylaxis
Puerperal
Putrefaction
Pyrogen
Sequelae
Seroprevalence
Vector
Vesiculobullous
Virulence

Although human beings are continually exposed to a vast array of microorganisms in the environment, only a small proportion of those microbes are capable of interacting with the human host in such a way that infection and disease result. With the steady advances being made in medicine, people are living longer, but infection is still a frequent cause of hospital admission and remains an important cause of death, especially in the aging population.

From 1950 until 1980 the management of communicable infectious diseases was well under control, and *morbidity* and *mortality* from infectious diseases such as yellow fever, cholera, typhus, malaria, typhoid fever, and plague were no longer serious threats in the United States.

The widespread availability and use of antibiotics successfully treated tuberculosis, syphilis, gonorrhea, bacterial meningitis, scarlet fever, and rheumatic fever. Organized efforts to immunize all children lowered the incidence of vaccine-preventable diseases such as measles, mumps, rubella, diphtheria, tetanus, and poliomyelitis. More recently children have also been vaccinated against chickenpox (varicella), human papilloma virus (HPV), and hepatitis A and B.

Unfortunately, this period of reduced morbidity and mortality secondary to infectious disease did not last, and in the 1970s and 1980s new infectious agents appeared. *Legionella*, human immunodeficiency virus (HIV), antibiotic-resistant organisms, avian flu, and a resurgence of tuberculosis are examples of infectious processes that have returned focus to the prevention and treatment of infectious diseases. Infectious diseases have the ability to spread more rapidly throughout the world than in the past, facilitated by a combination of environmental disruption and increasing human mobility.

At the same time, infectious agents are suspected in disorders such as cancer (liver and cervical), gastric and duodenal ulcers, heart disease, mental illness, and autoimmune diseases.[23] In addition, an area of major public health concern is the continued emergence of antibiotic-resistant microorganisms that appear in hospitals and communities. The most common of these resistant bacteria are methicillin-resistant *Staphylococcus aureus* (MRSA); vancomycin-resistant enterococci (VRE), and multidrug-resistant *Mycobacterium tuberculosis*. In addition, certain *S. aureus* strains demonstrate various levels of resistance to vancomycin, which will make treatment of this organism difficult.

Multidrug resistance in *Pseudomonas aeruginosa* is increasing. Recent increases in the frequency and severity of *Clostridium difficile*–associated illness are correlated with the emergence of a hypervirulent *C. difficile* strain with increased resistance to the fluoroquinolones.[60]

Although a number of new infectious diseases have appeared in recent years, there has been a worldwide resurgence of long-standing diseases once thought to be well controlled. Among infectious diseases in the world, tuberculosis is the second leading cause of death in adults, killing 2 million people a year. Organisms travel on the shoes of tourists, in the ballast of cargo ships, within the confines of jetliners, and in the blood of human beings.

When natural systems are weakened or altered by ecologic stresses, such as pollution and weather disasters, they become more vulnerable to damage or destruction by invading organisms, which can result in the spread of infection. Opportunistic organisms take advantage of the weakened defenses.

All health care professionals must maintain a vigilant attitude to preventing infectious disease. This requires an understanding of the infectious process, the chain of transmission, and selected aspects of control. A basic understanding of these concepts is provided in this chapter, along with a discussion of a few infectious diseases.

SIGNS AND SYMPTOMS OF INFECTIOUS DISEASES

Clinical manifestations of infectious disease are many and varied depending on the etiologic agent (e.g., viruses, bacteria).

Systemic symptoms of infectious disease can include fever and chills, sweating, malaise, and nausea and vomiting. Changes in blood composition may occur, such as an increased number of leukocytes or a change in the types of leukocytes. Older adults may experience a change in mentation. When observing any person for early signs of infection, the physical therapist assistant (PTA) will most likely see one or only a few symptoms (Box 5.1).

BOX 5.1   Signs and Symptoms of Infectious Disease

- Fever, chills, malaise (most common early symptoms)
- Enlarged lymph nodes

Integumentary System
- Purulent drainage from abscess, open wound, or skin lesion
- Skin rash, red streaks
- Bleeding from gums or into joints; joint effusion or erythema

Cardiovascular System
- Petechial lesions
- Tachycardia
- Hypotension
- Change in pulse rate (may increase or decrease depending on the type of infection)

Central Nervous System
- Altered level of consciousness, confusion, seizures
- Headache
- Photophobia
- Memory loss
- Stiff neck, myalgia

Gastrointestinal System
- Nausea
- Vomiting
- Diarrhea

Genitourinary System
- Dysuria or flank pain
- Hematuria
- *Oliguria*
- Urgency, frequency

Upper Respiratory System
- Tachypnea
- Cough
- Dyspnea
- Hoarseness
- Sore throat
- Nasal drainage
- Sputum production
- Oxygen desaturation
- Decreased exercise tolerance
- Prolonged ventilatory support

A change in body temperature is a characteristic systemic symptom of infectious disease, but fever may accompany other noninfectious causes (Box 5.2). *Fever*, a sustained temperature above normal, can be caused by abnormalities of the hypothalamus, brain tumors, dehydration, or toxic substances affecting the temperature-regulating center of the hypothalamus. *Pyrogens* are substances that cause fevers. Certain protein substances and toxins can cause the set point of the hypothalamic thermostat to rise. This results in activation of the hypothalamus to conserve heat and increase heat production.

In infectious disease the endotoxins of some bacteria and the extracts of normal leukocytes are pyrogenic. They act to raise the thermostat in the hypothalamus, thus raising the body temperature. Fever patterns may differ depending on the specific infectious disease present and occur clinically on a continuum—from fever associated with an acute illness lasting 7 to 10 days, to sepsis and ongoing infection lasting longer than 10 days, to fever of unknown origin associated with a possible infectious origin lasting at least 3 weeks.

Neoplasm is another cause of fever. A general guideline of 102° F divides conditions into two groups: those that do not cause temperature elevations exceeding 102° F (39° C) and those that regularly cause the temperature to exceed 102° F. Table 5.1 reflects hospital data; the outpatient population is more likely to experience fever accompanied by generalized arthralgias and myalgias associated with a self-limiting illness or fever with localized symptom(s), such as a sore throat, cough, or right lower quadrant pain, as occurs with bacterial infection. Temperature elevation to 104° F (40° C) may cause *delirium* and seizures, particularly in children. An extremely high fever may damage cells irreversibly.

It is important to note that some people with serious infection do not initially develop fever but instead become *tachypneic, confused* or develop *hypotension*. Most often this situation occurs in older adults, individuals with a health care–associated infection (HAI), or immunocompromised persons.

Inflammation and its exudates may remain localized, permeate the tissue, or spread throughout the body via the blood or lymph. Infection can develop, as is the case with an *abscess*, a localized infection and inflammation with purulent exudate. Leukocytes form a wall around the organisms. The abscess deepens as more leukocytes are drawn into the area, more organisms are killed, and more necrotic tissue is dissolved. The exudate may eventually be broken down and resorbed by the body, in which case the inflammation and infection are resolved. Rupture of the abscess and drainage into other tissues can spread the infection to other areas of the body.

Rash with fever can result from an infectious process caused by any microbe that has successfully penetrated the stratum corneum and multiplied locally. Skin rashes may also occur with infection elsewhere in the body unrelated to local skin

disease. The most common types of skin lesions associated with infectious disease are *maculopapular* eruptions such as measles, nodular lesions, diffuse erythema (scarlet fever), *vesiculobullous* eruptions, herpes zoster, and *petechial* purpuric eruptions.

Red streaks radiating from an infection site in the direction of a regional lymph node may be associated with lymphangitis, which usually occurs as a result of an infectious agent entering the lymphatic channels from an abrasion or local trauma, wound, or infection. The red streak may be obvious, or it may be faint and easily overlooked, especially in dark-skinned people. Involved nodes are usually tender and enlarged (greater than 3 cm).

Inflamed lymph nodes can be associated with other infectious diseases and may be palpated by the PTA, especially in cervical, axillary, or inguinal areas. Palpation may appear to aggravate a primary spasm as if originating in the muscle, when in fact a lymph node under the muscle is the source of the symptom.

In acute infections, nodes are tender, asymmetrical, and enlarged. The overlying skin may be erythematous (red) and warm. Unilaterally warm, tender, enlarged, and fluctuant lymph nodes sometimes associated with elevated body temperature may be caused by pyogenic infections and require medical referral.

Supraclavicular and inguinal nodes are also common metastatic sites for cancer. Nodes involved with metastatic cancer are usually hard and fixed to the underlying tissue. Any suspicious

BOX 5.2 Common Causes of Fever in the Hospitalized Person

- Pneumonia
- Catheter-related infection
- Surgical wound infection
- Urinary tract infection
- Drugs
- Pulmonary emboli
- Infected pressure ulcers

TABLE 5.1 Most Common Causes of Prolonged Fever[a]

Type of Fever	Conditions
Temperature generally does not exceed 102° F	Catheter-associated bacteriuria
	Atelectasis
	Phlebitis
	Pulmonary emboli
	Dehydration
	Pancreatitis
	Myocardial infarction
	Uncomplicated wound infections
	Any malignancy
	Cytomegalovirus
	Hepatitis
	Infectious mononucleosis (Epstein–Barr virus)
	Subacute bacterial endocarditis
	Tuberculosis
Temperature regularly exceeds 102° F	Malignant hyperthermia (secondary to anesthesia)
	Transfusion reactions
	Urosepsis
	Intravenous line sepsis
	Prosthetic valve endocarditis
	Intraabdominal or pelvic peritonitis or abscess
	Clostridium difficile colitis
	Procedure-related bacteremia
	Nosocomial pneumonia
	Drug fever
	HIV infection
	Heat stroke
	Acute bacterial endocarditis
	Tuberculosis (usually disseminated or extrapulmonary)
	Lymphoma
	Metastasizing carcinoma to liver or central nervous system

[a]The evaluation of fever magnitude with the 102° F rule is most often done in the acute care setting. This is a general guideline that must be taken into consideration with other presenting factors.

lymph node changes in size greater than 1 cm, changes in shape, such as being matted together, or changes in consistency, such as becoming rubbery, or the presence of painless, enlarged lymph nodes must be evaluated by a physician. *Joint effusion,* usually of one joint (associated with infectious arthritis), can occur as a result of bacterial, mycobacterial, fungal, or viral etiologic agents.

AGING AND INFECTIOUS DISEASES

As a group, older adults are more susceptible to infectious diseases and experience increased morbidity and mortality compared with younger people; this is especially noted in the frail and debilitated older adult. This increased susceptibility is most likely multifactorial, encompassing immune function as well as comorbidities.

The immune system is complex and requires well-orchestrated adaptability and responsiveness. With aging, there are modest changes in cell-mediated or T-cell function with a decrease in the number of some types of T cells but an increase in the number of memory T cells. These memory cells, however, are slower to respond and require a stronger stimulus. *Extrinsic* factors apart from the immune system can lead to increased susceptibility to infection in the older adult. Atrophic skin is more easily damaged, decreased cough and gag reflexes make it more difficult to control secretions, and decreased bronchiolar elasticity and mucociliary activity contribute to the development of pneumonia.[14]

In many aging people, physical decline or psychologic impairment may result in indifference to personal hygiene and loss of manual dexterity, body mobility, or vision. This may lead to an increased risk for falls, with accompanying injuries and fractures. Many types of infections are seen in the aging adult, but early recognition of infection in the older adult is difficult because people underreport symptoms, the presentation is often vague or atypical, and symptoms are difficult to assess. The older adult may be unable to describe the present illness or history or list the medications being taken. A complete physical examination may be difficult because of the person's uncooperativeness, cognitive impairment, neurologic deficits, or physical impairments. Pain may be poorly localized or absent, or it may be confused with preexisting conditions, such as in septic arthritis in a client with degenerative joint disease.

Fever in older people may not be high enough to cause concern because the basal body temperature is low. A lower threshold for infection should be used, especially if the person is taking a medication that masks fever (e.g., oral temperature of 37.2° C [99° F] or 37.8° C [100° F]). Watch for any recent episodes of confusion, memory loss, or other change in mental status; these may be the first symptoms of infection.[117]

If the febrile response is absent in an older adult with a serious infection, it is a grave sign. Acute infections in the older adult may cause delirium or a sudden change in mental status. Chronic infections of the lungs, bone, skin, kidneys, and central nervous system (CNS) may cause mental status changes perceived as dementia.[83]

INFECTIOUS DISEASES

Definition and Overview

Infection is a process in which an organism establishes a parasitic relationship with its host. This invasion and multiplication of microorganisms produces an immune response and subsequent signs and symptoms. Such reproduction injures the host by causing cellular damage from microorganism-producing toxins or intracellular multiplication or by competing with the host's metabolism.

The host's immune response may compound the tissue damage; such damage may be localized or systemic. However, in some instances, microorganisms may be present in the tissues of the host yet not cause symptomatic disease. This process is called *colonization of organisms.* The person with colonization may be a carrier and transmit the organisms to others but does not have detectable symptoms of infection.

The development of an infection begins with transmission of an infectious organism and depends on a complex interaction of the pathogen, an environment conducive to transmission of the organism, and the susceptibility of the human host. Even after successful transmission of a pathogen, the host may experience more than one possible outcome.

The pathogen may merely contaminate the body surface and be destroyed by first-line defenses such as intact skin or mucous membranes that prevent further invasion. A subclinical infection may occur in which no apparent symptoms are evident other than an identifiable immune response of the host. A rise in the titer of antibody directed against the infecting agent is often the only detectable response. Antibiotic treatment is not necessary, although infection control procedures remain in force to prevent spreading the bacteria to others.

A third possible outcome is the development of a clinically apparent infection in which the host–parasite interaction causes obvious injury and is accompanied by one or more clinical symptoms. This outcome is called *infectious disease,* and ranges in severity from mild to fatal depending on the organism and the response and underlying health of the host.[43]

The period between the pathogen entering the host and the appearance of clinical symptoms is called the *incubation period.* This period may last from a few days to several months, depending on the causative organism and type of disease. Disease symptoms herald the end of the incubation period. A *latent* infection occurs after a microorganism has replicated but remains dormant or inactive in the host, sometimes for years. The host may harbor a pathogen in sufficient quantities to be shed at any time. The stage when an organism can be shed is called the *period of communicability.*

From this concept of communicability, a *communicable disease* can be defined as any disease whereby the causative agent may pass or be carried from one person to another directly or indirectly. It usually precedes symptoms and continues through part or all of clinical disease, sometimes extending to convalescence; but it is important to note that an *asymptomatic* host can still transmit a pathogen. The communicable period, like the incubation period and mode of transmission, varies with different pathogens and different diseases.[95]

Types of Organisms

A great variety of microorganisms are responsible for infectious diseases, including viruses, mycoplasmas, bacteria, rickettsiae, chlamydiae, protozoa, fungi (yeasts and molds), helminths (e.g., tapeworms), mycobacteria, and prions. All microorganisms can be distinguished by certain *intrinsic* properties such as shape, size, structure, chemical composition, antigenic makeup, growth requirements, ability to produce toxins, and ability to remain alive (viability) under adverse conditions such as drying, sunlight, or heat.

These properties provide the basis for identification and classification of the organisms. Knowledge of the properties permits diagnosis of a specific pathogen in specimens of body fluids, secretions, or exudates. All these properties are important to consider when looking for ways to interfere with the mechanisms of transmission.

Viruses are subcellular organisms made up only of a ribonucleic acid (RNA) or a deoxyribonucleic acid (DNA) nucleus covered with proteins. They are the smallest known organisms, visible only through an electron microscope. Viruses are completely dependent on host cells and cannot replicate unless they invade a host cell and stimulate it to participate in the formation of additional virus particles.

The estimated 400 viruses that infect human beings are classified according to their size, shape, or means of transmission. Viruses are not susceptible to antibiotics. However, antiviral medications can mitigate (moderate) the course of the viral illness. *Mycoplasmas* are unusual, self-replicating bacteria that have no cell wall components and very small genomes. For this reason, antibiotics that are active against bacterial cell walls have no effect on mycoplasmas. At present, mycoplasmas remain sensitive to some antibiotics. They require a strict dependence on the host for nutrition and sustenance and are able to pass through many bacteria-retaining filters or barriers because they are very small.[9]

Bacteria are single-celled microorganisms with well-defined cell walls that can grow independently on artificial media without the need for other cells. Bacteria can be classified according to shape. Spherical bacterial cells are called *cocci*, rod-shaped bacteria are called *bacilli,* and spiral bacteria are called *spirilla* or *spirochetes.*

Bacteria can also be classified according to their response to staining (gram positive, gram negative, or acid fast), motility (motile or nonmotile), tendency toward capsulation (encapsulated or nonencapsulated), and capacity to form spores (sporulating or nonsporulating). Bacteria can also be classified according to whether oxygen is needed to replicate and develop (aerobic) or whether they can sustain life in an oxygen-poor (anaerobic) environment. Anaerobic bacteria are organisms that require reduced oxygen tension for growth.

Normal human flora are primarily anaerobic, and disease can be produced when these normal organisms are displaced from their usual tissue sites (e.g., mouth, skin, large bowel, female genital tract) into other tissues or closed body spaces.[84] Other common anaerobic organisms include the spore-forming bacilli such as *Clostridium botulinum* or *Clostridium tetani* that thrive in a strictly anaerobic environment.

Rickettsiae are primarily animal pathogens that generally produce disease in human beings through the bite of an insect vector such as a tick, flea, louse, or mite. They are small, gram-negative, obligate intracellular organisms that often cause life-threatening infections. Like viruses, these microorganisms require a host for replication. *Chlamydiae* are smaller than rickettsiae and bacteria but larger than viruses. They, too, depend on host cells for replication, but unlike viruses they always contain both DNA and RNA and are susceptible to antibiotics.

Protozoa have a single cell unit or a group of nondifferentiated cells loosely held together. They have cell membranes rather than cell walls, and their nuclei are surrounded by nuclear membranes. Larger parasites include roundworms and flatworms. *Fungi* are unicellular to filamentous organisms possessing hyphae (filamentous outgrowths) surrounded by cell walls and containing nuclei. Fungi show relatively little cellular specialization and occur as yeasts (single-cell, oval-shaped organisms) or molds (organisms with branching filaments). Depending on the environment, some fungi may occur in both forms. Fungal diseases in human beings are called *mycoses.*

Prions are proteinaceous, infectious particles consisting of proteins but without nucleic acids. These particles are transmitted from animals to human beings and are characterized by a long latent interval in the host. When reactivated, they cause a rapidly progressive deteriorating state in the host.[28]

The Chain of Transmission

Infection begins with transmission of a pathogen to the host. Successful transmission depends on a pathogenic agent, a reservoir, a portal of exit from the reservoir, a mode (mechanism) of transmission, a portal of entry into the host, and a susceptible host. This sequence of events is called the *chain of transmission.*

Heath care–associated infections (HAIs) are infections that develop in hospitalized persons or persons admitted to a health care facility that were not present before admission. In the United States about 5% of people who enter a health care facility without infection will acquire a *nosocomial* infection. Transmission can be through any of the possible routes discussed in this section. Nosocomial infections or HAIs result in prolongation of hospital stays, increase in cost of care, significant morbidity, and mortality.

In 2002, the Centers for Disease Control and Prevention (CDC) reported 1.7 million HAIs that occurred in U.S. hospitals and more than 98,987 deaths associated with an HAI.[118] Most were caused by pneumonia, but other causes included urinary tract infections from indwelling urinary catheters, surgical site infections, and primary blood infections.

In general, increases in HAIs can be related to more frequent use of invasive devices for monitoring or therapy, more colonization and infection by multidrug-resistant organisms (both viral and bacterial), and greater debilitation and severity of illness of hospitalized clients who acquire these infections.

The increased use of invasive and surgical procedures, immunosuppressants, antibiotics, and the lack of handwashing predispose people to such infections and superinfections. At the same time, the growing number of personnel who come in contact with the client makes the risk of exposure greater.

Prevention is of critical importance in controlling HAIs. The concept of standard precautions emphasizes that all clients must be treated as though each one has a potential bloodborne, transmissible disease; thus all body secretions are handled with care to prevent disease. Handwashing has been cited as the easiest and most effective means of preventing HAIs and must be done routinely even when gloves are used.[11]

Pathogens

Humans coexist with many microorganisms in complex, mutually beneficial relationships. Even so, many organisms are parasitic, maintaining themselves at the expense of their host. Some parasites arouse a pathologic response in the host and are called *pathogens* or *pathogenic agents.* A pathogen is defined as any microorganism that has the capacity to cause disease.[82] As such, pathogens are ineffective parasites because they stimulate a disease response, which may harm the host and eventually kill the pathogen.

The ability of a pathogen to stimulate an immune response in the host varies greatly among organisms, depending on the site of invasion, the number of pathogenic organisms, and the dissemination of organisms in the body. The immune status of a person plays the largest role in determining the risk for infection and the ability of the host to combat organisms that have gained entry.

The *mode of action* of a pathogen refers to how the organism produces a pathologic process. Great variation exists among the various pathogens. Some intracellular pathogens, such as viruses, invade cells and interfere with cellular metabolism, growth, and replication, whereas others invade and cause hyperplasia and cell death. Still other organisms, such as the influenza virus, have the potential to alter their characteristics. This virus is capable of extensive gene rearrangements, resulting in significant changes in surface antigen structure. This ability allows new strains to evade host antibody responses directed at earlier strains.

Some viruses cause a persistent latent infection that can be reactivated in certain circumstances. HIV causes immunosuppression by destroying helper T lymphocytes. Some pathogens, such as the tetanus bacillus, produce a toxin that interferes with intercellular responses. Some bacteria, such as diphtheria and tetanus, secrete water-soluble *exotoxins* that are quickly disseminated in the blood, causing potentially severe systemic and neurologic manifestations. Larger parasites such as roundworms cause anemia and interfere with the function of the gastrointestinal (GI) system.

The characteristics of the organism and the susceptibility of the host influence the likelihood of a pathogen producing infectious disease and the type of disease produced. Not all pathogens have an equal probability of inducing disease in the same host population. *Principal* pathogens regularly cause disease in people with apparently intact defense systems.

Opportunistic pathogens do not cause disease in people with intact host defense systems but can clearly cause devastating disease in many hospitalized and immunocompromised clients.[81] Organisms that may be harmless members of normal flora in healthy people may act as virulent invaders in people with severe defects in host defense mechanisms.[53]

Pathogenicity, the ability of the organism to induce disease, depends on the organism's speed of reproduction in the host, the extent of damage it causes to tissues, and the strength of any toxin released by the pathogen. *Virulence* refers to the potency of the pathogen in producing severe disease and is measured by the case fatality rate. Virulence provides a quantitative measure of pathogenicity. The amount and destructive potential of released toxin are closely related to virulence.

Reservoir

A reservoir is an environment in which an organism can live and multiply, such as an animal, plant, soil, food, or other organic substance or combination of substances. The reservoir provides the essentials for survival of the organism at specific stages in its life cycle. Some parasites have more than one reservoir. Some parasites require more than one reservoir at different growth stages, and still others, such as most sexually transmitted organisms, require only a human reservoir.

Human and animal reservoirs can be symptomatic or asymptomatic carriers of the pathogen. A carrier maintains an environment that promotes growth, multiplication, and shedding of the parasite without exhibiting signs of disease. Hepatitis is a common example of this carrier state in human beings.

Portal of Exit

The portal of exit is the place from which the parasite leaves the reservoir. Generally, this is the site of growth of the organism and corresponds to the system of entry into the next host. For example, the portal of exit for GI parasites is usually the feces, and the portal of entry into a new host is the mouth. Exceptions include hookworm eggs, which are shed in the feces but enter through the skin of a person walking barefoot in soil containing hatched eggs.

Common portals of exit include secretions and fluids, excretions such as urine and feces, open lesions, and exudates such as pus from an open wound or ulcer. Some organisms, such as HIV, have more than one portal of exit. Knowledge of the portal of exit is essential for preventing transmission of a pathogen.

Mode of Transmission

For infection to be transmitted, the invading organism must be transported from the infected source to a susceptible host. Microorganisms are transmitted by several possible routes, and the same microorganism can travel by more than one route. The five main routes of transmission are contact, airborne, droplet, vehicle, and vector borne.

Contact transmission occurs directly or indirectly. Direct contact is the direct transfer of microorganisms that come into physical contact either by skin-to-skin contact or mucous membrane–to–mucous membrane contact.

Indirect contact involves transfer of microorganisms from a source to a host by passive transfer from an inanimate, intermediate object. Inanimate objects can include items such as the telephone, sphygmomanometer, bedside rails, tray tables, countertops, and other items that come in direct contact with the infected person, thus emphasizing the need for thorough handwashing at all times.

Airborne transmission occurs when disease-causing organisms are so small (less than 5 microns) that they are capable of floating on air currents within a room and remain suspended in the air for several hours. They are often propelled from the respiratory tract through coughing or sneezing. A host then inhales the particles directly into the respiratory tract.

Droplet transmission is different from airborne transmission because droplets are larger particles (greater than 5 microns) than airborne particles and they do not remain suspended in air but fall out within 3 feet of the source. They are produced when a person coughs or sneezes and then travel only a short distance. A common example of droplet-spread infection is influenza. Those people who are in closest proximity to the infected source have the highest risk for infection.[43]

Vehicle transmission occurs when infectious organisms are transmitted through a common source to many potential susceptible hosts.

Vector-borne transmission of infectious organisms involves insects and/or animals that act as intermediaries between two or more hosts. Lyme disease and Rocky Mountain spotted fever are examples of vector-borne diseases.

Portal of Entry

A pathogen may enter a new host by ingestion, inhalation, or bites or through contact with mucous membranes, percutaneously or transplacentally. Infectious diseases vary as to the number of organisms and the duration of exposure required to start the infectious process in a new host.

Host Susceptibility

Each person has his or her own susceptibility to infectious disease, and this susceptibility can vary throughout time. A susceptible host has personal characteristics and behaviors that increase the probability of an infectious disease developing.

Biologic and personal characteristics such as age, sex, ethnicity, and heredity influence this probability. General health and nutritional status, hormonal balance, and the presence of concurrent disease also play a role. Likewise, living conditions and personal behaviors such as drug use, diet, hygiene, and sexual practices influence the risk of exposure to pathogens and resistance once exposed.

Older adults in hospitals and long-term care facilities are already susceptible hosts, especially if poorly nourished. Immunosuppressive agents and corticosteroids decrease the body's ability to resist infection. Inadequate or absent handwashing or other breaches of aseptic technique result in spread of microorganisms from health care workers (HCWs) to clients and between individuals receiving health care.

Surfaces of equipment can become contaminated and then transmit microorganisms that cause infection. Incorrect isolation procedures such as leaving doors open to rooms in which airborne precautions are in effect or not using masks increase the risk of transmitting organisms that cause HAIs.

The presence of underlying medical disorders decreases T-cell– and B-cell–mediated immune function. Breaches of body integrity such as nasogastric and chest tubes, intubation, urinary catheters, and IV devices impair the body's defense mechanisms, decreasing the ability of the integumentary, GI, genitourinary, and respiratory systems to resist invasion by microorganisms.[117]

Lines of defense. Susceptibility is also influenced by the presence of anatomic and physiologic defenses, sometimes called *lines of defense.* The *first-line defenses* are external, such as intact skin and mucous membranes; oil and perspiration on skin; cilia in respiratory passages; gag and coughing reflexes; peristalsis in the GI tract; and the flushing action of tears, saliva, and mucus.

These first-line defenses act to inhibit invasion of pathogens and remove them before they have an opportunity to multiply. The chemical composition of body secretions such as tears and sweat, together with the pH of saliva, vaginal secretions, urine, and digestive juices, further prevents or inhibits growth of organisms. Compromise in any of these natural defenses increases host susceptibility to pathogen invasion.

Another important first-line defense is the normal flora of microorganisms that inhabit the skin and mucous membranes in the oral cavity, GI tract, and vagina. These organisms occur naturally and usually coexist with their host in a mutually beneficial relationship. They control the replication of potential pathogens through a mechanism called *microbial antagonism.*

The importance of this mechanism is evident when it is disturbed, as happens when extensive antibiotic therapy destroys normal flora in the oral or vaginal cavity, resulting in *Candida albicans* infection, an overgrowth of yeast. Some normal flora can become pathogenic under specific conditions such as immunosuppression or displacement of the pathogen to another area of the body.

Displacement of normal flora is a common cause of HAIs. This can occur when *Escherichia coli,* ordinarily normal flora in the GI tract, invade the urinary tract. The *second-line defense,* the inflammatory process, and the *third-line defense,* the immune response, share several physiologic components. These include the lymphatic system, leukocytes, and a multitude of chemicals, proteins, and enzymes that facilitate the internal defenses.

Once a microorganism penetrates the first line of defense, the inflammatory response is initiated. Inflammation is a local reaction to cell injury of any type whether from physical, chemical, or thermal damage or microbial invasion. As a response to microbial injury, inflammation is aimed at preventing further invasion by walling off, destroying, or neutralizing the invading organism.

The early inflammatory response is protective, but it can continue for sustained periods in some infections, leading to granuloma formation. The production of new leukocytes may be stimulated for weeks or months and is reflected in an elevated white blood cell count. Sustained inflammation can become chronic and result in destruction of healthy tissues. Extensive necrosis from persistent inflammation can increase tissue susceptibility to the infectious agent or provide an ideal setting for invasion by other pathogens.

The first- and second-line defenses are nonspecific—that is, they operate against all infectious agents in the same way. In contrast, the immune system responds in a specific manner to individual pathogens.

Control of Transmission

Much can be done to prevent transmission of infectious diseases, including the use of barriers and isolation; comprehensive immunizations, including the required immunization of travelers to or emigrants from endemic areas; drug *prophylaxis;* improved nutrition, living conditions, and sanitation; and correction of environmental factors.

Breaking the transmission chain at any of these links can help control transmission of infectious diseases. The link most *amenable* to control varies with the characteristics of the organism, its reservoirs, the type of pathologic response it produces, and the available technology for control. The general goal is to break the chain at the most cost-effective point or points—that is, the point at which the greatest number of people can be protected with available technology and the smallest amount of resources.

Isolation and barriers can be used to prevent the transmission of microorganisms from infected or colonized people to other unaffected people. In hospital or institutional settings, the purpose of isolating individuals or residents is to prevent the transmission of colonized or infectious microorganisms. New isolation guidelines for health care settings were published in 2007 by the CDC and the Hospital Infection Control Practices Advisory Committee (CDC 2007). The guidelines outline a two-tiered approach with specific recommendations categorized as Standard Precautions or Transmission-Based precautions.

Standard precautions assume any person may be contagious. These precautions continue to be the foundation for preventing the transmission of infectious organisms and include hand hygiene, wearing personal protective gear, and, new for these guidelines, respiratory hygiene/cough etiquette. Box 5.3 presents a list of what is considered infectious and safe waste. Boxes 5.4 and 5.5 present hand hygiene indications and technique.

Standard Precautions apply to all clients, whereas Transmission-Based Precautions apply to anyone with documented or suspected infection or colonization with highly transmissible or epidemiologically important organisms that require additional precautions (i.e., in addition to Standard Precautions) to prevent transmission.

Transmission-based precautions are defined according to the major modes of transmission of infectious agents (contact, airborne, and droplet) in the health care setting. Barrier precautions stipulate that gloves should be worn to touch any of the following: blood; all body fluids; secretions and excretions

BOX 5.3   Infectious and Safe Waste

Infectious Waste

- Blood and components
- All disposable sharps (used or unused)
- Urine, stool, or *emesis* if visibly contaminated with blood
- Vaginal secretions
- Semen
- Cerebrospinal fluid (CSF)
- Synovial fluid
- Pericardial fluid (mediastinal tubes)
- Amniotic fluid

Safe Waste

- Cotton balls, Band-Aids
- Latex gloves, masks, or other personal protective devices
- Nasal secretions
- Sputum
- Feces
- Urine
- Vomitus
- Tears
- Sweat

BOX 5.4   Indications for Handwashing and Hand Antisepsis

Wash hands with soap (microbial or nonantimicrobial) and water:

- When hands are visibly soiled with blood or body fluid
- Before eating
- After using the restroom
- After proven or suspected exposure to *Bacillus anthracis*

Decontaminate hands with alcohol-based rub:

- After exposure to body fluids or excretions but hands not visibly soiled
- After having direct contact with a client
- Before and after putting on gloves for client care
- Before and after putting on gloves for a nonsurgical procedure
- After contact with intact client skin
- After attending to a contaminated body site and before moving to a clean body site on the same client
- After contact with objects in client area

Data from Boyce JM, Pittet D, Healthcare Infection Control Practices Advisory Committee, et al.: Guideline for hand hygiene in health-care settings. Recommendations of the Healthcare Infection Control Practices Advisory Committee and the HICPAC/SHEA/APIC/IDSA Hand Hygiene Task Force. Society for Healthcare Epidemiology of America/Association for Professionals in Infection Control/Infectious Diseases Society of America, MMWR Recomm Rep 51:1–45, 2002.

BOX 5.5   Proper Hand-Hygiene Technique

Alcohol-Based Rubs

Using alcohol-based hand rubs may reduce contamination better than soap and water. Apply product in the palm of the hand and rub hands together, remembering to cover all areas of the hands, including the back of the hands and webs of the fingers, until dry.

Washing Hands with Soap and Water

Wet hands before beginning, then add soap. Rub hands together vigorously for at least 15 to 20 seconds, covering all areas of the hands and fingers. Rinse soap from hands and dry completely with a disposable towel. Turn the water off using the towel.

Special Considerations

Jewelry may sequester gram-negative organisms, but more studies are needed to determine whether this translates to increased transmission of the organisms.

Artificial nails or extenders may harbor high concentrations of coagulase-negative staphylococci and gram-negative rods. Although more studies are needed to determine whether artificial nails increase the likelihood of transmitting organisms, the Centers for Disease Control and Prevention (CDC) recommends that artificial nails or extenders not be worn when in contact with clients at high risk for infection.

Wear gloves if potentially coming into contact with blood, body fluids, mucous membranes, or nonintact skin.

For more information on hand hygiene and infection control, visit the websites for the CDC (http://www.cdc.gov) and the Association for Professionals in Infection Control and Epidemiology (http://www.apic.org).

Data from Boyce JM, Pittet D, Healthcare Infection Control Practices Advisory Committee, et al.: Guideline for hand hygiene in health-care settings. Recommendations of the Healthcare Infection Control Practices Advisory Committee and the HICPAC/SHEA/APIC/IDSA Hand Hygiene Task Force. Society for Healthcare Epidemiology of America/Association for Professionals in Infection Control/Infectious Diseases Society of America, MMWR Recomm Rep 51:1–45, 2002.

remains very small.[2,3] The potential increase in susceptibility to influenza and death from respiratory illness in high-risk people suggests that the influenza and pneumococcal vaccines should include these groups in standard immunization programs.[1]

Prophylactic antibiotic therapy may prevent certain infections and is usually reserved for people at high risk of exposure to dangerous organisms.[36]

Improved nutrition, living conditions, and *sanitation* through the use of disinfection, sterilization, and antiinfective drugs can inactivate multidrug resistant organisms such as *S. aureus.*

Two distinct strains of MRSA have become common causes of hospital- and community-acquired infections. MRSA usually develops when multiple antibiotics are used in the treatment of infection and in older adults who are debilitated, are having surgery or multiple invasive procedures, or are being treated in critical care units.

Correction of environmental factors, particularly water treatment; food and milk safety programs; and control of animals, vectors, rodents, sewage, and solid wastes, can best eradicate nonhuman environments (reservoirs) and thus control pathogens.

Other prevention methods in this category include proper handling and disposal of secretions, excretions, and exudates; isolation of infected clients; and quarantine of contacts.

The CDC has recommended specific transmission precautions based on knowledge of the transmission chain for individual infections. The precautions were designed to prevent transmission of pathogens among hospitalized people, HCWs, and visitors.

except sweat, regardless of whether these are visibly bloody; nonintact skin; and mucous membranes.

Immunization, by decreasing host susceptibility, can now control many diseases, including diphtheria, tetanus, pertussis, measles, mumps, rubella, some forms of meningitis, poliomyelitis, hepatitis A and B, pneumococcal pneumonia, influenza (certain strains), and rabies. Vaccines, which contain live but attenuated (weakened) or killed microbes, induce active immunity against bacterial and viral diseases by stimulating antibody formation.

These molecules lock onto specific proteins made by a virus or bacterium, which are often those proteins lodged in the microbe's outer coat. Once antibodies attach to an invading microbe, other immune defenses are evoked to destroy it. Side effects to immunization can occur, but the incidence of significant adverse effects of immunization among human beings

5.1 Special Implications for The PTA: Control of Transmission

The impact of infections cannot be underestimated in a physical therapy practice or rehabilitation setting. Infections, and especially HAIs, decrease patients' endurance and delay recovery and progression toward discharge or transfer to a more independent setting. We must do everything we can to halt the spread of organisms that can cause or contribute to infections leading to morbidity and mortality at all levels of care.

The CDC has set up guidelines for the care of all clients regarding precautions against the transmission of infectious disease. These should be used with all clients regardless of their disease status. Blood and all body fluids are potentially infectious and should be handled as such (see Box 5.3).

All clients receiving therapy may be asymptomatic hosts during the period of communicability. The careful use of precautionary measures severely limits the transmission of any disease. In addition, each hospital has transmission-based precautions organized according to categories of transmission routes to prevent the spread of infectious disease to others. Professionals must be familiar with these procedures and follow them carefully.

HCWs should be concerned about improving their resistance and decreasing their susceptibility to infectious diseases. Maintaining an adequate immunization status is one approach. Every HCW should be adequately immunized against hepatitis B, measles, mumps, rubella, polio, tetanus, diphtheria, and varicella. The most recent CDC recommendations for immunization of HCWs are given in Table 5.2.

Second to immunization, handwashing is the most effective disease-preventing measure anyone can practice. Despite compelling evidence that proper handwashing can reduce the transmission of pathogens to patients and clients and the spread of antimicrobial resistance, the adherence of HCWs to recommended hand hygiene practices remains unacceptably low.[113] A single hand can carry 200 million organisms, including bacteria, viruses, and fungi. It takes a full 5 minutes of handwashing to cleanse 99% of the bacteria from fingernails, thumbs, palm creases, and backs of the hands. The average wash-and-rinse in the hospital setting is less than 10 seconds, and the dominant hand is often underwashed.[121]

However, many HCWs experience severe hand irritation, with cracking and bleeding, as a consequence of frequent handwashing and glove use. Integumentary breakdown has major implications for nosocomial infection control and promotes the spread of bloodborne viruses. An alcohol-based hand rub requires less time, is microbiologically more effective than washing with soap and water, and is less irritating to the skin. Alcohol-based hand rubs can replace handwashing as the standard for hand hygiene in health care settings in all situations in which the hands are not visibly soiled.[111]

Alcohol hand rinses may increase compliance with hand disinfection and are as effective as soaps; but used without the added skin protection, alcohol has a significant drying effect, leading to the same skin problems associated with frequent washing.[58] The use of lotions after hand sanitation may also decrease cracking of skin and lead to a reduction in bacterial shedding from hands.[11,59]

Health Care–Associated Infections

PTAs can help prevent transmission of HAIs from themselves to others, from client to client, and from client to self by following these standard precautions and guidelines:

- Follow strict infection-control procedures. Make sure to identify each client's individual transmission precautions and procedures. When in doubt, ask the nursing staff regarding the status of the person in question.

- Strictly follow necessary isolation techniques. Doors must remain closed, especially in negative pressure rooms.
- Observe *all* clients for signs of infection (see Box 5.1), especially those people at high risk. Notify nursing or medical staff of these observations.
- Always follow proper handwashing technique or use an alcohol-based hand antiseptic, and encourage other staff members to do so as well. Take time to wash or disinfect hands before and after every client.
- Stay away from susceptible, high-risk clients when you have an obvious infection. Make arrangements for another therapist to treat that client until the contagious period has passed. If in doubt, consult a physician.
- Take special precautions with vulnerable clients—those with Foley catheters, mechanical ventilators, or intravenous lines and those recuperating from surgery. Specific tips for preventing infection in these situations are listed in Box 5.6.
- Avoid the use of acrylic nails, which harbor pathogens.[58]

Hydrotherapy and Therapeutic Pool Protocol

In the past, routine cultures of hydrotherapy and pool equipment were performed to identify and supposedly eliminate colonization of infectious bacteria. In this way, the spread of infection from equipment to client and from client to client was prevented, especially in the acute care setting.

Now, under the outcomes-based management philosophy, infection control is cost driven so that the outcome is managed, as long as the outcome is what was predicted and intended or is improving. For example, in the case of preventing the spread of infection through hydrotherapy or therapeutic pool equipment, good disinfection and cleaning procedures are practiced and monitored closely. This plan is both cost effective and accompanied by a high degree of safety.

Under outcomes-based management, when an infectious problem develops, the cause is traced back to the source and eliminated at that point.

When using hydrotherapy (e.g., pulsatile lavage with suction, whirlpool) for wound care, clients should be treated in a private treatment room with all walls and doors closed. Proper personal protective equipment, such as masks, gloves, and eyewear, must be worn by the PTA when treating the individual and cleaning hydrotherapy equipment. Whirlpool equipment should be cleaned before and after treatment.[51]

Home Health Care

Preventing spread of an infectious disease to the family, the home health PTA, and perhaps the community is a primary concern when preparing the client for return home. The PTA should work closely with the home health nurse and seek guidance if unsure how to handle a specific situation. A list of helpful hints for home health care includes the following[95]:

- Handwashing is the best protection against transmission of infectious diseases, and it is essential after providing direct care and before touching anything when gloves are removed.
- Staff should leave extraneous clothing and equipment outside the client's area and take in only items that are needed.
- Equipment needed on a regular basis, such as the blood pressure cuff and stethoscope, should be in the room at the beginning of home health care. Stethoscopes are often contaminated with staphylococci and are therefore a potential vector of infection. Such contamination poses a risk to people with open wounds such as burns. This contamination is greatly reduced by frequent cleaning with alcohol or nonionic detergent; cleaning with antiseptic soap is only 75% effective in reducing the bacterial count.[47]

- When it is no longer needed, equipment should be bagged or covered and taken to the appropriate area for decontamination and reprocessing. Disposable equipment should be contained, labeled, and discarded.
- The PTA should be adequately supplied with gloves, masks, gowns, and disposable plastic aprons. Some plastic bags of different sizes should be carried for the PTA's own use and to demonstrate to the client's family how to handle soiled linens and trash.
- Paper towels are useful when working in the client's area. Use them as a clean surface during care and to wipe your hands.
- Before going into the client's area, plan what to do and gather the items needed.
- It is important to remember that isolation or precautions can have a negative effect on the family. Help the family feel comfortable with the techniques needed for isolation. Encourage them to visit with the client and not just be with him or her during care.
- Should the client have a feces-borne infectious disease such as hepatitis A or salmonellosis, it is important to show the family how to bag and launder soiled linens. It is equally important to demonstrate how to bag and dispose of soiled paper products such as linen savers, which cannot be flushed down the toilet. Remind the family to wash their hands afterward, and the PTA should do so as well.
- If the client has hepatitis A or salmonellosis, the family and the client should be reminded not to handle raw food served to others, such as lettuce or tomatoes, until the physician determines the client is past the infectious stage.
- If a client with a bloodborne illness accidentally sustains a cut, any spilled blood on inanimate objects or surfaces should be cleaned off with household bleach and water. Razors and toothbrushes should not be shared.
- The PTA should practice self-protection at all times. Use good handwashing technique, and when in doubt, ask for assistance from other, more knowledgeable health care staff.

SPECIFIC INFECTIOUS DISEASES

Most infections are confined to specific organ systems. In this book, many of the important infectious disease entities are discussed in the specific chapter dealing with the affected anatomic area. Only the most commonly encountered infectious problems not covered elsewhere are included in this chapter.

Bacterial Infections
Clostridium Difficile

Overview. C. difficile ("C diff") infection, also known as *Clostridium difficile–associated disease* (CDAD), is becoming an important public health issue as a cause of nosocomial and community-based diarrhea. Once thought to be only associated with antibiotic use in medical settings, it is now also detected in healthy persons in the community without a history of antibiotic exposure. *C. difficile* is an anaerobic, spore-forming bacillus that can cause symptoms ranging from mild diarrhea to severe colonic inflammation leading to death. It is the only anaerobe that poses a health care–associated risk

CDAD is increasingly recognized among residents of long-term care facilities or persons in acute care or short-stay hospitals because of the high rates of antibiotic use.[61]

Incidence. CDAD rates and severity appear to be increasing rapidly in the United States and Canada and show no sign of decline.

Etiology, transmission, and risk factors. Transmission of C. difficile occurs primarily in health care facilities via the fecal–oral route after contamination of the hands of HCWs and patients with oral ingestion of the causative organism. Contamination of the patient care environment also plays an important role.[109] Nonhuman reservoirs such as water, raw vegetables, and

---

TABLE 5.2   Centers for Disease Control and Prevention Recommendations for Immunization of Health Care Workers

Vaccine	Schedule
Hepatitis B	Give recombinant vaccine (intramuscularly [IM]) in a three-dose series; obtain anti-HBs serologic testing 1–2 months after last dose.
Influenza	Annual influenza vaccination is recommended for all persons aged 6 months and older who have no medical contraindications; therefore, vaccination of all HCP who have no contraindications is recommended
Measles, mumps, rubella (MMR)	For anyone born in 1957 or later without serologic evidence of immunity or prior vaccination (adults born before 1957 generally are considered immune); contraindicated in pregnancy
Varicella zoster (chickenpox)	HCWs who have no serologic proof of immunity, prior vaccination, or history of chickenpox; contraindicated in pregnancy.
Tetanus and diphtheria (Td)	Recommended for all adults with booster every 10 years; tetanus prophylaxis advised for HCP in wound management; advised after needlestick injury. New Advisory Committee on Immunization Practices (ACIP) recommendations for Tdap (combined tetanus, diphtheria, and pertussis vaccine) in adults and HCP were released in 2011.[a]
Meningococcal	Not recommended routinely for all HCP; recommended for HCP in direct contact with respiratory secretions from infected persons without proper use of precautions; microbiologists who are routinely exposed to *Neisseria meningitidis*; postexposure prophylaxis advised.
Bacille Calmette–Guérin (BCG)	Not used in the United States as prophylaxis; foreign-born HCWs who have received this vaccine outside the United States must be aware that it does *not* provide lifelong immunity.

[a]Updated recommendations for use of tetanus toxoid, reduced diphtheria toxoid, and acellular pertussis (Tdap) vaccine from the advisory committee on immunization practices, 2010, MMWR Morb Mortal Wkly Rep 60:13–15, 2011. For more complete information visit the CDC Vaccines and Immunizations website (http://www.cdc.gov/vaccines), Immunization Action Coalition (IAC) website (http://www.immunize.org/acip), and check with the CDC for updates (http://www.cdc.gov/vaccines/hcp/acip-recs/vacc-specific/index.html). Data from Centers for Disease Control and Prevention: Immunization of health-care personnel: recommendations of the Advisory Committee on Immunization Practices (ACIP), 60(RR07):1–45, 2011. http://www.cdc.gov/mmwr/preview/mmwrhtml/rr6007a1.htm. Accessed June 23, 2014.

anti-HBs, Antibody to the surface antigen of the hepatitis B virus; *HCP,* health care provider; *HCWs,* health care workers.
HCWs should consult with their physicians for individual recommendations based on medical and other indications.

animals can also cause infection.[6] Tube feeding is also a risk factor.[32]

Age (65 years or older) is a definite risk factor, especially when linked with antibiotic use and residence in acute or long-term health care facilities, where exposure is increased through physical proximity of residents and their health care providers or admittance to a room that housed someone with CDAD during the previous 10 to 14 days.[21,32]

BOX 5.6   Tips for Preventing Infection

Chest Tube
- Prevent chest tube from kinking by carefully coiling the tubing on top of the bed and securing it to the bed linen, leaving room for the person to turn.

Tracheostomy
- Contact with secretions occurs with a tracheostomy; follow standard precautions. When direct contact is made and potential splash secondary to expelled secretions occurs, gown, mask, protective facewear, and gloves are needed.

Urinary Catheter
- Follow standard precautions for handwashing techniques.
- Do not allow the drainage bag spigot to come in contact with a contaminated surface.
- When the drainage tubing becomes disconnected, do not touch the ends of the tubing or catheter. Contact the nursing staff for reconnecting.
- Before turning, moving, or transferring a catheterized person, locate the proximal end of the tubing and either clamp it to the person's gown or hold it to allow necessary slack during movement. This will help prevent the catheter from accidentally and traumatically being pulled out.
- Whenever possible, avoid raising the drainage bag above the level of the person's bladder.
- If it becomes necessary to raise the bag during transfers, clamp the tubing but avoid prolonged clamping or kinking of the tubing (except during bladder conditioning).
- Avoid allowing large loops of tubing to dangle from the bedside, wheelchair, or walker.
- Drain all urine from tubing into the bag before the person exercises or ambulates.

Intravenous Devices
- If you have exudative lesions or weeping dermatitis, refrain from all direct contact with intravenous (IV) or invasive equipment until the condition resolves.
- Notify the nursing staff of any suspicious observations, such as if the IV device is not dripping at a steady rate (either none at all or flowing very fast), if the IV bag is empty, or if blood is flowing from insertion of the IV catheter tip into the person's body out into the IV line.

Nasogastric and Feeding Tubes
- Care must be taken to avoid excessive movement or pulling and tugging of these tubes.
- Wash your hands before and after touching the entry point of the tube into the body.

Hydrotherapy
- Hydrotherapy for wound care (pulsatile lavage with suction, whirlpool) should be performed in a private treatment room with all walls and doors closed.
- Proper personal protective equipment (PPE) must be worn when treating the client and/or cleaning hydrotherapy equipment.
- Whirlpool equipment should be cleaned before and after treatment.

Pathogenesis. Change in the protective flora of the enteric system induced by antibiotics may produce acute diarrhea by overgrowth and toxin production by *C. difficile.* Gastric acid constitutes a major defense mechanism against ingested pathogens. Loss of stomach acid has been associated with colonization of the normally sterile upper GI tract.

In the healthy person the *C. difficile* organism is inactive in the spore form. It is assumed that antibiotic-induced change in the competing intestinal flora promotes a conversion from a spore state to the vegetative forms, which then replicate and produce toxins, causing cellular damage of the intestinal mucosa and increased gut permeability.[8]

A more virulent strain of *C. difficile* is associated with more frequent and more severe disease with higher rates of toxic megacolon, shock, and even death.

Clinical manifestations. CDAD is easily recognized by persistent diarrhea associated with antibiotic use in conjunction with abdominal cramping and tenderness. Although loose stools are frequently associated with antibiotic use without infection, *C. difficile* infection is noted by watery diarrhea at least three times a day for 2 or more days. Severe disease can be manifested by fever, abdominal pain, ileus, sepsis, toxic megacolon, perforation, and/or sepsis.

Medical Management

Diagnosis and Treatment

Diagnosis is typically confirmed by identifying toxins in the stool of the infected individual. Colonoscopy identifying pseudomembranous lesions present late in the disease may help identify difficult-to-diagnose cases.

Standard treatment consists of prompt discontinuation of the antibiotic agent with administration of oral metronidazole (Flagyl), an antibiotic effective against anaerobic bacteria.

Prevention

Prevention of this HAI is imperative to reduce patient morbidity and mortality and reduce health care costs associated with infection control, medication, and excess hospital days.

CDAD is by and large an HAI disease and therefore most prevention and control efforts take place in the health care setting. Proven strategies include hand hygiene, environmental disinfection, barrier precautions, and antimicrobial stewardship.[102]

Contact precautions are recommended to prevent the transmission of *C. difficile* in the health care setting and consist of using private rooms or rooms shared by CDAD patients, using gloves and gowns for all contact, and using disposable equipment or cleaning equipment between uses with different patients.[35] Preventing oral ingestion of the *C. difficile* organism is important whenever suction devices are used in the oral cavity (mouth). A strong correlation has been noted between ventilator-associated pneumonia rates and CDAD rates in the critical care population, emphasizing again the importance of cleanliness of anything introduced into a patient's mouth and stomach.[101]

Staphylococcal Infections

Overview and incidence. Staphylococci bacteria are among the most common bacterial pathogens normally residing on the skin. Although there are more than 30 species of staphylococci, only a few are clinically relevant.

Staphylococci can be characterized as *coagulase* positive or negative. *S. aureus* is, almost without exception, the only significant staphylococcal species that is coagulase positive.

Several species of coagulase-negative bacteria may be pathogenic, but all are often collectively referred to as "coagulase-negative staph" (CoNS). These organisms are nonmotile and anaerobic. They are hardy and able to survive on inanimate objects for an extended period.

Staphylococci bacteria are the leading cause of nosocomial and community-acquired infections, accounting for about 13% of all hospital infections each year. This figure translates into approximately 2 million hospital infections annually, resulting in 60,000 to 80,000 deaths each year. Staphylococcal species are the most common cause of infections, affecting all ages and involving the blood, skin, lung, soft tissue, joints, and bones. They are a leading cause of infective endocarditis.

Risk factors. *S. aureus* spreads by direct contact with colonized surfaces or people. The most common location of human colonization of *S. aureus* is the nares (nasal passages), although the skin, axilla, perineum, vagina, and oropharynx can also be colonized.

Colonization occurs more frequently in individuals with diabetes who are insulin dependent, individuals who are HIV positive, clients receiving hemodialysis, IV drug users, and persons with chronic skin lesions. Individuals more likely to develop a staphylococcal infection include surgical and burn patients (from damaged skin); individuals with diabetes who require insulin (from needlesticks); anyone who is neutropenic; individuals with prosthetics, chronic skin disease, rheumatoid arthritis, or catheters; and people undergoing corticosteroid therapy.

Predisposing factors are multiple and varied, depending on disease location (Table 5.3).

Pathogenesis. *S. aureus* cannot invade through intact skin or mucous membranes; infection usually begins with inoculation of the organism through damaged skin. Once inside the body, the organism is a virulent pathogen, secreting membrane-damaging enzymes and toxins that harm host tissues. If the bacteria are then able to evade local host defenses, they can spread via the bloodstream to almost any location in the body. The bones, joints, kidney, lung, and heart valves are the most common sites of *S. aureus* infections.

Clinical manifestations. When *S. aureus* is *inoculated* into a previously sterile site, infection usually produces abscess formation. The abscesses range in size from microscopic to lesions several centimeters in diameter filled with pus and bacteria (Fig. 5.1).

Fever, chills, and symptoms associated with the affected area may accompany staphylococcal infection of any body part.

Acute *S. osteomyelitis,* usually in the bones of the legs, most commonly affects boys aged 3 to 10 years, most of whom have a history of infection or trauma. Osteomyelitis manifesting in the vertebrae affects adults older than age 50 years, often following staphylococcal infections of the skin or urinary tract, after prostatic surgery, or after pinning of a fracture. Clinical manifestations include abrupt onset of fever, shaking, chills, pain and swelling over the infected area, restlessness, and headache.

Staphylococcus-associated *skin infections* include cellulitis, boil-like lesions, and small macules that may develop into pus-filled vesicles. Associated symptoms may include mild or spiking fever and malaise.

5.2 Special Implications for the PTA: Staphylococcal Infections

Some organisms such as *Staphylococcus aureus* (and streptococci) are considered resident organisms because they are not easily removed by scrubbing and often can be cultured from the HCW's skin. Many HCWs carry *S. aureus* without *sequelae* and are able to shed organisms into nonintact skin areas of susceptible hosts, causing infections.

For the most part, good handwashing with soap or an alcohol-based rub is adequate in the therapy or home setting, but PTAs need to consistently educate family members and caregivers about infection control through handwashing and environmental management.

Antimicrobial soaps that contain chemicals to kill transient and some resident organisms may be recommended, although debate continues over questions of long-term resistance. The choice of using an antimicrobial soap or plain soap is usually based on the need to reduce and maintain minimal counts of resident organisms and to mechanically remove transient organisms such as *Pseudomonas, Escherichia coli, Salmonella,* or *Shigella*.

When working with people who are infected with drug-resistant, gram-positive cocci such as MRSA[62] or VRE, antimicrobial soap may be recommended because some studies have shown that these organisms persist on hands until an antimicrobial product is used.[15]

Anyone with an active, resistant infection should not be discharged from an inpatient setting. However, if such a case is encountered, the PTA must remember that these organisms are spread by contact. Therefore the same germicidal cleaning measures used in a hospital or institutional setting are required.

All equipment that comes in direct contact with a draining area needs to be cleaned with an approved germicidal product before and after use. Isolation is not required. American Physical Therapy Association infection control guidelines for hydrotherapy and physical therapy aquatic programs recommend that clients with MRSA may attend therapy programs provided the area of colonization can be contained. If it is in a wound, the drainage must be contained within the dressing without evidence of breakthrough.

Streptococcal Infections

Group A streptococci. *Streptococcus pyogenes,* the prototype of group A streptococci (GAS), is one of the most common bacterial pathogens of human beings of any age. It causes many diseases of diverse organ systems, ranging from skin infections to acute self-limited pharyngitis to postinfectious syndromes of rheumatic fever (Box 5.7).

GAS disease is typically transmitted via contact with respiratory droplets, although other, less common mechanisms have been identified, such as foodborne transmission. In health care settings, personnel may spread GAS after contact with clients who have infected secretions or may become infected themselves. The infected personnel subsequently acquire a variety of GAS-related illnesses. HCWs who are GAS carriers have infrequently been linked to sporadic outbreaks of surgical site, postpartum, or burn wound infection and to foodborne transmission of GAS-causing pharyngitis. Adherence to standard precautions or other transmission-based precautions can prevent nosocomial transmission of GAS to personnel. Restriction from client care activities and food handling is indicated for personnel with GAS.

Streptococcal pharyngitis. Streptococcal pharyngitis, commonly known as *strep throat,* occurs most commonly in children and accounts for 15% to 36% of all sore throats in children. It is also the only pharyngitis requiring antibiotic treatment. This organism often colonizes in throats of people

TABLE 5.3 Staphylococcal Infections

Type	Predisposing Factors
Bacteremia	Infected surgical wounds Abscesses Infected intravenous or intraarterial catheter sites, catheter tips Infected vascular grafts or prostheses Infected pressure ulcers Osteomyelitis Injection drug abuse Source unknown (primary bacteremia) Cellulitis Burns Immunosuppression Debilitating diseases (e.g., diabetes, renal failure) Infective endocarditis Cancer (leukemia) or neutropenia after chemotherapy or radiation
Pneumonia	Immunodeficiency (especially older adults and children [2 years old]) Chronic lung disease and cystic fibrosis Malignancy Antibiotics that kill normal respiratory flora but spare *Staphylococcus aureus* Viral respiratory infections, especially influenza Bloodborne bacteria spread to the lungs from primary sites of infections (e.g., heart valves, abscesses, pulmonary emboli) Recent bronchial or endotracheal suctioning or intubation
Enterocolitis	Broad-spectrum antibiotics as prophylaxis for bowel surgery or treatment of hepatic coma Elderly; newborn infants (associated with staphylococcal skin lesions)
Osteomyelitis	Hematogenous organisms (bloodborne) Skin trauma Infection spreading from adjacent joint or other infected tissues *Staphylococcus aureus* bacteremia Orthopedic surgery or trauma Cardiothoracic surgery Usually occurs in growing bones, especially femur and tibia of children younger than 12 years old Male sex
Food poisoning	Contaminated food
Skin infections	Decreased resistance Burns or pressure ulcers Decreased blood flow Skin contamination from nasal discharge Foreign bodies Underlying skin diseases such as eczema and acne Common in persons with poor hygiene living in crowded quarters

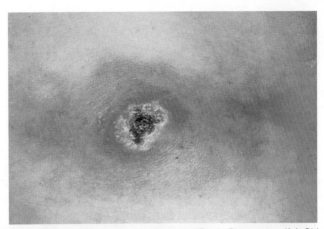

FIG. 5.1 *Staphylococcus* skin abscess. (From Braverman IM: Skin signs of systemic disease, ed 3, Philadelphia, 1998, Saunders.)

BOX 5.7 Streptococcal Infections

***Streptococcus Pyogenes* (Group A Streptococci)**
Suppurative
- Streptococcal pharyngitis
- Scarlet fever (scarlatina)
- Impetigo (streptococcal pyoderma)
- Streptococcal gangrene (necrotizing fasciitis)
- Streptococcal cellulitis
- Streptococcal myositis
- Puerperal sepsis (after vaginal delivery or abortion)
- Toxic shock syndrome (TSS)
- Pneumonia (rare)

Nonsuppurative
- Rheumatic fever
- Acute poststreptococcal glomerulonephritis

***Streptococcus Agalactiae* (Group B Streptococci)**
- Neonatal streptococcal infections
- Adult group B streptococcal infection

Streptococcus Pneumoniae
- Pneumococcal pneumonia
- Otitis media
- Meningitis
- Endocarditis

with no symptoms; up to 20% of schoolchildren may be carriers (pets may also be carriers).

The incubation stage is 1 to 5 days. Clinical manifestations vary but may include a fever, sore throat with pain on swallowing (may be severe), beefy red pharynx, edematous tonsils with exudate, swollen lymph nodes along the jaw line, generalized malaise and weakness, anorexia, and occasional abdominal discomfort (particularly in children). Up to 40% of affected children may have symptoms too mild for diagnosis.

Diagnosis is usually by rapid diagnostic kits, but if the results are negative, a throat culture (the gold standard) should be performed. Treatment is with antibiotics to avoid poststreptococcal syndromes.

Impetigo. Impetigo is principally caused by GAS, although other streptococcal or staphylococcal species may be involved. It occurs most commonly in children aged 2 to 5 years, especially in hot, humid weather. Predisposing factors include close contact in schools, overcrowded living quarters, poor skin hygiene, and minor skin trauma.

Colonization with GAS most often precedes the skin lesions, so good hygiene is essential. Small macules appear and rapidly develop into vesicles that become pustular and encrusted. Neither fever nor pain is typically a component of impetigo and if present suggests another diagnosis.

Scratching spreads infection, which may develop into lymphadenitis or cellulitis. Lesions often affect the face, although any area of the skin can be involved. Antibiotic treatment should cover both staphylococcal and streptococcal species.

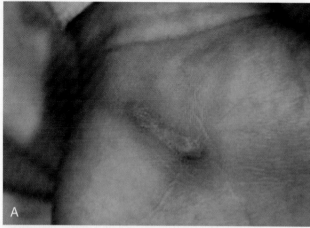

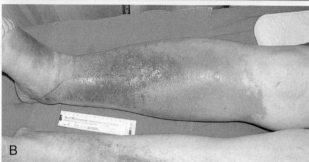

FIG. 5.2 Cellulitis and lymphangitis. (A) Infection in a wound is usually from streptococcal bacteria, but often in combination with *Staphylococcus*. Infection can be local without streaking (cellulitis), local infection with streaking toward the heart (lymphangitis or blood poisoning), or pus forming (boil or abscess). This boy stuck a needle into a burn blister on his palm the previous day. Note the redness and the streaking. (B) Erysipelas, a type of cellulitis, is more of a clinical diagnosis describing an infectious skin condition characterized by sharp, elevated, demarcated borders; redness; swelling; vesicles; bullae; fever; pain; and lymphadenopathy. Erysipelas affects the face and legs most often. It is almost always caused by group A streptococci but can be caused by *Staphylococcus*. (A, Courtesy Michael Engberson, Utah Mountain Biking. B, From Vinh DC, Embil JM: Rapidly progressive soft tissue infections. Lancet Infect Dis 5(8):501-513, 2005.)

Erysipelas. Streptococcal species and other organisms may cause a type of cellulitis that can lead to an acute infection of the skin accompanied by fever and chills. The skin may be very red, shiny, and swollen (Fig. 5.2). This type of cellulitis develops over a few hours; *bullae* may form in the affected areas after 2 to 3 days. The margins between normal and infected skin are well demarcated.

The most common areas affected include the face and legs, although erysipelas can occur anywhere. The disease is more common in women and may be especially severe in anyone with a debilitating condition.[41] Antibiotics that cover GAS are the treatment of choice but may need to be broadened to include staphylococcal species.

Streptococcal cellulitis. Streptococcal cellulitis, an acute spreading inflammation of the skin and subcutaneous tissues, usually results from infection of burns, wounds, or other breaks in the skin, although in some cases no entry site is noted. Recurrent episodes of cellulitis may occur in extremities in which lymphatic drainage has been impaired.

Lymphangitis may accompany cellulitis or may occur after clinically minor or unapparent skin infection. Lymphangitis is readily recognized by the presence of red, tender, linear streaks directed toward enlarged, tender regional lymph nodes. It is accompanied by systemic symptoms such as chills, fever, malaise, and headache.

Streptococcal necrotizing fasciitis. Necrotizing fasciitis (NF) is a serious infection that progresses rapidly along fascial planes, usually in the legs, causing severe tissue damage as it spreads. The classification of soft-tissue necrotizing infections has changed over the years, and NF was previously known as streptococcal gangrene. There are different types of NF caused by various organisms, but they often have overlapping features.

NF may be difficult to diagnose initially. Pain and fever are present, but the overlying skin often is without abnormalities. The infection spreads rapidly, causing edema and tenderness. Changes later occur in the skin as thrombosis of blood vessels occurs. The skin turns a dark red color with accompanying induration. Bullae form and fill with dark fluid. Later the skin becomes *friable* and turns a maroon or black color consistent with ischemia.

The bacteria produce several pyogenic endotoxins, causing severe breakdown of tissue in multiple organs. Affected individuals commonly experience toxic shock syndrome with hypotension, nausea, vomiting, and delirium. There is often renal and hepatic compromise as well as pulmonary infiltrates, leading to respiratory distress. The mortality rate is high, with 1 in 4 persons dying from the infection.[72]

Immediate surgery with aggressive debridement of all necrotic tissue along with appropriate intensive IV antibiotics are essential to save muscles and limbs.[92] Gram stain and culture of the site are essential to identify the organism(s) and antimicrobial susceptibility.

Streptococcal myositis. Streptococcal myositis is a rare but potentially life-threatening entity characterized by severe pain and inflammation in the affected muscle with few abnormalities of overlying skin. Typically blunt, nonpenetrating trauma or hematologic seeding of bacteria to the muscle leads to the infection. Two forms of streptococcal myositis have been reported. The first is a slower, less virulent process, whereas the second is more fulminant with systemic symptoms, high fever, bacteremia, and a high mortality rate.[110]

This condition can also be caused by other bacteria (usually *S. aureus*), mycobacteria, fungi, viruses, and protozoan forms. Clinical features of myositis and NF often overlap. Therapy includes aggressive surgical debridement and IV antibiotics.

Puerperal sepsis. *Puerperal* sepsis follows abortion or normal delivery when streptococci colonizing the woman or transmitted from medical personnel invade the endometrium and surrounding structures, lymphatics, and bloodstream. The resulting endometritis and septicemia may be complicated by pelvic cellulitis, septic pelvic thrombophlebitis, peritonitis, or pelvic abscess. Before the antibiotic era and the benefits of handwashing between clients were known, this disease was more common and associated with a high mortality rate.

5.3 Special Implications for the PTA: Streptococcal Infections Health care personnel can transmit and acquire streptococcal infections. Guidelines for preventing transmission must be followed at all times (see Boxes 5.3 and 5.4 and Table 5.2).

Group B streptococci. Group B streptococcal infection (*Streptococcus agalactiae*) is the leading cause of neonatal pneumonia, meningitis, and sepsis. More than 1000 neonatal infections with group B streptococci occur in the United States each year, and approximately 5% of the infants with the infection die. Group B streptococci are part of the normal vaginal flora and are found in more than 20% of women.[90]

Neonates who develop early infections may demonstrate hypotension, pneumonia, bacteremia, or meningitis. Late disease is acquired either at birth or from contact with the infected mother or other personnel. These babies demonstrate fever, bacteremia, meningitis, and pneumonia.[91]

Rapid administration of IV antibiotics is essential. The CDC recommends that pregnant women be screened for carriage of group B streptococci and appropriate antibiotics be given to prevent transmission to their babies.[79,90] A vaccine is under development that would reduce the number of women and babies exposed to antibiotics.

Streptococcus pneumoniae

Etiologic and risk factors. Pneumonia and other infections, such as sepsis, otitis media, and meningitis, can be caused by *Streptococcus pneumoniae* (see Box 5.7). This organism colonizes the oropharynx and nasopharynx and can be found in 5% to 10% of healthy adults and 20% to 40% of children. Once colonized, the host can develop illness related to *S. pneumoniae* when the organism spreads to the sinuses or eustachian tubes or when the bacteria are inhaled into the lungs. Hematogenous spread occurs, creating disease in other organs.

Transmission from person to person is by direct contact or inhalation of droplets of respiratory secretions. *S. pneumoniae* causes disease particularly in the very young and the old. It is the most common cause of community-acquired pneumonia. Pneumococcal pneumonia frequently follows influenza or viral respiratory infections and is often seen in clients with chronic diseases or immunosuppression and in alcohol abusers. Other risk factors are included in Box 5.8.

S. pneumoniae is the most common cause of meningitis in adults, infants, and toddlers. Head trauma, cerebrospinal fluid (CSF) leaks, otitis media, and sinusitis may precede pneumococcal meningitis, creating an extension of disease or opportunity for direct infection.[14]

Clinical manifestations. Clinical manifestations of pneumonia include acute onset of fever, chills, pleuritis with pleuritic chest pain, and dyspnea with productive cough or purulent sputum that may be blood tinged. Because pneumococcal disease occurs most commonly in the very young and the very old, the presenting features will vary.

Older adults may have only a slight cough or delirium but lack a fever. Complications from pneumococcal pneumonia may include empyema (about 2% of cases), bacteremia, sepsis, or meningitis. Infection of the meninges stimulates a robust inflammation, leading to increased intracranial pressure and brain edema with headache, nausea and vomiting, mental status changes, stiff neck, and fever.

BOX 5.8 Risk Factors for Pneumococcal Disease

- Age
  - Children younger than 2 years old
  - Adults 65 years old or older
- Recent episode of influenza or viral respiratory infection
- Chronic illness
  - Diabetes mellitus
  - Heart disease
  - Pulmonary disease
  - Renal disease
  - Liver disease
- Immunosuppression
  - Human immunodeficiency virus (HIV)
  - Multiple myeloma
  - Leukemia
  - Lymphoma
  - Hodgkin's disease
  - Transplant recipients
  - Chronic use of corticosteroids
- Neurologic impairment (cerebrospinal fluid [CSF] leak)
- History of alcoholism

The disease progresses rapidly over 24 to 48 hours, and mortality rate is high without treatment. Septic arthritis can occur in a natural or prosthetic joint or in joints damaged by rheumatoid arthritis; underlying chronic joint disease may delay diagnosis.

Diagnosis, treatment, and prevention. Diagnosis of pneumococcal disease is by laboratory examination of sputum, cerebrospinal fluid, or blood with Gram stain and culture of the organism. Treatment is with antibiotics that are effective against local pneumococcal strains and take into consideration resistance patterns in the community. A 13-valent pneumococcal polysaccharide conjugate vaccine became available for young children and infants in 2010.[121]

Currently, the 23-valent pneumococcal polysaccharide vaccine is available for adults.[121] Immunization for pneumococcal disease is available and is recommended in specific circumstances as defined by the CDC (see Box 5.8).[80] Adults age 65 years or older should receive one dose of the vaccine. Individuals 19 to 64 years with defined conditions such as immunocompromise, HIV infection, asplenia, chronic liver or renal dysfunction, pulmonary disorders (chronic obstructive pulmonary disease [COPD]), and diabetes mellitus should be vaccinated.

Overall the rate of antibiotic-resistant invasive pneumococcal infections has decreased for all ages. As a bonus, the use of vaccines against pneumococcal bacteria in children has also reduced the rate of pneumococcal disease in adults because fewer bacteria are passed from children to adults.[44,49]

Pseudomonas

Overview. *P. aeruginosa* is a major opportunistic pathogen and one of the most common hospital- and nursing home–acquired (nosocomial) pathogens. *Pseudomonas* is uncommon in community-acquired infections and healthy individuals. The organism infrequently colonizes human beings, but it can cause disease, particularly in the hospital environment, where it is associated with pneumonia, wound infections,[93] urinary tract disease, and sepsis in debilitated people.

Burns, urinary catheterization, cystic fibrosis, chronic lung diseases, *neutropenia* associated with chemotherapy, and diabetes

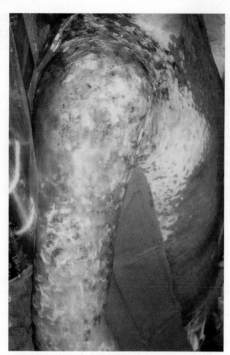

FIG. 5.3 *Pseudomonas*. Blue-green color in a burn wound indicates infection by *Pseudomonas aeruginosa*. (From VanMeter KC, Hubert RJ: Gould's pathophysiology for the health professions, ed 5, St. Louis, 2014, Saunders. Courtesy Judy Knighton, Ross Tilley Burn Center, Sunnybrook and Women's College Health Center, Toronto, Ontario, Canada.)

all predispose to infections with *P. aeruginosa*. It thrives on moist environmental surfaces, making swimming pools, whirlpool tubs, respiratory therapy equipment, flowers, endoscopes, and cleaning solutions prime targets for growth.

This organism produces several virulence factors and is inherently antibiotic resistant. Spread of the organism in a health care setting is by contact, typically from a reservoir as described previously. HCWs have been known to pass the organism on their hands or under fingernails.[11]

Pathogenesis. *P. aeruginosa* produces an array of proteins that allow it to attach to, invade, and destroy host tissues while avoiding host inflammatory and immune defenses. Injury to epithelial cells uncovers surface molecules that serve as binding sites for *P. aeruginosa*.

Many strains of this pathogen produce a proteoglycan that surrounds the bacteria, protecting them from mucociliary action, complement, and phagocytes. The organism releases extracellular enzymes that facilitate tissue invasion and are partially responsible for the necrotizing lesions associated with *Pseudomonas* infections.

Clinical manifestations. Signs and symptoms of *Pseudomonas* infection vary with the site of infection and the state of host defenses.[78] If the host has the capacity to respond to the invading bacteria with neutrophils, an acute inflammatory response results.

The *Pseudomonas* organism often invades small arteries and veins, producing vascular thrombosis and hemorrhagic necrosis, particularly in the lungs and skin. Blood vessel invasion predisposes to bacteremia, dissemination, and sepsis. This bacterium causes infections of the respiratory tract (pneumonia), bloodstream, CNS, skin (Fig. 5.3) and soft tissues, bone and joints, and other parts of the body.

Respiratory tract infections. *P. aeruginosa* is one of the most common causes of health care–acquired pneumonia.[84] The infection may be primary (contained to the lungs), or the organism may cause a bacteremia with metastasis of infection. Primary pneumonia is most often seen in clients with a predisposing history of chronic lung disease, congestive heart failure, or acquired immunodeficiency syndrome (AIDS) who are in a health care setting.

Signs and symptoms are typical of pneumonias seen with other organisms and include dyspnea, fever, productive cough, low oxygenation, elevated white cell count, and delirium. Chronic infections with *Pseudomonas* are noted in children or young adults with cystic fibrosis. Over time there is chronic progression of symptoms with acute exacerbations of disease. Clients typically experience mucous plugging and airway inflammation, which predispose to *P. aeruginosa* infection. The bacteria then contribute to further mucous plugging and cause a reaction, leading to bronchiectasis and atelectasis. Episodes of pneumonia are seen more frequently as more lung is damaged and becomes fibrotic.

Bacteremia. Bacteremia may occur without prior pneumonia and is an important cause of serious, life-threatening bloodstream infections in clients with neutropenia. *P. aeruginosa* bacteremia is typically acquired in the hospital and may be primary, with no identifiable source, or secondary to a focal infected site.

As with other *Pseudomonas* infections, bacteremia is rapidly progressive without treatment, with high morbidity and mortality rates. Clients experience fever, tachypnea, tachycardia, hypotension, and delirium, which can lead to renal failure, acute respiratory distress syndrome, and death.

Central nervous system infections. *Pseudomonas* infections of the CNS result from extension from a contiguous structure such as the ear, mastoid, or paranasal sinus; direct inoculation into the subarachnoid space or brain by means of head trauma, surgery, or invasive diagnostic procedures; and bacteremic spread from a distant site of infection such as the urinary tract, lung, or endocardium.

The clinical manifestations of *Pseudomonas* meningitis are like those of other forms of bacterial meningitis and include fever, headache, stiff neck, nausea, and confusion. The onset of disease may be acute and occur suddenly or may be more gradual and insidious.

Skin and soft tissue infections. *Pseudomonas* disease of the skin and mucous membranes can result from primary or metastatic foci of infections. Common predisposing factors for primary skin and soft tissue infections are a breakdown in the integument, especially resulting from surgery, burns, trauma, and pressure ulcers; whirlpool use; and chemotherapy-induced neutropenia.

The wound is hemorrhagic and necrotic and rarely may have a characteristic fruity odor (sweet, grape-like odor) with a blue-green exudate that forms a crust on wounds (see Fig. 5.3). *Pseudomonas* burn wound sepsis is a dreaded complication of extensive third-degree burns and is characterized by multifocal black or dark-brown discoloration of the burn eschar; degeneration of the underlying granulation tissue with rapid eschar separation and hemorrhage into subcutaneous tissue; edema, hemorrhage, and necrosis of adjacent healthy tissue; and erythematous nodular lesions on unburned skin.

Systemic manifestations may include fever, hypothermia, disorientation, hypotension, or leukopenia. The diagnosis is based on clinical signs and symptoms; biopsy of the burn site, which demonstrates evidence of invading bacteria; and culture positive for *Pseudomonas*.

Bone and joint infections. *Pseudomonas* infections of the bones and joints result from spreading from other sites or extension from contiguous sites of infection. Contiguous infections are usually related to penetrating trauma, surgery, or overlying soft tissue infections.

P. aeruginosa is the most common cause of osteochondritis of the foot following a puncture wound. Infection involves the cartilage of the small joints and the bones of the foot. Typically, the person experiences early improvement in pain and swelling after a puncture wound only to have the symptoms recur or worsen several days later. The average duration of symptoms before diagnosis is several weeks; fever and other systemic signs are usually absent. An area of superficial cellulitis is evident on the plantar surface of the foot, or there may merely be tenderness to deep palpation.

Bloodborne *Pseudomonas* from injection drug use or pelvic surgery appears to have a preference for fibrocartilaginous joints such as the symphysis pubis.[86] Vertebral osteomyelitis caused by *P. aeruginosa* is occasionally associated with complicated urinary tract infections and genitourinary surgery or instrumentation.

This disease occurs most often in older adults and involves the lumbosacral spine. Physical signs include local tenderness and decreased range of motion in the spine; fever and other systemic symptoms are relatively uncommon. Mild neurologic deficits may be present.

Other pseudomonas infections. *Pseudomonas* is noted to cause disease of the external ear, which may be benign (e.g., "swimmer's ear") or malignant with an invasion of bone, soft tissue, and cartilage. Infection of the cornea causes bacterial keratitis or corneal ulcers.

Native heart valves or prosthetic valves can become infected, causing endocarditis. *P. aeruginosa* is the most common cause of health care–acquired urinary tract infections, often arising from urinary catheters, instrumentation, or surgery. The prostate or kidney stones may harbor the bacteria, resulting in recurrent infections.

5.4 Special Implications for the PTA: Pseudomonas Infections Reservoirs for *Pseudomonas aeruginosa* are most often medical equipment or moist areas in the health care setting, such as sinks. However, the source of some outbreaks has been traced to HCWs' hands or nails.[119] *P. aeruginosa* can be removed from the skin by following proper hand hygiene guidelines, which prevents further spread of the organism.[10,87] Proper cleaning of any equipment in contact with mucous membranes or a moist environment is absolutely critical.[65]

Viral Infections
Bloodborne Viral Pathogens

The bloodborne viruses that most endanger HCWs are the bloodborne pathogens hepatitis B virus (HBV), hepatitis C virus (HCV), and HIV. In 1991 the U.S. Congress passed the Bloodborne Pathogens Standard, prepared by the Occupational Safety and Health Administration (OSHA) and written to help eliminate or minimize occupational exposure to HBV, HCV, HIV, and other bloodborne pathogens.[114]

The guidelines are based on the use of standard precautions, including appropriate handwashing and barrier precautions, to reduce contact with body fluids potentially contaminated by these viruses. The use of safety devices and techniques to reduce

the handling of sharp instruments can help in the reduction of significant contact with body fluids, particularly blood or blood-containing fluids.[120]

5.5 Special Implications for the PTA: Bloodborne Viral Pathogens

Hepatitis B
Nosocomial transmission of HBV is a serious risk for HCWs. The risk of acquiring HBV infection from occupational exposure is dependent on the degree of exposure to blood and the presence of HBV e antigen (HBeAg) from the source. Yet the rate of development of hepatitis from a needlestick was only 1% to 6%.

HBV can be transmitted to HCWs via percutaneous injuries or by direct or indirect contact with blood from an infected client. Blood contains the highest amount of infected particles and is the most efficient means of transmission. HBV in blood is able to survive up to 1 week on environmental surfaces. Preexposure HBV vaccination of HCWs who are at risk is strongly recommended and can prevent acquisition of HBV (see Table 5.2).[18] Once an HCW has been exposed, postexposure prophylaxis (PEP) should then be given if the HCW is unvaccinated or nonresponsive to previous vaccine.

Studies have shown that the combination of HBV immunoglobulin (HGIB) and HBV vaccine is 85% to 95% effective in preventing HBV compared with either agent alone. Data show that HGIB and the HBV vaccine are effective as single PEP for preventing clinical disease in occupational exposures (70% to 75%).

The OSHA bloodborne pathogen standard mandates that HBV vaccine and HGIB be made available, at the employer's expense, to all HCWs with potential occupational exposure. In addition, strict adherence to handwashing and standard precautions is critical in prevention of the transmission of hepatitis-contaminated body fluids. Transmission is also prevented by use of barriers during sexual activity and by not sharing personal or other items that may have blood on them.

Hepatitis C Virus
Hepatitis C virus (HCV) is the most common etiologic agent in cases of non-A, non-B hepatitis in the United States. *Seroprevalence* studies among HCWs have shown a significant association between acquisition of disease and health care employment, specifically client care or laboratory work. Accidental exposures (needlesticks or cuts with sharp instruments) are the highest risk vehicle for transmission to HCWs from people with acute or chronic HCV infection.

The incubation period for HCV is 6 to 7 weeks, and nearly all individuals with acute infection will have chronic (more than 3 to 6 months' duration) HCV infection and the potential for transmission to others over an extended period.

Currently no vaccine against HCV is available, and no PEP can be recommended. PEP with immunoglobulin or antiviral agents does not appear to be effective in preventing HCV infection.[114]

Strict adherence to handwashing and standard precautions is critical in prevention of transmission of hepatitis-contaminated body fluids. Transmission is also prevented by use of barriers during sexual activity and by not sharing personal or other items that may have blood on them.

Herpesviruses

Overview and definition. The term *herpes* is derived from the Greek word *herpein*, which means "to creep." The word refers to the tendency for this type of viral infection to become chronic, latent, and recurrent.

All herpesviruses are morphologically similar, but the biologic and epidemiologic features of each are distinct. Subclinical primary infection with the herpesviruses is more common than clinically symptomatic illness, and each type then persists in a latent state for the rest of the life of the host.

With the herpes simplex virus (HSV) and varicella-zoster virus (VZV), the virus remains latent in sensory ganglia, and, on reactivation, lesions appear in the distal sensory nerve distribution. Severe or fatal illness may occur in infants and the immunocompromised.

Herpes Simplex Viruses Types 1 and 2

See Table 5.4.

Incidence, etiologic factors, and risk factors. Approximately 70% of Americans older than 12 years of age harbor HSV-1, which is usually responsible for cold sores; 20% older than 12 years of age have HSV-2, the principal cause of genital herpes.[89]

Both strains can infect any visceral organ or mucocutaneous site, and HSV-1 can be transmitted to the genital area during oral sex. HSV creates a significant health risk because infection with these viruses increases the risk of infection with HIV and increases production of the human immunodeficiency virus once an individual has been infected.

Intermittent, asymptomatic shedding is common, and the typical time of transmission is during shedding, usually the period immediately preceding appearance of sores. Sexual contact during asymptomatic periods is less likely to result in transmission of the virus than when sores are present. However, because people with genital herpes are more likely to engage in sexual contact when they are free of sores, the rate of asymptomatic transmission is still significant.

Infants born to women with genital herpes can be infected with HSV when they pass through an infected birth canal. The virus can also be passed to other regions of the body by hand contact, particularly in people who are immunosuppressed.

Pathogenesis. Even though HSV-1 and HSV-2 produce different clinical symptoms, both virus types primarily affect the oral mucocutaneous (cold sores and mouth sores) and genital areas (genital herpes). Primary infection occurs through a break in the mucous membranes of the mouth, throat, eye, or genitals or via minor abrasions in the skin. Initial infection can be asymptomatic, although minor localized vesicular lesions may be evident.

The virus will multiply locally and enter the peripheral sensory nerves. The virus will then migrate to the CNS and reside there. The virus will be with the host for his or her lifetime and may trigger symptoms periodically.

Various disturbances such as physical or psychologic stress can disrupt the delicate balance of latency, and reactivation of the latent virus occurs. The virus travels back down sensory nerves to the surface of the body and replicates, forming new lesions. Although painful, most recurrent infections resolve spontaneously.

Clinical manifestations. Primary HSV-1 (first episode) typically affects the mouth and oral cavity, causing vesicles in the mouth, throat, and around the lips. Vesicles typically open to form moist ulcers after several days. Systemic symptoms such as fever, myalgias, and malaise can accompany the lesions. Symptoms and lesions resolve within 3 to 14 days.

HSV-2 is most often acquired through sexual contact. Primary HSV-2 causes vesicles to form in the genitourinary tract. Lesions are usually painful, small, grouped, and vesicular, with possible burning and itching. The blister-like lesions break and weep after a few days, leaving ulcer-like sores that usually crust over and heal in 1 to 3 weeks.

Genital ulcers may occur on the genital area, cervix, buttocks, rectum, urethra, or bladder, causing vaginal and urethral discharge, *dysuria,* cervicitis, proctitis, and tender inguinal adenopathy. Systemic symptoms occasionally noted include headache, malaise, myalgias, and fever.

HSV can be responsible for other infections. Viral meningitis from HSV is caused by inflammation of the meninges surrounding the brain. This occurs more commonly from HSV-2 than HSV-1. Aseptic meningitis may develop 3 to 12 days after the appearance of lesions. Typical symptoms are headache, nausea, stiff neck, and fever. An association has also been established between HSV-1 and Bell's palsy.

Herpetic keratitis (ulceration of the cornea from infection) is the most common cause of corneal blindness in the United States. Onset is acute, accompanied by blurred vision, conjunctivitis, and pain. Despite treatment, recurrences are common and cause scarring, making this a chronic disease. Prophylactic acyclovir may reduce recurrences and long-term scarring.[73]

Recurrences of HSV-1 or HSV-2 increase during pregnancy but do not appear to affect the fetus. Primary infection with HSV during pregnancy can occasionally cause visceral dissemination in the mother and possible transmission to the fetus. Neonatal herpes may also occur from unknown shedding in the mother's genital tract at the time of delivery. If untreated, babies develop visceral dissemination or infection of the CNS, with an 80% mortality rate.[13] Cesarean section reduces the risk of neonatal herpes in mothers known to be shedding the virus.

5.6 Special Implications for the PTA: Herpes Simplex Virus Recurrent disease is best treated with acyclovir, and recurrent genital disease requires barrier precautions during sexual activity in addition to medication. Although herpes simplex is contagious, health care–associated transmission is rare. However, it has been reported in some high-risk areas such as nurseries, intensive care units, burn units, and other areas where immunocompromised individuals might be placed.

Transmission of herpes simplex virus (HSV) occurs primarily through contact with lesions or with virus-containing secretions such as saliva, vaginal secretions, or amniotic fluid. Exposed areas of skin, particularly when minor cuts, abrasions, or other skin lesions are present, are the most likely sites of viral entry. The incubation period of HSV is 2 to 14 days.

HCWs can protect themselves from acquiring HSV by adhering to standard precautions and handwashing before and after all client contact and by the use of appropriate barriers such as a mask, gloves, or gauze dressing to prevent hand contact with the lesion.

During the prodromal stage of herpes simplex, the levator scapulae becomes vulnerable to activation of its trigger points by mechanical stresses that are usually well within its tolerance. However, a stiff neck syndrome can develop a day or two before the fully developed symptoms of herpes simplex.

Careful questioning regarding previous history of herpes, presence of prodromal symptoms, and observation for the development of a new outbreak of sores during the episode of care will help the PTA in making an accurate judgment of the client's presentation.

Varicella Zoster Virus (Herpesvirus Type 3)

Incidence. VZV is human herpesvirus 3 (HHV-3) and is known as *chickenpox* or *shingles.* Before the availability of the varicella vaccine, primary or first-infection VZV accounted for about 3 to 4 million cases of chickenpox per year in the United States.

TABLE 5.4	**Most Common Sexually Transmitted Infections[a]**			
Infection	**Incidence**	**Transmission**	**Clinical Manifestations**	**Treatment[b]**
Human papillo-mavirus (HPV) infection (genital warts)	6.2 million new cases per year	Unprotected sexual contact; condoms do not provide 100% protection because the virus can be spread by contact with an infected part of the genitals not covered by a condom; vertical transmission from mother to newborn with vaginal delivery (rare)	Often asymptomatic; warts on the vulva, anal region, vagina, cervix, mouth, penis, scrotum, or groin: 1–6 months after sexual contact with infected person; *in women:* abnormal pap smear, HPV can cause cervical cancer	Can be removed using topically applied chemicals, cryotherapy, or surgical therapies; recurrence not uncommon
Chlamydia	1 million new cases per year	Unprotected vaginal or anal intercourse; infection transmitted from infected mother to infant during delivery	*In men:* none or urethritis with discharge or burning with urination *In women:* none or vaginal discharge with pus or mucus; pain; burning during urination; can cause pelvic inflammatory disease (PID) and infertility if untreated; eye infections and respiratory tract infections in newborn	Can be cured with antibiotics; partner must be treated as well; PID may require additional treatment
Herpes simplex virus 2 infection (genital herpes)	1 million new cases per year 45 million carriers	Oral, genital, or anal sex; kissing or touching an infected area where there is a break in the skin; can be spread by asymptomatic person; transmission from mother to child during vaginal birth	None or vesicular (blisterlike) lesions on the genitals, vagina, cervix, anal region, mouth, or throat; can cause serious complications if untreated	Cannot be cured, but healing can be accelerated and recurrence of outbreaks can be reduced with antivirals; partner must be informed
Gonorrhea ("the clap")	330,000 new cases per year	Unprotected oral, vaginal, or anal sex; transmission to baby during delivery	*In men:* urethritis with discharge, frequent urge to urinate, and pain during urination; may be asymptomatic *In women:* none or slight vaginal discharge and difficulty or pain during urination; pelvic pain; vaginal bleeding between periods; PID *Both:* arthritis (if untreated)	Can be cured with antibiotics, although some strains are drug resistant
Hepatitis B	73,000 new cases per year	Infected blood; sexual contact; occupational needlesticks; sharing of needles; infection of baby during delivery	May be asymptomatic; jaundice, arthralgias, dark urine, anorexia, nausea, abdominal pain, cirrhosis, liver failure, liver cancer, clay-colored stools, fever	Can be prevented with hepatitis B vaccine In unvaccinated people, hepatitis B immune globulin (HBIG) and hepatitis B vaccine given as postexposure prophylaxis; antiviral agents are used but relapse on cessation of treatment is common
Syphilis (secondary)	See *Syphilis (primary)*		Flulike symptoms, lymphadenopathy, mucocutaneous lesions and rash occurring 6–12 weeks to 1–2 years after infection (but has a wide range of clinical symptoms)	
Syphilis (latent)			None; asymptomatic	
Syphilis (late; can occur up to 20 years after second stage)			Cardiovascular and central nervous system damage	
HIV/AIDS	42,000 new cases per year; half caused by sexual contact	Exposure to blood or blood products; exposure to body fluids (blood, semen, vaginal secretions, breast milk); sexual contact; shared needles in injection drug users; transmission from mother to child during vaginal delivery or breast-feeding	Widespread illness from immune system decline; may not develop symptoms for 10 years or more after infection	Cannot be cured, but combined antiviral therapy can prolong life for many people
Syphilis (primary)	8000 new cases per year (primary and secondary combined); overall incidence has been increasing since 2000	Unprotected sexual contact; sexual contact with exudates of skin and mucous membranes of infected person; transplacental infection of fetus if mother is infected; can be transmitted through blood transfusions[c]	Painless sore at site of infection (genitals, mouth) occurring 3–8 weeks after infection	Can be cured with antibiotics in primary, secondary, and latent stages; late-stage disease may cause irreversible damage

[a]Listed in descending order by incidence.
[b]All sexually transmitted diseases can be prevented by sexual abstinence and mutually monogamous sex between two uninfected partners. The Centers for Disease Control and Prevention has come under criticism from the medical community for not stressing this point in their prevention programs for young people.
[c]Data from Chin J: Control of communicable diseases manual, ed 17, Washington, DC, 2000, APHA Press.
Data from Centers for Disease Control and Prevention: Sexually transmitted disease surveillance, 2004, Atlanta, 2005, U.S. Department of Health and Human Services.

Approximately 10% to 20% of the population develops the secondary, or reactivation, form of VZV, resulting in herpes zoster or shingles. Approximately 300,000 cases of shingles occur in the United States every year and cause significant pain and disability. Adults older than 50 years and anyone who is immunocompromised are at greatest risk. Young adults such as college students living in dormitories are at increased risk for VZV as either chickenpox (first time) or shingles (recurrence).

Pathogenesis. Like other herpesviruses, VZV has the capacity to persist in the body as a latent infection after the primary infection. VZV is acquired from contact with infected airborne droplets into the respiratory tract or by direct contact with vesicular fluid to the respiratory tract or eye.

The virus is believed to initially multiply at the site of entry, with subsequent viremia occurring 4 to 6 days after infection. The virus then disseminates to other organs such as the liver, spleen, and sensory ganglia and further replicates in the viscera, followed by a secondary viremia with viral infection of the skin and mucosa. The incubation period is 14 to 16 days from exposure with a range of 10 to 21 days. This may be prolonged in immunocompromised people. VZV is present in white blood cells up to 5 days before the rash is present, and individuals can be contagious a day or two before the appearance of the rash. Individuals remain contagious until the lesions have crusted.[6]

Clinical manifestations. Disease manifestations are either chickenpox (varicella) or shingles (herpes zoster). Primary VZV is virtually always symptomatic. Second episodes of chickenpox are uncommon unless the child is younger than 1 year old at the time of the first episode. A mild warning symptom consisting of fever and malaise may precede the onset of the rash in adults, whereas in children the rash is often the first sign of disease.

The rash is classically described as a "dewdrop on a rose petal," with a vesicle on an erythematous base. The lesions begin as macules that quickly progress to papules, vesicles, and then pustules before crusting. VZV usually appears first on the scalp and moves to the trunk and then the extremities. Successive crops appear over several days, with lesions present in several stages of evolution at any one time.[6]

The generalized pattern of eruption without specific dermatome distribution distinguishes varicella from herpes zoster (Fig. 5.4). Shingles in the adult manifests as blister-like lesions that erupt along dermatomes, with the highest concentration of lesions on the trunk corresponding with dermatomes from T3 to L3 (Fig. 5.5). Pain and itching are common symptoms during the eruption of the vesicles.

Complications of varicella occur more often in adults, infants, and the immunocompromised. Adults are more likely to develop pneumonitis and CNS involvement than are healthy children. The immunocompromised can develop pneumonitis and encephalitis. The most common complication in persons with VZV is secondary bacterial skin infections.[118]

Shingles also can lead to chronic, often debilitating nerve pain called *postherpetic neuralgia* (PHN), lasting years or even a lifetime and often resulting in significant morbidity and reduction in quality of life. Pain, hyperalgesia, and allodynia are typical of PHN.[30] Examples of allodynia include pain from the touch of clothing (touch allodynia) or pain that occurs from a draft of warm or cold air on the skin (thermal allodynia).

When contracted during the first or second trimesters of pregnancy, varicella carries a low risk of congenital malformations. However, if a mother develops varicella within 5 days

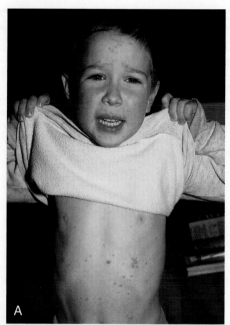

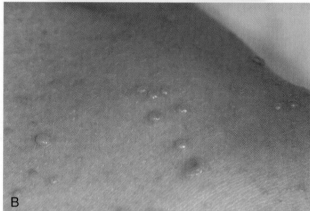

FIG. 5.4 (A) Early onset of varicella (chickenpox) in a young child. Painful itching can cause severe distress. Note the lesions on face and trunk. (B) Varicella (chickenpox) with the more characteristic rash classically described as a "dewdrop on a rose petal," with a vesicle on an erythematous base. (A, Courtesy Catherine Goodman. B, From Lemmi FO, Lemmi CAE: Physical assessment findings CD-ROM, Philadelphia, 2000, Saunders.)

before delivery to 2 days after delivery, the newborn is at risk for serious disseminated disease.

Prevention. The varicella vaccine is recommended for all adults who lack evidence of immunity, especially persons who have close contact with individuals at high risk for severe disease and complications.

Adults who are at high risk for exposure and transmission should also receive the vaccine. Children aged 12 to 18 months should routinely receive the vaccine. Currently the varicella vaccine is available with the measles, mumps, and rubella (MMR) vaccine.

It is also recommended that all children who have not developed immunity by the age of 13 years be vaccinated (see Table 5.2).[6] Because the vaccine is a live attenuated vaccine, it is contraindicated in pregnant women, those who may become pregnant within 4 weeks of receiving the vaccine, and individuals with HIV infection or other immunosuppressed states.

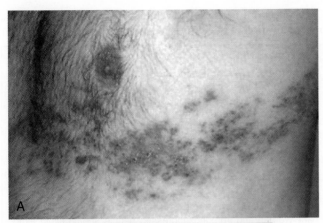

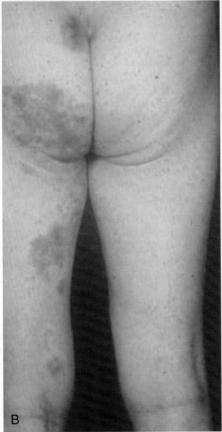

FIG. 5.5 Herpes zoster (shingles). Small grouped vesicles occur along the cutaneous sensory nerve, forming pustules that crust over. Reactivation of varicella-zoster virus (VZV), the dormant chickenpox virus, is the underlying cause of this condition. (A) Commonly seen on the trunk, these outbreaks can occur anywhere along the dermatome of the affected nerve. (B) Lesions appear unilaterally and do not cross the midline. Usually external, these lesions can occur internally as well. Pain is often severe and can become chronic, a condition called *postherpetic neuralgia*. (A, From Walsh TD, Caraceni AT: *Palliative medicine*, Philadelphia, 2009, Saunders. B, Courtesy Mary Lou Galantino, Stockton University, Galloway, New Jersey.)

There has been a progressive decline in the incidence of chickenpox and hospitalizations from complications since the varicella vaccine became available in 1995.[25,26] The first shingles

vaccine (Zostavax; zoster vaccine live) has been approved for adults aged 60 years and older. Among people who get shingles despite being vaccinated, it can reduce the disease's severity.

5.7 Special Implications for the PTA: Varicella Zoster Virus Varicella is highly contagious. The period of communicability extends from 1 to 2 days before the onset of the rash through the first 4 to 5 days or until all lesions have formed crusts. Immunocompromised individuals with progressive varicella are probably contagious during the entire period new lesions continue to appear.

Nosocomial transmission of VZV is well known. Sources for nosocomial exposures include clients or residents, HCWs, and visitors—including children—with either varicella or zoster. It is generally advisable to allow only HCWs who are immune to varicella to take care of clients with VZV.

Because of the possibility of transmission to and development of severe illness in high-risk clients, HCWs with localized zoster should not take care of such clients until all lesions are dry and crusted. However, they may take care of others if they cover their lesions.

When unvaccinated, susceptible HCWs are exposed to varicella, they are potentially infectious 10 to 21 days after exposure, and exclusion from duty is indicated from day 10 through day 21 after the last exposure or until all lesions are dry and crusted.

Any patient or client suspected of having herpes zoster (shingles) requires immediate medical attention. Reports of prodromal pain, symptoms, or onset of rash are red flags to warrant immediate diagnosis and early treatment. Early intervention can reduce morbidity.

Infectious Mononucleosis (Herpesvirus Type 4)

Overview. Infectious mononucleosis is an acute infectious disease caused by the Epstein–Barr virus (EBV), a member of the herpesvirus family. It primarily affects young adults and children although it may be seen at any age. It is usually so mild in children that its presence often goes unnoticed.

Incidence, etiologic factors, and risk factors. Infection with EBV is common in the United States, with 95% of people aged 35 to 40 years having been infected. When an adolescent or young adult becomes infected with EBV, 35% to 50% of the time he or she will develop infectious mononucleosis. Both genders are affected equally. Incidence varies seasonally among college students but not among the general population. The reservoir of EBV is limited to human beings, and transmission is through contact with oral secretions, blood, or transplanted organs infected with the virus. Because people carry EBV in the saliva during the acute infection and for an indefinite period afterward, it is sometimes called the "kissing disease."

Pathogenesis and clinical manifestations. The virus characteristically produces fever, sore throat, and tender cervical lymphadenopathy; headache, malaise, and abdominal pain may also be present. The incubation period is about 4 to 6 weeks.

Temperature fluctuations occur throughout the day, peaking in the evening. There is often an increase in the white blood cell count with an elevation in atypical lymphocytes. The spleen may enlarge to two to three times its normal size, causing left upper quadrant pain with possible referral to the left shoulder and left upper trapezius region. Affected individuals are at risk for splenic rupture, and care should be taken to avoid trauma. Both the peripheral nervous system and CNS can be involved.

Symptoms subside about 6 to 10 days after onset of the disease but may persist for weeks. Symptoms from EBV-related infectious mononucleosis rarely last longer than 4 months.

Studies support an association between infectious mononucleosis and the subsequent development of multiple sclerosis in both adults and children.[5,27,56] Young people who have had a strong immune response to the EBV are twice as likely to develop multiple sclerosis in adulthood. Scientists suspect this strong immune response could cross-react with brain substances, causing the brain to attack its own myelin in genetically susceptible individuals, as opposed to the idea that the virus actually enters the brain.[27,97]

5.8 Special Implications for the PTA: Infectious Mononucleosis Infectious mononucleosis is probably contagious before symptoms develop until the fever subsides and the oral and pharyngeal lesions disappear. Although infectious mononucleosis appears to be only mildly contagious, adherence to standard precautions—especially good handwashing and avoidance of shared dishware or food items with other people—is essential for preventing HCWs from contracting this condition.

The person with infectious mononucleosis should be cautioned against engaging in excessive activity, especially contact sports, which could result in splenic rupture or lowered resistance to infection. Usually this guideline is appropriate for a period of at least 1 month.

Any soft tissue mobilization or myofascial techniques necessary in the left upper quadrant, especially up and under the rib cage, must take into consideration the enlarged liver and/or spleen; indirect techniques away from the spleen are indicated.

Cytomegalovirus (Herpesvirus Type 5)

Overview and incidence. Cytomegalovirus (CMV, herpesvirus type 5) is a commonly occurring DNA herpesvirus. It increases in frequency with age. One percent of newborns have it, and four out of five adults older than 35 years of age have CMV. There are few symptoms or complications for the majority of people who are infected with the virus after birth. However, for unborn babies or the immunocompromised the consequences can be severe or life-threatening.

Etiologic and risk factors. CMV is transmitted by human contact with infected secretions such as urine, breast milk, feces, blood, semen, and vaginal and cervical secretions. It may also be transmitted through the placenta. The virus can be acquired from transplanted organs and rarely via blood transfusions. Like other herpesviruses, CMV can remain dormant to evade detection and persists in multiple organs.

Pathogenesis and clinical manifestations. CMV probably spreads through the body via lymphocytes or mononuclear cells, where it produces inflammatory reactions. Complications include diffuse interstitial pneumonitis leading to respiratory distress syndrome, hepatitis, adrenalitis, intestinal ulcerations, and calcifications around ventricles in neonatal CNS infections.

In normal adolescents or adults the infection is usually asymptomatic or manifests as an infectious mononucleosis–like illness with a self-limiting course.[24] Unlike infectious mononucleosis from EBV, CMV rarely causes pharyngitis or adenopathy. The course of the illness for the fetus ranges from mild splenomegaly or hepatitis to disease. Approximately 10% to 15% of those infected are born with the complications of hearing loss, vision impairment, or varying degrees of mental retardation, and the infection is deadly for 20% to 30% of affected neonates. Even up to 10% of infected babies born without symptoms go on to demonstrate varying degrees of hearing, mental, or coordination problems during the first few years of life.

In immunosuppressed people, particularly transplant recipients and those with HIV, various syndromes develop with

CMV infection. Primary CMV infection can be more serious, but reactivation of the virus is more common in this group.[87]

5.9 Special Implications for the PTA: Cytomegalovirus Other practice patterns depend on organ systems involved and clinical presentation.

The two principal reservoirs of CMV in health care institutions are (1) infants and young children and (2) immunocompromised individuals, but HCWs who provide care to these high-risk populations have a rate of primary CMV that is no higher than among personnel without such client contact.

CMV transmission appears to occur directly, either through close, intimate contact with contaminated secretions or through excretions, especially saliva or urine.[24] Transmission by the hands of HCWs or individuals with the virus has also been suggested. Pregnant women and immunosuppressed people should avoid exposure to confirmed or suspected CMV infection. Pregnant women or women of childbearing age need to be counseled regarding the risks and prevention of transmission of CMV, but no data show that HCWs can be protected from infection by transfer to areas with less contact with individuals who have been diagnosed with CMV.

Clients with CMV infection should be encouraged to wash their hands thoroughly and frequently to prevent spreading it. It is especially important to impress this on young children. As difficult as it may be, the child should not be allowed to kiss others, and parents and others should also avoid kissing the affected child.

Herpesviruses Types 6, 7, and 8

Primary HHV-6 is common in children, with 90% infected by the age of 2 years. Although the condition is classically described as 3 to 5 days of high fever followed by a macular rash on the neck and trunk (roseola), children more commonly develop a fever, runny nose, and fussiness.[52] Its occurrence in adults is more complicated and associated with immunocompromised states such as AIDS and lymphoma.

Viral Respiratory Infections

Viral respiratory infections are common problems in health care settings. Many viral pathogens can cause respiratory infections, but influenza and respiratory syncytial virus (RSV) are associated with significant morbidity and mortality rates.

Influenza

Each year in the United States influenza viruses cause serious illness and even death, especially in young children with chronic diseases, immunocompromised adults, and the frail elderly. Influenza is caused by influenza viruses A or B and occurs in epidemics between late fall and early spring. The mode of transmission is from person to person by inhalation of aerosolized virus or direct contact. Health care–associated transmission of influenza has been reported in acute and long-term health care facilities and has occurred from clients to HCWs, from HCWs to clients, and among HCWs. The incubation period is usually 1 to 4 days (average of 2 days).

Influenzas A and B resemble some other respiratory illnesses. The onset is usually abrupt, with high fever, chills, malaise, muscular aching, headache, sore throat, nasal congestion, and nonproductive cough. The fever lasts about 1 to 7 days (usually 3 to 5). Children often manifest nausea, vomiting, and otitis media. The infection can progress rapidly in the first few days, causing pneumonia and respiratory failure, particularly in high-risk groups. Secondary bacterial pneumonia may also develop, usually 5 to 10 days after the onset of viral symptoms, particularly in older adults.

Medical Management

Prevention

Vaccination is recommended before the beginning of each influenza season for people over age 50; people with chronic heart or lung disease, diabetes, renal dysfunction, or immunosuppression; pregnant women; nursing home residents; employees of medical or long-term care facilities; and HCWs (see Table 5.2).

Vaccination against influenza is associated with reduced hospitalization rates and shorter hospital stays for pneumonia, diabetes, heart disease, and stroke in adults age 65 or older who are immunized. Mortality rates are also lower for all causes during influenza season in older adults who are immunized.[67,68] A live attenuated influenza vaccine is also available. It is given intranasally to healthy persons 5 to 49 years of age who are not in contact with immunosuppressed individuals and do not have chronic medical problems.[81]

Treatment

Influenza antiviral agents can be given in conjunction with vaccine during institutional outbreaks of influenza.

Antiviral agents used to treat influenza help decrease the duration and severity of signs and symptoms. Treatment must be initiated within the first 2 days of the illness and benefits those at high risk for complications. Resistance to these antivirals does occur, and the CDC monitors and recommends specific, effective treatment for each season.[42]

Many people with influenza prefer to rest in bed; analgesics and a cough medicine mixture are often used.

Prognosis

The duration of the uncomplicated illness is 3 to 7 days, and the prognosis is usually very good in previously healthy people.

Most fatalities related to influenza are caused by bacterial and viral pneumonia.[41] The mortality rate is low except in debilitated individuals. People at greatest risk for influenza-related complications are (1) individuals older than 65, (2) residents of chronic health care facilities such as nursing homes, (3) people with chronic pulmonary or cardiovascular disease, and (4) people with diabetes mellitus.[114]

Respiratory Syncytial Virus

RSV is the leading cause of lower respiratory tract infections in children worldwide.[123] In the United States, between 75,000 and 125,000 hospitalizations related to RSV occur among children younger than 1 year old, and 1.5 million outpatient visits occur in children younger than age 5 years.[19]

Reinfection is common in adults and older children and manifests as mild upper respiratory tract infection and tracheobronchitis. In addition, infants with congenital heart disease, intensive care unit clients, those with cystic fibrosis, and older adults are at high risk for serious and complicated RSV.

Nosocomial transmission of RSV occurs among clients, visitors, and HCWs. RSV is present in large numbers in the respiratory secretions of children with symptomatic RSV infections. It can be transmitted through large droplets during close contact with such individuals or indirectly by hands or *fomites* that are contaminated with RSV. Hands can become contaminated through touching or handling of fomites or respiratory secretions and can transmit RSV by touching the nose or eyes.

Usually people shed the virus for 3 to 8 days, but young infants may shed the virus for as long as 3 to 4 weeks. Signs include low-grade fever, tachypnea, and wheezing. Hyperinflated lungs, decreased gas exchange, and increased work of breathing are also often present, and otitis media is a common complication.

Rapid diagnosis of RSV may be made by viral antigen identification of nasal washings using an enzyme-linked immunosorbent assay (*ELISA*). Treatment consists of hydration, humidification of inspired air, and ventilatory support as needed.

Avoidance of exposure to tobacco smoke, cold air, and air pollutants is also beneficial to long-term recovery from RSV bronchiolitis. A number of vaccines to prevent this infection are currently being studied, but because the immune response is neither durable nor complete, it has been a difficult task.[39,48]

5.10 Special Implications for the PTA: Viral Respiratory Infections

Influenza

HCWs must follow the guidelines in Table 5.2 regarding prevention of transmission of influenza, both for themselves and their clients. Recommendations for immunization must be reviewed and acted on individually. Because the immunization for influenza does not provide immunity for the entire year or for all strains of influenza, common sense must prevail in the case of an HCW who suspects he or she has early signs and symptoms of influenza.

Influenza can cause substantial morbidity and mortality among persons age 65 or older and among adults age 50 or older who have chronic illnesses. Anyone in these two groups is vulnerable to the serious complications of influenza. Routine influenza vaccination has been associated with reductions in influenza-associated and all-cause mortality during influenza season.[67] Despite the benefits of vaccination, utilization remains below target rates. PTAs can be instrumental in reducing morbidity and mortality rates by encouraging clients in these two groups to get a flu shot each year and to get one themselves.

MISCELLANEOUS INFECTIOUS DISEASES

Prostheses and Implant Infections

Implantation of any device of any synthetic material[94] into the body can give rise to serious life-threatening infections. Multiple reoperations carry a higher risk of infection.

Likewise, as the population ages, an increasing number of primary and revision arthroplasties are being done. Early detection of infection or other problems can reduce complications and morbidity associated with these devices. Anyone with implants of any kind with onset of increasing musculoskeletal symptoms (especially in the area of the surgery) must be screened for the possibility of infection.

Lyme Disease
Definition and Overview

Lyme disease is an infectious multisystemic disorder caused by the tick-borne spirochete *Borrelia burgdorferi*. It was first recognized in 1976 when a group of children in Lyme, Connecticut, developed an unusual type of arthritis and a bull's-eye rash.[107] Some of these children also had a history of tick bites.

In the United States the disease is transmitted to human beings only by the deer or black-legged tick in the northeastern (from Massachusetts to Maryland) and north central United States

(Wisconsin and Minnesota) and by the western black-legged tick, found on the western coast of northern California and Oregon. The ticks are extremely small, measuring approximately 1 to 2 mm.

Incidence

Lyme disease has become the most prevalent vector-borne infectious disease in the United States.[64] In 1982, when the CDC began national surveillance, only 229 cases were reported, whereas in 2006 a total of 19,931 cases were brought to medical attention.[7]

In the United States Lyme disease is often seen in the late spring and summer months when the tick nymphs are most active and human outdoor activities are greatest.

Pathogenesis

Human beings generally acquire the infection from tick nymphs when they attach to the skin to feed. After approximately 36 hours, the bacteria from an infected tick are passed into the host when a tick injects spirochete-laden saliva into the host.[76] Most commonly, however, the tick falls off or is removed before the bacteria are injected into the host's bloodstream.

After incubating for 3 to 32 days, the spirochetes cause an inflammatory response, resulting in characteristic skin lesions at the site of the tick bite The human host activates an immune response, producing cytokines and antibodies against the bacteria. Despite the host's response and if untreated, *B. burgdorferi* can survive for years in certain areas of the body by genetically adapting and inhibiting host immune responses.[105]

Clinical Manifestations

Lyme disease can be described as an imitator because its signs and symptoms mimic those of many other diseases. Symptoms vary widely and may not develop for as long as 1 month after a bite; in some cases, symptoms do not develop at all. Clinical manifestations of the infection occur in three stages.

Stage 1, the early, localized stage, usually occurs within days after a tick bite. About 80% of affected individuals have a red, slowly expanding rash (Fig. 5.6).[104] Not all people with the disease develop the telltale rash, and because early symptoms are often mild, some people may remain undiagnosed and untreated. The rash resolves spontaneously without treatment within an average of 4 weeks. Flulike symptoms suggestive of early dissemination such as fatigue, chills, fever, headache, lethargy, myalgias, or arthralgias may also develop early in the course of the infection and may be the presenting symptoms for anyone without a rash.

Stage 2, disseminated infection, occurs within days to weeks after the spirochete spreads, particularly to the nervous system, heart, and joints. Neurologic symptoms may be the first to arise and occur in 15% of all cases,[103] most commonly with mild headache, stiff neck, and difficulty with mentation; cranial neuropathies, particularly Bell's palsy; and radiculopathies (Box 5.9). Even in people who remain untreated, neurologic symptoms may improve or resolve.[105]

About half of those diagnosed may go on to develop painful Lyme arthritis, characterized by unilateral inflammation and swelling in the large joints, especially the knees.[104] Migratory musculoskeletal pain in joints, bursae, tendons, muscle, and bone may occur in one or a few locations at a time, often lasting only hours or days in a given location. Weeks to months later, untreated people often have intermittent or chronic monarticular (one joint) or oligoarticular (affecting only a few joints) arthritis.

Stage 3, late persistent infection, may become apparent weeks to months after the initial infection. In the United States about 60% of individuals left untreated develop stage 3 symptoms,

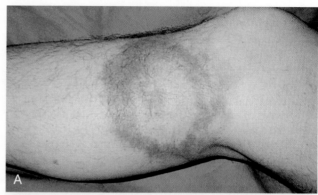

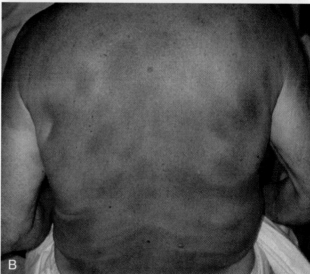

FIG. 5.6 Examples of erythema migrans associated with Lyme disease. (A) Many sources describe a characteristic bull's-eye rash with Lyme disease. (B) However, a wide range of skin reactions labeled as erythema migrans may occur with Lyme disease, as shown. Some skin rashes may be so minor as to be ignored or go unnoticed by the affected individual. (A, From Swartz MH: Textbook of physical diagnosis: history and examination, ed 7, Philadelphia, 2014, Saunders. B, From Nadelman RB: Erythema migrans. Infect Dis Clin North Am 29(2):211–239, 2015.)

BOX 5.9   Neurologic Manifestations of Lyme Disease

- Facial nerve palsy (Bell's palsy)
- Cognitive impairment (e.g., forgetfulness, decreased concentration, personality changes)
- Inflammation of the brain, spinal cord, or nerves
  - Cranial neuritis
  - Encephalitis
  - Encephalomyelitis
  - Encephalopathy
  - Meningitis
  - Radiculoneuropathies

---

characterized by intermittent arthritis associated with marked pain and swelling, especially in the large joints (Fig. 5.7). Rarely, affected individuals may go on to develop erosions or permanent joint abnormalities.[108]

Postinfection syndromes. Several syndromes involving persistent symptoms despite antibiotic treatments have been reported. One such syndrome, called *post-Lyme syndrome* or

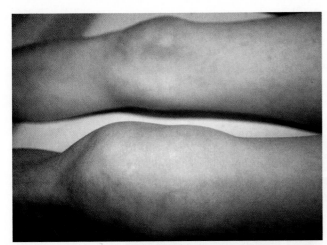

FIG. 5.7 Swollen knee of a youth with Lyme arthritis. (From Hochberg MC, Silman AJ, Smolen JS, et al., editors: Rheumatology, ed 6, Philadelphia, 2015, Mosby.)

chronic Lyme disease, resembles fibromyalgia or chronic fatigue syndrome. Affected individuals describe disabling fatigue, severe headache, diffuse muscle or joint pain, cognitive difficulties, and sleep abnormalities.[102] Symptoms may begin with the infection or emerge soon after treatment and persist for months to years. Debate continues as to whether these patients ever had an active infection with *B. burgdorferi*.[96,106] About 10% of the people who have Lyme arthritis will continue to have joint symptoms for months to years after treatment. Although evidence of the spirochete exists in the synovial fluid before treatment, posttreatment joint fluid is often negative for infection.

5.11 Special Implications for the PTA: Lyme Disease Box 5.10 provides specific strategies available for Lyme disease prevention.

Chronic arthritis is the most widely recognized result of untreated Lyme disease in the United States. Lyme arthritis does not affect the joints bilaterally, though both sides may be affected alternately.

The condition has been called *chronic* because episodes can last months, occurring intermittently over a period of 1 to 3 years. Permanent joint damage and cartilage destruction can occur if there is excessive use during the inflammatory period. Range-of-motion and strengthening exercises are important but must be carried out carefully and without overexertion.

Nervous system abnormalities can develop weeks, months, or even years after an untreated infection. These symptoms often last for weeks or months and may recur. The PTA may treat such a client at any time during the course of symptomatic presentation.

Frequent assessment of neurologic function and level of consciousness is important for anyone with known Lyme disease. Any signs of cardiac or neurologic abnormality must be reported to the physician immediately. Both upper- and lower-extremity peripheral nerve problems can occur and are managed as any neuropathy from other causes.

It has been hypothesized that people with symptoms of multiple sclerosis that respond to antibiotics may have been bitten by ticks years ago. Along the same lines, the question has been raised as to whether Lyme disease triggers fibromyalgia, because symptoms consistent with fibromyalgia and chronic fatigue syndrome develop in individuals with clear-cut Lyme disease, even after adequate treatment. To date no biologic relationship has been proven between these conditions and Lyme disease.[53]

BOX 5.10 Prevention of Lyme Disease

These precautions are advised for people living in tick-infested areas:

- Avoid tick-infested areas, especially in May, June, and July (check with local health departments or park services for the seasonal and geographic distribution in your area).
- Walk along cleared or paved surfaces rather than through tall grass or wooded areas.
- Wear long-sleeved shirts, long pants tucked into socks, and closed shoes (no part of foot exposed).
- Wear light-colored clothing to make it easy to detect ticks.
- Always check for ticks after being outdoors. If ticks are removed within 36 hours of attachment, the risk of infection decreases significantly.
- Shower as soon as possible after being outdoors. Ticks take several hours to attach themselves to the skin and can be washed away first.
- Wash clothing worn outdoors immediately and use a dryer (heat kills the ticks). If no access to laundry facilities is available, the clothing should not be stored in the bedroom, or if camping, the clothing should not be stored in the same area where people are sleeping.
- If bitten by a tick, remove the tick immediately by grasping it as close to the skin as possible with tweezers and tugging gently. Do not twist or turn the tweezers; pull straight away from the skin. Do not use petroleum jelly, fingernail polish or a hot match to remove ticks.
- To lessen the chance of contact with the bacterium, do not crush the tick's body or handle the tick with bare hands. Clean the bite area thoroughly with soap and water, then swab the area with an antiseptic to prevent bacterial infection.
- Whenever possible, save the tick in a glass jar for identification should symptoms develop.
- If living in an area in which deer ticks are common, keep the weeds and grass around the house mowed. Consider using wood chips where lawns meet forested areas. Ticks are less able to survive in a dry environment.
- Use flea and tick collars on pets; brush and examine them carefully after they have been outdoors. People can use insecticides such as permethrin or insect repellents containing diethyltoluamide (DEET).[a]

[a]The use of such chemicals may be objectionable to some people because they may cause neurotoxicity in children. Alternative methods are available.

Sexually Transmitted Infections
Overview and Incidence

Each year 19 million Americans contract a sexually transmitted disease (STD) or sexually transmitted infection (STI), and it is estimated that at least one out of every four sexually active people (56 million Americans) is carrying an infection other than HIV. It is likely that the incidence of STDs and STIs is underreported for several reasons.

Physicians may fail to report STD cases to local health departments despite being mandated to do so. Physicians also rely on patients to notify their sexual partners, who may or may not be tested and/or treated.[10] Syphilis, once thought to be trending toward elimination, has steadily increased in incidence since 2000, particularly in black men and men who have sex with men.[22,85] Although the incidence of gonorrhea has reached an all-time low in the United States, chlamydia and human papillomavirus (HPV) remain significant health problems.

STDs and STIs are spread primarily through sexual contact but in some cases may also be spread by sharing infected needles or by transmission from mother to child during vaginal childbirth. Many STDs and STIs are easily treated and cured, but others remain chronic. More than 50 different STDs and STIs have been described; only the most common ones are included here (see Table 5.4).

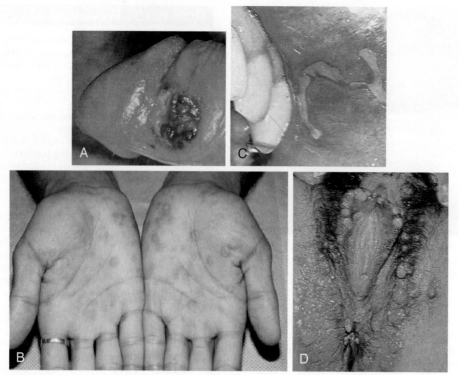

FIG. 5.8 Clinical manifestations of syphilis. Many sexually transmitted infections present with lesions of the skin and/or genitals. Each one presents differently based on the stage of the disease. (A) Chancre in primary syphilis on the penis. (B) Palmar lesions of a coppery color in secondary syphilis. (C) Mucous patch of the mouth in secondary syphilis. (D) Genital lesions called condylomata lata in a female patient (secondary syphilis). (A, C, and D, From Forbes CD, Jackson WF: Color atlas and text of clinical medicine, London, 2003, Mosby. B, From Trager JD: Sexually transmitted diseases causing genital lesions in adolescents, Adolesc Med Clin 15:323–352, 2004.)

Etiologic and Risk Factors

All groups of people are potentially at risk for STDs and STIs, but women, teens, men who have sex with men, and minorities have been disproportionately affected. Young people under the age of 18 are considered at greatest risk for getting an STD, but, in fact, the over-50 population is also at risk.

Although 25% of all STDs and STIs occur in people younger than 25 years old, numerous surveys of healthy adults have verified that older people are sexually active and less likely to practice safe sex. Risk factors vary but most often include multiple sex partners, a partner with a known risk factor, a history of a blood transfusion from 1977 to 1984, failure to use a condom (or use it properly) during sexual intercourse, and sharing needles during illicit drug use.

Pathogenesis and Clinical Manifestations

STDs and STIs are caused by bacteria, viruses, and occasionally parasites and may have a considerable latency period when the infectious organism lies dormant before triggering symptomatic presentation.

Clinical manifestations vary according to the STD present (Fig. 5.8; see also Table 5.4). STDs and STIs may be completely asymptomatic and therefore are less likely to be diagnosed until serious problems develop. Complications of STDs and STIs are more severe and more frequent in women than in men. Once infected, women are more susceptible to reproductive cancers, infertility, and contracting other STDs and STIs.

Medical Management

Prevention

Prevention is the most important key to managing STDs and STIs. The only prevention that is 100% effective is abstinence and/or a mutually monogamous sexual relationship (single partner) between two uninfected people. For those who are sexually active, condoms, properly used, are able to reduce the transmission of STDs spread by mucosal fluid.

Condoms do not cover all surfaces and only protect the skin they cover, however, and therefore are less likely to protect against diseases acquired from skin-to-skin contact such as syphilis, HPV infection, and HSV infection.[123] Genital warts are contagious; avoid touching them.

Pregnant women should have blood tests for syphilis and HBV. Pregnant women should also be tested for gonorrhea, chlamydia, HPV, and HIV. Those with recurrent genital herpes and open sores benefit from cesarean delivery to protect the child.

Drug users, especially injection drug users, can prevent transmission of disease best by discontinuance of drugs, but in most cases this is not immediately realistic. Programs have been set up to help reduce needle sharing by providing needle exchange centers and street education programs aimed at teaching more sterile practices.

Screening, Diagnosis, Treatment, and Prognosis

STDs and STIs can often be identified by the clinical manifestations, but various screening tests are also available. With the advent of urine-based testing, more frequent screening has been successful in both women and men.

HPV infection is another prevalent STD that has been found to cause cervical cancer in women. Because HPV slowly creates cellular changes before the development of cancer, recommendations for screening have been published.

Although HPV is most often acquired in younger clients, older women continue to be at risk, so testing should take risk factors into consideration.[38]

Antibiotics can cure some STDs and STIs (see Table 5.4), although some may be drug resistant. Limiting the number of sexual partners, practicing abstinence, and practicing safe sex (proper use of condoms) are recommended to prevent the transmission of disease. Intercourse during an active infection dramatically increases the risk of transmitting STDs and STIs.

When working with clients with active disease, following contact precautions, washing hands frequently, and avoiding touching the affected areas are essential practices. A vaccine is now available for HBV, and vaccines against HPV, HIV, and herpes are under investigation. The prognosis varies with each STD, but symptoms can be minimized and complications prevented with treatment. Without treatment, serious complications can occur, such as infertility, chronic pelvic pain, ectopic pregnancy and miscarriage, cardiovascular disease, CNS impairment, blindness, cervical cancer, and even death.

5.12 Special Implications for the PTA: Sexually Transmitted Diseases and Infections Any PTA treating men or women with clinical presentation of pelvic, buttock, hip, or groin pain of apparently unknown cause must be prepared to ask the client about history of STDs and STIs. If there is any suspicion that the clinical manifestations may be correlated to an STD, the client must be further evaluated by a physician.

Infections in Drug Users

Drug use in the United States continues to be a significant health problem, with over 19.5 million people, or 8.2% of the population, found to be using drugs in 2003. Serious illnesses such as HIV and hepatitis are transmitted with injection drug use. Drug users as a whole also have a higher incidence of bacterial infections because of the various drugs used, the route and sites of administration, and preparation of the drug. Each of these factors determines risk for infection and the likelihood of specific bacterial infections.[37]

IV use of black-tar heroin causes sclerosis of the veins and leads to "skin popping," or injecting the drug subcutaneously. Continued injection into the same site creates a necrotic environment. NF with toxic shock syndrome can result from the spread of a clostridial infection.[63]

Drug users, particularly IV drug users, vary the site of administration. Local abscess formation or infections are seen in unusual places because of the sites of injection (the femoral vein, or "groin hit," and the neck, or "pocket shot"). Osteomyelitis may develop in the sternoclavicular, sacroiliac, or vertebral spine. Septic arthritis is often seen in the knees.

Environmental factors frequently contribute to infections. Some users may lick the skin or needle before injecting, leading to polymicrobial infections. Others crush tablets between their teeth or blow clots out of needles before reusing. Sharing of needles and paraphernalia is also common.[37] Because of these habits, drug users are more likely to develop certain types of bacterial infections with specific organisms.

Drug users are more likely to develop a respiratory tract infection than are nonusers, and respiratory infections, particularly pneumonia, are the most common infection in drug users. Damage to cells from inhaling drugs and chronic cigarette use (many drug users also smoke) may lead to inability to clear secretions. Aspiration may occur because of decreased mental alertness.

Musculoskeletal infections may occur in unusual places, as discussed earlier. Flora from the skin is the most common pathogen. The infection may be subtle, with mild fever and pain.[37]

5.13 Special Implications for the PTA: Infections in Drug Addicts Being aware of the signs of substance abuse or drug addiction and the patterns of infection associated with drug addiction may assist the PTA in recognizing early signs of infection requiring medical evaluation and treatment. Any PTA involved in wound care management, needle electromyography, or other high-risk practice techniques who has not already been immunized against HBV should be vaccinated.

REFERENCES/SUGGESTED READINGS

To enhance this text and add value for the reader, references and suggested readings are included on the companion Evolve site that accompanies this textbook. The reader can view the source and access it online whenever possible.

6

Oncology

1. Review concepts of normal cell division and differentiation; review medical terminology for cellular organization in tissue.
2. Identify the risk factors for genetic mutations that alter normal cell division, differentiation, cell maturation and apoptosis to create neoplasm, and recognize the role of the immune system in fighting neoplasm.
3. Understand classifications, grading, and definition of benign and malignant. Understand that benign growths are not always harmless.
4. Understand the process of metastasis, including the connection between angiogenesis and metastasis, and the "downstream" factors that affect likelihood of locations for metastatic growths.
5. Explore the role of therapeutic exercise as a prevention modality for cancer.

OUTLINE

VOCAB BUILDERS

Angiogenesis	Dysplasia	Metaplasia
Antioncogenes	Hematopoietic	Metastasis
Apoptosis	Hyperplasia	Neoplasm
Benign	Hypertrophy	Oncogenes
CAM	In situ	Paraneoplastic
Differentiation	Malignant	

Cancer is a term that refers to a large group of diseases characterized by uncontrolled cell proliferation and spread of abnormal cells. Other terms used interchangeably with *cancer* are *malignant neoplasm, tumor, malignancy,* and *carcinoma.* According to the American Cancer Society (ACS), about 5% of cancer is genetic, whereas 95% is related to other factors.

DEFINITIONS

Differentiation

Normal tissue contains cells of uniform size, shape, maturity, and nuclear structure. *Differentiation* is the process by which normal cells undergo physical and structural changes as they develop to form different tissues of the body. Differentiated cells specialize in different physiologic functions.

In malignant cells, differentiation is altered and may be lost completely so that the malignant cell may not be recognizable in relationship to its parent cell. When a tumor has completely lost identity with the parent tissue, it is considered to be undifferentiated (anaplastic). In this case it may become difficult or impossible to identify the malignant cell's tissue of origin. Generally, the less differentiated a tumor becomes, the faster the *metastasis* (spread) and the worse the prognosis.

Dysplasia

A variety of other tissue changes can occur in the body. Some of these changes are *benign,* whereas others denote a malignant or premalignant state. *Dysplasia* is a general category that indicates a disorganization of cells in which an adult cell varies from its normal size, shape, or organization. It may reverse itself or may progress to cancer.

Metaplasia

Metaplasia is the first level of dysplasia. It is a reversible and benign but abnormal change in which one adult cell changes from one type to another.

Although metaplasia usually gives rise to an orderly arrangement of cells, it may sometimes produce disorderly cellular patterns. Anaplasia (loss of cellular differentiation) is the most advanced form of metaplasia and is a characteristic of malignant cells only.

Hyperplasia

Hyperplasia refers to an increase in the number of cells in tissue, resulting in increased tissue mass. This type of change can be a normal consequence of physiologic alterations such as increased breast mass during pregnancy, wound healing, or bone callus formation. Neoplastic hyperplasia, however, is the increase in cell mass because of tumor formation and is an abnormal process. The presence of such types of hyperplastic breast tissue increases the risk of later development of breast cancer.[85]

Tumors

Tumors, or neoplasms, are abnormal growths of new tissue that serve no useful purpose and may harm the host organism by competing for vital blood supply and nutrients. These new growths may be benign or malignant and primary or secondary.

A primary tumor arises from cells that are normally local to the given structure, whereas a secondary tumor arises from cells that have metastasized from another part of the body. For example, a primary neoplasm of bone arises from within the bone structure itself, whereas a secondary neoplasm occurs in bone as a result of metastasized cancer cells from another or (primary) site.

Carcinoma in situ refers to preinvasive, premalignant epithelial tumors of glandular or squamous cell origin. These tumors have not broken through basement membranes of the squamous cells and occur in the cervix, skin, oral cavity, esophagus, bronchus, and breast. Carcinoma in situ that affects glandular epithelium is most common in the cervix, breast, stomach, endometrium, large bowel, and prostate gland. How long the characteristic cell disorganization and atypical changes last before becoming invasive is variable for different cancers.

CLASSIFICATIONS OF NEOPLASM

A neoplasm can be classified on the basis of cell type, tissue of origin, degree of differentiation, anatomic site, or whether

TABLE 6.1   Classification of Neoplasms by Cell Type of Origin

Tissue of Origin	Benign	Malignant
Epithelial Tissue		
Surface epithelium (skin) and mucous membrane	Papilloma	Squamous cell, basal cell, and transitional cell carcinoma
Epithelial lining of glands or ducts	Adenoma	Adenocarcinoma
Pigmented cells (melanocytes of basal layer)	Nevus (mole)	Malignant melanoma
Connective Tissue and Muscle		
Fibrous tissue	Fibroma	Fibrosarcoma
Adipose	Lipoma	Liposarcoma
Cartilage	Chondroma	Chondrosarcoma
Bone	Osteoma	Osteosarcoma
Blood vessels	Hemangioma	Hemangiosarcoma
Smooth muscle	Leiomyoma	Leiomyosarcoma
Striated muscle	Rhabdomyoma	Rhabdomyosarcoma
Nerve Tissue		
Nerve cells	Neuroma	
Glia		Glioma or neuroglioma
Ganglion cells	Ganglioneuroma	Neuroblastoma
Nerve sheaths	Neurilemoma	Neurilemic sarcoma
Meninges	Meningioma	Meningeal sarcoma
Retina		Retinoblastoma
Lymphoid Tissue		
Lymph nodes		Lymphoma
Spleen		
Intestinal lining		
Hematopoietic Tissue		
Bone marrow		Leukemias, myelodysplasia, and myeloproliferative syndromes
Plasma cells		Multiple myeloma

it is benign or malignant. A benign growth is usually considered harmless and does not spread to or invade other tissue. Certain benign growths, recognized clinically as tumors, are not truly neoplastic but represent overgrowth of normal tissue elements. However, benign growths can become large enough to distend, compress, or obstruct normal tissues and to impair normal body functions, as in the case of benign central nervous system (CNS) tumors. These tumors can cause disability and even death.

When tumors, benign or malignant, are classified by cell type, they are named according to the tissue from which they arise (Table 6.1). The five major classifications of normal body tissue are epithelial, connective and muscle, nerve, lymphoid, and *hematopoietic* tissue. Not all tissue types fit into one of these five categories, thus requiring a miscellaneous category for other tissues such as the tissues of the reproductive glands, placenta, and thymus.

Epithelium covers all external body surfaces and lines all internal spaces and cavities. The skin, mucous membranes, gastrointestinal tract, and lining of the bladder are examples of epithelial tissue. The functions of epithelial tissues are to protect, excrete, and absorb. Cancer originating in any of these epithelial tissues is called a *carcinoma*. Tumors derived from glandular tissues are called adenocarcinomas.

Connective tissue consists of elastic, fibrous, and collagenous tissues such as bone, cartilage, and fat. Cancers originating in connective tissue and muscle are called *sarcomas*.

Nerve tissue includes the brain, spinal cord, and nerves and consists of neurons, nerve fibers, dendrites, and a supporting tissue composed of glial cells. Tumors arising in nerve tissue are named for the type of cell involved. For example, tumors arising from astrocytes are called *astrocytomas*. Tumors arising in nerve tissue are often benign, but because of their critical location they are more likely to be harmful than benign tumors in other sites.

Malignancies originating in lymphoid tissues are called *lymphomas*. Lymphomas can arise wherever lymphoid tissue is present. The most common sites to find lymphoid malignancies are the lymph nodes and spleen. However, lymphomas can appear in other parts of the body such as the skin, CNS, stomach, small bowel, bone, and tonsils.[29]

Hematopoietic malignancies include leukemias, multiple myeloma, myelodysplasia, and the myeloproliferative syndromes.

Staging and Grading
Staging

Staging is the process of describing the extent of disease at the time of diagnosis to aid treatment planning, predict clinical outcome (prognosis), and compare the results of different treatment approaches. The stage of disease at the time of diagnosis reflects the rate of growth, the extent of the neoplasm, and the prognosis. A simplified way to stage cancer is as follows:

- Stage 0: Carcinoma in situ (premalignant, preinvasive)
- Stage I: Early stage, local cancer
- Stage II: Increased risk of spread because of tumor size
- Stage III: Local cancer has spread but may not be disseminated to distant regions
- Stage IV: Cancer has spread and disseminated to distant sites

In some cases, cancer may be staged as II or III depending on the spread of the specific type of cancer. For example, in Hodgkin's disease, stage II indicates lymph nodes are affected on one side of the diaphragm. Stage III indicates affected lymph nodes above and below the diaphragm.

The tumor, node, metastases (TNM) system is used most often for solid tumors and has been adapted for other types of tumors. Some cancers do not have a staging system (e.g., brain cancer), and some can be staged using more than one system. The International Union Against Cancer is the universally accepted staging system, and it incorporates the TNM classification of malignant tumors.

It is important to realize that the TNM staging system is simply an anatomic staging system that describes the anatomic extent of the primary tumor, as well as the involvement of regional lymph nodes and distant metastases. Revisions to the TNM staging system are made as the understanding of the natural history of tumors at various sites improves with advancing technology. In the TNM classification scheme, tumors are staged according to the following basic components (Box 6.1):

- Tumor (T) refers to the primary tumor and carries a number from 0 to 4.
- Regional lymph nodes (N) represents regional lymph node involvement and is also ranked from 0 to 4.
- Metastasis (M) is zero (0) if no metastasis has occurred or 1 if metastases are present.

BOX 6.1   TNM Staging System

T: Primary Tumor

TX	Primary tumor cannot be assessed
T0	No evidence of primary tumor
TIS	Carcinoma in situ (confined to site of origin)
T1, T2, T3, T4	Progressive increase in tumor size and involvement locally

N: Regional Lymph Nodes

NX	Nodes cannot be assessed
N0	No metastasis to regional lymph nodes
N1, N2, N3	Increasing degrees of involvement of regional lymph nodes

M: Distant Metastasis

MX	Presence of distant metastasis cannot be assessed
M0	No distant metastasis
M1	Distant metastasis

Note: Extension of primary tumor directly into lymph nodes is considered metastasis to lymph nodes. Metastasis to a lymph node beyond the regional ones is considered distant metastasis.

Numbers are used with each component to denote the extent of involvement; for example, T0 indicates undetectable, and T1, T2, T3, and T4 indicate a progressive increase in size or involvement.[98]

Clinical staging is performed indirectly by observation of the person before the tumor is treated or removed. The pathologic stage is determined by direct examination of the tumor by the pathologist once it has been removed and is considered a more accurate reflection of the tumor and its spread. Not all tumors are resected or excised, so pathologic staging is not always available. Pathologic staging may underestimate the true stage for individuals who received adjuvant treatment before surgery.

Grading

Grading of tumor tissue is done by the pathologist using different grading for different types of tumors. For example, the Bloom–Richardson (or Nottingham) scale is used in breast cancer, the Gleason score in prostate cancer, and the Fuhrman scale in grading cancers of the kidney. Each grading method may use a different numerical score or scale, but generally the lower the value, the lower the grade of tumor and the better differentiation of tissue within the tumor. A highly scored/scaled tumor is considered a high-grade tumor with poor cellular differentiation and a tendency to metastasize early. Staging is more predictive than grading.

INCIDENCE

Estimates of worldwide incidence, mortality, and prevalence of 26 cancers are available from the International Agency for Research on Cancer (IARC). Geographic variations among 20 large areas of the world are studied. The most recent report published in 2011 identified a 12.7 million incidence of new cases and 7.6 million deaths. Rate of survivorship in developing countries is less than one-half of those of developed countries because of late diagnosis and lack of availability of care. Most of the international variation is a result of known or suspected risk factors related to lifestyle or environment. The IARC has been researching and providing a database of global cancer estimates (GLOBOCAN) for the last 30 years.[61,132]

The most commonly diagnosed cancers are lung, prostate, breast, and colorectal; the most prevalent cancer in the world is lung cancer and accounts for the highest number of cancer deaths worldwide.[61] The ACS publishes annual cancer statistics and estimates cancer trends (Fig. 6.1). Each year the ACS calculates estimates of the number of new cancer cases and expected cancer deaths in the United States and compiles the most recent data on cancer incidence, mortality, and survival.[61]

Based on statistical estimates, in the year 2014 the ACS predicted about 1.46 million new cases of invasive cancer in the United States and approximately 585,720 cancer-related deaths. This figure did not include most skin cancers, which were expected to affect 1 million people per year.[61]

It is estimated that at least one in three people will be diagnosed with some form of invasive cancer in their lifetime and that three of five people will be cured and/or survive 5 years after cancer treatment. However, cancer is still the second leading cause of death in the United States, exceeded only by heart disease. Poor health and nutrition habits, continued smoking, ozone destruction, and a long-term lack of exercise among many people continue to be discussed as contributors to the overall rise of this disease.[113]

Trends in Cancer Incidence and Survival

Overall incidence of cancer peaked in 1990 and has declined in the last decade by an average of 1.1% annually, with a 1.4% decline in cancer death rates. In 2003 and 2004, the rate doubled to 2% per year, largely attributed to smoking cessation among men. The latest drop in cancer deaths occurred across all four major cancer types.

Survival rates for cancer are on the rise, increasing from 50% to 64% over the last 30 years. Cancer prevention strategies may reduce the incidence of cancer occurrence and recurrence.[10]

Gender-Based Incidence

Among men, the most common cancers are predicted to be cancers of the prostate, lung and bronchus, and colon and rectum. Among women, the three most commonly diagnosed cancers are expected to be cancers of the breast, lung and bronchus, and colon and rectum.

The largest decreases in deaths occurred among men, who bear the heaviest overall cancer burden, and colorectal cancer in particular. Officials have attributed the steady downward trend to improved vigilance among Americans, who are benefiting from early screening and advances in treatment, as well as smoking less, improving their diets, and exercising more.

For 2004 to 2008, overall cancer incidence declined 0.6% per year in men and was stable in women. In the same period, death rates decreased 1.8% in men and 1.6% in women. Breast cancer alone accounted for approximately 235,030 new cancer cases in women in 2014 compared with 178,400 in 2007.[119,146]

The decline in rates of breast cancer deaths has been attributed in part to increased mammography but also to more aggressive therapy; overall decline in deaths among women may also be the result of the recent falloff in hormone replacement therapy.

Likewise, improved screening, detection, and treatment of prostate cancer have resulted in a decline in the death rate associated with this type of cancer. About a dozen cancers continue to rise in incidence or mortality, including melanoma, non-Hodgkin's lymphoma, thyroid cancer, esophageal cancer, breast cancer, and lung cancer in women.

Estimated New Cases

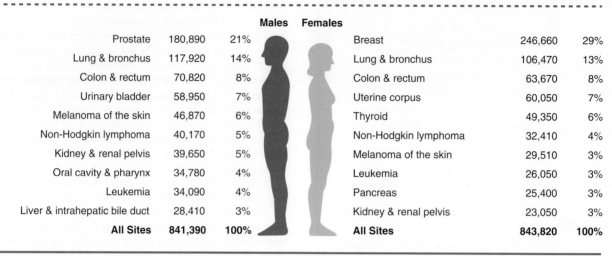

	Males			Females		
Prostate	180,890	21%	Breast	246,660	29%
Lung & bronchus	117,920	14%	Lung & bronchus	106,470	13%
Colon & rectum	70,820	8%	Colon & rectum	63,670	8%
Urinary bladder	58,950	7%	Uterine corpus	60,050	7%
Melanoma of the skin	46,870	6%	Thyroid	49,350	6%
Non-Hodgkin lymphoma	40,170	5%	Non-Hodgkin lymphoma	32,410	4%
Kidney & renal pelvis	39,650	5%	Melanoma of the skin	29,510	3%
Oral cavity & pharynx	34,780	4%	Leukemia	26,050	3%
Leukemia	34,090	4%	Pancreas	25,400	3%
Liver & intrahepatic bile duct	28,410	3%	Kidney & renal pelvis	23,050	3%
All Sites	**841,390**	**100%**	**All Sites**	**843,820**	**100%**

Estimated Deaths

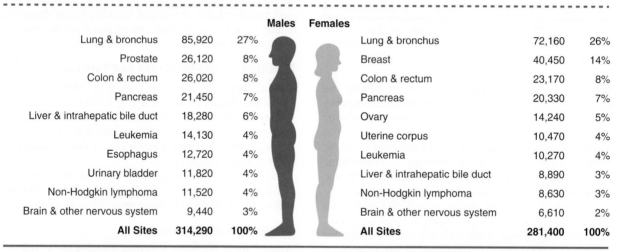

	Males			Females		
Lung & bronchus	85,920	27%	Lung & bronchus	72,160	26%
Prostate	26,120	8%	Breast	40,450	14%
Colon & rectum	26,020	8%	Colon & rectum	23,170	8%
Pancreas	21,450	7%	Pancreas	20,330	7%
Liver & intrahepatic bile duct	18,280	6%	Ovary	14,240	5%
Leukemia	14,130	4%	Uterine corpus	10,470	4%
Esophagus	12,720	4%	Leukemia	10,270	4%
Urinary bladder	11,820	4%	Liver & intrahepatic bile duct	8,890	3%
Non-Hodgkin lymphoma	11,520	4%	Non-Hodgkin lymphoma	8,630	3%
Brain & other nervous system	9,440	3%	Brain & other nervous system	6,610	2%
All Sites	**314,290**	**100%**	**All Sites**	**281,400**	**100%**

FIG. 6.1 Estimated new cancer cases *(top)* and estimated cancer deaths *(bottom)*, 2016, in the United States (percent distribution of sites by gender). (From Siegel RL, Miller KD, Jemal, A: Cancer statistics, 2016, CA Cancer J Clin 66:7–30, 2016.)

ETIOLOGY

The cause of cancer varies, and causative agents are generally subdivided into two categories: those of endogenous (genetic) origin and those of exogenous (environmental or external) origin. It is likely that most cancers develop as a result of multiple environmental, viral, and genetic factors working together to disrupt the immune system, along with failure of an aging immune system to recognize and scavenge cells that have become less differentiated.

Certain cancers show a familial pattern, giving people a hereditary predisposition to cancer. The most common cancers showing a familial pattern include prostate, breast, ovarian, and colon cancers. Research efforts have been directed at finding genes associated with various cancers that could identify high-risk individuals for screening and early detection.

The ACS estimates that 50% of all cancers are caused by one or more of nearly 500 different cancer-causing agents.[113] Etiologic agents capable of initiating the malignant transformation

of a cell (i.e., carcinogenesis) are called *carcinogens*. The study of viruses as carcinogens is one of the most rapidly advancing areas in cancer research today.

Researchers now have evidence that viruses play a role in the pathogenesis of cervical carcinomas, some hepatomas, Burkitt's lymphomas, nasopharyngeal carcinomas, adult T-cell leukemias, and, indirectly, many Kaposi's sarcomas.[29] Viruses, such as the human immunodeficiency virus, the causative agent of acquired immunodeficiency syndrome, weaken cell-mediated immunity, resulting in malignancies.

Chemical agents (tar, soot, asphalt, and dyes) and physical agents (radiation and asbestos) may cause cancer after close and prolonged contact. Most people affected by chemical agents are industrial workers. Radiation exposure is usually from natural sources, especially ultraviolet radiation from the sun, which can cause changes in deoxyribonucleic acid (DNA) structure that lead to malignant transformation. Basal and squamous cell carcinomas and malignant melanoma are all linked to ultraviolet exposure.

Some drugs, such as cancer chemotherapeutic agents, are in themselves carcinogenic. Cytotoxic drugs, including steroids, decrease antibody production and destroy circulating lymphocytes. Cancer clients treated with chemotherapy are at risk for future development of leukemia and other cancers.

Hormones have been linked to tumor development and growth. Other types of cancer occurring in target or hormone-responsive tissues include ovarian and prostate cancers.

Excessive alcohol consumption is associated with cancer of the mouth, pharynx, larynx, esophagus, and pancreas. It can also indirectly contribute to liver cancer. The possible association between alcohol and breast cancer is under investigation. The pathophysiologic link remains unclear, but researchers postulate that alcohol influences the metabolism of estrogen, and increased estrogen exposure is a known risk factor for breast cancer.

RISK FACTORS

Advancing age is one of the most significant risk factors for cancer. In addition to age and the carcinogens described earlier in the chapter, predisposing factors also influence the host's susceptibility to various etiologic agents (Box 6.2).

Nine modifiable risk factors are responsible for more than one-third of cancer deaths worldwide: tobacco, alcohol, obesity, inactivity, diet and nutrition, unsafe sex, urban air pollution, indoor smoke from household fuels, or contaminated injections in health care settings. Of these, smoking and alcohol consumption are the most damaging. This means that even without the potential benefits of early detection and treatment, at least one-third of cancer deaths are preventable.[28,131]

Aging

Being over 50 years of age is a significant risk factor for the development of cancer, but cancer is not an inevitable consequence of aging. The association between cancer and aging is becoming more common because of the aging of the general population. According to the Surveillance, Epidemiology, and End Results (SEER) Program report for 2002 to 2006, the median age for all races and gender at time of primary diagnosis is approximately 66. The median age is expected to increase over the next several decades.[36] The risk of multiple diseases (comorbidity) also increases with age, creating limitations in the life expectancy of individual aging adults and enhancing the likelihood of treatment complications.

Older people may be more susceptible to cancer simply because they have been exposed to carcinogens longer than younger people. The effects of age on immune function and host defense are being studied to determine what the association is between cancer and age. Factors such as accumulated nonlethal damage to DNA by free radicals, increased proinflammatory factors, and age-associated declines in DNA repair are important.[35] People aged 65 or older have a risk of cancer development much greater than the risk in younger persons, and some cancers in the older adult population seem to be biologically different from those in younger people. For example, the poor prognosis for older adults with acute leukemia is not just because of poor tolerance of aggressive chemotherapy but is more likely associated with resistance to chemotherapy.[56]

All the highest incidence cancers affect older adults in larger numbers. In both men and women over 65 years of age, cancers of the colon and rectum, stomach, pancreas, and bladder

BOX 6.2   Cancer Risk Factors

- Advancing age
- Previous cancer
- Lifestyle or personal behaviors
  - Tobacco use
  - Diet and nutrition (high fat, low fiber)
  - Obesity
  - Alcohol use
  - Sexual and reproductive behavior
  - Physical inactivity
- Type 2 diabetes
- Exposure to viruses
  - Human papillomavirus
  - Epstein–Barr virus
  - Hepatitis B virus
  - Hepatitis C virus
  - Herpesvirus 8
- *Helicobacter pylori*
- Exposure to hormones (e.g., estrogen, testosterone)
- Geographic location and environmental variables
- Previous cancer treatment (e.g., radiotherapy)
- Gender (either, depending on cancer)
- Ethnicity (type depends on cancer)
- Lower socioeconomic status
- Occupation
- Heredity (family history of cancer)
- Presence of precancerous lesions or polyps
- Stress
- Inflammatory bowel disease

account for two-thirds to three-fourths of the total number of these malignancies. More than 65% of lung cancers and 50% of non-Hodgkin's lymphomas occur in older men and women, 77% of cases of prostate cancer occur in men older than 65, and 48% of breast cancer cases and 46% of ovarian cancer cases occur in women older than 65.[145]

As previously mentioned, malignancies of the lung, colon and rectum, breast, and prostate account for the highest number of cancer deaths in the United States. Malignancies of the pancreas, stomach, ovary, and bladder and non-Hodgkin's lymphomas are also major causes of cancer deaths. For each of these cancers, more than one-half of the cancer deaths occur in persons older than 65.[145]

Lifestyle

Lifestyle or personal behaviors, such as tobacco use, poor diet and nutrition, alcohol use, and certain sexual and reproductive behaviors, are cited as risk factors for the development of cancer. Lifestyle-related risk factors for cancer combined with cancer-causing substances in the environment and the presence of genes that increase the risk of cancer account for 70% of the total risk for developing cancer.

Tobacco

Both epidemiologic and experimental data support the conclusion that tobacco is carcinogenic and remains the most important cause of cancer. Tobacco use accounts for approximately 30% of cancer deaths, with lung cancer now the leading cancer causing deaths in both genders.[31] Cigarette smoking is related to nearly 90% of all lung cancers, and accumulating evidence suggests that cigarette smoking increases the incidence of cancer of the bladder and pancreas and to a lesser extent the kidney, larynx, oral cavity, and esophagus.

Diet and Nutrition

The major role of diet and nutrition in affecting cancer risk is well established.[3,14,127] Consumption of a poor diet may blunt the immune system's natural defense mechanisms against genetic damage caused by long-term exposure to an environmental carcinogen. Diet and nutrition can directly influence various hormonal factors affecting growth and differentiation in the carcinogenic process. A healthful diet is thought to act, at least in part, to detoxify carcinogens and to inhibit certain processes in carcinogenesis, particularly at the stage of growth and spread.

Differences in certain dietary patterns among populations explain a proportion of cancers. These dietary patterns in combination with physical inactivity contribute to obesity and metabolic consequences such as increased levels of growth factor, insulin, estrogen, and possibly testosterone.

Obesity and type 2 diabetes are risk factors for breast, prostate, and colorectal cancer. Excess weight also contributes to cancers of the uterus, kidney, esophagus, pancreas, and gallbladder.[16,88]

It is estimated that approximately one-third of cancer mortality in developing countries may result from dietary causes.[6,137] The intake of cured, pickled, smoked, salted, and preserved food has been conclusively linked to stomach cancer, and it is suspected that there is a correlation between the amount of fat in the diet and the incidence of colorectal cancer in the United States.[16] There is a similar correlation between excessive red meat consumption and prostate, colon, and/or rectal cancer.[67] Epidemiologic data also suggest links between fat intake and prostate and ovarian cancers, although not all findings are consistent.[52]

Reduction of cancer risks for most epithelial tumors, especially colorectal cancer, has been demonstrated repeatedly in the presence of increased dietary intake of fresh fruits and vegetables and fiber. High cruciferous vegetable consumption may reduce bladder cancer risk and the risk of non-Hodgkin's lymphoma.[77,147] Although the role of fruits and vegetables and their antioxidant qualities in reducing free radicals that contribute to cancer of various sites has been proved, a recent report suggests that the recommendation to eat an abundance of fruits and vegetables to reduce cancer risk may be overstated.

Cancer and cancer treatment can cause profound metabolic and physiologic alterations affecting the body's needs for adequate nutritional intake. Gastrointestinal side effects of treatment can lead to loss of appetite and weight loss accompanied by malnutrition. All the major treatment modalities can adversely affect how the body digests, absorbs, and uses food. Preserving lean body mass is an important goal of nutritional care for survivors, especially during active cancer treatment.[110]

The use of nutritional supplements and antioxidants remains controversial. Until more evidence is available that suggests more benefit than harm, the Institute of Medicine suggests it is prudent for cancer survivors receiving chemotherapy or radiation therapy (RT) to avoid exceeding more than 100% of the daily value for antioxidant-type vitamins during the treatment phase.[59]

Alcohol

Alcohol consumption has been linked to increased rates of cancer of the mouth, pharynx, larynx, esophagus, liver, breast, and probably colon. In people who have been diagnosed with cancer, alcohol intake could also affect the risk for new primary cancers of these sites. Alcohol intake can increase the circulating levels of estrogens, theoretically increasing the risk for breast cancer recurrence.[107,121]

With tobacco use, alcohol interacts with smoke synergistically, increasing the risk of malignant tumors by acting as a solvent for the carcinogenic smoke products and thus increasing the absorption of carcinogens.

Sexual and Reproductive Behaviors

Sexual and reproductive behaviors are linked to the risk of developing various cancers. For example, the risk of developing cervical cancer is linked with early sexual intercourse and multiple partners. Pregnancy and childbearing seem to be protective against cancers of the endometrium, ovary, and breast. Prolonged lactation may also have a significant impact in the reduction of breast cancer risk by reducing the cumulative exposure of breast tissue to estrogen.[52]

Hormonal Exposure

Hormonal exposure is a factor for women. For example, prolonged exposure to estrogen is a risk factor for estrogen-sensitive breast cancer.

Prolonged use of estrogen hormone replacement therapy for relief of menopausal symptoms has been linked with increased rates of breast cancer. Data from the Women's Health Initiative resulted in a halt to the routine use of estrogen and progestin in combination (Prempro) in 2002 and estrogen alone (Premarin) in 2004. When hormone users were compared with a placebo group, it was clear that the hormone users were experiencing more breast cancer, heart disease, stroke, and blood clots. Estrogen showed some benefit, but it was not enough to outweigh the risks.[142]

Growth factors and hormones, such as estrogen and testosterone, are considered risk factors linked with cancers other than breast and prostate. A growing body of recent literature indicates that along with its essential role in growth and development, growth hormone may play a role in the development and progression of cancer.[90]

Geographic Location and Environmental Variables

The incidence of different types of cancer varies geographically. People living in rural areas are less likely to use preventive screening services or to exercise regularly. Colon cancer is more prevalent in urban than in rural areas, but in rural areas, especially among farmers, skin cancer is more common. Lack of availability of specialty care is a possible contributing issue for this group of people.

The greater susceptibility of certain geographic areas within the United States is probably related to exposure to different carcinogens.[24] The increased incidence of cancer found in urban areas may be related to the increased pool of minorities, increased poverty represented in this group, lack of local smoking ordinances, and diet.[93]

Occupational or environmental exposure to chemicals, fibers, radon, and air pollution is a risk factor for lung and hematologic cancers. Researchers are investigating the possible causal relationship between environmental exposure and the increased incidence of childhood cancers. According to the seventh report on the Biological Effects of Ionizing Radiation issued by the National Academy of Sciences, exposure to even low-dose imaging radiology (including computed tomography [CT] scans) can result in the development of malignancy.

Exposure to medical x-rays is linked with leukemia, thyroid cancer, and breast cancer. There is a 1 in 1000 chance of developing cancer from a single CT scan of the chest, abdomen, or pelvis. The latency period for leukemias is 2 to 5 years and for solid tumors is 10 to 30 years.[128]

Ethnicity

Despite advances in cancer diagnosis, treatment, and survival, racial and ethnic minorities are disproportionately affected by cancer. Poverty has emerged as a significant factor influencing poor cancer outcomes for all races, especially among minorities.[99] Inequities in insurance status adversely affect low-income families, preventing individual members from obtaining screening, access to high-quality care, or the entire range of cancer care available.[120]

In particular, racial disparities exist between Caucasians and other groups, especially African Americans. Overall, incidence of and mortality from cancer are 10% higher in African Americans than in Caucasians.[13,120] Studies have shown that equal treatment yields equal outcomes among individuals with equal disease.[8,76] At present, this increased incidence is attributed to preventable risk factors such as the absence of early screening, delayed diagnosis, and smoking and diet. The number of African American men who smoke is decreasing, but the incidence of lung cancer and other smoking-related diseases remains high, possibly because black men tend to smoke cigarettes with a higher tar and nicotine content. The incidence rates of prostate cancer in black men are at least 50% higher than rates in men of other ethnic groups.[61]

Lung cancer is the leading cause of cancer death among African American women. The number of African American women aged 45 to 54 years who have died from lung cancer has increased 30% over the last two decades.[139] The number of African American women of all ages who have died from breast cancer has risen nearly 20% over the last 25 years. Breast cancer is the second leading cause of death for African American women. Colorectal cancer has increased in both African American men and women; African American women are twice as likely to develop cervical cancer and nearly three times as likely to die of it as other women; African American men have the world's highest rate of prostate cancer.[63]

Some specific forms of cancer affect other ethnic groups at rates higher than the national average, for example, stomach and liver cancers among Asian American populations and colorectal cancer among Alaska Natives. African Americans have a lower incidence of bladder cancer but higher mortality rates compared with Caucasians.[133] The incidence of and mortality rates for esophageal cancer are twice as high for African Americans than for Caucasians.[11]

Differences among ethnic groups represent a challenge to understand the reasons and an opportunity to reduce illness and death while improving survival rates. Hispanic people originate from 23 different countries with a wide range of diversity. Racial variations exist in tumor growth, susceptibility, and treatment response. For example, Latino populations have a different drug resistance gene expression than non-Latino whites.[83]

Hispanics have lower incidence and death rates than non-Hispanic whites for all cancers combined, but the risk increases with the duration of U.S. residence. Cancer is the leading cause of death among U.S. Hispanics. The association between infectious agents (e.g., hepatitis B virus, *Helicobacter*

pylori) and cancer may account for higher rates of stomach, liver, uterine cervix, and gallbladder cancers but lower screening rates, differences in lifestyle and dietary patterns, and genetic factors are highly prevalent risk factors.[118,147]. Asian Americans have a unique situation in that they are the only racial or ethnic group to experience cancer as the leading cause of death, with proportionately more cancer of infectious origin than any other minority group. Cultural barriers to intervention exist, such as overcoming resistance to physician visits, reducing tobacco use, and increasing exercise.[20]

Newer federal legislation, the Patient Protection and Affordable Health Care Act (Public Law 111-148 and 111-152), signed into law in 2010 and upheld by the Supreme Court in 2012, provided the authority for preventive screening for certain cancers (breast, cervical, and colorectal). It also provided insurance coverage for those with a preexisting chronic condition, such as cancer, traditionally denied in the past. Elements of the law will be incorporated over the next few years until 2020.

Precancerous Lesions

Precancerous lesions and some benign tumors may undergo later transformation into cancerous lesions and tumors. Common precancerous lesions include pigmented moles, burn scars, senile keratosis, leukoplakia, and benign adenomas or polyps of the colon or stomach. All such lesions need to be examined periodically for signs of changes.

Stress

Recent research suggests a strong link between stress and cancer. Chronic physical or emotional stress can cause hormonal or immunologic changes or both, which in turn can facilitate the growth and proliferation of cancer cells. There is substantial evidence from both healthy populations and people with cancer that links psychologic stress with immune downregulation. Distress and depression are associated with two important processes for carcinogenesis: poorer repair of damaged DNA and alterations in programmed cell death.

Both aging processes and psychologic stress affect the immune system; in fact, the effects of stress and age are interactive. Psychologic stress can both mimic and exacerbate the effects of aging. Older adults often show greater immunologic impairment from stress compared with younger adults.[48] Conversely, the possibility that psychologic interventions and social support may enhance immune function and survival is under further investigation.[65] Psychologic modulation of immune function is now a well-established phenomenon. Psychoneuroimmunology and psychoneuroendocrinology research focuses on how the brain and body communicate with each other in a multidirectional flow of information that consists of hormones, neurotransmitter-neuropeptides, and cytokines.[136]

Proponents of psychooncology suggest that advances in mind–body medicine research combined with healthy nutrition and lifestyle choices can have a significant impact on health, health maintenance, disease, and prevention of disease, including cancer.[64,136]

PATHOGENESIS

Early in the study of cancer the concept that neoplasia originates in a single cell by acquired genetic change was proposed and remains today the view of cancer pathogenesis most supported by experimental evidence. This hypothesis, called the *somatic mutation theory,* was first substantiated when investigations of tumors confirmed that tumor cells are characterized by chromosomal abnormalities, both numeric and structural.

The discovery that chromosomal aberration is one of the basic mechanisms of tumor cell proliferation laid the foundation of modern cancer cytogenetics (the study of chromosomes in cancer). Chromosomal changes can include addition or deletion of entire chromosomes or translocations, deletions, inversions, and insertions of parts of chromosomes. Translocations occur when two or more chromosomes exchange material and are common in leukemias and sarcomas. Deletions or losses of chromosomal material are common in epithelial adenocarcinomas of the large bowel, lung, breast, and prostate. Chromosomal deletions may lead to neoplastic development when a tumor suppressor gene is lost. Chromosomal inversions and insertions are less common but still cause abnormal placement of genetic material.[105]

Two functionally different classes of cancer-relevant genes have been detected: (1) the dominant oncogenes and (2) the recessive tumor suppressor genes. Exactly how these chromosomal changes contribute to the malignant process remains unclear. Chromosomal rearrangements may lead to oncogene activation or may create a deranged oncogene template that codes for an abnormal protein product.

Another proposed mechanism suggests that chromosomal changes inactivate a tumor suppressor gene through chromosomal deletion. Loss of tumor suppressor genes is suspected because chromosomal regions found to be consistently missing in tumor cells have been observed in carcinomas of the lung, breast, bladder, and kidney.

Another genetic suppressor of cell growth and division also plays a part in the aging process. As cells divide and grow older, there is continuous progressive shortening of the end portions of the chromosomes or telomeres of those cells. Studies of human fibroblasts and other human tissues have shown a very close association between the development of cancer and the overproduction of the enzyme telomerase. When this enzyme is present, it prevents the telomeres from shortening, thus lengthening the lifespan of the cell indefinitely. Telomerase has been found to be present in more than 85% of human cancer cells but is absent in most normal human tissues.[89,108,134]

Although much remains to be learned about the cascade of genetic changes for every kind of cancer, increasing understanding may suggest a means for interrupting the genetic events leading to cancer and for diagnosing the early stages of tumorigenesis.

Current Theory of Oncogenesis

The study of viruses in tumors has led researchers to discover small segments of genetic DNA called *oncogenes.* Oncogenes, also called *cancer-causing genes,* have the ability to transform normal cells into malignant cells, independently or incorporated with a virus. Oncogenes are thought to be the abnormal counterparts of protooncogenes, which aid in regulating biologic functions, such as cell division, in normal cells.

Oncogenes force a cell to grow even when its surroundings contain none of the cues that normally provoke growth. Oncogenes are hyperactivated versions of normal cellular growth-promoting genes. By releasing strong, unrelenting growth-stimulating signals into a cell, oncogenes can drive cell growth ceaselessly.

Researchers also discovered a group of regulatory genes, originally called *antioncogenes* and now called *tumor suppressor genes,* which have the opposite effect of oncogenes. When activated, tumor suppressor genes can regulate growth and inhibit carcinogenesis. Tumor suppressor genes are the "brakes" to the "stuck accelerator" of the activated oncogene.

Tumor Biochemistry and Pathogenesis

Carcinogenesis is the process by which a normal cell undergoes malignant transformation. Usually, it is a multistep process, involving progressive changes after genetic damage to or alteration of cellular DNA through the development of hyperplasia, metaplasia, dysplasia, carcinoma in situ, invasive carcinoma, and metastatic carcinoma in that order.[79] These discrete stages in tumor development suggest that a single altered gene pushes a cell only part of the way down the path to actual malignancy. The process is completed when multiple, successive changes occur in distinct cellular genes, including activation or overexpression of oncogenes and loss or mutation of tumor suppressor genes.

The number of genetic events required for conversion of normal cells to malignant cells is still debated, but, at least in the case of many solid tumors, this number may be as great as seven or eight. This high number of genetic events may imply that genetic instability occurs during cancer progression.[79] This requirement for multiple changes creates an important protective mechanism against cancer. If a small number of genetic changes sufficed to transform a normal cell into a malignant one, multiple tumors would develop easily.

INVASION AND METASTASES

Malignant tumors differ from benign tumors in their ability to metastasize or spread from the primary site to other locations in the body. Metastasis occurs when cells break away from the primary tumor, travel through the body via the blood or lymphatic system, and become trapped in the capillaries of organs. From there, they infiltrate the organ tissue and grow into new tumor deposits. Cancer can also spread to adjacent structures and penetrate body cavities by direct extension.

Patterns of metastasis differ from cancer to cancer. Although there is no clear explanation of the exact mechanism of metastasis, certain cancers tend to spread to specific organs or sites in the body in a predictable manner (Table 6.2). The five most common sites of metastasis are the lymph nodes, liver, lung, bone, and brain. The spread of cancer may be influenced by a variety of host factors such as the aging or dysfunctional immune system, increasing age, hormonal environment, pregnancy, and stress. Factors that may slow the spread of metastasis include radiation, chemotherapy, anticoagulants, steroids, and other antiinflammatory agents.

Seed Versus Soil Theory of Metastasis

Some cancers favor certain sites of metastasis over others so that metastases occur only if the cancer cell (the seed) finds a favorable microenvironment at the site of the host (the soil). Certain tumor cells seem to have specific affinity for certain organs.

Studies in the 1990s showed that there is cross-talk between metastatic cells and the organ microenvironment. Host cells secrete growth factors that prompt tumor cell replication and allow the tumor to take over the host. Angiogenesis, the process by which blood vessels from preexisting vessels grow into the solid tumor, is one way that tumor cells take over for their own gain.[37]

TABLE 6.2   Pathways of Cancer Metastases

Primary Cancer	Mode of Dissemination	Location of Primary Metastases
Breast	Lymphatics Blood (vascular or hematogenous)	Bone (shoulder, hips, ribs, and vertebrae); CNS (brain and spinal cord) Lung, pleural cavity, liver
Bone	Blood	Lung, liver, bone, then CNS
Cervical (cervix)	Local extension and lymphatics Blood	Retroperitoneal lymph nodes, bladder, rectum; paracervical, parametrial lymphatics CNS (brain), lung, bone, liver
Colorectal	Direct extension Peritoneal seeding Blood	Bone (vertebrae and hip) Peritoneum Liver, lung
Ewing's sarcoma	Blood	Lung, bone, bone marrow
Kidney	Lymph Blood	Pelvis, groin Lung, pleural cavity, bone, liver
Leukemia		Does not really metastasize: causes symptoms throughout body
Liver	Blood	CNS (brain)
Lung (bronchogenic sarcoma)	Blood Blood Direct extension, lymphatics	CNS (brain and spinal cord) Bone (ribs first then disseminated) Mediastinum (tissue and organs between the sternum and vertebrae such as the heart, blood vessels, trachea, esophagus, thymus, and lymph nodes)
Lung (apical or Pancoast's tumors)	Direct extension Blood	Eighth cervical and first and second thoracic nerves within the brachial plexus CNS (brain and spinal cord), bone
Lymphoma	Blood Lymphatics	CNS (spinal cord) Can occur anywhere, including skin, visceral organs
Malignant melanoma	No typical pattern	Can occur anywhere; skin and subcutaneous tissue; lungs; CNS (brain); liver; GI tract; bone
Nonmelanoma skin cancer	Usually remain local without metastases; local invasion	Bones underlying involved skin; brain
Osteogenic sarcoma (osteo-sarcoma)	Lymphatics Blood	Lymph nodes, lungs, bone, kidneys, CNS (brain)
Ovarian	Direct extension into abdominal cavity; peritoneal fluid through the abdomen Lymphatics	Nearby organs (bladder, colon, rectum, uterus, and fallopian tubes) Liver, lungs; regional and distant (spread beyond the abdomen is rare)
Pancreatic	Blood	Liver
Prostate	Lymphatics	Pelvic and vertebral bones Bladder, rectum Distant organs (lung, liver, and brain)
Spinal cord	Local invasion; dissemination through the intervertebral foramina	CNS (brain and spinal cord)
Stomach, gastric	Blood Local invasion	Liver, vertebrae, abdominal cavity (intraperitoneum)
Thyroid	Direct extension Lymphatics Blood	Bone; nearby tissues of neck Regional lymph nodes (neck, upper chest, and mediastinum) Distant (lung and bone)

CNS, Central nervous system; *GI*, gastrointestinal.
Adapted from Goodman CC, Snyder TE: Differential diagnosis for physical therapists: screening for referral, ed 5, St. Louis, 2013, Saunders.

Traditional cancer treatment targets the seed, whereas today's research is focused on approaches that target the soil, making the sites of metastasis unsuitable for the growth of cancer cells. Treatment that is optimal in the primary organ may not work in the metastatic sites.[84]

Incidence of Metastasis

Approximately 30% of clients with newly diagnosed cancers have clinically detectable metastases. At least 30% to 40% of the remaining clients who are clinically free of metastases harbor occult (hidden) metastases. Unfortunately, most people have multiple sites of metastatic disease, not all of which are apparent at any one time. The formation of metastatic colonies is a continuous process, commencing early in the growth of the primary tumor and increasing with time.

Even metastases have the potential to metastasize; the presence of large, identifiable metastases in a given organ can be accompanied by a greater number of micrometastases that have been disseminated more recently from the primary tumor or the metastasis. The size variation in metastases and the dispersed anatomic location of metastases can make complete surgical removal of disease impossible and limit the effective concentration of anticancer drugs that can be delivered only to tumor cells in metastatic colonies.

Mechanisms of Metastasis

For rapidly growing tumors, millions of tumor cells are shed into the vascular system each day. Only a very small percentage of circulating tumor cells initiate metastatic colonies, because most cells that have invaded the bloodstream are quickly

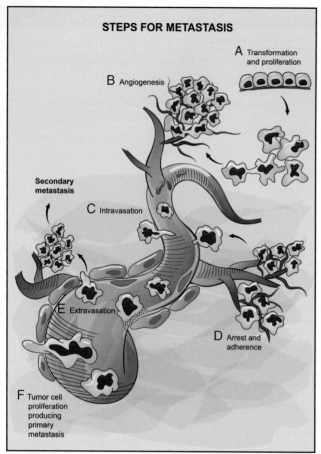

STEPS FOR METASTASIS

A Transformation and proliferation

B Angiogenesis

Secondary metastasis

C Intravasation

E Extravasation

D Arrest and adherence

F Tumor cell proliferation producing primary metastasis

FIG. 6.2 Major mechanisms of metastasis. To metastasize, tumor cells must gain several unique biologic properties such as invasive growth (A), induction of vascular growth (B), vascular invasion (C), adherence to endothelial cells or thrombosis of peripheral sinusoids (D), continuation of invasive growth with extravasation (E), and formation of primary and secondary metastatic foci (F). Not all tumor cells develop all the abilities shown here; some cell clones may subspecialize and create only angiogenesis; others may invade and move on. (From Czerniak B: Dorfman and Czerniak's bone tumors, Philadelphia, 2016, Saunders.)

eliminated. Classic isotope studies have shown that 99% of circulating potentially tumorigenic cells are killed by blood vessel turbulence within 24 hours.[37,38,45] Metastasis of the remaining 1% requires a good deal of coordination between the cancer cells and the body (Fig. 6.2).

The greater the number of invasive tumor cells in the bloodstream, the greater is the probability that some cells will survive to form metastases. Metastasis is more likely to occur via the veins as opposed to the arteries because the cancer cannot break through the arterial wall. The major challenge in treating cancer is not eradicating the primary tumor, because surgery or radiation is effective in these early cases. Eradicating metastases, often already present at the time of diagnosis, is the key factor for cancer cure.

A complicated series of tumor–host interactions resulting in a metastatic colony is called the *metastatic cascade* and is similar for all tumor cells. Once a primary tumor is initiated and starts to move by local invasion, then blood vessels from preexisting vessels grow into the solid tumor, a process called *tumor angiogenesis* (see Fig. 6.2). As a normal physiologic process, angiogenesis is crucial to tissue growth, repair, and maintenance.

The ability of a tumor to grow beyond a very small mass (1 to 2 mm) depends on its ability to gain access to an adequate supply of blood and in some cases the presence of hormonal factors. The supply of blood allows the tumor to obtain essential nutrients, such as oxygen, and to eliminate metabolic waste products, such as carbon dioxide and acids. The blood supply to tumors is provided by growth of new capillaries and larger vessels into the tumor mass from the blood supply of adjacent normal tissues.

Clinical Manifestations of Metastasis

Metastatic spread usually occurs within 3 to 5 years after initial diagnosis and treatment of malignancy, although some low-grade lesions can reappear as long as 15 to 20 years later. Therefore it is very important to conduct a thorough past medical history as part of any client interview. Metastases are most common in areas of the body that provide an environment rich in nutrition to the colonized tumor cells, such as the lung, brain, liver, and bone; metastases can be found in other areas as well

Pulmonary System (Lungs)

Pulmonary metastases are the most common of all metastatic tumors because venous drainage of most areas of the body is through the superior and inferior venae cavae into the heart, making the lungs the first organ to filter malignant cells. Parenchymal metastases are asymptomatic until tumor cells have obstructed bronchi, resulting in pulmonary symptoms, or until tumor cells have expanded and reached the parietal pleura, in which pain fibers are stimulated.

A dry, persistent cough is often the first symptom of pulmonary metastases. Pleural pain can indicate pleural invasion, and shortness of breath (dyspnea) usually occurs in the presence of a malignant pleural effusion. If hemoptysis occurs, there is usually bronchial tissue invasion either by a primary lung malignancy or metastatic disease.[130]

Hepatic System (Liver)

Liver metastases are among the most ominous signs of advanced cancer. The liver filters blood coming in from the gastrointestinal tract, making it a primary metastatic site for tumors of the stomach, colorectum, and pancreas. Symptoms include abdominal and/or right upper quadrant pain, general malaise and fatigue, anorexia, early satiety and weight loss, and sometimes low-grade fevers.

Skeletal System (Bone)

Primary bone tumors, such as osteogenic sarcoma, metastasize initially to the lungs, whereas in a large proportion of cases cancer metastasizes first to the bone, often with a poor prognosis. Bone is one of the three most favored sites of solid tumor metastasis, indicating that the bone microenvironment provides fertile ground for the growth of many tumors. Although lung, breast, and prostate are the three primary sites responsible for most metastatic bone disease, tumors of the thyroid and kidney, lymphoma, and melanoma can also metastasize to the skeletal system.

Bone metastases may be the osteolytic type, marked by areas of decreased bone density, or osteoblastic, appearing as areas of dense scarring and increased bone density. Osteolytic metastases predominate in lung, kidney, and thyroid cancer; breast metastases are primarily osteolytic but can be osteoblastic and prostate metastases are usually but not always osteoblastic. The axial skeleton is most commonly involved with spread to the spine, pelvis, ribs, proximal femurs, proximal humeri, and skull.[81]

The primary symptom associated with bone metastases is pain. Pain is usually deep and worsened by activity, especially weight bearing. Disabling pathologic fractures, especially of the vertebral bodies and proximal ends of the long bones, may occur in up to half of the people with osteolytic metastases and are sometimes one of the first signs of a malignant process.[49]

Hypercalcemia (abnormally high concentration of blood calcium) is a frequent complication of neoplastic disease and is associated with bony metastases, particularly osteolytic lesions, as a result of increased bone resorption. The presence of tumor cells in the bone disturbs the balance between new bone formation and bone resorption, resulting in abnormal bone remodeling.

Carcinoma cells secrete a variety of factors that stimulate tumor growth and osteoclast recruitment and activation. Osteoclasts are bone cells that break down bone tissue. Although more than 80% of people with hypercalcemia have bony metastasis, the severity of the hypercalcemia does not correlate with the extent of the bony disease.

Central Nervous System

Brain. Many primary tumors may lead to CNS metastases. Lung carcinomas account for approximately half of all metastatic brain lesions. Breast carcinoma and malignant melanoma also commonly metastasize to the brain. Metastatic disease in the brain is life-threatening and emotionally debilitating. Metastatic brain tumors can increase intracranial pressure, obstruct the normal flow of cerebrospinal fluid, change mentation and contribute to cognitive impairment, and reduce sensory and motor function.

Clinical manifestations of brain metastases depend on the location, either in the brain or outside the brain in the bony cranium exerting compression externally. Primary tumors of the CNS rarely develop metastases outside the CNS despite the highly invasive capacity of these tumors.

Tumor cells traveling from the lung via the pulmonary veins and carotid artery can result in metastases to the CNS. Lung cancer is the most common primary tumor to metastasize to the brain. Any neurologic sign may be the presentation of a silent lung tumor.[49]

Spinal cord. Metastatic involvement of the vertebrae may result in epidural spinal cord compression. In addition, severe, destructive osteolytic lesions can lead to fracture and fragility of one or more vertebral bodies. In such cases, compression of the cord occurs as a result of the subsequent deformity.[80] Spinal cord and nerve root compression cause either insidious or rapid loss of neurologic function. This compression phenomenon occurs in approximately 5% of people with systemic cancer and is most often caused by carcinoma of the lung, breast, prostate, or kidney. Lymphoma and multiple myeloma may also result in spinal cord and nerve root compression.

The earliest neurologic symptoms include gradual onset of distal weakness and sensory changes, including numbness, paresthesias, and coldness. The client with spinal cord symptoms caused by metastatic epidural disease and resultant compression may have only transient symptoms with proper medical treatment. More than 95% of people with spinal cord compression complain of progressive central or radicular back pain, often aggravated by recumbency, weight bearing, sneezing, coughing, or Valsalva's maneuver. Sitting often relieves it.

Lymphatic system. Cancer-related surgery or radiation treatment affecting the lymph nodes may result in dysfunction of the lymphatic system manifesting as lymphedema. It has a wide range of onset from weeks to years from the initial insult to the lymphatic system.

Diagnosis of Metastasis

Metastases usually reproduce the cellular structure of the primary growth well enough to enable a pathologist to determine the site of the primary tumor. For example, bone metastases from a carcinoma of the thyroid not only exhibit a microscopic structure similar to that of the original tumor but also may produce thyroid hormone. Sometimes symptoms of a cancer will manifest in the metastatic site rather than the site of origin.

Cancer Recurrence

Disease-free survival describes the time between diagnosis and recurrence or relapse. Recurrences may be local, regional, disseminated, or a combination of these. The most important predictors of recurrent cancer are the stage at the time of initial therapy and the histologic findings. Recurrence of cancer may be first recognized by the return of systemic symptoms.

CLINICAL MANIFESTATIONS

Local and Systemic Effects

Most cancers in their earliest stages are asymptomatic but treatable if found. Most primary site cancers cause certain symptoms that are recognizable causes for suspicion or concern. For example, endometrial cancer causes abnormal bleeding so often that it is usually detected in its early stages. Laryngeal cancer causes hoarseness, which is also an early sign. However, lung cancer is usually quite extensive before it causes enough symptoms to warrant investigation, as is true with breast cancer if it is a deeply buried tumor that is difficult to palpate. Most cancer is detected early and can be cured or successfully treated.

As the cancer progresses, symptoms characteristic of the involved organ or tissue may start to develop. With advanced cancer, nausea, vomiting, and retching accompanied by anorexia and subsequent weight loss are common as a result of the malignant process and its treatment. Nausea, vomiting, and retching is especially prevalent in association with lung carcinoma, hypernephroma, and pancreatic carcinoma.

Anorexia has been attributed to tumor production of tumor necrosis factor (TNF), which is a protein also called cachectin. Small amounts of TNF are beneficial in promoting wound healing and preventing tumors, but uncontrolled production is accompanied by symptoms of fever, weight loss, and tissue damage that can cause more problems than the benefits provided.

Cancer-related anorexia or cachexia (CAC) is a complex phenomenon in which metabolic abnormalities, cytokines produced by the host immune system, circulating tumor-derived factors, decreased food intake, and possibly other unknown factors all contribute. Profound muscle loss is prominent in CAC syndrome as a result of decreased protein synthesis and abnormal muscle proteolysis.

Later, the rapid growth of the tumor encroaches on healthy tissue, causing destruction, necrosis, ulceration, and hemorrhage and producing many local and systemic effects. Pain may occur as a late symptom caused by infiltration, compression, or destruction of nerves. With advanced or stage IV cancer, the presentation systemically involves muscular weakness, anemia, and coagulation disorders.

Fever may be seen with cancer in the absence of infection and is produced either by white blood cells inducing a pyrogen (an agent that causes fever) or by direct tumor production of a pyrogen. Continued spread of the cancer may lead to gastrointestinal, pulmonary, or vascular obstruction. Secondary infections frequently occur as a result of the host's decreased immunity and can lead to death.

Cancer Pain
Overview
One of the most common symptoms of cancer is pain, affecting 50% to 70% of clients in its early stages and 60% to 90% of clients in late stages of the disease. It is estimated that 1.1 million Americans experience cancer-related pain annually.[21] Alternately stated, pain occurs in approximately one-quarter of adults with newly diagnosed malignancies, one-third of individuals undergoing treatment, and three-quarters of all people with advanced disease.[47,125]

Depression and anxiety may increase the person's perception of pain or may be the result of the cancer pain. Symptoms often go unreported or underreported because clients are reluctant to take the pain medication prescribed. An unfounded fear of tolerance, addiction, or adverse effects from pain medication may result in underreporting of painful symptoms with subsequent inadequate cancer pain control and unnecessary pain-induced loss of function. Likewise, physicians may hesitate to provide adequate pain medications based on this misconception of client addiction.

Etiology and Pathogenesis
The cause of cancer pain is multifaceted, and the characteristics of the pain depend on the tissue structure, as well as on the mechanisms involved (Table 6.3). Some pain is caused by pressure on nerves or by the displacement of nerves. Microscopic infiltration of nerves by tumor cells can result in continuous, sharp, stabbing pain generally following the pattern of nerve distribution. Ischemic pain (throbbing) may also result from interference with blood supply or from blockage within hollow organs.

A common cause of cancer pain is metastasis of cancer to bone. Lung, breast, prostate, thyroid, and the lymphatics are the primary sites responsible for most metastatic bone disease. Bone metastasis results in increased release of prostaglandins and cytokines and subsequent bone destruction caused by breakdown and resorption. Bone pain may be mild to intense. Movement, weight bearing, and ambulation exacerbate painful symptoms from bone destruction. Pathologic fractures with resultant muscle spasms can develop; in the case of vertebral involvement, nerve pain may also occur. Pain may also result from diagnostic or therapeutic procedures such as surgery, RT, or chemotherapy.

Clinical Manifestations
Signs and symptoms accompanying mild to moderate superficial pain may include hypertension, tachycardia, and tachypnea (rapid, shallow breathing) as the result of a sympathetic

TABLE 6.3	**Common Patterns of Pain Referral**	
Pain Mechanism	**Lesion Site**	**Referral Site**
Somatic	C7, T1-T5 vertebrae	Interscapular area, posterior shoulder
	Shoulder	Neck, upper back
	L1, L2 vertebrae	SI joint and hip
	Hip joint	SI joint and knee
	Pharynx	Ipsilateral ear
	TMJ	Head, neck, heart
Visceral	Diaphragmatic irritation	Shoulder, lumbar spine
	Heart	Shoulder, neck, upper back, TMJ
	Urothelial tract	Back, inguinal region, anterior thigh, and genitalia
	Pancreas, liver, spleen, gallbladder	Shoulder, midthoracic or low back
	Peritoneal or abdominal cavity (inflammatory or infectious process)	Hip pain from abscess of psoas or obturator muscle
Neuropathic	Nerve or plexus	Anywhere in distribution of a peripheral nerve
	Nerve root	Anywhere in corresponding dermatome
	CNS	Anywhere in region of body innervated by damaged structure

CNS, Central nervous system; *SI,* sacroiliac; *TMJ,* temporomandibular joint.
From Goodman CC, Snyder TE: Differential diagnosis for the physical therapist: screening for referral, ed 5, St. Louis, 2013, Saunders.

nervous system response. In severe or visceral pain, a parasympathetic nervous system response is more characteristic, with hypotension, bradycardia, nausea, vomiting, tachypnea, weakness, or fainting.

Spinal cord compression from metastases may cause radicular back pain, leg weakness, and unilateral loss of bowel or bladder control. Back pain may precede the development of neurologic signs and symptoms. The presence of jaundice in association with an atypical presentation of back pain may indicate liver obstruction and/or liver metastasis. Signs of nerve root compression may be the first indication of a cancer, in particular lymphoma, multiple myeloma, or cancer of the lung, breast, prostate, or kidney.

Pain Control
Pain management and control may depend on its underlying cause. For example, epidural metastases with impending spinal cord compression require treatment with steroids, radiation, chemotherapy, or neurosurgery. Abdominal pain caused by obstruction of the hollow organs requires evaluation for surgical intervention.[30]

Treatment approaches depend on whether the individual is experiencing acute or chronic pain. The hope is to begin by gaining control of the pain during the acute phase and then to sustain that pain relief while minimizing side effects.

Before the start of therapy, the physician determines the underlying pain mechanism and diagnoses the pain syndrome.

Pain control measures used include narcotic and nonnarcotic analgesics; chemotherapy or RT or both; surgery; nerve blocks; or other, more invasive pain control measures such as intraspinal opioids, rhizotomy, or cordotomy. Appropriate opioid selection may be difficult and depends on the individual's pain intensity and any current analgesic therapy. Morphine, hydromorphone, fentanyl, and oxycodone are the opioids commonly used in the United States. A balance between analgesia and side effects might be achieved by changing to an equivalent dose of an alternative opioid. This approach, known as opioid rotation, is now a widely accepted technique used to address poorly responsive pain.[102]

Several methods of continuous infusion that are widely used in clinical practice include around-the-clock administration, as-needed administration, and patient-controlled analgesia (PCA). Around-the-clock administration is provided to chronic pain patients for continuous pain relief. A rescue dose should be provided as a subsequent treatment for patients receiving these controlled-release medications. Rescue doses of short-acting opioids should be provided for pain that is not relieved by sustained-release or controlled-release opioids.

Opioids administered on an as-needed basis are for patients who have intermittent pain with pain-free intervals. The as-needed method is also used when rapid dose escalation is required.

The PCA technique allows a person to control a device that delivers a bolus of analgesic "on demand" (according to and limited by parameters set by a physician). This system permits the person to self-administer a premeasured dose of analgesic by pressing a button that activates a pump syringe containing the analgesic. Clinical studies report that people using PCA effectively maintain comfort without oversedation and use less drug than the amount normally given by intramuscular injection.

Nonpharmacologic modalities, such as massage, acupuncture, imagery and hypnosis, reflexology, relaxation training, and other forms of complementary therapies, are based on client preference and clinical judgment of what is best when integrative medicine or health care is practiced. Complementary therapies can lessen procedural pain and distress even among children, especially when fear, anxiety, and tension heighten pain perception.[30,73,127]

Whereas severe cancer pain is treated pharmaceutically, mild to moderate joint and muscle pain can be addressed by the rehabilitation professional. Pain elimination through the use of medication may not be possible without accompanying severe loss of function, which is an undesirable outcome.

Noninvasive physical agents, such as cryotherapy, thermotherapy, electrical stimulation, immobilization, exercise, massage, biofeedback, and relaxation techniques, may be effective in pain management. Much debate exists about the safety and efficacy of massage therapy for individuals with cancer, especially anyone with lymphedema or at risk for developing lymphedema.[23] A review of data included in the *Cochrane Database of Systematic Reviews* suggests that conventional care for people with cancer can safely incorporate massage therapy, although individuals with cancer may be at higher risk for adverse events. There is no evidence that massage therapy can spread cancer, although direct pressure over a tumor is usually discouraged.[23]

The strongest evidence for the benefits of massage is stress and anxiety reduction. Research regarding the use of massage for pain control and management of other symptoms is promising. Massage therapists may advocate the use of massage to reduce constipation, improve immune system function, help promote postoperative wound healing, and reduce scar tissue formation, as well as to help release metabolic waste by improving circulation. Modifications to massage may be necessary to prevent potential harm such as bleeding, fracture, or increased pain when individuals with cancer receiving massage have a coagulation disorder such as a low platelet count or when receiving warfarin, heparin, or aspirin therapy. Similar precautions are required for anyone with cancer metastases to the bones. Massage should be avoided over open or healing wounds or radiation dermatitis.[23]

People with cancer may also experience pain because of nerve damage. This damage can be caused directly by tumor invasion or indirectly as a side effect of cytotoxic drug therapy. The treatment of neuropathic pain remains a dilemma because conventional analgesic drugs do not always provide relief.

Management of pain in people with cancer who live in long-term care facilities remains an ongoing concern. Consistent, daily pain is prevalent among nursing home residents with cancer and is frequently untreated, particularly among older and minority clients.[12] For individuals with difficult-to-control chronic pain, complementary therapies can help, even if only by reducing the level of analgesics required to maintain pain control.

Cancer-Related Fatigue

Much has been written about cancer-related fatigue (CRF) and its impact on clients. CRF is a distressing, persistent, and subjective sense of tiredness or exhaustion related to cancer or cancer treatment that is not proportional to recent activity and interferes with usual functioning.[43] CRF syndrome is a collection of symptoms with multiple characteristics and problems. Fatigue is a nearly universal symptom in all people receiving chemotherapy, radiotherapy, and treatment with biologic response modifiers (BRMs); reduced physical performance and fatigue are universal after bone marrow transplantation (BMT).

Up to 30% of cancer survivors report a loss of energy for years after cessation of treatment. For many people with cancer, fatigue is severe and imposes limitations on normal daily activities.[18] Many people's perceptions are that fatigue is more distressing than pain or nausea and vomiting, which can be managed with medication for most clients.

Fatigue should be screened, assessed, and managed according to clinical practice guidelines, which have been published for CRF.[43] All individuals should be screened for fatigue at their initial visit, at regular intervals during and after cancer treatment, and as clinically indicated. Fatigue should be recognized, evaluated, monitored, documented, and treated promptly for all age groups, at all stages of disease, during and after treatment. Clients and their families should be informed that management of fatigue is an integral part of total health care.[43]

Using a numeric rating scale, fatigue can be rated as mild (1 to 3), moderate (4 to 6), or severe (7 to 10).[100,114] Children can be asked if they are "tired" or "not tired." Fatigue that causes distress or interferes with daily activities or functioning should be treated according to its severity and the presence of other treatable factors known to contribute to fatigue. Clients should be reassured that treatment-related fatigue is not necessarily an indicator of disease progression. It may be the result of anemia, deconditioning, or the presence of certain cytokines. There may be contributing psychosocial factors such as anxiety, depression, and disrupted sleep pattern. Despite the prevalence of CRF, the exact mechanisms involved in its pathophysiology are unknown. Likewise, the cause of fatigue in posttreatment disease-free individuals is unclear and likely multifactorial. Findings together point to a chronic inflammatory process involving T cells as a possible fatigue-inducing mechanism.[43]

Paraneoplastic Syndromes
Overview and Definition

In addition to the local effects of tumor growth, cancer can produce systemic signs and symptoms that are not direct effects of either the tumor or its metastases. When tumors produce signs and symptoms at a site distant from the tumor or its metastasized sites, these remote effects of malignancy are collectively referred to as *paraneoplastic* syndromes.

Although malignant cells frequently lose the function, appearance, and properties associated with the normal cells of the tissue of origin, in some cases they can acquire new cellular functions uncharacteristic of the originating tissue. For example, tumors in nonendocrine tissues sometimes acquire the ability to produce and secrete hormones that are distributed by the circulation and act on target organs at a site other than the location of the tumor. Malignancy is often associated with a wide variety of musculoskeletal disorders, which may be the presenting symptoms of an occult tumor. Although musculoskeletal symptoms often result from direct invasion by the malignancy or its metastases into bone, joints, or soft tissue, they may also occur without invasion as a result of the paraneoplastic disorders, including well-recognized syndromes, as well as less well-defined disorders referred to as *cancer arthritis*.[123]

Incidence

Previously, paraneoplastic syndromes occurred in 10% to 20% of all cancer clients, but this figure may be increasing because of greater physician awareness and the availability of serodiagnostic tests for some syndromes.

Etiology and Pathogenesis

The causes of paraneoplastic syndromes are not well understood.

Clinical Manifestations

The paraneoplastic syndromes are of considerable clinical importance because they may accompany relatively limited neoplastic growth and provide an early clue to the presence of certain types of cancer. Nonspecific symptoms, such as neurologic changes, anorexia, malaise, diarrhea, weight loss, and fever, may be the first clinical manifestations of a paraneoplastic syndrome. Even these types of nonspecific symptoms occur as a result of the production of specific biochemical products by the tumor itself.

Gradual, progressive muscle weakness may develop over a period of weeks to months. The proximal muscles (especially of the pelvic girdle) are most likely to be involved; the weakness does stabilize. Reflexes of the involved extremities are present but diminished. Proximal leg weakness is most often associated with small cell carcinoma of the lung.

Muscular and cutaneous disorders associated with malignancy are presented in Table 6.4.

MEDICAL MANAGEMENT OF CANCER

Prevention

The goal of *Healthy People 2020* is to reduce the number of new cancer cases, as well as the illness, disability, and death caused by cancer.[19] Evidence suggests that several types of cancer can be prevented and that the prospects for surviving cancer continue to improve. The ACS estimates that half of all cancer deaths in the United States could be prevented if Americans adopted a healthier lifestyle and made better use of available screening tests. The ability to reduce cancer death rates depends in part on the existence and application of various types of resources.

First, the means to provide culturally and linguistically appropriate information on prevention, early detection, and treatment to the public and to health care professionals are essential. Second, mechanisms or systems must exist for providing people with access to state-of-the-art preventive services and treatment. Third, a mechanism for maintaining continued research progress and for fostering new research is essential. Combining genetic screening for cancer predisposition in the general population and selecting individualized targeted chemoprevention may dramatically reduce cancer rates in the future.[62]

Studying older adults who do not develop cancer may help identify the genetic changes associated with age-resistant protective mechanisms. Genetic information that can be used to improve disease prevention strategies is emerging for many cancers and may provide the foundation for improved effectiveness in clinical and preventive medicine services.

Primary Prevention

Prevention is the first key to the management of cancer. Primary prevention may include screening to identify high-risk people and subsequent reduction or elimination of modifiable risk factors. Physical activity and weight control also can contribute to cancer prevention.

Chemoprevention, the use of agents to inhibit and reverse cancer, has focused on diet-derived agents. More than 40 promising agents and agent combinations are being evaluated clinically as chemopreventive agents for major cancer targets, including breast, prostate, colon, and lung cancer.[63] In addition, low-dose aspirin intake and nonsteroidal antiinflammatory

---

TABLE 6.4 Muscular and Cutaneous Disorders Associated with Malignancy

Muscular or Cutaneous	Disorders
Muscular	Amyloidosis
	Amyotrophic lateral sclerosis
	Polymyositis
	Lambert–Eaton myasthenic syndrome (LEMS)
	Myasthenia gravis
	Metabolic myopathies
	Primary neuropathic diseases
	Type II muscle atrophy
Cutaneous	Acanthosis (diffuse thickening)
	Dermatomyositis
	Extramammary Paget's disease
	Nigricans (blackish discoloration; changes in skin pigmentation)
	Pemphigus vulgaris (water blisters)
	Pruritus (itching)
	Pyoderma gangrenosum (eruption of skin ulcers)
	Reactive erythemas (skin redness)

Data from Gilkeson GS, Caldwell DS: Rheumatologic associations with malignancy, J Musculoskelet Med 7:70, 1990; Cohen PR: Cutaneous paraneoplastic syndromes, Am Fam Physician 50:1273-1282, 1994.

drug (NSAID) intake have shown promising results in the prevention of gastrointestinal cancers.

Research focusing on a cancer vaccine to wake up the immune system with a warning that cancer is present and stimulate an immune response against cancer cells is being investigated in clinical studies, although currently no known specific immunization prevents cancer in general. The most promising vaccines are for malignant melanoma and prostate cancer; vaccines for cancer viruses are already in use.[40]

The person's own tumor cells can be obtained during surgery, radiated to inactivate them, and then reinfused. This stimulates the immune system to react and make antibodies against these specific cells. The vaccine specifically evokes the activity of killer T cells to directly target and destroy tumors in all vaccine recipients. A vaccine given on an outpatient basis would be less dangerous than surgery and less toxic than other cancer treatments such as chemotherapy and RT.

Secondary Prevention

Secondary prevention aimed at preventing morbidity and mortality uses early detection[43] and prompt treatment (Table 6.5). Some drugs, such as tamoxifen (Nolvadex), are used in both

TABLE 6.5	Early Detection of Cancer		
Cancer Site	**Population**	**Test or Procedure**	**Frequency**
Breast	Women age >20 years	BSE	Beginning in their early 20s, women should be told about the benefits and limitations of BSE; any new breast symptoms should be reported to a health professional; women who choose to do BSE should receive instruction; their techniques should be reviewed by a qualified health care professional; it is acceptable for women to choose not to do BSE or to do BSE irregularly
		Clinical breast examination	For women in their 20s and 30s, CBE should be part of a periodic health examination, preferably at least every 3 years; asymptomatic women aged 40 years old or older should continue to receive a CBE as part of a periodic health examination, preferably annually
		Mammography	Begin annual mammography at age 40; CBE should be performed first
Colorectal	Men and women age >50 years	Fecal occult blood test (FOBT) or fecal immunochemical test (FIT), or	Annual, starting at age 50
		Flexible sigmoidoscopy, or	Every 5 years, starting at age 50 years
		FOBT and flexible sigmoidoscopy, or	Annual FOBT (or FIT) and flexible sigmoidoscopy every 5 years, starting at age 50
		Double contrast barium enema (DCBE), or	DCBE every 5 years, starting at age 50
		Colonoscopy	Colonoscopy every 10 years, starting at age 50
Prostate	Men age >5	Digital rectal examination (DRE) and prostate-specific antigen (PSA) test	PSA test and DRE should be offered annually, starting at age 50, for men who have a life expectancy of at least 10 more years
Cervix	Women age >18	Pap test	Cervical cancer screening should begin approximately 3 years after a woman begins having vaginal intercourse, but no later than 21 years of age; screening should be done every year with conventional Pap tests or every 2 years using liquid-based Pap tests; at or after age 30 years, women who have had three normal test results in a row may get screened every 2–3 years with cervical cytology alone, or every 3 years with a human papillomavirus DNA test plus cervical cytology; women aged >70 years who have had three or more normal Pap test results and no abnormal Pap test results in the last 10 years and women who have had a total hysterectomy may choose to stop cervical cancer screening
Endometrial	Women, at menopause	At the time of menopause, women at average risk should be informed about risks and symptoms of endometrial cancer and should be strongly encouraged to report any unexpected bleeding or spotting to their physicians	
Cancer-related checkup	Men and women age >20	On the occasion of a periodic health examination, the cancer-related checkup should include examination for cancers of the thyroid, testicles, ovaries, lymph nodes, oral cavity, and skin, as well as health counseling about tobacco, sun exposure, diet and nutrition, risk factors, sexual practices, and environmental and occupational exposures	

BSE, Breast self-examination; *CBE,* clinical breast examination; *DCBE,* double contrast barium enema; *DRE,* digital rectal examination; *FOBT,* fecal occult blood test; *FIT,* fecal immunochemical test; *PSA,* prostate-specific antigen.
Data from the American Cancer Society Guidelines for the Early Detection of Cancer, www.cancer.org.

primary and secondary prevention of breast cancer. Tamoxifen has been approved by the U.S. Food and Drug Administration as a preventive agent in women at high risk for possible development of breast cancer.[138] The preliminary results of a randomized trial comparing tamoxifen with placebo in women considered at high risk for breast cancer suggested that the risk of breast cancer in this group of high-risk women could be decreased by approximately 50% with the administration of tamoxifen.[85]

Multifactor risk reduction is an important part of secondary prevention for people diagnosed with cancer who are at risk for recurrence. This is especially true because the adverse effects of several risk factors are cumulative, and many risk factors are interrelated.

Tertiary Prevention

Tertiary prevention focuses on managing symptoms, limiting complications, and preventing disability associated with cancer or its treatment.

Diagnosis

Medical history and physical examination are usually followed by more specific diagnostic procedures. Useful tests for the early detection and staging of tumors include laboratory values, radiography, endoscopy, isotope scan, CT scan, mammography, magnetic resonance imaging (MRI), and biopsy. Advances in nuclear medicine have made it possible to examine images of organs, structures, and physiologic or pathologic processes and detect the distribution of radiopharmaceuticals according to their uptake and metabolism.

Tissue Biopsy

Biopsy of tissue samples is an important diagnostic tool in the study of tumors. Tissue for biopsy may be taken by curettage (Pap smear), fluid aspiration (pleural effusion, lumbar puncture, or spinal tap), fine needle aspiration (breast or thyroid), dermal punch (skin or mouth), endoscopy (rectal polyps), or surgical excision (visceral tumors and nodes).

An open biopsy consists of making an incision and removing a portion of the abnormal tissue. The amount removed depends on the abnormality, but it is usually a piece of tissue about 1 inch in diameter.

Needle biopsy uses a large-diameter needle to take a core or plug of tissue. An incisional biopsy takes a slice or wedge of the lesion but does not attempt to remove the entire pathologic structure. Excisional biopsy (also referred to as a *lumpectomy*) removes the tumor and a perimeter of normal tissue or "margins." The goal is to remove enough tissue to get negative margins when the tissue sample is examined under a microscope by a pathologist.

Stereotactic mammotome biopsy of the breast uses digital x-ray studies of the breast taken from two angles to locate the abnormality seen on the mammogram. A computer then calculates the proper angle and depth of insertion of a core biopsy needle. This needle is inserted into the breast, using local anesthesia, and multiple (a dozen or more) core specimens are removed. These cores are then sent to the pathologist for diagnosis. Sentinel lymph node (SLN) biopsy has become a standard diagnostic procedure to assess lymph node status of various tumors and to assess staging. A blue dye is injected around the cancerous tumor. The dye flows through the ducts, and the first node or nodes it reaches is identified as the sentinel

or sentinels. An incision is made over the nodes, and the blue-stained sentinel node or nodes (one to three) are removed and analyzed. Information regarding the lymphatic drainage from the cancer can directly impact on surgery. SLN biopsy has reduced the number of unnecessary axillary dissections in breast cancer. The status of axillary nodes is the most important prognostic factor in breast cancer and in determining the medical management.

Tumor Markers

Tumor markers, substances produced and secreted by tumor cells, may be found in the blood serum. The level of tumor marker seems to correlate with the extent of disease. A tumor marker is not diagnostic itself but can signal malignancies. Carcinoembryonic antigen (CEA) is one tumor marker that may indicate malignancy of the large bowel, stomach, pancreas, lungs, and breasts. CEA and other serum titers, such as cancer antigen (CA) 125 (ovarian), CA 27-29 (breast), and prostate-specific antigen (PSA), may be valuable during chemotherapy to evaluate the extent of response and detect tumor recurrence.

Treatment

Changes in the health care system have shifted much of cancer care to ambulatory and home settings. The medical management of cancer may be curative or palliative (care that provides symptomatic relief but does not cure). Major therapies that are the focus of curative cancer treatment at this time include surgery, radiation, chemotherapy, biotherapy, angiogenesis therapy, and hormonal therapy.

New tests called *gene-profiling assays* are now available that can predict fairly accurately what certain tumors will do and how best to treat them. Research has shown that tumors, like any other living tissue, contain genetic information that can be read with increasing accuracy. The goal is to analyze the genetic makeup of the tumor, then choose the specific treatment most likely to be effective given that gene profile, while avoiding exposing the person to toxic therapies that might not be helpful or necessary. Two gene-profiling tests are already available for breast cancer; others are being evaluated for non-Hodgkin's lymphoma, head and neck cancer, prostate cancer, kidney cancer, melanoma, and ovarian cancer.

The future of oncologic care may rest on the model of individualized (tailored) therapy based on a pretreatment assessment of each individual's organ reserves, physical condition, and cognitive function. Identifying predictive factors of successful outcome will help assess who could benefit from more aggressive treatment and have the greatest chance for successful outcomes.[9,35] When curative measures are no longer possible or available, palliative treatment may include radiation, chemotherapy, physical therapy, medications, acupuncture, chiropractic care, alternative medicine, and hospice care.

Complementary and Alternative Medicine

Many people are seeking help in the cure and palliation of cancer through complementary and alternative medicine (CAM) therapies, such as acupuncture, hypnosis, mind–body techniques, massage, music, yoga, meditation, and other methods, to improve physical and mental well-being.[2,30] Conventional treatments do not always relieve symptoms of pain, fatigue, anxiety, and mood disturbance. Some people cannot tolerate the side effects of conventional treatment. CAM has received consumer attention and concern on the part of those who provide conventional or standard medical therapy.

The ACS has published a guide to help consumers make these kinds of treatment decisions[2] and has provided some direction for health care professionals.[135] Major research institutions and universities are beginning to investigate the effectiveness of these types of interventions for cancer. A new movement toward integrative medicine combining the best of complementary modalities with mainstream conventional therapies has been launched.

Major Treatment Modalities

Cancer treatment depends on an understanding of the biology of metastasis and how tumor cells interact with the micro-environment of different organs for effective therapies to be designed.[37] Each of the curative therapies described here may be used alone or in combination, depending on the type, stage, localization, and responsiveness of the tumor and on limitations imposed by the person's clinical status.

Surgery, once a mainstay of cancer treatment, is now used most often in combination with other therapies. Surgery may be used curatively for tumor biopsy and tumor removal or palliatively to relieve pain, correct obstruction, or alleviate pressure. Surgery can be curative in persons with localized cancer, but 70% of clients have evidence of micrometastases at the time of diagnosis, requiring surgery in combination with other treatment modalities to achieve better response rates. Adjuvant therapy used after surgery eradicates any residual cells.

Radiation therapy. RT (or XRT), also known as *radiotherapy*, plays a vital role in the treatment of cancer. It is used to destroy the dividing cancer cells by destroying hydrogen bonds between DNA strands within the cancer cells while damaging resting normal cells as little as possible. Recent advances in RT have primarily involved improvements in dose delivery.

Radiation consists of two types: ionizing radiation and particle radiation. Both types have the cellular DNA as their target; however, particle radiation produces less skin damage. The goal is to ablate as many cancer cells as possible while sparing surrounding normal tissues. Radiation is given over a period of weeks to capture cells at each stage of the cell cycle.

Radiation treatment approaches include external beam radiation and intracavitary and interstitial implants. Radiation may be used preoperatively to shrink a tumor, making it operable while preventing further spread of the disease during surgery. After the surgical wound heals, postoperative doses prevent residual cancer cells from multiplying or metastasizing.

Modern radiology has advanced to include site-specific techniques that take into account complex tissue contours and irregular shapes, visceral movement, digestion, and the effect of respiration on the lungs when the lungs are the target organ. Intensity-modulated RT (IMRT) now allows for sculpting the radiation field and dose to match the area being irradiated.

Normal and malignant cells respond to radiation differently, depending on blood supply, oxygen saturation, previous irradiation, and immune status. Cells most affected by chemotherapy and radiation have the greatest oxygenation and are the fast-producing cells (e.g., hair, skin). Generally, normal cells recover from radiation faster than malignant cells; damaged

cancer cells cannot self-repair. Success of the treatment and damage to normal tissue also vary with the intensity of the radiation.

Although a large single dose of radiation has greater cellular effects than fractions of the same amount delivered sequentially, a protracted schedule allows time for normal tissue to recover in the intervals between individual sublethal doses.[15]

Challenges with radiation treatment still remain because of the inability to identify microscopic disease with accuracy. Immobilizing patients and keeping them completely still for the duration of treatment are also difficult. Weight loss associated with treatment alters body geometry, requiring further corrections in dosimetry.

Chemotherapy. Chemotherapy includes a wide array of chemical agents to destroy cancer cells. It is particularly useful in the treatment of widespread or metastatic disease, whereas radiation is more useful for treatment of localized lesions. Chemotherapy is used in eradicating residual disease, as well as inducing long remissions and cures, especially in children with childhood leukemia and adults with Hodgkin's disease or testicular cancer

Chemotherapy (and RT) kills most of the billion or more cells in each cubic centimeter of tumor tissue. However, cytotoxic therapies do not always eradicate every tumor cell for several reasons. Unlike normal cells, cancer cells are genetically unstable and replicate inaccurately. As the tumor grows, multiple subpopulations of cells with different biologic characteristics develop. Some of the cells will be resistant to treatment. After the treatment-sensitive cells have been eliminated, the resistant cells may divide rapidly, recreating a tumor that is now resistant to the therapy.[124]

Almost all chemotherapy agents kill cancer cells by affecting DNA synthesis or function, a process that occurs through the cell cycle. Each drug varies in the way this occurs within the cell cycle. Chemotherapy interferes with the synthesis or function of nucleic acid, targeting cells in the growth phase, and therefore does not kill all cells.

Chemotherapeutic drugs can be given orally, subcutaneously, intramuscularly, intravenously, intracavitarily (into a body cavity such as the thoracic, abdominal, or pelvic cavity), or intrathecally (through the sheath of a structure, such as through the sheath of the spinal cord into the subarachnoid space) or by arterial infusion, depending on the drug and its pharmacologic action and on tumor location. Administration in any form is usually intermittent to allow for bone marrow recovery between doses.

"Chemobrain," sometimes called "chemo fog" or "brain fog," refers to problems with memory, attention, and concentration reported by many people who have been treated with chemotherapy.

Not all chemotherapy recipients develop problems with cognitive or mental function, but if it does happen, the effects can last several years. MRIs of brain structures have shown temporary shrinkage in the brain structures that are responsible for cognition and awareness. Shrinkage may be a possible physiologic explanation for chemotherapy-related cognitive difficulties.[58]

Biotherapy. Biotherapy, sometimes referred to as *immunotherapy* or *immune-based therapy*, relies on BRMs to change or modify the relationship between the tumor and host by strengthening the host's biologic response to tumor cells.

Much of the work related to BRMs is still experimental, so the availability of this type of treatment varies regionally within the United States.

Other forms of biotherapy include bone marrow or stem cell transplantation, monoclonal antibodies, colony-stimulating factors, and hormonal therapy. BMT or peripheral stem cell transplantation is used for cancers that are responsive to high doses of chemotherapy or radiation. These high doses kill cancer cells but are also toxic to bone marrow; BMT provides a method for rescuing people from bone marrow destruction while allowing higher doses of chemotherapy for a better anti-tumor result.

BMT was a technique developed to restore the marrow in people who had sustained lethal injury to that site because of bone marrow failure, destruction of bone marrow by disease, or intensive chemical or radiation exposure. The transplant product is a very small fraction of the marrow cells called *stem cells.* These cells occur in the bone marrow and also circulate in the blood and can be harvested from the blood of a donor by treating the donor with an agent or agents (e.g., granulocyte colony-stimulating factor) that cause a release of larger numbers of stem cells into the blood and collecting them by hemapheresis. Because blood (peripheral site), as well as marrow, is a good source of cells for transplantation, the term *stem cell transplantation* has replaced the general term for these procedures.

Antiangiogenic therapy. Antiangiogenic therapy shows promise as a strategy for cancer treatment. Research has shown that the one common area of vulnerability of all cells in any phase of growth is the nonnegotiable need for oxygen. Tumor cells cannot survive without oxygen and other nutrients transported by the blood.[115]

Antiangiogenic therapy may be able to put a stop to pathologic angiogenesis, the process by which a malignant tumor develops new vessels and the primary means by which cancer cells spread. Treatment with antiangiogenesis factors (approved for use in the United States) focuses on blocking the general process of tumor growth by cutting off the tumor's blood supply rather than on the destruction of an already formed cancerous mass.[39] In the future, antiangiogenic agents may be used as maintenance therapy to control cancer much the same way that medications are used to control hypertension or hyperlipidemia. It is expected that different mutations in cancer will require individualized therapy based on current knowledge of specific tumors, their patterns of resistance, and response to angiogenesis inhibitors.[10]

Hormonal therapy. Hormonal therapy is used for certain types of cancer shown to be affected by specific hormones. For example, tamoxifen, an antiestrogen hormonal agent, is used in breast cancer to block estrogen receptors in breast tumor cells that require estrogen to thrive.

The luteinizing-releasing hormone leuprolide is now used to treat prostate cancer. With long-term use, this hormone inhibits testosterone release and tumor growth.

Effects of Cancer Treatment

Long-term effects of cancer treatment are problems that affect multiple systems. The physical therapist assistant (PTA) must take this into consideration when planning intervention and offering patient/client education.

With improved survival rates, we expect to see more delayed reactions and long-term sequelae to today's cancer treatment modalities. With improved survival and longevity, we also may see an increased prevalence of cancer recurrence in the future. This may mean worsening of symptoms such as peripheral neuropathy or lymphedema from second and third rounds of treatment. In time, with the identification of genetic traits of cancer, treatment may become more specific to the cancer cells and less toxic to healthy cells and tissue, eventually reducing and maybe even eliminating side effects experienced by many of today's cancer survivors.

Prognosis

Thirty years ago a cancer diagnosis was often a death sentence; survivors referred to themselves as "victims." Cancer is no longer considered a death sentence, and many survivors return to the mainstream of family life, community activities, and work. Medical treatment is often provided in outpatient settings, making it possible to work during treatment.[53]

Today, there are 10 million cancer survivors in the United States; 65% of all people diagnosed with cancer have a 5-year survival rate, which means that the chance of a person recently diagnosed with cancer being alive in 5 years is 65% of the chance of someone not diagnosed with cancer. Generally, increased survival rates occur with screening and early detection, especially for cancers that do not have a highly effective treatment such as melanoma. Prognosis is influenced by the type of cancer, the stage and grade of disease at diagnosis, the availability of effective treatment, the response to treatment, and other factors related to lifestyle such as smoking, alcohol consumption, diet, and nutrition. Despite advances in early diagnosis, surgical techniques, systemic therapies, and patient care, the major cause of death from cancer is metastases that are resistant to therapy.[37]

The prognosis is poor for anyone with advanced, disseminated cancer. Researchers continue to search for the mechanisms responsible for cancer metastases and chemotherapeutic failure and develop new strategies to circumvent drug resistance. Generally, the earlier cancers are found, the simpler treatment may be and the greater likelihood there is of a cure.

The term *no evidence of disease* may be used when all signs of the disease have disappeared after treatment but before 5 years have elapsed. There are no signs of the disease using current tests. If the response is maintained for a long period, the term *durable remission* may be used (Box 6.3). The person who is alive and without evidence of disease for at least 5 years after diagnosis is considered cured. The terms *survival* and *cure* do not always portray the functional status of a cancer survivor. Many people considered cured are left with physical limitations and movement dysfunctions that interfere with their daily lives.

Even without complete remission, cancer can be controlled to provide longer survival time and improved quality of life (QOL), but these factors are not reflected in survival rates. Survival rates for many cancers have increased from 1960 to the present, but not all cancers have been characterized by this increase. For example, whereas survival rates for Hodgkin's disease and prostate, testicular, and bladder cancers have increased by at least 25%, the survival rates for cancers of the oral cavity and pharynx, liver, pancreas, esophagus, and colon have decreased or increased less than 5% during the same period.

BOX 6.3   Definitions of Cancer Treatment Outcomes

Cure

- The disease is gone and there is no sign of it reappearing; individual must have been in complete remission for at least 5 years (or more) from the time of treatment to be considered "cured."
- Cancer recurrence or the onset of a new type of cancer is still possible; in theory the chances of cancer recurrence or new cancer for a person who has been cured are no higher than in someone who has not had cancer.

Complete Remission

- All signs of disease have disappeared after treatment, although this does not mean there are no cancer cells present and it does not mean the person is cured. CR may be referred to as *no evidence of disease*. After several years this state may be referred to as *durable remission* until 5 years have passed, at which point the individual is considered cured.

Partial Remission

- Primary tumor has been reduced to half its original size after treatment; also known as *partial response*.

Improvement

- Size of primary tumor has been reduced, but tumor remains more than half its original size.

Advanced Disease

- Disease has spread to more than one location; staging is used to describe the extent of disease.

Stable Disease

- No change with treatment; the cancer is not increasing or decreasing in size, extent, severity, or symptoms.

Refractory

- Cancer is resistant, does not respond to treatment, and continues to progress; also referred to as *treatment failure, resistant cancer*, or *disease progression*.

Relapse

- Cancer returns after treatment or a period of improvement either in the first place it started or in another place.

Survival Rate

- The percentage of people in a study or treatment group who are alive for a given period of time after diagnosis. This is commonly expressed as *1-year, 5-year*, or *10-year survival rate*, referring to the chances of being alive in 1 year, 5 years, or 10 years compared with the chances of someone who has not been diagnosed with cancer.

Prognostic Index

- Used as a measure of risk for relapse, the prognostic index is not a predictor for death.

CR, Complete remission; *PR*, partial remission.

6.1 Special Implications for the PTA: Oncology and Cancer

Role of the Physical Therapist Assistant in Cancer Treatment

Treatment for cancer has improved over the past 20 years but often results in functional deficits caused by tissue resection or segmental bone, joint, or limb amputation. Treatment can result in severe disfigurement; cancer is the major cause of amputation in children. Site-specific cancer issues and side effects of radiotherapy, chemotherapy, and bone marrow or stem cell transplantation often require physical therapy intervention and education.[92,96]

At the present time, standard protocols do not exist for problems associated with cancer and cancer treatment encountered by the rehabilitation team including the physical therapist assistant (PTA). Indications and precautions for oncology patients are wide ranging, varied, or nonexistent regarding cardiovascular training, stretching, weight training, other exercise, or intervention by the PTA for any of the problems associated with this condition and its treatment.

Weakness, inflexibility, osteoporosis, risk of falls, altered or diminished breathing patterns, and lymphedema are just a few of the challenges faced by many of our cancer clients.

Many experts in the field of cancer treatment suggest automatic referral to a physical therapy team once the diagnosis of cancer has been made instead of waiting until radiation-induced fibrosis causes disabling contractures, for example. Psychosocial-spiritual issues (e.g., loss, grief, and anger) require consideration during planning of an effective therapeutic approach.[96] The psychosocial-spiritual status and cultural beliefs can be a driving factor in successful outcomes. Engaging the individual in honest discussion, listening to concerns or feelings, and sharing rehabilitation needs to set mutually achievable goals will enhance outcomes.[7,135]

As medical innovations help people with cancer live longer, there has been a shift in the way we approach cancer treatment. Shifting from the search for a cure to managing the disease as a chronic condition necessitates a more comprehensive and integrated management approach.[106] There is greater emphasis on maximizing function and improving quality of life (QOL) with a more holistic approach throughout the various phases of intervention and management.

The PTA will be involved in all phases of care, including prevention, restoration, support, and palliative care. Prevention lessens the impact of anticipated disability through education and training. Restorative care focuses on restoring physical function as much as possible. Supportive care assists clients in coping with the condition while maintaining maximal functional capacity. Palliative care provides comfort during function and activities of daily living to minimize dependence while offering emotional support.[70]

Benign Tumors

The PTA may be asked by clients to observe unusual skin lesions or aberrant tissue such as unusual moles, ganglion, fibromas, or lipomas. A general screening examination is required with history, age, and risk factors taken into consideration. The asymmetry, border, color, diameter (ABCD) skin cancer screening examination can be used with documentation of findings for any skin changes.

Benign fatty (lipoma) or fibrous tumors (fibroma) commonly located in the subcutaneous tissues can be located anywhere in the body. Lipomas are found most often in locations where fat accumulates, such as the abdomen, thighs, upper arms, back, and breast. These masses are usually round or oval, soft, lumpy, and easily moveable. They may be small (pea size) or as large as 3 to 4 inches across. Palpation reveals defined borders and a mass that is not fixed but moves readily with pressure along the edge.

These benign tumors are usually painless but can be tender when palpated. Many people who discover the lump are understandably concerned about cancer. Any suspicious integumentary or soft tissue mass must be evaluated medically, especially in the client with any additional risk factors. Only a pathologist can diagnose or rule out cancer in these types of lesions.

Side Effects of Cancer Treatment

Table 6.6 compares the potential side effects associated with the major treatment modalities discussed in this section.

The ACS provides an online guide to drugs used in the treatment of cancer with common side effects listed.[115] The National Comprehensive Cancer Network offers a number of clinical practice guidelines for cancer in general and for specific types of cancer.[135] The ACS offers suggestions for optimizing the preservation of fertility for men and women after cancer therapy.[4]

Each individual will experience and report discomfort in a slightly different way. The occurrence of symptoms is a stressor of its own, sometimes initiating a response of fear behaviors and distress. Individual perception of symptoms includes whether the person notices a change in how he or she usually feels or behaves, intensity of the symptoms, and the impact of both the presence and intensity of symptoms on daily activities, function, and QOL. Response to symptom distress includes physiologic, psychologic, sociocultural, and behavioral components. The most common and often distressing side effect of cancer and cancer-related treatment is fatigue. The PTA can be very instrumental in offering information and ideas about energy conservation and can help the client set priorities, pace himself or herself, and delegate activities and responsibilities as well as provide labor-saving devices and ideas. Scheduling activities at times of peak energy is important, as is a structured daily routine that focuses on one activity at a time. The importance of socializing, relaxing, and finding quiet moments of pleasure cannot be emphasized enough. Exercise to improve functional capacity, increase activity tolerance, manage stress, and improve mood is an integral part of fatigue management.

Physical Therapy Ongoing Assessment

In a physical therapy practice, anyone with a previous history of cancer, with known cancer risk factors, and/or over the age of 40 should be screened for red flags suggestive of cancer. The physical therapist (PT) and PTA are key professionals in offering education for risk-factor modification and cancer prevention. For the individual with a current diagnosis of cancer, an ongoing health assessment is important in providing the optimal exercise program. Recommended rehabilitation protocols during medical intervention with consideration for the specific cancer treatment are available for PTs and PTAs to consider.[39,146]

Cardiovascular and pulmonary tests and measures—including heart rate; breath sounds and respiratory rate, pattern, and quality; blood pressure; aerobic capacity test; and pulse oximetry—establish a baseline for reference in developing an exercise program. This is especially important with the aging demographics of cancer survivors. The older people are when diagnosed with cancer, the greater the likelihood of other problems being present, such as heart disease, hypertension, stroke, diabetes, osteoporosis, and so on.

Observe for and document any cluster of signs and symptoms of accompanying health conditions or comorbidities from cancer or cancer treatment such as hypoxia, decreased peripheral vascular supply, deep vein thrombosis, hypercalcemia, fluid or electrolyte imbalances, anemia, hypertension, integumentary changes, infection, and so on.

Integumentary, neuromuscular, musculoskeletal, and neurologic assessment should include but is not limited to observation of skin characteristics and condition (including lymph node palpation); anthropometrics; functional strength testing; assessment of range of motion and flexibility; arousal, attention, and orientation tests; evaluation of cranial and peripheral nerve integrity; tests of motor function; assessment of deep tendon and postural reflexes; and evaluation of sensory condition.[46,97]

The risk of falling is one of the more serious sequelae of both the local effects of cancer and the systemic consequences of cancer treatment. Weakness, pain, fatigue, orthostatic hypotension, peripheral neuropathy, decreased bone density (osteoporosis), and diminished flexibility, in various combinations, may result in falls. Anyone with metastasized cancer to the spine or long bones may fracture these bones in a fall, which can result in serious, long-term disability.

Higher incidences of osteoporosis and osteopenia are found in individuals with cancer. Management of long-term bone health is an important aspect of comprehensive cancer care.[129]

Fall prevention and education about falls are important aspects of the rehabilitation or exercise program. Assessment of the home environment is essential in providing a fall-prevention program.

In addition, the PTA must observe each client individually, possibly selecting an assistive device in appropriate cases. A wheelchair may be necessary for someone who experiences dizziness, weakness, fatigue, or signs of disorientation.

Precautions

The PTA must practice standard precautions carefully to help the individual undergoing cancer treatment avoid infection. Closely monitoring blood and vital signs and observing for signs of infection, bleeding, or arrhythmias are important. The PTA should contact the PT and physician when the client exhibits fever or a cluster of constitutional symptoms, unusual fatigue or tiredness, irregular heartbeat or palpitations, chest pain, unusual bleeding, or night pain.[104] Radiated tissue must be treated with care to avoid local trauma; extreme temperatures must be avoided, management of lymphedema may be required, and specific guidelines for the use of physical agents must be followed.[96]

Many people undergoing cancer treatment are using complementary and alternative herbs or supplements that can have an adverse effect when combined with radiation or chemotherapy. If the client perceives disapproval, this information may not be relayed to the appropriate health care professional. By being open and nonjudgmental and inviting more discussion about the use of these techniques, the PTA may be able to bring to light potential risks involved. The client should be advised that most herbal or natural supplements and complementary interventions are designed to support, not replace, traditional medical interventions that have been proved effective.

Oncologic Emergencies

Oncology patients/clients can present complex challenges for the PT and PTA. Treatment regimens and their potential side effects top the list of important considerations during the PTA's intervention. Early recognition of potential emergencies, such as superior vena cava syndrome (SVCS), tumor lysis syndrome (TLS), emergent spinal cord compression, severe thrombocytosis, and other conditions, is extremely important in reducing morbidity and mortality.[126]

Most of these conditions are uncommon or rare, making knowledge of them even more important so the PTA does not miss early clinical manifestations. Each one is typically associated with a particular type of cancer; knowing the patterns of potentially serious problems linked with individual cancers can help the PTA conduct surveillance with appropriate clients. For example, SVCS associated with small cell lung cancer and lymphoma is caused by mediastinal metastasis and central lung lesions compressing the superior vena cava. Presentation of SVCS is insidious, with dilated neck veins and facial and arm lymphedema. Treatment may be palliative if the malignancy causing the compressive force is not curable; curative chemotherapy for lymphoma is the exception.[126]

TLS occurs often in high-grade non-Hodgkin's lymphoma but may become clinically apparent in only a small number of affected individuals. TLS occurs in people with myeloproliferative disorders, such as leukemia and lymphoma, when chemotherapy causes lysis of a massive number of cells in a short period of time. Acute renal failure may occur from the deposition of potassium, phosphate, and uric acid from the cell lysis.[126,135] Symptoms of TLS are most common 6 to 72 hours after chemotherapy begins. The PTA may hear reports of and observe muscle weakness and cramping from TLS. In addition, the PTA must monitor for arrhythmias, decreased blood pressure, and tachycardia during activity.

Spinal cord compression affects up to 30% of individuals with disseminated cancer from lung, breast, prostate, multiple myeloma, and colon. The thoracic spine is targeted most often, followed by the lumbosacral region. Back pain, muscle weakness, gait changes, or other signs and symptoms of cord compression may develop slowly or may progress rapidly; prognosis is better with slow onset.

Many individuals undergoing treatment for cancer are thrombocytopenic (have low platelet levels). Severe thrombocytopenia (<5000 cells/mm^3) increases the risk of spontaneous bleeding The PTA may be instrumental in preventing intracranial bleeds and falls for anyone with this complication.

Physical Agents

Various forms of electric, electromagnetic, and other energy sources to relieve symptoms and side effects of cancer, as well as to slow, halt, or destroy tumors, have been investigated. Some physical modalities have the capacity to break down cell membrane barriers and stimulate changes in transmembrane potentials, which can trigger growth and development of abnormal tissue.[27]

The use of physical agents in people who have cancer is summarized in Table 6.7.[95] Heat modalities should not be used in people undergoing radiation because the thermal effect may enhance the effect of the radiation. Risk for modality use based on stage of medical management is listed in Box 6.4.

The application of therapeutic ultrasound over tumors is contraindicated (especially continuous ultrasound), presumably because it is believed that there is an increased risk of metastasis.[127] Studies conducted on mice have shown that a tumor given large doses of ultrasound will spread because of increasing blood supply to the area.[54,69,117]

The concern that electrical and thermal modalities can increase blood flow and possibly increase micrometastases in humans has not yet been proved in clinical studies. As a general guideline, some PTAs caution that people with cancer should not be treated with electrical or deep-heating thermal physical agents (ultrasound in particular), even at a site distant from the neoplasm, because the effect of ultrasound on micrometastases is not known.

Low-level laser treatment has recently been approved by the U.S. Food and Drug Administration for the treatment of postmastectomy lymphedema. The laser-beam pulses produce photochemical reactions at the cellular level, influencing the course of metabolic processes, reducing the volume of the affected arm, extracellular fluid, and tissue hardness.[17]

The use of low-level laser treatment over areas in which carcinoma was originally found has not been investigated. Prior carcinoma remains a contraindication to the use of laser therapy.[36] Research in this area is needed.

There may come a time in the client's situation when palliation, especially pain control, is more important than the risk of metastasis with the use of some modalities. However, this must still be determined based on clinical presentation, potential risks, and benefits. For example, if a tumor is impinging or even wrapped around a nerve, ultrasound over the site may increase tumor growth, causing further nerve compression.

Sexual Issues

Sexual dysfunction is a frequent side effect of cancer treatment, especially in adults with cancer of the reproductive organs and after Hodgkin's disease. The most common problems include loss of desire for sexual activity, erectile dysfunction in men, and dyspareunia in women. Unlike many other physiologic side effects, sexual problems do not tend to resolve within the first year or two of disease-free survival but remain constant.[112]

PTAs are often in a unique position to assist people with sexual concerns because of their repeated close contact with the affected individual. Sexual function is an important aspect of QOL and requires a brief assessment. In oncology settings, it is often helpful to designate and train a member of the team as the expert on sexuality issues.[112]

The PTA who is comfortable and knowledgeable in discussing sexual issues may be able to provide more focused assistance to the individual who is trying to adjust to changes in sexual style and practices as a result of the illness.

Palliative and Hospice Care

When curative measures have been exhausted and a cure is no longer possible or available, symptom management or palliative care may be offered. Palliative care is given to improve the QOL for people who have a serious or life-threatening disease. The goal is to prevent symptoms; side effects caused by treatment of the disease; and psychologic, social, and spiritual problems related to the disease or its treatment.

According to the guidelines of the World Health Organization,[144] the term *terminally ill patient* refers to individuals with cancer whose life expectancy is less than 90 days. Individual hospice agencies may use time periods other than 90 days as their qualification standard.

Although the cost of hospice may be covered by private insurance or by the client or family out of pocket, Medicare has three key eligibility criteria as follows:

- The patient's doctor and the hospice medical director use their best clinical judgment to certify that the patient is terminally ill with a life expectancy of 6 months or less, if the disease runs its normal course.
- The patient signs a statement choosing to receive hospice care rather than curative treatments for his or her illness.
- The patient enrolls in a Medicare-approved hospice program.

Palliative care for the terminally ill is aimed at improving the QOL of both the individual and family members. The primary goal is to decrease the physical and psychologic suffering of the individual while providing spiritual and emotional support. Every effort is made to help the individual achieve as full a life as possible, with minimal pain, discomfort, and restriction. Many medications, especially morphine, are used for pain control. Emphasis of hospice care is toward emotional and psychologic support for the client and the family, focusing on death as a natural end to life.[57]

Physical therapy may enhance the QOL of individuals receiving palliative care, as well as dying individuals receiving hospice care. Disability in individuals with advanced cancer often results from bed rest, deconditioning, and neurologic and musculoskeletal complications of cancer or cancer treatment. Weakness, pain, fatigue, and dyspnea are common symptoms.

Physical therapy intervention aims to improve level of function and comfort. Physical function and independence should be maintained as long as possible to improve QOL and reduce the burden of care for the caregivers.[74] Pain management and relief, positioning to prevent pressure ulcers and aid breathing, endurance training and energy conservation, home modification, and family education are just a few of the services the PTA can offer hospice clients and families. The PTA is an important team member in helping clients remain functional and retain dignity and control at the end of life.[103]

At the present time there is very little evidence that rehabilitation interventions can affect function and symptom management in individuals who are terminally ill. Clinical experience suggests that the application of rehabilitation principles is likely to improve their care.[109]

TABLE 6.6   Side Effects of Cancer Treatment

Surgery	Radiation	Chemotherapy	Biotherapy	Hormonal Therapy	Transplant (Bone Marrow, Stem Cell)
Fatigue	Fatigue	Fatigue	Fever	Hypertension	Severe bone marrow suppression
Disfigurement	Radiation sickness	GI effects	Chills	Steroid-induced diabetes	Mucositis
Loss of function	Immunosuppression	Anorexia	Nausea	Myopathy (steroid-induced diabetes)	Nausea and vomiting
Infection	Decreased platelets	Nausea	Vomiting	Weight gain	Graft-versus-host disease (allogenic graft only)
Increased pain	Decreased white blood cells	Vomiting	Anorexia	Hot flashes	Delayed wound healing
Deformity	Infection	Constipation	Fatigue	Impotence	Venoocclusive disease
Bleeding	Fibrosis	Anxiety and depression	Fluid retention	Decreased libido	Infertility
Scar tissue	Burns	Fluid, electrolyte imbalance from GI effects	CNS effects	Vaginal dryness	Cataract formation
Fibrosis	Mucositis	Hepatotoxicity	Slowed thinking		Thyroid dysfunction
	Diarrhea	Hemorrhage	Memory problems		Growth hormone deficiency
	Edema	Bone marrow suppression	Inflammatory reactions at injection sites		Osteoporosis
	Hair loss	Anemia	Anemia		Secondary malignancy
	Ulceration, delayed wound healing	Leukopenia (infection)	Leukopenia		
	CNS or PNS effects	Neutropenia	Altered taste sensation		
	Malignancy	Decreased bone density with ovarian failure[108a]			
		Muscle weakness			
		Skin rashes			
		Neuropathies			
		Hair loss			
		Sterilization			
		Stomatitis, mucositis (oral, rectal, vaginal)			
		Sexual dysfunction			
		Weight gain or loss			

CNS, Central nervous system; *GI*, gastrointestinal; *PNS*, peripheral nervous system.

TABLE 6.7   Common Physiologic Effects and Uses of Physical Agents and Modalities

Superficial Heating Agents: Hot Packs, Paraffin Baths, Infrared Lamps, Fluidotherapy, Local Immersion, Monochromatic Near-Infrared Photo Energy

Potential Benefits	Contraindications (Do Not Use)	Effectiveness[a]
Increases blood flow to affected area Increases metabolism Reduces pain, muscle spasm, chronic inflammation Increases relaxation, increases ROM Provides mild heat (<40°C) to trunk; vigorous heat (>40°C) to extremities	Over dysvascular tissue (after radiation therapy) and with people who are insensate to temperature or pain in application area Over areas of bleeding or hemorrhage (i.e., if there has been long-term corticosteroid therapy or chemotherapy) Over an acute injury or inflammation Presence of thrombophlebitis Directly over a tumor Over open wounds (except whirlpool at warm temperature)	Heat and stretch may decrease pain and muscle spasm in abnormal tissue; modulates pain and facilitates relaxation (gating effect) Not effective with deep cancer pain or bone pain (NSAIDs used) Under investigation; some reports of adverse response (e.g., burns) when used beyond recommended duration because of insensate, avascular conditions

Deep Heating Agents: Diathermy, Ultrasound, Full-Body Immersion Hydrotherapy

Potential Benefits	Contraindications (Do Not Use)	Effectiveness[a]
Increases extensibility of collagen tissue (scar tissue, tendons) (ultrasound) Reduces pain and muscle spasm Increases range of motion Alters threshold of nerve conduction Provides mild heat (<40°C) to trunk; vigorous heat (>40°C) to extremities Increases metabolism	Over growing epiphyses Over areas of acute hemorrhage (long-term use of corticosteroids or NSAIDs) Over acute injury or inflammation Over insensitive skin; dysvascular or irradiated skin Over tumors (unless trained in hyperthermia) Over implants (devices such as pacemakers or defibrillators, insulin pumps, morphine pumps, breast implants, plastic components, joint prosthetics—ultrasound over joint) Over reproductive organs; lumbosacral, pelvic, and lumbar regions if pregnant	Acute stage: there is a cancer treatment used for tumor hyperthermia to kill tumor tissue, administered at greater than therapeutic doses Advanced cancer or terminal stage: not indicated over tumor; this will increase tumor growth, often increasing the severity of symptoms such as pain

Cryotherapy: Cold Packs, Ice Massage, Cold Hydrotherapy or Baths, Vapocoolant Spray, Cold Compression

Potential Benefits for Acute Musculoskeletal Trauma	Contraindications (Do Not Use)	Effectiveness[a]
Reduces acute inflammation or inhibits edema, muscle spasm, spasticity (transient decrease of spasticity) Alters threshold of nerve conduction Decreases metabolism Decreases blood flow with later increase in blood flow	Over dysvascular tissue (after radiation therapy) and with people who are insensate to temperature or pain in application area When transient increase of blood pressure might be dangerous (monitor anyone with hypertension) When wound healing is delayed If nerve injury has occurred (applies especially to irradiation-induced or chemotherapy-induced nerve injury) If Raynaud's disease or peripheral vascular disease is present (exacerbated by chemotherapy)	Acute stage or advanced cancer: tumor treatment is supercooled at below therapeutic temperatures for local, superficial tumor destruction (e.g., liquid nitrogen for precancerous skin lesions) Immediate postchemotherapy cancer treatment: cold packs (cold cap) to head are suggested to reduce hair loss Chronic stage and cured or in remission: used for usual indications for cold therapy Occasionally selected by clients for pain relief; must be monitored by health or personal caregiver Treatment of pain in advanced cancer: not as acceptable to some for comfort care

Mechanical Agents: Traction (Sustained or Intermittent, Mechanical or Manual, Spinal or Peripheral)

Potential Benefits	Contraindications (Do Not Use)	Effectiveness[a]
Improves motion and mobility in clients with degenerative joint disease, joint hypomobility, or herniated disks	Structural disease (tumor, infection) Acute injury Positive vertebral artery test Positive alar ligament test	Effective when there has not been previous radiation therapy to spine

External Compression (Mechanical or Manual: Jobst Pump, Lympha Press, Wright Linear Pump, Garments, Bandages)

Potential Benefits	Contraindications (Do Not Use)	Effectiveness[a]
Reduces edema or lymphedema and pain secondary to edema or lymphedema; improves ROM problems related to edema	Difficulty tolerating treatment (impaired circulation) Phlebitis, DVT, thrombosis in area to be compressed Compression setting should not be greater than 45 mm Hg	Acute stage: may not be indicated Immediate postcancer treatment, advanced or terminal stage, chronic stage or cured: not indicated for lymphedema management unless cleared of cancer metastasis or recurrence or new cancer in region(s) to be treated

Hydrotherapy with Agitation (Agitation and Local Immersion Hydrotherapy)

Potential Benefits	Contraindications (Do Not Use)	Effectiveness[a]
Depending on temperature, same as for superficial heat and/or cold in region to be immersed Wound healing—stimulates circulation to promote healing; removes exudates and necrotic tissue Facilitates exercise Relaxation; pain control	Depending on water temperature, same as for superficial heat and/or cold in region to be immersed Agitation should be minimized with painful open lesions, severely traumatized tissue, or recent skin grafts Risk of cross-infection must be controlled, especially for immunocompromised clients	Same as for superficial heat in region to be immersed

Electrical Stimulation: Neuromuscular Electrical Nerve Stimulation and Functional Electrical Stimulation

Potential Benefits	Contraindications (Do Not Use)	Effectiveness[a]
Reduces or eliminates muscle spasm Minimizes disuse atrophy Strengthens weak but innervated muscle Increases circulation secondary to muscle pump Functions as a substitute orthotic	If there is a potential for pathologic fracture in the area Any type of implanted devices (see previous list) Severe cardiopulmonary insufficiency Active phlebitis, DVT, thrombosis in area to be treated	Wound healing: high-voltage pulsed current, low-intensity direct (microcurrent) Strengthening Increased endurance

TENS and Electrical Stimulation at Acupuncture Points

Potential Benefits	Contraindications (Do Not Use)	Effectiveness[a]
Partial or complete alleviation of pain Acute pain Postoperative incisional pain Chronic pain Phantom pain Peripheral neuropathy pain Postherpetic neuralgia Advanced malignancy (but not over tumor)	Any type of implanted electronic device (pacemaker, insulin pump, morphine pump, defibrillator) Not useful in control of generalized pain or deep bone pain Occasional allergic reactions to gel or adhesive Decreased effectiveness over time	Advantages over narcotic analgesics: few side effects, relatively inexpensive and easy to use Allows interpersonal interaction and is controlled by the client During treatment (chemotherapy): effective as an antiemetic for nausea and vomiting Immediately after treatment: postoperative pain and chronic pain control for 2–4 months

[a]Safe if cleared for possible cancer recurrence, metastasis, or new cancer in area or areas to be treated and if the sensation and circulation in the area or areas to be treated are not impaired.

DVT, deep vein thrombosis; *NSAID,* nonsteroidal antiinflammatory drug; *ROM,* range of motion; *TENS,* transcutaneous electrical nerve stimulation.
Courtesy Lucinda Pfalzer, PT, PhD, University of Michigan, 2001. Used with permission.

BOX 6.4 **Risks for Modality Use Based on Stage of Medical Management**

Acute Stage

- Medical diagnosis and treatment for new or newly recurrent cancer.
- Potential for disseminated cancer until the medical diagnostic process is completed (except cases of local cancer).
- Stage I cancer: Local disease, usually receives a local treatment (e.g., surgery and/or radiation therapy).
- Stage II cancer: Option of local treatment (surgery and radiation therapy) without systemic therapy (e.g., chemotherapy); higher risk of metastases or recurrence.
- Stage III cancer: Systemic therapy, often chemotherapy; the process of micrometastasis is unlikely in someone responding to chemotherapy.
- Risk: high risk; thermal agents should not be used during or in close time proximity to radiation or chemotherapy; general contraindications and precautions apply (e.g., insensate or dysvascular tissue with decreased sensation or decreased blood flow).

Subacute Stage

- Immediately after cancer treatment; may extend 6 to 12 months depending on treatment intervention (e.g., surgery, chemotherapy, radiation); hormone therapy (e.g., tamoxifen or aromatase inhibitors for breast cancer) continues for 5 years.
- Acute side effects or toxicities from treatment (e.g., radiation or chemotherapy) begin to subside.
- Risk: high risk; thermal agents should not be used during or in close time proximity to radiation or chemotherapy; general contraindications and precautions apply (e.g., insensate or dysvascular tissue with decreased sensation or decreased blood flow).

Chronic Stage

- Remission or recurrence may occur from 6 to 12 months up to 5 years or more after cancer treatment.
- Chronic states of cancer with risk of death for people living with cancer metastases or advanced disease.
- Risk of recurrence decreases over time, so the likelihood of recurrence diminishes the further the client is from the time of diagnosis and treatment. Risk is as follows:
  - Stage I[a]: No restrictions on use of physical agents or modalities in the absence of clinical signs or symptoms of potential recurrence or new cancer; client has had recent medical checkup including testing for cancer (e.g., bone scan, serum markers) with negative findings; general contraindications and precautions apply (e.g., insensate or dysvascular tissue with decreased sensation or decreased blood flow).
  - Stage II[a]: Moderate-risk to low-risk group; same restrictions as stage I.
  - Stage III[a]: Moderate-risk group; same restrictions as stage I.
  - Stage IV[a] (advanced): High-risk group; caution should be taken over any painful area or mass; thermal agents should not be used during or in close proximity to radiation or chemotherapy; general contraindications and precautions apply.

Statistically Cured Stage

- Remission more than 5 years after cancer treatment.
- Statistical risk of recurrence is minimal.
- Return to lifetime risk of cancer as an individual statistical measure.
- Risk: Low-risk group; no restrictions on use of physical agents or modalities in the absence of clinical signs or symptoms of potential recurrence or new cancer; general contraindications and precautions apply.

Courtesy Lucinda Pfalzer, PT, PhD, University of Michigan, 2001. Used with permission.
[a]At the time of diagnosis.

CANCER, PHYSICAL ACTIVITY, AND EXERCISE TRAINING

Investigators have begun extensive research in the area of exercise and cancer. As with the prevention and management of heart disease, obesity, osteoporosis, and diabetes, exercise plays an important role in relation to cancer. The results of studies are varied and wide ranging and complicated by the fact that exercise can be aerobic, strength training, flexibility, balance training, and conditioning or any combination of these forms. Each type of exercise has its own physiologic and psychologic benefits in the normal, healthy adult population.

The effects of each type of exercise on individuals with cancer are being investigated in many studies. In addition, not all cancers are alike or affect the body in the same way; cancer exercise benefits may vary based on cancer type, stage, type of treatment, changes made by treatment, and so on. Exercise appears to be safe, but long-term outcomes have not been reported. Some types of exercise have been shown to be detrimental to the immune system, and this must be considered.

Exercise as a Cancer Prevention Strategy

Physical activity is defined as body movement caused by skeletal muscle contraction that results in quantifiable energy expenditure. Exercise is distinguished from other types of physical activity by the fact that the intensity, duration, and frequency of the activity are specifically designed to improve physical fitness.

Based on available data, a role for exercise in specifically reducing cancer risk has been shown for breast and colorectal cancer, with more equivocal evidence for others such as melanoma, lung, and prostate cancers.[116] The exact amount of exercise needed to prevent cancer is debatable. It is currently not known what would be most beneficial for which cancers, at which stage of disease or treatment.[55] The ACS advises moderate habitual physical activity as a potentially protective measure against certain types of neoplasms, particularly tumors of the colon and the female reproductive tract. The activity should cause a slight increase in heart rate and breathing lasting 30 minutes, at least 5 days a week.

Exercise-induced changes in the activity of macrophages, natural killer cells, lymphokine-activated killer cells, neutrophils, and regulating cytokines suggest that immunomodulation may contribute to the protective value of exercise.[78,143]

Exercise for the Person with Cancer

Exercise programs also appear to have a beneficial influence on the clinical course of cancer, at least in the early stages of the disease. Researchers theorize that exercise can regulate production of certain hormones that when unregulated may spur tumor growth.

With 10 million Americans alive today who have been through the cancer experience, it is important to develop interventions to enhance immune function, prevent or minimize muscle wasting (thus counteracting the detrimental physiologic effects of cancer and chemotherapy), and maintain QOL after cancer diagnosis. Physical activity and exercise training are interventions that address a broad range of QOL issues, including physical, functional, psychologic, spiritual, emotional, and social well-being.[26]

Studies examining the therapeutic value of exercise for people with various cancers during primary cancer treatment suggest that exercise is safe and feasible, improving physical functioning and some aspects of QOL.[25,66,111]

Screening and Assessment

Medical screening should be conducted with all clients before their participation in an exercise program.[5] This type of screening is especially important for people with cancer who receive various levels of treatment that can affect the physiologic response to exercise. For example, fatigue is a common symptom of nearly every form of cancer treatment.

The therapist will need to take a detailed history of treatment administered to date, examine laboratory results, and distinguish between fatigue from deconditioning and fatigue from medical interventions to determine the most effective and efficient approach to rehabilitation. The medical history should also look for conditions not related to cancer, such as hypertension, diabetes, coronary artery disease, and preexisting orthopedic conditions. The person's current physical condition, condition before disease onset, and age are also important variables.[141]

The PTA must understand the stages of the disease and know the type and timing of the medical intervention, especially for radiation and chemotherapy. The body's physiologic response to these agents may alter the normal training response and affect tolerance for exercise and compliance with exercise programs. Cognitive rehabilitation techniques may be needed to improve patient/client compliance, function, and QOL.[41]

Cardiac dysfunction months to years after chemotherapy can result in left ventricular failure, cardiomyopathy, and/or congestive heart failure. These conditions may affect the client's ability to exercise. Signs and symptoms of subclinical cardiac conditions may develop with the initiation of an exercise program. Careful history taking and clinical assessment may result in early detection and intervention, potentially reducing morbidity.

Auscultation to screen for abnormal lung or heart sounds is important to identify any precautions or contraindications to exercise. The individual is not likely to be able to sustain exercise levels if there are any physiologic abnormalities present. Medical consultation may be required before a training program is initiated.

Monitoring Vital Signs

Monitoring physiologic responses to exercise is important in the immunosuppressed population. Exercise intensity may be difficult to determine by training heart rate because some people have inappropriate heart responses to exercise and large physiologic changes on a day-to-day basis from disease and treatment.

Baseline testing is important to determine safe guidelines and to provide a starting place against which to measure improvement and to identify the individual's functional exercise level. A hypertensive response to exercise is common among individuals with cancer and those who are undergoing cancer treatment. Starting an aerobic training program is not advised if such a response is observed during testing.[104]

Exercise intensity can be guided by heart rate ranges based on oxygen consumption or metabolic equivalent levels. The therapist can use test results to prescribe a program starting at approximately 60% of the individual's maximum level. The PTA uses prior exercise levels, prior exercise capabilities, baseline function, and individual abilities even when using the predictive formula, because each client may respond differently (unpredictably).[104]

The PTA (or client) should always monitor oxygen saturation with pulse oximetry and should monitor heart rate (for arrhythmias), pulse rate, breathing frequency, and blood pressure before, during, and after the treatment session. The Borg Rating of Perceived Exertion (RPE) scale or other scales can be used to determine level of symptom distress or severity. The RPE scale is also used when the client is taking cardiac medications that blunt heart rate response to exercise or when other conditions and comorbidities are present that may prevent the use of target heart rate formulas.

Watch closely for dyspnea, pallor, sweating, and fatigue, which are all early signs of cardiopulmonary complications of cancer treatment. The activity level of someone with anemia also may require adjustment. This client may have elevated pulse and respiratory rates because of hypoxia, with increased cardiac output resulting from the body's effort to maintain an adequate oxygen supply.

Exercise during and after Chemotherapy or Radiation Therapy

Bone marrow suppression is a common and serious side effect of many chemotherapeutic agents and can be a side effect of RT. Therefore it is extremely important to take a client history of current or past RT dosages and to monitor the hematologic values in clients receiving these treatment modalities.

The PTA must review these values before any type of vigorous exercise or activity is initiated. Current guidelines recommend that individuals undergoing chemotherapy or RT should not exercise within 2 hours of the treatment because increases in circulation may attenuate (alter or change) the effects of the treatment.[42] Although this recommendation is not based on evidence-based research, it is a guideline followed by the National Institutes of Health because of the physiologic effects of moderate to vigorous physical activity and exercise on the redistribution of cardiac output and blood flow to the working muscle. In the case of both RT and chemotherapy, there is a potential to enhance treatment toxicity with the shift in blood flow.

Moderate-intensity aerobic exercise has been shown to maintain erythrocyte levels during radiation treatment (of breast cancer).[34] Physical activity can also improve mood and reduce anxiety and mental stress for people undergoing chemotherapy. Independence and QOL improve as functional ability improves.[32,33,101] A helpful guideline to indicate when aerobic exercise is contraindicated in chemotherapy clients is given in Box 6.5. Keep in mind these values are primarily educated estimates based on clinical consensus; there is a need for further research and stronger evidence to support these values.[94]

Older adults, especially older adults with bone disease or significant comorbidities and impairments, such as arthritis or peripheral neuropathies, still need help with balance, strength, and coordination to remain safe from falls and injuries.

Exercise for Cancer-Related Fatigue

Fatigue related to cancer treatment is common and disabling for many people. People in cancer treatment are often advised to rest after chemotherapy, but aerobic exercise and physical activity have been shown to help improve energy level and stamina, reduce fatigue, reduce nausea, increase muscle mass,

BOX 6.5   **Winningham Precautions to Aerobic Exercise in Chemotherapy Clients[a]**

Platelet count	<50,000/mL
Hemoglobin	<10 g/dL
White blood cell count	<3000/mL; 10,000 with fever (no exercise)
Absolute granulocytes	<500/mL

Modified from Winningham ML, MacVicar MG, Burke CA: Exercise for cancer patients; guidelines and precautions. Phys Sportsmed 14:125–134, 1986.

[a]Single threshold values are not usually clinically relevant but provide a general guideline. For example, hemoglobin levels have the most variability from client to client; protocols vary from center to center.

BOX 6.6   **Symptomatic Precautions during Exercise Testing or Training**

Anyone with cancer experiencing any of the following (especially brought on or exacerbated by exercise) should contact his or her physician:
- Fever
- Extreme or unusual tiredness or fatigue
- Unusual muscular weakness
- Irregular heartbeat, chest palpitations, or chest pain
- Sudden onset of dyspnea
- Leg pain or cramps
- Unusual joint pain
- Recent-onset or new-onset back, neck, or bone pain
- Unusual bruising, nosebleeds, or bleeding from any other body opening
- Sudden onset of nausea during exercise
- Rapid weight gain or weight loss
- Severe diarrhea or vomiting
- Disorientation, confusion, dizziness, or light-headedness
- Blurred vision or other visual disturbances
- Skin pallor or unusual skin rash
- Night pain

Data from Drouin J, Pfalzer LA: Aerobic exercise guidelines for the person with cancer. Acute Care Perspect 10:18–24, 2001.

and increase daily activities without increasing fatigue. The use of exercise as an adjunct intervention for CRF is gaining favor as an effective strategy.[122]

Exercise combined with improved nutrition for CRF and deconditioning has also been reported successful in demonstrating significant improvements in the 6-minute walk test distance, the squat test, and fatigue level.[86]

Clients undergoing chemotherapy and RT who are experiencing CRF and who are already on an exercise program may need to exercise temporarily at a lower intensity and progress at a slower pace; the goal is to remain as active as possible. For sedentary individuals, low-intensity activities, such as stretching and brief, slow walks, can be implemented and slowly advanced.[15]

However, it can be difficult to convince someone who is extremely tired that exercise will improve his or her symptoms. The PTA may have to begin with discussions over a period of time about the importance of exercise. This is especially important if the person is significantly deconditioned.

Symptoms of fatigue, headache, and lethargy begin in most people when hemoglobin falls to 12 g/dL. Mild to moderate graded exercise is possible for many people at this level. Symptoms become more pronounced when hemoglobin decreases to 10 g/dL, reducing exercise capacity.

People with cancer are advised to contact their physician if any of the abnormal responses listed in Box 6.6 develop.

Prescriptive Exercise

Types, limitations, and precautions of prescriptive exercise intervention in the treatment of cancer, especially cancer pain, are being studied. The programs under study vary in length from 6 weeks for individuals going through RT to 6 months for those in chemotherapy and the entire duration of BMT. The exercise interventions vary somewhat but most include progressive programs of 15- to 30-minute sessions, 3 to 5 days a week, at an intensity equal to 60% to 80% of maximum heart rate (RPE 11 to 14).

The frequency and duration of exercise are determined by the clinical status of the person. If weight training is prescribed, high-repetition, low-weight circuit programs that do not exceed an RPE of 14 are recommended.[71]

Individuals who exercised more than 60 minutes per day were more likely to report higher levels of fatigue, suggesting a maximum effective dose for individuals receiving adjuvant chemotherapy. No serious adverse events were reported in any of the studies, although anyone in the high-risk category with serious comorbidities was excluded, and most exercise programs were flexible and symptom limited.

The reported outcomes of these and other studies show that exercise has a powerful effect on CRF, with fatigue levels reported as 40% to 50% lower in exercising participants. Exercise reduces fatigue and emotional distress and improves QOL.

Without exception, all of these studies showed lower levels of fatigue and emotional distress as well as decreased sleep disturbance in people who exercised during treatment compared with controls or with baseline scores in single-group designs. Not all people with cancer are able to participate in aerobic exercise. People who ambulate less than 50% of the time or who are confined to bed and those who fatigue with mild exertion may not be candidates for aerobic exercise.[140] Range-of-motion exercises and gentle resistive work until tolerance for activity improves are still important. Some people may become easily fatigued with minimal exertion. Energy-conservation techniques and work simplification (Box 6.7) may be necessary for the person with chronic fatigue and for those whose functional status is declining. Therapeutic exercise should be scheduled during periods when the person has the highest level of energy.

Generalized weakness associated with cancer treatment can be more debilitating than the disease itself. Whenever possible, exercise, including strength training and cardiovascular training, is an essential component for many people with cancer. Improving strength and endurance aids in countering the effects of the disease and the effects of medical interventions. Increased physical activity may increase the homeostatic sleep drive to increase nighttime sleep and may help relieve CRF.[22]

Interval exercise or a bedside exercise program may be preferred at first. Interval exercise may be the only treatment possible in this circumstance. This is performed during frequent but short sessions throughout the day with work–rest intervals beginning at the person's level of tolerance. This may be no more than 1 minute of exercise activity followed by 1 minute of rest, then 1 minute of exercise, and so on. As the person's endurance level increases, the duration of work may be increased and the interval of rest decreased.

Modified from Hamburgh RR: Principles of cancer treatment. Clin Manage 12:37–41, 1992.

Exercise and Lymphedema

In the past, PTAs were cautioned to carefully design a program that did not cause or exacerbate cancer-related complications such as edema. It was advised that repetitive or strenuous exercise would increase the production of lymph fluid, and lymphedema would be the result because lymph nodes were removed during surgery, damaged by RT, or invaded by the tumor, leaving scar tissue that prevented normal lymph drainage. In fact, it is now known that exercise activates muscle groups and joints in the affected extremity and does not induce lymphedema.[50,51] Resistance training has not been shown to adversely affect lymphedema.[1]

Exercise and Advanced Cancer

With improved detection and treatment, more and more people are living with cancer as a controllable chronic disease or in advanced stages of cancer. There is insufficient research on exercise in such individuals to make specific recommendations for physical activity and exercise. In such cases PTAs are advised to prescribe exercise based on individual needs and abilities.

General training precautions for warm-up and cool down should be followed while monitoring for abnormal heart rate or blood pressure responses and observing each individual for pathologic symptomatic responses (e.g., hypertension, chest pain, onset of wheezing, claudication or leg cramps, shortness of breath, dizziness or fainting). Clients should be encouraged to remain adequately hydrated at all times unless medically directed otherwise.

Compromised skeletal integrity, especially in the presence of muscle wasting, increases the risk of fracture and may prevent weight-bearing activities. Aerobic exercise may have to begin with non–weight-bearing exercise, such as cycling, rowing, or

Data from Doyle C: Nutrition and physical activity during and after cancer treatment: an American Cancer Society guide for informed choices. CA Cancer J Clin 56:323–353, 2006.

swimming, with a gradual return to weight-bearing activities whenever possible to prevent loss of bone density. People with severe muscle weakness may tolerate cycling better than walking.[91] Interval exercise may be used with a goal of increasing the exercise time and decreasing the rest.[91]

Exercise for Cancer Survivors

Being sedentary is a risk factor for several of the most common types of cancer. Survivors tend to decrease levels of physical activity and exercise during and after completion of their treatment, especially if they were sedentary before their cancer diagnosis.[60] Low-intensity exercise can seem like high-intensity exercise for these individuals. In addition, some therapies reduce exercise capacity because of cardiopulmonary, neurologic, and musculoskeletal impairments. Until studies verify these findings, it is assumed that the beneficial effects of activity and exercise on cardiovascular health, bone strength, lean body mass, and balance also apply to cancer survivors.

The type, frequency, duration, and intensity of exercise should be individualized based on the survivor's age and previous fitness level, the type of cancer and cancer treatment, and the presence of any additional comorbidities. Some specific guidelines are available in Box 6.8.

Until results of systematic studies are available, the ACS recommends at least 30 to 60 minutes of moderate to vigorous physical activity at least 5 days per week to reduce the risk of cancer, cardiovascular disease, and diabetes.[67,72] There is no reason to think these recommendations would not benefit cancer survivors. Survivors should be educated to understand that any exercise has a linear benefit, with increasing health benefit with higher volume of physical activity. People should be cautioned that extremely high levels of exercise might increase the risk for infections and exercise-related injuries.[82]

CHILDHOOD CANCER

Incidence and Overview

Each year approximately 8400 children in the United States are diagnosed with cancer; approximately 2000 deaths of children

19 years old or younger are attributed to cancer.[91] With recent advances in treatment, 79% of children with cancer will survive 5 years or more. Cancer is the second leading cause of death in children 1 to 14 years of age.[61,75] Treatment-related deaths have declined as a result of advances in clinical supportive care that maximize the benefits and minimize the side effects of cancer therapy.

The types of cancers that occur in children vary greatly from those seen in adults. Leukemias, particularly acute lymphocytic leukemia (ALL); lymphomas; brain tumors; embryonal tumors; and soft tissue sarcomas are the most common pediatric malignancies, whereas adenocarcinomas are more common in adults.[68,75]

Other differences that must be taken into account when treating the child with cancer include the stage of growth and development, stage of psychosocial and cognitive development, and emotional response of the child to the illness and its treatment. The immaturity of the child's organ systems often has important treatment implications.

Types of Childhood Cancers

The most common pediatric malignancies are ALL, non-Hodgkin's lymphoma, Hodgkin's disease, and primary CNS tumors.

ALL, the most common childhood malignancy, accounts for almost one-third of all pediatric cancers. Caucasian boys are affected most often, and although the exact cause is unknown, radiation, chromosomal abnormalities, viruses, and congenital immunodeficiencies have all been associated with an increased incidence of leukemia. Wilms' tumor, a malignancy that may affect one or both kidneys, occurs in children under the age of 14 and is slightly more prevalent in girls than in boys. Epidemiologic research suggests an increased incidence in children of men exposed to lead or hydrocarbons. Recently an association between Wilms' tumor and chromosomal abnormalities has been established. This chromosomal anomaly is an autosomal dominant trait requiring evaluation of other family members.

Neuroblastoma is the most common extracranial solid tumor in children and the most commonly diagnosed neoplasm during the first year of life. Approximately 500 new cases are diagnosed annually in the United States, and the incidence is higher among whites than nonwhites. Neuroblastoma can originate anywhere along the sympathetic nervous system, but more than half of the tumors occur as an abdominal mass. Other common sites include the posterior mediastinum, pelvis, and neck. If the bone marrow is involved, bone pain may occur. Rhabdomyosarcoma is the most common soft tissue sarcoma and the seventh leading cause of cancer in children. This tumor, which is more prevalent in boys than girls, originates from the same embryonic cells that give rise to striated muscle. The peak incidence is at age 2 to 5 years, and a second peak occurs at 15 to 19 years, with much improved survival rates with early detection and treatment today. The most common tumor sites include the head and neck, genitourinary tract, and extremities.

Late Effects and Prognosis

As advances in cancer therapy improve, the prognosis of children with malignancies continues to improve. Over the past 25 years there have been significant improvements in the 5-year survival rate for many childhood cancers. From 1974 to 1996, 5-year survival rates among children for all cancer sites combined improved from 56% to 75%.[91] With increasing survival rates, there is a growing concern about the late effects of disease and treatment.

The term *late effects* refers to the damaging effects of surgery, radiation, and chemotherapy on nonmalignant tissues, as well as to the social, emotional, and economic consequences of survival. These effects can appear months to years after treatment and can range in severity from subclinical to clinical to life-threatening. Fortunately, not all children experience such effects, but those who do often end up in the rehabilitation setting.

Late effects have been identified in almost every organ system. Treatment involving the CNS can cause deficits in intelligence, hearing, and vision. Treatment involving the CNS, head and neck, or gonads can cause endocrine abnormalities such as short stature, hypothyroidism, or delayed secondary sexual development. Surgery and radiation involving the musculoskeletal system have been associated with defects such as kyphosis, scoliosis, and spinal shortening. Finally, the child who has received radiation or chemotherapy has a 10-fold greater chance of developing a second malignancy than a child who has never had cancer.

REFERENCES/SUGGESTED READINGS

To enhance this text and add value for the reader, references and suggested readings are included on the companion Evolve site that accompanies this textbook. The reader can view the source and access it online whenever possible.

7

The Integumentary System

CHAPTER OBJECTIVES

1. Describe primary pathology in the integumentary system.
2. Describe integumentary system manifestations of other systemic pathologies.
3. Discuss thermal injuries, including classifications of burns.
4. Discuss signs and symptoms of skin ulceration, including vascular, neuropathic, and pressure-related ulcers.
5. Discuss integumentary red flags, such as signs and symptoms of skin cancers, cellulitis, and spread of infections to lymph system.

OUTLINE

VOCAB BUILDERS

Bullous	Lund–Browder	Telangiectasia
Curettage	Neurofibromatosis	Turgor
Desquamation	Pemphigus	Unna's boot
Discoid	Pruritus	Urticaria
Eschar	PUVA	Xerosis
Excoriated	Rule of nines	
Langerhans cells	Slough	

Skin is the largest body organ, constituting 15% to 20% of the body weight and consisting of three primary layers (Fig. 7.1). The dermis is more distinctly divided into two separate layers, referred to as the *papillary dermis* and the *reticular dermis*. The structures included in each layer are listed in Table 7.1.

The skin differs anatomically and physiologically in different areas of the body, but the overall primary function of the skin is to protect underlying structures from external injury and harmful substances. The skin is primarily an insulator, but it has many other functions, including holding the organs together, sensory perception, contributing to fluid balance, controlling temperature, absorbing ultraviolet (UV) radiation, metabolizing vitamin D, and synthesizing epidermal lipids.

SKIN LESIONS

Definition and Incidence

Approximately one in every four people who consults a physician has a skin disorder. Skin lesions can occur as a result of a wide variety of etiologic factors (Box 7.1). Lesions of the skin or skin manifestations of systemic disorders can be classified as *primary* or *secondary* lesions.

The primary lesion is the first lesion to appear on the skin and has a visually recognizable structure (e.g., macule, papule, plaque, nodule, tumor, wheal, vesicle, pustule). When changes occur in the primary lesion, it becomes a secondary lesion (e.g., scale, crust, thickening, erosion, ulcer, scar, excoriation, fissure, atrophy). These changes may result from many factors,

including scratching, rubbing, medication, natural disease progression, or processes of healing.

Birthmarks, commonly caused by a nevus (pl., nevi), may involve an overgrowth of one or more of any of the normal components of skin, such as pigment cells, blood vessels, and lymph vessels. Birthmarks may be classified as pigment cell (e.g., Mongolian spot, café-au-lait spot), vascular (e.g., port-wine stain, strawberry hemangioma), epidermal (e.g., epidermal nevus, nevus sebaceus), or connective tissue (e.g., juvenile elastoma, collagenoma) birthmarks.

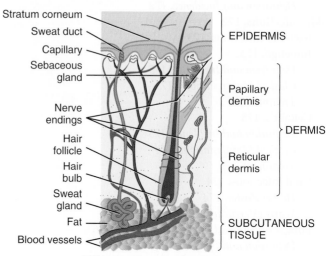

FIG. 7.1 Overall skin structure.

Most birthmarks do not require treatment. Vascular birthmarks may be removed with laser therapy for cosmetic reasons. The presence of six or more café-au-lait spots over 5 cm in length necessitates medical investigation, because these may be diagnostic of *neurofibromatosis* or Albright's syndrome. Mongolian spots (blue–black macules) are found over the lumbosacral area in 90% of Native American, African American, and Asian infants and can easily be mistaken for a large bruise by uninformed individuals (Fig. 7.2).

SIGNS AND SYMPTOMS

Pruritus (itching) is one of the most common manifestations of dermatologic disease and is a symptom of underlying systemic disease in up to 50% of people with generalized itching, especially among the chronically ill and older populations.[74] It can lead to damage if scratching injures the skin's protective barrier, possibly resulting in increased inflammation, infection, and scarring. Many systemic disorders can cause pruritus, most commonly diabetes mellitus, drug hypersensitivity, and hyperthyroidism. In the case of pruritus, regardless of the cause, the physical therapist assistant (PTA) can offer some practical suggestions to help soothe skin, ease the itching, and prevent skin damage (Box 7.2). *Bullous* skin lesions, including blisters, are associated with risk of exposure to human immunodeficiency virus (HIV). Standard precautions must be used while treating anyone with skin lesions or burns.[15]

Urticaria, more commonly known as *hives,* is a vascular reaction of the skin marked by the appearance of smooth, slightly elevated patches (wheals). These are redder or paler than the surrounding skin and are often accompanied by severe itching. These eruptions are usually an allergic response to drugs or infection and rarely last longer than 2 days but may exist in a chronic form, lasting more than 3 weeks or, rarely, months to years. There is approximately a 50% reduction in numbers of mast cells responsible for urticaria in intrinsically aged skin.

TABLE 7.1   **Skin Structure**

Layer	Structure[a]	Function
Epidermis	Stratum corneum	Protection (from trauma, microbes); barrier (prevents fluid, electrolyte, and chemical loss)
	Keratinocytes (squamous cells)	Synthesis of keratin (skin protein)
	Langerhans cells	Antigen presentation; immune response
	Basal cells	Epidermal reproduction
Dermis	Collagen, reticulum, elastin	Skin proteins; skin texture
	Fibroblasts	Collagen synthesis for skin strength and wound healing
	Macrophages	Phagocytosis of foreign substances, initiates inflammation and repair
	Mast cells	Provide histamine for vasodilation and chemotactic factors for inflammatory responses
	Lymphatic glands	Removal of microbes and excess interstitial fluids; provide lymphatic drainage
	Blood vessels	Provide metabolic skin requirements; thermoregulation
	Nerve fibers	Perception of heat and cold, pain, itching
Epidermal appendages	Eccrine unit	Thermoregulation by perspiration
	Apocrine unit	Production of apocrine sweat; no known significance
	Hair follicles	Production; cavity enclosing hair
	Nails	Protection; mechanical assistance
	Sebaceous glands	Produce sebum (oil to lubricate skin)
Subcutaneous tissue	Adipose (fat)	Energy storage and balance; trauma absorption

[a]Understanding the structure of the integument is important in wound management. Knowing why a wound closes the way it does is an essential assessment tool.
Data from Black JM, Hawks JH, editors: Medical-surgical nursing: clinical management for positive outcomes, ed 8, St. Louis, 2009, Saunders.

BOX 7.1   **Causes of Skin Lesions**

- Contact with injurious agents (e.g., chemical toxins)
- Contact with infective organisms
- Reaction to medication
- Physical trauma
- Hereditary factors
- Reaction to allergens
- Reaction to radiotherapy
- Systemic origin (e.g., diseases with a cutaneous manifestation; arterial insufficiency)
- Burns (thermal, electrical, chemical, inhalation)
- Neoplasm (paraneoplastic syndrome)

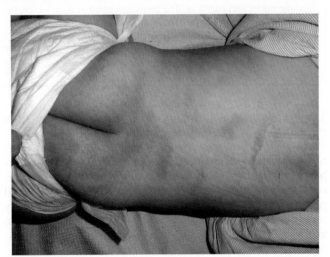

FIG. 7.2 Mongolian spots (congenital dermal melanocytosis). Mongolian spots are common among people of Asian, East Indian, Native American, Alaskan American, African, and Latino or Hispanic heritage. They are also present in about 1 in 10 fair-skinned infants. Bluish gray to deep brown to black skin markings, they often appear on the base of the spine, on the buttocks and back, and even sometimes on the shoulders, ankles, or wrists. Mongolian spots may cover a large area of the back. When the melanocytes are close to the surface, they look deep brown. The deeper they are in the skin, the more bluish they look, often mistaken for signs of child abuse. These spots "fade" with age as the child grows and usually disappear by age 5. (Courtesy Dr. Dubin Pavel, 2004.)

BOX 7.2　Skin Care Strategies

Reduce Pruritus

- Avoid scratching.
- Keep fingernails trimmed short to prevent damage in case of unconscious or nighttime scratching.
- Bathe with nondrying, fragrance-free or unscented soap or other agent when indicated.
- Use soothing bath products such as Aveeno Oatmeal, mineral oil, cottonseed oil, or cornstarch (make a paste with 2 cups cornstarch and 4 cups warm water) added to warm—not hot—bath water.
- Scleroderma: Apply cooling agents, such as menthol or camphor (e.g., contained in Sarna lotion), to the affected areas.
- Psoriasis: Try skin preparations such as creams containing capsaicin, chaparral, or aloe (some advocate the use of pure aloe). Do not apply hot-pepper creams on broken skin.
- Discuss with your physician the possible use of an alphahydroxy acid (AHA) product or other prescription cream containing urea to dissolve the outer layer of skin and get rid of the dead scales.
- Second rinse all clothing and bedding to remove residual laundry soap; avoid the use of fabric softeners.
- Wear open-weave, loose-fitting, cotton-blend fabrics to allow air to circulate and minimize perspiration, thereby reducing the risk of pruritus; avoid rough, wool, or tightly woven fabrics.
- Avoid temperature extremes that can trigger itching secondary to vasodilation and increased cutaneous blood flow. Avoid hot water (baths or hot tubs) for the same reason.
- Take antihistamines to reduce itching according to physician recommendation.
- Take a shower or bath immediately after swimming; wash with mild soap to remove any residual chlorine or chemicals from the skin.

Reduce Inflammation

- Apply topical steroids (available as lotion, solution, gel, cream, or ointment) to affected areas twice daily or as directed. Topical steroids are used to reduce skin inflammation, relieve itching, and control flare-ups of dermatitis and psoriasis. The proper preparation depends on the location and severity of the lesions and should not be applied to normal skin.
- Apply tar preparations (available as lotion, solution, gel, cream, ointment, or shampoo) to affected skin as directed. (Some tar preparations can be added to bath water.) The antiinflammatory properties of tars are not as fast-acting as topical steroids, but the effect is longer lasting and they have fewer side effects.
- Tar preparations should not be used on acutely inflamed skin because this may cause burning or irritation.

Maintain Skin Hydration

- Bathing has been discouraged because of its alleged drying effect, but some skin care professionals advocate the use of long soaks in a warm (not hot) bath for 15 to 20 minutes, suggesting that soaking for 15 to 20 minutes allows the stratum corneum to become saturated with water.
- Others recommend only showers or brief baths. Both groups agree that drying of the skin is the result of failure to immediately apply the appropriate occlusive moisture, thereby allowing evaporation to occur. Avoid vigorous or brisk towel drying, because this removes more water from the skin and increases vasodilation; gently and quickly pat dry. Immediately (within 2 to 4 minutes of leaving the bath) apply an appropriate emollient or prescribed topical agent.

Avoid Sun (Light) Exposure

- Wear sun-protective clothing with tightly woven material covering as much of the body as possible (e.g., long sleeves, long pants, neckline with a collar, hat with broad brim, UVA/UVB protective sunglasses).
- Avoiding sitting near a window at work or for prolonged periods of time.
- Avoid outdoor activities during peak sunlight hours (10:00 a.m. to 4:00 p.m. in most time zones but may vary geographically). Limit sun exposure during nonpeak hours.
- Avoid fluorescent lighting or reflected sunlight.
- Wear sunscreen daily and year round, even if driving inside an automobile or on cloudy days.
- Apply sunscreen 30 to 60 minutes before sun exposure to ensure maximum absorption. Sunscreen preparations must provide a minimum ultraviolet B sun protection factor (SPF) of 30 plus an ultraviolet A sunscreen for anyone with a current skin condition or who is at risk for skin cancer. A sunscreen of SPF 15 is considered adequate for anyone else who does not meet this criterion.
- Reapply every 2 hours if you are in the water or perspiring. Sunscreens are not recommended for infants under 6 months of age.
- Do not increase sun exposure because you are wearing a sunscreen. High SPF has been shown to lead to increased time spent in the sun by 25%. Sunscreen is most effective against squamous cell carcinoma.

This explains the relative rarity of urticaria in the older adult population.

Rash is a generalized term for an eruption on the skin, most often on the face, trunk, axilla, and groin, and is often accompanied by itching. As such, a rash can manifest on a continuum anywhere from erythema to macular lesions to a raised papular appearance. Rashes typically occur as a secondary response to some primary agent such as exposure to the sun, allergens, irritants, or medications or in association with systemic disease.

The most common rashes are diaper rash, drug rash, heat rash, and butterfly rash (a cutaneous reaction across the nose and adjacent areas of the cheeks in the pattern of a butterfly, most often encountered in systemic lupus erythematosus [SLE]; see Fig. 7.8). Rash appearing on the breast—especially a rash on the areola or nipple with or without accompanying symptoms of itching, soreness, or burning—may be a sign of Paget disease of the nipple, a rare form of breast cancer.

Blisters (vesicles or bullae) are fluid-containing elevated lesions of the skin with clear watery or bloody contents. They can occur as a manifestation of a wide variety of diseases. Blisters may be primarily associated with diseases of a genetic or autoimmune origin or may be secondary to viral or bacterial infections of the skin (e.g., herpes simplex, impetigo), local injury to the skin (e.g., burns, ischemia, pressure, dermatitis), or drug administration (e.g., penicillamine, captopril).[13] Blisters associated with underlying neoplasm, called *paraneoplastic pemphigus,* may be the first sign of underlying malignancy. Blisters may be associated with a variety of skin conditions, such as frostbite, dermatitis, burns, pressure, or malignancy, or may possibly occur as a side effect of medications. All blisters should be opened and debrided, except hemorrhagic frostbite blisters and stable, noninfected arterial and heel blisters, which subsequently should be monitored carefully for signs of infection or deep injury.

Although an intact blister is theoretically sterile, few blisters are substantial enough to remain intact for long. Blister fluid will "set" into a gelatinous film if debridement is delayed. In a burn, this film is the beginning of eschar and is an ideal culture medium for bacteria.

Blister fluid impairs normal function of neutrophils and lymphocytes, which reduces the effectiveness of local immunity. Blister fluid also contains arachidonic acid metabolites that increase the inflammatory response and retard the fibrinolytic process. All these effects delay healing of the wound.[66]

Xeroderma is a mild form of ichthyosis or excessive dryness of the skin characterized by dry, rough, discolored skin with the formation of scaly *desquamation* (shedding of the epithelium in small sheets). This problem is accentuated by dry climates and by the use of drying skin cleansers, soaps, disinfectants, and solvents.

Other symptoms—such as unusual spots, moles, cysts, fibromas, nodules, swelling, or changes in nail beds—may frequently be observed, because more than half of all people have some basic skin problem at some point in their lives. Any unusual spot that has appeared recently or changed since its initial appearance should be documented and brought to the physician's attention. On the legs, varicosities and stasis changes from poor venous return may be signaled by changes in skin pigmentation, skin *turgor*, and skin texture. Edema of the lower extremities can be a sign of multiple systemic illnesses, such as heart, kidney, or liver disease.

7.1 Special Implications for the PTA: Skin Lesions Any time a client reports signs or symptoms of skin lesions, further evaluation is necessary, and documentation and possible medical referral may be required. The PTA must remain alert to any skin changes that may indicate the onset or progression of a systemic condition.

Any rash on the breast, regardless of whether it's symptomatic or accompanied by other symptoms, raises the suspicion of Paget disease and must be examined by a medical doctor. Blisters of unknown cause may be the first sign of underlying malignancy requiring immediate medical evaluation.

Certain skin lesions should be examined by a physician because of their premalignant status; these may include actinic keratosis (slightly raised, red, scaly papules) or sebaceous cysts (enclosed cysts in the dermis). Seborrheic keratosis can be moved with friction and may bleed, causing alarm, but this is not a malignancy; however, the PTA must avoid contact with the skin in that area.

When examining the skin and documenting the presence of a skin disorder, note the location, size, and any irregularities in skin color, temperature, moisture, ulceration, texture, thickness, mobility, edema, turgor, odor, and tenderness (Box 7.3). If more than one lesion is present, note the pattern of distribution: localized or isolated; regional; general; or universal (total), involving the entire skin, hair, and nails. Note whether the lesions are unilateral or bilateral, note whether they are symmetric or asymmetric, and note the arrangement of the lesions (clustered or linear configuration), especially if they occur as a result of contact with clothing, jewelry, or another external object.

Special care must always be taken when working with the older adult. It is essential to avoid shear and friction forces during treatment, particularly during repositioning. Extreme caution is also necessary whenever using electrical or thermal modalities (heat or cold) with older people.

Decreased circulation, reduced subcutaneous adipose tissue, and altered metabolism create a situation in which initial skin resistance to electricity or poor dissipation of heat or cold can lead to tissue damage. Extra toweling and close supervision are necessary to prevent complications. Use appropriate dressings and skin moisturizers for treatment intervention, and avoid using adhesives.

AGING AND THE INTEGUMENTARY SYSTEM

Definition and Incidence

The skin undergoes numerous changes that can be seen and felt throughout the life span. The most obvious changes occur first during puberty and again during older adulthood. Hormone

---

BOX 7.3   Documentation of Skin Lesions

Characteristics
- Size (measure all dimensions)
- Shape or configuration
- Color
- Temperature
- Tenderness, pain, or pruritus
- Texture
- Mobility; skin turgor
- Elevation or depression
- Pedunculation (stemlike connections)

Exudates
- Color
- Odor
- Amount
- Consistency

Pattern of Arrangement
- Annular (rings)
- Grouped
- Linear
- Arciform (bow-shaped)
- Diffuse

Location and Distribution
- Generalized, localized, or universal
- Region of the body; unilateral or bilateral; symmetric or asymmetric
- Patterns (dermatomal, flexor or extensor, random, related to clothing lines)
- Discrete or confluent (running together)

Modified from Hill MJ: Skin disorders, St. Louis, 1994, Mosby.

---

changes during puberty stimulate the maturation of hair follicles, sebaceous glands, and apocrine and eccrine units in certain body areas. Mild acne, perspiration and body odor, freckles (promoted by sun exposure), and pigmented nevi (moles) are common occurrences.

During adolescence and adulthood, the use of birth control pills or pregnancy may result in temporary changes in hair growth patterns or hyperpigmentation of the cheeks and forehead known as *melasma* or *pregnancy mask*. Other hormonal abnormalities may result in excessive facial and body hair in women (androgen-related). Hormonal and genetic changes also produce male-pattern baldness (alopecia). Smoking is an independent causative factor of facial wrinkles.[18]

The skin exhibits changes that denote the onset of senescence (the process or condition of growing old). These changes may be caused by the aging process itself (intrinsic aging), the cumulative effects of exposure to sunlight (photoaging), or environmental factors (extrinsic aging). As aging occurs, both structural and functional changes occur in the skin, resulting clinically in diminished pain perception, increased vulnerability to injury, decreased vascularity, and a weakened inflammatory response.

Visible indications of skin changes associated with aging include gray hair, balding and loss of secondary sexual hair, and increased facial hair. For women, excessive facial hair may occur along the upper lip and around the chin. Women may also experience balding after menopause. Men frequently develop increased facial hair in the nares, eyebrows, and helix of the ear.

Other common age-related integumentary changes include lax skin, vascular changes (e.g., decreased elasticity of blood vessel walls, angiomas), dermal or epidermal degenerative changes, and wrinkling. Wrinkling signifies loss of elastin fibers, weakened collagen, and decreased subcutaneous fat and is accelerated by smoking and excessive sun exposure.

Blood vessels within the reticular dermis are reduced in number, and the walls are thinned. This compromises blood flow and appears physiologically as pale skin and an impaired capacity to thermoregulate, a possible contributing factor to the increased susceptibility of older individuals to hypothermia and hyperthermia. Many other benign changes may occur, including seborrheic keratoses (raised brown or black wartlike growths), lentigines (liver spots, unrelated to the liver but rather secondary to sun exposure), and skin tags (small flesh-colored papules).

A primary factor in the loss of protective functions of the skin is the diminished barrier function of the stratum corneum (outermost layer of the epidermis; see Fig. 7.1). As this layer becomes thinner, the skin becomes translucent and paper thin, reacting more readily to minor changes in humidity, temperature, and other irritants. There are fewer melanocytes, with decreased protection against UV radiation.

The epidermis is also one of the body's principal suppliers of vitamin D, which is produced when the hormone 7-dehydrocholesterol is exposed to sunlight. At 65 years of age, the levels of that hormone are only about 25% of what they were in youth, contributing to vitamin D deficiency and, because vitamin D plays a vital role in building bone, to osteoporosis as well.

It is generally agreed that one of the major and important contributions to skin aging, skin disorders, and skin diseases is the oxidative damage that occurs to the skin as a result of environmental exposures and endogenous (within the skin itself) factors.

The skin is rich in lipids, proteins, and deoxyribonucleic acid (DNA), all of which are extremely sensitive to the oxidation process. Scientists are striving to understand the mechanisms involved in skin oxidation and the skin defense systems in order to understand skin aging and the mechanisms involved in various pathologic processes of the skin.[43]

7.2 Special Implications for the PTA: Aging and the Integumentary System The PTA must remain alert to all skin changes, because age-associated blunting of vascular and immune responses may make skin findings more subtle in older adults than in younger clients with similar disorders. Vascular changes affecting thermoregulation and wound healing require careful consideration when planning therapy intervention.

Likewise, loss of collagen increases susceptibility to shearing force trauma, increasing the risk for pressure ulcers. Wound healing is impaired in intrinsically aged compared with young skin in that the rate of healing is appreciably slower, but paradoxically the resultant scar is usually more cosmetically acceptable.[26]

Skin diseases and symptoms caused by skin disorders are exceedingly common among the older population. Although these disorders are not usually life threatening, they may provoke anxiety and psychologic distress. Often the client has not brought these concerns to the attention of a physician, and the PTA is the first health care professional to observe the skin lesion.

It is important to ask about physical findings in other parts of the body (e.g., the client may not mention genital lesions or may be unaware of the significance of other symptoms). All dermatologic lesions must be examined by a physician, and anyone with evidence of sun damage, particularly those with actinic keratoses, should have a full skin examination annually.

COMMON SKIN DISORDERS

Atopic Dermatitis

Definition and Incidence

Atopic dermatitis (AD) is a chronic inflammatory skin disease. It is the most common type of eczema, frequently already present during the first year of life and affecting more than 10% of children.

AD is considered an early manifestation of atopy that appears before the development of allergic rhinitis or asthma. The word *atopic* (from *atopy*) refers to a group of three associated allergic disorders: asthma, allergic rhinitis (hay fever), and AD. There is usually a personal or family history of allergic disorders present, and AD is often associated with food allergies as well.

Etiologic and Risk Factors

The exact cause of AD is unknown, although recent studies have demonstrated the complex interrelationship of genetic, physical environment, skin barrier, pharmacologic, psychologic, and immunologic etiologic factors that contribute to the development and severity of AD.[46,91]

The pathomechanisms associated with AD are also unknown but most likely include both immediate and cellular immune responses. Two possibilities include the release of inflammatory mediators by autoallergens and the release of proinflammatory cytokines by autoreactive T cells in response to autoallergens mediated by immunoglobulin E (IgE).[88]

AD is often associated with increased levels of serum IgE and with sensitization to food allergens.[79] Some foods may be responsible for exacerbations of skin inflammation, but their pathogenic role must be clinically assessed before an avoidance diet is recommended.[36] *Xerosis* (abnormal dryness) associated with AD is usually worse during periods of low humidity and over the winter months in northern latitudes.

Compared with normal skin, the dry skin of AD has a reduced water-binding capacity, higher transepidermal water loss, and a decreased water content. Rubbing and scratching of itchy skin are responsible for many of the clinical changes seen in the skin. Hands frequently in and out of water make the condition worse.

Clinical Manifestations

AD begins in many people during infancy in the form of a red, oozing, crusting rash classified as acute dermatitis. As the child grows, the chronic form of dermatitis results in skin that is dry, thickened, and brownish-gray in color (lichenified). The rash tends to become localized to the large folds of the extremities as the person becomes older. It is found mainly on flexor surfaces such as the elbows and knees, neck, sides of the face, eyelids, and backs of the hands and feet. Hand and foot dermatitis can become a significant problem for some people.

Xerosis and pruritus are the major symptoms of AD and cause the greatest morbidity with severely excoriated lesions, infection, and scarring. Viral, bacterial, and fungal secondary skin infections may cause further changes in the skin. *Staphylococcus aureus* is the most common bacterial infection, resulting in extensive crusting with serous weeping, folliculitis (inflammation of hair follicles), pyoderma (pus), and furunculosis (boils).

Diagnosis, Treatment, and Prognosis

Although no cure exists, AD often resolves spontaneously, and more than 90% of cases of AD can be effectively controlled through proper management. The goal of medical therapy is to break the inflammatory cycle that causes excess drying, cracking, itching, and scratching.

Personal hygiene, moisturizing the skin, avoidance of irritants, topical pharmacology, and systemic medications (e.g., antibiotics, antihistamines, and, rarely, systemic corticosteroids) are treatment techniques currently available. *S. aureus,* known to colonize the skin of people with AD, may exacerbate skin lesions, and infection with this organism needs to be treated with antibiotics. Advancing knowledge in understanding the immunologic basis of this disease will continue to result in effective new local and systemic treatments in the decade to come.[57,80]

7.3 Special Implications for the PTA: Atopic Dermatitis The PTA may be instrumental in providing client education that results in avoiding factors that precipitate or exacerbate inflammation and then teaching proper management techniques for flare-ups. Daily care (hydration and lubrication) of the skin is important, and applications (two or three times daily) of emollients that occlude the skin to prevent evaporation and retain moisture should be recommended.

Creams or ointments containing petrolatum or lanolin may be used unless the person is sensitized to lanolin (see the section on contact dermatitis), and those that contain urea or lactic acid improve the binding of water in the skin and prevent evaporation. In the case of skin redness, the skin lesion must be identified first because of possible fungal origin requiring an antifungal preparation.

Understanding the individual disease pattern and identifying exacerbating factors are crucial to effective management of this disorder. It is important to identify and eliminate triggers that cause the AD to flare.

Older clients should be encouraged to bathe with tepid water using a nondrying, fragrance-free or unscented soap or other agent when indicated. Emollients must be applied to the body within 5 minutes after showering or bathing, especially in dry winter weather, to prevent further skin drying.

Dermatitis must be considered a precaution, if not a contraindication, to some treatment modalities used by PTAs. The use of water, alcohol, or any topical agents containing alcohol should be avoided. Use topical agents such as ultrasound gel and mobilization creams carefully and observe for any skin reaction. A nonreactive response does not guarantee the client will not react when such agents are subsequently applied in future interventions. Caution and careful observation are encouraged.

Contact Dermatitis
Definition and Incidence

Contact dermatitis can be an acute or chronic skin inflammation caused by exposure to a chemical, mechanical, physical, or biologic agent. It is one of the most common environmental skin diseases occurring at any age. As people age, they may develop delayed cell-mediated hypersensitivity to a variety of substances that come in contact with the skin.

Common sensitizers include nickel (found in jewelry and many common foods), chromates (used in tanning leathers), wool fats (particularly lanolin, found in moisturizers and skin creams), rubber additives, topical antibiotics (typically neomycin and bacitracin),[82] and topical anesthetics, such as benzocaine or lidocaine.[28] Dermatitis of unknown cause is more commonly diagnosed in the older population.

A small percentage of the population is allergic to silicone. The PTA is most likely to see this reaction in a sensitized person with an amputation using a silicone type of interface in a prosthetic device (designed to reduce shear, decrease repetitive stress, and absorb shock). Silicone sheets used for scar reduction in the postburn population may also result in an episode of contact dermatitis.

Clinical Manifestations

Intense pruritus (itching), erythema (redness), and edema of the skin occur 1 to 2 days after exposure in previously sensitized persons. Clinical manifestations begin at the site of exposure but then extend to more distant sites. These conditions may progress to vesiculation, oozing (watery discharges), crusting, and scaling. If these symptoms persist, the skin becomes thickened, with prominent skin markings and pigmentation changes. Older people have a less pronounced inflammatory response to standard irritants than do younger persons.

Diagnosis, Treatment, and Prognosis

If contact dermatitis is suspected, the client should be referred to a physician. A detailed history and careful examination are frequently all that are needed to make the diagnosis. It may be necessary to perform patch testing to identify the causative agent.

Primary treatment is removal of the offending agent; treatment of the skin is secondary. The client should be instructed to avoid contact with strong soaps, detergents, solvents, bleaches, and other strong chemicals. The involved skin should be lubricated frequently with emollients. Topical anesthetics or steroids (topical or sometimes systemic) or both may be prescribed. For those people unable to avoid known allergens, immunosuppressant therapies (including phototherapy) can be helpful.[3]

Acute lesions usually resolve in 3 weeks; chronic lesions persist until the causative agent has been removed.

7.4 Special Implications for the PTA: Contact Dermatitis The therapy professional should always consider the client's reactions to external substances. This is of particular importance when applying any cream, topical agent, or solution. Various modalities used within the profession may involve causative substances (e.g., whirlpool additives, ultrasound gels, self-sticking electrode pads).

Whirlpools should be used rarely and with no additives. The client's skin must always be examined before and after intervention for the appearance of any adverse reactions. The client should be instructed to report any discomfort or unusual findings during or after treatment to the PTA.

The person with contact dermatitis associated with the use of a silicone sleeve or interface with a prosthetic device should be cautioned about the use of soaps that do not include a rinsing agent. Many antibacterial and antiperspirant soaps leave particles on the surface of the skin that act as a barrier on the skin's surface against bacterial invasion. A rash or blister may occur in patchy areas corresponding to pressure points when the friction of the interface drives the soap particles back into the skin.[8]

There are several care plans for this type of contact dermatitis. The use of alcohol-based lubricants or soaps, antifungal or antibacterial soaps without a rinsing agent, and lanolin should be avoided. Soap-free cleansing agents or a soft soap should be used for daily cleansing, and a petroleum-based ointment can be applied to the limb before putting on the liner.

Water-based ointments should be avoided when using urethane liners, because these can cause the normally tacky urethane to adhere to the skin so that when the liner is removed, bits of skin may be pulled off as well. Alcohol-based lubricants or soaps should also be avoided with urethane products because these components act as a solvent on urethane, increasing the stickiness of the urethane.[8]

Eczema and Dermatitis
Definition

Eczema and *dermatitis* are terms that are often used interchangeably to describe a group of disorders with a characteristic appearance. Eczema or dermatitis is a superficial inflammation of the skin caused by irritant exposure, allergic sensitization (delayed hypersensitivity), or genetically determined idiopathic factors.

Many types of dermatitis are represented according to these major etiologic categories (e.g., allergic dermatitis, irritant dermatitis, seborrheic dermatitis, nummular eczema, AD, stasis dermatitis).

Eczema or dermatitis has three primary stages. This condition can manifest in any one of the three stages, or the three stages may coexist. *Acute dermatitis* is characterized by extensive erosions with serous exudate or by intensely pruritic, erythematous papules and vesicles on a background of erythema.

Subacute dermatitis is characterized by erythematous, *excoriated* (scratched or abraded), scaling papules or plaques that are either grouped or scattered over erythematous skin. Often the scaling is so fine and diffuse that the skin acquires a silvery sheen.

Chronic dermatitis is characterized by thickened skin and increased skin marking (called *lichenification*) secondary to rubbing and scratching; excoriated papules, fibrotic papules, and nodules (prurigo nodularis); and postinflammatory hyperpigmentation and hypopigmentation.

Incidence and Etiologic Factors

Dermatitis is a common skin disorder in older people. It may be caused by hypoproteinemia, venous insufficiency, allergens, irritants, or underlying malignancy, such as leukemia or lymphoma. Because older people often take multiple medications, dermatitis from drug–drug interaction can occur. The normal aging process with the flattened epidermal–dermal junction and loss of dermis results in skin fragility, which contributes to the development of skin tears and dermatitis.

Stasis Dermatitis

Stasis dermatitis is the development of areas of very dry, thin skin and sometimes shallow ulcers of the lower legs primarily as a result of venous insufficiency. The client commonly has a history of varicose veins or deep vein thrombosis.

The process of stasis dermatitis begins with edema of the leg as a result of slowed venous return. As the venous insufficiency continues, the tissue becomes hypoxic from inadequate blood supply. This poorly nourished tissue begins to necrose.

The clinical manifestations include itching, a feeling of heaviness in the legs, brown-stained skin, and open shallow lesions. The lesions are very slow to heal because of a lack of oxygenated blood. Gait training is an important part of compression, the gold standard, in the treatment of stasis dermatitis. Compression hose work well in the recumbent position, but ambulation with the muscular contract-relax cycle pushes the venous return within the compressive field.

Environmental Dermatoses

It is well documented that exposure to various environmental chemicals and to physical stimuli is capable of inducing adverse cutaneous responses. Common environmental skin diseases seen in a therapy practice may include irritant and allergic dermatitis, acne lesions, pigmentary changes (hyperpigmentation, hypopigmentation, absence of pigment), photosensitivity reactions, scleroderma, infectious disorders, and cutaneous malignancy. Each of these environmentally induced skin conditions is discussed separately in this chapter.

Rosacea
Definition and Incidence

Rosacea[a] is a chronic facial disorder of middle-aged and older people. Although it is a form of acne, it is differentiated by age, the presence of a large vascular component (erythema, telangiectasis), and usually the absence of comedones.

An acneiform rosacea can occur, with papules, pustules, and oily skin. No known cause or factor has been identified to explain the pathogenesis of this disorder. It is currently considered a condition with vascular and inflammatory components in the presence of an altered innate immune response.[14] A statistically significant incidence of migraine headaches accompanying rosacea has been reported.

Clinically, the cheeks, nose, and chin (sometimes the entire face) may have a rosy appearance marked by reddened skin. This benign but obvious condition is most common in people with fair skin who flush easily. Sun, hot weather, and humidity can all trigger flare-ups; the condition is worse in the summer.

The affected person reports burning or stinging with episodes of flushing that come and go, but the condition may worsen over time, causing lasting redness, pimples, telangiectasias, or nasal hypertrophy (rhinophyma). Inflammatory papules are prominent, and there may be pustules. It is not uncommon to have associated ophthalmic disease, including blepharitis and keratitis.

Medical management aimed at the inflammatory papules, pustules, and surrounding erythema may include topical or systemic therapy. Rosacea tends to be a persistent condition that can be controlled with drugs. Chronic rosacea has long been treated by pulsed dye lasers. A newer system, the intense pulsed light (IPL) system, allows deeper and wider-area treatments.[73]

Rosacea associated with *Helicobacter pylori*–induced gastritis can be effectively treated by addressing the underlying problem. Although therapists do not treat this condition, clients with other diagnoses often manifest this condition also. Clients with this condition should see a physician for adequate medical treatment.

SKIN INFECTIONS

Many bacterial, viral, fungal, and other parasitic skin infections encountered by the PTA are not the primary focus of intervention but rather occur in clients who are hospitalized or being treated for some other condition. Many of these skin disorders are contagious (Table 7.2) and require careful handling by all health care professionals to avoid spreading the infection and becoming contaminated.

Sources of infection differ depending on the disease and mode of transmission. Predisposing factors to skin infections include decreased resistance, dehydrated skin, burns or pressure ulcers, decreased blood flow, contamination from nasal discharge, poor hygiene, and crowded living conditions. Only the most common skin infections encountered in the therapy or rehabilitation setting are discussed further in this section.

---

[a] For further information contact the National Rosacea Society, Barrington, Illinois, 1-847-382-8971 or www.rosacea.org.

TABLE 7.2 Infections of the Skin

Type of Infection	Transmission
Bacterial	
Impetigo contagiosa	Contagious
Pyoderma	Contagious
Folliculitis (pimple, boil)	Contagious; minimal chance of spread
Cellulitis	Contagious[a]
Viral	
Verrucae (warts)	Contagious; autoinoculable[b]
Verruca plantaris (plantar wart)	Contagious; autoinoculable
Herpes simplex	
Type 1: cold sore, fever blister	Contagious
Type 2: genital lesion	Contagious
Varicella-zoster virus (herpes zoster; shingles)	Contagious; chickenpox can occur in anyone not previously exposed
Fungal	
Tinea corporis (ringworm)	Person to person Animal to person Inanimate object to person
Tinea capitis (affects scalp)	Person to person Animal to person
Tinea cruris (jock itch)	Person to person
Tinea pedis (athlete's foot)	Transmission to other people rare despite general opinion to the contrary
Candidiasis	Person to person; sexually transmitted during birth from colonized vagina to neonatal oropharynx
Other	
Scabies	Person to person; sexually transmitted during birth from colonized vagina to neonatal oropharynx Inanimate object to person
Lice	Same as scabies

[a]Technically cellulitis is contagious, but from a practical point of view the chances of it spreading are very low, and transmission would require a susceptible host—for example, an open cut on the therapist's hand coming in contact with blood or pus from the client's open wound.
[b]Capable of spreading infection from one's own body by scratching.

Bacterial Infections

Normally the skin harbors a variety of bacterial flora, including the major pathogenic varieties of staphylococci and streptococci. The degree of their pathogenicity depends on the invasiveness and toxigenicity of the specific organisms, the integrity of the skin, the barrier of the host, and the immune and cellular defenses of the host. Organisms usually enter the skin through abrasions or puncture wounds of the hands.

In the therapist's practice, periwound care requires cleaning away from the wound opening to avoid introducing bacteria from the surrounding skin into the wound. Clinical infection develops 3 to 7 days after inoculation. Septicemia can develop if treatment is not provided or if the person is immunocompromised.

People at risk for the development of bacterial infections include children and adults who are immunocompromised, such as occurs with acquired or inherited immunodeficiency; anyone in a debilitated physical condition; those undergoing immunosuppressive therapy; and those with a generalized malignancy, such as leukemia or lymphoma.

All these factors emphasize the importance of careful hand-washing before and after caring for infected people and their lesions and cleanliness to prevent spread of infection.

Some conditions (e.g., impetigo) are easily spread by self-inoculation, therefore the affected person must be cautioned to avoid touching the involved area. Follicular lesions should not be squeezed because this will not hasten the resolution of the infection and may increase the risk of making the lesion worse or spreading the infection.

Impetigo
Definition and Incidence

Impetigo is a superficial skin infection commonly caused by staphylococci or streptococci. It is most commonly found in infants, young children 2 to 5 years of age, and older people. Predisposing factors include close contact in schools, overcrowded living quarters, poor skin hygiene, anemia, malnutrition, and minor skin trauma. It can be spread by direct contact, environmental contamination, or an arthropod vector. Impetigo often occurs as a secondary infection in conditions characterized by a cutaneous barrier broken to microbes, such as eczema or herpes zoster excoriations.

Clinical Manifestations

Small macules (flat spots) rapidly develop into vesicles (small blisters) that become pustular (pus-filled). When the vesicle breaks, a thick yellow crust forms from the exudate, causing pain, surrounding erythema, regional adenitis (inflammation of gland), cellulitis (inflammation of tissue), and itching.

Scratching spreads infection, a process called *autoinoculation*. Lesions frequently affect the face, heal slowly, and leave depigmented areas. If infection is extensive, malaise, fever, and lymphadenopathy may also be present. A less common presentation occurs with few isolated bullae.

Treatment

Single small lesions can often be managed by soaking them for 10 minutes with drying agents (Burow's solution). Oral antibiotics are regularly used to treat impetigo. Rarely, extensive lesions require systemic antibiotics to reduce the risk of glomerulonephritis and to prevent this contagious condition from spreading. A skin swab culture may be necessary to determine the contaminating organism.

Cellulitis
Definition and Incidence

Cellulitis is a rapidly spreading acute inflammation with infection of the skin and subcutaneous tissue that spreads widely through tissue spaces. *Streptococcus pyogenes* or *Staphylococcus* is the usual cause of this infection in adults and *Haemophilus influenzae* type B in children, although other pathogens may be responsible. Clients at increased risk for cellulitis include older adults and people with lowered resistance from diabetes, malnutrition, steroid therapy, and the presence of wounds or ulcers.

Other predisposing factors include the presence of edema or other cutaneous inflammation or wounds (e.g., tinea, eczema, burns, trauma). Venous insufficiency or stasis, thrombophlebitis, surgery, substance abuse, immunocompromise (e.g., HIV infection, chemotherapy, autoimmune diseases, chronic use of immunosuppressants), and lymphedema also predispose individuals to this condition. There is a tendency for recurrence, especially at sites of lymphatic obstruction.

Cellulitis usually occurs in the loose tissue beneath the skin, but it may also occur in tissues beneath mucous membranes or around muscle bundles. The skin is erythematous, edematous, tender, and sometimes nodular. Cellulitis can develop under the skin anywhere but affects the extremities most often.

Clinical Manifestations

Erysipelas, a surface cellulitis of the skin, affects the upper dermis and is characterized by patches of skin that are red and painful with sharply defined borders and that feel hot to the touch. Red streaks extending from the patch indicate that the lymph vessels have been infected. Facial cellulitis involves the face, especially the cheek or periorbital or orbital tissues; the neck may also be affected. Pelvic cellulitis involves the tissues surrounding the uterus and is called *parametritis*.

Treatment

Intravenous (IV) antibiotic infusion is the primary treatment. Oral antibiotics can be effective if the infection is caught early; individuals who are susceptible to recurrent cellulitis may have a prescription for oral antibiotics on hand (or at least a prescription that can be filled at the first sign of infection). The PTA can draw around the red area and take photos to look for progression. If there are signs of progression and/or new onset of constitutional symptoms (especially fever), the person must be seen by medical personnel immediately. Good nutrition and hydration are advised to help fight infection, repair tissue, and remove bacteria and their byproducts. Extensive cellulitis requires surgical debridement of the necrotic tissue. Lymphangitis may occur if cellulitis is untreated, and gangrene, metastatic abscesses, and sepsis can result.

Viral Infections

Viruses are intracellular parasites that produce their effect by using the intracellular substances of the host cells. Viruses are composed only of DNA or ribonucleic acid (RNA)—not both, usually enclosed in a protein shell, and are unable to provide for their own metabolic needs or to reproduce themselves.

After a virus penetrates a cell of the host organism, it sheds the outer shell and disappears within the cell, where the nucleic acid core stimulates the host cell to form more virus material from its own intracellular substance. In a viral infection the epidermal cells react with inflammation and vesication (as in herpes zoster) or by proliferating to form growths (warts).

Herpes Zoster

Definition and incidence. Herpes zoster, or shingles, is a local disease brought about by the reactivation of *varicella-zoster virus* (VZV), the same virus that causes a systemic disease called *varicella* (chickenpox). The initial infection with VZV is common during childhood. Shingles may occur and recur at any age, although peak incidence occurs from ages 50 to 70 years.

An estimated 300,000 episodes of zoster occur annually. Of these episodes, 95% are first occurrences and 5% are recurrences. By age 80 years, almost 15% of persons will have experienced at least one episode of zoster.[2] The disease is usually brought on by an immunocompromised state, such as occurs with stress, advancing age, underlying malignancy, organ transplantation, or acquired immunodeficiency syndrome (AIDS).

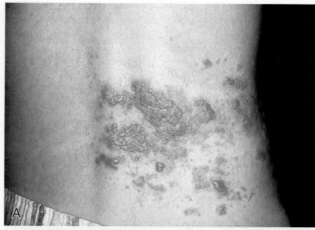

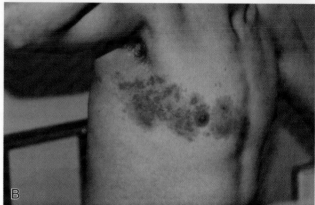

FIG. 7.3 Herpes zoster (shingles). (A) Lesions appear unilaterally along the path of a spinal nerve. (B) Eruptions involving the T4 dermatome. (A, From Bennett JE, Dolin R, Blaser MJ: Mandell, Douglas, and Bennett's principles and practice of infectious diseases, ed 8, Philadelphia, 2015, Saunders. B, Courtesy David Effron, MD. In Marx J, Hockberger R, Walls R: Rosen's emergency medicine: concepts and clinical practice, ed 8, Philadelphia, 2014, Saunders.)

Clinical manifestations. The vesicular eruption of zoster generally occurs unilaterally in the distribution of a specific dermatome supplied by a dorsal root or extramedullary cranial nerve sensory ganglion. Most often this involves the trunk or the area of the fifth cranial nerve; 2 to 4 days before the eruption the affected person may have some warning (prodromal symptoms) that the virus has become reactivated, especially in repeat incidences.

Early symptoms of pain and tingling along the affected spinal or cranial nerve dermatome are usually accompanied by fever, chills, malaise, and gastrointestinal (GI) disturbances; 1 to 3 days later, red papules are seen along a dermatome (Fig. 7.3). The lesions most commonly spread unilaterally around the thorax or vertically over the arms or legs.

Herpes papules rapidly develop into vesicles that vary in size and may be filled with clear fluid or pus. The vesicles are confined to the distribution of the infected nerve root and begin to dry 5 days after eruption, with gradual, progressive healing over the next 2 to 4 weeks.

Postherpetic neuralgia, or pain in the area of the recurrence that persists after the lesions have resolved, is a distressing complication of zoster with no adequate therapy currently available. Incidence of postherpetic neuralgia increases sharply in people over the age of 60 years and may last as long as 1 year after the episode of zoster. Children are unaffected by postherpetic pain.

In the adult, severe neuralgic pain can occur in peripheral areas innervated by the nerves arising in the inflamed root ganglia. The pain may be constant or intermittent and vary from light burning to a deep visceral sensation. The cause of postherpetic neuralgia is not fully understood. Scarring and degenerative changes involving the nerve trunks, ganglia, and skin may be important factors. The incidence of scarring and hyperpigmentation is much higher in older adults.

Occasionally herpes zoster involves the cranial nerves, especially the trigeminal and geniculate ganglia or the oculomotor nerve. Geniculate zoster may cause vesicle formation in the external auditory canal, ipsilateral facial palsy, hearing loss, dizziness, and loss of taste. Trigeminal ganglion involvement causes eye pain and possibly corneal and scleral damage with loss of vision.

In rare cases, herpes zoster leads to generalized central nervous system (CNS) infection, muscle atrophy, motor paralysis (usually transient), acute transverse myelitis, and ascending myelitis. More often, generalized infection causes acute retention of urine and unilateral paralysis of the diaphragm.

Diagnosis. Diagnosis is usually based on clinical examination and recognition of the skin lesions with accompanying systemic signs of infection. Laboratory diagnosis may include culture and histologic examination of a skin biopsy specimen.

Differentiation of herpes zoster from localized herpes simplex requires staining of antibodies from vesicular fluid and identification using a fluorescent monoclonal antibody test that is very sensitive and specific. A variety of serologic tests for the varicella antibody are available for individuals who are uncertain whether they have had childhood varicella.

Treatment. There is no curative agent for shingles, but supportive treatment to relieve itching and neuralgic pain is provided. The use of systemic corticosteroids within the first week of eruption may abort the attack and appears to reduce both the acute symptoms and the risk of postherpetic neuralgia in older persons.

Hospitalized clients with varicella-zoster should be placed in isolation rooms, and personnel entering the room should wear gowns, gloves, and masks. Eye involvement in zoster requires ophthalmologic evaluation and treatment.

A live varicella virus vaccine (Varivax) is available for use in persons 12 months of age or older who have not had varicella. The Advisory Committee on Immunization Practices (ACIP) also recommends the vaccine for use in susceptible persons after exposure to varicella. Data from the United States and Japan collected in a variety of settings indicate that varicella vaccine is effective in preventing illness or modifying the severity of illness if used within 3 days—and possibly up to 5 days—of exposure.[2]

The vaccine provides long-lasting (but not lifelong) immunity, with an 80% to 85% efficacy. Vaccine breakthrough cases are common but mild. Persons develop fewer lesions (usually less than 50) and lack systemic symptoms (such as fever).

Prognosis. Overall prognosis is good unless the infection spreads to the brain (rare). Most people recover completely, with the possible exception of scarring and, with corneal damage, visual impairment. Occasionally, intractable pain associated with neuralgia may persist for months or years. Persons who develop postherpetic neuralgia may require further medical intervention.

7.5 Special Implications for the PTA: Herpes Zoster Adults with herpes zoster (shingles) are infectious to persons who have not had chickenpox, and the person with shingles can develop shingles more than one time. For this reason, therapy staff who have never had chickenpox should receive the vaccination; complications and morbidity associated with adult onset of varicella warrant this precaution.

Any female PTA who is pregnant or planning a pregnancy should be tested for immune status if unsure about her previous history of chickenpox (varicella). This is especially important because transmissibility of the virus occurs 2 to 3 days before symptoms develop; immunocompromised clients with shingles are probably contagious during the entire period new lesions are appearing until all lesions are crusted over.

This means anyone receiving intervention by a PTA may be an asymptomatic host during the period of communicability; self-exposure and further transmission to others can occur without the PTA's awareness.

Susceptible health care workers with significant exposure to varicella should be relieved from direct client contact from day 10 to day 21 after exposure. If workers develop chickenpox, varicella lesions must be crusted before such workers return to direct client contact.

The Centers for Disease Control and Prevention (CDC) has set up guidelines for the care of all clients regarding precautions for the transmission of infectious skin diseases. These standard precautions should be used with all clients regardless of their disease status.

All skin lesions are considered potentially infectious and should be handled as such. The careful use of these precautionary measures severely limits the transmission of any disease. In addition, each hospital has isolation precautions organized according to categories of disease to prevent the spread of infectious disease to others. Every health care professional must be familiar with these procedures and follow them carefully. See also the section on isolation procedures in Chapter 5.

Neither heat nor ultrasound should be used on a person with shingles, because these modalities can increase the severity of the person's symptoms. Relaxation techniques may be useful for the person with severe herpetic pain. In the case of unresolved postherpetic neuralgia, the individual may benefit from a program of chronic pain management.

Warts (Verrucae)

Definition and incidence. Warts are common, benign viral infections of the skin and adjacent mucous membranes caused by human papillomaviruses (HPVs). The incidence of warts is highest in children and young adults, but warts can occur at any age. Transmission is probably through direct contact, but autoinoculation is possible.

Clinical manifestations. Warts may appear singly or as multiple lesions with thick white surfaces containing many pointed projections. Clinical manifestations depend on the type of wart and its location. The most common wart (verruca vulgaris) is referred to as such and appears as a rough, elevated, round surface most frequently on the extremities, especially the hands and fingers. Plantar warts are slightly elevated or flat, occurring singly or in large clusters referred to as *mosaic warts*, primarily at pressure points of the feet.

Diagnosis. Diagnosis is usually made on the basis of visual examination. Plantar warts can be differentiated from corns and calluses by certain distinguishing features. Plantar warts obliterate natural lines of the skin, may contain red or black capillary dots that are easily discernible if the surface of the wart is shaved down with a scalpel, and are painful on application of pressure. Both plantar warts and corns have a soft, pulpy core surrounded by a thick callous ring; plantar warts and calluses are flush with the skin surface.

Treatment. Some warts respond to simple treatment, and some disappear spontaneously. Warts can be chronic or recurrent. Many treatment regimens are available. The specific choice of treatment method is influenced by the location of the wart or warts, size and number of warts, presence of secondary infection, amount of tenderness present on palpation, age and gender of the client, history of previous treatment, and individual compliance with treatment. Over-the-counter salicylic acid preparations (e.g., DuoFilm, Wart-Off, Clear Away, and other wart-removing compounds) applied topically may be used to induce peeling of the skin.

Cryotherapy is performed with either liquid nitrogen or solid carbon dioxide. This procedure is widely used as the cosmetically preferred treatment choice, but it is painful. The procedure causes epidermal necrosis; the area dries and peels off together with the wart.

Acids in liquid form or as a paste (salicylic acid, lactic acid) can be painted on warts daily, removed after 24 hours, and reapplied. This treatment choice is not recommended for areas where perspiration is heavy, for areas likely to get wet, or for exposed body parts where patches are cosmetically undesirable. Acid therapy requires a commitment from the client or family to perform it on a daily basis.

Electrodesiccation and *curettage* of warts are widely used for common warts and occasionally for plantar warts. High-frequency electric current destroys the wart and is followed by surgical removal of dead tissue at the base with application of an antibiotic ointment and bandage for 48 hours. Atrophic scarring may occur, and the recurrence rate is 20% to 40%.

The use of mechanical (nonthermal) ultrasound has been advocated by some in the treatment of plantar warts, but this has not been widely accepted by the medical community.

Fungal Infections (Dermatophytoses)
Definition and Incidence
Fungal infections such as ringworm are caused by a group of fungi that invade the stratum corneum, hair, and nails.[28] These are superficial infections by fungi that live on—not in—the skin and are confined to the dead keratin layers, unable to survive in the deeper layers. Because the keratin is being shed (desquamated) constantly, the fungus must multiply at a rate that equals the rate of keratin production to maintain itself; otherwise the organisms would be shed with the discarded skin cells.

Fungal infections will spread without treatment; antifungal creams are available over the counter, but diagnosis is required to identify the skin lesion.

Ringworm (Tinea Corporis)
Dermatophytoses, or fungal infections of the hair, skin, or nails, are designated by the Latin word *tinea,* with further designation related to the affected area of the body (see Table 7.2). Tinea corporis, or ringworm, has no association with worms but rather is marked by the formation of ring-shaped pigmented patches covered with vesicles or scales that often become itchy (Fig. 7.4). Transmission can occur directly through contact with infected lesions or indirectly through contact with contaminated objects, such as shoes, towels, or shower stalls.

Diagnosis can be made through laboratory examination of the affected skin. Treatment for any type of ringworm requires

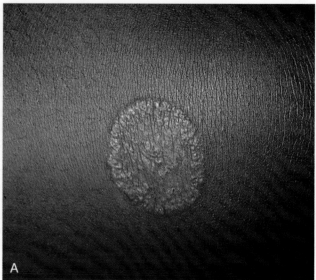
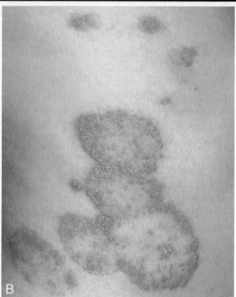

FIG. 7.4 Tinea corporis (ringworm). (A) Scales forming circular lesions with clear centers are characteristic of tinea corporis (ringworm). (B) Most adults and children have multiple lesions that are hyperpigmented in Caucasians and depigmented in dark-skinned people. The lesions occur most often on the face, chest, abdomen, and back of the arms. (From Zitelli BJ, McIntire SC, Nowalk AJ: Zitelli and Davis' atlas of pediatric physical diagnosis, ed 6, Philadelphia, 2012, Saunders.)

maintaining clean, dry skin and applying antifungal powder or topical agent as prescribed.

Treatment. Treatment with the drug griseofulvin may take weeks to months to complete and should be continued throughout the prescribed dosage schedule even if symptoms subside. Possible side effects of this agent include headache, GI upset, fatigue, insomnia, and photosensitivity. Prolonged use of this drug requires monitoring of liver function. Oral medication is reserved for clients with more involved cases. Because ringworm can be acquired by animal-to-human transmission (see Table 7.2), all household pets must be examined for the presence of ringworm as well. Other sources of infection include seats with headrests (e.g., theater seats,

seats on public transportation, or other public seats that can be shared).

Athlete's Foot (Tinea Pedis)

Tinea pedis, or athlete's foot, causes erythema, skin peeling, and pruritus between the toes that may spread from the interdigital spaces to the sole. Severe infection may result in inflammation, with severe itching and pain on walking. Some individuals develop a strong foot odor as well. Athlete's foot, often observed by the PTA, should be discussed with the client. Although the client may consider this condition a nuisance or a minimal problem that does not require medical attention, it can be an entry point for bacterial infections, especially in older adults. Keeping athlete's foot under control is an important way to prevent cellulitis, a bacterial infection in the legs, and is especially important in the presence of diabetes.[29]

Clean, dry socks and adequate footwear (well-ventilated, properly fitting) are important. After the feet are washed and dried thoroughly between the toes, antifungal cream or powder (the latter to absorb perspiration and prevent excoriation) can be applied.

A history of antibiotic use, yeast infections (candidiasis, including intestinal yeast), and other risk factors for *candidiasis* may contribute to athlete's foot. If symptomatic treatment including topical preparations does not eradicate the problem, treatment of intestinal yeast may be required.

7.6 Special Implications for the PTA: Fungal Infections The infectious nature of fungal infections requires specific hygienic measures common to all infectious conditions. Affected persons should not share hair care products (e.g., combs, brushes, headgear), clothes, or other articles that have been in proximity to the infected area. Affected persons must use their own towels and linens.

Because fungal infections are superficial (living on the skin), the PTA is advised to avoid shaving body hair for the application of electrodes or other adhesives. Cutting the hair closely will avoid providing microscopic nicks that can give entrance for the transmission of surface pathogens.

Other Parasitic Infections

Some parasitic infections of the skin are caused by insect and animal contacts. Contact with insects that puncture the skin for the purpose of sucking blood, injecting venom, or laying their eggs is relatively common. Substances deposited by insects are considered foreign to the host and may create an allergic sensitivity in that individual and produce pruritus, urticaria, or systemic reactions of a greater or lesser degree, depending on the individual's sensitivity.

Scabies

Definition and incidence. Scabies (mites) is a highly contagious skin eruption caused by a mite, *Sarcoptes scabiei.* It is a common public health problem with an estimated prevalence of 300 million cases worldwide. The female mite burrows into the skin and deposits eggs that hatch into larvae in a few days.

Scabies is easily transmitted by skin-to-skin contact or by contact with contaminated objects, such as linens or shared inanimate objects. Infections with human T-cell leukemia or lymphoma virus 1 (HTLV-1) and HIV are associated with scabies.[13] Mites can spread rapidly among members of the same household, nursing home, or institution, but the inflammatory response and itching do not occur until approximately 30 to 60 days after initial contact.

Clinical manifestations. The symptoms include intense pruritus (worse at night), usually excoriated skin, and the burrow, which is a linear ridge with a vesicle at one end. The mite is usually found in the burrow, commonly in the interdigital web spaces, flexor aspects of the wrist (volar surface), axillae, waistline, nipples in females, genitalia in males, and umbilicus. Intense scratching can lead to severe excoriation and secondary bacterial infection. Itching can become generalized secondary to sensitization.

Diagnosis and treatment. The mite can be excavated from one end of a burrow with a needle or a scalpel blade and examined under a microscope. In long-standing cases, a mite may not be found. At that point treatment is based on a presumptive diagnosis.

Treatment has traditionally been with a scabicide—usually a lotion or cream containing permethrin or lindane—applied to the entire body from the neck down. Single oral-dose therapy with ivermectin (Stromectol) is an effective treatment for this infestation. Permethrin is generally the treatment of choice for head lice and scabies because of its residual effect and because toxicity and absorption are minimal. Ivermectin may be reserved for cases in which permethrin fails[17]; further research is advocated regarding the safety and effectiveness of ivermectin.

7.7 Special Implications for the PTA: Scabies If a hospitalized person has scabies, prevent transmission to self and others by practicing good handwashing technique and by wearing gloves when touching the affected person and a gown when in close contact. Observe wound and skin precautions for 24 hours after treatment of scabies. Gas-autoclave blood pressure cuffs or other pieces of equipment used with the affected person before using them on other people. All linens and toweling used must be isolated after use until the person is noninfectious. If the person is treated anywhere outside the hospital room (e.g., on a plinth or treatment mat), the area must be thoroughly disinfected after each session.

In using a scabicide, the individual must understand that *no* area can be missed. After 24 hours, the affected person should bathe. All bed linens and clothes must be laundered in hot water or drycleaned. Other household members and those in close contact with the affected person should be treated. A second application of the cream or lotion may need to be applied 7 days later. The same procedure is followed.

Itching may persist for 1 to 2 weeks after treatment until the stratum corneum is replaced, but lesions on the forearms or legs can be occluded with *Unna's boots* to eliminate the scratch–itch cycle. Widespread bacterial infections require additional treatment with systemic antibiotics.

Pediculosis (Lousiness)

Definition and incidence. Pediculosis is an infestation by *Pediculus humanus,* a very common parasite infecting the head, body, and genital area. Transmission is from one person to another, usually on shared personal items, such as combs, lockers, clothes, or furniture. Lice are not carried or transmitted by pets. School-age children are easily infected, as are people who live in overcrowded surroundings and older adults who have poor personal hygiene, depend on others for care, or live in a nursing home.

P. humanus var. *capitis,* the head louse, is transmitted through personal contact or through shared hairbrushes or shared headwear. Severe itching accompanied by secondary eczematous changes develops, and small grayish or white nits (eggs) are usually seen attached to the base of the hair shafts.

Pediculus corporis, the body or clothes louse, produces intense itching, which in turn results in severe excoriations from scratching and possible secondary bacterial infections. The lice or nits are generally found in the seams of the affected individual's clothing.

Pediculus pubis (Phthirus pubis), the pubic or crab louse, is usually transmitted by sexual contact but can be transferred on clothing or towels. The lice and nits are usually found at the base of the pubic hairs. Sometimes dark brown particles (louse excreta) may be seen on underclothes.

Treatment. Traditional treatment has been with the appropriate cleaning solution (e.g., shampoo or soap containing permethrin) specific to the type of louse present. As with scabies, single oral-dose therapy of ivermectin (Stromectol) is an effective treatment for this infestation (see previous section on scabies).

7.8 Special Implications for the PTA: Pediculosis (Lousiness) The PTA must always be conscious of the personal hygiene of all clients. Anyone can get pediculosis (lice) regardless of age, socioeconomic status, or status of personal cleanliness. Wear gloves while carefully inspecting the head of any adult or child who scratches excessively. Look for bite marks, redness, and nits or movement that indicates a louse. If exposure to lice occurs, treatment for the client as well as the PTA may be required, depending on the exposure level. Use the same precautions outlined earlier in the section on scabies.

All combs and brushes should be soaked in the cleaning agent, and clothing must be boiled, dry cleaned, or washed in a machine (hot cycle). The seams of the clothing should be pressed with a hot iron. Carpets, car seats, pillows, stuffed animals, rugs, mattresses, upholstered furniture, and similar objects that come in contact with the affected person must be vacuumed or cleaned thoroughly with hot water and the cleaning agent. Any item that cannot be cleaned can be stored in a sealed plastic bag for 2 to 3 weeks until all lice have been killed.

SKIN CANCER

The American Cancer Society (ACS) estimates that skin cancers are the most prevalent form of cancer, eventually affecting nearly all Caucasian people older than 65 years of age. Skin cancer is the most rapidly increasing cancer in the United States, with over 1 million new cases of nonmelanoma (primarily basal and squamous cell) skin cancer diagnosed annually in the United States. There is no evidence that this epidemic has peaked.

Solar radiation (exposure to midrange-wavelength UVB radiation) causes most skin cancers, and protection from the sun during the first two decades of life significantly reduces the risk of skin cancer (Box 7.4). The melanoma rate is rising most rapidly in persons younger than 40 years of age, and melanoma is now the most common cancer in women aged 25 to 29 years and second only to breast cancer in the age group from 30 to 34 years.

In this chapter, skin cancer is discussed in three broad categories: benign, premalignant, and malignant. Malignant lesions

---

BOX 7.4   Important Trends in Skin Cancer

Incidence
- More than 1 million cases per year with the majority being the highly curable basal or squamous cell cancers; not as common is the most serious skin cancer (malignant melanoma), with an estimated 62,000 new cases per year.

Mortality
- Incidence: 3.5 million cases per year, with an estimated 68,720 new cases per year. Mortality: Total estimated deaths in 2009 were 11,150. Among those, 8650 are from malignant melanoma and 2500 are from other skin cancers.

Risk Factors
- Excessive exposure to ultraviolet radiation from the sun; fair complexion; occupational exposure to coal tar, pitch, creosote, arsenic compounds, and radium; chronic immunosuppression. Skin cancer is negligible in blacks because of heavy skin pigmentation.

Warning Signals
- Any unusual skin condition, especially a change in the size or color of a mole or other darkly pigmented growth or spot.

Prevention and Early Detection
- Avoid sun when ultraviolet light is strongest (e.g., between 10 a.m. and 4 p.m.); use sunscreen preparations. Basal and squamous cell skin cancers often form a pale, waxlike, pearly nodule or a red, sharply outlined patch. Melanomas are usually dark brown or black; they start as small molelike growths that increase in size, change color, become ulcerated, and bleed easily from a slight injury.

Treatment
- There are four methods of treatment: surgery, electrodesiccation (tissue destruction by heat), radiation therapy, and cryosurgery (tissue destruction by freezing). For malignant melanomas, wide and often deep excisions and removal of nearby lymph nodes are required.

Survival
- For basal cell and squamous cell cancers, cure is virtually ensured with early detection and treatment. Malignant melanoma, however, metastasizes quickly; this accounts for a lower 5-year survival rate for white people with this disease.

---

of the skin are considered as either melanoma or nonmelanoma. Kaposi's sarcoma (KS), which occurs in the skin, is not included in these categories and is discussed separately in this chapter.

Benign skin lesions such as seborrheic keratosis or nevi (moles) do not usually undergo transition to malignant melanoma or require treatment. Although most moles remain benign skin lesions, when malignant melanoma does occur, it often arises from a preexisting mole derived from pigment cells (melanocytes) of the skin.

Keratoacanthomas do require treatment. Precancerous lesions, such as actinic keratosis or Bowen's disease, may progress to malignancy and must be carefully evaluated. The most common types of (nonmelanoma) malignant skin cancer are basal cell carcinoma and squamous cell carcinoma.

These carcinomas occur twice as often in Caucasian men as in Caucasian women, and the incidence increases steadily with age. A third type of malignant skin cancer (also affecting Caucasian men more than Caucasian women), malignant melanoma, is the most serious skin cancer, resulting in early metastasis and possible death.

Benign Tumors
Seborrheic Keratosis
Seborrheic keratosis is a hereditary benign proliferation of basal cells occurring most frequently after middle age and manifesting as multiple lesions on the chest, back, and face. The lesions also often appear after hormonal therapy or inflammatory dermatoses. The areas are waxy, smooth, or raised lesions that vary in color from yellow to beige to dark brown or black. Their size varies from barely palpable to large verrucous (wartlike) plaques. These tumors are usually left untreated unless they itch or cause pain. Otherwise, cryotherapy with liquid nitrogen is an effective treatment.

Nevi (Moles)
Nevi are pigmented or nonpigmented lesions that form from aggregations of melanocytes beginning early in life. Most moles are pale brown, black, or flesh-colored and may appear on any part of the skin. They vary in size and thickness, occurring in groups or singly.

Nevi seldom undergo transition to malignant melanoma, but as previously mentioned, when malignant melanoma does occur, it often arises from a preexisting mole; the chances of cancerous transformation are increased as a result of constant irritation. Any change in size, color, or texture of a mole; bleeding; or excessive itching should be reported to a physician.

Precancerous Conditions
Actinic Keratosis
Actinic keratosis (also known as *solar keratosis*) is a skin disease resulting from many years of exposure to the sun's UV rays. The damage caused by overexposure to sunlight results in abnormal cell growth, causing a well-defined, crusty, or sandpaper-like patch or bump that appears on chronically sun-exposed areas of the body (e.g., face, ears, lower lip, bald scalp, dorsa of hands and forearms).

The base may be light or dark, tan, pink, red, or a combination of these, or it may be the same color as the skin. The scale or crust is horny, dry, and rough; it is often recognized by touch rather than sight. Occasionally it itches or produces a pricking or tender sensation. The skin abnormality or lesion develops slowly to reach a size that is most often 3 to 6 mm. It may disappear only to reappear later. Often there are several actinic keratoses present at one time.

Actinic keratosis affects nearly 100% of the older Caucasian population. It is most common in fair-complexioned, blue- or green-eyed, middle-aged men with a history of sun exposure (solar radiation). The number of lesions that develops is directly related to heredity and lifetime exposure to the sun.

There is a known risk of malignant degeneration and subsequent metastatic potential in neglected lesions. Almost half of the estimated 5 million current cases of skin cancer began as actinic keratosis lesions. It is important that this condition be diagnosed properly because it is often difficult to distinguish a large or hypertrophic actinic keratosis from a squamous cell carcinoma. A biopsy may be indicated.

Not all keratoses need to be removed. The decision about treatment protocol is based on the nature of the lesion, the number of lesions, and the age and health of the affected person. Treatment may be with 5-fluorouracil (5-FU, Efudex), a topical antimetabolite that inhibits cell division, or masoprocol cream; cryosurgery using liquid nitrogen; or curettage by electrodesiccation (superficial tissue destruction through the use of bursts of electrical current).

These clients should be advised to avoid sun exposure and use a high-potency (sun protection factor [SPF] 15) sunscreen 30 to 60 minutes before going outside. SPF 30 is recommended for people of fair complexion. Sunscreens are not recommended for infants under 6 months of age. Infants should be kept out of the sun or shaded from it. Fabric with a tight weave, such as cotton, is suggested.

Some conditions call for more invasive treatments, such as laser resurfacing (outer layers of the skin are vaporized) or chemical peels (outer layers are burned off via chemical solution). In June 2000 the U.S. Food and Drug Administration (FDA) approved the use of photodynamic treatment of actinic keratosis of the face and scalp using a topical application (Levulan Kerastick) followed by exposure to a nonlaser blue light source. This is a painful and involved treatment requiring application of Levulan 16 hours before exposure to the light source.

Bowen's Disease
Bowen's disease can occur anywhere on the skin (exposed and unexposed areas) or mucous membranes (especially the glans penis in uncircumcised males). It causes a persistent, brown to reddish brown, scaly plaque with well-defined margins. Often the person has a history of arsenic exposure in youth. Multiple lesions have been associated with an increased number of internal malignancies and therefore require close follow-up. Treatment is with surgical excision and topical 5-fluorouracil.

Malignant Neoplasms
Basal Cell Carcinoma
Definition and incidence. Basal cell carcinoma is a slow-growing surface epithelial skin tumor originating from undifferentiated basal cells contained in the epidermis. This type of carcinoma rarely metastasizes beyond the skin and does not invade blood or lymph vessels but can cause significant local destruction.

Until recently, this tumor rarely appeared before age 40 years and was more prevalent in blond, fair-skinned males. In people younger than 30, more women than men develop skin cancer associated with the use of indoor tanning booths with concentrated doses of UV radiation. Basal cell carcinoma is the most common malignant tumor affecting Caucasians, with a reported 100,000 new cases each year; African Americans and Asians are rarely affected.

Prolonged sun exposure and intermittent sun exposure are the most common causes of basal cell carcinoma, but immunosuppression (e.g., organ transplant recipients, individuals who are HIV positive), genetic predisposition, and, rarely, the site of vaccinations are other possible causes. Immunosuppressed organ transplant recipients are more likely to develop squamous cell carcinoma, whereas HIV-infected adults are far more likely to have basal cell carcinoma.

These lesions are seen most frequently in geographic regions with intense sunlight in people with outdoor occupations and on those areas most exposed: the face and neck. Dark-skinned people are rarely affected because their basal cells contain the pigment melanin, a protective factor against sun exposure. Anyone who has had one basal cell carcinoma is at increased risk for developing others. Recurrences of previously treated lesions are possible, usually within the first 2 years after initial treatment.

Clinical manifestations. Basal cell carcinoma typically has a pearly or ivory appearance, has rolled edges, and is slightly

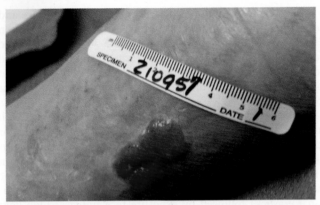

FIG. 7.5 Chronic venous ulcer. Basal cell carcinoma can also mimic a chronic venous ulcer, potentially causing a delay in diagnosis. Biopsy is required to make the definitive medical diagnosis. (Courtesy Harriett B Loehne, PT, DPT, CWS, FCCWS, Archbold Center for Wound Management, Thomasville, GA, 2006. Used with permission.)

elevated above the skin surface, with small blood vessels on the surface (*telangiectasia*).

The nodule is usually painless and slowly increases in size and may ulcerate centrally. More than 65% of basal cell carcinomas are found on the head and neck. Other locations are the trunk, especially the upper back and chest.

They also can appear similar to Bowen's disease, chronic venous ulcer (Fig. 7.5), or squamous cell carcinoma in a flatter, scaling lesion, usually on the trunk or extremities.

Diagnosis and treatment. Diagnosis by clinical examination of appearance must be confirmed via biopsy and histologic study. Treatment depends on the size, location, and depth of the lesion and may include curettage and electrodesiccation, chemotherapy, surgical excision, and irradiation.

Mohs' micrographic surgery is the gold standard treatment in which the specimen is excised, frozen-sectioned, and examined for positive margins while the client waits, thus ensuring clean margins before complex repairs are performed. Irradiation is used if the tumor location requires it and in older or debilitated people who cannot tolerate surgery.

Radiation therapy is generally contraindicated in persons younger than 50 years of age because of the risk of recurrence and the development of secondary radiation-induced tumors of the skin. Radiotherapy can be followed by chronic skin ulcers that are difficult to close, much less heal. Some radiation-induced ulcers open on and off for years, and some develop 10 to 20 years after the radiation therapy.[77]

If the tumor is identified and treated early, local excision or even nonexcisional destruction is usually curative. Skin grafting may be required in cases in which large areas of tissue have been removed. A new experimental treatment called *photodynamic therapy* (PDT) is being investigated in the treatment of superficial nonmelanoma skin cancers. This technique requires the administration of a drug that induces photosensitivity, followed in 48 to 72 hours by exposure to light that helps outline the tumor. The tumor cells concentrate this drug so as to allow selective destruction of the cancer cells when exposed to a laser light of 630 nm.[41,85]

Tretinoin has proven effective in preventing UV-induced lesions and can be considered for high-risk basal or squamous cell carcinoma patients, as well as those with actinic keratosis (note that this is off-label use).[72] Topical imiquimod was approved by the FDA in 2004 for individuals who have superficial basal cell carcinoma.[23]

Cytokine therapy, including interferon (IFN) and interleukin, is a type of systemic immunotherapy used to treat skin cancer. Both cytokines mentioned here have been FDA approved for metastatic melanoma.[69]

Prognosis. If left untreated, basal cell lesions slowly invade surrounding tissues over months and years, destroying local tissues such as bone and cartilage, especially around the eyes, ears, and nose.

Squamous Cell Carcinoma

Definition and incidence. Squamous cell carcinoma is the second most common skin cancer in Caucasians, usually arising in sun-damaged skin such as the rim of the ear, the face, the lips and mouth, and the dorsa of the hands. It is a tumor of the epidermal keratinocytes and rarely occurs in dark-skinned people.

Squamous cell tumors may be one of two types: in situ (confined to the site of origin) and invasive (infiltrate surrounding tissue). *In situ* squamous cell carcinoma is usually confined to the epidermis but may extend into the dermis. Common premalignant skin lesions associated with in situ carcinomas are actinic keratosis and Bowen's disease (see earlier section).

Invasive squamous cell carcinoma can arise from premalignant lesions of the skin, including sun-damaged skin, actinic dermatitis, scars, whitish discolored areas (leukoplakia), radiation-induced keratosis, tar and oil keratosis, and chronic ulcers and sinuses.

As with basal cell carcinoma, fair-skinned people have a higher incidence of squamous cell carcinoma. This particular type of tumor has a peak incidence at 60 years of age and affects men more than women.

Predisposing factors associated with squamous cell carcinoma include cumulative overexposure to UV radiation (e.g., outdoor employment or residence in a warm, sunny climate), burns, presence of premalignant lesions such as actinic keratosis or Bowen's disease, radiation therapy, ingestion of herbicides containing arsenic, chronic skin irritation and inflammation, exposure to local carcinogens (tar, oil), and hereditary disease such as xeroderma pigmentosum and albinism.

Organ transplant recipients who are chronically immunosuppressed are at risk for the development of recurring squamous cell carcinoma. Rarely, squamous cell carcinoma may develop at the site of a smallpox vaccination, psoriasis, or chronic discoid lupus erythematosus.

Clinical manifestations. Squamous cell lesions are more difficult to characterize than basal cell tumors. The squamous cell tumor has poorly defined margins because the edge blends into the surrounding sun-damaged skin.

This type of carcinoma can be present as an ulcer, a flat red area, a cutaneous horn, an indurated plaque, or a nodule. It may be red to flesh-colored and surrounded by scaly tissue. More than 80% of squamous cell carcinomas occur in the head and neck region.

Malignant transformation of any chronic wound can occur. *Marjolin's ulcer* is the term given to aggressive epidermoid tumors that arise from areas of chronic injury and form squamous cell carcinomas. Healed burn wounds are common sites, but any chronic wound can transform into a malignancy.

Usually lesions on unexposed skin tend to be more invasive and more likely to metastasize, with the exception of lesions on the lower lip and ears. Carcinoma at these sites tends to metastasize early, beginning with the process of induration and inflammation of the lesion. Metastasis can occur to the regional lymph nodes, producing characteristic systemic symptoms of pain, malaise, fatigue, weakness, and anorexia.

Diagnosis, treatment, and prognosis. An excisional biopsy provides definitive diagnosis and staging of squamous cell carcinoma. Other laboratory tests may be appropriate, depending on the presence of systemic symptoms. The size, shape, location, and invasiveness of a squamous cell tumor and the condition of the underlying tissue determine the treatment method selected. A deeply invasive tumor may require a combination of techniques. As with all benign, premalignant, or malignant skin lesions, sun protection is vitally important (see Box 7.2).

All the major treatment methods have excellent rates of cure; generally the prognosis is better with a well-differentiated lesion in an unusual location.

Malignant Melanoma

Definition. Malignant melanoma is a neoplasm of the skin originating from melanocytes or cells that synthesize the pigment melanin. The melanomas occur most frequently in the skin but can also be found in the oral cavity, esophagus, anal canal, vagina, or meninges or within the eye. The clinical varieties of cutaneous melanoma are classified into four types[4]:

1. *Superficial spreading melanoma* is the most common type of melanoma and accounts for 75% of cutaneous melanomas. It can occur on any part of the body, especially in areas of chronic irritation, the legs of females between the knees and ankles, or the upper back in both genders. It is usually diagnosed in people 20 to 60 years of age. It usually arises in a preexisting mole as a brown or black, raised patch with an irregular border and variable pigmentation (red, white, and blue; brown-black; black-blue). It is usually asymptomatic. Itching and bleeding may occur with advanced lesions.

2. *Nodular melanoma* is the most aggressive form and can be found on any part of the body with no specific site preference. Men 60 and older are affected more often than women. It is frequently described as a small, uniformly and darkly pigmented papule (may be grayish) that appears suddenly but enlarges quickly; it accounts for approximately 15% of cutaneous melanomas. This type invades the dermis and metastasizes early.

3. *Lentigo maligna melanoma* is a less common type of lesion occurring predominantly on sun-exposed areas, especially the head, neck, and dorsa of hands or under the fingernails, in the 50- to 80-year-old age group, accounting for 10% of cutaneous melanomas. This lesion looks like a large (3- to 6-cm), flat freckle with an irregular border containing varied pigmentation of brown, black, blue-black, red, and white found in a single lesion. These lesions enlarge and become progressively irregularly pigmented over time. Approximately one-third develop into malignant melanoma and therefore bear careful watching.

4. *Acral lentiginous melanoma* is a relatively uncommon form of melanoma accounting for 5% of all cutaneous melanomas. It is the most common form of melanoma in dark-skinned people (e.g., Africans, Asians). These lesions usually have flat, dark-brown portions with raised bumpy areas that are predominantly brown-black or blue-black. Most common areas include low-pigment sites where hair is absent, such as the palms of the hands, soles of the feet, nail beds of fingers and toes, and mucous membranes.

Incidence. Malignant melanoma accounts for up to 5% of all cancers, with a lifetime probability of developing melanoma at 1 in 36 for men and 1 in 55 for women. This has increased dramatically from a 1 in 1500 risk of developing melanoma in the 1930s.

Epidemiologists report that the incidence of melanoma is doubling every 10 to 20 years and call this a *melanoma epidemic.* The ACS estimated 76,250 new cases of malignant melanoma in 2012,[81] accounting for 9180 deaths, more than from any other skin disorder. The peak incidence is 40 to 60 years. The incidence is rising in younger age groups, but the disorder remains rare in children before adolescence.

Most people who develop melanoma have blond or red hair, fair skin, and blue eyes; are prone to sunburn; and are of Celtic or Scandinavian ancestry. These risk factors are believed to be linked to variations in a gene called *MC1R* that assists in producing melanin pigment to help protect the skin against UV rays.[30,65] Not all UVB radiation (280 to 320 nm) but all UVA radiation (320 to 400 nm)—the type produced by sun lamps—may promote skin cancer. For these reasons, the use of tanning devices is considered a significant risk factor for the development of skin cancer. In fact, the risk of melanoma reportedly increases 75% when the use of tanning devices starts before age 30. The greater the frequency and intensity of exposure, the greater the risk. The risk is even higher for individuals using high-intensity or high-pressure devices.[45]

Clinical manifestations. Melanoma can appear anywhere on the body, not just on sun-exposed areas. Common sites are the head and neck in men, the legs in women, and the backs of people exposed to excessive UV radiation. Up to 70% arises from a preexisting nevus. Any change in a skin lesion or nevus (increased size or elevation; bleeding; soreness or inflammation; changes in color, pigmentation, or texture) must be examined for melanoma.

Diagnosis. Early recognition of cutaneous melanomas can have a major impact on the surgical cure of this disease. The ACS suggests a monthly self-examination. A skin biopsy with histologic examination can distinguish malignant melanoma from other lesions, determine tumor thickness, and provide staging.

There are several techniques for staging skin cancer. The Breslow method measures the thickness of the melanoma; the thinner the melanoma, the better the prognosis. Melanomas less than 1 mm in depth generally have a very small chance of spreading. A second system (Clark levels) evaluates the layers of skin that are invaded by the melanoma to determine the appropriate stage.

A third method of staging, TNM, combines both previously described methods. Depending on the depth of the tumor invasion and metastatic spread, other testing procedures may be used, including baseline laboratory studies, a bone scan for metastasis, or computed tomography (CT) scan for metastasis to the chest, abdomen, CNS, and brain.

Diagnostic accuracy will continue to improve as digitized images of lesions can be analyzed, enabling the physician to determine whether a biopsy is needed. Computer-aided microscopic examination of biopsy slides may lead to better diagnosis, and teledermatology will give additional assistance in melanoma diagnosis. This technology makes it possible to compress digital images of suspicious lesions and transmit them electronically anywhere in the world, making consultation easier.[68]

Treatment. Neither cryosurgery with liquid nitrogen nor electrodesiccation is used to treat melanoma, although they are among the acceptable procedures for squamous cell and basal cell tumors. The treatment of choice for melanoma without evidence of distant metastatic spread is surgical excision. Surgery is combined with postoperative adjuvant radiation therapy and/or chemotherapy when there is evidence of regional spread. Surgery is not usually recommended for tumors that have metastasized to distant sites.[54]

Previously, surgical excision of the primary lesion site may have been accompanied by removal of regional lymph nodes (regional lymphadenectomy), but sentinel node biopsy (see Chapter 6) has been shown to be a reliable diagnostic tool for selecting individuals to undergo lymph node dissection, thereby reducing the extent of surgery for those who do not need this procedure.[7,55]

There is considerable debate about the use of sentinel node biopsy in staging melanoma at this time. Some studies report that this type of biopsy is highly reliable in experienced hands but is a low-yield procedure in most thin melanomas,[11,94] whereas others argue against its use except in clinical trials[86] and claim that there is not enough evidence to support the current combined use of sentinel node biopsy and systemic IFN for melanoma.[59]

Surgeons are now able to use aggressive surgical approaches on a more selective basis and therefore decrease treatment-related complications and disfigurement without compromising surgical goals. This change in treatment approach came as a result of the knowledge that the recurrence rate for people with melanoma clinically localized to the skin correlates directly with tumor thickness or depth of invasion, whereas the prognosis for people whose disease has spread to the regional lymph nodes depends primarily on the number of nodes that have tumors.[70]

Deep primary lesions may warrant adjuvant chemotherapy and biotherapy to eliminate or reduce the number of tumor cells, but there is no role at present for chemotherapy or radiation therapy as the initial treatment. Radiation therapy is used for metastatic disease to reduce tumor size and provide palliative relief from painful symptoms; it does not prolong survival time.

Prognosis. Malignant melanoma is a more serious problem than other skin cancers because it can spread quickly and insidiously, becoming life threatening at an earlier stage of development. It is essentially 100% curable if detected early, however.

The prognosis for all types of melanoma depends primarily on the tumor's thickness and depth of invasion, not on the histologic type. The thinner or more superficial the tumor, the better the prognosis. For example, melanoma lesions less than 0.76 mm deep carry an excellent prognosis (5-year survival rate is 90%), whereas deeper lesions (more than 0.76 mm) carry the risk for metastasis (5-year survival rate is 65% with local metastasis; 30% to 35% when distant metastases are present). Metastases to the brain, lungs, bones, liver, and CNS are universally fatal.

7.9 Special Implications for the PTA: Malignant Melanoma Health care professionals should be alert to the potential signs of skin cancer during observation and inspection of any client. The PTA should not become overly concerned about small pink spots on the client's skin, because other common skin conditions, such as eczema, psoriasis, and seborrheic dermatitis, are prevalent in more than half of all people at some time in their lives.

One should look for abnormal spots, especially in sun-exposed areas, that are rough in texture, are persistently present, and bleed on minimal contact or with minimal friction. Keep in mind that seborrheic keratosis commonly bleeds; once diagnosed, this bleeding should not cause undue alarm.

Any change in a wart or mole (color, size, shape, texture, ulceration, bleeding, itching) should be inspected by a physician. The Skin Cancer Foundation advocates the use of the ABCD method for early detection of melanoma and examination of dysplastic (abnormal in size or shape) moles (Box 7.5).

Other signs and symptoms that may be important include irritation and itching; tenderness, soreness, or new moles developing around the mole in question; or a sore that keeps crusting and does not heal within 6 weeks. For any client with a previous history of skin cancer, emphasize the need for continued close follow-up to detect recurrence early. Education on the effects of UV radiation and taking precautions (Box 7.6) can dramatically reduce the incidence of skin cancer.

If surgery included lymphadenectomy, the PTA may be involved in minimizing lymphedema or treating residual lymphedema. Wound management may involve care of a skin graft and the associated donor site; the donor site may be as painful as the tumor excision site and just as much at risk for infection. Standard precautions are essential for the postoperative as well as the immunosuppressed client.

For the dying client, hospice care may include pain control and management. It is important that pain relief not be delayed until after pain occurs but rather that a schedule of analgesia to prevent pain or to prevent an increase in pain level be instituted. Wound management must include standard of care unless the client declines it.

BOX 7.5   ABCD Method of Early Melanoma Detection

A: Asymmetry: uneven edges, lopsided in shape, one half unlike the other
B: Border: irregularity, irregular edges scalloped or poorly defined edges
C: Color: black, shades of brown, red, white, pink, occasionally blue
D: Diameter: Larger than a pencil eraser

BOX 7.6   Guidelines for Prevention of Skin Cancer

- Avoid peak hours of sunlight.
- Wear close-woven protective clothing.
- Use a sunscreen of sun protection factor (SPF) 15 or higher.
- Teach children sun protection.
- Do not work on getting a tan.
- Do not patronize tanning salons.
- Examine your skin regularly.
- If you notice any changes, see your physician promptly.

Kaposi's Sarcoma

Definition and incidence. KS is a malignancy of vascular tissue that manifests as a skin disorder. In the past, this tumor was most commonly seen in older men of Mediterranean or Eastern European origin, especially men of Jewish or Italian ancestry (now referred to as *classic KS*).

The sudden emergence of this malignancy in the Western world is directly related to AIDS-associated immunodeficiency, and the incidence has risen dramatically along with the incidence of AIDS *(epidemic KS)*. KS may also occur in kidney transplant recipients taking immunosuppressive drugs.

Research in the mid-1990s confirmed that KS is caused by a herpesvirus infection. Human herpesvirus 8 (HHV-8) or KS-associated herpesvirus (KSHV) is present in all AIDS-related KS and has been linked to all four forms of KS (classic, iatrogenic, endemic [African], HIV associated); however, only iatrogenic KS and HIV-associated KS have been shown to be linked to impairment of the host immune response. This universal detection of KSHV or HHV-8 suggests a central role for the virus in the development of KS and common etiologic factors for all KS types.[38] Genetic or hereditary predisposition may be a factor in the classic form.

Clinical manifestations. This neoplasm involves the skin and mucous membranes as well as other organs and can lead to tumor-associated edema and ulcerations. Classic KS occurs commonly on the lower extremities, and the affected areas are red, purple, or dark blue macules that slowly enlarge to become nodules or ulcers. Itching and pain in the lesions that impinge on nerves or organs may occur, and the legs become edematous as the sarcoma progresses, causing lymphatic obstruction. The lesions may spread by metastasis through the upper body to the face and oral mucosa.

Unlike classic forms of the disease, AIDS-associated KS is a multicentric entity that appears on the upper body (including face, chest, and neck) but can occur on the legs. It frequently involves lymph nodes, the lungs, and the GI tract; it may be the first manifestation of AIDS.

Early lesions are faint pink and can easily be mistaken for bruises or nevi and be ignored. Systemic involvement may manifest with one or more signs and symptoms, including weight loss (10% of body weight), fever of unknown origin in which temperature exceeds 100° F (37.8° C) for more than 2 weeks, chills, night sweats, lethargy, anorexia, and diarrhea. Pulmonary involvement may be characterized by dyspnea, cough, chest pain, and hemoptysis (in order of prevalence).

Diagnosis and treatment. Diagnosis is by skin biopsy using a highly sensitive and specific test for this neoplasm. A CT scan may be performed to detect and evaluate possible metastasis. Dermatologic manifestations of KS can be alarming, but it is visceral involvement associated with AIDS KS that is most life-threatening.

New antiretroviral therapies, in particular the protease inhibitors, appear to be changing the clinical course of KS, however. It is now possible to see a complete resolution and control of KS with the use of these new agents. As researchers continue to unravel the pathogenesis of KS, new treatment modalities will target its pathogenic pathways.

Chemotherapy remains an integral part of treatment, and new agents are becoming available. Experimental therapies that are being evaluated in ongoing clinical trials include angiogenesis inhibitors, pregnancy hormone (human chorionic gonadotropin), photodynamic therapy, isotretinoin, antiviral medications ganciclovir and foscarnet, retinoic acid derivatives, and immune modulators such as interleukin-12.[22,96]

7.10 Special Implications for the PTA: Kaposi's Sarcoma KS skin lesions in the AIDS client are not contagious, and the health care provider need have no fear of transmission of KS or HIV through daily contact with the client. Standard Precautions must be followed whenever providing care for clients with KS to prevent the spread of infection to the client.

Prevention of skin breakdown and wound management is the usual focus of intervention. Clients receiving radiation therapy must keep the irradiated skin dry to avoid possible breakdown and subsequent infection.

SKIN DISORDERS ASSOCIATED WITH IMMUNE DYSFUNCTION

Psoriasis

Definition and Incidence

Psoriasis is a chronic, inherited, recurrent inflammatory but noninfectious dermatosis characterized by well-defined erythematous plaques covered with a silvery scale (Fig. 7.6). There are several types of psoriasis, including plaque, guttate, erythrodermic, and pustular psoriasis.

Psoriasis occurs equally in both genders and most commonly in young adults (mean age of onset is 27 years) but can occur at any point in a person's life and, once present, becomes a chronic condition that may go in and out of remission. Although psoriasis can occur in infancy, it is uncommon in children under the age of 6 years. It is uncommon among African Americans but affects 1% to 2% of the Caucasian population; more than 6 million Americans are affected, with more than 100,000 classified as having severe cases.

The cause of psoriasis is unknown, but it appears to be hereditary—that is, the tendency to develop psoriasis is genetically determined. Researchers have discovered a significantly

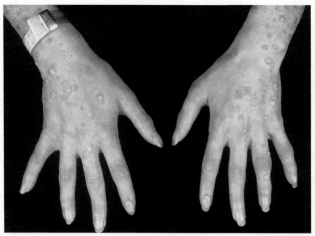

FIG. 7.6 Deforming arthritis of the hands in a person with psoriasis (psoriatic arthritis). (From McIntosh N, Helms PJ, Smyth RL, et al, editors: Forfar and Arneil's textbook of pediatrics, ed 7, Edinburgh, 2008, Churchill Livingstone.)

higher-than-normal incidence of certain human leukocyte antigens (HLAs) in families with psoriasis, suggesting a possible immune disorder.

Although psoriasis is believed to be genetically linked, it may be triggered by mechanical, UV, and chemical injury; various infections (especially by β-hemolytic streptococci); prescription drug use; psychologic stress; smoking; and pregnancy and other conditions causing endocrine changes.[60]

Cold weather and severe anxiety or emotional stress tend to aggravate psoriasis. Flare-ups are often related to specific systemic and environmental factors but may be unpredictable. New epidemiologic studies present evidence that both smoking and drinking have an influence on psoriasis, suggesting that simple modifications in lifestyle may reduce both the prevalence and the severity of psoriasis.[35]

Clinical Manifestations

Psoriasis appears as erythematous papules and plaques covered with silvery scales. The lesions in ordinary cases have a predilection for the scalp, chest, nails, elbows, knees, groin, skin folds, lower back, and buttocks. The occurrence may vary from a solitary lesion to countless patches covering large areas of the body in a symmetric pattern. Two clearly distinguishing features are the tendency for this condition to recur and to persist.

Lesions that develop at the site of a previous injury are known as the *Koebner phenomenon*. Flare-ups are more common in the winter as a result of dry skin and lack of sunlight. As is true for many skin ailments, the severity of psoriasis varies over time, and its exacerbations and remissions often correlate with stress levels and mental outlook.

The most common subjective complaints are itching and occasionally pain from dry, cracked, encrusted lesions. In approximately 30% of cases, psoriasis spreads to the fingernails, producing small indentations and yellow or brown discoloration. In severe cases, the accumulation of thick, crumbly debris under the nail causes it to separate from the nail bed (nail dystrophy).

Approximately 10% of people with psoriasis (usually moderate to severe) develop arthritic symptoms referred to as *psoriatic arthritis*. Psoriatic arthritis usually affects one or more joints of the fingers or toes, or sometimes the sacroiliac joints, and may progress to spondylitis. These clients report morning stiffness that lasts more than 30 minutes.

Joint symptoms show no consistent linkage to the course of the cutaneous manifestations of psoriasis but rather demonstrate remissions and exacerbations similar to those of rheumatoid arthritis. No other systemic effects of psoriasis have been reported, but hyperuricemia (gout) is fairly common in clients, precipitated by treatment with methotrexate and as a result of nucleic acid turnover caused by cellular breakdown in lesions of psoriasis.[95]

Diagnosis

Diagnosis depends on the history, clinical presentation, and, if needed, skin biopsy to identify psoriatic changes in skin or rule out other causes for the lesions. Typically the serum uric acid level is elevated because of accelerated nucleic acid degradation but without the corresponding gout usually associated with increased uric acid levels. Psoriasis must be distinguished from eczema, seborrheic dermatitis, and lichenlike papules.

Treatment

In the absence of a cure, the goal of treatment is to maximize remission and lessen outbreaks. Psoriasis therapy is highly individualized and often determined by trial and error because different people respond to different treatments. Psoriasis does not spread, and early treatment does not prevent the condition from progressing.

New options exist that adequately suppress the disease process and help provide better control of the psoriasis through the use of a combination of therapies. Various forms of local or systemic treatment routinely offered fall into five general categories: (1) topical preparations, (2) phototherapy, (3) antimetabolites, (4) oral retinoid therapy, and (5) immunosuppressants. New biologic systemic drugs for moderate to severe psoriasis are now available.[44]

Topical treatment of psoriasis is usually the first line of therapy, and therapeutic agents include corticosteroids, synthetic vitamin D_3, vitamin A analogs (retinoids), occlusive ointments (e.g., petroleum jelly, salicylic acid preparations, urea-containing topical ointments), oatmeal baths and emollients to relieve pruritus, and occasionally tar preparations.

Corticosteroids are the most commonly prescribed therapy for psoriasis but should be used sparingly because of the incidence of side effects, which have increased with the use of the superpotent fluorinated preparations. Only weak preparations, such as 0.5% or 1.0% hydrocortisone, should be used on the face, perineum, or other sensitive areas (e.g., the flexor surfaces of the arms, abdomen).

The major concerns with all corticosteroid preparations are dermal atrophy, skin fragility, fast relapse times, and, in rare cases, adrenal suppression resulting from systemic absorption. See also the section on corticosteroids in Chapter 2.

Crude coal tar, one of the oldest remedies for psoriasis, is assumed to work by an antimitotic effect (helps retard rapid cell production). This treatment consists of the daily application of 2% to 5% crude coal tar combined with a tar bath and UV light. The disadvantages of this treatment are the extended time commitments required by the client and the associated mess. Products (e.g., gels, creams, bath additives) with liquor carbonis detergens, an extract of crude coal, are also used to facilitate healing.

Exposure to UV light (phototherapy), such as UVB or natural sunlight, also helps retard rapid cell production. Widespread involvement may improve with whole-body irradiation with UV light. *PUVA* refers to the combination of an orally administered photosensitizing drug plus exposure to 1 to 1.5 hours of UVA radiation. It is more effective for the thick plaque type of psoriasis, pustular psoriasis, and generalized erythroderma.

Prognosis

Psoriasis usually recurs at intervals and lasts for increasingly longer periods, but treatment advances bring relief during flareups in approximately 85% to 90% of cases. Spontaneous cure is uncommon, and the risk of infection is high because of the greater-than-normal amounts of staphylococci present on psoriatic plaques.

People with psoriasis who are HIV positive are at high risk for infection from self-inoculation. As many as 20% of clients who develop psoriatic arthritis may sustain early and severe joint damage with accompanying deformity and disability.

7.11 Special Implications for the PTA: Psoriasis

Physical therapy and occupational therapy are key components in the treatment of moderate to severe psoriasis, with desired outcomes based on minimizing functional limitations.

Client instruction and direct intervention to provide skin care should emphasize the following: (1) steroid cream application must be in a thin film, rubbed gently into the skin until all the cream disappears; (2) all topical medications, especially those containing anthralin and tar, should be applied with a downward motion to avoid rubbing them into the hair follicles causing inflammation (folliculitis); (3) medication should be applied only to the affected lesions, avoiding contact with normal surrounding skin; and (4) gloves must be worn when applying the cream because anthralin stains and injures the skin.

After application, the client must dust himself or herself with powder to prevent anthralin from rubbing off on the clothes. Mineral oil followed by soap and water can be used to remove the anthralin; the skin should never be rubbed vigorously, but a soft brush can be used to remove the scales.

Any side effects, especially allergic reactions to anthralin; atrophy and acne from steroids; and burning, itching, and nausea, must be reported to the physician immediately. Squamous cell epithelioma may develop from PUVA. Cytotoxins from methotrexate therapy may cause hepatic or bone marrow toxicity; methotrexate may be teratogenic (harmful to fetal development) and should not be prescribed for women who are pregnant, trying to become pregnant, or breast feeding.

Other immunosuppressants, when used over a long period, have a cumulative effect and therefore the potential to cause serious side effects, such as poor wound healing, high blood pressure, kidney damage, and many other complications (see the section on immunosuppressants in Chapter 2).

Relaxation techniques and stress management are valuable tools whose use should be encouraged on a daily basis but especially during periods of exacerbation.

Psoriatic Arthritis

Clinically, psoriatic arthritis differs from rheumatoid arthritis in the more frequent involvement of the distal interphalangeal joints, asymmetric distribution of affected joints, presence of spondyloarthropathy (including the presence of both sacroiliitis and spondylitis), and characteristic extraarticular features (e.g., psoriatic skin lesions, iritis, mouth ulcers, urethritis, colitis, aortic valve disease).

Joints are less tender in psoriatic arthritis, which may lead to underestimation of the degree of inflammation. Pain and stiffness of inflamed joints are usually increased by prolonged immobility and alleviated by physical activity. Evidence of inflammation is pain on stressing the joint, tenderness at the joint line, and the presence of effusions.

The increasing use of nuclear magnetic resonance imaging (MRI) techniques, with their ability to delineate cartilage and ligamentous structures and to identify edema, is providing a radical improvement in ascertainment of musculoskeletal abnormalities associated with this disease. It is expected that in the decade to come new information about this aspect of the disease will offer greater information and improved treatment regimens.[92]

Psychologic Considerations

Psoriasis can result in psychologic problems because the skin lesions may cause the person to feel contagious and untouchable. In addition, ongoing treatment may not work, and the smell of some topical preparations and the stain may add to the psychologic reaction. Assure the client that psoriasis is not contagious. Flare-ups can be controlled with treatment, and stress control can help prevent recurrences. Relaxation techniques, group counseling, stress management, and medications to treat depression or anxiety may be suggested.

Cutaneous Lupus Erythematosus

Overview and Incidence

Lupus erythematosus is a chronic inflammatory disorder of the connective tissues. It appears in several forms, including cutaneous lupus erythematosus, which primarily affects the skin, and SLE, which affects multiple organ systems (including the skin) with considerably more morbidity and associated mortality. *Lupus* is the Latin word for "wolf," referring to the belief in the 1800s that the skin erosion of this disease was caused by a wolf bite. The characteristic rash of lupus is red, hence the term *erythematosus*.

The subsets of lupus erythematosus (LE) involving the skin include chronic cutaneous LE, acute cutaneous LE, and subacute cutaneous LE. Only the skin-related components of LE are discussed in this chapter. See also the section on SLE in Chapter 4.

Chronic cutaneous LE, formerly known as *discoid lupus*, is marked by chronic skin eruptions on sun-exposed skin that can lead to scarring and permanent disfigurement if left untreated. A systemic disorder does not usually develop, but in 5% to 10% of cases SLE does develop later; conversely, discoid lesions occur in 20% of people with SLE.[75] It is estimated that approximately 60% of persons with chronic cutaneous LE are women in their late twenties or older. The disease is rare in children.

Acute cutaneous LE occurs in 30% to 50% of clients who have SLE and includes malar erythema, widespread erythema, and bullous lesions. Association with systemic disease is highest in acute cutaneous LE, with virtually all clients meeting the American College of Rheumatology criteria for SLE (see Chapter 4).

The exact cause of cutaneous LE is unknown, but evidence suggests an autoimmune defect. There appear to be interrelated immunologic, environmental, hormonal, and genetic factors involved. Smoking is considered a risk factor for the development of the discoid lesions associated with chronic cutaneous LE and for resistance to treatment with antimalarial agents in this subgroup.[20,39]

Just how the sun causes skin rash flare-ups remains unknown. One theory is that the DNA of people with lupus becomes more antigenic (able to induce a specific immune response) when exposed to sunlight. This antigenicity causes accelerated antigen–antibody reactions and thus more deposition of immune complexes in the skin at the dermal–epidermal junction. The photosensitivity is most commonly associated with LE and not other rheumatologic diseases.

Clinical Manifestations

Discoid lesions (*chronic cutaneous LE*) can develop from the rash typically seen in lupus and become raised, red, smooth plaques with follicular plugging and central atrophy. The raised edges and sunken centers give them a coinlike appearance. Although these lesions can appear anywhere on the body, they usually erupt on the face, scalp, ears, neck, and arms or any part of the body that is exposed to sunlight. Lesions more typical of systemic lupus, discussed in Chapter 4, are shown in Fig. 7.7.

Hair tends to become brittle, and scalp lesions can cause localized alopecia (bald patches). Facial plaques sometimes assume the classic butterfly pattern, with lesions appearing on the cheeks and the bridge of the nose. The rash may vary in severity from a sunburned appearance to *discoid* (plaque-like) lesions. These lesions can occur in the absence of other

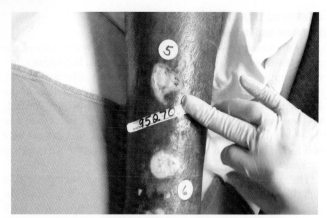

FIG. 7.7 The lesions here are typical of *systemic* lupus found on the lower extremities. They are ulcerated, punched-out wounds with necrotic bases. *Discoid* lupus lesions are usually found on the face and scalp and are raised, flat, coin-shaped wounds. (Courtesy Harriett B Loehne, PT, DPT, CWS, FCCWS, Archbold Center for Wound Management, Thomasville, GA, 2006. Used with permission.)

lupus-related symptoms and tend to leave hypopigmented and hyperpigmented scars that can become a cosmetic concern.

The most recognized skin manifestation of SLE *(acute cutaneous LE)* is the classic butterfly rash over the nose, cheeks, and forehead (Fig. 7.8) commonly precipitated by exposure to sunlight (UV rays). This classic rash over the nose and cheeks occurs in a large percentage of affected people, but rash can occur on the scalp, neck, upper chest, shoulders, extensor surface of the arms, and dorsum of the hands. These rashes begin abruptly and last from hours to days. They may be precipitated by sun exposure and often coincide with a flare-up of systemic disease.[75]

Other skin manifestations may point to the presence of vasculitis (inflammation of cutaneous blood vessels) leading to infarctive lesions in the digits, necrotic leg ulcers, or digital gangrene.

Acute cutaneous LE is usually accompanied by other symptoms of SLE, commonly including malaise, overwhelming fatigue, arthralgia, fever, arthritis, anemia, hair loss, Raynaud's phenomenon, and urologic symptoms associated with kidney involvement.

Diagnosis and Treatment

The client history and appearance of the rash itself are diagnostic. Skin biopsy of the discoid lesions may be performed. The client must report any changes in the lesions to the attending physician. Drug treatment consists of topical, intralesional, or systemic medication.

Potential side effects of systemic therapy (antimalarial agents) for chronic cutaneous LE include diarrhea, nausea, myopathy, cardiomyopathy, and anemia. The lesions resolve spontaneously in 20% to 40% of affected individuals or may cause hypopigmentation or hyperpigmentation, atrophy, and scarring. Discoid lesions are not life threatening (unless accompanied by complications of SLE) but are associated with psychologic distress and altered quality of life.

Skin lesions require topical treatment, maintaining an optimal wound environment (moist enough to allow tissue healing but not swamplike) while preventing further deterioration or infection. Most often, topical corticosteroid creams are used. The disease process can cause loss of skin integrity and subsequent loss of function.

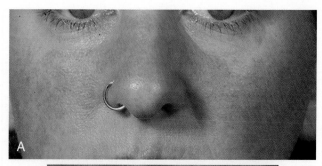

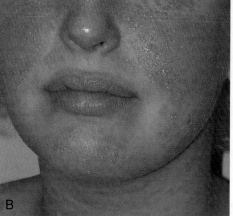

FIG. 7.8 (A) Butterfly rash of systemic lupus erythematosus across the bridge of the nose and the cheeks. (B) In some cases the rash covers a larger portion of the face, including the lips and chin. (A, From Herrick AL, Andrew JG, Funk L, et al.: Orthopaedics and rheumatology in focus, Edinburgh, 2010, Churchill Livingstone. B, From Bolognia JL, Jorizzo JL, Schaffer JV: Dermatology, ed 3, Philadelphia, 2012, Saunders.)

Clients with any form of cutaneous lupus should avoid prolonged exposure to the sun, fluorescent lighting, and reflected sunlight. They are encouraged to wear protective clothing, use sun-screening agents, and avoid engaging in outdoor activities during periods of intense sunlight (see Box 7.2).

Prognosis

The survival rate has improved dramatically in recent years, although death can occur from renal failure when there is kidney involvement causing progressive changes in the glomeruli; cardiac involvement with deposition of immune complexes in the coronary vessels, myocardium, and pericardium; or cerebral infarct.

7.12 Special Implications for the PTA: Cutaneous Lupus Erythematosus Clients with LE with skin involvement require careful assessment, supportive measures, and emotional support. Skin lesions should be checked thoroughly at each visit. The client should be urged to get plenty of rest, follow energy conservation guidelines, and practice good nutrition.

The PTA can be instrumental in teaching and assisting with skin care and prevention of skin breakdown, range-of-motion (ROM) exercises, prevention of orthopedic deformities, ergonomic and postural training, and relief of joint pain associated with SLE. Persons with LE exposed to the long-term effects of corticosteroids should be followed carefully. See specific side effects and the section on corticosteroids and 2.5 Special Implications for the PTA: Corticosteroids in Chapter 2. See also the section on SLE and 4.6 Special Implications for the PTA: Systemic Lupus Erythematosus in Chapter 4.

Systemic Sclerosis

Definition and Incidence

Systemic sclerosis (SSc, progressive systemic sclerosis [PSS], scleroderma) is a diffuse connective tissue disease that causes fibrosis of the skin, joints, blood vessels, and internal organs. SSc is a chronic disease, lasting for months, years, or a lifetime, and is classified according to the degree and extent of skin thickening.

The presence of a distinctive, widespread vascular lesion characterized by endothelial abnormalities as well as by proliferative reaction of the vascular intima was a significant factor in changing terminology from *scleroderma* to *systemic sclerosis*. General clinical vernacular still refers to this condition as *scleroderma*, although that term simply refers to thickening or hardening of the skin.

There are two distinct subtypes: systemic scleroderma and localized scleroderma (Box 7.7). *Systemic scleroderma* can take one of three forms: limited (lSSc), diffuse (dSSc), and an overlap form with either diffuse or limited skin thickening.

Limited cutaneous SSc was previously known as the *CREST syndrome* from its manifestations (*calcinosis, Raynaud's phenomenon, esophageal dysmotility, sclerodactyly, telangiectasia*). Persons with this form of SSc have a much lower incidence of serious internal organ involvement, although pulmonary hypertension and esophageal disease are not uncommon. Skin tightness is limited to the hands and face (excluding the trunk).

Although the diffuse form is less common than the limited form, it is by far the more debilitating because of the more frequent renal and pulmonary involvement. Some measurable degree of heart, lung, or kidney involvement, or any combination of these, can be found in the majority of people with SSc.

Diffuse scleroderma is characterized by involvement of all body parts, including the skin. In most people this involvement tends to progress slowly, if at all; but if involvement is to become severe, it tends to do so early, within the first 5 years. The severity of the disease depends on the number of organs affected and the extent of the effect.

Localized scleroderma affects primarily the skin in one or many different areas without visceral organ involvement and is therefore a benign form of this disease. Localized scleroderma should not be confused with limited cutaneous scleroderma. The latter is a form of systemic rather than localized disease.

There is further differentiation of localized scleroderma: *morphea* is characterized by hard, oval patches on the skin, generally on the trunk. These patches are usually white with a purple ring around them. *Linear* refers to the bandlike lesions that occur in the areas of the arms, legs, and forehead. The bones and muscles beneath these areas may also be affected. Ultimately, ROM and a child's growth are greatly affected. Linear scleroderma often occurs in childhood.

The annual incidence of SSc based on epidemiologic studies of hospital records and death certificates is 10 to 20 cases per 1 million, affecting approximately 400,000 Americans. SSc affects women two to three times more often than men, with the female/male ratio peaking at 15:1 during the childbearing years.

The cause of scleroderma is reportedly unknown. However, several groups suggest that scientific evidence accumulated over the last 50 years strongly points to SSc as an acquired disease triggered by bacteria (*Mycoplasma*).[9,47] It has also been suggested that an autoimmune mechanism is the underlying cause because specific autoantibodies occur in the sera of these clients. Other possible triggers suggested include cytomegalovirus (CMV; increased levels of anti-CMV antibodies present in scleroderma) or immune reactions to viral or environmental factors.[40]

Clinical Manifestations

The three stages in the clinical development of scleroderma are the *edematous stage,* the *sclerotic stage,* and the *atrophic stage.* In the edematous stage, bilateral nonpitting edema is present in the fingers and hands and, rarely, in the feet. The edema can progress to the forearms, arms, upper chest, abdomen, back, and face. After a few weeks to several months, edema is replaced by thick, hard skin.

The replacement of edema takes place in the sclerotic stage, when the skin becomes tight, smooth, and waxy and seems bound down to underlying structures. Accompanying changes include a loss of normal skin folds, decreased flexibility, and skin hyperpigmentation and hypopigmentation.

The skin changes may stabilize for periods (years) and may then either progress to the third stage or soften and return to normal. Actual atrophy of skin may occur, particularly over joints at sites of flexion contractures, such as the proximal interphalangeal joints and the elbows. Such thinning of the skin contributes to the development of ulcerations at these sites. Softening and return to normal of the skin may occur to some extent. Improvement typically begins centrally, so that the last areas to become classically involved are the first to show regression.

BOX 7.7   Classification of Scleroderma

Systemic Sclerosis

Limited (75% to 80%)
- Symmetric skin thickening
- Restricted to distal extremities and face
- Slow progression of skin changes
- Late development of visceral involvement
- CREST syndrome
- Relatively good prognosis (≥70% survival at 10 years)

Diffuse (15% to 20%)
- Symmetric skin thickening
- Widespread, affecting distal and proximal extremities, face, trunk
- Rapid progression of skin changes
- Early appearance of visceral involvement (GI tract, lungs, heart, kidneys)
- Overall poor prognosis (40% to 60% survival at 10 years)

Overlap (5% to 10%)
- Either diffuse or limited skin thickening
- Associated with one or more connective tissue diseases (e.g., systemic lupus erythematosus, dermatomyositis)

Localized Scleroderma
- Morphea
- Single or multiple plaques of skin fibrosis without systemic disease
- Linear
- Single or multiple fibrotic bands involving skin deeper tissues

CREST, Calcinosis, Raynaud's phenomenon, esophageal dysmobility, sclerodactyly, telangiectasia; *GI,* gastrointestinal.

BOX 7.8   Characteristics Likely to Be Seen in Clients with Systemic Sclerosis Early and Late in the Disease Course

Early (≤5 Years)

Limited Disease
- Rapidly progressive
  - Renal crisis (5%)
  - Interstitial lung disease (severe in 10%–15% of cases)
- Slowly progressive
  - Reynaud's phenomenon
  - Cutaneous ulceration
  - Esophageal dysmotility

Diffuse Disease
- Rapidly progressive
  - Skin thickening
  - Heart involvement (severe in 10%–15%)
  - Interstitial lung disease (severe in 15%)
- Renal crisis (15%–20%)
  - Contractures, joint pain
  - Cutaneous ulcerations
  - Esophageal dysmotility
  - Gastrointestinal complications

Late (>5 Years)

Limited Disease
- Slowly progressive
  - Reynaud's phenomenon
  - Cutaneous ulcerations
  - Esophageal dysmotility
  - Gastrointestinal complications
- Very late
  - Pulmonary artery hypertension
  - Biliary cirrhosis

Diffuse Disease
- Improvement
  - Skin thickening
  - Musculoskeletal pain
- Slowly progressive
  - Heart, lung, kidney involvement
  - Reynaud's phenomenon
  - Esophageal dysmotility
  - Gastrointestinal complications

Modified from Clements PJ: Systemic sclerosis: natural history and management strategies, J Musculoskelet Med 11:43–50, 1994.

Not all people pass through all the stages. Subcutaneous calcification (calcinosis) is a late-developing complication that is considerably more frequent in lSSc. Sites of trauma are often affected, such as the fingers, forearms, elbows, and knees. These calcifications vary in size from tiny deposits to large masses ulcerating the overlying skin.

Raynaud's phenomenon. Scleroderma affects everyone in a different fashion. Each previously mentioned form affects the body in different ways (Box 7.8). Raynaud's phenomenon is very often the first manifestation of SSc, preceding the onset of all the other signs and symptoms of the disease by months or years.[25] It appears almost universally in lSSc and in approximately 75% of cases of dSSc.

Raynaud's phenomenon is characterized by sudden blanching, cyanosis, and erythema of the fingers and toes as the walls of the blood vessels that supply the hands and feet become narrowed, making it difficult for the blood to pass through. Closure of the muscular digital arteries, precapillary arterioles, and arteriovenous shunts of the skin causes the hands or feet to become white and numb and then bluish in color as blood flow remains blocked.

As the spasm eases and blood flow returns (approximately 10 to 15 minutes after the triggering stimulus has ended), rewarming occurs and the fingers or toes become red and painful. This cycle is initiated in response to stress or exposure to cold. Progressive phalangeal resorption may shorten the fingers, and compromised circulation resulting from abnormal thickening of the arterial intima may cause slowly healing ulcerations on the tips of the fingers or toes that may lead to gangrene.[90]

Skin. Other symptoms include pain, stiffness, and swelling of the fingers and joints. Skin thickening produces taut, shiny skin over the entire hand and forearm. As tightening progresses, contractures may develop. Flexion contractures are especially severe in people with dSSc.

Facial skin may also become tight and inelastic, and the face takes on a stretched and masklike appearance, with thin lips and a pinched nose. Peripheral nervous system involvement affects nerve terminals, reducing sensory fibers in SSc skin. Neuropeptides released by sensory nerve endings are reduced, resulting in vasoconstriction in the skin.

Neuromusculoskeletal system. Most persons with dSSc have disuse atrophy of muscle because of limited joint motion secondary to skin, joint, or tendon involvement. A small percentage of people may have overlap syndromes and demonstrate marked weakness and inflammatory myopathy indistinguishable from polymyositis or dermatomyositis.

Some individuals develop myositis or erosive arthropathy that complicates the joint retraction induced by skin fibrosis. SSc also targets the peripheral nervous system with distal mononeuropathy of the median nerve as a frequent and early feature.[24] Neuropathy from carpal tunnel syndrome is also common.

Polyarthralgias affect both small and large joints and are especially frequent early in dSSc; polyarthritis is unusual. Tenosynovial involvement with inflammation and fibrosis of the tendon sheath or adjacent tissues is characterized by the presence of carpal tunnel syndrome and by coarse, leathery friction rubs palpated during motion over the extensor and flexor tendons of the fingers, distal forearms, knees, ankles, and other sites. These friction rubs are found almost exclusively in persons with dSSc, and their presence signifies a poorer overall clinical outcome.[90]

Viscera. GI motility dysfunction affects the esophagus and anorectal regions, causing frequent reflux, heartburn, dysphagia, and bloating after meals. Other effects include abdominal distention, diarrhea, constipation, and malodorous, floating stools. In advanced disease, cardiac and pulmonary fibrosis develops.

Cardiac involvement can be manifested as myocardial disease, pericardial disease, conduction system disease, or arrhythmias. Pulmonary involvement is characterized by impaired diffusing capacity for carbon monoxide. Kidney involvement and scleroderma renal crisis are now considered rare because of the introduction of angiotensin-converting enzyme (ACE) inhibitors.[24]

Other. Nearly 50% of adults with scleroderma report other symptoms, such as major depression, sexual dysfunction, trigeminal neuralgia, hypothyroidism, dental involvement, and corneal tears.

Diagnosis

Early diagnosis and accurate staging of visceral involvement are fundamental for appropriate management and therapeutic approach to this disease, but diagnosis can be delayed because there is no single laboratory test diagnostic for SSc. A thorough physical examination and history are the first steps to a definitive diagnosis.

Treatment

Presently there is no cure for SSc. A global vision of SSc is necessary for this multisystem disease, and each treatment program is individualized to manage the specific disease process. Treatment ranges from merely symptomatic for a person with only limited skin involvement after 5 years to aggressive treatment for a person with early, diffuse skin involvement.

When organ involvement occurs, it most often develops early in the disease course, and in the acute phase it requires aggressive management. The program may include medications (e.g., immunosuppressants, penicillamine, antiinflammatory drugs), exercises, joint protection techniques, skin protection techniques, and stress management.

Treatment of the pulmonary complications (pulmonary hypertension, interstitial lung disease) remains difficult. Home blood pressure monitoring can screen for acute hypertension signaling a renal crisis; treatment with ACE inhibitors may be lifesaving.

Prognosis

The prognosis in SSc principally depends on early diagnosis; the intensity and rapidity of involvement of the lungs, heart, gut, and kidneys; and appropriate medical management. A model to predict mortality based on a combination of three factors (proteinuria, elevated erythrocyte sedimentation rate [ESR], low carbon monoxide diffusing capacity) has been reported to have an accuracy of more than 80% in predicting mortality. The absence of these three factors is associated with 93% survival.[6]

Spontaneous recovery is common in children, but approximately 30% of clients with SSc die within 5 years of onset. Persons with dSSc who have lived beyond the 5-year mark with no significant visceral involvement are unlikely to experience such organ involvement. Those in whom significant visceral disease developed early can expect a slowing in its progression or at least a stabilization of its course. This 5-year mark is also a time when skin softening begins and musculoskeletal aches and pains begin to ease.

When started early, treatment with ACE inhibitors now prevents previously fatal complications (acute hypertension, renal failure). Aggressive treatment of early interstitial lung disease may further survival.[27] Localized scleroderma may reach an end point beyond which the disease does not progress.

7.13 Special Implications for the PTA: Systemic Sclerosis
Itching can be a major problem in dSSc, and excoriation from scratching can cause open wounds susceptible to infection. The PTA can offer some simple suggestions to soothe skin, ease the itching, and prevent skin damage (see Box 7.2).

Local management of digital tip ulcers may include an occlusive dressing to promote wound healing and protect against trauma and infection. Commercial occlusive dressings are particularly helpful with larger noninfected ulcers.

Infected ulcers are treated with a trial of oral antistaphylococcal antibiotics and may require surgical debridement of necrotic tissue. Local skin care requires avoidance of excessive bathing or using moisturizing creams containing glycerin.

Muscle

Myositis (muscle inflammation) is treated with corticosteroids and sometimes requires the addition of immunosuppressive drugs, whereas fibrotic myopathy (fibrotic tissue laid down within the muscle) is best managed with strengthening and ROM exercises. The efficacy of using soft tissue mobilization or similar techniques has not been investigated. Caution must be used when attempting such treatment, because the skin of these people is usually very sclerosed and sensitive to pressure. Aquatic therapy is an excellent choice for clients with this condition.

Joints and Tendons

Joint and tendon sheath involvement is common and may be treated successfully with nonsteroidal antiinflammatory drugs (NSAIDs). In early dSSc, tenosynovitis can be very painful, limiting joint movement. In addition to NSAIDs, early aggressive therapy is important in preventing or minimizing contractures.

For clients with scleroderma, regular exercise will assist with keeping the skin and joints flexible, maintaining better blood flow, and preventing contractures. Active and passive stretching exercises are necessary but difficult in the presence of extreme pain.

Analgesia is required to optimize participation in an exercise program. Protecting swollen and painful joints from stresses and strains is also an important factor. This may require teaching ways to carry out activities of daily living (ADLs) without causing strain on the joint or joints.

Lightweight splints may be necessary to provide joint protection. Dynamic splinting has not been found effective in preventing flexion contractures. Carpal tunnel syndrome, which often occurs before the diagnosis of scleroderma, usually responds well to conservative treatment without requiring surgery.

Exercise

Practice patterns in this area will vary depending on the form of cardiovascular or pulmonary involvement manifested. When cardiopulmonary involvement occurs, intervention must take into consideration the effects of this disease on the individual's activity and lifestyle. The client's primary diagnosis and primary intervention may be integument- or orthopedics-related, but functional limitations may be present secondary to systemic involvement (e.g., decreased aerobic capacity, endurance, and overall general physical condition secondary to cardiovascular and/or pulmonary involvement).

Psychologic Considerations

Persons with early dSSc with or without organ involvement are often anxious because their bodies are changing rapidly and in unexpected ways. They may not understand the grave nature of the disease.

Because persons with dSSc are at greatest risk for early visceral disease and early mortality, education about the disease is important, as is identifying where they are in the natural history of SSc. They should be encouraged to take their blood pressure at home at least three times per week, because this is the best method of screening for acute hypertension.

Polymyositis and Dermatomyositis
Definition

Polymyositis and dermatomyositis are the two most common idiopathic inflammatory diseases of muscle. Other types of inflammatory muscle disease have been distinguished, but no satisfactory classification of the idiopathic inflammatory myopathies exists; however, histologic analysis allows differentiation among the types of dermatomyositis.[5] They are diffuse, inflammatory myopathies that produce symmetric weakness of striated muscle, primarily the proximal muscles of the shoulder and pelvic girdles, neck, and pharynx. These related illnesses belong to the family of rheumatic diseases. These diseases often progress slowly, with frequent exacerbations and remissions.

Incidence

Polymyositis and dermatomyositis are not very common in the United States, affecting approximately 5 to 10 persons per 1 million; the incidence appears to be increasing. Myositis can affect people of any age, but mostly adults 45 to 65 and children 5 to 15 years old are affected. Twice as many women as men are affected, with the exception of dermatomyositis associated with malignancy, which is most common in men over age 40 years.

The cause of these conditions remains unknown, although there appears to be some autoimmune mechanism whereby the T cells inappropriately recognize muscle fiber antigens as foreign and attack muscle tissue.

Clinical Manifestations

Symmetric proximal muscle weakness is the dominant feature of these diseases, although it is variable in its onset, progression, and severity. In some people, symptoms appear suddenly, progress rapidly, and quickly result in a bedridden state, sometimes necessitating ventilatory assistance and tube feeding.

More typically, malaise and weight loss develop insidiously over months or even years, with some people either unable to identify the onset of the disease or unaware of the gradual disability developing. Fatigue, rather than weakness, is a commonly reported symptom, but close questioning usually reveals functional losses indicating weakness as well. Pain is not a key feature of these diseases in the adult population, although aching muscles are not uncommon. Muscle wasting is observed in long-standing or severe cases.

Cardiac involvement is not uncommon and contributes significantly to mortality. Nearly half of all people with polymyositis or dermatomyositis have arrhythmias, congestive heart failure, conduction defects, ventricular hypertrophy, or pericarditis.

Pulmonary disease (progressive pulmonary fibrosis) can result from weakness of the respiratory muscles, intrinsic lung pathologic conditions, or aspiration. Swallowing difficulties, nasal regurgitation, and esophageal dysphagia and reflux are common, especially in severe cases.

Polymyositis. Polymyositis begins acutely or insidiously with muscle weakness, tenderness, and discomfort. The proximal muscles of the shoulder and pelvic girdle are affected more often than the distal muscles, usually in a symmetric pattern, but asymmetry is common.

The legs are affected more often than the arms, and the anterior thigh is more frequently involved than the posterior thigh. Initially the muscles may be slightly swollen, but as the disease progresses muscular atrophy and induration become more noticeable, reflecting the deposition of fibrous tissue. Some persons have a mild peripheral neuropathy with loss of deep tendon reflexes.

Early signs of muscle weakness may include impaired functional status, such as difficulty climbing stairs, getting up from a chair, reaching into an overhead cupboard, combing the hair, or lifting the head from a pillow; difficulty with balance; or a tendency to fall, often resulting in a fracture.

Other muscular effects may include decreased deep tendon reflexes, contractures, arthralgias, arthritis, an inability to move against resistance (e.g., pushing open a heavy door, opening a car door), proximal dysphagia (difficulty swallowing), and dysphonia (difficulty speaking).

Dermatomyositis. When a rash is associated with polymyositis, it is referred to as *dermatomyositis*. A characteristic purplish rash appears on the eyelids (heliotrope erythema), accompanied by periorbital edema (puffy eyelids). The rash may progress to the anterior neck, upper chest and back, shoulders, and arms and may appear around the nail beds. Gottron's papules (red or violet, smooth or scaly patches) may appear on the knuckles, elbows, knees, or medial malleoli.

Although the disease usually begins with erythema and swelling of the face and eyelids, cutaneous manifestations can develop concomitantly with muscle involvement or even afterward with proximal muscle weakness manifested as reaching overhead, difficulty getting up out of a chair, going up stairs, shortness of breath, and difficulty swallowing. The cutaneous lesions of dermatomyositis are nearly always present by the time proximal muscle weakness manifests itself. In some persons, muscle involvement is minimal, whereas in others it may progress to wasting and contractures associated with extreme disability.[95]

Diagnosis

The diagnosis of myositis is often difficult because it resembles closely several other diseases and the pathologic manifestation can be localized, sometimes resulting in nondiagnostic biopsies. The physician must rule out internal malignancy first, requiring appropriate medical testing. The presence of progressive, symmetric weakness is a hallmark diagnostic finding.

Laboratory studies to evaluate muscle enzymes, biopsy to assess muscle fibers, and electromyography (EMG) to measure the electrical activity of the muscles are all necessary to properly diagnose myositis.

Treatment

The treatment must be individualized; the components include medication, exercise, and rest. High-dose daily oral systemic corticosteroid therapy is the usual initial pharmacologic treatment for polymyositis or dermatomyositis. Steroids reduce the inflammation, shorten the time to normalization of muscle enzymes, and reduce morbidity. Persons who do not respond well to steroids or who are unable to tolerate the high dosages required may be treated with immunosuppressive drugs.

Prognosis

The adult prognosis varies depending on age and progression of the disease process, but overall prognosis has improved with the introduction of systemic glucocorticoid therapy. At present, 85% of people with dermatomyositis can be expected to survive. Approximately 50% are left with residual weakness and have persistently elevated serum creatine kinase (CK) levels or experience a relapse when corticosteroids are reduced, and 20% are substantially disabled.

Generally, the prognosis is worse with visceral organ involvement, and death occurs from associated malignancy, respiratory disease, or heart failure. Side effects of therapy (corticosteroids, immunosuppressants) contribute to long-term morbidity. The prognosis for children is guarded if the disease is left untreated; it progresses rapidly to disabling contractures and muscular atrophy.

7.14 Special Implications for the PTA: Polymyositis and Dermatomyositis Physical therapy plays a pivotal role in the management of myositis. Manual muscle testing and tests of functional abilities are useful tools in following disease progression and therapeutic response over a long period. The individualized exercise program can help improve muscle strength and function.[31] Aerobic exercise testing may be a useful functional assessment tool in some cases.[89]

It is suggested that the medication regimen be well established before exercise is begun. In the early stages of treating myositis, the muscle fibers are fragile and could be damaged further, causing rhabdomyolysis (disintegration of muscle fibers) from exercises and other forms of therapy.

The PT/PTA team treating a client with myositis should keep in close contact with the physician, who will be using physical examination and laboratory tests to determine the most opportune time for initiating a graded exercise program (i.e., when muscle enzyme levels fall to acceptable levels, indicating effective medical intervention). Often heat, whirlpools, and massages are very effective adjunctive treatments. Pool therapy may be initiated sooner than other forms of exercise.

Early goals are to preserve functional mobility and ADL skills. If the person is confined to bed, protection from foot drop and contractures and prevention of pressure ulcers are essential. If the client has a skin rash, the PTA should caution about the possibility of infection from scratching. If antipruritic medications do not relieve severe itching, tepid sponges or compresses can be applied (see also Box 7.2). If the client is receiving corticosteroids, observe for side effects (weight gain, acne, edema, hypertension, purplish stretch marks [striae], easy bruising).

Long-term use of steroids lowers resistance to infection, may induce diabetes, causes myopathy and/or neuropathy, and is associated with loss of potassium in the urine and gastric irritation (see the section on corticosteroids in Chapter 2). If side effects are marked, advise against abruptly discontinuing corticosteroids until the client consults the physician first. A low-sodium diet will help prevent fluid retention.

Progressive pulmonary fibrosis complicates dermatomyositis and polymyositis in 10% of adults. During the acute phase of illness, clients must be closely monitored for signs of respiratory weakness that requires ventilatory assistance and for overwhelming infection that can lead to circulatory collapse.[5]

THERMAL INJURIES

Cold Injuries

Definition and Incidence

Cold injuries result from overexposure to cold air or water and occur in two major forms: localized injuries (e.g., frostbite) and systemic injuries (e.g., hypothermia). Untreated or improperly treated frostbite can lead to gangrene and may necessitate amputation, requiring therapy and rehabilitation. Hypothermia is a medical emergency and is not discussed in detail here.

Cold injuries, once almost exclusively a military problem, are becoming more prevalent among the general population, especially in athletes using localized cryotherapy or participating in outdoor sports. Frostbite results from prolonged exposure to dry temperatures far below freezing.

The risk of serious cold injuries is increased by lack of insulating body fat, old age, homelessness, drug or alcohol use, cardiac disease, psychiatric illness, motor vehicle problems, or smoking when combined with unplanned circumstances leading to cold exposure without adequate protective clothing.[83]

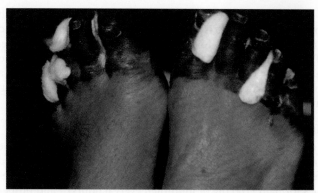

FIG. 7.9 Frostbite of the feet. Blackened areas in the photo show tissue necrosis and gangrene, the result of deep frostbite that extends beyond the subcutaneous tissue. (From Auerbach PS: *Wilderness medicine,* ed 5, St. Louis, 2007, Mosby.)

Clinical Manifestations

Cold-induced injuries can be local or systemic. Severe cold affects all organ systems and especially the central nervous and cardiovascular systems. Many biologic reactions and pathways become distorted or slowed at low body core temperatures. Low body shell temperature can interfere with athletic ability by weakening and slowing muscle contractions, by delaying nerve conduction time, and by facilitating injury.[76]

Typically an initial vasoconstriction in the skin will protect body parts from a drop in core temperature, but when tissue temperature drops to 35.6° F (2° C), ice crystals form in the tissues and expand extracellular spaces, resulting in localized cold injuries. With compression of cells, cell membranes rupture, interrupting enzymatic and metabolic activities.

Additional injury occurs with thawing when increased capillary permeability accompanies the release of histamine, resulting in aggregation of red blood cells and microvascular occlusion. Research into the pathophysiology of cold injuries has revealed marked similarities in inflammatory processes to those seen in thermal burns and ischemia-reperfusion injury.[56]

Frostbite may be deep or superficial. Superficial frostbite affects the skin and subcutaneous tissue, especially of the face, ears, extremities, and other exposed body areas. Although it may go unnoticed at first, after return to a warm place, frostbite produces burning, tingling, numbness, swelling, and a mottled, blue-gray skin color.

When the affected area begins to rewarm, the person will feel pain and numbness followed by hypoesthesia. Deep frostbite extends beyond subcutaneous tissue and usually affects the hands or feet. The skin becomes white until it has thawed and then turns purplish blue. Deep frostbite produces pain, blisters, tissue necrosis, and gangrene (Fig. 7.9).

Diagnosis

Diagnosis is usually made based on the history and presenting symptoms; measures to prevent and treat general hypothermia are taken before management of the local frostbite injuries. Evidence of the role of thromboxanes and prostaglandins in cold injuries has resulted in more active approaches in the medical treatment of frostbite wounds, including the use of vasodilators, thrombolysis, and hyperbaric oxygen.[56]

Triple-phase bone scans can be used to distinguish between tissue that is irreversibly destined for necrosis and tissue that is at risk for necrosis but potentially salvageable. These improvements in radiologic assessment have led to earlier surgical intervention to provide at-risk tissue with a new blood supply and preserve both function and length in an extremity.[83]

Treatment

In a localized cold injury, treatment consists of rewarming the injured part without rubbing or massaging the area to avoid further tissue damage, and supportive measures (e.g., analgesics for pain [200 mg of ibuprofen every 6 hours][64] and proper positioning to avoid weight bearing with gauze between the toes to prevent maceration). More severe and deeper injuries should not be thawed until medical treatment can be given in a hospital.

The management of blisters is still somewhat controversial, but current practice indicates that clear blisters (shallow injury) should be aspirated; hemorrhagic blisters (deep injury) should not be debrided to avoid desiccation and infection of underlying deep tissue[37] (see the section on skin lesions and 7.1 Special Implications for the PTA: Skin Lesions).

All frostbitten areas should be treated with topical aloe vera cream. Foam dressings may be applied to maintain a moist wound bed, absorb drainage, and provide protection. A bed cradle may be needed to keep the weight of bedcovers off the affected part or parts.

In the case of a developing compartment syndrome a fasciotomy may be performed to increase circulation by lowering edematous tissue pressure. If gangrene occurs, amputation may be necessary. Smoking causes vasoconstriction and slows healing; the client should be advised to quit smoking, at least during the recovery period.

Prognosis

The prognosis depends on the extent of localized cold injury and development of any complications, such as compartment syndrome, necrosis, or gangrene. Rapid triage and treatment of frostbite can lead to dramatic improvements in outcome and prognosis.[64] Long-term effects may include increased sensitivity to cold, burning and tingling on reexposure to cold, and increased sweating of the affected area.

Future cold injuries may be prevented through the use of windproof, water-resistant, many-layered clothing; moisture-wicking socks; a head covering; mittens instead of gloves; and heat-generating devices (except for those with peripheral neuropathy) in pockets or battery-operated socks.

7.15 Special Implications for the PTA: Cold Injuries Local cold injury subsequent to prolonged exposure may not be seen in a therapy practice until complications such as necrosis and gangrene result in amputation. Whirlpool with gentle agitation directed away from the affected area may be prescribed as part of the rewarming procedure. Water temperature is based on tissue temperature and should be determined in conjunction with the medical staff.

Use of cryotherapy as a modality among the general population can result in localized tissue damage requiring documentation (e.g., filing an accident report) and possible medical evaluation and treatment. Massage may cause further tissue damage and should not be carried out until local tissue has healed.

Burns

Definition and Incidence

Injuries that result from direct contact with or exposure to any thermal, chemical, electrical, or radiation source are termed *burns*. Burn injuries occur when energy from a heat source is transferred to the tissues of the body. The depth of injury is a function of temperature or source of energy (e.g., radiation) and duration of exposure.

The severity of burn injury is assessed with respect to the risk of infection, mortality, and cosmetic or functional disability.[63] Factors that influence injury severity include burn depth, burn size (percentage of total body surface area [TBSA]), burn location, age, general health, and mechanism of injury. Burn depth can be divided into categories based on the elements of the skin that are damaged (Fig. 7.10). Most burn wounds that require medical intervention are a combination of partial- and full-thickness burns.

Burn size is determined by one of two techniques: the rule of nines (Fig. 7.11) and the Lund–Browder method (Figs. 7.12 and 7.13). The *rule of nines* is based on the division of the body into anatomic sections, each of which represents 9% or a multiple of 9% of the TBSA. This is an easy method to quickly assess the percentage of TBSA injured and is most commonly used in emergency departments where the initial evaluation takes place.

The *Lund–Browder* method modifies the percentages for body segments and provides a more accurate estimate of burn size according to age. For the most accurate estimate of burn size, the burn diagram should be confirmed after the initial wound debridement.[49]

In the United States approximately 1.4 to 2 million burn injuries occur each year, 70,000 people are hospitalized with severe injuries, and 7500 are fatalities. Extensive autografts are required in over 1500 third-degree burns and 40,000 second-degree burns every year.

Burn injuries are the third leading cause of accidental death in all age groups. Males tend to be injured more frequently than females, except for the older population (older than 70 years).[62]

Etiologic Factors

Burn injuries are categorized according to their mechanism of injury: thermal, chemical, electrical, or radiation. *Thermal* burns are caused by exposure to or contact with sources such as flames, hot liquids, steam, semisolids (tar), or hot objects.

Chemical burns are caused by tissue contact with or ingestion, inhalation, or injection of strong acids, alkalis, or organic compounds. Chemical burns can result from contact with certain household cleaning agents and various chemicals used in industry, agriculture, and the military.

Electrical burns are caused by heat that is generated by the electrical energy as it passes through the body. Electrical burns can result from contact with exposed or faulty electrical wiring, high-voltage power lines, or lightning.

Radiation burns are the least common burn injury and are caused by exposure to a radioactive source. These types of injuries have been associated with the use of ionizing radiation in industry or with therapeutic radiation sources in medicine. A sunburn from prolonged exposure to UV rays is also considered a type of radiation burn.

Risk Factors

Data collected from the National Burn Information Exchange indicate that 75% of all burn injuries result from the actions of

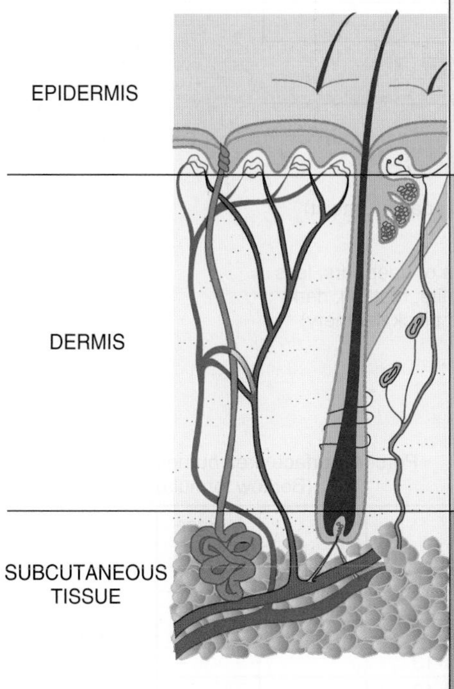

		CAUSE	APPEARANCE	SENSATION	COURSE
EPIDERMIS	SUPERFICIAL BURN First-degree burn	Sunburn Ultraviolet exposure Brief exposure to flash, flame, or hot liquids	Mild to severe erythema; skin blanches with pressure; dry, no blisters; edema variable amount	Painful Hyperesthetic Tingling Pain eased by cooling	Discomfort lasts about 48 hours Desquamation in 3-7 days
DERMIS	PARTIAL-THICKNESS BURN Second-degree burn	Superficial: Scalding liquids, semiliquids (oil, tar), or solids Deep: Immersion scald, flame	Large thick-walled blisters covering extensive area (vesiculation) Edema; mottled red base; broken epidermis; wet, shiny, weeping surface	Painful Sensitive to cold air	Superficial partial-thickness burn heals in 14-21 days Deep partial-thickness burn requires 21-28 days for healing Healing rate varies with burn depth and presence or absence of infection
SUBCUTANEOUS TISSUE	FULL-THICKNESS BURN Third-degree or fourth-degree burn	Prolonged exposure to: Chemical, electrical, flame, scalding liquids, steam	Variable (e.g., deep red, black, white, brown) Dry surface Edema Fat exposed Tissue disrupted	Little or no pain Insensate	Full-thickness dead skin suppurates and liquefies after 2-3 weeks Spontaneous healing may be impossible but small areas may be left alone to form scarring without grafting (called secondary intent) Requires removal of eschar and subsequent split- or full-thickness skin grafting Hypertrophic scarring and wound contractures likely to develop without preventive measures

FIG. 7.10 Burn injury classification according to depth of injury. This information is important to review because it will help determine the practice pattern to use when making a physical therapy diagnosis. A *partial-thickness* burn involves loss of epidermis and/or a portion of the dermis. Because part of the dermis is intact and that is where the regenerating elements are, a partial-thickness wound has the ability to heal via epithelialization. A *full-thickness* burn involves total destruction of the epidermis and dermis and cannot heal independently without granulation and contraction, sometimes requiring a flap or skin graft procedure.[38]

the injured person, occurring most often in the home. Children younger than 3 and adults older than 70 are at the highest risk for burn injury.

Risk factors include inadequate adult supervision (in the case of children), psychomotor disorders (e.g., impaired judgment, impaired mobility, drug or alcohol use), rural location, mobile home residence, occupation, lack of smoke detectors, fireworks, and misuse of cigarettes.[12,52,53]

Safety recommendations for prevention of burn injuries while showering have been made, including nonlever water handles, limited-temperature devices on water heaters, and curtains rather than cubicles for easy escape.[87]

Clinical Manifestations

Appearance, sensation, and course of injury of superficial, partial-thickness, and full-thickness burns are outlined in Fig. 7.10. Burn location influences injury severity in that burns of certain areas of the body are commonly associated with specific complications. For example, burns of the head, neck, and chest frequently have associated pulmonary complications.

Burns involving the face may have associated corneal abrasions. Burns of the hands and joints can result in permanent

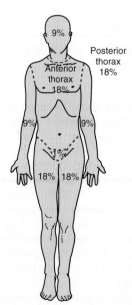

FIG. 7.11 The rule of nines provides a quick method for estimating the extent of a burn injury.

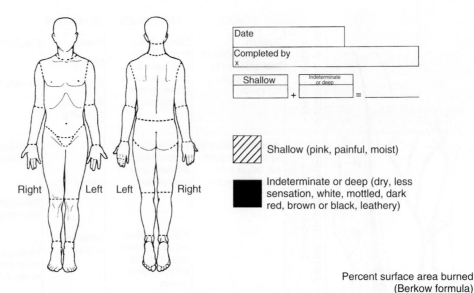

Percent surface area burned
(Berkow formula)

Area	1 Year	1 to 4 Years	5 to 9 Years	10 to 14 Years	15 to 18 Years	Adult	Shallow	Indeterminate or deep
Head	19	17	13	11	9	7		
Neck	2	2	2	2	2	2		
Ant. trunk	13	13	13	13	13	13		
Post. trunk	13	13	13	13	13	13		
R. buttock	2½	2½	2½	2½	2½	2½		
L. buttock	2½	2½	2½	2½	2½	2½		
Genitalia	1	1	1	1	1	1		
R. U. arm	4	4	4	4	4	4		
L. U. arm	4	4	4	4	4	4		
R. L. arm	3	3	3	3	3	3		
L. L. arm	3	3	3	3	3	3		
R. hand	2½	2½	2½	2½	2½	2½		
L. hand	2½	2½	2½	2½	2½	2½		
R. thigh	5½	6½	8	8½	9	9½		
L. thigh	5½	6½	8	8½	9	9½		
R. leg	5	5	5½	6	6½	7		
L. leg	5	5	5½	6	6½	7		
R. foot	3½	3½	3½	3½	3½	3½		
L. foot	3½	3½	3½	3½	3½	3½		
Total								

FIG. 7.12 A sample chart for recording the extent and depth of a burn injury using the Lund–Browder formula.

physical and vocational disability requiring extensive therapy and rehabilitation. Circumferential burns of extremities may produce a tourniquet-like effect and lead to total occlusion of circulation.

Theoretically, with a full-thickness burn the nerve endings have been destroyed and no pain should be associated with this type of injury. However, most full-thickness burns occur with superficial and partial-thickness burns in which nerve endings are intact and exposed. Excised *eschar* (dead tissue) and donor sites expose nerve fibers as well. As peripheral nerves regenerate, painful sensation returns. Consequently, people with burn injuries often experience severe pain that is related to the size and depth of the burn.

The clinical course of the (major) burn client can be divided into three phases: the emergent and resuscitation phase, the acute phase, and the rehabilitation phase. The *emergent period* begins at the time of injury and concludes with the restoration of capillary permeability, usually 48 to 72 hours after injury.

The *resuscitation period* begins with initiation of fluid resuscitation measures and ends when capillary integrity returns to near-normal levels and the large fluid shifts have decreased. The *acute phase* of recovery begins when the person is hemodynamically stable, capillary permeability is restored, and diuresis has begun, usually 48 to 72 hours after the initial injury occurred. The acute phase continues until wound closure is achieved.

The *rehabilitation phase* represents the final phase of burn care, often overlaps the acute care phase, and lasts well beyond the period of hospitalization. This phase focuses on gaining independence through achievement of maximal functional recovery.

Infection is the most common and life-threatening complication of burn injuries. Burn wound infections can be classified

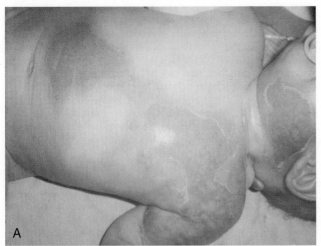

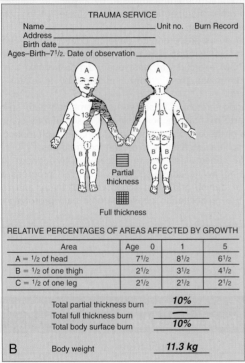

TRAUMA SERVICE

Name _____ Unit no. _____ Burn Record
Address _____
Birth date _____
Ages–Birth–7½. Date of observation _____

RELATIVE PERCENTAGES OF AREAS AFFECTED BY GROWTH

Area	Age 0	1	5
A = ½ of head	7½	8½	6½
B = ½ of one thigh	2½	3½	4½
C = ½ of one leg	2½	2½	2½

Total partial thickness burn	*10%*
Total full thickness burn	
Total body surface burn	*10%*
Body weight	*11.3 kg*

FIG. 7.13 (A) Pediatric scald burn. (B) Corresponding Lund–Browder chart. (Courtesy Katherine S. Harris, PT, MS, PhD, Quinnipiac University, Hamden, CT.)

on the basis of the causative organism, the depth of invasion, and the tissue response.

Individuals with extensive burns and in whom wound closure is difficult to achieve are at greatest risk for infection and other complications. Inhalation injury with major burns and added staphylococcal septicemia are often fatal.[21] The multiple organ system response that occurs after a burn injury may result in multiple organ dysfunction syndrome and death (see Chapter 2).

Hypertrophic scarring is a second complication that is not life threatening but is associated with considerable morbidity and potential lifelong disfigurement. Children and African Americans are at greatest risk for hypertrophic scarring, presumably because of the abundance of collagen in these groups. Aging Caucasian adults with wrinkled, loose skin have little to no hypertrophic scarring because of the absence of collagen.

Treatment

The PTA may be involved in wound care for minor burns consisting of cleansing; removal of any damaging agents (e.g., chemicals, tar); debridement of loose, nonviable tissue; and application of topical antimicrobial creams or ointment and a sterile dressing. Blister management usually includes debridement of the blister. Although the blister fluid is theoretically sterile, most blisters break, and the fluid is an ideal medium for bacteria.[71]

Instructions for home care include observation for clinical manifestations of infection and active ROM exercises to maintain normal joint function, decrease edema formation, and decrease possible scar formation.

Treatment of major burns includes lifesaving measures (ABCs: *a*irway, *b*reathing, *c*irculation) immediately after the injury, followed by restorative care (e.g., infection control, wound care, skin grafts, pain management) during the acute phase until wound closure is achieved. PTAs are closely involved early in the acute phase of recovery to maximize functional recovery and cosmetic outcome.

Therapeutic interventions include wound management—irrigation, debridement, advanced wound dressings—positioning and immobilization after skin grafting to prevent unwanted movement and shearing of grafts, scar and contracture prevention and management, exercise, ambulation, and ADLs. Elasticized garments help reduce scar hypertrophy and may be worn for months to 2 years after hospitalization.

Bioengineered temporary biologic dressings may be used to minimize fluid and protein loss from the burn surface, prevent infection, and reduce pain. Types of temporary grafts include *allografts* (homografts), which are usually cadaver skin; *xenografts* (heterografts), which are typically pigskin; and *biosynthetic grafts,* which are a combination of collagen and synthetics. To treat a full-thickness burn, an *autograft* (the person's own skin) may be required.

The transplanted skin graft will be used intact over areas where appearance or joint movement is important, but the graft may be meshed (fenestrated) to cover up to three times its original size. Several new permanent skin substitutes are being used to aid in replacing dermal thickness and to assist in coverage of large surface area injuries.[61] Cultured skin is usually used in conjunction with allograft dermis.

Prognosis

Burn care has improved in recent decades, resulting in a lower mortality rate for victims of burn injuries. Current techniques of burn wound management, such as effective topical antimicrobials and early burn wound excision, have significantly reduced the overall occurrence of invasive burn wound infections.[63]

The client's age affects the severity and outcome of the burn. Mortality rates are higher for children younger than 4 and for clients older than 65, although survival rates after burns have improved significantly for children. At present most children, even children with large burns, should survive.[78] Survival rate for older clients is 70%, with at least 60% of those individuals becoming fully functional 6 months after hospital discharge.[52]

Factors such as obesity, alcoholism, and cardiac disorders affecting general health—especially disorders that impair peripheral circulation, such as peripheral vascular disease—increase the complication and mortality rates for adults with burns.

Delay in amputation results in prolonged hospital stay, delayed rehabilitation, and a higher mortality rate. Early amputation is associated with a 14% mortality rate compared with a 50% mortality rate for cases of delayed amputation. Earlier identification of nonsalvageable limbs may decrease infectious complications and improve chances of survival.[97]

7.16 Special Implications for the PTA: Burns In light of statistics showing that the population over 70 years old is at highest risk of burn injury, prevention of burn accidents, especially in this population, is an important part of client education. Additional resources for the PTA are available.[10,58,66,93]

Reviewing simple cooking precautions may be helpful—for example, do not leave burners in use unattended, do not use high heat, do not wear clothing with loose sleeves or belts (especially bathrobes), use front burners whenever possible, and avoid leaning over front burners when using back burners.

Most PTAs do not begin to treat the burn client until the acute phase (as soon as the person is physiologically stable), continuing intervention through much of the rehabilitation phase. However, initiating bedside intervention before the person is medically stable is ideal for reducing morbidity and functional loss.

Initial treatment interventions encourage deep breathing and facilitate lung expansion; promote wound healing; reduce dependent edema formation and promote venous return; prevent or minimize deformities and hypertrophic scarring; increase range of motion (ROM), strength, and function; increase independence in daily activities and self-care; and encourage emotional and psychologic well-being. Specific compression, lymphatic movement, debridement, and wound care procedures are beyond the scope of this book; the reader is referred to other texts for more detailed information.[10,32,51,66,84]

Throughout the acute and rehabilitation phases of burn care, the PTA must remain alert to the development of medical complications, such as ileus, gastric ulcers, respiratory distress, infection, and impaired circulation. Monitor vital signs (e.g., heart rate, blood pressure, oxygen saturation levels) to ensure the person can tolerate therapy. Notify the nursing staff of any new or unusual findings observed during assessment and intervention (Table 7.3).

Laboratory values will change with a burn, especially a full-thickness burn. It is important to review the values before treatment interventions to be aware of response to treatment and possible mental status changes.

Clients with burns with acute renal failure and abnormal sodium, potassium, chloride, and magnesium values are candidates for hemodialysis. Abnormal BUN (blood urea nitrogen) can be a reflection of decreased renal function or fluid intake. A client may respond to physical therapy treatment with a decreased mental status. Because of the increased metabolism and catabolic state, clients will experience increased weakness.

Wounds will not heal optimally unless protein status, reflected in prealbumin, is addressed; protein status will be affected by the catabolic state. Glucose must be monitored because of the same metabolic situation.

Regular inspection of the wound must be made; any change in wound appearance must be reported. The amount of body surface area exposed during wound care must be minimized to prevent hypothermia, because heat is lost in open wounds and after hydrotherapy by evaporation. Hydrotherapy treatment must be limited to 30 minutes or less with water temperature in the 98° to 102° F (36.7° to 38.9° C) range if a whirlpool is used. External heat shields or radiant heat lamps can provide a source of external heat.

Clients excluded from hydrotherapy are generally those who are hemodynamically unstable and those with new grafts. In recent years, hydrotherapy has been challenged, and alternative methods are being advocated (e.g., shower versus tub).[48] Pulsed lavage with suction (PLWS) (Fig. 7.14) is an ideal intervention for irrigation and debridement, allowing treatment in the Burn Unit of appropriate areas without disturbing new grafts.[48]

People with burns are at high risk for infection because of the significant loss of skin barrier and impaired immune response. Infection control techniques must be practiced carefully at all times. Skin donor sites require the same care and precautions as other partial-thickness wounds in order to promote healing and prevent infection.

Arrange any therapy that is likely to elicit a pain response to coincide with medications (allow 30 minutes for oral, 10 minutes for intramuscular [IM], 3 to 5 minutes for intravenous [IV] administration). Combining relaxation techniques, music therapy, distraction, and other techniques for pain modulation may be helpful. Burned areas must be maintained in positions of physiologic function within the limits imposed by associated injuries, grafting, and other therapeutic devices (see Table 7.4 for positioning recommendations).

Burned areas are prone to develop contractures, necessitating close assessment of ROM and muscle strength. Encourage active ROM exercises at least every 2 hours while the person is awake unless this is contraindicated by a recent grafting procedure.

Prolonged stretching is sometimes combined with splinting or orthoses to maintain motion. Splinting is sometimes controversial because of the lack of evidence validation, although most clinicians employ splints successfully to prevent contractures.[67]

Provide honest, positive reinforcement throughout intervention, being aware that each individual will progress through stages of denial, grief, and acceptance of injury and recovery. During the rehabilitation phase, chronic pain protocols may be helpful.

TABLE 7.3 Assessing Medical Complications in the Burn-Injured Adult

System	Complications
Urinary	Visible red or dark brown urine (catheter)
Respiratory	Signs of respiratory distress
	Restlessness
	Confusion
	Labored breathing
	Tachypnea (>24 respirations/min)
	Dyspnea
	Pao_2 <90 mm Hg; O_2 <95%
Peripheral vascular	Pulses absent on palpation
	Capillary refill (unburned area) >2 sec
	Numbness or tingling
	Increased pain with active range-of-motion exercises
	Increased edema, changes in skin color
Infection	Discoloration of wounds or drainage, odor, delayed healing
	Headache, chills, anorexia, nausea
	Increased pain
	Change in vital signs
	Paralytic ileus, confusion, restlessness, hallucinations
Gastrointestinal	Paralytic ileus (painful, distended abdomen)
	Stress-induced gastric ulcer (epigastric pain, abdominal distention, loss of appetite, nausea)

MISCELLANEOUS INTEGUMENTARY DISORDERS

Integumentary Ulcers

Integumentary ulcers can be caused by a variety of underlying disorders, including diabetes, arterial insufficiency, radiation damage, SSc, vasculitis, and prolonged pressure.

Pressure Ulcers

Definition and incidence. A pressure ulcer (formerly called *bedsore, decubitus ulcer*) is a lesion caused by unrelieved pressure resulting in damage to underlying tissue. Pressure ulcers usually occur over bony prominences, such as the heels, sacrum, ischial tuberosities, greater trochanters, elbows, and scapula, and are staged to classify the degree of tissue damage observed (Box 7.9).

Wounds cannot be backstaged. Once a pressure ulcer has been designated as stage II, III, or IV, it will always remain classified the same for documentation. As the lesion fills with granulation tissue and closes with epithelial tissue, grafts, or flaps, it should be documented as *healing* stage II, III, or IV (still using the original deepest level noted). Nursing homes no longer are required to backstage pressure ulcers for reimbursement purposes.

It should be noted that this staging classification is only for pressure ulcers. Other types of ulcers, such as vascular (arterial, venous) ulcers are designated as partial or full thickness. Neuropathic ulcers are staged using Wagner classifications (Table 7.5). The term *neuropathic ulcer* is used interchangeably with *diabetic ulcer*, but a diabetic ulcer is really a neuropathic ulcer in someone with diabetes. Neuropathic ulcers can occur in anyone with loss of sensation (e.g., alcoholic neuropathy, peripheral neuropathy).

It is estimated that 2.5 million[1] people develop pressure ulcers each year, including 500,000 people in nursing homes and another 400,000 people with neuropathy.

Pressure ulcers are viewed as high-volume, high-risk problems in most health care settings. In long-term care facilities, regulatory agencies have designated the development of pressure ulcers as an indicator of quality of care provided to clients.[19]

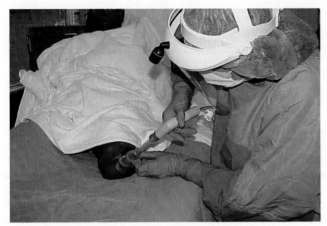

FIG. 7.14 Personal protective equipment (PPE) worn during treatment with pulsed lavage with suction (PLWS). (Courtesy Harriett B. Loehne, PT, DPT, CWS, FCCWS, Archbold Center for Wound Management, Thomasville, GA, 2006. Used with permission.)

TABLE 7.4	Therapeutic Positioning for the Burn-Injured Client	
Burned Area	**Therapeutic Position**	**Positioning Techniques**
Neck		
Anterior	Extension	No pillow; small towel roll beneath cervical spine to promote neck extension
Circumferential	Neutral toward extension	No pillow
Posterior or asymmetric	Neutral	No pillow
Shoulder, axilla	Arm abduction to 90–110 degrees	Splinting; arms positioned away from body and supported on arm troughs; elbow splint
Elbow	Arm extension	Elbow splint; elbow(s) positioned in extension with slight bend at elbow (≤10 degrees of elbow flexion)
		Arms supported on arm troughs with the forearm in slight pronation
Hand		
Wrist	Wrist extension	Hand splint
Metacarpophalangeal (MCP) joints	MCP flexion at 90 degrees	Hand splint
Proximal or distal interphalangeal (PIP, DIP) joints	PIP or DIP extension	Hand splint
Thumb	Thumb abduction	Hand splint with thumb abduction
Web spaces	Finger abduction	Web spacers of gauze, foam, or thermoplastics to decrease webbing formation
Hip	Hip extension	Supine with the head of bed flat and legs extended
		Trochanter roll to maintain neutral rotation (toes pointing toward ceiling)
		Prone positioning
Knee	Knee extension	Supine with knees extended and toes pointing toward ceiling
		Prone with feet extended over end of mattress
		Sitting with legs extended and elevated
		Knee splint
Ankle	Neutral	Padded footboard
		Ankle positioning devices (avoid position of ankle inversion or eversion)
		Suspend heels (lying and sitting) to prevent pressure ulcer

Modified from Black JM, Hawks JH, editors: Medical-surgical nursing: clinical management for positive outcomes, ed 8, St. Louis, 2009, Saunders.

BOX 7.9   Pressure Injury Stages

Stage 1 Pressure Injury: Nonblanchable erythema of intact skin

Intact skin with a localized area of nonblanchable erythema, which may appear differently in darkly pigmented skin. Presence of blanchable erythema or changes in sensation, temperature, or firmness may precede visual changes. Color changes do not include purple or maroon discoloration; these may indicate deep tissue pressure injury.

Stage 2 Pressure Injury: Partial-thickness skin loss with exposed dermis

Partial-thickness loss of skin with exposed dermis. The wound bed is viable, pink or red, moist, and may also present as an intact or ruptured serum-filled blister. Adipose (fat) is not visible and deeper tissues are not visible. Granulation tissue, *slough*, and eschar are not present. These injuries commonly result from adverse microclimate and shear in the skin over the pelvis and shear in the heel. This stage should not be used to describe moisture associated skin damage (MASD) including incontinence associated dermatitis (IAD), intertriginous dermatitis (ITD), medical adhesive related skin injury (MARSI), or traumatic wounds (skin tears, burns, abrasions).

Stage 3 Pressure Injury: Full-thickness skin loss

Full-thickness loss of skin, in which adipose (fat) is visible in the ulcer and granulation tissue and epibole (rolled wound edges) are often present. Slough and/or eschar may be visible. The depth of tissue damage varies by anatomical location; areas of significant adiposity can develop deep wounds. Undermining and tunneling may occur. Fascia, muscle, tendon, ligament, cartilage and/or bone are not exposed. If slough or eschar obscures the extent of tissue loss this is an Unstageable Pressure Injury.

Stage 4 Pressure Injury: Full-thickness skin and tissue loss

Full-thickness skin and tissue loss with exposed or directly palpable fascia, muscle, tendon, ligament, cartilage, or bone in the ulcer. Slough and/or eschar may be visible. Epibole (rolled edges), undermining and/or tunneling often occur. Depth varies by anatomical location. If slough or eschar obscures the extent of tissue loss this is an unstageable pressure injury.

Unstageable Pressure Injury: Obscured full-thickness skin and tissue loss

Full-thickness skin and tissue loss in which the extent of tissue damage within the ulcer cannot be confirmed because it is obscured by slough or eschar. If slough or eschar is removed, a Stage 3 or Stage 4 pressure injury will be revealed. Stable eschar (i.e., dry, adherent, intact without erythema or fluctuance) on an ischemic limb or the heel(s) should not be removed.

Deep Tissue Pressure Injury: Persistent nonblanchable deep red, maroon, or purple discoloration

Intact or nonintact skin with localized area of persistent nonblanchable deep red, maroon, purple discoloration or epidermal separation revealing a dark wound bed or blood-filled blister. Pain and temperature change often precede skin color changes. Discoloration may appear differently in darkly pigmented skin. This injury results from intense and/or prolonged pressure and shear forces at the bone–muscle interface. The wound may evolve rapidly to reveal the actual extent of tissue injury, or may resolve without tissue loss. If necrotic tissue, subcutaneous tissue, granulation tissue, fascia, muscle, or other underlying structures are visible, this indicates a full-thickness pressure injury (Unstageable, Stage 3 or Stage 4). Do not use DTPI to describe vascular, traumatic, neuropathic, or dermatologic conditions.

Used with permission of the National Pressure Ulcer Advisory Panel, April 2016.

TABLE 7.5   Wagner's Ulcer Grade Classification

Grade	Characteristics
0	Preulcerative lesions; healed ulcers; presence of bony deformity
1	Superficial ulcer without subcutaneous tissue involvement
2	Penetration through the subcutaneous tissue; may expose bone, tendon, ligament, or joint capsule
3	Osteitis, abscess, or osteomyelitis
4	Gangrene of digit
5	Gangrene of foot necessitating disarticulation

This classification scheme for ulceration is used for neuropathic ulcers and does not represent pressure ulcers. It is included here for comparison with the stages of pressure ulcers.

Data from Wagner REW: The dysvascular foot: a system for diagnosis and treatment, Foot Ankle 2:64–122, 1981.

Etiologic and risk factors. Pressure ulcers are caused by unrelieved pressure that results in damaged skin, muscle, and underlying tissue, usually over bony prominences. The primary causative factors for the development of pressure ulcers are (1) interface pressure (externally), (2) friction (rubbing of the skin against another surface), (3) shearing forces (two layers sliding against each other in opposite directions, causing damage to the underlying tissues), (4) maceration (softening caused by excessive moisture), (5) decreased skin resilience (e.g., dehydration), (6) malnutrition, and (7) decreased circulation.

Pressure contributes to other types of ulcers (e.g., arterial, venous, neuropathic), and likewise, the underlying cause of the other types of ulcers can contribute to the development of pressure ulcers. However, pressure ulcers are a separate entity from these other types of ulcers.

Intrinsic factors most commonly associated with pressure ulcer development include decreased sensation, impaired mobility or activity levels, incontinence, diaphoresis, impaired nutritional status, and altered levels of consciousness. Extrinsic factors include pressure, shear, friction, and moisture.

Bed- and chair-bound clients and those with impaired ability to reposition themselves should be assessed for additional factors that increase the risk of developing pressure ulcers. These factors include decreased mobility or immobility; hip or femoral fractures; contractures; increased muscle tone; loss of sensation; incontinence; obesity; nutritional factors; chronic disease accompanied by anemia, edema, renal failure, or sepsis; and altered level of consciousness. Nutritional factors may include malnutrition or inadequate nutrition leading to weight loss and subsequent reduction of subcutaneous tissue and muscle bulk.

Pressure is the external factor causing ischemia and tissue necrosis. Continuous pressure on soft tissues between bony prominences and hard or unyielding surfaces compresses capillaries and occludes blood flow. Normal capillary blood pressure at the arterial end of the vascular bed averages 32 mm Hg.

That pressure may be exceeded when tissues are externally compressed, reducing blood supply to—and lymphatic drainage of—the affected area.[33,34] Shearing (when the skin layers move in opposite directions) is the intrinsic factor that contributes to ripping or tearing of blood vessels, further damaging the integument.

If the pressure is relieved, a brief period of rebound capillary dilation (called *reactive hyperemia*) occurs and no tissue damage develops. If the pressure is not relieved, the endothelial cells lining the capillaries become disrupted by platelet aggregation, forming microthrombi that occlude blood flow and cause anoxic necrosis of surrounding tissues. Necrotic tissue predisposes to bacterial invasion and subsequent infection, preventing healthy granulation. Muscle and tendon tissue can tolerate less pressure loading than skin before incurring ischemic damage.[50]

In the case of neuropathic ulcers associated with diabetes, the primary pathogenesis is the absence of protective sensation combined with high pressure. The absence of protective sensation indicates a high risk for pressure ulcers on the feet; diabetic ulcers are typically present on the soles of the feet.

Clinical manifestations. Pressure ulcers usually occur over bony prominences and often in a circular pattern shaped like an inverted volcano, with the greatest tissue ischemia at the apex next to the bone, or they may assume the shape of objects causing the pressure, such as tubing or clamps. Irregular patterns indicate additional shearing forces or other contributing factors.

Sacral ulcers are often large, undermined, and deep to the bone because the tissue mass over the sacrum is thin and erodes easily to the deep tissues. Pressure ulcers are manifested at the surface as the deeper tissues die, so a stage I ulcer can become a stage III or IV ulcer quickly without further injury.

The wounds can be described, measured, and categorized with respect to surface area, exudates, and type of wound tissue. PTAs may want to use the PUSH Tool to assess and document pressure ulcers. This tool is available from the National Pressure Ulcer Advisory Panel (NPUAP; http://www.npuap.org). When present, infection can be localized and self-limiting or can progress to sepsis. Proteolytic enzymes from bacteria and macrophages dissolve necrotic tissues and cause a foul-smelling discharge that appears like, but is not, pus.

Necrosis associated with pressure ulcers is not painful, but the surrounding tissue is often painful in individuals who do not have loss of sensation from spinal cord trauma or neuropathy. Trauma to the tissues produces an acute inflammatory response with hyperemia, fever, and increased white blood cell count.

Diagnosis. Prevention is the key to this condition (Box 7.10), starting with assessment of people at high risk for the development of pressure ulcers. In fact, risk prediction should be an ongoing assessment carried out by all health care professionals. In addition to the Braden Scale (Table 7.6) or Norton Scale (Table 7.7), laboratory data on hemoglobin, hematocrit, prealbumin, total protein, and lymphocytes should be assessed by all health care professionals involved.

The diagnosis is reached by looking at the location of the wound and the type of tissue response. The pressure ulcer is then staged. If there is evidence of infection, the wound is cleaned with isotonic saline and debrided if necrosis is present, and then viable tissue is cultured (not a swab specimen of the exudates or necrotic tissue).

The definition of infection is invasion into viable tissue. Cultures of the organisms that have invaded the tissue causing the infection must be determined following these procedures. Clinical practice of wound cultures must be careful to avoid culturing wound exudate contaminants, of which there are usually a minimum of three per wound.[42]

BOX 7.10   Guidelines for Prevention of Pressure Ulcers in Adults

- All clients at risk should have a systematic skin inspection at least once each day, with particular attention paid to the bony prominences. Results of skin inspection should be documented (see Box 7.3).
- Clean skin at the time of soiling and at routine intervals. Individualize the frequency of skin cleaning according to need and client preference. Avoid hot water, and use a mild cleaning agent that minimizes irritation and dryness of the skin. During the cleaning or wound care process, minimize the force and friction applied to the skin. Ideal is the use of disposable perineal cloths, impregnated with dimethicone.
- Minimize environmental factors leading to skin drying, such as low humidity (<40%) and exposure to cold. Treat dry skin with moisturizers.
- Do *not* perform massage over reddened areas. Perform indirect soft tissue mobilization techniques or massage the tissue around and toward the area with caution.
- Minimize skin injury caused by friction and shear forces through proper positioning, transferring, and turning techniques. Reduce friction injuries by the use of moisturizers, transparent film dressings, skin sealants, and protective padding.
- Maintain current activity level, mobility, and range of motion. Evaluate the potential for improving the person's mobility and activity status and institute rehabilitation efforts.
- Monitor and document interventions and outcomes.
- If abnormal (<20), order prealbumins one or two times weekly and have dietitian follow to optimize nutrition.
- Reposition any person in bed who is assessed to be at risk of developing pressure ulcers at least every 2 hr if consistent with overall treatment goals.
- For persons in bed, use positioning devices such as pillows or foam wedges to keep bony prominences (e.g., knees, ankles) from direct contact with one another.
- Provide persons in bed who are completely immobile with devices that completely relieve pressure on the heels—that is, *suspend* the heels.
- Do not use doughnut-type devices.
- When a side-lying position is used in bed, avoid positioning directly on the greater trochanter.
- Maintain the head of the bed at the lowest degree of elevation (30- to 35-degree lateral incline) consistent with medical conditions and other restrictions, except at mealtimes. Limit the amount of time the head of the bed is elevated.
- Use lifting devices, such as a trapeze, hydraulic lift, slide board, or linen, to move (rather than drag) persons in bed who cannot assist during transfers and position changes.
- Place any person assessed to be at risk for developing pressure ulcers, when lying in bed, on a pressure-redistribution surface, such as foam, air loss, gel, or water mattress.
- Avoid uninterrupted sitting in any chair or wheelchair for any person at risk of developing a pressure ulcer. Reposition the person, shifting the points under pressure at least every hour, or put him or her back to bed if consistent with overall management goals. Persons who are able should be taught to shift weight every 15 minutes.
- For chair-bound persons, use a pressure-redistribution device. Do not use doughnut-type devices.

Modified from Panel on the Prediction and Prevention of Pressure Ulcers in Adults: Pressure ulcers in adults: prediction and prevention, Clinical Practice Guidelines, CPR Publication No. 92-0050, Rockville, MD, 1992, Agency for Health Care Policy and Research, U.S. Public Health Service.

Treatment. Prevention and removing the causative factor are the first step in the treatment intervention for pressure ulcers. Preventing shear and friction forces requires education of the client and primary caretakers. The pressure ulcer is cleansed

TABLE 7.6 The Braden Scale for Predicting Pressure Sore Risk

Sensory perception (ability to respond to discomfort)	*Completely limited* Unresponsive to painful stimuli, because of either unconsciousness or severe sensory impairment, which limits ability to feel pain over most of body surface	*Very limited* Responds only to painful stimuli (but not verbal commands) by opening eyes or flexing extremities Cannot communicate discomfort verbally OR Has a sensory impairment that limits the ability to feel pain or discomfort over half of body surface	*Slightly limited* Responds to verbal commands by opening eyes and obeying some commands but cannot communicate discomfort or needs OR Has some sensory impairment that limits ability to feel pain or discomfort in one or two extremities	*No impairment* Responds to verbal commands by obeying Can communicate needs accurately Has no sensory deficit that would limit ability to feel pain or discomfort
Moisture (degree to which skin is exposed to moisture)	*Very moist* Skin kept moist almost constantly by perspiration and urine Dampness detected every time patient is moved or turned Linen must be changed more than one time each shift	*Occasionally moist* Skin frequently, but not always, kept moist Linen must be changed two or three times over 24 hr	*Rarely moist* Skin is rarely moist more than three or four times per week, but linen does require changing at that time	*Never moist* Perspiration and incontinence are never a problem; linen changed at routine intervals only
Activity (degree of physical activity)	*Bed-fast* Confined to bed	*Chair-fast* Ability to walk severely impaired or nonexistent; must be assisted into chair or wheelchair Is confined to chair or wheelchair when not in bed	*Walks occasionally* Walks occasionally during day but for very short distances, with or without assistance Spends majority of each shift in bed or chair	*Walks frequently* Walks a moderate distance at least once every 1–2 hr during waking hours
Mobility (ability to change and control body position)	*Completely immobile* Makes occasional slight changes in position without assistance	*Very limited* Makes occasional slight changes in position without help but unable to make frequent or significant changes in position independently	*Slightly limited* Makes frequent although slight changes in position without assistance but unable to make or maintain major changes in position independently	*No limitations* Makes major and frequent changes in position without assistance
Nutrition (usual food intake pattern)	*Very poor* Never eats a complete meal Rarely eats more than one-third of any food offered Intake of protein is negligible Takes even fluids poorly Does not take a liquid dietary supplement OR Is NPO or maintained on clear liquids or IV feeding for more than 5 days	*Probably inadequate* Rarely eats a complete meal and generally eats only about half of any food offered Protein intake is poor Occasionally will take a liquid dietary supplement	*Adequate* Eats over half of most meals Eats moderate amount of protein source one or two times daily Occasionally will refuse a meal Will usually take a dietary supplement if offered OR Is on tube feeding or TPN, which probably meets most nutritional needs	*Excellent* Eats most of every meal Never refuses a meal Frequently eats between meals Does not require a dietary supplement
Friction and shear	*Problems* Requires moderate to maximum assistance in moving Complete lifting without sliding against sheets is impossible Frequently slides down in bed or chair, requiring frequent repositioning with maximum assistance Spasticity, contractures, or agitation leads to almost constant friction	*Potential problem* Moves freely independently or requires minimum assistance Skin probably slides against bed sheets or chair to some extent when movement occurs Maintains relatively good position in chair or bed most of the time but occasionally slides down	*No apparent problem* Moves in bed and in chair independently and has sufficient muscle strength to lift up completely during move Maintains good position in bed or chair at all times	

IV, Intravenous; *NPO*, nothing by mouth; *TPN*, total parenteral nutrition.
Key: A score of 15 to 16 (15 to 18 if >75 years old) indicates minimum risk; 13 to 14, moderate risk; ≤12, high risk.

TABLE 7.7 Norton Scale

NAME_____   DATE_____

Physical Condition	Mental Condition	Activity	Mobility	Incontinent	Total Score
Good 4	Alert 4	Ambulant 4	Full 4	Not 4	
Fair 3	Apathetic 3	Walk/help 3	Slightly limited 3	Occasional 3	
Poor 2	Confused 2	Chair-bound 2	Very limited 2	Usually/urine 2	
Very bad 1	Stupor 1	Bed 1	Immobile 1	Doubly 1	

Key: The Norton Scale is a summated rating scale made up of five subscales scored from 1 to 4 (1 for low level of functioning and 4 for highest level functioning), for total scores that range from 5 to 10. The subscales measure functional capabilities of the person that contribute to their risk in developing pressure ulcers. A lower Norton Scale score indicates lower levels of functioning and therefore higher levels of risk for pressure ulcer development. A score of 5 to 14 rates the client "at risk."
Modified from Norton D, McLaren R, Exton-Smith AN: An investigation of geriatric nursing problems in the hospital, National Corporation for the Care of Old People (now the Centre for Policy on Ageing).

thoroughly. Healing will occur optimally when the ulcer is kept moist.

Topical antibiotics (e.g., Polysporin, Neosporin, bacitracin, Bactroban, MetroGel) can be effective on local infections without systemic involvement to control bacterial concentration, being mindful of allergic reactions, especially to neomycin and bacitracin. Antiseptics are not recommended because these are cytotoxic.

Some physicians continue to advocate the initial use of wet-to-dry dressing for debridement (application of open wet dressing, allowing it to dry on the ulcer, and mechanically debriding exudate by removal of the dressing). Because there is a risk of removing viable tissue, damaging new granulation tissue, and bleeding with this procedure, it is not acceptable for debridement if any viable tissue is evident and should be used only rarely. Wet-dry is not permissible as a dressing change order—only for debridement.[3,41]

The use of antiseptics such as hydrogen peroxide or povidone iodine (cadexomer iodine is an excellent antimicrobial dressing choice) is not recommended because these are cytotoxic and can be damaging to granulation tissue. Hyperbaric oxygen therapy (HOT) has not been approved for pressure ulcers except when osteomyelitis is present that has failed systemic antibiotic treatment or there are complications from a flap or graft.

Successful healing requires continued adequate redistribution of pressure (e.g., turning, positioning, support surfaces) and absence of infection. The presence of necrotic tissue in a wound may provide an optimal environment for bacteria to grow, hence the importance of removing necrotic material from a wound as rapidly as possible.

Therapeutic intervention may include hydrotherapy, electrical stimulation, ultrasound, debridement (autolytic, enzymatic, mechanical, sharp), or any combination of these. An appropriate wound dressing is then applied to provide an optimal wound environment.

Large, deep pressure ulcers may require sharp or surgical debridement of necrotic tissue and opening of deep pockets for drainage. A slower method of debridement is the use of proteolytic enzymes. A variety of skin-grafting techniques may be used if the wound requires surgical closure.

In stage III ulcers, undamaged tissue near the wound is rotated to cover the ulcer. In stage IV ulcers, musculoskeletal flaps (a single unit of skin with its underlying muscle and vasculature) and a variety of other skin-grafting techniques may be used effectively to close the wound.

Bioactive human dermal tissue capable of interacting with the wound bed is now available commercially for use in pressure and neuropathic ulcer wound management.

These skin substitutes derived from living human tissue (human fibroblasts) represent an important advance in the treatment of burns and skin ulcers, including neuropathic foot ulcers, venous ulcers, and pressure ulcers.

Prognosis. Most clients have multiple complicating medical factors that contribute to poor wound closure. Each client responds differently to a course of therapy. Provided there is no infection, there is a good blood supply, the pressure has been eliminated or redistributed, and the client is not malnourished and has no medical complications, the wound should heal successfully. The presence of any of these factors alters the prognosis negatively.

> **7.17 Special Implications for the PTA: Pressure Ulcers** The PTA plays a pivotal role in the prevention and management of pressure ulcers. The PTA is an expert not only in the delivery of therapeutic modalities but also in appropriate positioning, management of tissue load (mechanical factors acting on the tissues), and good mobility, all of which are essential to the success of the intervention.
>
> High-risk clients should be identified using the Braden Scale or Norton Scale (see Tables 7.6 and 7.7), but all clients in the health care delivery system should be evaluated for risk levels and reassessed at least every 3 months for changes in status (or when there is a change in medical status).
>
> Anyone with a history of pressure ulcers is considered at high risk, requiring a prevention protocol immediately. Acute care clients should be reassessed daily or at least weekly, on transfer to another unit or floor, and with changes in medical status.
>
> The high-risk client will need frequent position changes, at least every 2 hours in bed, and at least every hour while sitting, every 15 minutes if the client can move himself or herself. Using all turning surfaces, position the client at a 35-degree oblique angle when he or she is side-lying (Fig. 7.15).
>
> Elevate the head of the bed to no greater than 30 degrees when the client is supine; if the head of the bed is elevated beyond 30 degrees (e.g., for eating, watching television, nursing care, or therapy intervention) the duration of this position needs to be limited to minimize both pressure and shear forces. A trapeze bar, turning sheet, or transfer board can be used to prevent shearing injury to the skin during movement or position change. Frequent shifting of body weight prevents ischemia by redistributing the weight and allowing blood to recirculate.
>
> Static or dynamic pressure-redistribution devices using air, gel or water, foam, or other substances are commercially available, but the PTA must be aware that the material covering these devices can also create heat and friction, contributing to pressure. Redistributing pressure on the skin must be accompanied by adequate fluid and nutrition intake (see also Box 7.10). Doughnut cushions should never be used, because they can cause tissue ischemia and new pressure ulcers.
>
> The person who is incontinent presents an additional challenge to keeping the skin clean and dry. Stool or urine becomes an irritant and places the person at additional risk for skin breakdown. Contamination of an already existing wound by wound drainage, perspiration, urine, or feces is also a concern for the incontinent and immobile population.
>
> Fecal containment products are available for use in the case of acute diarrhea or fecal incontinence when these conditions contribute to the development of ulcers. New products for urinary or fecal incontinence are available to help prevent skin maceration from backflow of urine or feces. These include skin barriers, ointments, and fecal incontinence systems.
>
> Cleaning should be carried out using a mild agent that minimizes irritation and dryness of the skin. Avoid harsh alkali soaps, alcohol-based products that can cause vasoconstriction, tincture of benzoin (may cause painful erosions), and hexachlorophene (may irritate the CNS). The force and friction applied to the skin should be minimized during cleaning or wound care. The use of a disposable, no-rinse, perineal cloth that is impregnated with a barrier ingredient is ideal.

Pigmentary Disorders
Definition and Incidence

Skin color or pigmentation is determined by the deposition of melanin, a dark polymer found in the skin, as well as in the hair, ciliary body, choroid of the eye, pigment layer of the retina, and certain nerve cells.

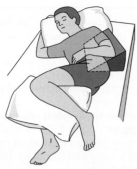

FIG. 7.15 Following the "rule of 30s" (head position at 30 degrees), bed positioning should include side-lying at oblique angles, usually described as a 30- to 45-degree side-lying position to either side. (Courtesy National Pressure Ulcer Advisory Panel.)

Melanin is formed in the melanocytes in the basal layer of the epidermis and is regulated (dispersion and aggregation) through the release of melatonin, a pineal hormone.

Hyperpigmentation is the abnormally increased pigmentation resulting from increased melanin production. *Hypopigmentation* is the abnormally decreased pigmentation resulting from decreased melanin production.

Pigmentary disorders (either hyperpigmentation or hypopigmentation) may be primary or secondary. Secondary pigmentary changes occur as a result of damage to the skin, such as irritation, allergy, infection, excoriation, burns, or dermatologic therapy, such as curettage, dermabrasion, chemical peels, or freezing with liquid nitrogen.

The formation and deposition of melanin can be affected by external influences such as exposure to heat, trauma, solar or ionizing radiation, heavy metals, and changes in oxygen potential. These influences can result in hyperpigmentation, hypopigmentation, or both. Local trauma may destroy melanocytes temporarily or permanently, causing hypopigmentation, sometimes with hyperpigmentation in surrounding skin.

Other pigmentary disorders may occur from exposure to exogenous pigments, such as carotene, certain metals, and tattooing inks. Carotenemia occurs as a result of excessive carotene in the blood, usually from ingesting certain foods (e.g., carrots, yellow fruit, egg yolk). It may also occur in diabetes mellitus and in hypothyroidism. Exposure to metals such as silver can cause argyria, a poisoning marked by a permanent ashen gray discoloration of the skin, conjunctivae, and internal organs. Gold, when given long term for rheumatoid arthritis, can also cause pigmentary changes.

Clinical Manifestations

Hyperpigmentation. Primary disorders in the hyperpigmentation category include pigmented nevi, Mongolian spots, juvenile freckles (ephelides), lentigines (also called *liver spots*) from sun exposure, café-au-lait spots associated with neurofibromatosis, and hypermelanosis caused by increased melanocyte-stimulating hormone (e.g., Addison's disease).

Secondary hyperpigmentation most commonly occurs after another dermatologic condition, such as acne (e.g., postinflammatory hyperpigmentation seen in dark-skinned people). *Melasma*, a patterned hyperpigmentation of the face, can occur as a result of steroid hormones, estrogens, and progesterones,

such as occurs during pregnancy and in 30% to 50% of women taking oral contraceptives. Secondary hyperpigmentation may also develop as a phototoxic reaction to medications, oils in perfumes, and chemicals in the rinds of limes, other citrus fruits, and celery.

Hypopigmentation and depigmentation. The disorder most commonly seen by a PTA in the hypopigmentation or depigmentation category is vitiligo. In *vitiligo*, pigment cells (melanocytes) are destroyed, resulting in small or large circumscribed areas of depigmentation often having hyperpigmented borders and enlarging slowly. This condition may be associated with hyperthyroidism, hypothyroidism, pernicious anemia, diabetes mellitus, Addison's disease, and carcinoma of the stomach.

Hypopigmentation can also occur on African American skin from the use of liquid nitrogen. Intraarticular injections of high concentrations of corticosteroids may also cause localized temporary hypopigmentation.

Blistering Diseases
Definition and Incidence
On occasion, blistering diseases may be seen in a therapy practice when severe enough to warrant localized treatment intervention (wound management). Blisters occur on skin and mucous membranes in a condition called *pemphigus*, which is an uncommon intraepidermal blistering disease in which the epidermal cells separate from one another. This disease occurs almost exclusively in middle-aged or older adults of all races and ethnic groups.

The exact cause of blistering diseases is unknown, but they may occur as a secondary event associated with viral or bacterial infections of the skin (e.g., herpes simplex, impetigo) or local injury of the skin (e.g., burns, ischemia, dermatitis), or they may be drug induced (e.g., penicillamine, captopril). In other diseases, blistering of the skin occurs as a primary autoimmune event characterized by the presence of autoantibodies directed against specific adhesion molecules of the skin and mucous membranes.[16]

Clinical Manifestations

Blistering diseases are characterized by the formation of flaccid bullae, or blisters. These bullae appear spontaneously, often on the oral mucous membranes or scalp, and are relatively asymptomatic. Erosions and crusts may develop over the blisters, causing toxemia and a mousy odor. The lesions become extensive, and the complications of the disease, especially infection, can lead to great toxicity and debility. Disturbances of electrolyte balance are also common because of fluid losses through the involved skin in severe cases. See the section on fluid and electrolyte balance in Chapter 2.

Treatment

Medical management may include hospitalization (with bed rest, IV antibiotics and feedings) when the disease is severe. In other cases, treatment may be with corticosteroids (e.g., prednisone) and local measures. The course of this disorder tends to be chronic in most people, and high-dose corticosteroids can mask the signs and symptoms of infection. If untreated, this condition is usually fatal within 2 months to 5 years as a result of infection. In the case of paraneoplastic pemphigus, early diagnosis and treatment of the underlying neoplasm are imperative.

Cutaneous Sarcoidosis

Sarcoidosis is a multisystemic disorder characterized by the formation of granulomas, inflammatory lesions containing mononuclear phagocytes usually surrounded by a rim of lymphocytes. These granulomas may develop in the lungs, liver, bones, or eyes and may be accompanied by skin lesions.

Subcutaneous nodules around the knee and elbow joints may occur in association with pulmonary or cardiac involvement and resolve in response to systemic corticosteroids. In the United States sarcoidosis occurs predominantly among African Americans, affecting twice as many women as men. Acute sarcoidosis usually resolves within 2 years. Chronic, progressive sarcoidosis, which is uncommon, is associated with pulmonary fibrosis and progressive pulmonary disability.

REFERENCES/SUGGESTED READINGS

To enhance this text and add value for the reader, references and suggested readings are included on the companion Evolve site that accompanies this textbook. The reader can view the source and access it online whenever possible.

The Endocrine and Metabolic Systems

VOCAB BUILDERS

A1c test
Acetone
Adrenergic
Amyloidosis
Anabolism
Brittle diabetes
Catabolism
Catecholamine
Chvostek's sign
Diuretics
Endorphins
Exophthalmos
Fowler's position
Gangrene
Glucocorticoid
Graves' disease
Hemochromatosis
Hirsutism perfusion
Hyponatremia
Metastasis
Myxedema achlorhydriaiatrogenic
Neuroendocrine theory of aging
Osteophyte
Polydipsia nocturia
Rhabdomyolysis
Somogyi effect
Suppurative
Tetany
Thyroid storm
Toxemia
Trousseau sign
Turgor

ENDOCRINE SYSTEM

The endocrine system is composed of various glands located throughout the body (Fig. 8.1). These glands are capable of synthesis and release of special chemical messengers called *hormones,* which are transported by the bloodstream to the cells and organs on which they have a specific regulatory effect (Table 8.1). The endocrine system and the nervous system control and integrate body function to maintain homeostasis. Whereas the nervous system sends its messages along nerve fibers, eliciting swift and selective neural responses, the endocrine system sends its messages in the form of hormones via the bloodstream.

Hormonal effects have a slower onset than neural effects, but they maintain a longer duration of action. The actions of the endocrine system may be localized to one area or generalized to all the cells of the body.[97] The endocrine system has the following five general functions:

1. Differentiation of the reproductive system and the central nervous system (CNS) of the developing fetus
2. Stimulation of sequential growth and development during childhood and adolescence
3. Coordination of the male and female reproductive systems
4. Maintenance of optimal internal environment throughout the life span
5. Initiation of corrective and adaptive responses when emergency demands occur[98]

The endocrine system meets the nervous system at the hypothalamic-pituitary interface. The hypothalamus integrates the endocrine and autonomic nervous systems and controls the function of endocrine organs by neural and hormonal pathways. Although the communicative and integrative roles of the endocrine and nervous systems are similar, the precise ways in which each system functions differ.

Hypothalamic Control

Neural pathways connect the hypothalamus to the posterior pituitary, providing the hypothalamus direct control over both the anterior and the posterior portions of the pituitary gland (Fig. 8.2). Disorders of the hypothalamic-pituitary partnership are manifested clinically, usually either by syndromes of hormone excess or deficiency or by visual impairment from optic nerve compression because of the location of the hypothalamus and pituitary.

Neural stimulation to the posterior pituitary provokes the secretion of two effector hormones: antidiuretic hormone (ADH) and oxytocin. The hypothalamus also exerts hormonal control at the anterior pituitary through releasing and inhibiting factors. Hypothalamic hormones stimulate the pituitary to release tropic (stimulating) hormones. At the same time, effector hormones are released or inhibited, affecting the adrenal cortex, thyroid, and gonads. Endocrine pathology develops as a result of dysfunction of releasing, tropic, or effector hormones or when defects occur in the target tissue.

In addition to hormonal and neural controls, a negative feedback system regulates the endocrine system. The mechanism may be simple or complex. Simple feedback occurs when the level of one substance regulates the secretion of a hormone. For example, low serum calcium levels stimulate parathyroid hormone (PTH) secretion; high serum calcium levels inhibit it. Complex feedback loops occur through the hypothalamic-pituitary–target organ axis. Steroid therapy disrupts the hypothalamic-pituitary-adrenal (HPA) axis by suppressing secretion of cortisol. Steroid treatment is necessary for some conditions, but problems can occur when withdrawal of the external steroid occurs too rapidly or abruptly. The result can be life-threatening adrenal insufficiency, because the HPA axis does not have enough time to recover sufficiently to stimulate cortisol secretion.

Hormonal Effects

In response to the hypothalamus, the *posterior pituitary* secretes oxytocin and ADH. Oxytocin stimulates contraction of the uterus and is responsible for the milk letdown reflex in lactating women. ADH controls the concentration of body fluids by alteration of the permeability of the kidney's distal convoluted tubules and collecting ducts to conserve water. The secretion of ADH depends on plasma volume and osmolality as monitored by hypothalamic neurons. Circulatory shock and severe hemorrhage are the most powerful stimulators of ADH; other stimulators include pain, emotional stress, trauma, morphine, tranquilizers, certain anesthetics, and positive-pressure breathing.

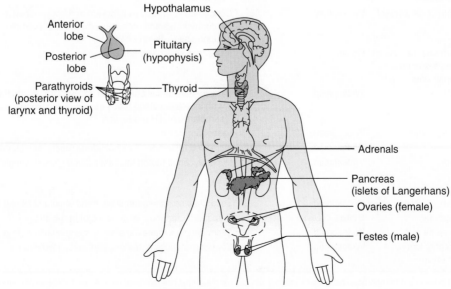

FIG. 8.1 Endocrine glands.

The *anterior pituitary* secretes prolactin, which stimulates milk production, and human growth hormone (HGH), which affects most body tissues. HGH stimulates growth by increasing protein synthesis and fat mobilization and by decreasing carbohydrate use. Hyposecretion of HGH results in dwarfism; hypersecretion causes gigantism in children and acromegaly in adults.

The *thyroid gland* secretes the thyroid hormones thyroxine (T_4) and triiodothyronine (T_3). Thyroid hormones, necessary for normal growth and development, act on many tissues to regulate our basal metabolism and to increase metabolic activity and protein synthesis. Deficiency of thyroid hormone causes varying degrees of hypothyroidism, from a mild, clinically insignificant form to a life-threatening coma. Hypersecretion of thyroid hormone causes hyperthyroidism and, in extreme cases, causes thyrotoxic crisis. Excessive secretion of thyroid-stimulating hormone (TSH) from the pituitary gland causes thyroid gland hyperplasia, resulting in goiter in chronic iodine deficiency states.

The *parathyroid glands* secrete PTH, which regulates calcium and phosphate metabolism. PTH elevates serum calcium levels by stimulating resorption of calcium and phosphate from bone, reabsorption of calcium and excretion of phosphate by the kidneys, and, by combined action with vitamin D, absorption of calcium and phosphate from the gastrointestinal (GI) tract.

Hyperparathyroidism results in hypercalcemia; hypoparathyroidism causes hypocalcemia.

The *endocrine pancreas* produces glucagon from the alpha cells and insulin from the beta cells. Glucagon, the hormone of the fasting state, releases stored glucose to raise the blood glucose level. Insulin, the hormone of the nourished state, facilitates glucose transport, promotes glucose storage, stimulates protein synthesis, and enhances free fatty acid uptake and storage. Insulin deficiency causes diabetes mellitus (DM); insulin

TABLE 8.1   Endocrine Glands: Secretion, Target, and Action*

Gland	Hormone	Target	Basic Action
Pituitary			
Anterior lobe	Somatotropin (GH)	Bones, muscles, organs	Retention of nitrogen to promote protein *anabolism*
	TSH	Thyroid	Promotes secretory activity
	FSH	Ovaries, seminiferous tubules	Promotes development of ovarian follicle, secretion of estrogen, and maturation of sperm
	Luteinizing hormone	Follicle, intestinal cell	Promotes ovulation and formation of corpus luteum, secretion of progesterone, and secretion of testosterone
	Prolactin (luteotropic hormone)	Corpus luteum, breast	Maintains corpus luteum and progesterone secretion; stimulates milk secretion
	ACTH	Adrenal cortex	Stimulates secretory activity
Posterior lobe	ADH	Distal tubules of kidney	Reabsorption of water
	Oxytocin	Uterus	Stimulates contraction
Thyroid	T_4 and T_3	Widespread	Regulate oxidation of body cells and growth metabolism; influence gluconeogenesis, mobilization of fats, and exchange of water, electrolytes, and protein
	Calcitonin	Skeleton	Calcium and phosphorus metabolism
Parathyroids	PTH	Bone, kidney, intestinal tract	Essential for calcium and phosphorus metabolism and calcification of bone
Adrenal			
Cortex	Mineralocorticoids (aldosterone)	Widespread, primarily kidney	Maintains fluid-electrolyte balance; reabsorbs sodium chloride; secretes potassium
	Glucocorticoids (cortisol)	Widespread	Concerned with food metabolism and body response to stress; preserves carbohydrates and mobilizes amino acids; promotes gluconeogenesis; suppresses inflammation
	Sex hormone (testosterone, estrogen, progesterone)	Gonads	Influences secondary sex characteristics
Medulla	Epinephrine	Widespread	Cardiac; myocardial stimulation, tachycardia, dysrhythmias; vasoconstriction with increased blood pressure; increased blood glucose via glycolysis; stimulates ACTH production
	Norepinephrine	Widespread	Vasoconstriction
Pancreas	Insulin	Widespread	Increased utilization of carbohydrate, decreased blood glucose
	Glucagon	Widespread	Hyperglycemic factor; increases blood glucose via glycogenolysis
Gonads			
Ovaries	Estrogen	Widespread	Secondary sex characteristics; maturation and sexual function
	Progesterone	Uterus, breast	Preparation for and maintenance of pregnancy
Testes	Testosterone	Widespread	Secondary sex characteristics; maturation and normal sex function
Adipose tissue	Adiponectin, leptin, angiotensin	Widespread	Control metabolism, hunger, and vasoconstriction

*When reading a client's chart, it is important to know basic hormone functions or effects that may impact therapy treatment. At least 30 different hormones have been identified, but only those most common to therapy clients are included here.

ACTH, Adrenocorticotropic hormone; *ADH,* antidiuretic hormone; *FSH,* follicle-stimulating hormone; *GH,* growth hormone; *PTH,* parathyroid hormone; T_3, triiodothyronine; T_4, thyroxine; *TSH,* thyroid-stimulating hormone.

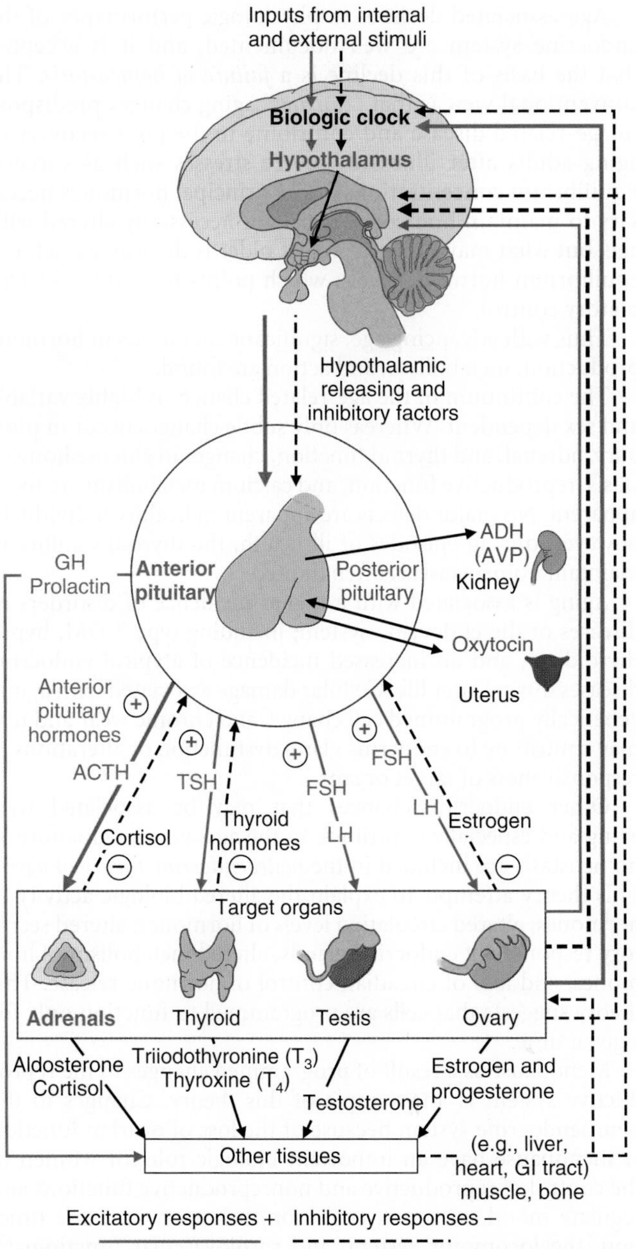

FIG. 8.2 Control of the endocrine system by the nervous system. One example of the complex feedback loops described in the text is highlighted here. The hypothalamus controls the pituitary gland through releasing and inhibiting factors. The anterior lobe of the pituitary gland then releases tropic (stimulating) hormones that act on target glands (thyroid, adrenals, and gonads). Endocrine pathology occurs when dysfunction occurs in releasing, tropic, or effector hormones or when defects occur in the target tissue. The anterior pituitary controls adrenocorticotropic hormone (ACTH), thyroid-stimulating hormone (TSH), growth hormone (GH), prolactin, follicle-stimulating hormone (FSH), and luteinizing hormone (LH). The posterior pituitary controls oxytocin and antidiuretic hormone (ADH [AVP]).

excess can be exogenous or may result from a tumor of the beta cells. Whatever the cause of excess insulin, hypoglycemia is the result.

The *adrenal cortex* secretes mineralocorticoids, glucocorticoids, and sex steroids. Aldosterone, a mineralocorticoid, regulates the reabsorption of sodium and the excretion of potassium by the kidneys and is involved intimately in the regulation of blood pressure. An excess of aldosterone can result primarily from hyperplasia or secondarily from many conditions, such as congestive heart failure or cirrhosis. The *adrenal medulla* is an aggregate of nervous tissue that produces the catecholamines epinephrine and norepinephrine, which are involved in the fight-or-flight response. The *testes* and *ovaries* are also endocrine glands responsible for synthesizing and secreting hormones.

Adipose tissue can be classified as an endocrine gland because it secretes several hormones responsible for metabolism, hunger, vasoconstriction, and cellular growth and development. The concept of adipose tissue as an endocrine organ is quite new, but it is clear that molecules secreted into the bloodstream by fat, such as adiponectin and leptin, act on target organs at distant sites.

Endocrine Pathology

Dysfunctions of the endocrine system are classified as hypofunction or hyperfunction. The source of hypofunction and hyperfunction may be inflammation or tumor originating in the hypothalamus, the pituitary gland, or other endocrine glands. Inflammation may be acute or subacute but is usually chronic, which results in glandular hypofunction. Chronic endocrine abnormalities are common health problems necessitating lifelong hormone replacement for survival.

Ectopic hormone production is the production and secretion of hormone or hormone-like substances from a source other than the normal source of the hormone. For example, some endocrine gland tumors can metastasize and produce excess hormone from new tumor sites.

Neuroendocrine Response to Stress

The concept that stress of any kind (emotional, physical, psychologic, or spiritual) may influence immunity and resistance to disease has been the subject of investigation for many years. The endocrine system, together with the immune and nervous systems, mounts an integrated response to stressors. Only a brief review of the neuroendocrine response to stress contributing to disease is presented in this section.

Hormones of the neuroendocrine system affect components of the immune system,[32] and mediators produced by immune components regulate the neuroendocrine response. The sympathetic nervous system is aroused during the stress response and causes the medulla of the adrenal gland to release catecholamines, such as epinephrine, norepinephrine, and dopamine, into the bloodstream. Simultaneously, the anterior pituitary gland releases a variety of hormones, including ADH, prolactin, GH, and adrenocorticotropic hormone (ACTH).

Catecholamines

Catecholamines are organic compounds that play an important role in the body's physiologic response to stress. Their release at sympathetic nerve endings increases the rate and force of muscular contraction of the heart, increasing cardiac output; constricts peripheral blood vessels, resulting in elevated blood pressure; elevates blood glucose levels by hepatic and skeletal glycogenolysis; and promotes an increase in blood lipids by increasing the *catabolism* (breakdown) of fats.

Glycogenesis is the splitting of glycogen, a starch, yielding glucose. The well-known metabolic effects of adrenal catecholamines prepare the body to take physical action in the fight-or-flight phenomenon. Stressors commonly associated with catecholamine release include exercise, thermal changes, and acute emotional states.

Cortisol

Cortisol is the principal glucocorticoid hormone released from the adrenal cortex and also known as *hydrocortisone* when synthesized pharmaceutically. Cortisol has multiple functions but it primarily regulates the metabolism of proteins, carbohydrates, and lipids to cause an elevation in blood glucose level. These effects on glucose level and fat metabolism result in increased blood glucose and plasma lipid levels and promote the formation of ketone bodies when insulin secretion is insufficient.

Cortisol is essential to norepinephrine-induced vasoconstriction and other physiologic phenomena necessary for survival under stress. The production of glucose promoted by cortisol provides a source of energy for body tissues, and the pooling of amino acids from proteins may ensure amino acid availability for protein synthesis at sites in which replacement is critical, such as muscle or cells of damaged tissue.

Another effect of cortisol is that of dampening the body's inflammatory response to invasion by foreign agents. This anti-inflammatory protective mechanism helps preserve the integrity of body cells at the site of the inflammatory response and provides the basis for the major therapeutic use of this steroid. Cortisol also inhibits fibroblast proliferation and function at the site of an inflammatory response and accounts for the poor wound healing, increased susceptibility to infection, and decreased inflammatory response often seen in individuals with chronic glucocorticoid excess.

Other Hormones

Other hormones, such as endorphins, GH, prolactin, and testosterone, may be released as part of the response to stressful stimuli. *Endorphins,* a term derived from *endogenous* and *morphine,* are a group of opiate-like structures produced naturally by the body at neural synapses in the CNS. These hormones serve to modulate the transmission of pain perceptions by raising the pain threshold and producing sedation and euphoria.

As its name implies, *growth hormone* stimulates and controls the rate of skeletal and visceral growth by directly influencing protein, carbohydrate, and lipid metabolism. GH levels increase in the blood after a variety of physically or psychologically stressful stimuli such as surgery, fever, physical exercise, or the anticipation of exhausting exercise, cardiac catheterization, electroshock therapy, or gastroscopy.[10]

Prolactin stimulates the growth of breast tissue and sustains milk production in postpartum mammals. Prolactin levels in plasma increase with a variety of stressful stimuli, but they show little change after exercise. *Testosterone,* a hormone that regulates male secondary sex characteristics and sex drive (libido), decreases after stressful stimuli such as anesthesia, surgery, marathon running, and acute illness. Decreased testosterone during these circumstances restrains growth and reproduction to preserve energy for protective responses.[10]

Aging and the Endocrine System[33,71]

The exact effects of aging on the endocrine system are not clear. In particular, the question of whether changes in endocrine function are a cause of aging or a natural consequence of aging remains unresolved. The endocrine system has not been implicated as the direct cause of aging.

Age-associated declines in physiologic performance of the endocrine system are well documented, and it is accepted that the basis of this decline is a *failure of homeostasis*. The conventional view is that "normal" aging changes predispose to age-related disease and contribute to the poor recovery of aging adults after illness or severe stresses such as surgery. Equilibrium concentrations of the principal hormones necessary to maintain homeostasis are not necessarily altered with age, but what may differ as we get older is the way we achieve equilibrium hormone levels, which points to changes in regulatory control.

Thus with advancing age, significant alterations in hormone production, metabolism, and action are found.

The continuum of the age-related changes is highly variable and sex dependent. Whereas only subtle changes occur in pituitary, adrenal, and thyroid function, changes in glucose homeostasis, reproductive function, and calcium metabolism are more apparent. No major defects are apparent in healthy individuals; however, during episodes of ill health, the thyroid's ability to maintain homeostasis is often limited.[33]

Aging is associated with a higher incidence of disorders or diseases of the endocrine system, including type 2 DM, hypothyroidism, and an increased incidence of atypical endocrine diseases during later life. Cellular damage associated with aging, genetically programmed cell change, and chronic wear and tear may contribute to endocrine gland dysfunction or alterations in responsiveness of target organs.

Other endocrine changes that may be associated with aging and especially contribute to the age-associated failure in homeostasis are included in the *neuroendocrine theory of aging*. This theory attempts to explain the altered biologic activity of hormones, altered circulating levels of hormones, altered secretory responses of endocrine glands, altered metabolism of hormones, and loss of circadian control of hormone release. This theory suggests that cells are programmed to function only for a given time.

Menopause as a result of programmed changes in the reproductive system is an example of this theory. Changes in the neuroendocrine system because of the loss of ovarian function at menopause have an important biologic role for women in the control of reproductive and nonreproductive functions and regulate mood, memory, cognition, behavior, immune function, the locomotor system, and cardiovascular functions.[123] It is thought that neural signals are altered during middle age, leading to cessation of reproductive cycles, and that the complex interplay of ovarian and hypothalamic or pituitary pacemakers becomes increasingly dysfunctional with aging, ultimately resulting in menopause.[123]

In addition, as the nervous system ages, a progressive reduction takes place in the body's capacity to maintain homeostasis in the face of environmental stress. Thus although the initial response to a stressful stimulus may be appropriate, as the body ages the response is more likely to be persistent and ultimately inappropriate or even harmful.[37]

Anatomic Changes with Aging

The *pituitary gland* undergoes both anatomic and histologic changes associated with aging. The blood supply is reduced, and a higher incidence of adenomas and cysts is developed during later life.

The *thyroid gland* becomes relatively smaller and fibrotic, and its position becomes lower lying with age. As with the pituitary gland, blood supply to the thyroid gland is decreased. Secretion of thyroid hormones may diminish with age.

The *parathyroid gland* demonstrates tissue changes with advancing age, but no major change is apparent in PTH levels. Hyperparathyroidism occurs primarily in persons older than age 50. It is rarely caused by parathyroid carcinoma.

The *adrenal glands* have more fibrous tissue with aging, but because of compensatory feedback mechanisms, no relative alteration is apparent in functional cortisol levels. The most common cause of hypercortisolism occurs with the use of corticosteroids for medical conditions.

Changes in the *reproductive glands* have been shown clearly to have physiologic effects, most notably on the cardiovascular system, the skeleton, muscle mass, and libido.[111]

Hormonal Changes with Aging

The female reproductive system undergoes changes as part of the normal aging process. Menopause leads to changes in the genitourinary tract, accelerates the loss of minerals from bone, and leads to an alteration in the lipid composition in the mature woman. Male hormones have been linked to preservation of bone and muscle mass and to an increased tendency toward developing certain diseases during later life.

Loss of body hair, changes in the skin's collagen content and thickness, an increase in the percentage of body fat, a decrease in lean body mass, a decrease in bone mass, and a decrease in protein synthesis are signs of endocrinopathy that may be associated with decreased GH levels.[71] With the decline of GH secretion, sleep cycles are disrupted, and the potential for depression, fibromyalgia, and other disorders associated with sleep deprivation is now recognized.[156]

As mentioned, interactions between the endocrine and immune systems also influence the aging process. Declining hormonal levels are accompanied by increased activity of tumor suppressor genes in the aging population unless these genes have been mutated so that suppressor function is lost. In the presence of decreased hormonal levels, loss of tumor suppressor genes accounts for the increased probability of tumors with advancing age, again demonstrating the link between the endocrine and immune systems.[71]

All of these changes have an increasing effect on humans because the average life span has increased, meaning a greater part of women's lives will be lived in a hypoestrogenic state. Men and women alike will experience a decline in GH secretion, increased exposure to mutagens, and a greater possibility of the loss of tumor suppressor genes.[123]

Musculoskeletal Signs and Symptoms of Endocrine Disease

Signs and symptoms of endocrine pathology vary, depending on the gland affected and whether the pathology is a result of an excess (hyperfunction) or insufficiency (hypofunction) of hormonal secretions.[59]

Growth and development of connective tissue structures are influenced strongly and sometimes controlled by various hormones and metabolic processes. When these processes are altered, structural and functional changes can occur in various connective tissues, producing musculoskeletal signs and symptoms in addition to other systemic signs and symptoms of endocrine dysfunction (Table 8.2).

The physical therapist assistant (PTA) must be aware that clients with an underlying but undiagnosed endocrine disorder

TABLE 8.2 Signs and Symptoms of Endocrine Dysfunction	
Neuromusculoskeletal	**Systemic**
Rheumatic-like signs and symptoms	Excessive or delayed growth
Muscle weakness	Polydipsia
Muscle atrophy	Polyuria
Myalgia	Mental changes (nervousness, confusion, depression)
Fatigue	
Carpal tunnel syndrome	Changes in hair (quality and distribution)
Synovial fluid changes	
Periarthritis	Changes in skin pigmentation
Adhesive capsulitis (diabetes mellitus)	Changes in distribution of body fat
Chondrocalcinosis	
Spondyloarthropathy	Changes in vital signs (elevated body temperature and pulse rate, increased blood pressure)
Diffuse idiopathic skeletal hyperostosis	
Osteoarthritis	Heart palpitations
Osteoporosis	Increased perspiration
Osteonecrosis	Kussmaul's respirations (deep, rapid breathing)
Hand stiffness	
Arthralgia	Dehydration or excessive retention of body water
Pseudogout	

may initially present a musculoskeletal problem and that clients with established endocrine disorders are not cured by hormonal replacement or suppression. Rather, they may develop progression of musculoskeletal impairment in response to hormone fluctuations.

Rheumatoid arthritis can be an indicator of an underlying endocrine disease. Early rheumatic symptoms, such as myalgias and arthralgias, are common with a number of endocrine diseases. DM is associated with a variety of rheumatic syndromes such as the stiff hand syndrome and limited joint motion syndrome. Although rheumatic symptoms can appear suddenly in people with an endocrine disorder, an insidious onset is much more common.

Muscle weakness, atrophy, myalgia, and *fatigue* that persist despite rest may be early manifestations of thyroid or parathyroid disease, acromegaly, diabetes, Cushing's syndrome, or osteomalacia. In endocrine disease, most proximal muscle weakness is usually painless and may be unrelated to either the severity or the duration of the underlying disease. However, when true demonstrative weakness occurs, proximal muscle weakness is related to the severity and duration of the underlying endocrine problem. Any compromise of muscle energy metabolism aggravates and perpetuates trigger points such as are associated with myofascial pain syndrome or tender points in muscle associated with fibromyalgia syndrome (FMS).

Carpal tunnel syndrome (CTS) resulting from median nerve impairment at the wrist is a common finding in people with certain endocrine and metabolic conditions such as acromegaly, diabetes, pregnancy, and hypothyroidism. Any increase in the volume of contents of the carpal tunnel impinges on the median nerve. In endocrine disorders, CTS is frequently bilateral, which is one characteristic that may distinguish it from overuse syndromes and other causes of CTS.

Tenosynovitis (inflammation of the tendon sheaths) occurs with some infectious processes and many musculoskeletal conditions. Fluid infiltrating the tunnel may soften the transverse carpal ligament, which can make the bony arch flatten and compress the nerve.[57] Thickening of the transverse carpal ligament also may occur with systemic disorders such as acromegaly or myxedema.

CTS in persons with diabetes represents one form of diabetic neuropathy caused by ischemia-related microvascular damage of the median nerve. This ischemia then causes increased sensitivity to even minor pressure exerted in the carpal tunnel area.[68] Vitamin B_6 deficiency, repetitive activities, and obesity may also be factors in the development of CTS for the person with diabetes.[1,40]

CTS occurring during pregnancy may be caused by extra fluid and/or fat, diabetes, vitamin deficiencies, or other causes unrelated to the pregnancy itself. The fact that many women develop CTS at or near menopause may suggest that the soft tissues about the wrist may be affected in some way by hormones.[25]

Periarthritis (inflammation of periarticular structures including the tendons, ligaments, and joint capsule) and *calcific tendinitis* occur most often in the shoulders of people who have endocrine disease. *Chondrocalcinosis* is the deposition of calcium salts in the joint cartilage; when accompanied by attacks of goutlike symptoms, it is called *pseudogout*. In 5% to 10% of people with chondrocalcinosis, an associated underlying endocrine or metabolic disease, such as hypothyroidism, hyperparathyroidism, or acromegaly, occurs.[52] People diagnosed with fibromyalgia also may have altered thyroid function[91] and shoulder impingement secondary to chondrocalcinosis. *Spondyloarthropathy* (disease of joints of the spine) and *osteoarthritis* occur in individuals with various endocrine or metabolic diseases. *Hand stiffness,* hand pain, and arthralgias of the small joints of the hand may occur with endocrine and metabolic diseases. Flexor tenosynovitis with stiffness is a common finding in persons with hypothyroidism. This condition often accompanies CTS.[90]

8.1 Special Implications for the PTA: Overview of Endocrine and Metabolic Disease Disorders of the endocrine and metabolic systems may cause recognizable clinical signs and symptoms (see Table 8.2). Clients with a variety of endocrine and metabolic disorders report symptoms of fatigue, muscle weakness, and occasionally muscle or bone pain. Painless muscle weakness associated with endocrine and metabolic disorders usually involves proximal muscle groups. In most cases the person who has received a diagnosis of an endocrine or metabolic disorder has undergone a combination of clinical and laboratory tests. This person may be in the care of a therapy professional for some other unrelated musculoskeletal problem that can be affected by symptoms associated with hormone imbalances.

Individuals with other clinical presentations of musculoskeletal symptoms, such as CTS, rheumatoid arthritis, or adhesive capsulitis, may be referred to therapy without accurate diagnosis of the underlying endocrine pathology. In addition, a lack of progress in therapy should signal the possibility of a systemic origin of musculoskeletal symptoms.

SPECIFIC ENDOCRINE DISORDERS

Pituitary Gland

The pituitary gland, or hypophysis, is a small oval gland located at the base of the skull in an indentation of the sphenoid bone (see Figs. 8.1 and 8.2). It is often referred to as the *master gland* because of its role in regulating other endocrine glands. It is

joined to the hypothalamus by the pituitary stalk and is influenced by the hypothalamus through releasing and inhibiting factors. The pituitary consists of two parts: the anterior pituitary and the posterior pituitary lobes. The anterior pituitary secretes six different hormones (ACTH, TSH, luteinizing hormone [LH], follicle-stimulating hormone [FSH], HGH, and prolactin; see Fig. 8.2).

The posterior pituitary is a downward offshoot of the hypothalamus and contains many nerve fibers; it produces no hormones of its own. The hormones ADH (also called *vasopressin*) and oxytocin are produced in the hypothalamus and then stored and released by the posterior pituitary. Transmitter substances, such as acetylcholine and norepinephrine, are thought to activate release of these substances by the posterior pituitary gland when they are stimulated by nerve impulses from the hypothalamus.[10]

Anterior Lobe Disorders

Disorders of the pituitary gland occur most frequently in the anterior lobe and are most often caused by tumors, pituitary infarction, genetic disorders, and trauma. The three principal pathologic consequences of pituitary disorders are hyperpituitarism, hypopituitarism, and local compression of brain tissue by expanding tumor masses.[11]

Hyperpituitarism

Overview. Hyperpituitarism is an oversecretion of one or more of the hormones secreted by the pituitary gland, especially GH, resulting in acromegaly or gigantism. It is caused primarily by a hormone-secreting pituitary tumor, typically a benign adenoma. Other syndromes associated with hyperpituitarism include Cushing's disease, amenorrhea, and hyperthyroidism.

Cushing's disease is one form of Cushing's syndrome and results from oversecretion of ACTH by a pituitary tumor, which in turn results in oversecretion of adrenocortical hormones. Pituitary tumors produce both systemic effects and local manifestations.

Systemic effects include the following:

1. Excessive or abnormal growth patterns, resulting from overproduction of GH
2. Amenorrhea, galactorrhea (spontaneous milk flow in women without nursing), and gynecomastia and impotence in men
3. Overstimulation of one or more of the target glands, resulting in the release of excessive adrenocortical, thyroid, or sex hormones

Local pituitary tumors produce symptoms as the growing mass expands within the bony cranium. Local manifestations may include visual field abnormalities, headaches, and somnolence (sleepiness).

Gigantism and acromegaly. Gigantism, an overgrowth of the long bones, and acromegaly, increased bone thickness and hypertrophy of the soft tissues, result from GH-secreting adenomas of the anterior pituitary gland. Although GH-producing tumors that cause these conditions are rare, they are the second most common type of hyperpituitarism. Gigantism develops in children before the age when the epiphyses of the bones close; people who develop gigantism may grow to a height of 9 feet. Gigantism develops abruptly, whereas acromegaly develops slowly.

Acromegaly is a disease of adults and develops after closure of the epiphyses; the bones most affected are those of the face, jaw, hands, and feet. In adults, acromegaly occurs equally among men and women and usually from age 30 to 50 years.[11] Both conditions are characterized by the same skeletal abnormalities because hypersecretion of GH produces cartilaginous and connective tissue overgrowth, resulting in coarsened facial features; protrusion of the jaw; thickened ears, nose, and tongue; and broad hands, with spadelike fingers (Fig. 8.3).

Acromegaly-induced myopathy with muscle weakness and reduced exercise tolerance may be more common than previously appreciated. The pathologic or physiologic reason for this weakness has not been determined. Alterations in muscle size and strength in individuals with acromegaly are an accepted association.

Medical Management

Diagnosis, Treatment, and Prognosis

Timely diagnosis and appropriate treatment are imperative in reducing this potentially disabling chronic and progressive condition.[46] Long-term follow-up of disease activity and comorbidities is recommended, with management rather than cure being the primary goal.[45] Quality of life is often below reference values for the normal population of the same age.[162]

Drugs are now available that effectively normalize levels of GH and prolactin and decrease pituitary tumor size.[45] Drug therapy has replaced surgery in most cases of prolactin-secreting adenomas, but surgery is still the treatment of choice for pituitary adenomas that cause acromegaly.

8.2 Special Implications for the PTA: Hyperpituitarism

Postoperative Care

Ambulation and exercise are encouraged within the first 24 hours after surgery. Coughing, sneezing, and blowing the nose are contraindicated after surgery, but deep breathing exercises are encouraged. Postoperatively, vital signs and neurologic status must be closely monitored. Any alteration in level of consciousness or visual acuity, falling pulse rate, or rising blood pressure may signal an increase in intracranial pressure resulting from intracranial bleeding or cerebral edema and must be reported immediately.

The nursing staff members monitor blood glucose levels often because GH levels fall rapidly after surgery. The PTA is advised to consult with nursing staff to determine the possible need for blood glucose monitoring during or after exercise. The therapist should be familiar with signs and symptoms and special implications of hypoglycemia.

Tumors causing visual changes may require the therapist to consciously remain within the client's visual field. Unexpected mood changes can occur, requiring patience and understanding on the part of health care workers. Although surgical removal of the tumor and/or pituitary gland prevents permanent soft tissue deformities, bone changes already present do not change.

Orthopedic Considerations

Skeletal manifestations, such as arthritis of the hands and osteoarthritis of the spine, may develop with these conditions. Osteophyte formation and widening of the joint space as a result of increased cartilage thickening may be seen on radiographs. CTS is seen in up to 50% of people with acromegaly.

About half of individuals with acromegaly have thoracic and/or lumbar back pain. X-ray studies demonstrate increased intervertebral disk spaces and large osteophytes along the anterior longitudinal ligament. The PTA may be called on to provide a program that promotes maximum joint mobility, muscle strength, and functional skills. Assistance with activities of daily living may be an important aspect of intervention.

Acromegaly

Anyone with acromegaly should be screened for weakness, changes in joint mobility, and poor exercise tolerance. Skeletal abnormalities associated with acromegaly are usually irreversible. Joint symptoms are controlled with aggressive medical intervention with surgery, pharmacologic treatment, and in some cases pituitary irradiation in an attempt to normalize hormonal levels. Improvement of joint pain, crepitus, and range of motion has been reported with the newer drug therapy.[151]

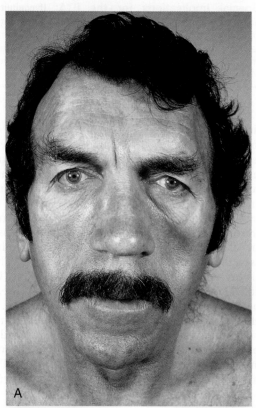

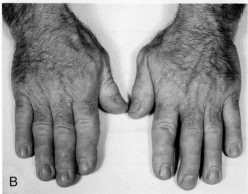

FIG. 8.3 Acromegaly (hyperpituitarism). Acromegaly occurs as a result of excessive secretion of growth hormone after normal completion of body growth. The resulting overgrowth of bone in the face, head (A), and hands (B) is pictured here. (From Glynn M, Drake WM: Hutchison's clinical methods: an integrated approach to clinical practice, ed 23, Edinburgh, 2012, Elsevier.)

Hypopituitarism. Hypopituitarism (also *panhypopituitarism* and *dwarfism*) is rare and results from decreased or absent hormonal secretion by the anterior pituitary gland. *Panhypopituitarism* refers to a generalized condition caused by partial or total failure of all six of the anterior pituitary's vital hormones.

Clinical manifestations are dependent on the age at onset and the hormones affected (Box 8.1). More than 75% of the pituitary must be obliterated before symptoms develop. Treatment for hypopituitarism involves removal (if possible) of the causative factor, such as tumors, and lifetime replacement of the missing hormones.

8.3 Special Implications for the PTA: Hypopituitarism

Although rarely encountered in a therapy setting, the client with hypopituitarism may report symptoms associated with hormonal deficiencies until hormone replacement therapy is complete. The PTA may observe weakness, fatigue, lethargy, apathy, and orthostatic hypotension.

Posterior Lobe Disorders

Diabetes insipidus. Diabetes insipidus, a rare disorder, involves a physiologic imbalance of water secondary to ADH deficiency. Injury or loss of function of the hypothalamus, the neurohypophyseal tract, or the posterior pituitary gland can result in diabetes insipidus (Box 8.2).

Because the major functions of ADH are to promote water resorption by the kidney and to control the osmotic pressure of the extracellular fluid, when ADH production decreases, the kidney tubules fail to resorb water. The end result is excretion of large amounts of dilute urine. Unlike urine in DM, which contains large amounts of glucose, urine in diabetes insipidus is dilute and contains no glucose. Other clinical manifestations include polydipsia (excessive thirst), nocturia (excessive urination at night), and dehydration (e.g., poor tissue *turgor*, dry mucous membranes, constipation, muscle weakness, dizziness, and hypotension). Fatigue and irritability may develop secondary to sleep disruption and in association with nocturia.

8.4 Special Implications for the PTA: Diabetes Insipidus

The PTA must be alert for possible serious side effects of any type of ADH administration. ADH stimulates smooth muscle contraction of the vascular system (causing increased blood pressure), the GI tract (causing diarrhea), and the coronary arteries (causing angina or myocardial infarction).[68]

Increases in blood pressure can cause additional serious problems in some people, particularly those with hypertension or coronary artery disease (CAD) and cerebrovascular disease.

Syndrome of inappropriate antidiuretic hormone secretion. Syndrome of inappropriate ADH (SIADH) is a disorder associated with excessive release of ADH, which disturbs fluid and electrolyte balance, resulting in a water imbalance. SIADH has a wide variety of causes, including pituitary damage resulting from infection or trauma.

BOX 8.1   Clinical Manifestations of Hypopituitarism

Growth Hormone Deficiency
- Short stature
- Delayed growth
- Delayed puberty

Adrenocortical Insufficiency
- Hypoglycemia
- Anorexia
- Nausea
- Abdominal pain
- Orthostatic hypotension

Hypothyroidism (see also Table 8.4)
- Tiredness
- Lethargy
- Sensitivity to cold
- Menstrual disturbances

Gonadal Failure
- Secondary amenorrhea
- Impotence
- Infertility
- Decreased libido
- Absent secondary sex characteristics (children)

Neurologic Signs (Produced by Tumors)
- Headache
- Bilateral temporal hemianopia
- Loss of visual acuity
- Blindness

BOX 8.2   Causes of Diabetes Insipidus

- Intracranial or pituitary neoplasm
- Metastatic lesions (e.g., breast or lung cancer)
- Surgical hypophysectomy or other neurosurgery
- Skull fracture or head trauma (damages the neurohypophyseal structures)
- Infection (e.g., meningitis, encephalitis)
- Granulomatous disease
- Vascular lesions (e.g., aneurysm)
- Idiopathic cause
- Autoimmune; heredity cause
- Drugs or medications (e.g., phenytoin; alcohol)
- Nephrogenic diabetes insipidus (congenital; drug induced)

Tumors can cause unregulated production of ADH, leading to severe sodium depletion (*hyponatremia*) with resultant lethargy, nausea, anorexia, and generalized weakness. Mild hyponatremia causes increased thirst, muscle cramps, and lethargy. Rapid onset of SIADH can result in coma, convulsions, or death.[148] SIADH can be triggered by the stress of surgery, many systemic disorders, and certain medications. SIADH is the opposite of diabetes insipidus, so treatment of diabetes insipidus with vasopressin can lead to SIADH if excessive amounts are administered. When serum osmolality (a measure of the number of dissolved particles per unit of water) falls, a feedback mechanism causes inhibition of ADH, which promotes increased water excretion by the kidneys to raise serum osmolality to normal. When this feedback mechanism fails and ADH levels are sustained, fluid retention results. Ultimately, serum sodium levels fall, resulting in hyponatremia and water intoxication.[68]

Correction of life-threatening sodium imbalance is the first aim of treatment, followed by correction of the underlying cause. If SIADH is caused by malignancy, success in alleviating water retention may be obtained by surgical resection, irradiation, or chemotherapy. Otherwise, treatment for SIADH is symptomatic and includes restriction of water intake, careful replacement of sodium chloride, and administration of *diuretics*.

> **8.5 Special Implications for the PTA: Syndrome of Inappropriate Antidiuretic Hormone Secretion** Anyone at risk for SIADH should be monitored for sudden weight gain or fluid retention and changes in urination and fluid intake. Observe for headache, lethargy, muscle cramps, restlessness, irritability, convulsions, or weight gain without visible edema.
>
> Continued need for sodium and fluid restrictions may be necessary for the person discharged to home or who is in a facility other than the acute care setting (hospital). People with unresolved SIADH should avoid the use of aspirin or nonsteroidal antiinflammatory agents without a physician's approval because these drugs can increase hyponatremia.
>
> Each individual must be evaluated to determine the most appropriate plan of care, ranging from bed mobility and transfers to range-of-motion exercises to a program of strengthening and conditioning.[148]
>
> In the acute care setting, fluid restrictions must be noted and followed. This may require some coordination and scheduling for the patient who may need water in association with his or her exercise program. Patients on fluid restriction must also be monitored for urinary output. Any change in mental status, motor coordination, or energy level should be recorded and reported for consideration by the medical and nursing staff.

Thyroid Gland

The thyroid gland is located in the anterior portion of the lower neck, below the larynx, on both sides of and anterior to the trachea (see Fig. 8.1). The primary hormones produced by the thyroid are T_4, T_3, and calcitonin. Both T_3 and T_4 regulate the metabolic rate of the body and increase protein synthesis. Calcitonin has a weak physiologic effect on calcium and phosphorus balance in the body. Thyroid function is regulated by the hypothalamus and pituitary feedback controls and by an intrinsic regulator mechanism within the gland.[62]

Both thyroid hormones travel from the thyroid via the bloodstream to distant parts of the body, in which they activate genes that regulate body functions. When the hypothalamus senses that circulating levels have dropped, it signals the pituitary gland, which sends TSH to the thyroid to trigger the release of thyroid hormones.

Susceptibility to thyroid disease is largely determined by the interaction of genetic makeup, age, and sex. Approximately 27 million Americans have been diagnosed with thyroid disease; many other people are undiagnosed because the signs and symptoms are so nonspecific. The risk of thyroid disease increases with age but is difficult to detect in adults over 60 because it typically masquerades as other illnesses such as heart disease, depression, or dementia. Women, particularly those with a family history of thyroid disease, are much more likely to have thyroid pathology than men. Although most thyroid conditions cannot be prevented, they respond well to treatment.

Thyroid hormone acts on nearly all body tissues, so excessive or deficient secretion affects various body systems. Alterations in thyroid function produce changes in nails, hair, skin, eyes, GI tract, respiratory tract, heart and blood vessels, nervous tissue, bone, and muscle.[62]

Women may notice disturbances in mood and in menstrual cycles. Menstrual irregularity, worsening premenstrual syndrome, new onset of depression later in life, postpartum depression (after pregnancy and birth), anxiety syndromes, and excessive fatigue have been reported by many women with thyroid dysfunction.

Both hyperthyroidism and hypothyroidism can adversely affect cardiac function. Sustained tachycardia in hyperthyroidism and sustained bradycardia with cardiac enlargement in hypothyroidism can result in cardiac failure. Both conditions affect the general rate of metabolism, the muscular system, the nervous system, the GI system, and, as mentioned, the cardiovascular system.

Hyperthyroidism

Definition and overview. Hyperthyroidism is an excessive secretion of thyroid hormone. Excessive thyroid hormone creates a generalized elevation of body metabolism, the effects of which are manifested in almost every system.

The most common form of hyperthyroidism is the autoimmune condition known as *Graves' disease*. Like most thyroid conditions, hyperthyroidism affects women more than men (4:1), especially women aged 20 to 40 years.

Etiologic and risk factors. Hyperthyroidism may result from both immunologic and genetic factors. Graves' disease, the most common form of hyperthyroidism, is most likely autoimmune in development, and although it is more common in women with family histories of thyroid abnormalities, major risk factors have not been identified.

Hyperthyroidism also may be caused by the overfunction of the entire gland, as in Graves' disease, or less commonly by hyperfunctioning of a single area.

Pathogenesis. Because the action of thyroid hormone on the body is stimulatory, hypermetabolism results with increased sympathetic nervous system activity. The excessive amounts of thyroid hormone stimulate the cardiac system. This excess thyroid hormone secretion leads to tachycardia, increased stroke volume, and increased peripheral blood flow. The increased metabolism also leads to a negative nitrogen balance, lipid depletion, and a resultant state of nutritional deficiency.

Clinical manifestations. Because hyperthyroidism is caused by an excess secretion of thyroid hormone, the clinical picture of Graves' disease is in many ways the opposite of that of hypothyroidism. The classic symptoms of Graves' disease are mild symmetric enlargement of the thyroid (goiter), nervousness, heat intolerance, weight loss despite increased appetite, sweating, diarrhea, tremor, and palpitations. Hyperthyroidism may induce atrial fibrillation, precipitate congestive heart failure, and increase the risk of underlying CAD for myocardial infarction.

Exophthalmos (abnormal protrusion of the eyes; Fig. 8.4) is considered most characteristic but is absent in many people with hyperthyroidism and may worsen after adequate treatment of the hyperthyroid state. Many other symptoms are common because this condition affects many body systems

(Table 8.3). Emotions are adversely affected by the increased metabolic activity within the body. Moods may be cyclic, ranging from mild euphoria to extreme hyperactivity or delirium and depression, which may persist even after successful treatment of hyperthyroidism.[18] Excessive hyperactivity may be associated with extreme fatigue.

Hyperthyroidism in older adults is notorious for causing atypical or minimal symptoms.[153] Signs and symptoms are not the usual ones and may be attributed to aging. Many older people actually appear apathetic instead of hyperactive. Cardiovascular abnormalities, as described previously, are much more common in older adults.

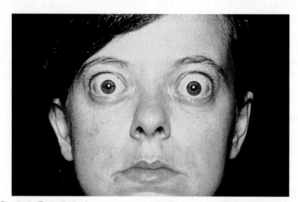

FIG. 8.4 Exophthalmos, or protruding eyes. This is a forward displacement of the eyeballs associated with thyroid disease. Because the eyes are surrounded by unyielding bone, fluid accumulation in the fat pads and muscles behind the eyeballs causes protruding eyes and a fixed stare. Without treatment of the underlying cause, the client with severe exophthalmos may be unable to close the eyelids and may develop corneal ulceration or infection, eventually resulting in loss of vision. Note the lid lag; the upper eyelid rests well above the limbus (edge of the cornea where it joins the sclera), and white sclera is visible. This is evident when the person moves the eyes from up to down. Physical therapy is not recommended in these cases until after the endocrine problem is resolved. Then therapeutic intervention with ultrasound, joint mobilization, stretching, and strengthening may be indicated to treat any residual dysfunction. (From Ignatavicius DD, Workman ML: Medical-surgical nursing: patient-centered collaborative care, ed 8, St Louis, 2016, Elsevier.)

Neuromuscular manifestations. Chronic periarthritis also is associated with hyperthyroidism. Inflammation that involves the periarticular structures, including the tendons, ligaments, and joint capsule, is termed *periarthritis*. This syndrome is characterized by pain and reduced range of motion. Calcification, whether periarticular or tendinous, may be seen on x-ray studies. Both periarthritis and calcific tendinitis can occur most often in the shoulder in clients who have undiagnosed, untreated, or inadequately treated endocrine disease. The involvement can be unilateral or bilateral and can worsen progressively to become adhesive capsulitis, or frozen shoulder. Acute calcific tendinitis of the wrist also has been described in such clients. Although antiinflammatory agents may be needed for acute symptoms, chronic periarthritis usually responds to treatment of the underlying hyperthyroidism.

Proximal muscle weakness (most marked in the pelvic girdle and thigh muscles) accompanied by muscle atrophy, known as *myopathy*, can occur in cases of undiagnosed, untreated, or inadequately treated hyperthyroidism. The PTA may first notice problems with coordination or balance or notice weakness of the legs, causing a client difficulty in ambulating, rising from a chair, or climbing stairs.[43]

Respiratory muscle weakness can manifest as dyspnea. The pathogenesis of the weakness is still a subject of controversy; muscle strength seems to return to normal in 6 to 8 weeks after medical treatment, with a slower resolution of muscle wasting. In severe cases, normal strength may not be restored for months.

Medical Management

Prevention

There is no way to prevent Graves' disease. Early screening can help determine whether someone is at risk. Two simple blood tests can be conducted, one to measure TSH and the second for antithyroid antibodies. Testing should be done by age 40 years, especially in the presence of a positive family history.

Diagnosis

Diagnosis is based on clinical history, physical presentation, examination findings, and laboratory test results.

TABLE 8.3	Systemic Manifestations of Hyperthyroidism				
Central Nervous System Effects	**Cardiovascular and Pulmonary Effects**	**Musculoskeletal Effects**	**Integumentary Effects**	**Ocular Effects**	**Genitourinary Effects**
Tremors	Increased pulse rate, tachycardia, palpitations	Muscle weakness and fatigue	Capillary dilation (warm flushed, moist skin)	Exophthalmos	Polyuria (frequent urination)
Hyperkinesis (abnormally increased motor function or activity)	Increased cardiac output	Muscle atrophy	Heat intolerance	Weakness of the extraocular muscles (poor convergence, poor upward gaze)	Amenorrhea (absence of menses)
Nervousness	Increased blood volume	Chronic periarthritis	Onycholysis (separation of the fingernail bed)	Sensitivity to light	Female infertility
Emotional lability	Dysrhythmias (especially atrial fibrillation)	Myasthenia gravis	Easily broken hair and increased hair loss	Spasm and retraction of the upper eyelids, lid tremor	Increased risk of spontaneous miscarriage
Weakness and muscle atrophy	Weakness of respiratory muscles (breathlessness, hypoventilation)		Hard purple area over the anterior surface of the tibia with itching, erythema, and occasionally pain		Gynecomastia (males)
Increased deep tendon reflexes	Increased respiratory rate				

Modified from Goodman CC, Snyder TE: Differential for physical therapists screening for referral, ed 5, St. Louis, 2013, Saunders.

Treatment

The three major forms of therapy are (1) antithyroid medication, (2) radioactive iodine (RAI), and (3) surgery. Most endocrine specialists would now recommend RAI as first-line therapy in anyone older than 18 years of age who is not pregnant. Some physicians treat patients as young as 12 because long-term studies have shown no increased incidence of thyroid cancer or leukemia in people receiving such treatment.[157]

Iodine-131 therapy takes several months before it is effective. Typically, everyone who receives RAI becomes hypothyroid and requires thyroid hormone replacement for the rest of their lives. Use of antithyroid drugs is also effective and is the usual choice of therapy during pregnancy and for children younger than 12. Partial or subtotal thyroidectomy is an effective way to treat hyperthyroidism caused by Graves' disease. The ideal surgical treatment leaves a small portion of the functioning thyroid gland to avoid permanent hormone replacement. Surgical treatment is effective in most cases.

8.6 Special Implications for the PTA: Hyperthyroidism

Any time a PTA observes a client's neck and finds unusual swelling, enlargement with or without symptoms of pain, tenderness, hoarseness, or dysphagia (difficulty swallowing), notification to the supervisory PT is required. For the client requiring lifelong thyroid hormone replacement therapy, nervousness and palpitations may develop with overdosage. A small number of people experience fever, rash, and arthralgias as side effects of antithyroid drugs. The physician should be notified of these or any other unusual symptoms, because it may be possible to use an alternative drug.

Monitoring Vital Signs

Monitoring vital signs is important to assess cardiac function if the involved person is an older adult,[153] has CAD, or has symptoms of dyspnea, fatigue, tachycardia, and/or arrhythmia. If the heart rate is more than 100 beats/minute, check the blood pressure and pulse rate and rhythm frequently. The person with dyspnea is most comfortable sitting upright or in a high *Fowler's position* (head of the bed raised 18 to 20 inches above a level position with the knees elevated).

Because clients with Graves' disease may experience heat intolerance, they should avoid exercise in a hot aquatic or pool physical therapy setting. Exercise in a warm pool would be safe and would not be contraindicated as long as the person's temperature was monitored.

Postoperative Care

Postoperatively, observe for signs of hypoparathyroidism (muscular twitching, tetany, numbness and tingling around the mouth, fingertips, or toes), a complication that results from the accidental removal of the parathyroid glands during surgery. Symptoms can develop 1 to 7 days after surgery.

Any health care worker in contact with clients who have undergone radioiodine therapy must follow necessary precautions. Saliva is radioactive for 24 hours after iodine-131 therapy; health care professionals in contact with clients while they are coughing or expectorating must take precautions.

Side Effects of Radioiodine Therapy

Radioiodine therapy has few immediate side effects. Rarely, anterior neck tenderness may develop 7 to 10 days after therapy, consistent with radiation-induced thyroiditis.[130] The potential exists for worsening hyperthyroidism soon after radioiodine therapy, secondary to inflammation and release of stored thyroid hormone in the bloodstream. Older adults and anyone with cardiac disease usually are pretreated with antithyroid agents before receiving radioiodine to prevent this occurrence.

The major adverse reaction from radioiodine is iatrogenic hypothyroidism. This development is so characteristic that it is considered an inevitable consequence of therapy rather than a side effect. Hypothyroidism develops in at least 50% of all cases treated with radioiodine therapy within the first year after therapy, with a gradual increased incidence thereafter. This complication necessitates lifelong follow-up with close monitoring of thyroid function.

Hyperthyroidism and Exercise

Hyperthyroidism is associated with exercise intolerance and reduced exercise capacity, although the exact relationship is unknown. Cardiac output is either normal or enhanced during exercise in the hyperthyroid state, and blood flow to muscles is augmented during submaximal exercise. However, proximal muscle weakness with accompanying myopathy is characteristic in individuals with Graves' disease and may affect exercise capability.

Impaired cardiopulmonary function (more noticeable in older people with hyperthyroidism) also may affect exercise capacity.

Fatigue as a result of the hypermetabolic state and rapid depletion of nutrients may affect exercise capacity.[42] With perceived exertion or exercise tolerance used as a guide, exercise parameters (frequency, intensity, and duration) remain the same for the person treated for hyperthyroidism as for anyone who does not have this condition.

Ultrasound and Iontophoresis

The benefit of physical therapy intervention in the treatment of endocrine-induced calcific tendinitis has not been proved. Some experts advocate waiting until after the endocrine problem is resolved before initiating a plan of care. Therapeutic intervention with ultrasound, joint mobilization, stretching, and strengthening may be indicated to treat any residual dysfunction.

Hypothyroidism

Definition and etiologic factors. Hypothyroidism (hypofunction) refers to a deficiency of thyroid hormone in the adult that results in a generalized slowed body metabolism; it is the most common disorder of thyroid function in the United States and Canada. More than 50% of cases occur in families in which thyroid disease is present.

Like diabetes, hypothyroidism can be categorized as type I (hormone deficient) and type II (hormone resistant). The condition has traditionally been classified as either primary or secondary. *Type I* or *primary hypothyroidism* occurs as a result of reduced functional thyroid tissue mass or impaired hormonal synthesis or release. *Type II* or *secondary hypothyroidism* accounts for a small percentage of all cases of hypothyroidism and occurs as a result of inadequate stimulation of the gland because of pituitary or hypothalamic disease.

Incidence. Hypothyroidism is about four times more prevalent in women than in men. Although hypothyroidism may be congenital and therefore present at birth, the highest incidence occurs from age 30 to 60 years. More than 95% of all people with hypothyroidism have the primary form of the disease.[68]

Pathogenesis. In type I or primary hypothyroidism, the loss of thyroid tissue leads to decreased secretion of thyroid hormone. Whenever the body perceives an inadequate amount of thyroid hormone, the pituitary releases more and more

TSH in an effort to stimulate thyroid hormone production. The result is an elevated TSH level in the blood when thyroid function is low.

Decreased levels of thyroid hormone lead to an overall slowing of the basal metabolic rate. This slowing of all body processes leads to bradycardia, decreased GI tract motility, slowed neurologic functioning, a decrease in body heat production, and achlorhydria (absence of hydrochloric acid from gastric juice). Lipid metabolism also is altered by hypothyroidism with a resultant increase in serum cholesterol and triglyceride levels and a concomitant increase in arteriosclerosis and coronary heart disease. Thyroid hormones also play a role in the production of red blood cells, with the potential for the development of anemia.

Type II or secondary hypothyroidism is most often the result of failure of the pituitary gland to synthesize and release adequate amounts of TSH.

Clinical manifestations. As with all disorders affecting the thyroid and parathyroid glands, clinical signs and symptoms associated with hypothyroidism affect many systems of the body (Table 8.4). Typically, the early clinical features of hypothyroidism are vague and ordinary—fatigue, mild sensitivity to cold, mild weight gain resulting from fluid retention, forgetfulness, depression, and dry skin or hair—so they escape detection.

As the disorder progresses, myxedema and its associated signs and symptoms appear. *Myxedema* is a result of an alteration in the composition of the dermis and other tissues, causing connective tissues to become thickened, causing a nonpitting, boggy edema, especially around the eyes, hands, and feet and in the supraclavicular fossae. Thickening of the tongue and the laryngeal and pharyngeal structures, hoarseness, and slurred speech occur as a result of myxedema.[166]

Other clinical manifestations associated with hypothyroidism may include decreasing mental stability; dry, flaky, inelastic skin; dry, sparse hair; hoarseness; upper eyelid droop; and thick, brittle nails. Cardiovascular involvement leads to decreased cardiac output, slow pulse rate, and signs of poor peripheral circulation. Other possible effects of hypothyroid function are anorexia, abdominal distention, menorrhagia, decreased libido, infertility, ataxia, intention tremor, and nystagmus.

Neuromuscular symptoms are among the most frequent manifestations of hypothyroidism seen in a therapy practice. Flexor tenosynovitis with stiffness can accompany CTS in persons with hypothyroidism. Most people with CTS associated with hypothyroidism do not require surgical treatment because symptoms of median nerve compression respond to thyroid replacement therapy.

A wide spectrum of rheumatic symptoms occurs in people with hypothyroidism. A subset of fibromyalgia with muscle aches and tender points may be seen early; replacement therapy with thyroid hormone eliminates the symptoms, which aids in the diagnosis of the underlying cause of this form of fibromyalgia. An inflammatory arthritis indistinguishable from rheumatoid arthritis may be seen. The arthritis predominantly involves the small joints of the hands. Generally, the arthritis resolves with normalization of the thyroid hormone levels.[100]

Proximal muscle weakness can occur in persons with hypothyroidism, sometimes accompanied by pain. Trigger points are frequently detected on examination, and diffuse muscle tenderness may be the major finding. Muscle weakness is not always related to either the severity or the duration of hypothyroidism; it can be present several months before a medical diagnosis of hypothyroidism is made. Deep tendon reflexes show delayed relaxation time (i.e., prolonged reflexes), especially in the Achilles tendon.[43]

TABLE 8.4   Systemic Manifestations of Hypothyroidism

Central Nervous System Effects	Musculoskeletal Effects	Cardiovascular Effects	Hematologic Effects	Respiratory Effects	Integumentary Effects	Gastrointestinal Effects	Genitourinary Effects
Slowed speech and hoarseness	Proximal muscle weakness	Bradycardia	Anemia	Dyspnea	Myxedema (periorbital and peripheral)	Anorexia	Infertility
Slow mental function (loss of interest in daily activities, poor short-term memory)	Myalgias	Congestive heart failure	Easy bruising	Respiratory muscle weakness	Thickened, cool, and dry skin	Constipation	Menstrual irregularity, bleeding (menorrhagia)
Fatigue and increased sleep	Trigger points	Poor peripheral circulation (pallor, cold skin, intolerance to cold, hypertension)			Scaly skin (especially elbows and knees)	Weight gain disproportionate to caloric intake	
Headache	Stiffness	Severe atherosclerosis, hyperlipidemia			Carotenosis (yellowing of the skin)	Decreased protein metabolism (retarded skeletal and soft tissue growth)	
Cerebellar ataxia	Carpal tunnel syndrome	Angina			Coarse, thinning hair	Delayed glucose uptake	
Depression	Prolonged deep tendon reflexes (especially Achilles)				Intolerance to cold	Decreased glucose absorption	
Psychiatric changes	Subjective report of paresthesias without supportive objective findings				Nonpitting edema of hands and feet		
	Muscular and joint edema				Poor wound healing		
	Back pain				Thin, brittle nails		
	Increased bone density						
	Decreased bone formation and resorption						

Modified from Goodman CC, Snyder TE: Differential diagnosis for physical therapists: screening for referral, ed 5, St. Louis, 2013, Saunders.

Medical Management

Diagnosis

Specific testing of TSH levels is the most sensitive indicator of primary hypothyroidism. TSH levels are always elevated in primary hypothyroidism.

Serum cholesterol, alkaline phosphatase, and triglyceride levels also can be significantly elevated in the presence of hypothyroidism.

Treatment

The goals of treatment for hypothyroidism are to (1) correct thyroid hormone deficiency, (2) reverse symptoms, and (3) prevent further cardiac and arterial damage. If treatment with lifelong administration of synthetic thyroid hormone preparations is begun soon after symptoms appear, recovery may be complete.

8.7 Special Implications for the PTA: Hypothyroidism

In the case of myxedematous hypothyroidism, distinctive changes in the synovium can occur, resulting in a viscous noninflammatory joint effusion. When these hypothyroid clients have been treated with thyroid replacement therapy, some have experienced attacks of acute pseudogout caused by the crystals in the periarticular joint structures. Without medical treatment, this condition can lead to permanent joint damage.

Calcium pyrophosphate dihydrate deposition disease (pseudogout) usually affects larger joints, but symptomatic involvement of the spine with deposition of crystals in the ligamentum flavum and atlantooccipital ligament can result in spinal stenosis and subsequent neurologic syndromes.[127] Effective treatment of pseudogout may include joint aspiration to relieve fluid pressure, steroid injection, and nonsteroidal antiinflammatories.[140] Although the synovium contains noninflammatory joint effusion, crystals may loosen, resulting in crystal shedding into the joint fluid, causing an inflammatory response.

The role of the PTA is similar to his or her role in the treatment of rheumatoid arthritis. Muscular complaints (aches, pain, and stiffness) associated with hypothyroidism are likely to develop into persistent myofascial trigger points. Clinically, any compromise of the energy metabolism of muscle aggravates and perpetuates trigger points. These do not resolve just with specific physical therapy intervention; they also require thyroid replacement therapy.[137]

Hypothyroidism and Fibromyalgia

The correlation between hypothyroidism and FMS continues to be investigated.[92] Despite the correlation between hypothyroidism and FMS, thyroid dysfunction is seen at least three times more often in women with rheumatoid arthritis than in women with similar demographic features with noninflammatory rheumatic diseases such as osteoarthritis and fibromyalgia.[95] Studies have shown an association between hypothyroidism and fibromyalgia.

These clients are particularly weather conscious and have muscular pain that increases with the onset of cold, rainy weather.[140]

Hypothyroidism and Medication

Clients with cardiac complications are started on small doses of thyroid hormone because large doses can precipitate heart failure or myocardial infarction by increasing body metabolism, myocardial oxygen requirements, and, consequently, the workload of the heart. Carefully observe for chest pain and tachycardia. Report any signs of hypertension or congestive heart failure in the older adult. After thyroid replacement therapy begins, watch for symptoms of hyperthyroidism

Hypothyroidism and Exercise

Activity intolerance, weakness, and apathy secondary to decreased metabolic rate may require developing increased tolerance to activity and exercise once thyroid replacement therapy has been initiated. Increased activity and exercise are especially helpful for the client who is constipated secondary to slowed metabolic rate and decreased peristalsis. Exercise-induced myalgia leading to *rhabdomyolysis* (disintegration of striated or skeletal muscle fibers with acute edema and excretion of myoglobin in the urine) has been reported in untreated or undiagnosed hypothyroidism. Rhabdomyolysis also could occur possibly as a result of poor drug compliance in combination with other aggravating factors such as exercise.[88,133]

Goiter

Goiter, an enlargement of the thyroid gland, may be a result of lack of iodine, inflammation, or tumors (benign or malignant). Enlargement also may appear in hyperthyroidism, especially Graves' disease. Goiter occurs most often in areas of the world in which iodine, which is necessary for the production of thyroid hormone, is deficient in the diet (Fig. 8.5).

Thyroglobulin is the large molecule. When iodine is absent, only the thyroglobulin is made by the gland. Because the thyroglobulin molecule is large, its increased production causes rapid glandular growth, and a marked increase in overall glandular mass occurs called a *colloid goiter*.[62] With the use of iodized salt and iodine-containing binders in commercial foods, this problem almost has been eliminated in the United States and Canada. Although the younger population in the United States may be goiter free, aging adults may have developed goiter during their childhood or adolescent years and may still have clinical manifestations of this disorder.

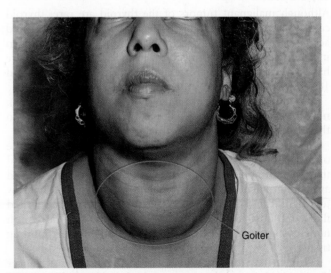

FIG. 8.5 Goiter. The enlarged thyroid gland appears as a swelling of the anterior neck. This condition results from a low dietary intake of iodine and is rare in Canada and the United States but may be seen in other parts of the world. (From Ignatavicius DD, Workman ML: Medical-surgical nursing: patient-centered collaborative care, ed 8, St Louis, 2016, Elsevier.)

Increased neck size may be observed, and when the thyroid increases to a certain point, pressure on the trachea and esophagus may cause difficulty breathing, dysphagia (difficulty swallowing), and hoarseness. Compression of the upper airway can be a fatal complication. Surgical intervention is essential when the trachea is compromised.

Thyroiditis

Thyroiditis, inflammation of the thyroid, may be classified as *acute suppurative* (pus forming and very rare), *subacute granulomatous* (uncommon), and *lymphocytic* or *chronic* (Hashimoto's thyroiditis). Acute and subacute thyroiditis are uncommon conditions caused by bacterial and viral agents, respectively. Infected glands are painful and associated with systemic symptoms of fever and hyperthyroidism. Several varieties of related autoimmune causes of thyroiditis exist, such as Hashimoto's (lymphocytic) thyroiditis and postpartum thyroiditis. These types of thyroiditis are generally painless, with only a rare case of Hashimoto's thyroiditis causing pain. Only the most common form of Hashimoto's thyroiditis is discussed further.

Hashimoto's (chronic) thyroiditis affects women more frequently than it does men (10 : 1) and is most often seen in the 30- to 50-year-old age group. The disorder has an autoimmune basis, and genetic predisposition appears to play a role in the cause. Hashimoto's thyroiditis causes destruction of the thyroid gland. It is one of the most common causes of hypothyroidism in women older than 50.

Signs of chronic thyroiditis usually include painless symmetric or asymmetric enlargement of the gland and an irregular surface, which occasionally causes pressure on the surrounding structures. This pressure may subsequently cause dysphagia and respiratory distress.

The course of Hashimoto's thyroiditis varies. Most people see a decrease in the size of the goiter and remain stable for years with treatment.

Thyroid Cancer

Although malignant tumors of the thyroid are rare, thyroid cancer makes up more than 90% of all endocrine cancers and accounts for 63% of deaths from endocrine cancer, with an increasing incidence worldwide.[13] In the United States, there has been a significant increase to 60,220 new cases in 2013 and 1850 deaths.[135]

Thyroid cancer affects women more than men (2 : 1 ratio), mainly from ages 40 to 60. A past medical history of radiation to the head, neck, or chest is the most obvious risk factor.

The usual presentation of thyroid cancer is the appearance of a hard, painless nodule on the thyroid gland or a gland that is multinodular. Most palpable nodules of the thyroid are benign adenomas and rarely become malignant or grow to a significant size to cause pressure against the trachea. Red flag symptoms include vocal cord paralysis, cervical lymph node dysfunction, and fixation of the nodule to surrounding tissues.[29,64]

Women have more thyroid nodules and more thyroid cancer than men. However, the presence of a thyroid nodule in a man is regarded with greater suspicion for cancer. Thyroid cancer is diagnosed by fine-needle aspiration biopsy. Treatment usually involves removal of all or part of the thyroid. Neck resection of involved lymph nodes may be done for metastases to the neck. Radioactive ablation of remaining thyroid tissue is standard practice for most thyroid cancers. External radiation may be used in some situations. Major postoperative complications may involve damage to the laryngeal nerve, hemorrhage, and hypoparathyroidism.[110]

Most thyroid cancers are treatable; however, disease recurrence and *metastasis* may occur in as many as 20% of affected individuals.[13] Individuals treated for thyroid cancer require long-term follow-up to detect recurrent disease, which can manifest years after initial therapy.[80]

8.8 Special Implications for the PTA: **Thyroid Cancer** A thyroid neoplasm can be the incidental finding in persons being treated for a musculoskeletal condition involving the head and neck. Most thyroid nodules are benign, but as mentioned previously, any time a PTA observes an asymptomatic nodule or unusual swelling or enlargement in the client's neck, hoarseness, dyspnea, or dysphagia (difficulty swallowing), a medical referral is required.

Individuals treated for head and neck cancers can have complex, difficult-to-treat problems secondary to cancer treatment. Proper stretching to prevent loss of motion of the head, neck, and jaw is important, especially if fibrosis has impaired eating and swallowing.

Parathyroid Glands

Two parathyroid glands are located on the posterior surface of each lobe of the thyroid gland. These glands secrete PTH, which regulates calcium and phosphorus metabolism.

PTH exerts its effect by the following:
1. Increasing the release of calcium and phosphate from the bone (bone demineralization)
2. Increasing the absorption of calcium and excretion of phosphate by the kidneys
3. Promoting calcium absorption in the GI tract[68]

Disorders of the parathyroid glands may come to the PTA's attention because these conditions can cause periarthritis and tendinitis. Both types of inflammation may be crystal induced, with formation of periarticular or tendinous calcification.

Hyperparathyroidism

Definition and incidence. Hyperparathyroidism is a disorder caused by overactivity of one or more of the four parathyroid glands that disrupts calcium, phosphate, and bone metabolism. Women are affected more than men (2 : 1), usually after age 60. Hyperparathyroidism is frequently overlooked in the over-60 population. Symptoms in the early stages for this group are subtle and easily attributed to the aging process, depression, or anxiety. Eventually the symptoms intensify as the level of serum calcium rises, but this situation is accompanied by increased bone damage and other complications.

Etiologic and risk factors. Hyperparathyroidism is classified as primary, secondary, or tertiary. *Primary hyperparathyroidism* develops when one or more of the parathyroid glands enlarge, increasing PTH secretion and elevating serum (blood) calcium levels.

Secondary hyperparathyroidism occurs when the glands are hyperplastic from malfunction of another organ system. This

TABLE 8.5   Systemic Manifestations of Hyperparathyroidism

Early Central Nervous System Symptoms	Musculoskeletal Effects	Gastrointestinal Effects	Genitourinary Effects
Lethargy, drowsiness, paresthesias Slow mentation, poor memory Depression, personality changes Easily fatigued Hyperactive deep tendon reflexes Occasionally glove-stocking distribution sensory loss	Mild to severe proximal muscle weakness of the extremities Muscle atrophy Bone decalcification (bone pain, especially spine; pathologic fractures; bone cysts) Gout and pseudogout Arthralgias involving the hands Myalgia and sensation of heaviness in the lower extremities Joint hypermobility	Peptic ulcers Pancreatitis Nausea, vomiting, anorexia Constipation Abdominal pain	Renal colic associated with stones Hypercalcemia (polyuria, polydipsia, constipation) Kidney infections Renal hypertension

Modified from Goodman CC, Snyder TE: Differential diagnosis for physical therapists: screening for referral, ed 5, St. Louis, 2013, Saunders.

is usually the result of renal failure, but it also may occur with osteogenesis imperfecta, Paget disease, multiple myeloma, carcinoma with bone metastasis, laxative abuse, and vitamin D deficiency.

Tertiary hyperparathyroidism is seen almost exclusively in dialysis clients who have long-standing secondary hyperparathyroidism.

Pathogenesis and clinical manifestations. The primary function of PTH is to maintain a proper balance of calcium and phosphorus ions within the blood. PTH maintains normal blood calcium levels by increasing bone resorption and GI absorption of calcium. It also maintains an inverse relationship between serum calcium and phosphate levels by inhibiting phosphate reabsorption in the renal tubules.

Abnormal PTH production disrupts this balance. Excessive circulating PTH leads to bone damage, hypercalcemia, and kidney damage (Table 8.5). In fact, hyperparathyroidism is the most common cause of hypercalcemia, which can lead to nervous system, musculoskeletal, metabolic, and cardiovascular problems.

Bone damage. Oversecretion of PTH causes excessive osteoclast growth and activity within the bones. Osteoclasts are active in promoting resorption of bone, which then releases calcium into the blood, causing hypercalcemia. This calcium loss leads to bone demineralization, and in time the bones may become so fragile that pathologic fractures, deformity, and compression fractures of the vertebral bodies occur.

Hypercalcemia. As excessive PTH secretion results in bone resorption and hypercalcemia as just described, excessive calcium in the urine eventually develops because the excessive filtration of calcium overwhelms this renal mechanism.

Kidney damage. As serum calcium levels rise in response to excessive PTH levels, large amounts of phosphorus and calcium are excreted and lost from the body. Excretion of these compounds occurs through the renal system, leaving deposits of calcium phosphate within the renal tubules.

Some people with hyperparathyroidism may be completely asymptomatic, but even seemingly asymptomatic clients with elevated serum and PTH levels have been found to have paresthesias, muscle cramps, and loss of pain and vibratory sensation in a glove-stocking distribution. Others develop a wide range of symptoms as a result of skeletal disease, renal involvement, GI tract disorders, and neurologic abnormalities.

Medical Management

Diagnosis

The diagnosis of hyperparathyroidism depends on measurement of PTH levels in persons found to be hypercalcemic.

Treatment and Prognosis

Treatment for primary hyperparathyroidism is surgical removal (parathyroidectomy). Minimally invasive parathyroidectomy is advised even for individuals with mild elevation in calcium because of the risk for more serious complications of hyperparathyroidism such as renal failure, osteoporosis, and early death.

The prognosis is good if the condition is identified and treated early. Untreated, hyperparathyroidism exacerbates many conditions among older adults, such as osteoporosis and CAD.

8.9 Special Implications for the PTA: Hyperparathyroidism

The PTA is likely to see skeletal, articular, and neuromuscular manifestations associated with hyperparathyroidism. Chronic low back pain and easy fracturing resulting from bone demineralization may be compounded by marked muscle weakness and atrophy, especially in the legs.[68]

Acute Care

Clients with osteopenia are predisposed to pathologic fractures and must be treated with caution to minimize the risk of injury. Take every safety precaution, assisting carefully with walking, keeping the bed at its lowest position, raising the side rails, and lifting the immobilized person carefully to minimize bone stress. Schedule care to allow the person with muscle weakness recovery time and rest between all activities.

Postoperative Care

Postoperatively, after parathyroidectomy, the person should use a semi-Fowler's position with support for the head and neck to decrease edema, which can cause pressure on the trachea. Observe for any signs of mild tetany, such as reports of tingling in the hands and around the mouth.

Early ambulation (although uncomfortable) is essential, because weight bearing and pressure on bones speed up recalcification. The use of light ankle weights or light weight-resistive elastic for the lower extremities provides tension at the musculotendinous-bone interface, accomplishing the same response. The physician first must approve the same type of exercise program for the upper extremities, because care must be taken not to disturb the surgical site.

Hypoparathyroidism

Definition. Because the parathyroid glands primarily regulate calcium balance, hypoparathyroidism causes hypocalcemia and produces a syndrome opposite that of hyperparathyroidism, with abnormally low serum calcium levels, high serum phosphate levels, and possible neuromuscular irritability (*tetany*; Box 8.3).

Etiologic factors and incidence. Iatrogenic (acquired) causes include accidental removal of the parathyroid glands during thyroidectomy or anterior neck surgery. Variations in location and color in addition to the minute size of parathyroid glands make identification difficult and may result in glandular damage or accidental removal during thyroid removal or anterior neck surgery. Idiopathic causes affect children nine times as often as adults and affect twice as many women as men. Like Graves' disease and Hashimoto's thyroiditis, idiopathic hypoparathyroidism may be an autoimmune disorder with a genetic basis.

Pathogenesis. PTH normally functions to increase bone resorption to maintain a proper balance between serum calcium and phosphate. When parathyroid secretion of PTH is reduced, bone resorption and GI tract absorption slow, serum calcium levels fall, and severe neuromuscular irritability develops. Calcifications may form in various organs such as the eyes and basal ganglia.

Clinical manifestations. Mild hypoparathyroidism may be asymptomatic, but it usually produces hypocalcemia and high serum phosphate levels that affect the CNS and other body systems (Table 8.6). The most significant clinical consequence of hypocalcemia associated with hypoparathyroidism is neuromuscular irritability. In people with chronic hypoparathyroidism, this neuromuscular irritability may result in tetany.

BOX 8.3   Characteristics of Hyperparathyroidism and Hypoparathyroidism

Hyperparathyroidism

- Increased bone resorption
- Elevated serum calcium levels
- Depressed serum phosphate levels
- Hypercalciuria and hyperphosphaturia
- Decreased neuromuscular irritability

Hypoparathyroidism

- Decreased bone resorption
- Depressed serum calcium levels
- Elevated serum phosphate levels
- Hypocalciuria and hypophosphaturia
- Increased neuromuscular activity, which may progress to tetany

From Black JM, Matassarin-Jacobs E, editors: Medical surgical nursing, ed 5, Philadelphia, 1997, Saunders.

Acute (overt) tetany begins with a tingling in the fingertips, around the mouth, and occasionally in the feet. This tingling spreads and becomes more severe, producing painful muscle tension, spasms, grimacing, laryngospasm, and arrhythmias.

Medical Management

Diagnosis
Diagnosis of this condition is based on history, clinical presentation, examination, and laboratory values (low serum calcium, high serum phosphate, or low or absent urinary calcium).

Treatment
Treatment is directed toward elevation of serum calcium levels as rapidly as possible with intravenous calcium, prevention or treatment of convulsions, and control of laryngeal spasm. Treatment of chronic hypoparathyroidism with pharmacologic management is accomplished more gradually than treatment for an acute situation.

Prognosis
Full recovery from the effects of hypoparathyroidism is possible when the condition is diagnosed early, before the development of serious complications. Unfortunately, once formed, cataracts and brain calcifications are irreversible.

8.10   Special Implications for the PTA: Hypoparathyroidism
Chronic Hypoparathyroidism

For the person with chronic hypoparathyroidism, observe carefully for any minor muscle twitching or signs of laryngospasm because these may signal the onset of acute tetany. Chronic tetany is less severe, usually affects one side only, and may cause difficulty with gait and balance. Gait training and prevention of falls are key components of a therapy program.

Chronic hypoparathyroidism can lead to cardiac complications that necessitate careful monitoring.

Home Health Care

Lifelong medication, dietary modifications, and medical care are required for the person with chronic hypoparathyroidism. If hypophosphatemia persists, cheese and milk should be omitted from the diet because they have a high calcium content. Other foods high in calcium but low in phosphorus are encouraged.

Adrenal Glands

The adrenals are two small glands located on the upper part of each kidney (see Fig. 8.1). Each adrenal gland consists of two relatively discrete parts: an outer cortex and an inner medulla. The outer cortex is responsible for the secretion of steroid hormones that regulate fluid and mineral balance, called *mineralocorticoids;* steroid hormones are responsible for controlling the metabolism of glucose, called *glucocorticoids;* and sex hormones are called *androgens.*

The centrally located adrenal medulla secretes epinephrine and norepinephrine, which exert widespread effects on vascular tone, the heart, and the nervous system, and affects glucose metabolism. Together, the adrenal cortex and medulla are major factors in the body's response to stress.

TABLE 8.6   Systemic Manifestations of Hypoparathyroidism

Central Nervous System Effects	Musculoskeletal Effects[a]	Cardiovascular Effects[a]	Integumentary Effects	Gastrointestinal Effects
Personality changes (irritability, agitation, anxiety, depression) Convulsions	Hypocalcemia (neuromuscular excitability and muscular tetany, especially involving flexion of the upper extremity) Spasm of intercostal muscles and diaphragm, compromising breathing Positive *Chvostek's sign*	Cardiac arrhythmias Eventual heart failure	Dry, scaly, coarse, pigmented skin Tendency to have skin infections Thinning of hair, including eyebrows and eyelashes Fingernails and toenails become brittle and form ridges	Nausea and vomiting Constipation or diarrhea Neuromuscular stimulation of the intestine (abdominal pain)

[a]The PTA should be aware of musculoskeletal and cardiovascular effects, which are the most common and important.

Glandular hypofunction and hyperfunction characterize the major disorders of the adrenal cortex. Underactivity of the adrenal cortex results in a deficiency of glucocorticoids, mineralocorticoids, and adrenal androgens. Overactivity results in excessive production of the same hormones.

Adrenal Insufficiency

Hypofunction of the adrenal cortex can originate from a disorder within the adrenal gland itself (primary adrenal insufficiency), or it may result from hypofunction of the pituitary-hypothalamic unit (secondary adrenal insufficiency).[140] Adrenocortical insufficiency, whether primary or secondary, can be either acute or chronic.

Primary adrenal insufficiency (Addison's disease)

Definition and overview. Addison's disease is a condition that occurs as a result of a disorder within the adrenal gland itself; insufficient cortisol is released from the adrenal glands, causing a wide range of problems. It was named for the physician who first studied and described the associated symptoms. Adrenal insufficiency affects about 4 adults in 100,000 each year in the United States. Both sexes are affected, but the incidence is slightly higher in women than in men. Addison's disease can occur anytime across the life span, with a preponderance of cases occurring during middle age (40 to 60 years old).

Etiologic factors. At one time, most causes of Addison's disease occurred as a complication of tuberculosis, but now most cases are considered idiopathic or autoimmune. Because more than half of all people with idiopathic Addison's disease have circulating autoantibodies that react specifically against adrenal tissue, this condition is considered to have an autoimmune basis.

Risk factors. Surgery (including dental procedures); pregnancy (especially with postpartum hemorrhage); accident, injury, or trauma; infection; salt loss resulting from profuse diaphoresis (hot weather or with strenuous physical exertion); or failure to take steroid therapy in persons who have chronic adrenal insufficiency can cause acute adrenal insufficiency.

Pathogenesis and clinical manifestations. This adrenal gland disorder results in decreased production of cortisol (a glucocorticoid) and aldosterone (a mineralocorticoid). Glucocorticoid deficiency causes widespread metabolic disturbances, with resultant hypoglycemia and liver glycogen deficiency. The person grows weak, exhausted, and hypotensive, and develops anorexia, weight loss, nausea, and vomiting. Emotional disturbances can develop, ranging from mild neurotic symptoms to severe depression. Glucocorticoid deficiency also diminishes resistance to stress.

In anyone who has previously been diagnosed with Addison's disease, acute symptoms, such as severe abdominal pain, low back or leg pain, severe vomiting, diarrhea, and hypotension, may develop quickly in response to triggers such as trauma, infarction, or infection. Chronic adrenal insufficiency with chronic cortisol deficiency causes increases in skin and mucous membrane pigmentation. Persons with Addison's disease may have a bronzed or tanned appearance, which is the most striking physical finding with primary adrenal insufficiency (not present in all people with this disorder). This change in pigmentation may vary in the Caucasian population from a slight tan or a few black freckles to an intense generalized pigmentation. Members of darker-skinned races may develop a slate-gray color that is obvious only to family members.

Aldosterone deficiency causes numerous fluid and electrolyte imbalances. Aldosterone normally promotes conservation of sodium and therefore conserves water and excretion of potassium. A deficiency of aldosterone causes increased sodium excretion, dehydration hypotension (low blood pressure causing orthostatic symptoms), and decreased cardiac output affecting heart size (decrease in size). Other clinical effects include decreased tolerance for even minor stress, poor coordination, fasting hypoglycemia, and a craving for salty food. Addison's disease may also retard axillary and pubic hair growth in females, decrease the libido, and in severe cases cause amenorrhea (absence of menstruation).[165]

Medical Management

Diagnosis and Prognosis

Diagnosis of Addison's disease depends primarily on blood and urine hormonal tests. Decreased serum cortisol levels are the hallmark of Addison's disease.

Complications from Addison's disease, such as hyponatremia, hypoglycemia, hyperkalemia, hypercalcemia, and metabolic acidosis, will be apparent in the blood chemistry values obtained.

Treatment

Acute adrenal insufficiency is treated by replacing fluids, electrolytes, glucose, and cortisol while identifying the underlying cause of the problem. Medical management for chronic adrenal insufficiency is primarily pharmacologic, consisting of lifelong administration of synthetically manufactured corticosteroids and mineralocorticoids. If untreated, Addison's disease is ultimately fatal. Adrenal crisis requires immediate hospitalization and treatment.

8.11 Special Implications for the PTA: Primary Adrenal Insufficiency (Addison's Disease) With pharmacologic therapy, listlessness and exhaustion should gradually lessen and disappear, making exercise possible. Stress should be minimized with physical activity, and exercise progressed very gradually per individual tolerance. Too much stress of any kind can put the client into an "addisonian crisis" as the body is unable to meet the cortisol demand caused by the extra "stress" of exercise.

Aquatic physical therapy may be contraindicated for anyone with Addison's disease. The heat and humidity of the pool environment causes the body to require more cortisol so that blood vessels can respond to increase blood pressure and cool the body down. The PTA should monitor vital signs in anyone with Addison's disease, especially when initiating and progressing an exercise program. Even small changes in medication dose can create a medical emergency in people with Addison's disease. Watch for any signs of an impending crisis such as dizziness, nausea, profuse sweating, elevated heart rate, and tremors or shaking.

Any signs of infection, such as sore throat or burning on urination, should be reported to the physician.

Steroid-induced psychosis can occur but often has some of the same symptoms as addisonian crisis. There can be personality changes as the affected individual becomes suspicious, confused, and irritable. Slurred speech and difficulty moving with poor motor planning and motor incoordination may be compounded by severe exhaustion. The PTA is encouraged to be sensitive to clients experiencing medication-induced psychosis; what may appear as a lack of motivation or poor compliance or noncompliance may require compassion, understanding, and patience until the medical condition is under control and the client can begin to make progress. The PTA must monitor and help the client monitor fatigue or periods of adrenal insufficiency to avoid the return of psychotic symptoms.

If steroid replacement therapy is inadequate or too high, changes in amounts of sodium and water are observed. Persons receiving glucocorticoid alone may need mineralocorticoid therapy if signs of orthostatic hypotension or electrolyte abnormalities develop. Older adults may be more sensitive to the side effects of steroid therapy, such as osteoporosis, hypertension, and diabetes, when these conditions already exist.

Anyone with identified Addison's disease should wear an identification bracelet and carry an emergency kit containing dexamethasone or hydrocortisone. Steroids administered in the late afternoon or evening may cause stimulation of the CNS and insomnia in some people. Anyone reporting sleep disturbances should be encouraged to discuss this with the physician.

Secondary adrenal insufficiency. Secondary adrenal insufficiency is caused by other conditions outside the adrenals, such as hypothalamic or pituitary tumors, removal of the pituitary, or other causes of hypopituitarism, or too-rapid withdrawal of corticosteroid drugs. Steroid therapy must be discontinued gradually so that pituitary and adrenal function can normalize.

Clinical manifestations of secondary disease are somewhat different from symptoms of primary adrenal insufficiency. Whereas most symptoms of primary adrenal insufficiency arise from cortisol and aldosterone deficiency, symptoms of secondary disease are related to cortisol deficiency only. Because the gland is still intact, aldosterone is secreted normally, but there is deficient cortisol secretion. Arthralgias, myalgias, and tendon calcification can occur, which resolve with treatment of the underlying condition.

As with primary adrenal insufficiency, treatment involves replacement of ACTH and monitoring for fluid and electrolyte imbalances. Too much cortisol replacement can result in the development of Cushing's syndrome (see next section).

Adrenocortical Hyperfunction

Hyperfunction of the adrenal cortex can result in excessive production of glucocorticoids, mineralocorticoids, and androgens. The three major conditions of adrenocortical hyperfunction are Cushing's syndrome (glucocorticoid excess), Conn's syndrome or aldosteronism (aldosterone excess), and adrenal hyperplasia (adrenogenital syndrome). This last condition is rare and congenital and is not discussed further in this text.

Cushing's syndrome

Definition and overview. Hypercortisolism is a general term for an excess of cortisol in the body. This condition can occur as a result of hyperfunction of the adrenal gland, an excess of corticosteroid medication, or an excess of ACTH. ACTH secreted by the pituitary has a key role in cortisol release. When the hypothalamus senses low ACTH levels in the blood, it stimulates ACTH secretion, which in turn stimulates the adrenal glands to release cortisol. When blood cortisol levels are adequate or elevated, the hypothalamus and pituitary release less ACTH.

Hypercortisolism resulting from adrenal gland oversecretion is *Cushing's syndrome*. When the hypercortisolism results from oversecretion of ACTH from the pituitary, the condition is called *Cushing's disease*. The clinical presentation is the same for both conditions.[98]

Etiologic factors and incidence. Cushing's disease results from pituitary adenomas, which secrete an excess of ACTH, causing overstimulation of a normal adrenal gland.

PTAs are more likely to treat people who have developed medication-induced Cushing's syndrome. This condition occurs after these individuals have received large doses of cortisol (also known as *hydrocortisone*) or cortisol derivatives. These steroids are administered for a number of inflammatory and other disorders such as asthma or rheumatoid arthritis. Cushing's syndrome occurs mainly in women, with an average age at onset of 20 to 40 years, although it can be seen in people up to age 60 years.

Pathogenesis and clinical manifestations. Cushing's syndrome involves excess cortisol release from the adrenal glands. When the normal function of the glucocorticoids becomes exaggerated, a wide range of physiologic responses can be triggered, including hyperglycemia, hypertension, proximal muscle wasting, and osteoporosis (Table 8.7).

Cortisol has a key role in glucose metabolism and a lesser part in protein, carbohydrate, and fat metabolism. Cortisol also helps maintain blood pressure and cardiovascular function while reducing the body's inflammatory responses. Overproduction of cortisol causes liberation of amino acids from muscle tissue with resultant weakening of muscle and elastic tissue. The end result may include a protuberant abdomen (Fig. 8.6) with purple striae (stretch marks), poor wound healing, thinning of the skin, generalized muscle weakness, and marked osteoporosis that is made worse by an excessive loss of calcium in the urine. In severe cases of prolonged Cushing's syndrome, muscle weakness and demineralization of bone may lead to pathologic fractures and wedging of the vertebrae, kyphosis, osteonecrosis (especially of the femoral head), bone pain, and back pain.

TABLE 8.7   Pathophysiology of Cushing's Syndrome

Physiologic Effect	Clinical Result
Persistent hyperglycemia	"Steroid diabetes"
Protein tissue wasting	Weakness as a result of muscle wasting; capillary fragility resulting in ecchymoses; osteoporosis as a result of bone matrix wasting
Potassium depletion	Hypokalemia, cardiac arrhythmias, muscle weakness, renal disorders
Sodium and water retention	Edema and hypertension
Hypertension	Predisposes to left ventricular hypertrophy, congestive heart failure, cerebrovascular accidents
Abnormal fat distribution	Moon-shaped face; dorsocervical fat pad; truncal obesity, slender limbs, thinning of the skin with striae on the breasts, axillary areas, abdomen, and legs
Increased susceptibility to infection; lowered resistance to stress	Absence of signs of infection; poor wound healing
Increased production of androgens	Virilism in women (e.g., acne, thinning of scalp hair, hirsutism or abnormal growth and distribution of hair)
Mental changes	Memory loss, poor concentration and thought processes, euphoria, depression ("steroid psychosis")

The effect of increased circulating levels of cortisol on the muscles varies from slight to marked. Muscle wasting can be so extensive that the condition simulates muscular dystrophy.

Medical Management

Diagnosis
Although there is a classic cushingoid appearance in persons with hypercortisolism (see Fig. 8.6), diagnostic laboratory studies, including measurement of urine and serum cortisol, are used to confirm the diagnosis.

Treatment and Prognosis
Treatment to restore hormone balance and reverse Cushing's syndrome or disease may require radiation, drug therapy, or surgery, depending on the underlying cause. For individuals with muscle wasting or who are at risk for muscle atrophy, a high-protein diet may be prescribed. Prognosis depends on the underlying cause and the ability to control the cortisol excess.

Conn's syndrome
Definition and overview. Conn's syndrome, or primary aldosteronism, occurs when an adrenal lesion results in hypersecretion of aldosterone, the most powerful of the mineralocorticoids. Its primary role is to conserve sodium, and it also promotes potassium excretion. The major cause of primary aldosteronism (an uncommon condition present most often in women aged 30 to 50 years) is a benign aldosterone-secreting tumor called *aldosteronoma*.[53]

Secondary hyperaldosteronism also can occur as a consequence of pathologic lesions that stimulate the adrenal gland to increase production of aldosterone.

Pathogenesis and clinical manifestations. Aldosterone affects the tubular reabsorption of sodium and water and the excretion of potassium and hydrogen ions in the kidneys. This leads to the development of hypernatremia (excess sodium in blood, indicating water loss exceeding sodium loss), hypervolemia (fluid volume excess, increase in the volume of circulating fluid or plasma in the body), hypokalemia (low blood levels of potassium), and metabolic alkalosis. With the hypervolemia and hypernatremia, the blood pressure increases, often to very high levels. This hypertension can lead to cerebral infarctions and renal damage.

Hypokalemia results from excessive urinary excretion of potassium, causing muscle weakness; intermittent, flaccid paralysis; paresthesias; or cardiac arrhythmias. This excessive urinary excretion of potassium (hypokalemia) leads to polyuria and resulting polydipsia (excessive thirst). DM is common because hypokalemia interferes with normal insulin transport.

Medical Management

Diagnosis, Treatment, and Prognosis
Diagnosis of primary hyperaldosteronism is based on elevations in serum and urine aldosterone study findings and computed tomography (CT) scanning of the abdomen for evidence of unilateral and sometimes bilateral adenomas of the adrenal gland.[53]

The goals of treatment are to reverse hypertension, correct hypokalemia, and prevent kidney damage. Without early diagnosis and treatment, renal complications from long-term hypertension may be progressive. Pharmacologic treatment to increase sodium excretion and treat the hypertension and hypokalemia is a nonsurgical alternative.

8.12 Special Implications for the PTA: Conn's Syndrome The PTA treating someone with hyperaldosteronism, primary or secondary, may observe signs of tetany and hypokalemia-induced cardiac dysrhythmias, paresthesias, or muscle weakness. If these are encountered in an acute care setting, the medical team is usually well aware of such symptoms and is working to establish a fluid-electrolyte balance. When such signs and symptoms are observed in the outpatient setting, the client must seek medical attention.

Adipose Tissue
One does not normally think of fat as endocrine tissue. In fact, adipose tissue can be classified as the largest endocrine organ in the body. This revelation occurred only a few years ago. Before that time, fat was viewed as a storage site for energy, with little other function. Now it is clear that neurotransmitters and glucose (along with other molecules) directly act on adipocytes to induce the release of a number of different proteins collectively termed *adipokines* (or adipocytokines) that can act locally as autocrine hormones or through the bloodstream as endocrine hormones.[60]

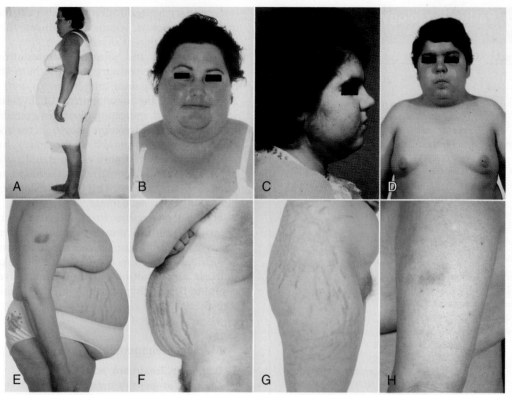

FIG. 8.6 Clinical features of Cushing's syndrome. (A) Central and some generalized obesity and dorsal kyphosis in a 30-year-old woman with Cushing's disease. (B) Same woman as in A, showing moon facies (round face), *hirsutism* (hair growth), and enlarged supraclavicular fat pads. (C) Facial rounding, hirsutism, and acne in a 14-year-old girl with Cushing's syndrome. (D) Central and generalized obesity and moon facies in a 14-year-old boy with Cushing's syndrome. (E and F) Typical central obesity with visible abdominal striae ("stretch marks") seen in a 41-year-old woman and 40-year-old-man with Cushing's syndrome. (G) Striae in a 24-year-old woman with congenital adrenal hyperplasia treated with excessive doses of dexamethasone as replacement therapy. (H) Typical bruising and thin skin of Cushing's syndrome. In this case the bruising has occurred without obvious injury. (From Melmed S, Polonsky KS, Larsen PR, et al., editors: Williams textbook of endocrinology, ed 13, Philadelphia, 2016, Elsevier.)

Some of the factors released by adipocytes function to maintain the balance of energy. However, others have roles that are beyond the conservation of energy, including the induction of vasoconstriction (angiotensin), inflammation (leptin), or angiogenesis. Research supporting the role of adipocytes in the secretion of molecules that are transported in the blood has only recently begun. Thus this concept is very new to both researchers and professionals in the health care field. One of the reasons that the role of adipose tissue in health and disease has been difficult to describe is the fact that fat from different parts of the body functions in various ways. In mammals, adipose tissue is divided into two categories: brown and white. Brown fat is a very specialized tissue that is important in thermoregulation, converting energy from food into heat.[21] Infants have more brown fat; thus they are more sensitive to temperature changes, especially the cold. The amount of brown fat decreases into adulthood, but some does remain in specific locations throughout the life span. The activity of the adipocytes in brown fat is closely regulated by the sympathetic nervous system.

White fat is the classic adipose tissue responsible for storage of triglycerols to provide a long-term reservoir of energy for the body.[152] In terms of the role of white fat as an endocrine organ, the secretion of adipokines by white visceral tissue is stressed, yet it is important to remember that the major stimulating agent from adipocytes is fatty acids, which are used as a source of energy.

Obesity

Obesity is the most common nutritional disorder in the Western world and has been categorized as a disease process by the U.S. Social Security Administration.[154] Their policy describes obesity as a "complex, chronic disease characterized by excessive accumulation of body fat."

Obviously there is a direct correlation with adipose cells and obesity—more adipose tissue results in a more obese person. However, obesity is a multifactorial problem related to both behavior and biology. The role of fat cells to send signals to the brain that are translated as feelings of hunger or satiation has only recently been uncovered.

Leptin, the first adipokine identified, acts on the hypothalamus to alter hunger, with increased levels of leptin acting as a hunger depressor. In humans and in animal models, the level of leptin highly correlates with the levels of adipose tissue.[93] Animals that lack the ability to make leptin are extremely obese and develop diabetes. If the animals are treated with leptin, there is a subsequent reduction in the animal's food intake and substantial weight loss.[113]

In human obesity, which has many causes, the role of leptin in hunger is not as clear. As a person becomes more obese, the leptin levels increase, which is the opposite of the expected result. It appears that the target receptors for leptin become less sensitive with increasing amounts of fat.[60]

It is now thought that leptin's role in appetite regulation is more important in reduced-calorie situations. When calories are restricted and weight loss is occurring, leptin levels decrease. Historically, when humans had to gather their own food, this signal to the brain was important to stave off starvation. Leptin's role in hunger for persons who have sufficient calorie intake is unclear.

Obesity and cancer. The link between obesity and cancer in humans has been apparent for years and continues to be borne out by statistics.[56,61] In a major study undertaken in Austria, obesity in men was associated with a high risk of colon cancer and pancreatic cancer. In women, there was a weak positive association between increasing body mass index (BMI) and all cancers combined and strong associations with non-Hodgkin's lymphoma and uterine cancer.[122] In addition, the incidence of breast cancer was positively associated with high BMI but only after 65 years of age. Along with the greater risk of developing cancer in the obese, the outcome for obese cancer patients is significantly worse compared with the lean cancer patient in terms of recurrence of the cancer, malignancy, and life span.[69,118]

Although the epidemiologic data strongly link some cancers with obesity, the physiologic mechanisms are only beginning to be elucidated. Leptin has been identified as a major adipokine linking prostate cancer with obesity.[8] Along with an increase in leptin levels in obese men, a decrease in the adiponectin levels is also associated with prostate cancer.[17]

In studies in men, low plasma adiponectin levels resulted in a higher risk of colorectal cancer.[163] At the cellular level, leptin has been shown to cause increased proliferation and precancerous changes in cultured colon epithelial cells.[48]

Obesity has been associated with an increased risk of breast cancer and a reduced survival rate in women with invasive breast cancer.[119] Obese women have higher levels of plasma leptin,[69] and high levels of leptin have been found in some types of breast cancer.[54] The exact mechanism by which leptin would induce breast cancer growth is unknown.

The number of newly identified adipokines continues to grow. The field of adipose endocrinology is in its infancy and will expand our understanding of the dynamic role of fat in health and disease.

Type 2 Diabetes Mellitus

Although type 2 DM is discussed later in this chapter, the role of adipose tissue is presented here. Although excess white fat in any location may lead to the progression of diabetes, it is the fat surrounding the viscera and the hepatic circulation that is most important.

It is interesting to note that even abdominal obesity has subcategories. Magnetic resonance imaging and CT scans indicate that some people carry abdominal weight in the subcutaneous region, but the distribution of fat around the organs is minimal. These people appear to have little insulin resistance. In contrast, when intraabdominal fat accumulates around the organs (visceral fat; Fig. 8.7), insulin resistance quickly follows.[51] The

molecular link between abdominal fat and insulin resistance has been identified as the adipokine adiponectin, which is released into the circulation by adipocytes.

Adiponectin increases insulin sensitivity in muscle and liver and increases free fatty acid oxidation in muscle tissues along with other cell types.[60] As the level of adiponectin decreases, the risk of insulin resistance increases. Conversely, if insulin-resistant mice are given extra adiponectin, their glucose tolerance improves and the insulin resistance is reduced.[167]

Inflammation

An interesting observation led to the discovery of an additional role for adipose tissue. Obesity is associated with a systemic low-grade inflammation. This observation led to the idea that adipocytes released compounds into the blood to cause the inflammation. Eventually, it was determined that leptin activates many members of the inflammatory pathway, including CD4+ and CD8+ T lymphocytes, causing proliferation of the cells.[89]

Leptin can also activate natural killer cells.[168] Within the white fat of obese people, macrophages are known to infiltrate and produce local proinflammatory molecules. With weight loss there is a decrease in the number of macrophages within adipose tissue and a decrease in the local inflammation. Thus leptin works locally in the adipose tissue.

However, it also has an effect on distant tissues. Leptin links the immune and inflammatory processes to the neuroendocrine system. In addition to playing a key role in modulating T cells, it also is important in autoimmune conditions such as autoimmune encephalomyelitis, type 1 diabetes, bowel inflammation, and rheumatoid arthritis.[110]

In obesity, leptin is not the only adipokine to induce widespread inflammation. White fat is characterized by an increased production and secretion of a wide range of inflammatory molecules, which may have local and systemic effects. Visceral adipose tissue is again the site of much of the inflammatory secretion.

Adipocytes from visceral fat produce large amounts of monocyte chemoattractant protein 1, an adipokine directly involved in cellular remodeling of the heart.

In contrast to leptin, adiponectin has an antiinflammatory action. It has been shown to be protective against atherosclerotic events in large vessels.[144] In addition, adiponectin levels rise with long-term physical exercise, accompanied by a reduction in inflammatory mediators in the blood.[107] However, this antiinflammatory role may be tissue specific, as recent evidence suggests that high adiponectin levels may be involved in the chronic inflammation associated with arthritis.[38]

8.13 Special Implications for the PTA: Adipose Tissue Fat accumulated in the lower body (subcutaneous fat) results in a pear-shaped figure, whereas fat in the abdominal area (visceral fat) produces more of an apple shape. Specific genes have been identified that help dictate the number of fat cells and where they are located. This process is also influenced by hormonal production.

Visceral fat produces cytokines that increase the risk of cardiovascular disease (CVD) by promoting insulin resistance and low-level chronic inflammation. Excess abdominal fat has also been linked to colorectal cancer, hypertension, and memory loss. But the good news is that visceral fat can be reduced with diet and exercise. The PTA can offer education and guidance in this area of prevention and management.

Increasing physical activity and exercise to 1 hour daily may be ideal, but benefits have been observed with even 30 minutes of daily, moderate activity. Twice-weekly strength training has also been shown to prevent increases in body fat percentage and attenuate increases in abdominal fat in at least one study of overweight or obese women.[132]

The PTA can help individual clients assess BMI, waist-to-hip ratio, and waist circumference. BMI helps identify people whose weight increases their risk for several conditions such as heart disease, stroke, and diabetes. It can be misleading in individuals who are very muscular or very tall.

Waist-to-hip ratio is measured by dividing the waist measurement at its narrowest point by the hip measurement at its widest point. This marker of abdominal fat is more accurate than the BMI. The risk for heart disease and stroke begins to rise at a ratio of 0.8.

The waist circumference may be the simplest way to measure abdominal fat. A tape measure is placed around the waist at about the level of the navel. Waist measurement greater than 33 for women indicates rising risk, and 35 or higher is considered high risk. A large waist correlates with diabetes risk. The relationship between waist circumference and health risk may vary by ethnic group.[83,126]

Pancreas (Islets of Langerhans)

The pancreas lies behind the stomach, (see Fig. 8.1). It has two functions, acting as both an endocrine gland (secreting the hormones insulin and glucagon) and an exocrine gland (producing digestive enzymes). The cells of the pancreas that function in the endocrine capacity are the islets of Langerhans.

The islets of Langerhans have three major types of functioning cells: (1) the alpha cells produce glucagon, which increases the blood glucose levels by stimulating the liver and other cells to release stored glucose (glycogenolysis); (2) the beta cells produce insulin, which lowers blood glucose levels by facilitating the entrance of glucose into the cells for metabolism; and (3) the delta cells produce somatostatin, which is believed to regulate the release of insulin and glucagon (Table 8.8).[68]

Diabetes Mellitus

Definition and overview. DM is a chronic, systemic disorder characterized by hyperglycemia (excess glucose in the blood) and disruption of the metabolism of carbohydrates, fats, and proteins. Insulin, produced in the pancreas, normally maintains a balanced blood glucose level. DM is characterized as a group of metabolic diseases resulting from defects in the secretion of insulin, action of insulin, or both. The chronic hyperglycemia of DM is associated with long-term damage and dysfunction and impairment of tissues and organs, especially the eyes, kidneys, nerves, heart, and blood vessels.

The majority of cases of DM fall into two large categories: type 1 and type 2. In type 1 DM (previously called *insulin-dependent DM [IDDM]* or *juvenile-onset DM*), the cause of hyperglycemia is an absolute deficiency of insulin production and secretion.

Most individuals with type 1 DM can be identified by evidence showing an autoimmune process occurring in the islet

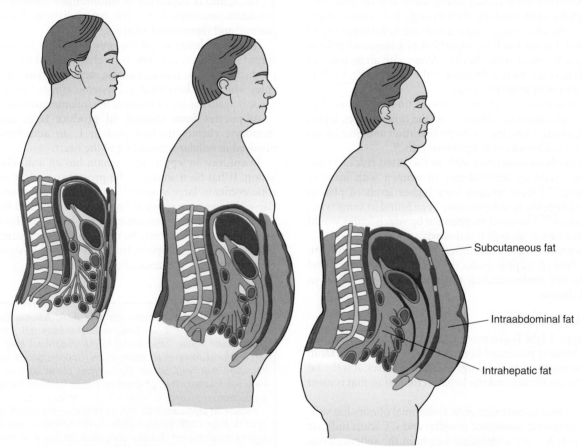

Subcutaneous fat

Intraabdominal fat

Intrahepatic fat

FIG. 8.7 Abdominal adipose tissue (fat) can accumulate as subcutaneous, intraabdominal, or intrahepatic (fatty lobules throughout the liver). The body has an almost unlimited capacity to store fat. Central obesity has been linked with serious health consequences (e.g., cardiovascular disease, insulin resistance, diabetes mellitus).

TABLE 8.8 Regulation of Glucose Metabolism

Gland	Regulating Function
Pancreas	
Alpha cells (islets of Langerhans)	Secrete glucagon; increase blood glucose level
Beta cells (islets of Langerhans)	Secrete insulin (glucose-regulating hormone); decrease blood glucose level
Gamma cells (islets of Langerhans)	Secrete somatostatin; regulate the release of insulin and glucagon
Adrenal Gland	
Medulla: epinephrine	Responds to stress; epinephrine stimulates liver and muscle glycogenolysis to increase the blood glucose level
Cortex: glucocorticoids	Increase blood glucose levels by promoting the flow of amino acids to the liver, where they are synthesized into glucose
Anterior Pituitary	
ACTH	Increases blood glucose levels
HGH	Limits storage of fat; favors fat catabolism; inhibits carbohydrate catabolism, raising blood glucose levels
Thyroid	
T_3 and T_4	May raise or lower blood glucose levels

ACTH, Adrenocorticotropic hormone; *HGH,* human growth hormone.

TABLE 8.9 Differences Between Types of Diabetes Mellitus[a]

Features	Type 1 (Ketosis Prone)	Type 2 (Not Ketosis Prone)
Age at onset	Usually <20 years	Usually >40 years
Proportion of all cases	<10%	>90%
Type of onset	Abrupt (acute or subacute)	Gradual
Etiologic factors	Possible viral or auto-immune, resulting in destruction of islet cells	Obesity-associated insulin resistance
HLA association	Yes	No
Insulin antibodies	Yes	No
Bodyweight at onset	Normal or thin, obesity uncommon	Majority are obese (80%)
Endogenous insulin production	Decreased (little or none)	Variable (above or below normal)
Ketoacidosis	May occur	Rare
Treatment	Insulin, diet, and exercise	Diet, oral hypoglycemic agents, exercise, insulin, and weight control

[a]This table does not reflect changes in our understanding of a "hybrid" form of diabetes referred to as *type 1.5* or *maturity-onset diabetes of the young.*
HLA, Human leukocyte antigen.
Modified from Goodman CC, Snyder TE: Differential diagnosis in physical therapy, ed 5, St. Louis, 2013, Saunders.

TABLE 8.10 Blood Glucose Levels

Fasting Plasma Glucose Test	Two-Hour Oral Glucose Tolerance Test
Normal: <100 mg/dL	Normal: <139 mg/dL
Prediabetes: 100-125 mg/dL	Prediabetes: 140-199 mg/dL
Diabetes: >125 mg/dL	Diabetes: ≥200 mg/dL

cells of the pancreas along with specific genetic markers. People with type 1 DM are prone to hyperglycemia; they require exogenous insulin to maintain life.

Type 2 DM (previously called *non–insulin-dependent DM [NIDDM]* or *adult-onset DM*) is a much more prevalent form of diabetes, and the cause is a combination of cellular resistance to insulin action and an inadequate insulin secretory response. Type 2 DM usually can be controlled with diet, exercise, and oral hypoglycemic agents. In some cases, however, people with type 2 DM do require insulin replacement.[25] A comparison of the primary differences between the two types of diabetes is shown in Table 8.9.

In recent years the lines between type 1 and 2 DM have begun to blur. An autoimmune type of diabetes that begins in middle to late adulthood has been identified. In addition, with increased obesity, type 2 DM is being diagnosed in younger and younger children.[155] The exact classification of these "hybrid" types of diabetes is still being sorted out. It is important to understand that the characteristics of type 1 and 2 diabetes are not mutually exclusive and should be considered along a spectrum of attributes of the disease.

Prediabetes. Prediabetes occurs when the body cannot use glucose the way it should. After food is ingested, carbohydrates are converted into glucose. The pancreas releases insulin to help move the glucose into the cells to be used for energy. In someone with prediabetes, this process is not completed because either the body cells do not recognize all of the insulin (decreased insulin sensitivity) or the cells stop responding to the action of insulin (increased insulin resistance).

With less glucose moving into the cells, the blood glucose levels start to rise. This is the beginning of a condition referred to as *prediabetes*. In prediabetes the blood glucose levels are higher than normal but not quite high enough to be considered diabetes (Table 8.10). Many people with prediabetes have hypertension and dyslipidemia. The trio of comorbidities increases the risk of developing type 2 diabetes and heart disease.

Other types and categories of diabetes mellitus. In addition to the main categories of type 1 and type 2 DM, other rare specific types of DM exist:
- Genetic beta cell defects
- Genetic defects in insulin action
- Disorders of the exocrine pancreas such as injury, neoplasm, cystic fibrosis, or infection
- Other endocrinopathies
- Drug- or chemical-induced DM
- Uncommon forms of immune or genetically associated syndromes
- Infections

Gestational diabetes mellitus. *Gestational DM* is defined as any degree of glucose intolerance recognized with the onset of pregnancy. Approximately 6 weeks or more after pregnancy ends, the woman should be reclassified into one of the other categories, depending on whether or not her glucose tolerance resolves. She

BOX 8.4 Risk Factors for Type 1 and Type 2 Diabetes Mellitus

Type 1 DM Risk Factors
- Presence of type 1 diabetes in a first-degree relative (sibling or parent)

Type 2 DM Risk Factors
- Positive family history
- Ethnic origin: African American, Native American, Hispanic, Asian American, Pacific Islander
- Obesity
- Increasing age (≥45 years old)
- Habitual physical inactivity; sedentary lifestyle
- Previous history of GDM or delivery of babies weighing more than 9 lb
- Presence of other clinical conditions associated with insulin resistance (e.g., polycystic ovary syndrome)
- History of vascular disease
- Previously identified IFG or IGT
- Hypertension (>140/90 mm Hg in adults)
- HDL cholesterol level 35 mg/dL and/or triglyceride level ≥250 mg/dL
- Cigarette smoking

DM, Diabetes mellitus; *GDM;* gestational diabetes mellitus; *HDL,* high-density lipoprotein; *IFG,* impaired fasting glucose; *IGF,* impaired glucose tolerance.

could be reclassified as normal if no glucose intolerance remains after the pregnancy is completed. Gestational DM accompanies approximately 4% of all pregnancies.

Most women who have gestational DM return to normal glucose metabolism after pregnancy.[25] However, with time, these women will likely be diagnosed with type 2 DM.[146]

Incidence and prevalence. According to the American Diabetes Association, more than 14.6 million Americans have been diagnosed with diabetes, and approximately 6.2 million more people have undiagnosed cases. In addition to the 20.8 million Americans with diabetes (7% of the entire U.S. population), 41 million have prediabetes.

Diabetes, with its severe complications of heart disease, stroke, kidney disease, blindness, and loss of limbs, is the most common endocrine disorder, ranked as a leading cause of death from disease in the United States. It is the leading cause of blindness and renal failure in adults.[49,103]

African Americans, Native Americans, Hispanic Americans, Mexican Americans, and Asian Americans are 1.5 to 2 times more likely to develop DM than are white Americans, with increasing incidence associated with advancing age. Nearly one-half of all Americans with DM are older than 60, and nearly one-fourth of the U.S. population over age 65 has diabetes[30]; males and females are affected equally.

Approximately 90% of all cases of DM are type 2. Type 1 DM and secondary causes account for the remaining 10%. Since the mid-1970s, the incidence of diabetes has steadily increased as a result of prolonged life expectancy; increased incidence of obesity; and reduced mortality resulting in increased live births to people with type 1 DM, whose children are predisposed to future development of type 1 DM.

Etiologic and risk factors. Risk factors for type 1 and type 2 DM have been identified (Box 8.4). In addition, lifestyle factors, such as watching 2 or more hours of television daily, skipping breakfast, drinking a daily carbonated beverage, and having a waist measurement larger than 35 inches for women and 40 inches (a sign of abdominal fat) for men, may be linked with type 2 diabetes.

More television (sedentary lifestyle) is often linked with less activity, which can lead to weight gain. Eating nonnutritious snacks while watching television and/or drinking soda adds extra empty calories, which can also result in weight gain. Eating fast food more than twice a week raises the risk of obesity and the likelihood of becoming resistant to insulin.

High stress can interfere with the body's ability to make insulin and process glucose; cortisol is a key factor in glucose metabolism and stress is linked with elevated cortisol levels. Stress can also interrupt sleep, and sleep disturbances may be linked with an increased risk of developing insulin resistance. Other lifestyle and risk factors under investigation for diabetes include consuming processed meat (e.g., bacon, hot dogs, and lunch meat) and major depressive disorders.

Type 1 diabetes mellitus. Type 1 DM results from cell-mediated autoimmune destruction of the beta cells of the pancreas and is a condition of absolute insulin deficiency. People with autoimmune destruction of beta cells are also prone to other autoimmune disorders such as Graves' disease, Hashimoto's thyroiditis, Addison's disease, vitiligo, autoimmune gastritis, and pernicious anemia.[81]

In type 1 DM, the rate of beta cell destruction is rapid in some people (mainly infants and children) and slow in others (mainly adults). Even though immune-mediated diabetes commonly occurs in childhood and adolescence, it can occur at any age, even late in life. Both genetic and environmental factors are associated with autoimmune destruction of the beta cell, although the environmental relationship is still poorly defined.[25]

In about 10% of cases of type 1 DM, no definable cause exists. Some individuals in this category (usually of African or Asian origin) have permanent hypoinsulinemia and are prone to ketoacidosis but have no evidence of autoimmunity. Their need for insulin replacement is usually inconsistent. Up to 20% of women with type 1 DM have some kind of eating disorder that predisposes them to further complications with glucose control. Binge eating and use of intense, excessive exercise are common in preteen, teenage, and young women with type 1 DM.[28,58] The emphasis on weight control, dietary habits, and food at a time when poor self-esteem, stress, and altered image occur in young women with type 1 DM may contribute to an increased risk of eating disorders.[94]

Type 2 diabetes mellitus. Type 2 DM is a form of diabetes in which individuals have insulin production but have difficulty with effective insulin action at the cellular level. People with type 2 DM may not need insulin treatment to survive but need other forms of therapy to prevent hyperglycemia and its resulting complications.

Type 2 DM is associated with obesity. In fact, obesity-dependent diabetes in childhood is now referred to as *diabesity* and is considered an inflammatory metabolic condition. Both insulin resistance and defective insulin secretion appear very prematurely in obese individuals, and both worsen similarly toward diabetes.[131]

Most people with type 2 DM are obese and sedentary; these two risk factors cause some degree of insulin resistance. At least 80% of all persons with type 2 DM are obese, and the remaining 20%, who are not obese by traditional weight criteria, may have an increased percentage of body fat distribution, particularly in the abdominal area.[25]

Type 2 diabetes was originally called *late-* or *adult-onset diabetes* because it primarily occurred in people 60 years old or older. Starting in the early 1990s, a trend toward the development of type 2 DM in children and adolescents was observed.

Excess body fat and sedentary lifestyle are the key risk factors contributing to the development of type 2 DM in younger population groups. Cigarette smoking may also be a risk factor. Smokers exhibit a significantly increased incidence of diabetes compared with people who have never smoked.[50]

People with this form of diabetes may have normal or elevated insulin levels, but the insulin produced is ineffective because the cells do not allow insulin to attach. Insulin secretion also is impaired, and the beta cells are unable to secrete increased amounts of insulin when needed. People with type 2 DM are at increased risk for developing vascular complications. The risk of developing this form of diabetes increases with age, obesity, low cardiorespiratory fitness, and lack of exercise.[164] Type 2 DM occurs more frequently in women with prior gestational DM and in individuals with hypertension or dyslipidemia. Its frequency varies in different racial or ethnic groups.

Pathogenesis. Insulin is a hormone secreted by the beta cells of the pancreas that transports glucose into the cell for use as energy. It assists in storing glucose in the cells as glycogen. It also stimulates protein synthesis and free fatty acid storage in the fat deposits. In DM, insulin is either insufficient in amount (type 1) or ineffective in action (type 2).

Insulin deficiency compromises the body tissues' access to essential nutrients for fuel and storage.[140] When glucose levels are elevated normally (e.g., after eating a meal), beta cells increase secretion of insulin to transport and dispose of the glucose into peripheral tissues, lowering blood glucose levels and reestablishing blood glucose homeostasis. Normally, after a meal, the blood glucose level rises. The liver takes up a large amount of this glucose for storage or for use by other tissues such as skeletal muscle and fat. When insulin is deficient or its function is impaired, the glucose in the general circulation is not used by the muscles or fat, and it is not stored in the liver; thus it continues to accumulate in the blood. Because new glucose has not been deposited in the liver, the liver produces more glucose and releases it into the general circulation, which increases the already elevated blood glucose level (Fig. 8.8).[124,140]

When a true deficiency of insulin exists, such as in type 1 DM, the following three major metabolic problems exist: (1) decreased use of glucose (as described), (2) increased fat mobilization, and (3) impaired protein use. Cells that require insulin for transporting glucose inside the cell, such as in skeletal muscle, cardiac muscle, and adipose tissue, are affected most. Nerve tissue, erythrocytes, and the cells of the intestines, liver, and kidney tubules, which do not require insulin for glucose transport, are affected the least.

In an attempt to restore balance and normal levels of glucose, the kidney excretes the excess glucose, resulting in glucosuria (sugar in the urine). Glucose excreted in the urine causes excretion of increased amounts of water. The conscious person becomes extremely thirsty and drinks large amounts of water (polydipsia).

Increased fat mobilization occurs because the body can rely on fat stores for energy when glucose is not available. The process of fat metabolism leads to the formation of breakdown products called *ketones,* which accumulate in the blood and are excreted through the kidneys and lungs. Ketones can be measured in the blood and the urine to indicate the presence of diabetes. They interfere with acid-base balance by producing hydrogen ions. The pH can fall, and the affected person can develop metabolic acidosis.

After the renal threshold for ketones is exceeded, the ketones appear in the urine as *acetone* (ketonuria). When large amounts

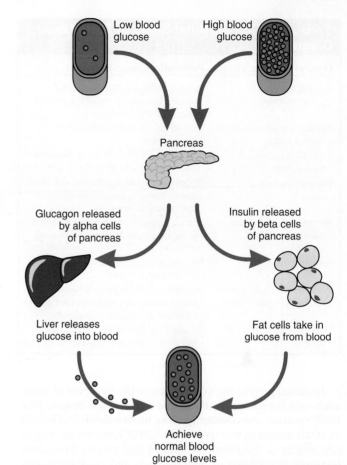

FIG. 8.8 Endocrine function of the pancreas. Type 2 diabetes can promote excess sugar release from the liver, render the pancreas incapable of producing sufficient insulin, and dampen the effects of insulin on muscle and fat. Normally after intake of food, the stomach transforms food into glucose, which then enters the bloodstream. Rising blood glucose levels signal beta cells in the pancreas to release insulin. The insulin transports glucose into the cell and sets up a cascade of events (e.g., increased rate of glucose use and adenosine triphosphate generation, conversion of glucose to glycogen, increase in protein and fat synthesis) that eventually results in a decline in blood glucose concentration and restoration of homeostasis. When the blood glucose levels drop (such as occurs in a hypoglycemic state or when fasting), alpha cells in the pancreas produce glucagon, which increases the blood glucose levels by stimulating the liver and other cells to release stored glucose (a process called *glycogenolysis*). The blood glucose concentration rises, thus restoring the proper balance and returning the body to a state of homeostasis. Either beta cell dysfunction or insulin resistance can disrupt this process, resulting in decreased plasma insulin and ultimately hyperglycemia.

of glucose and ketones are excreted, fluid and electrolyte loss through the kidneys increases. Sodium, potassium, and other critical electrolytes are lost in the urine, resulting in severe dehydration and electrolyte deficiency and worsening acidosis. When fats are used for a primary source of energy, the body lipid level can rise to five times the normal amount. This elevated level can lead to atherosclerosis and its subsequent cardiovascular complications.

TABLE 8.11 Cardinal Signs of Diabetes at Diagnosis

Clinical Manifestations	Pathophysiologic Bases
Polyuria (excessive urination, types 1 and 2)	Water is not reabsorbed from renal tubules because of osmotic activity of glucose in the tubules
Polydipsia (excessive thirst, types 1 and 2)	Polyuria causes dehydration, which causes thirst
Polyphagia (excessive hunger, type 1)	Starvation secondary to tissue breakdown causes hunger
Weight loss (type 1)	Glucose is not available to the cells; body breaks down fat and protein stores for energy; dehydration
Recurrent blurred vision (types 1 and 2)	Chronic exposure of the lenses and retina to hyperosmolar fluids causes blurring of vision
Ketonuria (type 1)	Fatty acids are broken down, so ketones are present in urine
Weakness, fatigue, and dizziness (types 1 and 2)	Dehydration leads to postural hypotension; energy deficiency and protein catabolism contribute to fatigue and weakness
Often asymptomatic (type 2)	Physical adaptation often occurs because rise in blood glucose is gradual

Impaired protein use occurs because the transport of amino acids, which make up proteins, into cells requires insulin. Normally, proteins are constantly being broken down and rebuilt. Without insulin to transport amino acids, contributing to protein synthesis, the balance is altered and protein breakdown increases. Breakdown of body proteins and resultant protein loss diminish the tissue's ability to repair itself.

Because the person with type 2 DM continues to produce and use some amount of insulin, the metabolic problems are not as severe. People with type 2 DM are not prone to ketoacidosis. They are, however, still at great risk for hyperglycemic osmotic diuresis, dehydration, shock, and loss of electrolytes.[140]

Clinical manifestations

Pathophysiology of diabetic complications. The long-term presence of DM affects the large blood vessels (macrovasculature), small blood vessels (microvasculature), and nerves throughout the body. The chronic hyperglycemia of diabetes results in the accelerated atherosclerosis that affects arteries that supply the heart, brain, and lower extremities.

Diabetes is also associated with the development of diabetes-specific microvascular pathology in the retina, renal glomerulus, and peripheral nerve. As a result, diabetes is a leading cause of blindness, kidney failure, and a variety of debilitating neuropathies.

Hyperglycemia causes abnormalities in blood flow and increased vascular permeability, and with time, microvascular cell loss and progressive capillary occlusion occur.

Neuropathy in diabetes presumably results from an increased accumulation of sorbitol, a byproduct of improper glucose metabolism, in the nerve cells. This accumulation then results in abnormal fluid and electrolyte shifts and nerve cell dysfunction. The combination of this metabolic derangement and the diminished vascular perfusion to nerve tissues contributes to the severe problem of diabetic neuropathy.

Cardinal signs and symptoms. In type 1 diabetes, symptoms of marked hyperglycemia include polyuria, polydipsia, weight loss with polyphagia, and blurred vision (Table 8.11). These symptoms occur as a result of the inability of the body to use glucose appropriately and the resulting dehydration and starvation of body tissues. In type 1 DM the use of fats and proteins for energy causes severe hunger, fatigue, and weight loss.

People with type 2 diabetes also may have some of these cardinal signs and symptoms, but the aging population may not recognize the abnormal thirst or frequent urination as abnormal for their age. The person with type 2 diabetes frequently goes undiagnosed for many years because onset of type 2 DM is often gradual enough that the classic signs of hyperglycemia are not noticed. It is more common that affected individuals may experience visual blurring, neuropathic complications (e.g., foot pain), infections, and significant blood lipid abnormalities. Type 2 DM is commonly diagnosed while the client is hospitalized or receiving medical care for another problem.

Atherosclerosis. Because of the hyperglycemia and increased fat metabolism associated with type 1 DM, atherosclerosis begins earlier and is more extensive among people with diabetes than in the general population. Atherosclerotic changes in large blood vessels, caused by lipid accumulation and thickening of vessel walls, result in decreased vessel lumen size, compromised blood flow, and ischemia to adjacent tissues. Consequently, people with diabetes have a much higher risk of myocardial infarction, stroke, and limb amputation.

Atherosclerosis and the accompanying large-vessel changes result in cardiovascular and cerebrovascular changes, skin and nail changes, poor tissue perfusion, decreased or absent pedal pulses, and impaired wound healing. Atherosclerosis combined with peripheral neuropathy and the subsequent foot deformities increases the risk for ulceration of skin and underlying tissues and limb amputation.

Individuals with undiagnosed type 2 DM are at significantly higher risk for CAD, stroke, and peripheral vascular disease than the population without diabetes. Screening of the type 2 at-risk population is essential in the prevention and treatment of diabetes-related complications. In addition, all individuals with diabetes should be aware of the strong and consistent data regarding the risks of smoking and the exacerbation of atherosclerosis-related diabetic complications.

Clients and families should be consistently and continuously counseled and encouraged in smoking cessation. The combination of smoking and diabetes dramatically increases the risks related to atherosclerotic vessel disease, impaired wound healing, and the associated morbidity and mortality rates.[3]

Cardiovascular complications. CVD is the leading cause of mortality and morbidity in diabetes and accounts for approximately two-thirds of all deaths among the diabetic population.[25] People with diabetes have 1.5- to 4-fold increased risk of having CAD, stroke, and myocardial infarction.[25] Although diabetes has long been recognized as a potent and prevalent risk factor for ischemic heart disease caused by coronary atherosclerosis, only recently has it become associated with left ventricular dysfunction. This is a disease of a cardiac muscle itself and is called *diabetic cardiomyopathy*.[47]

Because of the presence of neuropathy, people with diabetes may have what is called "silent ischemia" or silent heart attack. They do not experience typical pain because of the damage to the nerves that occurs in diabetes.

Retinopathy and nephropathy. Diabetic retinopathy is a highly specific vascular complication in both persons with type

1 and those with type 2 DM, and its prevalence is correlated closely with duration and control of high blood glucose levels. After 20 years with DM, nearly all individuals with type 1 DM and more than 60% of those with type 2 DM have some degree of retinopathy.

Underlying microvascular occlusion of the retina resulting in progressive areas of retinal ischemia and tissue death causes diabetic retinopathy. Studies have established that intensive control of blood glucose level to consistent near-normal levels can prevent and delay the progression of diabetic retinopathy.[35]

Diabetes is now the leading cause of end-stage renal disease, which is kidney failure requiring dialysis or transplantation, in the United States and Europe.[104] Hardening and thickening of the cell basement membrane in the kidneys, which result in eventual destruction of critical renal filtration structures, cause diabetic nephropathy. The presence of small amounts of albumin in the urine is the earliest clinical evidence of nephropathy. The eventual destruction of the filtering ability of the kidney causes chronic renal failure and the need for permanent dialysis or renal transplantation.

Infection. Chronic, poorly controlled DM can lead to a variety of blood vessel and tissue changes that result in impaired wound healing and markedly increased risk of infections. Impaired vision and peripheral neuropathy contribute to the decreased ability of the person with diabetes to feel or see breaks in skin integrity and developing wounds. Vascular disease contributes to tissue hypoxia, which further decreases healing ability.

In addition, once pathogens are inside the body, they multiply rapidly because the increased glucose content in body fluids and tissues fosters bacterial growth. Because the blood supply to tissues is already compromised, white blood cells are not mobilized to the affected areas efficiently or adequately. Diabetes results in higher incidences of skin, urinary tract, vaginal, and other types of tissue infections.[68]

Musculoskeletal problems. Musculoskeletal complications are common, often involving the hands, shoulders, spine, and feet. CTS, Dupuytren's contracture, trigger finger, and adhesive capsulitis occur four times more often in people with diabetes than in those who do not have diabetes.[19,20] Available data show that more than 30% of people with type 1 or type 2 DM have some kind of hand or shoulder disease. More people with type 1 DM have musculoskeletal disorders than those with type 2 DM, and the degree of stiffness is greater with this type of diabetes. Although these disorders are not life-threatening, they can add significant functional impairment to a person's life.

Upper Extremity. In the hand, the syndrome of limited joint mobility (SLJM or LJM) and the stiff hand syndrome are unique to diabetes. SLJM is characterized by painless stiffness and limitation of the finger joints (Fig. 8.9). Flexion contractures typically progress to result in loss of dexterity and grip strength. SLJM is an underdiagnosed complication of diabetes, largely because this type of loss of hand range of motion is considered a common normal sign of aging.[59] The severity of this syndrome in diabetes is correlated with the duration of disease, duration and quantity of insulin therapy, and smoking. Joint contractures also may develop in larger joints, such as the elbows, shoulders, knees, and spine.

The stiff hand syndrome has a distinct pathogenesis and clinical presentation. It occurs uniquely with diabetes and is seen more frequently with type 1 DM and poor blood glucose control. Paresthesias, which eventually become painful, are accompanied by subcutaneous tissue changes such as stiffness and hardness.

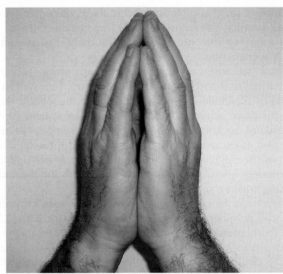

FIG. 8.9 The prayer sign. The individual is unable to press the palms flat against each other, which is a diagnostic sign of the syndrome of limited joint mobility in diabetic persons. Other conditions also may result in loss of extension with a positive prayer sign. (From Glynn M, Drake WM: Hutchison's clinical methods: an integrated approach to clinical practice, ed 23, Edinburgh, 2012, Elsevier.)

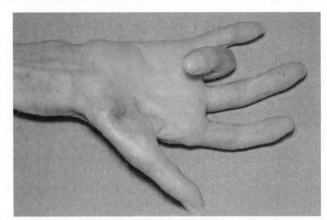

FIG. 8.10 Dupuytren's contracture. Painless nodules develop in the distal palmar crease, often in line with the ring finger, that slowly mature into a longitudinal cord that is readily distinguishable from a tendon. The skin overlying the nodules is usually puckered. The contracture may be symptomatic (painful), but with or without pain it results in impaired hand function. (From Monahan F, Sands JK: Phipps' medical-surgical nursing: health and illness perspectives, ed 8, St Louis, 2007, Mosby.)

Dupuytren's contracture is characterized by the formation of a flexion contracture, palmar nodules, and thickening band or cord of palmar fascia (Fig. 8.10), usually involving the third and fourth digits in the population with diabetes rather than the fourth and fifth digits in the population without diabetes. Pain and decreased range of motion are the primary presentation. Painless nodules develop in the distal palmar crease, often in line with the ring finger, which slowly mature into a longitudinal cord that is readily distinguishable from a tendon. In some cases, regression of symptoms does occur without intervention, although the underlying mechanism for this phenomenon remains unknown. Surgical excision has not been shown to be a reliable cure for the disease and is not recommended unless there is a contracture that is bothersome.

Flexor tenosynovitis is another rheumatologic condition that is more common in persons with diabetes. Tenosynovitis is caused by accumulation of fibrous tissue in the tendon sheath and can cause aching nodules along the flexor tendons and contracture. Locking of the digit, called *trigger finger,* can occur in flexion or extension and may be associated with crepitus or pain. In the population with diabetes, tenosynovitis is found predominantly in women and affects the thumb and the middle and ring fingers most often.

Diabetes is the systemic disease most often seen in connection with peripheral neuropathy of the hand, including CTS. The clinical presentation of CTS is the same for the person with diabetes as for the person without diabetes, although in diabetes CTS can be either a neuropathic process or an entrapment problem. Both neuropathy and compression within the carpal tunnel may exist together.

Adhesive capsulitis (also known as *frozen shoulder*) is characterized by diffuse shoulder pain and loss of motion in all directions, often with a positive painful arc test and limited joint accessory motions. The pattern is slightly different from that of typical adhesive capsulitis, in which regional tightness in the joint capsule primarily compromises external rotation, followed by loss of abduction and less often, internal rotation and flexion.

The pattern in diabetes is one of significant global tightness with external and internal rotation equally limited in the dominant shoulder, followed by limitations in abduction and hyperextension. External rotation and hyperextension are most limited in the nondominant shoulder, followed by internal rotation and abduction. The pathogenesis of the capsular thickening and adherence to the humeral head remains unknown. The long head of the biceps tendon may become glued down in its tendon sheath on the anterior humeral head.[147]

Adhesive capsulitis may be accompanied by vasomotor instability of the hand previously referred to as *reflex sympathetic dystrophy* but now classified as the complex regional pain syndrome. This condition is characterized by severe pain, swelling, and skin changes of the hand including thinning and shininess of the skin with loss of wrinkling and sometimes with increased hair growth.

Tendinopathy with thickening of the plantar fascia and Achilles tendon and tendo-Achilles tightening occurs as glucose deposits in tendons and ligaments result in loss of flexibility and rigid foot. In the diabetic population, loss of Achilles tendon flexibility, especially when combined with a flatfoot, increases pressure under the foot, adding to the compressive forces that contribute to ulcer formation.[55]

Spine. Diffuse idiopathic skeletal hyperostosis (DISH) is a condition of the spine seen most often in people with type 2 DM, although it can occur in a person who does not have diabetes. In DISH, osteophytes develop into bony spurs that may join to form bridges (Fig. 8.11). The thoracic spine most commonly is involved. Calcaneal and olecranon spurs may develop, and new bone may form around hips, knees, and wrists.

People with DISH may be asymptomatic or they may experience back pain and stiffness without limitations in range of motion. Dysphagia may develop if extensive cervical spine involvement occurs.

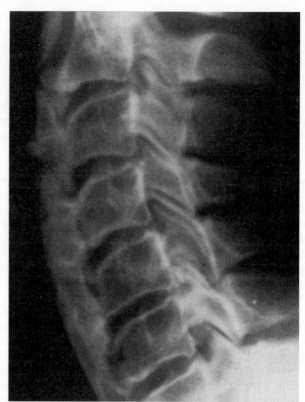

FIG. 8.11 Diffuse idiopathic skeletal hyperostosis (DISH), or ankylosing hyperostosis, associated with type 2 diabetes mellitus. DISH can occur with other conditions such as ankylosing spondylitis. Although the dense anterior bony bridging of the cervical vertebrae is pictured on this lateral roentgenogram, the thoracic spine most commonly is involved in diabetes. This type of DISH can be distinguished from ankylosing spondylitis by the preservation of sacroiliac joints, which are a site of typical involvement in ankylosing spondylitis. (From Kaye T: Watching for and managing musculoskeletal problems in diabetes, J Musculoskelet Med 11:25–37, 1994.)

Osteoporosis. Generalized osteoporosis usually develops within the first 5 years after the onset of DM and is more severe in persons with type 1 DM. It is hypothesized that bone matrix formation may be inadequate in the absence of normal circulating insulin levels. Results of bone density studies in persons with type 2 DM are conflicting, with some studies demonstrating decreased bone density and others indicating increased bone density.

As in any case of osteoporosis, regardless of the underlying cause, this condition places the person at greater risk for fractures. With the additional loss of sensation associated with diabetes, minor trauma easily produces injury. Microfractures can occur in already weakened bone and cartilage and may remain unrecognized because of the lack of pain appreciation.

Sensory, Motor, and Autonomic Neuropathy. Sensory, motor, and autonomic neuropathy associated with DM is a common phenomenon with known risk factors: long-standing diabetes, increased BMI, smoking, hypertension, and high triglycerides.

Neuropathy may affect the CNS, peripheral nervous system, or autonomic nervous system. The most common form of diabetic neuropathy is a sensory polyneuropathy, usually affecting the hands and feet and causing symptoms that range from mild tingling, burning, numbness, or pain to a complete loss of sensation (usually feet) and foot drop.

Sensory Neuropathy. Many people with diabetes suffer from *diabetic peripheral neuropathic pain* associated with nerve damage. Spontaneous pain, allodynia (painful response to stimuli that usually are not painful), hyperalgesia, and other unpleasant symptoms are common. Neuropathic pain often progressively increases in intensity throughout the day and is worse at night, significantly impairing sleep. Some individuals experience painful neuropathy called *insulin neuritis syndrome* at the beginning of therapy for diabetes; the feet are affected more often than the hands, and the condition is usually self-limiting.[158]

The loss of sensation in diabetic neuropathy predisposes joints to repeated trauma and progressive joint destruction. Chronic progressive degeneration of the stress-bearing portion of a joint associated with loss of proprioceptive sensation in the joint produces a condition called *Charcot's disease*, or *neuropathic arthropathy*. Diabetes is the most common cause of neuropathic joints.

Several stages of neuropathic arthropathy (Charcot's foot) occur involving bone destruction and absorption leading to dislocation and an unstable joint. Bone fragments and debris are deposited in the affected joint. Subluxation of the tarsal and metatarsal joints commonly results in a rocker-bottom foot deformity and a redistribution of pressure on the plantar surface of the foot with progressive ulceration. An acute neuropathic joint is swollen, warm, and edematous, but pain may be minimal because of the underlying altered sensation.

Left untreated, neuropathic changes can progress to complete destruction of the joint. The presence of autonomic neuropathy may hasten this process, because the blood vessels are unable to respond appropriately to even minor trauma.

Reduction of weight bearing, joint immobilization, and joint protection are important conservative treatment tools. Surgical fusion can be performed if all else fails, but joint replacement is contraindicated in this condition.[23,128]

Motor Neuropathy. Motor neuropathy is more common with long-standing disease and produces weakness and atrophy; bilateral but asymmetric proximal muscle weakness is called *diabetic amyotrophy*. This leads to bony deformities such as claw toes, severe flatfoot with valgus of the midfoot, or collapse of the longitudinal arch.

Autonomic Neuropathy. Autonomic neuropathy is sometimes referred to as *diabetic autonomic neuropathy* and affects nerves that innervate heart, lung, stomach, intestines, bladder, and reproductive organs. It may manifest itself through the loss of control of blood pressure, blood glucose levels, temperature, regulation of sweating, and blood flow in the limbs. Skin changes such as these can create more openings for bacteria to enter. Diabetic autonomic neuropathy may also lead to hypoglycemia because the patient does not feel the warning signs of sweating and palpations; the person's ability to manage the disease is impaired, and death may result.

Cardiovascular autonomic neuropathy is manifested by the lack of heart rate variability in response to deep breathing and exercise, exercise intolerance, persistent sinus tachycardia, bradycardia, and postural hypotension. Stress testing should be considered before starting an exercise program, especially in the older adult.[5]

Ulceration. Sensory neuropathy, occurring as a result of improper glucose metabolism and diminished vascular perfusion to nerve tissues, places the diabetic person at risk

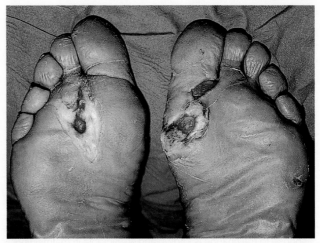

FIG. 8.12 Neurotrophic ulcers associated with diabetic neuropathy. (From Swartz MH: Textbook of physical diagnosis: history and examination, ed 7, Philadelphia, 2014, Saunders.)

for the development of ulcers. Diabetic foot ulcers are caused primarily by repetitive stress on the insensitive skin with increased pressure and/or shear or stress. Body weight and activity level may increase pressure and shear force.

The loss of autonomic nerve function eliminates the production of sweat, leaving the skin dry and inelastic. Changes in pressure and gait, fat atrophy, and muscle weakness are mechanical factors that, along with sensory neuropathy, influence the development of plantar skin abnormalities, especially ulceration.[12,139] Diabetes-induced changes in the skin are likely to contribute to ulceration with increased cross-linking, making the skin stiff. The areas most commonly affected by foot ulcers are the plantar areas of the metatarsal heads, the toes, and the plantar area of the hallux (Fig. 8.12). In Charcot's foot, the incidence of ulceration beneath the talus and navicular bones becomes more common because of the rigid rocker-bottom deformity.

Medical Management

Prevention

Prevention of obesity-related health problems, including type 2 diabetes, is a key focus of the medical community. PTAs play an important role in providing education on the beneficial effects of exercise combined with proper nutrition. Studies have clearly shown that people who incorporate physical activity and exercise into their daily lives are less likely to develop type 2 diabetes no matter what their initial weight. Adopting an activity program of 150 minutes weekly of moderate-intensity activity (e.g., brisk walking) similar to what the Surgeon General advises is a key prevention strategy.[77-79]

Screening

The American Diabetes Association recommends universal screening for type 2 diabetes at age 45, and if normal, repeat testing every 3 years. Testing should be considered in adults of any age who are overweight or obese and who have one or more additional risk factors (see Box 8.4).

Diagnosis

Diagnostic assessment may include a variety of testing procedures, such as plasma glucose, glucose tolerance test, and urine ketone levels, to name just a few. A diagnosis of diabetes is confirmed by symptoms of hyperglycemia and blood and urine glucose and ketone abnormalities.

Glucose Monitoring

Individuals using multiple daily insulin injections or an insulin pump should perform self-monitoring of blood glucose (SMBG) three or more times a day. It may also be useful for individuals using insulin injections that are less frequent, oral antidiabetes medications, or medical nutrition therapy. SMBG is also recommended when a new physical activity is introduced, such as occurs in an exercise or rehabilitation program, and should be continued until the individual's response to the change is known and predictable in maintaining stable blood glucose levels.[44] New insulins and easier blood glucose monitoring have improved the ability to obtain much tighter control of blood glucose levels with fewer fluctuations and reduced risk of hypoglycemia. There are several methods used to monitor glucose immediately and over time.

Frequent self-monitoring by performing a direct blood sampling (fingerstick or laser technique) provides immediate monitoring of blood glucose levels and is an important management tool in the long-term treatment of this disease. The development of noninvasive testing methods to monitor glucose levels without the use of fingersticks is underway. One device already commercially available (the GlucoWatch G2 Biographer [GW2B]) is worn like a watch and uses electrical currents to obtain interval measurements of glucose levels in the skin.

Other technology in use or being actively researched includes nocturnal alarms using a real-time glucose sensor to alert parents and children of hypoglycemic and hyperglycemic events while sleeping and, for adolescents and adults, glucose-sensing skin patches, tattoos, and contact lenses. The contact lens would allow the individual with diabetes to see changes in the color of the lens to give an indication of blood glucose levels.[7]

Treatment

There is no widely available cure for diabetes. The goal of overall care for persons with diabetes is control or regulation of blood glucose. Many large-scale studies have shown that tight glucose control reduces the risk of vascular complications in both type 1 and type 2 diabetes. Early identification and intervention are strongly linked with risk reduction of late complications.[86] Key standards and goals in the treatment and self-management of DM include the following:

- Blood pressure less than 130/80 mm Hg
- Total cholesterol less than 200 mg/dL (low-density lipoprotein less than 100 mg/dL)

Researchers continue to investigate drugs that would prevent the formation of fat cells, reducing the problem of obesity before type 2 DM can develop. Studies of the use of gene therapy as a treatment for both types of diabetes are ongoing. Experimental research is underway in the development of a vaccine for type 1 DM that may help stop the immune system attack of the insulin-producing beta cells of the pancreas.[158]

Type 1 Diabetes Mellitus

Type 1 DM requires insulin administration and dietary management to achieve tight (near-normal) blood glucose control. With no circulating insulin produced by the body, the effect of aerobic exercise in providing increased glycemic control for the person with type 1 DM may be limited. To date, studies of the effect of aerobic exercise in type 1 DM have shown mixed results.

The insulin dosage schedule varies depending on the individual's age, level of compliance, and severity of diabetes. Control over blood glucose levels dictates how "brittle" the diabetes is. *Brittle diabetes* is a term used when a person's blood glucose level often swings quickly from high to low and from low to high. The individual with wide glucose excursions is considered very brittle.

Poorly controlled diabetes is ideally treated with more frequent administration of insulin (e.g., four times per day), whereas other individuals may receive insulin once or twice daily, sometimes mixing different types of insulin.

Insulin Pump

An insulin pump, also known as *continuous subcutaneous insulin infusion (CSII)*, is now available to deliver fixed amounts of regular insulin continuously, more closely imitating the release of the hormone by the islet cells. This lightweight, pager-sized device is worn conveniently in a pocket or on a belt clip (Fig. 8.13); a waterproof design makes swimming possible.

The insulin pump offers many advantages such as flexible eating and exercising schedules, fewer episodes of severe hypoglycemia, and the convenience of taking insulin without the social consequences of public injections, to name a few.[27] Although this type of insulin administration provides better control, it has some disadvantages. It cannot detect and respond to changes in the blood glucose level, so the individual must continue to monitor glucose levels and make dosage adjustments. It cannot be removed for more than 1 hour, reactions to the needle are common, bleeding can occur at the sensor insertion site, and like any other mechanical device it is subject to malfunction. Insulin pump technology is improving every year; new "smart" features are added to the designs to simplify the tasks involved in delivering an insulin bolus. Implantable pump options that can dispense insulin in constant, steady pulses throughout the day are being tested. Penlike injection cartridges also are in use.[73]

Type 2 Diabetes Mellitus

Type 2 DM is most often treated with diet and exercise, sometimes in conjunction with oral hypoglycemic drugs; insulin occasionally is required. *Exercise* is a recognized therapy for the prevention of complications in type 2 DM. Numerous studies have shown a consistent positive effect of regular exercise training on carbohydrate metabolism and insulin sensitivity. Some of the beneficial effects include decreased need for insulin, prevention of CVD and obesity, management of hypertension, and reduction in very-low–density-lipoprotein cholesterol.[25,99]

A plant-based *diet* is becoming more widely known for its potential effects and benefits in the prevention and treatment of type 2 DM. The use of whole-grain or traditionally processed cereals and legumes has been associated with improved glycemic control in individuals with diabetes and in individuals who are insulin-resistant. Long-term studies have shown that whole-grain consumption reduces the risk of both type 2 diabetes and CVD.[70]

The combination of diet and exercise is more powerful than either one alone and may be even more effective than drugs for preventing type 2 DM. A low-fat, low-calorie diet with moderate exercise (30 minutes 5 times a week) has been shown to reduce new diabetes cases by 58% over a 3-year period.

Treatment of Long-Term Complications

Prevention of long-term complications is the goal for all clients with DM. Risk of complications is associated independently and additively with hyperglycemia and hypertension. Intensive treatment of both these risk factors is required to prevent and minimize the incidence of most complications.[145]

Medical treatment of long-term diabetic complications may include dialysis or kidney transplantation for renal failure and vascular surgery for large-vessel disease. Currently, the American Diabetes Association advises that people with diabetes take low-dose aspirin (75 to 162 mg) daily to help minimize risks such as heart attacks and strokes. New treatment guidelines from the American College of Physicians recommend the use of cholesterol-lowering drugs for anyone with diabetes and diagnosed CAD, even if cholesterol levels are normal.

Diabetic Ulcers

The PTA often is involved in prevention and wound care for diabetic ulcers, which may help prevent amputation. Early recognition and prompt management of wounds, ulceration, and Charcot's foot can facilitate healing. For example, a Centers for Disease Control study showed that people with diabetes who wore proper shoe protection had only a 20% recurrence rate of ulceration compared with an 80% rate for those without offloading.[141]

Offloading or pressure reduction is a key component for healing ulcers and preventing recurrence. The normal response to damaged areas is to spare them from pressure because they are painful. However, in the insensitive foot of a person with diabetes, this normal alteration of weight-bearing surface, pressure, and duration does not take place, resulting in repetitive stress and injury with subcutaneous and cutaneous necrosis and skin breakdown.

Interventions include debridement, infection control, protective dressings, revascularization, proper nutrition, and client education. Active dressings, such as growth factors and living skin, are also in use. Topical application of growth factors on wounds without infection and with at least a minimal level of vascularization was introduced in the early 1990s and has progressed to include new techniques in skin transplantation.

Infrared light therapy has been applied to improve sensory impairment, reduce pain, and prevent and heal ulcers. Long-term studies are still needed to show whether the results can be sustained.[74,75,85,120]

The use of cool laser therapy as a revascularization therapy is now available. Cool laser uses a laser and catheter system to vaporize arterial blockages, restoring blood flow and promoting wound healing. Reduction in pain, improved circulation, and facilitation of wound healing may help prevent limb loss in this population.

Treatment of diabetic peripheral neuropathic pain has not been successful using any one single intervention technique. The ideal treatment is correcting the underlying condition of chronic hyperglycemia.

Transplantation

Research is being conducted on the use of transplanted pancreatic islet cells rather than the entire pancreas. The transplant recipient receives one or more infusions of pancreatic islet cells that include insulin-producing beta cells. Almost 500 people with type 1 diabetes have received islet transplants at 43 institutions worldwide in the last 5 years.[134]

High rates of insulin independence have been reported at 1 year in the leading islet transplant centers. Loss of insulin independence by 5 years occurs in the majority of recipients. Lifelong immunosuppression and its complications limit this treatment to candidates who have the most severe, unstable glycemic control despite optimal insulin therapy.[134]

Stem cell research may find a way for people to develop their own stem cells into islet cells and allow infusions without cell-rejection complications and the need for lifelong immunosuppression. An artificial pancreas contains a reservoir for insulin (which must be filled by the affected individual, typically through a tube in the abdomen) and an internal glucose monitor that continuously determines the plasma glucose level, automatically releasing the appropriate amount of insulin. Such instruments are expected to reach the market shortly.

Prognosis

Diabetes control depends on the proper interaction among the following three factors: (1) food, (2) insulin or oral medication to lower blood glucose, and (3) activity or exercise. When diabetes is regulated successfully, complications of hyperglycemia and hypoglycemia can be avoided with minimal disruption to a normal lifestyle. However, diabetes can be fatal even with medical treatment, or it can cause major permanent disabilities and seriously impair functional abilities. Studies have shown that type 2 DM raises a person's risk of dying from heart disease by two to three times.[143] Diabetes is the leading cause of new blindness and is a contributory cause to renal failure and peripheral vascular disease.

Regardless of the modality of treatment used for the person with type 1 or type 2 DM, recent studies have shown clearly that tight glucose control delays onset and progression of diabetic complications. The only apparent danger in maintenance of tight control is the greater possibility of hypoglycemia, particularly in those people with type 1 DM who receive frequent insulin administration.[25]

8.14 Special Implications for the PTA: Diabetes Mellitus

Client education is the key to therapeutic, nonsurgical treatment of the neuromusculoskeletal complications associated with DM. Extensive self-management is the focus of the educational program.

Exercise is a key component of the overall intervention plan.[25] The client must be taught the importance of assessing glucose levels before and after exercise and to judge what carbohydrate and insulin requirements are suitable for the activity or workout. People with diabetes and peripheral neuropathy have a high incidence of injuries (e.g., falls, fractures, sprains, cuts, and bruises) during walking or standing and a low level of perceived safety.

Complications of Insulin Therapy

Hypoglycemia

Insulin therapy can result in hypoglycemia (low blood glucose, also called an *insulin reaction*)[31]; tissue hypertrophy, atrophy, or both at the site of injection; insulin allergy; erratic insulin action; and insulin resistance. Symptoms of hypoglycemia are related to two body responses: increased sympathetic activity and deprivation of CNS glucose supply (Table 8.12). The clinical picture may vary from a report of headache and weakness to irritability and lack of muscular coordination (much like drunkenness) to apprehension, inability to respond to verbal commands, and psychosis.

Symptoms can occur when the blood glucose level drops to 70 mg/dL or less, although this value varies among those with diabetes and can be lower than 70 mg/dL before symptoms are elicited. In diabetes, an overdose of insulin, late or skipped meals, or overexertion in exercise may cause hypoglycemic reactions. Immediately provide carbohydrates in some form (e.g., fruit juice, honey, hard candy, or commercially available glucose tablets or gel); a blood glucose test should be performed as soon as the symptoms are recognized. The unconscious person needs immediate medical attention; to prevent aspiration, fluids should not be forced. Hospitalization is recommended when the following occur:

- The blood glucose is less than 50 mg/dL and/or the treatment of hypoglycemia has not resulted in prompt recovery of altered mental status.
- The individual has had seizures or is unconsciousness.
- A responsible adult cannot be with the person for the next 12 hours.

It is important to note that clients can exhibit signs and symptoms of hypoglycemia when their elevated blood glucose level drops rapidly to a level that is still elevated (e.g., 400 to 200 mg/dL). The rapidity of the drop is the stimulus for sympathetic activity–based symptoms; even though a blood glucose level appears elevated, affected individuals may still have symptoms of hypoglycemia.

When a person with diabetes mentions the presence of nightmares, unexplained sweating, and/or headache causing sleep disturbances, hypoglycemia may be indicated during nighttime sleep. These symptoms should be reported to the physician.

Erratic insulin action (i.e., low blood glucose followed by high blood glucose) can occur as a result of a variety of factors such as overeating, irregular meals, irregular exercise, irregular rest periods, chronic overdosage of insulin, emotional or psychologic stress, failure to administer insulin, or intermittent use of hyperglycemic or hypoglycemic drugs

Lipogenic Effect of Insulin

Frequent injections of insulin at the same site can cause thickening of the subcutaneous tissues and a loss of subcutaneous fat, resulting in a dimpling of the skin that is lumpy and hard or spongy and soft. These abnormal tissue changes may cause decreased absorption of the injected insulin and poor glucose control.

The client usually is instructed to choose an injection site that is easily accessible (e.g., thighs, upper arms, abdomen, or lower back) and relatively insensitive to pain (away from the midline of the body). Sites of injection should be rotated, and rotation within each area is recommended. An individual can rotate within an area using 1 inch of the surrounding tissue at a time. The client who is going to exercise should avoid injecting sites or muscles that will be exercised heavily that day because exercise increases the rate of absorption. Following a definite injection plan can help avoid tissue damage.

Even with an insulin pump the infusion site should be changed every 2 or 3 days or whenever the client's blood glucose is above 240 mg/dL for two tests in a row. Rotating insertion sites will help prevent infection and tissue damage.

Diabetic Ketoacidosis

The PTA must always be alert for signs of ketoacidosis (e.g., acetone breath, dehydration, weak and rapid pulse, progressing to polyuria, thirst, neurologic abnormalities, and stupor). Immediate medical care is essential. If it is not clear whether the symptoms are the result of hypoglycemia or hyperglycemia (Table 8.13), the health care worker is advised to administer fruit juice or honey. This procedure does not harm the hyperglycemic person but could

potentially save the hypoglycemic person. Everyone with diabetes should wear a medical alert identification tag.

Diabetes and Exercise

An overwhelming body of evidence now exists that acute muscle contractile activity and chronic exercise improve skeletal muscle glucose transport and whole-body glucose homeostasis in the person with type 2 DM.[136] Exercise helps to increase insulin sensitivity, thus lowering blood glucose levels. Increased insulin sensitivity allows the body to use the available blood glucose for the person with type 2 diabetes; an increase in insulin sensitivity can last 12 to 72 hours after exercise.

A program of planned exercise, including all the elements of fitness (flexibility, muscle strength, and cardiovascular endurance) can benefit persons with diabetes, especially those with type 2 DM. Exercise increases carbohydrate metabolism (which lowers the blood glucose level); aids in maintaining optimal body weight; increases high-density lipoproteins (HDLs); and decreases triglycerides, blood pressure, and stress and tension (Table 8.14).

Exercise and physical activity (even leisure-time physical activity and activity on the job) have been shown to independently reduce the risk of total and cardiovascular mortality of adults with type 2 diabetes. Exercise capacity is reduced by diabetes-related CVD, but exercise training is an excellent therapeutic adjunct in the treatment of diabetic CVD.[99]

The favorable association of physical activity with longevity occurs regardless of BMI, blood pressure, smoking habits, and total cholesterol levels.[65,66] Once again, the PTA can be very instrumental in client education on the importance of exercise for a wide range of reasons and benefits to the individual with diabetes.

General Exercise Considerations

For anyone with diabetes, type 1 or type 2, the exercise prescription must take into account any of the complications present, especially cardiovascular changes, autonomic and sensory neuropathy, and retinopathy.[169] Muscle damage, with accompanying insulin resistance and impaired glucose uptake and disposal, can occur when untrained individuals begin to exercise.[138] For this reason, clients with diabetes must start any new activity at a well-tolerated intensity level and duration, gradually increasing over a period of weeks or even months.[169]

For the person with type 1 DM in good control, sports in which hypoglycemia may be life-threatening (e.g., scuba diving, rock climbing, or parachuting) should be discouraged. Walking necessitates care toward proper footwear for the person who does not already have evidence of peripheral neuropathy.

Intermittent, high-intensity activities (e.g., racquetball, baseball) or contact sports (e.g., basketball, soccer) should be avoided to prevent trauma (especially to the feet or eyes). High-resistance strength-training programs should be limited to the young person with diabetes who has no diabetic complications. More specific recommendations for the long-distance runner and other athletes are available.[2,9,87,97,149]

Low-resistance strength training programs should be encouraged unless retinopathy is present (Box 8.5). Exercise involving jarring or rapid head motion may precipitate hemorrhage or retinal detachment. Outdoor activities must be evaluated carefully, taking into consideration the weather extremes (hot or cold) and the person's ability to maintain distal circulation. Stationary indoor equipment (many types are now available) may be the best overall choice.

Exercise Precautions

As positive as exercise is in the prevention and control of diabetes, the PTA must keep in mind that diabetes is a metabolic disorder with cardiovascular and circulatory implications. Blood flow to the skin and skeletal muscle, already reduced, can be further compromised by intense exercise, and recovery time is longer. All possible effects of exercise must be kept in mind when designing an exercise program. Strenuous exercise can have some serious side effects and is not recommended for most people with diabetes.[114]

Before beginning any exercise program, the person with diabetes should undergo a detailed medical evaluation with appropriate diagnostic studies. Screening should be done for the presence of vascular complications that may be worsened by the exercise program. The PTA can help by designing an exercise program that suits the individual's needs. Low-impact activities, such as walking, bicycling, and swimming, are good choices for anyone who has a loss of sensation in the feet. Strength training, especially upper body work, puts no additional strain on the feet. Resistance exercise training may help avoid insulin therapy, especially for overweight women with gestational DM.[15] Moderate-intensity resistive training also can improve mobility and strength in older adults with diabetes, potentially reducing the rate of mobility loss during aging.[14]

Diabetic Autonomic Neuropathy

Many people with diabetes may not be able to exercise intensely to a calculated heart rate because of preexisting heart conditions, deconditioning, age, neuropathies, arthritis, or other joint problems. Exercise may be contraindicated in anyone with a severe form of autonomic neuropathy (see Box 8.5), especially anyone with vasomotor instability, angina, and a history of myocardial infarction.[25] The PTA is advised to communicate and collaborate with the client, health care team, and physician when considering an exercise program for anyone with this problem.

Generally, individuals with autonomic neuropathy have a poor ability to perform aerobic exercise because of decreased maximal heart rate and increased resting heart rate. They also demonstrate a predisposition toward dehydration in the heat and poor exercise tolerance in cold environments.

People with diabetic autonomic neuropathy may have a higher resting heart rate but lower maximal heart rate, making exercise at safe levels more difficult. It may be better to use the percent of heart rate reserve, which is the difference between resting heart rate and maximum heart rate, as a valid measure in prescribing exercise intensity instead of the rating of perceived exertion scale, which relies on self-assessment of exertion.[26] Some people with autonomic neuropathy may have silent myocardial infarctions without angina. The first symptom may be shortness of breath resulting from congestive heart failure. Decrease in nerve innervation to the heart associated with this type of neuropathy may prevent a normal increase in heart rate with stress or exercise, requiring careful observation and monitoring of vital signs during exercise. Blood pressure regulation is altered with autonomic neuropathy; exercise can further stress the impaired system. Clients with autonomic neuropathy are prone to hypothermia, dehydration, and hypotension or hypertension.

Diabetes is associated with reduced tolerance to heat. Autonomic neuropathy may also include changes in thermoregulation with a decreased or altered ability to perspire. Exercise with a concomitant increase in core body temperature can lead to heat stroke.[116] Impairment of sweating has been demonstrated even with isometric exercise.[117] Proper hydration is essential, and precautions should be taken to avoid heat stroke. Valsalva's maneuver should be avoided.

Exercise in Type 1 Diabetes Mellitus

The person with type 1 DM tends to be thin, may be poorly nourished, and because of the islet cell deficiency always needs insulin supplementation for adequate control of blood glucose. Exercise can increase strength and facilitate maintenance of weight and provide other important benefits (see Table 8.14), but unfortunately

exercise has not been proven to provide increased glycemic control for the person with type 1 DM.

The person with well-controlled type 1 DM may commonly work out for approximately 30 to 45 minutes of sustained intense aerobic exercise without problems. Lack of adequate glycogen stores leads to impaired aerobic exercise endurance compared with the nondiabetic person.

Hypoglycemia is a common occurrence in persons with type 1 DM who are exercising. In those who do not have diabetes, plasma insulin levels decrease during exercise and insulin counter-regulatory hormones promote increased hepatic glucose production, which matches the amount of glucose used during exercise.

For the person with type 1 DM who is not insulin deficient because of administration of insulin, plasma insulin concentrations may not fall during exercise and may even increase if exercise occurs within 1 hour of insulin injection. These sustained insulin levels during exercise enhance peripheral glucose uptake and stimulate glucose use by exercising muscle. For this reason, insulin should not be injected into muscles or at sites close to areas involved in exercise within 1 hour of exercise. Moderate periods of exercise provide beneficial effects, but longer periods may result in hypoglycemia. Watch for symptoms such as sweating, shakiness, nausea, headache, and difficulty concentrating. The greatest risk of severe hypoglycemia occurs 6 to 14 hours after strenuous exercise. Muscle and hepatic glycogen must be restored during periods of rest. Insulin and caloric intake must be adjusted after strenuous exercise to avoid severe nocturnal hypoglycemia.

Exercise in Type 2 Diabetes Mellitus

In contrast, people with type 2 DM are often obese, and exercise is a major contributor in controlling hyperglycemia. Exercise can improve short-term insulin sensitivity and reduce insulin resistance, making it possible to prevent type 2 DM in those persons at risk and to improve glycemic control in those with diabetes.[137] These effects disappear a few days after exercise is discontinued. Long-term higher intensity exercise training (80% peak aerobic capacity) provides more enduring benefits to insulin action compared with low- or moderate-intensity exercise.[36]

Hypoglycemia is not as common a problem for the person with type 2 DM because insulin levels usually can be maintained. Control of blood glucose levels by lowering the medication dose or increasing carbohydrate intake (or both) before exercise can prevent hypoglycemia.

For anyone with diabetes, exercise should not be initiated if the blood glucose is 70 or less. Because one effect of exercise is the transfer of glucose in the cells, glucose levels should be checked again 2 hours after exercise. Vigorous exercise should not be undertaken within 2 hours before going to sleep at night because this is when exercise-induced hypoglycemia can occur with potentially fatal consequences.

Unplanned exercise can be dangerous for people taking insulin or oral hypoglycemic agents. During periods of exercise, muscles are stimulated to take up glucose to supply the fuel to the working muscles, causing blood glucose levels to fall abruptly. However, anyone with blood glucose levels at or near 300 mg/dL should *not* exercise because vigorous activity also can raise the blood glucose level by releasing stored glycogen. Exercise or therapy sessions should be scheduled to avoid peak insulin times and to avoid periods of fasting.

Balancing Insulin, Food, and Exercise

As mentioned, insulin should be injected in sites away from the part of the body involved in exercising. Because glucose can enter the cells without insulin during exercise, food should be eaten if the person is exercising more than usual. Conversely, when exercising less often, a lighter diet or more insulin is required.

Glucose levels should be monitored before and after exercise (or therapy activities), remembering that the effect of exercise can be felt up to 12 to 24 hours later. Clients taking insulin should have their own glucose monitoring devices.

After exercise, available glucose is important for the replenishment of muscle glycogen stores. Bouts of hypoglycemia can be delayed until hours after completion of exercise. The insulin-dependent person must regulate activity so that the rate of energy expenditure balances the amount and type of insulin and food intake. Women who are menstruating may need to increase their insulin during menses.

Exercise and the Insulin Pump

The normal metabolic response to exercise in a person who does not have diabetes is to decrease the release of insulin as muscles contract, causing the transport of more blood glucose into cells without insulin.

CSII therapy brings the exercising individual with diabetes a response as close to normal as possible. Anyone with diabetes who uses an insulin pump must make frequent insulin adjustments to mimic the normal metabolic response, maintaining a more normal glycemic control, especially during periods of higher intensity or longer duration exercise.[27]

Time of day, exercise intensity, and elevated starting blood glucose levels appear to affect the metabolic response and can result in hyperglycemia instead of the more usual hypoglycemia for several hours after exercise. Metabolic control can deteriorate with intense exercise even in people who have tightly controlled blood glucose levels. It is suggested that 30 minutes of mild to moderate exercise is possible 2 or 3 hours after breakfast when an insulin pump is used. One of the disadvantages of an insulin pump is that it can malfunction or become displaced without the person knowing it. Exercise can exacerbate the situation when insulin delivery has been unknowingly disrupted. Teach the client to be vigilant during exercise to maintain the integrity of the infusion site and to pay attention to any symptoms of thirst, nausea, weakness, or excessive urination.

Diabetes and Neuromusculoskeletal Complications

The treatment of musculoskeletal problems does not differ from treatment for these same conditions in the nondiabetic population. Early aggressive therapy for adhesive capsulitis usually results in restoration of functional motion, even though full range of motion may not be achieved.

Hand function can be maintained and disease progression delayed with hand therapy. Stiff hand syndrome does not always benefit from therapy, but treatment intervention should be tried. The client must understand the importance of a self-directed exercise program established by the therapy team to prevent recurrence of symptoms and to maintain functional outcomes.

Intervention for CTS must take into account the neuropathic and entrapment components in the person with diabetes. Nonsurgical efforts should be the focus of treatment.

Diabetes and Foot Care

Disorders of the feet constitute a source of increasing morbidity associated with diabetes. Foot problems are a leading cause of hospital admission in people with diabetes, and diabetes is the most common reason for lower limb amputation. Half of those cases are preventable with proper foot care.[139,158] Treatment of the underlying diabetes has little effect on any joint disease already present. The most beneficial interventions include stabilizing the joint, minimizing trauma, maintaining muscular strength, and performing daily foot care.

The PTA must teach each person with diabetes proper foot and skin care. Regular foot checks after exercise using a mirror to inspect all surface areas and between the toes is advised. Any areas of warmth, erythema, swelling, or skin changes must be evaluated carefully and immediately. The PTA is *advised to reinforce client education at each and every session.*

Diabetic Peripheral Neuropathy

The therapy team should assess for risk factors for amputation (e.g., previous ulcer or amputation) and for signs of diabetic neuropathy.

Health care professionals should provide clients with a monofilament for self-testing (Fig. 8.14). This test is an easily used clinical indicator for identifying people who are at risk for developing foot ulcers and requiring subsequent amputation. It can clearly demonstrate physiologic changes in peripheral nerve function. If the person cannot feel the monofilament when applied with slight pressure against the skin, there is an increased risk of ulceration. The results of this test provide a definitive idea of who can benefit most from preventive care, education, and prescription of appropriate therapeutic footwear.[105]

Decreased sensation in the feet associated with diabetic neuropathy can affect both the timing and quality of gait, requiring retraining. Gait and strength training are important in the management of large-fiber neuropathies when impaired vibration, depressed tendon reflexes, and shortening of the Achilles tendon occur.[160] Diabetes gait may occur independent of sensory impairment. Increased joint movement, wider stance, and slower pace demonstrated in some individuals with type 2 diabetes may be neurologic in origin and not related to muscle weakness or loss of sensation in the feet.[115]

Anyone with peripheral neuropathy is advised to avoid soaking the feet. There is a danger of burns, and prolonged exposure to warm water leaves the skin susceptible to fungal infections. Whirlpools are contraindicated and baths are not advised. Bathing and soaking remove the protective barrier from the skin and can lead to other infections, especially if there are fissures from dry skin caused by decreased circulation.

Moderate-intensity aerobic exercise may help prevent the onset of peripheral neuropathy. Exercise guidelines for people with diabetes and peripheral neuropathy have been changed to allow moderate-intensity weight-bearing exercise for individuals with peripheral neuropathy but no foot ulcers. Recent studies indicate that walking at moderate intensity does not increase risk of foot ulcer, including reoccurrence of ulcers in people with peripheral neuropathy.[84]

Neuropathic (Diabetic) Ulcers

All people with diabetes should have an annual comprehensive foot examination to identify risk factors predictive of neuropathic ulcers. The most common cause of neuropathic (diabetic) ulcers is excessive plantar pressure in the presence of sensory neuropathy and foot deformity. Neuropathic foot ulcers can occur anywhere pressure or shear force is applied to the foot (top, sides, or bottom). Many occur beneath the metatarsal heads and are the result of painless trauma caused by excessive plantar pressures during walking.[106]

The presence of corns or calluses is an indication that footwear fits poorly and should be carefully evaluated. Lacking an adequate insulin supply, the articular cartilage in the person with diabetes does not tolerate repetitive trauma, compression, and motion, making proper footwear all the more important.[119]

Note the location of any foot ulcerations for possible causes that can be corrected. For example, ill-fitting shoes may cause ulcers on the medial or lateral borders of the feet, whereas ulcers on top of the foot may be caused by deformities such as hammer (claw) toes.

The presence of a previous history of plantar ulceration may alert the PTA to the need to teach the client how to control activity levels to lessen shear forces on scars from previous ulcers.[16] Orthoses are often used to redistribute or move pressure away from a blister or other area of pressure. Soft, moldable orthoses are preferred to the rigid orthoses used by clients with other types of foot problems.

Total contact inserts (TCIs) and metatarsal pads can be used to reduce excessive plantar stresses, preventing skin breakdown and ulceration. The TCI reduces excessive pressures at the metatarsal heads by increasing the contact area of weight-bearing forces. Metatarsal pads act by compressing the soft tissues proximal to the metatarsal heads and relieving compression at the metatarsal heads.[106]

The prevention of foot problems before they begin is always the most effective method in offsetting the development of foot ulceration and infection and their potentially devastating effects. The use of proper footwear, proper cleaning and lubrication of the feet, safe removal of corns or calluses, and the removal of mechanical sources of foot pressure are critical components in the prevention of foot problems. Client education is a key component in the monitoring and detection of potential difficulties.[118]

Delayed Wound Healing

Because wound healing is impaired in the diabetic foot, surgery can be accompanied by increased risks of poor healing and infection.

The detrimental effects of cigarette smoking on wound healing and peripheral circulation are well documented. Smoking increases insulin resistance, worsens diabetes complications, and has a negative effect on prognosis. People with diabetes who smoke have a higher all-cause mortality rate than those who do not smoke.[142]

Smoking cessation is one of the two most important ways to reduce macrovascular complications in adults with diabetes, and control of hypertension is the other. The American Diabetes Association recommends that all health care providers routinely identify the smoking (tobacco use) status of clients with diabetes and offer cessation support and education.[4]

The U.S. Public Health Service Clinical Guideline[150] suggests health care providers use the 5 As: ask, assess, advise, assist, and arrange. A brief, nonconfrontational discussion of smoking cessation may help move the smoker to the next level of readiness. The clinician can help clients think about what will be better if they quit; moving the person to the contemplation stage doubles the chance of quitting during that time.[121]

Diabetes and Physical Agents

Insulin absorption is impaired or altered by smoking, injection site, thickness of skin fold (adipose tissue), exercise, subcutaneous edema, local subcutaneous blood flow, ambient and skin temperature, and local massage.[6,63]

Heat from the use of hot baths, whirlpools, saunas, or sun beds has been shown to accelerate the absorption of subcutaneous injections of insulin by increasing skin blood flow. To reduce the risk of hypoglycemia, local application of heat to the site of a recent insulin injection should be avoided. The use of cryotherapy (cold) with its effects of vasoconstriction and decreased skin blood flow would be expected to slow or delay insulin absorption from the injection site.

Diabetes and Menopause

As life expectancy increases, women are living a greater proportion of their lives in the postmenopausal phase, a time when the prevalence of type 2 diabetes also increases. The PTA should be aware that the consequences of CVD, osteoporosis, and cancer are more pronounced in women who have type 1 or type 2 diabetes, especially in women who have metabolic syndrome followed by the development of type 2 diabetes.

The transition from premenopause to postmenopause estrogen-deficient status is associated with the emergence of many features of the metabolic syndrome, such as central obesity (intraabdominal body fat), insulin resistance, and dyslipidemia, which are also known to be risk factors for CVD. The prevalence

of the metabolic syndrome increases with menopause and may partially explain the apparent acceleration of heart disease after menopause.[22]

As the woman with diabetes approaches menopause, changes in estrogen and progesterone affect how cells respond to insulin and therefore blood glucose levels. Menopause symptoms can mimic low blood glucose levels (e.g., moodiness or short-term memory loss).

Sleep disturbance and weight gain associated with menopause make it harder to control blood glucose levels. During the postmenopause years when female hormone levels remain low, insulin sensitivity may increase, with a drop in the expected blood glucose levels.[125]

Diabetes and Psychosocial Behavior

The PTA should keep in mind the psychologic and behavioral aspects of diabetes with regard to improving clinical outcomes. Common psychologic problems known to complicate diabetes management include poor self-esteem, impact on the family dynamics, family and social support, compliance and motivation, and eating disorders (particularly compulsive overeating); 20% to 40% of people with diabetes experience some level of depression, twice the rate of depression in people without diabetes.[41] Depression can negatively impact diabetes self-care. Exercise may help relieve depression.[82] It is also important to remember that symptoms of poor glycemic control, such as lethargy, look like symptoms of depression.

Diabetes and Aquatic Physical Therapy[24]

The Aquatics Section of the American Physical Therapy Association (APTA) has an annotated bibliography with relevant articles related to pool therapy, including the use of aquatics with medical conditions such as diabetes mellitus. This document is available through the Aquatics Section of the APTA.

Swimming may be a good choice to offer the individual with diabetes, once again taking care to provide meticulous foot care. Wearing boat shoes (specially designed shoes for water wear available in many local stores) can help prevent scraping the feet along the sides or bottom of the pool. Care must be taken to gently dry the feet, especially between the toes, after swimming, to prevent infection. Anyone with abrasions or open sores should not enter a swimming pool environment.

A rise in ambient (surrounding) temperature such as a client might experience in an indoor, warm, and humid pool setting also causes an increase in insulin absorption from subcutaneous injection sites. The insulin disappearance rate may be as much as 50% to 60% greater with an increase of 15° in ambient temperature.[76]

In addition, the ease of movement in the water allows increased activity without the same perceived intensity of exertion for the same amount of work performed outside the water. The combination of increased temperatures and increased activity can result in hypoglycemia. The PTA and client must work closely together to maintain a balance of activity, food intake, and insulin dosage.

When a client with diabetes begins aquatic physical therapy, both the time in the water and the intensity of exercise should be systematically progressed and monitored, with one of the parameters being increased with each session according to the client's tolerance. Before pool therapy, the client must not miss any meals or snacks and must measure blood glucose levels.

With careful management, the individual should be able to adjust food intake and exercise tolerance to avoid having to increase insulin dosage. Throughout the pool program, the PTA must closely monitor each individual with diabetes for any signs of hypoglycemia (see Table 8.12). The affected individuals must be cautioned to perform self-monitoring and to respond to the earliest perceived symptoms.

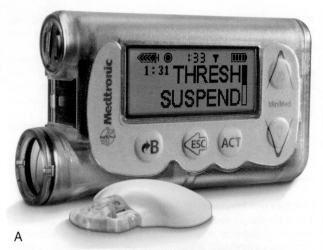

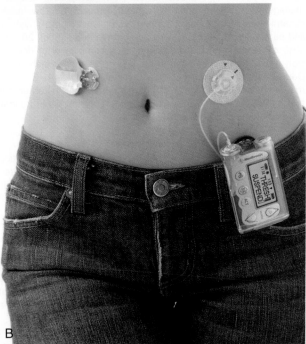

FIG. 8.13 (A) Programmable insulin pump (MiniMed 530G system). (B) Compact and worn like a pager, the programmable insulin pump delivers fixed amounts of insulin continuously, based on blood glucose levels determined by regular fingerstick glucose monitoring. The device includes the pump itself (including controls, processing module, and batteries), a disposable reservoir for insulin (inside the pump), and a disposable infusion set, including a cannula for subcutaneous insertion (under the skin) and a tubing system to interface the insulin reservoir to the cannula. (Reproduced with permission of Medtronic, Inc., Northridge CA.)

TABLE 8.12   Clinical Signs and Symptoms of Hypoglycemia

Sympathetic Activity (Increased Epinephrine)	Central Nervous System Activity (Decreased Glucose to Brain)
Pallor	Headache
Perspiration[a]	Blurred vision
Piloerection (erection of the hair)	Thickened speech
Increased heart rate (tachycardia)	Numbness of the lips and tongue
Heart palpitation	Confusion
Nervousness[a] and irritability	Emotional lability
Weakness[a]	Convulsion[a]
Shakiness, trembling	Coma
Hunger	

[a]Signs most often reported by clients.

TABLE 8.13   Comparison of Manifestations of Hypoglycemia and Hyperglycemia

Variable	Hypoglycemia	Hyperglycemia
Onset	Rapid (minutes)	Gradual (days)
Mood	Labile, irritable, nervous, weepy	Lethargic
Mental status	Difficulty concentrating, speaking, focusing, coordinating	Dulled sensorium, confused
Inward feeling	Shaky, hungry, headache, dizziness	Thirst, weakness, nausea, vomiting, abdominal pain
Skin	Pallor, sweating	Flushed, signs of dehydration
Mucous membranes	Normal	Dry, crusty
Respirations	Shallow	Deep, rapid (Kussmaul's respirations)
Pulse	Tachycardia	Less rapid, weak
Breath odor	Normal	Fruity, acetone
Neurologic	Tremors; late: dilated pupils, convulsion	Diminished reflexes, paresthesias
Blood Values		
Glucose	Low <50 mg/dL	High ≤250 mg/dL
Ketones	Negative	High, large
pH	Normal	Low: ≤7.25
Hematocrit	Normal	High
Urine Values		
Output	Normal	Polyuria (early) to oliguria (late)
Glucose	Negative	High
Ketones	Negative, trace	High

From Ignatavicius D, Workman M, et al: Medical-surgical nursing: patient centered collaborative care, ed 6, St. Louis, 2010, Saunders.

Insulin Resistance Syndrome

Insulin resistance, a generalized metabolic disorder in which the body cannot use insulin efficiently, appears to play a key role in metabolic syndrome. Although not everyone with insulin resistance has metabolic syndrome, most people with metabolic syndrome are also resistant to the action of insulin.

Obesity and insulin resistance are the underlying factors responsible for the diagnosis of metabolic syndrome. Several definitions of metabolic syndrome have been proposed, but all include insulin resistance or glucose intolerance, hypertension, dyslipidemia, and central obesity. For this reason, the term *insulin resistance syndrome* was suggested by the American College of Endocrinology and the American Association of Clinical Endocrinologists to more aptly describe the prediabetic state.[39]

TABLE 8.14 Benefits and Potential Risks of Exercise in People with Diabetes Mellitus

Benefits	Potential Risks[a]
Improves cardiovascular function	Hypoglycemia in people taking oral hypoglycemics or insulin
Improves maximum oxygen uptake	Worsening of hyperglycemia
Improves insulin binding and sensitivity	Cardiovascular disease, such as myocardial infarction, arrhythmias, excessive increases in blood pressure during exercise, postexercise orthostatic hypotension, or sudden death
Lowers insulin requirements (type 2 diabetes mellitus)	
Improves sense of well-being and quality of life	
Promotes other healthy lifestyle activities	
Increases carbohydrate metabolism	Microvascular disease, such as retinal hemorrhage or increased proteinuria
Improves blood glucose control[b]	
Reduces hypertension	Degenerative joint disease
May help with weight reduction	Orthopedic injury related to neuropathy
Improves lipid profile	
Reduces stress	

[a]These are potential risks over the long term. Generally, the benefits of regular exercise outweigh the risks.
[b]Not confirmed for insulin-dependent diabetes mellitus (type 1 diabetes mellitus).

BOX 8.5 Contraindications to Exercise in Diabetes Mellitus

- Poor control of blood glucose levels
- Unevaluated or poorly controlled associated conditions:
  - Retinopathy
  - Hypertension
  - Neuropathy (autonomic or peripheral)
  - Nephropathy
- Recent photocoagulation or surgery for retinopathy
- Dehydration
- Extreme environmental temperatures (hot or cold)

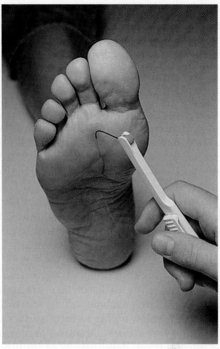

FIG. 8.14 Semmes-Weinstein monofilament testing for protective sensation. Performed if the client is suspected of having peripheral neuropathy or known diabetes with possible peripheral neuropathy. The 5.07 monofilament (calibrated to apply 10 g of force) has been adopted for screening in the diabetic population. The monofilament is applied perpendicular to the test site with enough pressure to bend the monofilament for 1 second. Abnormal response: client does not perceive the monofilament. Do not test over calloused areas. An initial foot screen should be performed on anyone with diabetes and at least annually thereafter. Anyone who is at risk should be seen at least four times a year to check the feet and shoes to help prevent foot problems from occurring. (From Ball JW, Dains JE: Seidel's guide to physical examination, ed 8, St Louis, 2015, Mosby.)

Regardless of the definition or criteria, most agree that obesity is the single modifiable factor that sets off the cascade. The syndrome is associated with alterations in the abdominal fat cells. With increased fat storage, these cells become distorted in shape, and the receptor site for insulin becomes "warped" or out of proper alignment, so the insulin molecule "key" no longer fits in the receptor. Insulin resistance makes it more difficult to lose weight because the cells are not getting enough fuel and the individual perceives hunger when adequate amounts of circulating glucose exist.

The affected individual may develop elevated blood pressure and problems with reactive hypoglycemia. When the excess insulin is suddenly used, glucose rushes into the cells and the blood glucose drops suddenly. This sequence creates intense sweet cravings, and the cycle repeats itself with increasing insulin resistance.[159]

The most important implications of recent research indicate that a diagnosis with a syndrome is not necessary to treat the individual risk factors. At this prediabetic stage, changes in lifestyle will have the greatest impact on halting any disease progression. In fact, it may be the only time in the disease progression in which changes in daily activity levels and nutritional status may have an impact.

8.15 Special Implications for the PTA: Insulin Resistance Syndrome or Metabolic Syndrome PTAs have a unique opportunity to address insulin resistance syndrome or metabolic syndrome through reasonable dietary advice and carefully prescribed exercise counseling. After assessment, the therapy team should guide individuals toward an activity program that includes near-daily exercise that is progressive to a weekly expenditure exceeding 1200 kilocalories of aerobic activity.[67]

The PTA can provide education regarding the importance of weight loss, exercise, and dietary changes needed to help control dyslipidemia and hypertension. With appropriate lifestyle changes, people can reduce their risk of CVD, prediabetic states, and diabetes.

The mechanisms responsible for the improvement in insulin sensitivity after exercise training have been studied extensively but are not fully understood. Research focusing on insulin resistance in skeletal muscle and in particular its relation to changes in aerobic fitness in type 2 diabetes is ongoing.[108,129]

Hyperglycemia

Two primary life-threatening metabolic conditions, diabetic ketoacidosis (DKA) and hyperosmolar hyperglycemic state (HHS), can develop if uncontrolled or untreated DM progresses to a state of severe hyperglycemia (greater than 300 mg/dL).[72]

Diabetic Ketoacidosis

Definition and overview. DKA is most commonly seen in type 1 diabetes when complications develop from severe insulin deficiency. About half of the people who require hospitalization for DKA develop this hyperglycemic emergency secondary to an acute infection or failure to follow their prescribed dietary or insulin therapy.[161]

Most episodes of DKA occur in persons with previously diagnosed type 1 DM. However, the condition may occur in new cases of type 1 and in persons with type 2 DM. It is characterized by the triad of hyperglycemia, acidosis, and ketosis.[140]

Etiologic factors. Any condition that increases the insulin deficit in a person with diabetes can precipitate DKA. Common causes of DKA include taking too little insulin; omitting doses of insulin; failing to meet an increased need for insulin because of surgery, trauma, pregnancy, stress, puberty, or infection; and development of insulin resistance caused by insulin antibodies. Other precipitating causes are listed in Box 8.6.

The most common precipitating factor is infection, which occurs in up to half of all cases and may seem like a trivial condition such as mild cellulitis or upper respiratory tract infection. Omission of insulin, either because of noncompliance or because people mistakenly believe that insulin is not required on sick days when they are not eating well, is another important and preventable cause of DKA.

In young individuals with type 1 DM, psychologic problems complicated by eating disorders may be a contributing factor in 20% of recurrent ketoacidosis. Factors that may lead to insulin omission in younger people include fear of weight gain with improved metabolic control, fear of hypoglycemia, rebellion from authority, and stress of chronic disease. In approximately 15% to 30% of cases, no identifiable cause of DKA can be determined.[140]

Pathogenesis. The initiating metabolic defect in DKA is an insufficient or absent level of circulating insulin. Insulin may be present, but not in a sufficient amount for the increase in glucose resulting from the stressor (see Box 8.6). Inadequate insulin creates a biologic state of starvation, which triggers the excess secretion of hormones, particularly glucagon, in an attempt to get more glucose to the cells and tissues. The abnormal insulin-to-glucagon ratio initiates a host of complex metabolic reactions, leading to hyperglycemia, acidosis, and ketosis.

When the body lacks insulin and cannot use carbohydrates for energy, it resorts to fats and proteins. The process of catabolizing fats for fuel gives rise to incomplete lipid metabolism, dehydration, metabolic acidosis, and electrolyte and acid-base imbalances.

Clinical manifestations. The signs and symptoms of DKA vary, ranging from mild nausea to frank coma (Table 8.15). Common symptoms are thirst, polyuria, nausea, and weakness that have progressed over several days. This condition also may develop quickly, with symptoms progressing to coma over the course of only a few hours. Other symptoms may include dry mouth; hot, dry skin; fruity (acetone) odor to the breath, indicating the presence of ketones; overall weakness, possible paralysis; confusion, lethargy, or coma; and deep, rapid respirations. Fever is seldom present even though infection is common. Severe abdominal pain, possibly accompanied by nausea and vomiting, easily mimics an acute abdominal disorder.

Medical Management

Diagnosis, Treatment, and Prognosis

Prevention of DKA through client education is the key to avoiding this serious condition. Once DKA is suspected, the diagnosis must be established quickly, with immediate treatment after diagnostic confirmation.

Treatment includes fluid administration, insulin therapy, and correction of metabolic abnormalities, in addition to correction of any underlying illnesses (e.g., infection). Before the discovery of insulin in the 1920s, DKA was almost universally fatal. This complication is still potentially lethal, with an average mortality rate of 5% to 10%.

BOX 8.6   Precipitating Causes of Diabetic Ketoacidosis[a]

- Inadequate insulin under stressful conditions
- Infection
- Missed insulin doses
- Trauma
- Medications
  - β-Blockers
  - Calcium-channel blockers
  - Pentamidine (NebuPent, Pentam)
  - Steroids
  - Thiazides (diuretics)
- Alcohol abuse (inability to manage insulin because of mentation change; alcoholic ketoacidosis)
- Hypokalemia
- Myocardial ischemia
- Surgery
- Pregnancy
- Pancreatitis
- Renal failure
- Stroke

[a]Listed in descending order.

8.16 Special Implications for the PTA: Diabetic Ketoacidosis

The PTA will be an active member of the health care team, emphasizing to anyone with type 1 DM the need for regular, daily SMBG; adherence to the diabetes management program; and early recognition of and intervention for mild ketosis. The PTA also must be able to recognize early signs and symptoms of DKA in addition to signs of infection, a major cause of DKA. The first sign of an infection in a foot or leg or an upper respiratory, urinary tract, or vaginal infection should be reported immediately to the physician.

DKA can cause major potassium shifts accompanied by muscular weakness that can progress to flaccid quadriparesis. The weakness is initially most prominent in the legs, especially the quadriceps, and then extends to the arms, with involvement of the respiratory muscles.

TABLE 8.15   Clinical Symptoms of Life-Threatening Glycemic States

Hyperglycemia		Hypoglycemia
Diabetic ketoacidosis (DKA)	Hyperosmolar hyperglycemic state (HHS)	Insulin shock
Gradual onset[a]	Gradual onset	Sudden onset
Headache	Thirst	Pallor
Thirst	Polyuria leading quickly to decreased urine output	Perspiration
Hyperventilation	Volume loss from polyuria leading quickly to renal insufficiency	Piloerection
Fruity odor to breath	Severe dehydration	Increased heart rate
Lethargy, confusion, coma	Lethargy, confusion	Palpitations
Abdominal pain and distention	Seizures	Irritability, nervousness
Dehydration	Coma	Weakness
Polyuria	Blood glucose level >250 mg/dL	Hunger
Flushed face	Arterial pH >7.30	Shakiness
Elevated temperature		Headache
Blood glucose level >250 mg/dL		Double or blurred vision
Arterial pH <7.30		Slurred speech
		Fatigue
		Numbness of lips, tongue
		Confusion
		Convulsion, coma
		Blood glucose level <70 mg/dL

[a]Less gradual than hyperosmolar hyperglycemic state.
Modified from Goodman CC, Snyder TE: Differential diagnosis for physical therapist, ed 5, St. Louis, 2013, Saunders.

Hyperosmolar Hyperglycemic State

HHS, a variation of DKA, is another acute complication of diabetes. It is characterized by extreme hyperglycemia (800 to 2000 mg/dL), mild or undetectable ketonuria, and the absence of acidosis. It is most common in older adults with type 2 DM.[68,72]

The precipitating factors of HHS may be similar to those of DKA, such as infections, inadequate fluid intake, medications (see Box 8.6), or stress. The major difference between HHS and DKA is the lack of ketosis with HHS. Because some residual ability exists to secrete insulin in type 2 DM, the mobilization of fats for energy is avoided. When adequate insulin is lacking, blood becomes concentrated with glucose. Because glucose molecules are too large to pass into cells, osmosis of water occurs from the interstitial spaces and cells to dilute the glucose in the blood, and eventually the cells become dehydrated. If not treated promptly, the severe dehydration leads to vascular collapse and death.

Clinical manifestations of HHS are polyphagia, polydipsia, polyuria, glucosuria, dehydration, weakness, changes in sensorium, coma, hypotension, and shock (see Table 8.15). Lactic acidosis also can develop if tissue perfusion is compromised.

Treatment is with short-acting insulin, electrolyte replacement, and careful fluid replacement to avoid congestive heart failure and intercerebral swelling in older adults, who often have other cardiovascular or renal disorders.

8.17 Special Implications for the PTA: Hyperosmolar Hyperglycemic State The PTA should be alert to any signs of HHS in the aging adult who may have a previous diagnosis of type 2 diabetes mellitus. Early recognition and treatment to restore fluid and electrolyte balance are important for a good prognosis in this condition.

METABOLIC SYSTEM

As noted earlier, the endocrine system works with the nervous system to regulate and integrate the body's metabolic activities. Metabolism is the physical and chemical (physiologic) processes that allow cells to use food to continually rebuild body cells and transform food into energy. Metabolism is broken down into two phases: the anabolic (tissue-building) and catabolic (energy-producing) phases. The *anabolic phase* converts simple compounds derived from nutrients into substances the body cells can use, whereas the *catabolic phase* is a consumptive phase in which these organized substances are reconverted into simple compounds with the release of energy necessary for the proper functioning of body cells.[62]

The body gets most of its energy by metabolizing carbohydrates, especially glucose. A complex interplay of hormonal and neural controls regulates the homeostasis of glucose metabolism. Hormone secretions of five endocrine glands dominate this regulatory function (see Table 8.8). The rate of metabolism can be increased by exercise, elevated body temperature, hormonal activity, and increased digestive action after the ingestion of food.

Fluid and Electrolyte Balance

Fluid and electrolyte balance is a key component of cellular metabolism. Homeostasis, maintaining the body's chemical and physical balance, involves the proper functioning of body fluids to preserve osmotic pressure, acid-base balance, and anion-cation balance. The goal of metabolism and homeostasis is to maintain the complex environment of body fluid that nourishes and supports every cell.

Body fluids, classified as intracellular and extracellular, contain two kinds of dissolved substances: those that dissociate (separate) in solution (electrolytes) and those that do not. The composition of these electrolytes in body fluids is electrically balanced, so the positively charged cations (sodium, potassium, calcium, and magnesium) equal the negatively charged anions (chloride, bicarbonate, sulfate, phosphate, and carbonic acid).

Although these particles are present in relatively low concentrations, any deviation from their normal levels can have profound physiologic effects.

Because many situations in the body cause both normal and abnormal fluid shifts, it is important to have a clear understanding of fluid compartments. The recognition of pathologic conditions, such as edema, dehydration, ketoacidosis, and various types of shock, can depend on the understanding of these concepts.

In the healthy body, fluids and electrolytes are constantly lost or exchanged between compartments. This balance must be maintained for the body to function properly. The amount used in these functions depends on such factors as humidity; body and environmental temperature; physical activity; metabolic rate; and fluid loss from the GI tract, skin, respiratory tract, and renal system. Normal balance is achieved through fluid intake and dietary consumption.

Acid-Base Balance

The proper balance of acids and bases in the body is essential to life. The body maintains the pH of extracellular fluid (fluid found outside cells) at 7.35 to 7.45 through a complex chemical regulation of carbonic acid by the lungs and base bicarbonate by the kidneys. The pH is essentially a measure of hydrogen ion concentration in body fluid. Nutritional deficiency or excess, disease, injury, or metabolic disturbance may interfere with normal homeostatic mechanisms and cause a lowering of pH called *acidosis* or a rise in pH called *alkalosis*.

Various bodily functions operate to keep the pH at a relatively constant level. Acid-base regulatory mechanisms include chemical buffer systems, the respiratory system, and the renal system. These systems interact to maintain a normal acid-base ratio of 20:1 bicarbonate to carbonic acid. The consequences of an acid-base metabolism disorder can result in many signs and symptoms encountered by the PTA.

Aging and the Metabolic System

Aging as measured by loss of physiologic function has not yet been defined precisely, so the distinction between usual, normal, and ideal metabolic changes remains undetermined. Studies of the aging population have shown that several physiologic parameters, such as body weight, basal metabolism, renal clearance, and cardiovascular function, decline with age. Protein-calorie nutritional status has pervasive effects on metabolic regulatory systems; nutritional status often declines with age, which contributes to metabolic dysfunction.[71]

Because the respiratory and renal systems are largely responsible for maintaining acid-base balance, changes in these systems associated with aging also impact metabolic function. Loss of muscle mass associated with aging can affect stroke volume capacity and oxidative metabolism.[112] The low-level metabolic acidosis that appears to occur in many people with advancing age may play a role in age-associated bone loss.

Mitochondria, the principal site of adenosine triphosphate (ATP) synthesis (also containing DNA and RNA), is the cellular site of energy production from oxygen and the principal site of free radical damage.[34]

Free radicals (unstable oxygen molecules robbed of electrons) attempt to replace their missing electrons by scavenging the body and taking electrons from healthy cells. They are generated as a result of normal metabolic activity, producing destructive oxidation of membranes, proteins, and DNA.

The formation of free radicals can be triggered by many exogenous (outside) factors such as cigarette smoke, air pollution, anticancer drugs, ultraviolet lights, pesticides and other chemicals, uncontrolled diabetes, radiation, and emotional stress. The major defenses against these destructive by-products of normal metabolism are the protective enzymes, which remove the free radicals and remove, repair, and replace cell constituents.

The use of antioxidants found naturally in fruits and vegetables or ingested in the form of nutritional supplements to counteract this process is believed to increase longevity but remains under scientific investigation.[101,102]

REFERENCES/SUGGESTED READINGS

To enhance this text and add value for the reader, references and suggested readings are included on the companion Evolve site that accompanies this textbook. The reader can view the source and access it online whenever possible.

9

The Cardiovascular System

CHAPTER OBJECTIVES

1. Recognize the role of the physical therapist assistant in primary, secondary, and tertiary prevention of cardiovascular pathology.
2. Recognize gender differences in cardiac physiology and pathology.
3. Recognize common cardiovascular pathologies and physical signs and symptoms of worsening cardiovascular status.
4. Recognize sternal precautions that may affect types of therapeutic activity included or excluded from postoperative cardiac plan of care.

OUTLINE

VOCAB BUILDERS

Angina pectoris	Dissecting aneurysm	Perfusion
Angiogram	Distention	PTCA
Claudication	Dyslipidemia	QT interval
Concomitant	Dyspnea	Recumbent
Cyanosis	Frank–Starling Law	Sequelae
Decision delay	Lumen	Sternal precautions
Diaphoresis	Palpitation	

The cardiovascular system functions in coordination with the pulmonary system to circulate oxygenated blood through the arterial system to all cells. The deoxygenated blood is then collected from the venous system and delivered to the lungs for reoxygenation (Fig. 9.1). Pathologic conditions of the cardiovascular system are varied, multiple, and complex. This chapter presents cardiovascular structure and function according to how diseases affect each individual part, including diseases of the heart muscle, cardiac nervous system, heart valves, pericardium, and blood vessels.

Other factors, such as surgery, pregnancy, and complications from other pathologic conditions, can also adversely affect the normal function of the cardiovascular system.

SIGNS AND SYMPTOMS OF CARDIOVASCULAR DISEASE

Cardinal symptoms of cardiac disease usually include chest, neck, or arm pain or discomfort; palpitations; dyspnea; syncope (fainting); fatigue; cough; and cyanosis. Edema and leg pain (*claudication*) are the most common symptoms of the vascular component of cardiovascular pathologic conditions. Symptoms of cardiovascular involvement should be reviewed by system as well (Table 9.1).

Chest pain or discomfort, defined as tightness or a pressure sensation, is a common presenting symptom of cardiovascular disease and must be evaluated carefully. Chest pain of systemic origin may be cardiac or noncardiac and may radiate to the neck, jaw, upper trapezius, upper back, shoulder, or arms (most commonly the left arm). Radiating pain down the arm is in the pattern of the ulnar nerve distribution. Noncardiac chest pain can be caused by an extensive list of disorders and is not covered in this text.

Cardiac-related chest pain may arise secondary to ischemia, myocardial infarction (MI), pericarditis, endocarditis, mitral valve prolapse (MVP), or aortic dissection with or without aneurysm. Location, frequency, intensity, and duration vary according to the underlying pathologic condition.

Chest pain is often accompanied by associated signs and symptoms such as nausea, vomiting, diaphoresis, dyspnea, fatigue, pallor, or syncope. Cardiac chest pain or discomfort can also occur when coronary circulation is normal, as in the case of anemia causing lack of oxygenation of the myocardium (heart muscle) during physical exertion, although this situation is uncommon.

Angina (see the section Angina Pectoris for more details) is chest pain or discomfort occurring when a heart muscle does not get enough oxygen, and it is a symptom of coronary artery disease (CAD). It usually starts behind the breastbone, but it may project in the arm, shoulder, neck, jaw, throat, and back. Angina is described as pressure, squeezing, or tightness in the chest. Some people may mistake it for indigestion. Shortness of breath, weakness, light-headedness, and sweating may occur.

Palpitations, the presence of an irregular, fast, or "extra" heartbeat, may also be referred to as arrhythmias or dysrhythmias, which may result from relatively benign causes such as MVP, caffeine, anxiety, exercise, or athlete's heart (an increase in left ventricular mass as a result of intensive training)[172] or a severe condition such as CAD, cardiomyopathy, complete heart block, ventricular aneurysm, atrioventricular valve disease, or mitral or aortic stenosis.

Palpitations have been described as a bump, pound, jump, flop, flutter, butterfly, or racing sensation of the heart. Associated symptoms may include light-headedness or syncope. The palpated pulse may feel rapid or irregular, as if the heart has skipped a beat. Some people report fluttering sensations in the neck rather than in the chest or thoracic area.

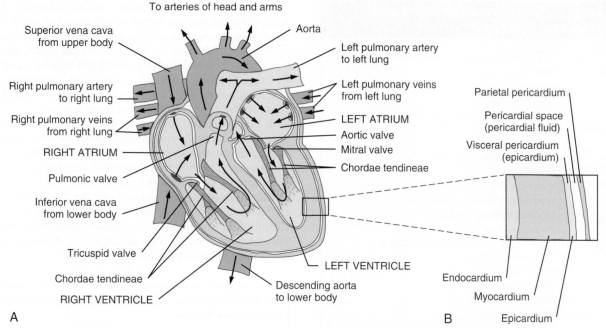

FIG. 9.1 (A) Structure and circulation of the heart. Blood flows from the superior and inferior venae cavae into the right atrium through the tricuspid valve to the right ventricle. The right ventricle ejects the blood through the pulmonic valve into the pulmonary artery during ventricular systole. Blood enters the pulmonary capillary system in which it exchanges the carbon dioxide for oxygen. The oxygenated blood then leaves the lungs via the pulmonary veins and returns to the left atrium. From the left atrium, blood flows through the mitral valve into the left ventricle. The left ventricle pumps blood into the systemic circulation through the aorta to supply all the tissues of the body with oxygen. From the systemic circulation, blood returns to the heart through the superior and inferior venae cavae to begin the cycle again. (B) Sagittal view of the layers of the heart wall.

Dyspnea, also referred to as *breathlessness* or *shortness of breath,* can be cardiovascular in origin, but it may also occur secondary to pulmonary pathologic conditions, trauma, fever, certain medications, or obesity. Early onset of dyspnea may be described as a sensation of having to breathe too much or as an uncomfortable feeling during breathing after exercise or exertion. Shortness of breath with mild exertion (dyspnea on exertion) can be caused by an impaired left ventricle that is unable to contract completely. The result is an abnormal accumulation of blood in the pulmonary vasculature, and pulmonary congestion and shortness of breath then ensue. With severe compromise of the cardiovascular or pulmonary system, dyspnea may occur at rest.

Dyspnea may be a predictor of death from cardiac or other causes. In a large study of over 17,000 adults, those with no history of CAD who had dyspnea had four times the risk of sudden death from cardiac causes compared with asymptomatic individuals. They also had twice the risk compared with participants already diagnosed with typical angina.[2]

The severity of dyspnea is determined by the extent of disease; the more severe the heart disease, the more readily episodes of dyspnea occur. More extreme dyspnea includes paroxysmal nocturnal dyspnea and orthopnea. Paroxysmal nocturnal dyspnea, which is sudden, unexplained episodes of shortness of breath, awakens a person sleeping in a supine position, because the amount of blood returning to the heart and lungs from the lower extremities increases in this position. This type of dyspnea frequently accompanies congestive heart failure (CHF).

During the day, the effects of gravity in the upright position and the shunting of excessive fluid to the lower extremities permit more effective ventilation and *perfusion* of the lungs,

keeping the lungs relatively fluid free, depending on the degree of CHF. *Orthopnea* is the term used to describe breathlessness that occurs during recumbency that is relieved by sitting upright, using pillows to prop the head and trunk. Orthopnea can occur anytime during the day or night.

Cardiac syncope (fainting or, in a milder form, light-headedness) can be caused by reduced oxygen to the brain when the heart's pumping ability becomes compromised. Conditions resulting in cardiac syncope include arrhythmias, orthostatic hypotension (sudden drop in blood pressure), aortic dissection, hypertrophic cardiomyopathy, CAD, vertebral artery insufficiency, and hypoglycemia. If the heart does not pump as much blood, then blood pressure drops low enough to cause fainting.

Predictors of cardiac syncope include a history of stroke or transient ischemic attacks, use of cardiac medication, and high blood pressure. Marginally associated risk factors also include lower body mass index (BMI), increased alcohol intake, and diabetes or elevated plasma glucose level. During the period of initiation and regulation of cardiac medications, side effects such as orthostatic hypotension may occur.

Noncardiac conditions, such as anxiety and emotional stress, migraine headaches, seizures, or psychiatric conditions, can cause hyperventilation and subsequent light-headedness.

Vasovagal syncope is a term that is used for a very strong parasympathetic response that leads to vasodilation throughout the body. It can occur after a prolonged period of sitting or standing. Normally in such a situation, blood tends to pool in the legs, requiring a heart rate and vasoconstriction sufficient to push the blood back to the heart. When vasovagal syncope occurs, it is because the heart rate slows and vessels dilate, causing hypotension and

TABLE 9.1 Cardiovascular Signs and Symptoms by System

System	Symptom
General	Weakness
	Fatigue
	Weight change
	Poor exercise tolerance
Integumentary	Pressure ulcers
	Loss of body hair
	Cyanosis (lips and nail beds)
Central nervous system	Headaches
	Impaired vision
	Light-headedness or syncope
Respiratory	Labored breathing, dyspnea
	Productive cough
Cardiovascular	Chest, shoulder, neck, jaw, or arm pain or discomfort (angina)
	Palpitations
	Peripheral edema
	Intermittent claudication
Genitourinary	Urinary frequency
	Nocturia
	Concentrated urine
	Decreased urinary output
Musculoskeletal	Muscular fatigue
	Myalgias
	Chest, shoulder, neck, jaw, or arm pain or discomfort
	Peripheral edema
	Intermittent claudication
Gastrointestinal	Nausea and vomiting
	Ascites (abdominal distention)

cerebral hypoperfusion with subsequent fainting and/or falling. Some individuals may experience this type of parasympathetic reaction when having blood drawn for testing or when donating blood. This type of syncope is not as serious as cardiac syncope (except as a potential source of injury from falling).

Fatigue provoked by minimal exertion indicates a lack of energy that may be cardiac in origin or it may occur secondary to neurologic, muscular, metabolic, or pulmonary pathologic conditions. Often fatigue of a cardiac nature is accompanied by associated symptoms, such as dyspnea, chest pain, palpitations, or headache.

Cough is usually associated with pulmonary conditions but may occur as a pulmonary complication of a cardiovascular pathologic condition. Left ventricular dysfunction, including mitral valve dysfunction as with resulting pulmonary edema, may result in a cough when aggravated by exercise, metabolic stress, supine position, or paroxysmal nocturnal dyspnea. The cough is often hacking and dry when associated with left ventricular dysfunction and failure, and may be productive of large amounts of frothy, blood-tinged sputum in full-blown pulmonary edema. In the case of CHF, cough develops because a large amount of fluid is trapped in the pulmonary tree, irritating the lung mucosa. A persistent, dry cough can develop as a side effect of some cardiovascular medications.

Cyanosis is a bluish discoloration of the lips and nail beds of the fingers and toes in the Caucasian population that accompanies inadequate blood oxygen levels. Look for gray color tones (instead of pink or red) along the gum line in the mouths of African Americans, Hispanics, or other dark-skinned individuals.

Although cyanosis can accompany cardiac, pulmonary, hematologic, or central nervous system (CNS) disorders, visible cyanosis most often accompanies cardiac and pulmonary problems.

Peripheral edema is the hallmark of right ventricular failure; it is usually bilateral and dependent and may be accompanied by jugular venous *distention,* cyanosis, and abdominal distention from ascites. Right upper quadrant pain, described as constant, aching, or sharp, may occur secondary to an enlarged liver with this condition. Right-sided heart failure and subsequent edema can also occur as a result of cardiac surgery, venous valve incompetence or obstruction, or cardiac valve stenosis.

Claudication, sometimes described as cramping or leg pain, is brought on by a consistent amount of exercise or activity. It develops as a result of peripheral vascular disease (PVD) (arterial or venous), often occurring simultaneously with CAD.[49] Claudication can be more functionally debilitating than other associated symptoms, such as angina or dyspnea, and may occur in addition to these other symptoms.

9.1 Special Implications for the PTA: Signs and Symptoms of Cardiovascular Disease

Evaluation and Monitoring

As part of the evaluation, the physical therapist will assess cardiac signs and symptoms, assess the degree of risk of an adverse cardiac event, assess the type and degree of impairment, and assess the level of disability and functional limitations.[61]

Older adults with cardiac impairment should be examined by a physician. Exercise testing to diagnose the specific level of pathology and impairment will aid the therapy team in prescribing an individual exercise program with specific parameters (mode, intensity, duration, and frequency) determined based on the results of examination and testing.[70]

In some cases, monitoring individuals closely and minimizing risk of an adverse event are a priority. If the individual is symptomatic, recommendations are given to minimize life-threatening risks; interventions are directed at the underlying impairments whenever possible.

As a general guideline, the physical therapist assistant (PTA) monitors the unstable cardiac client during initial exercise to keep intensity lower than the threshold at which cardiac symptoms appear. In other cases, when the degree of risk is low, the need for monitoring may be reduced accordingly, and treatment can be less conservative.[61]

Signs and Symptoms

Cervical disk disease and arthritic changes can mimic atypical *chest pain* requiring screening for medical disease. Pain of cardiac origin can be experienced in the shoulder because the heart (and diaphragm) are supplied by the C5 to C6 spinal segment, which refers visceral pain to the corresponding somatic area. Chest pain attributed to trigger points and other noncardiac causes is discussed in Chapter 11.[85]

Palpitations lasting for hours or occurring in association with pain, shortness of breath, fainting, or severe light-headedness or dizziness require medical evaluation. Palpitations in any person with a personal history of cardiac disease or a family history of unexplained sudden death necessitate medical referral. Clients describing palpitations or similar phenomena may not be experiencing symptoms of heart disease.

Palpitations can be considered physiologic (i.e., fewer than six occurring per minute may be considered within the normal function of the heart), or they may occur as a result of an overactive thyroid; secondary to caffeine sensitivity; as a side effect of some medications; during menopause when estrogen levels decline; and through the use of drugs, such as cocaine.

Encourage the client to report any such symptoms to the physician if they have not already been brought to the physician's attention.

Before referring the client to the physician, the PTA can help the client characterize the symptom or symptoms by asking a series of questions. Is the sensation long-lasting or transient? Palpitations that begin and end abruptly are more often true sustained arrhythmias. Episodes that gradually appear and disappear tend to be normal alterations in heart rhythm.

Does anything precipitate the symptom or symptoms? Eliminating possible triggers (e.g., caffeine) one at a time may reduce or eliminate palpitations. Is there an association between hormonal status and palpitations (e.g., onset or change in frequency associated with ovulation or start or stop of menstruation)? If exercise brings on the palpitations, ventricular tachycardia may be the underlying cause.

On the other hand, sometimes starting an exercise program reduces the frequency of palpitations. Some people find that deep breathing, coughing, or relaxation can stop the symptom when it begins. If fainting occurs with the palpitations and there is a family history of sudden death, there may be an inherited cardiomyopathy or primary arrhythmia.

Dyspnea may be a sign of poor physical conditioning, obesity, or asthma or allergies. Anyone who cannot climb a single flight of stairs without feeling moderately to severely winded or who awakens at night or experiences shortness of breath when lying down should be evaluated by a physician. Anyone with known cardiac involvement in whom progressively worse dyspnea develops must also notify the physician of these findings.

Dyspnea relieved by specific breathing patterns (e.g., pursed-lip breathing) or by specific body positions (e.g., leaning forward on arms to lock the shoulder girdle) is more likely to be pulmonary than cardiac in origin. Because breathlessness can be a terrifying experience, any activity that provokes the sensation is avoided, which quickly reduces functional activities. Pulmonary rehabilitation can favorably influence both exertional and clinically assessed dyspnea. The therapist and PTA are key in preventing this vicious circle and in delaying decline of function in people with cardiopulmonary disorders.

Syncope without any warning period of light-headedness, dizziness, or nausea may be a sign of heart valve or arrhythmia problems but rarely occurs as a result of myocardial ischemia. Sudden death can occur; therefore medical referral is recommended for any unexplained syncope, especially in the presence of heart or circulatory problems or if the client has any risk factors for heart attack or stroke.

Physical therapy orthopedic examination of the cervical spine may include vertebral artery tests for compression of the vertebral arteries, which can contribute to the development of syncope.

Athletes may experience neurocardiogenic syncope, a benign noncardiac cause of fainting in athletes. This disorder of autonomic cardiovascular regulation is precipitated by prolonged standing after exertion, a warm environment, or stress, or it may occur during or after exercise; it is not life-threatening. Fainting during exertion, however, should always be evaluated by medical personnel.

Fatigue beyond expectations during or after exercise, especially in a client with a known cardiac condition, must be closely monitored. It should be remembered that some medications prescribed for cardiac problems can also cause unusual fatigue symptoms. For the client experiencing fatigue without a prior diagnosis of heart disease, monitoring vital signs may indicate a failure of the blood pressure to rise with increasing workloads.

Peripheral edema in the form of a 3-lb or greater weight gain or gradual, continuous gain over several days with swelling of the ankles, abdomen, and hands and shortness of breath, fatigue, and dizziness may be a red flag symptom of CHF. When such symptoms persist despite rest, medical referral is required. Edema of a cardiac origin may require electrocardiographic monitoring during exercise or activity, whereas edema of peripheral origin requires medical treatment of the underlying cause.

Claudication is always accompanied by diminished peripheral pulses in the presence of vascular disease, usually accompanied by skin discoloration and trophic changes (e.g., thin, dry, hairless skin). Core temperature, peripheral pulses, and skin temperature should be assessed. Cool skin is more indicative of vascular obstruction; warm to hot skin may indicate inflammation or infection.

If persons with intermittent claudication have normal-appearing skin at rest, exercising the extremity to the point of claudication usually produces marked pallor of the skin over the distal one-third of the extremity. This postexercise cutaneous ischemia occurs in both upper and lower extremities and is caused by selective shunting of the available blood to the exercised muscle and away from the more distal parts of the extremity.

AGING AND THE CARDIOVASCULAR SYSTEM

Cardiovascular disease, especially coronary atherosclerosis, is the most common cause of hospitalization and death in the older population in the United States. With the aging of America, by the year 2030 nearly 50% of all Americans will be 45 years old or older. By that time the number of people 65 years old or older will have more than doubled, and the population 85 years old and older is expected to have tripled.[158] With this increase in the number of older persons, cardiovascular disease is likely to be even more of a major health problem in the future, because it accounts for over 80% of cardiovascular deaths in people aged 65 years and above.[123]

Specific Effects of Aging

Aging of the heart is associated with a number of typical morphologic, histologic, and biochemical changes, although not all observed changes with age are associated with deterioration in function. The high prevalence of hypertension and ischemic heart disease makes the distinction between normal aging changes and the effects of underlying cardiovascular disease processes difficult.

Disease-independent changes in the aging heart associated with a reduction in function include (1) reduction in the number of myocytes and cells within the conduction tissue, (2) the development of cardiac fibrosis, (3) a reduction in calcium transport across membranes, (4) lower capillary density, (5) decreases in the intracellular response to β-adrenergic stimulation, and (6) impaired autonomic reflex control of heart rate.[123]

Other characteristic changes, such as epicardial fat deposition and "brown atrophy" caused by intracellular lipofuscin deposits, appear to be signs of the aging process but without any obvious effects on function. The hearts of older persons, even fit, healthy, and active adults, pump less blood to the skin and require the heart of the older person to work much harder under the same circumstances (e.g., exercise in warm environments) than that of a younger person.

Although the specific organ changes associated with aging are discussed here, disease and lifestyle may have a greater impact on cardiovascular function than aging. Research now shows that even children need to control their modifiable risk factors for heart disease.

Heart studies of adolescents and young adults who have died from accidental causes demonstrate that heart disease begins earlier than formerly expected. Cholesterol deposits and blood vessel changes have been demonstrated in early adolescence, with substantial changes observed by age 30 years in some people.

As the arteries age, increased collagen and calcium content and progressive deterioration of the arterial media, combined with atherosclerotic plaque formation, result in stiff arterial walls, increased systolic blood pressure, and increased fatigue of arterial walls, all of which accelerate arterial damage, producing a self-perpetuating cycle.

Effects of Aging on Function

None of the changes described earlier has clinical relevance at rest but may have considerable consequences during cardio-vascular stress, such as occurs with increased flow, demand for acute autonomic reflex control, or severe disease. Physiologic aging is accompanied by a progressive decline in resting organ function. Consequently, the reserve capacity to compensate for impaired organ function, heat, drug metabolism, and added physiologic demands is impaired, and functional disability will occur more quickly and take longer to resolve.[167]

According to experts at the National Institute on Aging, age is the greatest risk factor for cardiovascular disease.[123,157] The heart also undergoes some changes associated with advancing age in individuals who do not exercise and who have risk factors for cardiac disease. Moderate thickening of the left ventricular wall and increased left atrial size occur as a result of myocyte enlargement (hypertrophy) or replacement by fibrous tissue. Decreased ventricular filling, compensated for by increased systolic blood pressure, occurs as a result of the changes in the ventricular wall. Left ventricular functioning is compromised in the presence of stress such as vigorous exercise or disease. Arrhythmia or hypertension may occur as a result.

The vasculature changes with aging as the arterial walls stiffen with age and the aorta becomes dilated and elongated. The incidence and severity of atherosclerosis do increase with aging, and this contributes to changes in vasculature function.

Calcium deposition and changes in the amount of and loss of elasticity in elastin and collagen most often affect the larger and medium-sized vessels.

Resting cardiac function shows minimal age-related changes. Changes in functional capacity are more apparent during exercise than at rest. The maximal heart rate or the highest heart rate during exercise does decline with age. This decline in maximal heart rate is reflected in the target zone heart rates for exercising senior citizens.

The *Frank–Starling law* states that the greater the myocardial fiber length (or stretch) is, the greater the fiber's force of contraction. The more the left ventricle fills with blood, the greater will be the quantity of blood ejected into the aorta. This is like a rubber band: the more it is stretched, the more strongly it recoils or snaps back. Thus a direct relationship exists between the volume of blood in the heart at the end of diastole (the length of the muscle fibers) and the force of contraction during the next systole.

Effects of Exercise on Aging

It is commonly accepted that a decline in maximal oxygen uptake and heart rate and reduced maximal cardiac output with aging occur during exercise, even in older athletes. These cardiovascular alterations parallel changes that occur with deconditioning or disuse, including the decrease in maximal oxygen intake and maximal cardiac output. These functions normalize with increased activity, and exercise can reverse some of the age-associated changes in the heart, at least partially,[123] supporting the hypothesis that age-related cardiovascular changes are simply the result of inactivity.

In older people, aerobic exercise training lowers heart rate at rest; reduces heart rate and levels of plasma catecholamine at the same absolute submaximal workload; improves heat tolerance[221]; and, at least in men, improves left ventricular performance during peak exercise.[197]

Finally, although the benefits of physical activity and exercise among older persons are becoming increasingly clear, the role of exercise stress testing and safety monitoring for older people who want to start an exercise program is unclear. Current guidelines regarding exercise stress testing may not be applicable to the majority of adults aged 75 years or older who are interested in restoring or enhancing their physical function through a program of physical activity and exercise.

GENDER DIFFERENCES AND THE CARDIOVASCULAR SYSTEM

Interest in gender differences in all of medicine but especially the cardiovascular system has come to the forefront in the new millennium.

Female hearts not only are smaller than male hearts but also are constructed differently and respond to age and hypertrophic stimuli differently. Structural differences in the mitral valve may explain why women are more prone to MVP than men. At puberty, a young woman's QT interval lengthens, and the woman with a long QT interval is at greater risk for a serious form of ventricular arrhythmia and sudden cardiac death, especially when taking drugs that prolong the QT interval.[25]

The *QT interval* is a measure of the duration of ventricular depolarization and repolarization. A prolonged period of time for depolarization may predispose a person to ventricular tachycardia.

Left ventricular mass increases with age in healthy women but remains constant in men. Under increased cardiac loading conditions this disparity between genders is even more obvious, especially in adults older than 50 years.[96] The risk for drugs other than cardiac and psychotropic ones to cause prolongation of the QT interval has recently been recognized. Women also have a three times greater risk of potentially fatal arrhythmias from some cardiac and psychotropic medications. It is anticipated that the list of drugs known to produce such effects will grow.[195] Complications from antiarrhythmic drug use are most common during the first 3 days or after a dosage increase.

Women also tend to have a higher incidence of bleeding episodes from thrombolytic agents. They also have different outcomes with surgery and *percutaneous transluminal coronary angioplasty (PTCA)*, with more repeat PTCAs, possibly because of smaller arteries, more advanced disease compared with men, or different tolerance to medications.[127] Women, in contrast to men, with premature coronary disease are at higher risk for developing vascular and ischemic complications after percutaneous coronary intervention.[126]

Coronary Artery Disease in Women

It was long believed that CAD was a more benign process in women, but this has been soundly disproved. A woman with angina postmenopausally has the exact same mortality as a man with angina in his sixties. CAD is the single leading cause of death and a significant cause of morbidity among women in the United States.

Certain characteristics and clinical conditions may place women at higher risk of CAD development or progression, including depression, being black, menopausal status, older age, and type 2 diabetes mellitus. In addition, being female may adversely influence the relative benefits of some risk-modification interventions in older adults (e.g., cholesterol lowering, sedentary behavior, smoking cessation).[108,234]

Underrecognition and underdiagnosis of CAD in women contribute to the high mortality rate,[147] and underuse of guideline-based preventive and therapeutic strategies for women probably contributes to their less favorable CAD outcomes.[239] Researchers are actively studying specific risk factors for women.

A new predictive model for women that combines newer risk markers with traditional risk factors and family history is being investigated. A family history of heart attack before age 60 has been added to the list of risk factors of which women should be aware.

Coronary Microvascular Dysfunction

A "stealth" form of heart disease called *coronary microvascular dysfunction* or *disease* has been identified in women. This type does not show up on *angiograms*. Classic signs of reduced blood flow to the heart (ischemia) are not present; instead there are false-positive stress test results. It may be that the tiny blood vessels to the heart become constricted, reducing blood flow.

Scientists suspect ischemia may have different effects on women compared with CAD (Table 9.2). It was previously believed that women with chest pain but clear arteries had an aggravating case of coronary microvascular syndrome, but it was not considered harmful.

Research in the Women's Ischemia Syndrome Evaluation (WISE) study, a federally funded investigation into ischemic heart disease in women, is ongoing to explain this phenomenon.[23,178,204,205] Autopsy comparisons of women and men have shown that women who die of heart attacks are more likely to have plaque buildup uniformly around the inside of the blood vessel, possibly as a result of chronic inflammation. Inflammation may not be the only cause of coronary microvascular dysfunction. Risk factors such as anemia and polycystic ovarian syndrome have been identified as well.[93] Women with this type of heart disease are at increased risk for heart attack, stroke, and reduced quality of life.

Gender Differences

Many studies have suggested that women with acute MI receive less aggressive therapy than men and have a poorer outcome when treatment is received. Until recently, women in all age groups have been less likely to undergo diagnostic catheterization than men, and this difference was especially pronounced among older women (more than 85 years old). Women have been less likely than men to receive preventive care such as drug treatment for lipid management; risk factor management through exercise, nutrition, and weight reduction; invasive treatments (revascularization procedures); and thrombolytic therapy within 60 minutes of heart attack (or stroke).[78,239]

Women delay longer than men before seeking help for symptoms of acute MI, which is referred to as *decision delay*, further compromising effective treatment and improved outcomes.[189] This is especially true given the evidence that first heart attacks in women may be more severe and that women are more likely to die in the first weeks and months after a heart attack.

For many years, women and minorities were underrepresented in studies conducted on heart disease and stroke, but this has changed over the last decade along with *concomitant* expansion of prevention and educational outreach programs for heart attack, stroke, and other cardiovascular diseases in women. The use of noninvasive testing in women was controversial because of a perception of diminished accuracy, limited female representation, and technical limitations.

Large observational studies now report marked improvements in the accuracy of results for women undergoing exercise treadmill, echocardiography, and nuclear testing as a result of expanding risk parameters in the test interpretations and improved diagnostic accuracy of such tests.[147] Because of technologic advances, improved surgical techniques, greater awareness of gender differences in heart disease, and increased funding for gender-based research, these trends are improving, and women now seem to do as well as men after surgical (revascularization) procedures to restore blood flow to the heart.

Although the American Heart Association reports a decline in death rates in women for CAD and stroke, women are still twice as likely as men to die within 1 year of having a heart attack, and women are at greater risk for second heart attacks and for disability because of heart failure.

Many women die of CAD without any warning signs, and by age 65 years one in four women has heart disease (the same proportion as in men). CAD claims the lives of nearly 250,000 women annually in the United States,[147] compared with 40,200 for breast cancer and 63,000 for lung cancer. Despite these statistics, misperceptions still exist that cardiovascular disease is not a real problem for women and that, despite the fact that some risk factors for CAD can be prevented, CAD is not curable. For these reasons, education and prevention[152] are vitally important to reduce risk of heart disease.

TABLE 9.2	Ischemic Heart Disease	
	Coronary Artery Disease	**Coronary Microvascular Disease**
Clinical presentation	Chest pain often described as "crushing" radiating to the left arm, jaw, upper back; can manifest differently in women (see Figs. 9.8 and 9.12)	Diffuse discomfort
		Extreme fatigue
		Depression
		Dyspnea
	Cold sweat, nausea	Older adult: confusion or increased confusion
Pathology	Plaque buildup extending in toward the blood vessel lumen	Microvascular constriction (narrowing of smaller coronary arteries); plaque deposited uniformly around inside of the artery walls
Diagnosis	Stress test, coronary angiography	Stress test,[a] functional vascular imaging (e.g., multidirectional CT scan of the heart, stress echocardiography, SPECT)
Treatment	Surgery (angioplasty, CABG) Medication (statins)	Medication (antihypertensives, antiinflammatories, and statins)

[a]Stress echocardiography uses ultrasound to produce images of the heart after an exercise stress test.
Data from Harvard Women's Health Watch: New view of heart disease in women, Harv Womens Health Watch 14:1–3, 2007.
CABG, Coronary artery bypass graft; *CT,* computed tomography (serves as a noninvasive angiogram; moves around the heart generating a three-dimensional image of the heart and coronary arteries); *SPECT,* single-photon emission computed tomography (injects a radioactive tracer into the bloodstream to chart the flow of blood in the heart and coronary vessels).

Coronary Artery Surgery and Women

The number of women undergoing coronary artery bypass graft (CABG; pronounced "cabbage") has continued to increase.[11,13] Women may experience more chest wall discomfort as a common side effect of CABG than men.

Women undergoing bypass surgery have a death rate about twice as high as that of men.[28] This has been attributed to the fact that women generally have smaller bodies, meaning smaller coronary arteries on which it may be technically more difficult to operate. Data from the WISE study also suggest that women may have both CAD and unrecognized microvessel disease, in which case opening the arteries is not sufficient.

Hormonal Status

Influence of Hormones on Coronary Artery Disease

Estrogen has been considered to have a cardioprotective benefit for women via a variety of mechanisms. It stimulates the formation of high-density lipoprotein (HDL; the good cholesterol), which carries plaque away from the artery wall and back to the liver to be broken down and excreted, while also stimulating low-density lipoprotein (LDL) receptors in the liver and possibly the blood vessel walls. These receptors bind the LDL (the bad cholesterol) and remove it from the circulation, preventing its damaging effects in plaque formation.

Estradiol acts as a calcium channel blocker to relax artery walls, which helps dilate the arteries, improves blood flow throughout the brain and body, and helps to reduce blood pressure. Estrogen maintains the normal balance of two chemicals that regulate clot formation. It also increases arterial wall production of prostacyclin, which improves blood flow and reduces platelet aggregation.

Another possible mechanism by which estrogen protects against heart disease before menopause is the release of a chemical stimulated by estrogen, which is responsible for dilating blood vessels to maintain normal pressure and flow. As women lose the biologically active estradiol, gender differences become gender similarities and the incidence of cardiovascular disease increases dramatically, matching the incidence among men within 10 years of menopause without hormone replacement therapy (HRT).

Hormone Replacement for Postmenopausal Women

The use of hormones for cardioprotection has been under investigation for many years. Because heart attacks tend to occur 10 years later in women than in men, it was assumed that the protective effect of estrogen was responsible. Exogenous (externally administered) estrogen has been reported to improve plasma lipid profiles, carbohydrate metabolism, and vascular reactivity, but it is surprising to note that hormonal therapy does not alter the progression of CAD or protect against MI or coronary death. The Heart and Estrogen/Progestin Replacement Study failed to demonstrate cardioprotection and even showed an early adverse outcome in women with documented CAD who received daily HRT. A woman's risk for heart disease increases when she becomes menopausal regardless of age or the means by which menopause occurs.

Oral Contraceptives

Studies show that women smokers over 35 years old who use oral contraceptives are much more likely to have a heart attack or stroke than nonsmokers who use birth control pills. In the last 20 years, cardiovascular complications in all women taking oral contraceptives have become less common because current contraceptives contain the lowest dose of estrogen possible without breakthrough bleeding.[15]

At this dose, the risk of thromboembolic disease is reduced to about 40 events per 100,000 women per year, approximately the same risk as in the general population.[41] However, much debate continues about the use of so-called *third-generation* (newest) *oral contraceptives* containing low doses of estrogen and a type of progestin known as *desogestrel*. Women taking this contraceptive are twice as likely to develop superficial venous blood clots compared with women taking second-generation oral contraceptives containing progestins, such as levonorgestrel and norethindrone. It is estimated that 425 ischemic strokes can be attributed to oral contraceptive use each year in the United States, even with the newer low-estrogen preparations.[83]

Hypertension in Women

More women than men eventually develop hypertension in the United States because of their higher numbers and greater longevity. White coat hypertension (rise in blood pressure when being evaluated by a physician or other health care worker) is more prevalent among women, and black women are more likely to have hypertension than black men.

Alcohol, obesity, and oral contraceptives are important causes of rise in blood pressure among women. Alcohol is known to have specific toxic effects on heart muscle fibers, and excessive alcohol consumption is increasing in women. Still, women are less likely than men to be identified as alcohol abusers at early stages of the illness and are less often referred for alcohol treatment until later stages of abuse, when cardiac and other severe complications have occurred.[227]

Cholesterol Concerns for Women

Total cholesterol is broken into HDL, or good cholesterol, which carries cholesterol away from the cells, and LDL, or bad cholesterol, which carries cholesterol to the cells. A helpful way to remember the function of these is to think of *HDL* as "*Healthy*" or beneficial cholesterol and *LDL* as "*Lousy*" or detrimental cholesterol. Lipoproteins are complexes that help dissolve, transport, and use the cholesterol molecule.

The National Heart, Lung, and Blood Institute estimates that more than half of all women over age 55 years need to lower their blood cholesterol. The recommended level for initiating treatment in women is less than 50 mg/dL and for men is less than 40 mg/dL.

After menopause, women have higher concentrations of total cholesterol than men do, but the significance of this finding remains unknown. Research results at this time suggest that women need higher levels of the HDL for protection against heart disease and that other blood markers, such as serum triglycerides and C-reactive protein (CRP), may play more meaningful roles in defining women's heart disease risk. Low levels of HDL cholesterol are predictive of CAD in women and appear to be a stronger risk factor for women older than 65 years than for men of the same age.[153]

DISEASES AFFECTING THE HEART MUSCLE

Ischemic Heart Disease

Coronary arteries carry oxygenated blood to the myocardium. When one of these arteries becomes narrowed or blocked, the areas of the heart muscle supplied by that artery do not receive sufficient oxygen and become ischemic and injured, and infarction may result. Major disorders of the myocardium caused by insufficient blood supply are collectively known as *ischemic heart disease, coronary heart disease* (CHD), or *coronary artery disease.*

Despite improved clinical care, heightened public awareness, and widespread use of health innovations, atherosclerotic diseases (resulting in narrowing of arteries) and their thrombotic complications remain the number one cause of mortality and morbidity in the United States.

An estimated 12 million persons in the United States have CAD. Each year approximately 220,000 fatal CAD events occur suddenly in unhospitalized people. Eleven million Americans who are alive today have a history of angina pectoris, MI, or both, and an estimated 2 million middle-aged and older adults (older than 75) have silent myocardial ischemia.[150]

Although CAD death rates in the United States have decreased since reaching a peak during the late 1960s, a decline in the incidence of coronary disease has not been achieved. In 1940 the rate of cardiovascular disease was 26.4 per 100,000 people, compared with 173.5 in 2000.[14]

The declining mortality rate does not apply to adults with diabetes and has been attributed to improvements in lifestyle (e.g., reduced smoking in men, improved treatment for lipid lowering, improved coronary care), whereas the increased incidence may be related to the increasing number of people who are surviving past age 65 years.

Arteriosclerosis

Arteriosclerosis is a group of diseases characterized by thickening and loss of elasticity of the arterial walls, and is often referred to as *hardening of the arteries.* Arteriosclerosis can be divided into three types: (1) atherosclerosis, in which plaques of fatty deposits form in the inner layer or intima of the arteries; (2) Mönckeberg's arteriosclerosis, involving the middle layer of the arteries with destruction of muscle and elastic fibers and formation of calcium deposits; and (3) arteriolosclerosis or arteriolar sclerosis, characterized by thickening of the walls of small arteries (arterioles). All three forms of arteriosclerosis may be present in the same person but in different blood vessels. Frequently the terms *arteriosclerosis* and *atherosclerosis* are used interchangeably, although technically atherosclerosis is the most common form of arteriosclerosis.

Atherosclerosis

Atherosclerosis, defined as thickening of the arterial wall through the accumulation of lipids, macrophages, T lymphocytes, smooth muscle cells, extracellular matrix, calcium, and necrotic debris, can affect any of the arteries in a condition known as *cardiovascular disease.*

When the arteries of the heart are affected it is referred to as *coronary artery disease* or *coronary heart disease;* when the arteries to the brain are affected, cerebrovascular disease develops. Atherosclerosis of blood vessels to other parts of the body can result in PVD, aneurysm, and intestinal infarction. Atherosclerosis as it affects the heart vessels is discussed in this section.

Etiologic and risk factors. In 1948 the U.S. government decided to investigate the etiologic factors, incidence, and pathologic findings of CAD by studying residents of a typical small town in the United States: Framingham, Massachusetts. In 1971 a second generation of adult children and their spouses of the original participants were added. Results from this ongoing research have identified important modifiable and nonmodifiable risk factors associated with death caused by CAD.

Modifiable risk factors that can be controlled are referred to now as "risk factors for which intervention has been shown to *reduce* incidence of CAD"; other risk factors that can be managed are now referred to as "risk factors for which intervention is *likely to reduce* incidence of CAD" or "risk factors for which intervention *might reduce* incidence of CAD." Some risk factors cannot be altered (nonmodifiable), such as those involving age, gender, family history of heart disease, ethnicity, and exposure to infectious agents (Table 9.3).

TABLE 9.3   Coronary Artery Disease Risk Factors

MODIFIABLE RISK FACTORS			NONMODIFIABLE RISK FACTORS	NEW PREDICTORS OF RISK FACTORS
Risk Factors for which Intervention has been Shown to Reduce Incidence of CAD	Risk Factors for which Intervention Is Likely to Reduce Incidence of CAD	Risk Factors for which Intervention Might Reduce Incidence of CAD		Risk Factors Under Investigation
Cigarette smoking	Obesity	Psychologic factors and emotional response to stress	Age	Elevated homocysteine (>15 μm/L)
Elevated total serum cholesterol level	Physical inactivity		>55 years (women)	C-reactive protein
Elevated LDL cholesterol level	Diabetes or impaired glucose tolerance; insulin resistance	Discriminatory medicine[a]	>45 years (men)	Fibrinogen
Hypertension	Low HDL	Oxidative stress	Male gender	Lipoprotein a; Lp(a) (>30 mg/dL)[b]
	<40 mg/dL (men)	Excessive alcohol consumption or complete abstinence	Family history; genetic determinants	Troponin T
	<50 mg/dL (women)	Elevated triglycerides	Ethnicity	Plasminogen activator inhibitor (marker for recurrence of MI)
	Hormonal status; oral contraceptives; hysterectomy or oophorectomy; menopause without hormone replacement (especially before age 40 years)	Sleep-disordered breathing	Infection (viral, bacterial)	D-dimer (fibrin)
	Thrombogenic factors	Poor nutrition		Dermatologic indicators
				Graying of the hair
				Thoracic hairiness
				Earlobe creases
				Male impotence
				Ankle/brachial blood pressure index (see Box 9.10)

CAD, Coronary artery disease; *HDL,* high-density lipoprotein; *LDL,* low-density lipoprotein; *MI,* myocardial infarction.
[a]Discriminatory medicine is not technically a risk factor for CAD but results in a different natural history for some individuals.
[b]Applies to whites and Asians but not to blacks.

As the Framingham study continues to gather and analyze new data, results are reported that help modify existing health risk appraisal models relating risk factors to the probability of developing CAD. With these new models, blood lipid levels; diabetes; and, in women, systolic blood pressure and cigarette smoking are emphasized once again as independent predictors of risk.

In a national sample of older women and men (65 to 84 years old), black and Mexican American women and black men were at the greatest risk for cardiovascular disease. These findings parallel a previously documented increased risk of cardiovascular disease among younger ethnic minority populations. Differences in socioeconomic status (as measured by educational level and family income) do not explain the higher prevalence of cardiovascular disease risk factors in these ethnic minority groups.[215]

A higher prevalence of certain risk factors in black women, particularly diabetes and obesity, may explain their increased risk of CAD, but ethnic differences in CAD for Hispanics remain unknown. The Newcastle Thousand Families Study confirmed that adult lifestyles are more important than socioeconomic variables,[124] but further research to identify ethnic differences in cardiovascular disease risk factors is needed.

Modification of risk factors that reduce the incidence of coronary artery disease. *Cigarette smoking* remains the leading preventable cause of CAD. Tobacco products increase heart rate and blood pressure; decrease the oxygen-carrying capacity of blood; increase poisonous gases and elements of the blood such as carbon monoxide, cyanide, formaldehyde, and carbon dioxide; cause narrowing of blood vessels; and increase the work of the heart.

Nicotine enhances the process of atherosclerosis by a direct effect on the blood vessel wall, increasing the circulating levels of fibrinogen and the tendency for plaque formation in the coronary arteries. Nicotine also increases the expression of LDL receptors on smooth muscle cells lining the plaque, priming the cells for the entry of LDL cholesterol. By-products of tobacco products in the blood act as potent oxidizing agents. This oxidation damages the intimal lining of the arterial walls, exposes collagen, and results in platelet aggregation. People who quit smoking will reduce their risk of CAD by half after 1 year and equalize their risk of CAD to that of a nonsmoker in 15 years.

Elevated total serum cholesterol levels (more than 200 mg/dL) place a person at greater risk for heart disease; this risk doubles when cholesterol levels exceed 240 mg/dL and the ratio of total cholesterol to HDL cholesterol is more than 4.5 (Table 9.4). It is now well known that therapy to lower LDL levels can stabilize, reduce, or even reverse the progression of atherosclerotic plaques and coronary stenosis and reduce recurrent cardiac episodes. Cholesterol levels are influenced by heredity, diet, exercise, alcohol consumption,[60,121] obesity, medications, menopausal status, thyroid function, and smoking. Impaired thyroid function is a cause of elevated cholesterol and arterial stiffness, especially in women older than 50 who smoke.[166,229]

Hypertension, or high blood pressure, causes the heart to work harder and may injure the arterial walls, making them prone to atherosclerosis. Epidemiologic studies document a strong association between high levels of both systolic and diastolic blood pressure and risk of CAD (and stroke) in both men and women.

Hypertension is aggravated by obesity and is associated with diabetes and regular alcohol use. It can be initiated or aggravated by the use of oral contraceptives, especially in women who smoke. Women who have undetected or uncontrolled hypertension are five times more likely to experience angina, heart attack, or sudden death than women with normal blood pressure. Weight reduction, dietary interventions, and pharmacologic intervention have important roles in the prevention and treatment of hypertension.

Modification of risk factors that are likely to reduce the incidence of coronary artery disease. Physical inactivity, sedentary lifestyle, and obesity are parallel, interrelated epidemics in the United States that contribute to increased risk of CAD.

Obesity alone can lead to CAD, because the excess weight makes the heart work harder to pump blood throughout the body. Obesity is commonly associated with diabetes mellitus, high blood pressure, and high fat levels. The prevalence of obesity has increased in both men and women in the United States in the past decade. More than half of adult Americans are overweight or obese, and more than half of this population is overweight with associated medical conditions.[159]

The U.S. Department of Health and Human Services has reported that 17% of children are obese, and the obesity rates in children ages 6 to 11 years increased 147% from 1971 to 1994.[50] Target body measurements (adults) for the prevention of heart disease are listed in Table 9.4. Increasing research and knowledge related to nutrition have led to the identification of several dietary factors that influence CAD risk. The epidemiologic evidence confirms that diets low in saturated fat and high in fruits, vegetables, whole grains, and fiber are associated with a reduced risk of CAD.

Physical inactivity is a major risk factor equal to cholesterol, cigarette smoking, and high blood pressure. Because a higher proportion of U.S. adults lead a sedentary lifestyle (60%) than

---

TABLE 9.4   Heart Disease Prevention Target Measurements[a]

Risk Factors	Targets
Body Measurements	
Body mass index: multiply your weight in pounds by 700, then divide that number by the square of your height in inches	18.5-24.0
Waist/hip ratio: divide your waist measurement in inches by your hip measurement in inches	≤0.8
Lipids, Lipoproteins	
Total cholesterol	<200 mg/dL
HDL cholesterol	≥40 mg/dL (men)[a] ≥50 mg/dL (women)[a]
LDL cholesterol	≤129 mg/dL (optimal: 100 mg/dL; <70 mg/dL for women at high risk for heart attack or stroke)
Triglycerides	200 mg/dL (<150 mg/dL)[b]
Total cholesterol/HDL ratio	<4.5
Blood pressure	See Table 9.8

[a]These target measures are for healthy adults without evidence of heart disease.
[b]The current standard for all adults is set at ≥35 mg/dL. Proposed targets of ≥40 mg/dL for men and ≥50 mg/dL for women are the new guidelines from the American Heart Association[199] and are developed for adults and children over age 2 (no upper age limit). Some experts recommend 55 mg/dL or higher for women, but this remains unproven and is under investigation.
HDL, High-density lipoprotein; *LDL*, low-density lipoprotein.

have hypertension (10%), have hypercholesterolemia (excessive cholesterol in the blood) (10%), or smoke one pack or more of cigarettes per day (18%), increasing the general population's physical activity level may have a greater effect on reducing the incidence of CAD than the modification of the other three risk factors.

Regular aerobic exercise lowers resting pulse rate and blood pressure, improves the ratio of good to bad cholesterol, and helps prevent and control diabetes and osteoporosis. The risk of heart attack and death from heart disease declines steadily as the frequency of vigorous exercise increases. Occasional exercise (one or two times per week) reduces the risk of heart attack by 36%, moderate exercise (three or four times per week) reduces it by 38%, and regular, vigorous exercise (five or more times per week) reduces it by 46%. The benefit of habitual exercise toward reducing heart attack was greatest in those who worked out for 11 to 24 minutes and did not change or increase further after 24 minutes of exercise.[5]

Impaired glucose metabolism (e.g., insulin resistance, hyperinsulinemia, glucose intolerance) is reported to be atherogenic. Diabetes mellitus, impaired glucose tolerance, and high-normal levels of glycated hemoglobin were powerful contributors to atherosclerotic cardiovascular events in the Framingham study.[246]

The association is complex, and the pathways by which elevated insulin adversely affects both CAD risk factors and the risk of developing CAD remain unknown. The risk for CAD in participants younger than 65 years was double in men and triple in women with diabetes compared with their nondiabetic counterparts. Individuals with type 2 diabetes mellitus have a risk of MI equivalent to that of someone without diabetes who has had a previous MI.

Diabetes confers the same risk of cardiovascular disease as aging 15 years.[30] Kidney disease accompanied by hypertension is a serious complication affecting the cardiovascular system in people with diabetes. More than 80% of persons who have diabetes die of some form of cardiovascular disease. Bypass surgery provides significantly better survival than angioplasty for individuals with diabetes in some subgroups. This may be attributed to the more extensive CAD in people with diabetes and the greater tendency for their arteries to restenose after angioplasty.

Low levels of HDL cholesterol (and high levels of triglycerides) produce twice as many cases of CAD as any other lipid abnormality; this effect is exaggerated in women (see Table 9.4). *Hormonal status* in the menopausal or postmenopausal woman is now known to be a likely contributing risk factor in the development of CAD.

Modification of risk factors that might reduce the incidence of coronary artery disease. *Psychologic factors and emotional stress* contribute significantly to the pathogenesis and expression of CAD. People who are negative, insecure, and distressed (type D personality) are three times more likely to experience a second heart attack than non-D types.[64]

Other personality traits likely to affect the heart are free-floating hostility associated with anger and a sense of time urgency (two major components of the type A personality). The long-held belief that anger can increase the risk of acute MI and can be an immediate trigger of heart attacks has been verified.[244]

The relationship between these entities and CAD can be divided into behavioral mechanisms in which psychosocial conditions contribute to a higher frequency of adverse health behaviors such as poor diet and smoking and direct stress-induced mechanisms. Personality traits are more difficult to change than other psychologic risk factors, such as depression or anxiety.[64]

Improved technologies and research demonstrate that acute mental or emotional stress triggers myocardial ischemia, promotes arrhythmogenesis, stimulates platelet function, and increases blood viscosity through hemoconcentration. Moderate to severe depression is associated with altered cardiac autonomic modulation including elevated heart rate, elevated norepinephrine, and reduced heart rate variability, which are known risk factors for cardiac morbidity and mortality.

In the presence of atherosclerosis in people with CAD, acute stress also causes coronary vasoconstriction. Hypersensitivity of the sympathetic nervous system to perceived adversity is an intrinsic characteristic among these individuals; in addition, the calming response of the parasympathetic nervous system is diminished in persons who are hostile, and the parasympathetic counterbalance does not stop the effects of adrenaline on the heart.

These emotions trigger the stress response, increasing blood pressure and heart rate and altering platelet function. Increasing evidence suggests that cognitive behavioral therapy and anger management may benefit cardiac clients by improving medical outcome.

Oxidative stress, or the oxidation of LDL particles as part of the atherosclerotic formation, is under active investigation. Oxidative stress is considered a significant risk factor for cardiovascular disease. However, antioxidant nutrients failed to provide benefits for cardiovascular disease in several human trials.

This apparent paradox between the role of antioxidants in reducing oxidative stress and the failure of many antioxidant supplementations warrants further research. Meanwhile, according to the current American Heart Association scientific statement, antioxidant vitamin supplements to prevent cardiovascular disease are not recommended.[133]

Moderate alcohol consumption decreases the risk of heart disease in some people. This is attributed to alcohol's beneficial effects on hemostasis, including platelet aggregation, coagulation factors, and the fibrinolytic system.[190] Alcohol intake increases activity of an enzyme that helps to keep blood flowing smoothly by initiating dissolving of clots (fibrinolysis). The highest levels of the endogenous t-PA protein have been found among daily consumers of red wine, and the lowest levels have been found among subjects who never (or rarely) consume alcohol.[3]

Although a small amount of alcohol taken daily with meals may elevate levels of HDL cholesterol, and although the bioflavonoids in red wine may reduce atherosclerosis, most researchers oppose recommending drinking as a public health measure to fight heart disease and stress that no one, particularly people with a personal or family history of alcohol abuse, should drink alcohol to improve cholesterol. It should always be remembered that heavy alcohol consumption and binge drinking increase risk of blood clot formation, cardiac arrhythmia, elevated blood pressure, and cardiovascular disease. Dietary supplements containing flavonoids and antioxidants are now available without the sugar in grape juice or the alcohol in wine.

The cardioprotective benefits appear to be effective only in men over age 45 years and women over age 55 years when limited to one or two drinks per day.[100] Greater concentrations of alcohol cause direct coronary artery constriction, which may explain the relationship between ethanol and sudden coronary ischemia that is seen clinically. In addition, the depressive effect of excessive alcohol on the function of myocardial cells decreases myocardial contractility and can be very disabling. Chronic abuse of alcohol is also related to a higher incidence of hypertension, which places greater stress on a heart already compromised by CAD. Chemical dependency is also associated with increased stress on the diseased heart.

Nonmodifiable risk factors. The risk of cardiovascular disease or CAD increases with *increasing age,* and the person older than 40 is more likely to become symptomatic. *Gender* as a nonmodifiable risk factor is reflected in the fact that heart disease is more prevalent among men; women generally experience heart attacks 10 years later than men, possibly because of the biologic protection factor provided premenopausally by estrogen.

By age 45 years, heart disease affects one woman in nine. By age 65 years, this ratio becomes one in three, more closely approximating rates among men. These statistics represent the outcome when no HRT is initiated, but as previously mentioned, the effectiveness of HRT in reducing morbidity and mortality associated with CAD is still under investigation.

A *family history* of cardiovascular disease (i.e., one or more members of the immediate family with the disease) is associated with increased incidence of heart disease. It is proposed that a mix of environmental and genetic factors leads to atherosclerosis of the coronary arteries in a complex, unpredictable, and unknown series of interactions. For selected individuals, genetic predisposition, especially abnormalities in lipoprotein metabolism, can play a very important role in the risk of developing atherosclerosis.

Certain *ethnicities* are a risk factor, and certain ethnic groups have a higher rate of heart disease. The risk of heart disease is highest among blacks, who are three times more likely to have extremely high blood pressure, which is a major risk factor for CAD, and who have a higher prevalence of other risk factors, such as diabetes mellitus, obesity, and cigarette smoking.

Native Americans have an unusually high rate of diabetes and obesity, although lower total and LDL cholesterol levels appear to offset the difference. Conflicting comparisons of CAD mortality between Mexican Americans and non-Hispanic whites have been reported. Despite their adverse cardiovascular risk profiles, especially a greater prevalence of diabetes, Mexican Americans are reported to have lower mortality rates from CAD. However, when death certificates are more carefully examined and coded, Mexican Americans have rates equal to or higher than those of non-Hispanic whites.[170] Hispanics are less likely than whites to receive catheterization and angioplasty procedures.[71]

Infections (bacterial and viral) as a cause of atherosclerosis and thereby CAD in some people have been supported by experimental and clinical data. This discovery came about as researchers identified the presence of a common virus (cytomegalovirus) in arterial plaque as a contributing factor to angioplasty failure. Atherosclerosis, now recognized as an inflammatory process, and injury to the inner layer of the artery may be triggered by acute or chronic infection, particularly in more susceptible disease states such as diabetes.

New predictors. Investigators may have identified markers for heart disease present in apparently healthy people, that is, components of blood or other factors that can help identify risk of CAD before symptoms develop (see Table 9.3). Serum cholesterol has been used for a long time, but many more potential predictors of risk are being examined. *Homocysteine* occurs naturally in blood and tissues and is more common in people with CAD. Elevated levels of homocysteine may be as much of a risk factor as high cholesterol or smoking.

High-sensitivity C-reactive protein, an acute-phase reactant that reflects low-grade systemic inflammation, is produced by the liver in response to trauma, tissue inflammation, and infection, and seems to predict hypertension, diabetes, heart attacks, and strokes before they occur.[185] People with even slightly elevated blood levels of CRP appear to be at increased risk for CAD and its complications regardless of age, gender, general health, or the presence of other CAD risk factors.

Cigarette smokers have elevated levels of CRP, and individuals experiencing a heart attack who have high levels of CRP have a slower than normal response to antithrombotic medication.

Fibrinogen, a blood protein essential for proper clotting, may predict first heart attacks (and strokes) in people with unstable CAD and is a risk factor for future cardiovascular problems in those who have not yet developed CAD.

Lipoprotein (a) (Lp[a]), an LDL cholesterol particle with an additional protein attached, slows the breakdown of blood clots. People with high levels of Lp(a) are at greater risk for MI than those with lower levels of Lp(a).

Erectile dysfunction (impotence) is a hemodynamic event that can warn of ischemic heart disease in some men. Researchers may eventually call impotence a "penile stress test" that can be as predictive as a treadmill exercise stress test.[165]

Metabolic syndrome has received increased attention within the last few years.[90] The term *metabolic syndrome* is most commonly used in the cardiovascular field. It can be viewed as an aggregation of multiple cardiovascular risk factors of endogenous origin in one individual. Until recently, metabolic syndrome has been considered a complex disorder with no single factor as a cause.[90]

Metabolic syndrome is a group of interrelated factors of metabolic origin or *metabolic risk factors* that appear to directly promote the development of atherosclerotic cardiovascular disease. Another group of factors, the *underlying risk factors,* can precipitate the metabolic syndrome.

Metabolic risk factors include *dyslipidemia,* elevated blood pressure, elevated plasma glucose, a prothrombotic state, and a proinflammatory state.[90] The most important *underlying risk factors* are abdominal obesity and insulin resistance; other associated conditions include physical inactivity, aging, hormonal imbalance, and genetic or ethnic predisposition.[90] Excess visceral fat is considered more strongly associated with metabolic syndrome than any other adipose tissue compartment.[47,103]

People with metabolic syndrome have a twofold increase in relative risk for cardiovascular events, and in individuals without established type 2 diabetes mellitus there is a fivefold increase in risk for developing diabetes compared with people without the syndrome.

Usually, metabolic syndrome is manifested in the presence of some degree of obesity and physical inactivity. In addition to the lifestyle changes (exercise and smoking cessation) drug therapy for risk factors may be required.

The primary goal of clinical management of metabolic syndrome is to reduce the risk for atherosclerotic cardiovascular disease. When encountering clients presenting with abdominal obesity, physical therapists and PTAs should appreciate that waist circumference may be associated with lipid abnormalities.[103]

A possible link has been recently demonstrated between psychosocial stressors from everyday life and metabolic syndrome. Employees with chronic work stress more than double the odds for developing the syndrome compared with those without the stress.[51]

Pathogenesis. The exact mechanism by which the development of cardiovascular disease or CAD can be explained has yet to be determined. Clinical and laboratory studies have shown that inflammation plays a major role in the initiation, progression, and destabilization of atheromas.

In the normal artery, the endothelial lining is tightly packed with cells that allow the smooth passage of blood and act as a protective covering against harmful substances circulating in the bloodstream. The normal endothelium presents a nonreactive surface to blood, but injury triggers the thrombotic process.

In the earliest stage of atherosclerosis, damage to arteries arises from a combination of factors. In some cases, the initial damage comes from LDL cholesterol that has been modified by free radicals. Free radicals are abundant in people who smoke and who have high blood pressure or diabetes. In other cases, high levels of homocysteine or bacteria may contribute to early damage of arterial linings.

Generally the most current theories include the following major events in the development of atherosclerotic plaque (Fig. 9.2): arterial wall damage occurs either from injury caused by harmful substances in the blood or by physical wear and tear as a result of high blood pressure. This injury to the blood vessel wall permits the infiltration of macromolecules (especially cholesterol) from blood through the damaged endothelium to the underlying smooth muscle cells. Naked collagen acts like flypaper for platelets, causing them to aggregate at the site of injury and plug up the wound.

The core of a coronary thrombus (clot) is composed of platelets, forming a so-called "white thrombus." Early stage plaque formations known as *fatty streaks* consist of foam cells (white blood cells coated with LDL particles, smooth muscle cells that move in from deeper layers of the artery wall, and platelets).

Cholesterol-filled plaques can take decades to form, sitting snugly in an artery wall for years. What makes a plaque break open and leak its contents into the bloodstream, causing a clot that can block an artery supplying the heart or brain, remains unknown. Experts speculate it could be a spike of high blood pressure or a surge of chemical messages that accompany anger, stress, or other intense emotion. It could be the result of cholesterol crystallization inducing cap rupture and/or erosion.[1,134]

Although platelet activation is a normal response to injury, in atherosclerosis, once the platelets adhere they also release chemicals that alter the structure of the blood vessel wall. What starts out as a small erosion in the wall can end up a swollen mound of platelets, muscle cells, and fibrous clots or a process called *proliferation*, which obstructs the flow of blood through the vessel.

After a thrombus forms and causes static or reduced blood flow in the vessel, the clot stabilizes with fibrin. This is commonly referred to as a *red thrombus* because of the presence of entrapped red blood cells. Within the thrombus is thrombin, which remains active and can activate platelets. Platelets also release a potent natural inhibitor of fibrinolysis that can lead to vessel spasm, further platelet aggregation, and thrombus formation or reocclusion. This

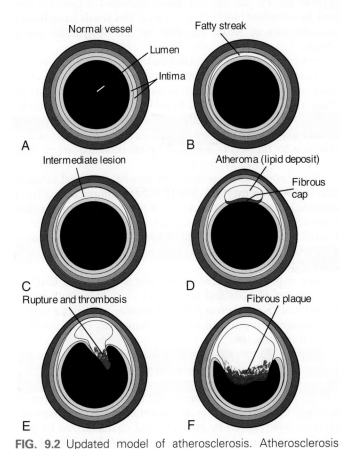

FIG. 9.2 Updated model of atherosclerosis. Atherosclerosis begins with an injury to the endothelial lining of the artery (intimal layer), which makes the vessel permeable to circulating lipoproteins. New technology using intravascular ultrasound shows the entire atherosclerotic plaque and has changed the way we view things. The traditional model held that atherosclerotic plaque in the blood vessel, particularly a coronary blood vessel, kept growing inward and obstructing flow until it closed off and caused a heart attack. This is not entirely correct. (A and B) It is more accurate to say that in the normal vessel, penetration of lipoproteins into the smooth muscle cells of the intima produces fatty streaks, and the start of a coronary lesion forms. (C and D) The coronary lesion grows outward first in a compensatory manner to maintain the open lumen. This is called *positive remodeling*. The blood vessel tries to maintain an open lumen until it can do so no longer. A little roof or "fibrous cap" separates the plaque from the inside of the lumen. A blood clot called an *intraplaque thrombosis* can form inside the plaque; the clot may never leave the plaque. (E) The plaque (atheroma) begins to build up, gradually pressing inward into the lumen with obstruction of blood flow and possible rupture and thrombus, potentially leading to myocardial infarction or stroke. Capped plaques are not as likely to rupture as the softer type packed with viscous cholesterol and white blood cells but only capped with a thin layer of collagen. (F) Vascular disease today is considered a disease of the wall. Some researchers like to say that the disease is in the donut, not the hole of the donut, and that is a new concept. (From Goodman CC, Snyder TEK: Differential diagnosis for physical therapists: screening for referral, ed 5, St. Louis, 2013, Saunders. Data from Horn HR: Insulin resistance, diabetes, and vascular disease: the rationale for prevention, April 2004. www.medscape.com/viewarticle/466799_2. Accessed August 25, 2016.)

cycle of injury, platelet activation, and lipid deposition can lead to complete blockage of a vessel and result in ischemia and necrosis of tissue supplied by the obstructed blood vessel.

Clinical manifestations. Atherosclerosis by itself does not necessarily produce symptoms. For manifestations to develop, there must be a critical deficit in blood supply to the heart or other structures supplied by affected blood vessels. For example, symptoms of CAD may not appear until the *lumen* of the coronary artery narrows by 75%. Then, pain and dysfunction referable to the region supplied by an occluded artery may occur.

When atherosclerosis develops slowly, collateral circulation develops to meet the heart's needs. Complications from atherosclerosis occur because it is a progressive disorder that results in more severe cardiac disease if it is not prevented or treated. Common *sequelae* of atherosclerosis affecting coronary arteries include angina pectoris, MI or heart attack, and sudden death.

Men experience angina as the first symptom of CAD in one-third of all cases and heart attack or sudden death in the majority of cases, whereas half of all women experience angina and remain asymptomatic or, in the remaining cases, manifest atypical symptoms.

Atypical symptoms of angina in women include breathlessness, pain in the left chest, upper abdominal pain, and back or arm pain in the absence of substernal chest pain. The pain may be more diffuse and is described as sharp or fleeting, unrelated to exercise, unrelieved by rest or nitroglycerin but relieved by antacids, and characterized by palpitations without chest pain. The pain may be repeated and prolonged. Chest pain in women with chronic stable angina is more likely to occur during rest, sleep, or periods of mental stress.

Medical Management

Prevention

Overwhelming evidence indicates that cardiovascular disease and CAD are largely preventable; therefore whenever possible, prevention of cardiovascular disease and CAD is the goal for everyone. Atherosclerosis is not a disease of middle to old age; it begins in adolescence and young adulthood and develops slowly but progressively throughout the body.

Preventing heart disease means controlling LDL before atherosclerosis gets a chance to do much damage. Reduction in the plasma level of LDL (at or below 100 mg/dL) throughout a person's life span by diet, exercise, and the use of statins or other cholesterol-lowering drugs is the proposed way to do this.[54]

Healthy People 2020[97] has identified the following goals for heart disease and stroke: improvement of cardiovascular health and quality of life through the prevention, detection, and treatment of risk factors; early identification and treatment of heart attacks and strokes; and prevention of recurrent cardiovascular events.

Health perceptions, health care–seeking behavior, and willingness to participate in long-term preventive therapies are significantly influenced by age and cultural and socioeconomic factors. Many physicians underestimate the life expectancy in older adults. For example, the average 65 year old can expect to live an additional 15 to 20 years and function independently for more than 70% of this time.

Adults older than 80 can expect to live 7 to 10 more years and function independently for half of that time. Older individuals are less likely to be referred to cardiac rehabilitation and exercise-training programs and less likely to attend than younger adults. Therefore preventive cardiology, including primary and secondary preventive efforts directed at the older adult, is important.[132]

Primary and secondary prevention programs are needed that are modified for the linguistic, cultural, and medical needs of people of all age groups and ethnic backgrounds but especially for older individuals of ethnic minorities who are at increased risk for cardiovascular disease.[215] Ethnic comparisons of health behaviors and prevalence of risk factors among teenagers support the need for health promotion intervention among urban ethnic teenagers.[68]

Women are less likely than men to receive health care advice on risk reduction while they are still healthy, even though they are more likely to die with the first heart attack. For this reason, new guidelines for prevention of heart disease in women were published in 2007 and updated in 2011.[153]

The bottom line is that even for people with a strong genetic component, modifying risk factors can slow the growth and spread of atherosclerotic plaque and reduce the risk of heart attack or stroke. The goal is to prevent cholesterol-filled plaque from rupturing, which is a key event that leads to the formation of blood clots that can block a coronary or carotid artery. Many people with significant nonmodifiable risk factors for heart disease but who follow a heart-healthy lifestyle live longer and in better health with better quality of life compared with those individuals who do not follow a heart-healthy plan.

Modification of Risk Factors

Modifying risk factors whenever possible can decrease the risk of cardiovascular disease and CAD, especially prevention or cessation of cigarette smoking, management of diabetes and hypertension, and modification of diet.

Changing dietary habits by reducing fat intake can result in regression and disappearance of fatty streaks consisting of lipid-laden macrophages, T lymphocytes, and smooth muscle cells before these components progress to form a fibrous plaque.

Dietary changes are recommended for everyone, including children and adults, because it is now recognized that blood vessel changes associated with heart disease begin as early as 15 years of age and that the progression of the lesions is strongly influenced by the same risk factors that predict risk of clinically manifested coronary disease in middle-aged adults.[213,247]

Exercise and Physical Activity

Exercise and physical activity, according to recommendations from the Centers for Disease Control and Prevention (CDC; i.e., moderate-intensity exercise for at least 30 minutes on most days of the week) have been shown to reduce the risk for coronary events, ischemic stroke,[102] metabolic syndrome and insulin resistance, and diabetes mellitus for men and women.[136,230]

The American College of Sports Medicine's position on the quantity and quality of exercise for developing and maintaining cardiorespiratory and muscular fitness and flexibility in healthy adults recommends aerobic endurance training at least 2 days per week at 50% or higher Vo_2 and for at least 10 minutes.

In recent years the view that physical activity has to be vigorous to achieve a reduction in risk of CAD has been under question. Substantial evidence supports the benefit of continued regular physical activity that does not need to be strenuous or prolonged and includes daily leisure activities, such as walking or gardening. Taking up regular light or moderate physical activity in middle or older age confers significant benefit for cardiovascular disease.[229]

The National Runners' Health Study reports that substantial health benefits occur (in men) at exercise levels that exceed the CDC guidelines, suggesting that intense exercise offers one set of benefits whereas lengthy exercise provides another.[245] Other studies report the benefits of shorter periods of physical activity in decreasing the risk of CAD as being equal to the benefits of one longer, continuous session of exercise, as long as the total caloric expenditure is equivalent.[87]

The effect of exercise on cholesterol has been documented, but it remains unclear which component of exercise is the underlying beneficial mechanism. Exercise frequency may be more important than intensity in improving HDL cholesterol and cholesterol ratios,[118] and resistive exercise training has been reported to raise HDL cholesterol levels, but studies in these areas have been limited.[84,174] Even so, many health benefits from physical activity can be achieved in shorter bouts at less intensity.[9]

More studies are required to identify the ideal prescriptive exercise. It is interesting to note that endothelial damage has been reported after intense aerobic exercise, raising additional questions about exercise for athletes with cardiovascular risk factors.[26] It is likely that in the future, different exercise regimens for specific heart disease risk factors will be individually prescribed.

Exercise alone, independent of weight loss or diet changes, can have significant beneficial effects on cardiovascular risk factors in overweight people with elevated cholesterol levels.[39] Exercise is the one single intervention with the ability to influence the greatest number of risk factors.

Researchers at the University of Texas using real-time three-dimensional echocardiography to compare the effects of medications with the effects of exercise on coronary artery perfusion declare exercise to be "the most powerful drug available in preventing cardiac events."[52] Exercise can lessen depression, anger, and stress, which frequently interfere with recovery, and heart attack survivors who follow the CDC exercise guidelines reduce their risk of a fatal second episode by up to 25%.[109]

Pharmacotherapy and Chemoprevention

Chemoprevention is an established method in the primary and secondary prevention of cardiovascular (and cerebrovascular) disease. Clinical trials have proven conclusively that both fatal and nonfatal coronary events and strokes can be prevented.[225] Pharmacologic management is used to reduce the risk of clotting, to treat hypertension and to decrease the serum cholesterol level when it exceeds 200 mg/dL.

Medications known as "statins" are now available and have been proven effective not only in lowering LDL levels and raising HDL levels but also in reducing cardiac events (primary and secondary prevention of MI). However, caution has to be exercised when a combination of drugs is used.

Low-dose aspirin, 75 to 81 mg/day, was found to be just as effective in prevention of cardiovascular disease as high doses that result in increased incidence of bleeding events, primarily related to gastrointestinal (GI) tract toxicity.[44] The American Heart Association now recommends low-dose aspirin therapy of 81 mg/day or 100 mg every other day for all women age 65 or older. Studies show that aspirin will not prevent heart attacks in low-risk women under age 65, but it may be considered for all women at risk for stroke who are not at increased risk for bleeding.

Treatment

Medical management is directed toward the specific blood vessel occlusion and depends on complications.

Surgery

Surgical management of atherosclerosis of the coronary arteries may include PTCA (Fig. 9.3), CABG (Fig. 9.4), and coronary stents (Fig. 9.5). The current generation of drug-coated stents are bare metal covered with a polymer (plastic) coating that holds and releases a drug to inhibit the growth of endothelial cells. Several companies are working on polymers that are more compatible with the body and less likely to trigger clots. Others are testing polymers that dissolve and disappear after a period of time.

Angioplasty is performed 10 times more often than bypass surgery; angioplasty combined with a stent reduces the incidence of restenosis, especially for people with diabetes, who

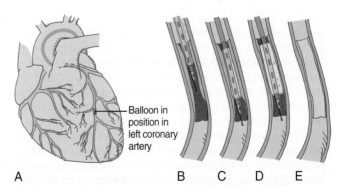

FIG. 9.3 Percutaneous transluminal coronary angioplasty can open an occluded coronary artery without opening the chest, which is an important advantage over bypass surgery. (A) Once coronary angiography has been performed to determine the presence and location of an arterial occlusion, a guide catheter is threaded through the femoral artery into the left coronary artery. (B) When the angiography shows the guide catheter positioned at the site of occlusion, the uninflated balloon is centered in the obstruction. (C) A smaller double-lumen balloon catheter is inserted through the guide catheter. (D) The balloon is inflated, compressing the plaque against the arterial wall, and deflated until the angiogram confirms a reduced pressure gradient in the vessel. (E) The balloon is removed, and the artery is left unoccluded.

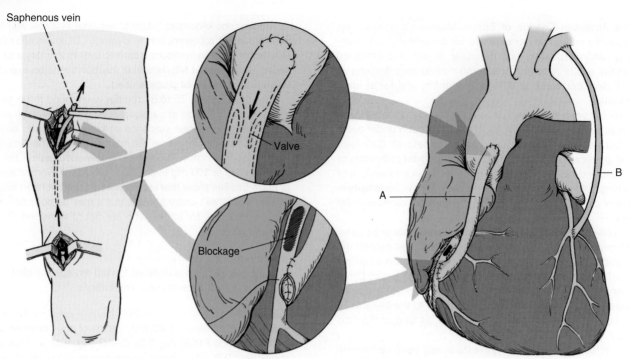

FIG. 9.4 Coronary artery bypass graft (CABG). This procedure involves taking a portion of a vein or artery from the chest or leg and grafting it onto the coronary artery. (A) A section of the saphenous vein is used as a graft to route blood around areas of blockage. (B) Bypassing the clogged vessel provides an alternative route for blood to reach the heart muscle. The internal mammary artery can be used as an alternate vein site for grafting. CABG has been a major surgery requiring a sternotomy but is being refined to possibly become an off-pump bypass grafting through a partial sternotomy. It is considered most effective in individuals who have several severely blocked coronary arteries and a previously damaged heart muscle or when repeated revascularization has failed. (From Black JM, Hawks JH, Keene AM: Medical-surgical nursing: clinical management for positive outcomes, ed 6, Philadelphia, 2001, Saunders.)

have a high restenosis rate when treated by standard balloon angioplasty.[226] The use of a combined antiplatelet treatment with aspirin and glycoprotein IIb/IIa receptor blockers (Table 9.5) is a standard pharmacologic regimen after coronary artery stenting for the prevention of thrombosis (*thrombosis* is the formation of a clot; *thrombus* is the clot). It is important to note that cardiovascular medications come with a variety of side effects (Table 9.6).

Intravascular ultrasound, a technology that combines echo with catheterization, may eventually allow diagnosis and therapy to be combined as the cardiologist uses a camera on the tip of a catheter to precisely target atherosclerotic blockage. In keeping with the new data on the time of day that cardiac events occur (i.e., thrombus formation is more likely to occur in the morning hours), researchers are now investigating the possibility that postoperative complications are related to the time the procedure takes place.[218]

Although surgical intervention has been a mainstay for the treatment of CAD, researchers are questioning the necessity of heart surgery and are studying the benefits of pharmacologic intervention combined with exercise and lifestyle changes. The role of exercise in the prevention of atherosclerosis has been discussed, but the role of exercise as a treatment modality is equally important.

Cardiac Rehabilitation

Cardiac rehabilitation exercise training consistently improves objective measures of exercise tolerance, without significant cardiovascular complications or other adverse outcomes. Appropriately prescribed and conducted exercise training is recommended as an integral component of the treatment of atherosclerosis and CAD.[4]

Results from the Stanford Coronary Risk Intervention Project conducted over 4 years demonstrated that intensive multifactor risk reduction favorably alters the rate of luminal narrowing in coronary arteries of men and women with CAD and decreases hospitalizations for clinical cardiac events. In cases of low-risk, stable CAD, aggressive lipid-lowering therapy is at least as effective as angioplasty in reducing the incidence of ischemic events.[40]

Numerous other trials have focused on the effect of diet-induced reductions in LDL cholesterol and the resultant changes in CAD. Restricting the intake of saturated fat and cholesterol has a favorable result in changing the course of coronary atherosclerosis.

In addition, dietary and lifestyle interventions slowed CAD progression, decreased the incidence and severity of angina, and reduced the number of cardiac events. Exercise-based

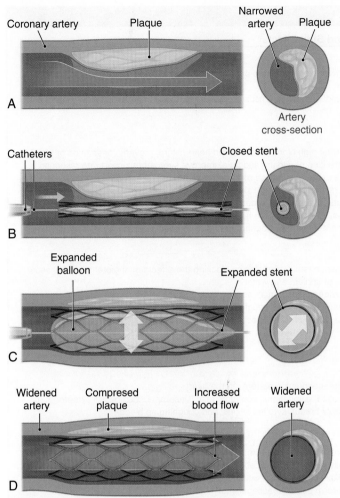

FIG. 9.5 Application of the coronary stent. (A) A severely occluded coronary artery. (B and C) Blocked coronary artery can be held open using a balloon-expandable device called a *coronary stent*. (D) Stent maintains an opened vessel, allowing blood to pass through freely. Biodegradable stents are under development to reduce or eliminate problems associated with metal stents.[228] Delivery of drugs or gene therapy to inhibit intimal hyperplasia and prevent postangioplasty restenosis is under investigation.[57,69] (© GettyImages.com.)

the blocked vessels, a process referred to as *therapeutic angiogenesis* or *biologic revascularization*.[163,247]

Genetic approaches will continue to identify genes and pathways involved in the predisposition to and pathophysiology of atherosclerosis. Targets for therapeutic intervention based on gene profiling continue to be the focus of research at this time.[148]

Complementary and Integrative Medicine

Alternative or complementary integrative medicine, sometimes referred to as *mind–body therapy,* and its effects on heart disease, blood pressure, lipid levels, morbidity, and mortality are under investigation. Such therapies include prayer or meditation and/or religious attendance at church or services; yoga, Tai Chi, and other forms of martial arts; acupuncture; social support and/or support groups; cognitive-behavioral therapy; imagery; hypnosis; physiologic quieting; relaxation techniques; music therapy; and others (Fig. 9.6).

Prognosis

The American Heart Association reports compelling scientific evidence that comprehensive risk factor interventions in people with cardiovascular heart disease extend overall survival, improve quality of life, decrease the need for interventional procedures, and reduce the incidence of subsequent MI. Even so, despite the well-documented benefit of preventive measures and cardiac rehabilitation, compliance with recommendations for reducing risk factors and usage rates of rehabilitation programs remain low, especially among women.[153]

Fatality rates for CAD remain low before age 35 years, but these figures increase exponentially until age 75 years, with men generally experiencing mortality at approximately twice the rate of women until age 65 years. Total CAD mortality in women after age 65 years now exceeds that of men.

Surgical procedures are considered safe, and although complications can occur, the rates of complications after CABG surgery have declined substantially in the last 15 years despite higher client risks. In the case of angioplasty, the risks of failure, reoperative procedures, and operative mortality are higher with advanced age, female gender, diabetes mellitus, elevated serum cardiac enzymes after the procedure, and impaired left ventricular dysfunction.[211]

cardiac rehabilitation is effective in reducing cardiac deaths, but the effect of exercise alone without a comprehensive cardiac rehabilitation intervention has not been evaluated.[111]

Gene Therapy

Gene therapy is one strategy with the potential to prevent some of the sequelae after arterial injury, induce growth of new vessels, or remodel preexisting vessels.[69] Several groups have injected a gene that makes a protein called *vascular endothelial growth factor.* When injected directly into the heart, this gene prompts the heart to sprout tiny new blood vessels to bypass

9.2 Special Implications for the PTA: Atherosclerosis (Cardiovascular Disease and Coronary Artery Disease) Other practice patterns may be necessary depending on the clinical manifestations and disease outcomes (see discussion of each specific disease). The therapist or PTA can be very instrumental in guiding individuals through a preoperative wellness program, including client education, risk factor reduction, and exercise program.

Postoperative Considerations

Cardiac rehabilitation (phases I to IV) is an important component of intervention for anyone treated medically for CHF, arrhythmias, unstable angina, CAD, MI, valvular disease, or heart transplantation.

TABLE 9.5   Common Cardiovascular Medications

Medications: Trade Names (Generic Names)	Indications and Side Effects[a]
α(Adrenergic) Blockers (-zosin) Cardura (doxazosin) Hytrin (terazosin) Minipress (prazosin)	**Indication:** To lower blood pressure by dilating peripheral blood vessels, reducing peripheral resistance **Side effects:** Headache, fatigue, nausea, weakness, drowsiness, palpitations,[b] dizziness,[c] fainting[c]
Angiotensin-Converting Enzyme Inhibitors (-pril) Capoten (captopril) Lotensin (benazepril) Vasotec (enalapril) Prinivil, Zestril (lisinopril) Altace (ramipril) Accupril (quinapril)	**Indications:** To treat high blood pressure and heart failure; prevent constriction of blood vessels and retention of sodium and fluid, improve sympathetic heart rate response during exercise in the early phase of MI to prevent heart failure **Side effects:** Persistent, dry cough; skin rash; loss of taste; weakness; headaches; palpitations[b]; swelling of feet or abdomen[b]; dizziness or fainting[c] (because of low blood pressure); numbness or tingling of the hands, feet, or lips; renal failure; may cause congenital cardiovascular defects if taken during the first trimester in pregnancy[58]
Angiotensin II Receptor Antagonists (-sartan) Atacand (candesartan) Avapro (irbesartan) Cozaar (losartan) Diovan (valsartan) Micardis (telmisartan) Teveten (eprosartan) Verdia (tasosartan)	**Indication:** To vasoconstrict arterioles by blocking the effects of angiotensin II, enhance renal clearance of sodium and water **Side effects:** Dizziness,[c] insomnia,[b] anxiety,[b] confusion,[b] stroke,[c] hypotension,[c] visual changes,[c] GI and GU effects,[b] cough,[b] upper respiratory infection,[b] myalgia, many other various but less common side effects
Antiarrhythmics Cardioquin (quinidine) Procan (procainamide) Rythmol (propafenone)	**Indication:** To alter conduction patterns in the heart **Side effects:** Nausea, palpitations, vomiting, rash,[b] insomnia,[b] dizziness,[c] symptoms of CHF (shortness of breath, swollen ankles, and coughing up blood)[c]
Anticoagulants (Antithrombotic) Coumadin (warfarin) Unfractionated heparin (Lovenox [enoxaparin]) Low molecular weight heparin (Fragmin [dalteparin], Orgaran [danaparoid], Normiflo [ardeparin]) Hirudin (Refludan [lepirudin])	**Indication:** To prevent blood clot formation **Side effects:** Easy bruising, joint or abdominal pain,[c] difficulty in breathing or swallowing,[c] paralysis,[c] unexplained swelling, unusual or uncontrolled bleeding,[c] rib and vertebral fractures (long-term use of anticoagulants)[45]
β-Blockers (-olol) Inderal (propranolol) Lopressor (metoprolol) Tenormin (atenolol) Kerlone (betaxolol) Cartrol (carteolol) Corgard (nadolol) Coreg (carvedilol) Levatol (penbutolol) Blocadren (timolol) Not registered (clinical trial status): bucindolol	**Indications:** To relax the blood vessels of the heart muscle by blocking sympathetic conduction at β-receptors on the SA node and myocardial cells, producing a decline in the force of contraction and a reduction in heart rate; decrease blood pressure, dysrhythmias, and angina; decrease myocardial oxygen demand **Side effects:** Insomnia, nausea, fatigue, slow pulse, weakness, increased cholesterol and blood glucose levels, nightmares,[b] depression,[b] sexual dysfunction,[b] asthmatic attacks,[c] dizziness[c]
Calcium-Channel Blockers (-pine) Procardia (nifedipine) Cardizem (diltiazem HCl) Calan, Verelan (verapamil) Norvasc (amlodipine) Plendil (felodipine) Cardene (nicardipine)	**Indications:** To dilate coronary arteries to lower blood pressure and suppress some arrhythmias **Side effects:** Fluid retention, palpitations, headache from vasodilation, flushes, rash,[b] dizziness[c]
Central Antiadrenergic Agents Aldomet (methyldopa) Catapres (clonidine) Wytensin (guanabenz) Tenex (guanfacine)	**Indication:** To lower high blood pressure by dilating the blood vessels **Side effects:** Drowsiness, depression, sexual dysfunction, fatigue, dry mouth, stuffy nose, fever, upset stomach, change in bowel habits, weight gain, fluid retention, dizziness[c]

TABLE 9.5 Common Cardiovascular Medications—cont'd

Medications: Trade Names (Generic Names)	Indications and Side Effects[a]
Digitalis Compounds (Cardiac Glycosides) Lanoxin (digoxin) Crystodigin (digitoxin)	**Indications:** To strengthen the heart's pumping force to increase cardiac output and decrease electrical conduction through the AV node; slows heart rate to allow heart to fill completely; too fast a heart rate does not give the heart enough time to fill completely, then the heart does not pump enough blood out to supply the body **Side effects:** Fatigue, lethargy, weakness, headache,[b] visual disturbances (blurred vision, yellow-green halos, blind spots in visual field or scotomata, and double vision),[b] cardiac disturbances (bradycardia and irregular heart rhythms),[c] hypotension,[b] anorexia, nausea, vomiting,[b] diarrhea,[b] CNS disturbance[b] (depression, irritability, confusion, restlessness, drowsiness, and seizures[c]), electrolyte disturbances (hypokalemia)[b]
Diuretics Thiazide diuretics (e.g., Hydrodiuril [hydrochlorothiazide]) Potassium-sparing diuretics (e.g., Aldactone [spironolactone]) Loop diuretics (e.g., Lasix [furosemide], Bumex [bumetanide], Demadex [torsemide])	**Indications:** To increase the excretion of sodium and water and control high pressure and fluid retention **Side effects:** Drowsiness, dehydration, electrolyte imbalances, gout, nausea, pain, hearing loss, blood glucose abnormalities, elevated cholesterol and lipoprotein levels, muscle cramps,[b] dizziness,[c] light-headedness[c]
Lipid-Lowering Drugs Lipitor (atorvastatin) Crestor (rosuvastatin) Mevacor (lovastatin) Zocor (simvastatin) Loscol (fluvastatin) Pravachol (pravastatin) Lopid (gemfibrozil) Questran (cholestyramine) Nia-Bid, Niacor, Nicobid (niacin) Zetia (ezetimibe)	**Indication:** To interfere with the metabolism of blood fats in various ways by lowering cholesterol, low-density lipoproteins, and/or triglyceride levels in the blood or by blocking the absorption of cholesterol that comes from food; non–lipid-lowering effects include improving endothelial function, producing antiproliferative actions on smooth muscle, and reducing platelet aggregation **Side effect:** Nausea, vomiting,[b] diarrhea,[b] constipation,[b] flatulence, abdominal discomfort, myalgia, increased liver enzymes; more rarely, statins can cause myositis or rhabdomyolysis (a debilitating muscle-wasting condition resulting in acute renal failure), peripheral neuropathy, sleep disturbances (insomnia, bad, or vivid dreams), or rash; statins may stimulate bone growth and reduce osteoporosis (under investigation)
Nitrates (Vasodilators) Nitrostat, Nitro-Bid (nitroglycerin) Iso-Bid, Isordil (isosorbide dinitrate)	**Indication:** For dilation of coronary arteries **Side effects:** Headache, dizziness,[b] orthostatic hypotension,[b] tachycardia[b]
Platelet Inhibitors (Antiplatelet) Aspirin Ticlid (ticlopidine) Plavix (clopidogrel) Glycoprotein IIb/IIa receptor blockers ("super aspirin") ReoPro (abciximab) Integrilin (eptifibadtide) Aggrastat (tirofiban)	**Indication:** To prevent platelet aggregation and subsequent clot formation **Side effects:** Gastric irritation (aspirin),[b] bleeding or hemorrhage,[c] leg or pelvic pain,[b] rash, atrial fibrillation,[c] tachycardia,[c] dizziness,[b] confusion[b]
Thrombolytics Streptokinase Urokinase Tissue-type plasminogen activator (t-PA) (Activase [alteplase], tenecteplase or TNKase [reteplase])	**Indication:** Used to break down and dissolve already formed blood clots **Side effects:** Bleeding (GI, GU, intracranial, and surface),[c] headache,[b] fever,[b] nausea,[b] low back pain[b]
Vasodilators Nitroglycerin Isosorbide dinitrate (Isordil, Iso-Bid)	**Indication:** To dilate the peripheral blood vessels (used in combination with diuretics) **Side effects:** Headache, drowsiness, nausea, vomiting, diarrhea, hair growth (minoxidil only), increased heart rate,[b] swollen ankles,[b] dizziness,[c] difficulty in breathing[c]
Human B-Type Natriuretic Peptide (Vasodilator, Diuretic; Genetically Engineered Form of Naturally Occurring Cardiac Hormone) Nesiritide (Natrecor)	**Indications:** Combination of effects including rapid dilation of arteries and veins; promotes diuresis; used in decompensated CHF and arrhythmias **Side effects:** Dose-related hypotension[b]

[a]The therapist is more likely to see potential side effects not otherwise present because these develop when the person is physically challenged. Any unusual signs or symptoms and potential side effects should be documented and reported to the prescribing physician.
[b]Document and call physician when possible.
[c]Call physician immediately; document findings.
AV, Atrioventricular; *CHF,* congestive heart failure; *CNS,* central nervous system; *GI,* gastrointestinal; *GU,* genitourinary; *MI,* myocardial infarction; *SA,* sinoatrial.

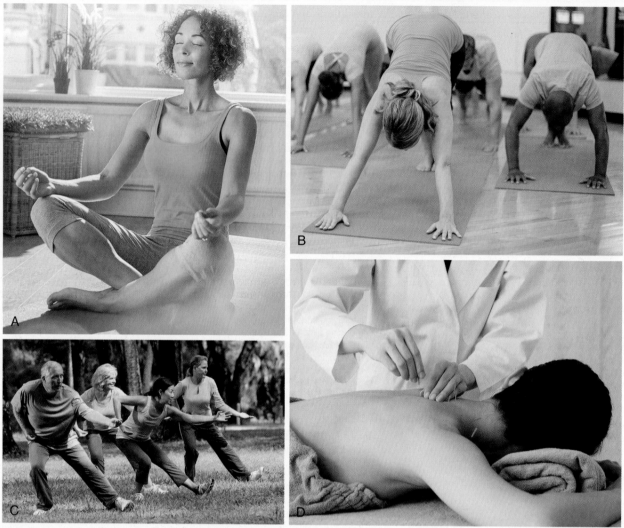

FIG. 9.6 Examples of mind-body therapies. (A) Meditation. (B) Yoga. (C) Tai chi. (D) Acupuncture. (Courtesy GettyImages.com.)

TABLE 9.6 Common Side Effects Associated with Cardiovascular Medications Requiring Adjustments to Physical Therapy Interventions
• Orthostatic hypotension
• Dizziness with position change
• Blunted exercise response
• Bradycardia, decreased resting heart rate
• Tachycardia (reflex)
• Fluid depletion/electrolyte imbalance
• Muscle weakness
• Fatigue
• Induction of new arrhythmias
• Peripheral edema

Courtesy Susan A. Queen, PT, PhD, Associate Professor Emeritus, University of New Mexico, Division of Physical Therapy, 2016.

This multidisciplinary program of education and exercise is designed to promote the development and maintenance of a desirable level of physical, social, and psychologic function in individuals with an acute cardiovascular illness.

Specific goals of cardiac rehabilitation include stratifying risk, improving emotional well-being and psychologic factors, reducing CAD risk factors, and decreasing symptoms. In addition, older adults often have reduced functional capacity and quality-of-life scores compared with younger CAD clients, making this an important goal for those individuals.[128,130]

Implementation of phase I physical therapy begins on days 1 to 3 after CABG or other surgery or an MI. Primary emphasis is on post-surgical mobilization; client education is essential given the presence of comorbidities and the need for individualized prescriptive exercise.

During this phase the therapist and PTA use and teach the client sternal precautions (Box 9.1)[106] and adjust the intensity of mobilization to optimize recovery from surgery and tissue injury, minimizing length of stay without compromising the client.[105]

Postoperative brachial plexus injury can occur after cardiac surgery that requires a sternotomy when prolonged sternal separation or asymmetric traction of the sternal halves causes nerve compression or overstretching. Uncomplicated cases are usually transient and do not require intervention. As cardiac operative techniques continue to improve and move toward noninvasive methods, this type of injury will become obsolete.

Home monitoring of symptoms for the first weeks after surgery is essential, following the guidelines in Box 9.2. The physician should be notified if the client experiences one or more of the signs and symptoms outlined. Transfusion is no longer a standard part of open heart surgery, so hematocrit levels are usually low (25% to 29%) after this procedure, requiring modification of exercise guidelines unless directed otherwise by the physician. Carotid artery disease is a risk factor for CNS complications after CABG surgery, requiring close monitoring for signs and symptoms of CNS involvement.

Discharge instructions for the cardiovascular surgical population may vary according to physician and institution, but some general guidelines apply (Box 9.3). The PTA can be helpful in teaching about unexpected symptoms and ways to manage them.

Reassurance and education are extremely important for clients who are emotionally distressed. Although these people are successful in improving their functional status and physical capacity, they are more likely to experience angina during activities of daily living and during exercise and to be less successful in returning to work.

Prescriptive Exercise

The known benefits of regular physical activity and exercise in both primary and secondary prevention of cardiovascular disease have been thoroughly documented. Exercise training increases cardiovascular functional capacity and decreases myocardial oxygen demand at any level of physical activity in apparently healthy people as well as in most people with cardiovascular disease.

Regular dynamic exercise is considered adjunctive therapy for lipid management, along with dietary management and reduction of excess weight, but must be maintained for the training effects to be sustained. Both short- and long-term endurance exercise can contribute to an improvement in blood lipid abnormalities.[7]

Although exercise and physical training have been shown to improve exercise capacity and recovery of autonomic nervous activity,[216] there is an increased risk that exercise may precipitate cardiovascular complications and silent symptoms of ischemia, arrhythmias, or abnormal blood pressure. Heart responses to exercise and fatigue necessitate special considerations for the formulation and execution of physical conditioning programs. Determining

---

BOX 9.1   Sternal Precautions

- It is important to know whether the chest has been closed; the skin may be sutured, but the underlying chest structures may not be closed.
- To observe/document chest wall stability at rest, the therapist places his or her hands on the client's chest and asks the client to cough. Observe chest movement; any type of asynchronous movement between the two chest sides is a sign of an unstable chest requiring sternal precautions. These precautions vary from center to center and sometimes from surgeon to surgeon based on the surgical procedure performed but usually include the following:
- No pulling up in bed during acute care is allowed; client must roll into side-lying position and use the top arm to assist in pushing up while allowing the feet to drop off the side of the bed as a pendulum-type of assist.
- Handheld assistance during mobilization may be required initially in place of assistive devices, such as walkers or canes.
- No pushing, pulling, or lifting more than 10 lb (some precautions list 5 lb) for 6 weeks postoperatively is allowed; this includes running the vacuum cleaner and lifting or pushing pets (or walking pets on a leash), furniture, bowling balls, doors, children, or anything that weighs more than 1 gallon of milk.
- No driving motorized vehicles (e.g., automobile, golf cart, or other similar large conveyance) for 4 weeks postoperatively (some centers require 6 to 8 weeks) is permitted; during this time, no sitting in the front seat of any vehicle and especially vehicles equipped with airbags.
- Full neck, shoulder, and torso range of motion may be permitted as long as the sternum is stable but not if a sternectomy with skin or muscle flap is present; presence of a flap limits range of motion to 90 degrees (flexion or abduction) or to the point of movement at the chest wall or rib cage.
- Avoid shoulder horizontal abduction with extreme external rotation.
- Progression is based on client tolerance and signs of wound healing; once the incision is fully healed, scar mobilization is permissible. The usual precautions for scar mobilization apply, including mobilizing the tissue in the direction of the scar before using any cross-transverse techniques and mobilizing toward the scar rather than away from the scar to avoid overstretching the healing tissue.
- Use of the more conservative precautions is advised with anyone who has diabetes mellitus, severe osteoporosis, or other equally compromising comorbidities.
- Woman with larger breasts are at higher risk for dehiscence post-sternotomy; however, more research is needed on using supportive undergarments to reduce sternal skin stress.[106]
- Sternal support or harness may be useful to treat pain associated with sternotomy wounds, especially during coughing.[143]

---

how heart rate and blood pressure respond to exercise forms the basis for an exercise prescription.

Frequent premature ventricular contractions are considered a contraindication to exercise unless approved by the physician. Indications for stopping an exercise test can be used as precautions during therapy or exercise (see Box 9.2).

PTAs in all settings are encouraged to read the complete American Heart Association Exercise Standards.[7] Lists of risks associated with resistance exercise in older adults and recommended guidelines for resistance exercise prescription in this population of cardiac rehabilitation clients are also available.[33]

Postoperative Exercise

People recovering from cardiac surgery, despite an excellent hemodynamic result, may be disabled by persistent left ventricular hypertrophy and years of presurgical restricted activity and deconditioning.

BOX 9.2 Indications for Discontinuing or Modifying Exercise

Symptoms

- New-onset or easily provoked anginal chest pain
- Increasing frequency, intensity, or duration of angina (unstable angina)
- Discomfort in the upper body, including chest, arm, neck, or jaw; chest pain unrelated to chest incision
- Fainting, light-headedness, dizziness
- Sudden, severe dyspnea
- Severe fatigue or muscle pain
- Nausea or vomiting
- Back pain during exercise
- Bone or joint pain or discomfort during or after exercise
- Severe leg claudication

Clinical Signs

- Pallor; peripheral cyanosis; cold, moist skin
- Staggering gait, ataxia
- Confusion or blank stare in response to inquiries
- Resting heart rate >130 beats/min or <40 beats/min
- >6 arrhythmias (irregular heartbeats; palpitations) per hour
- Frequent premature ventricular contractions
- Uncontrolled diabetes mellitus (blood glucose >250 mg/dL)
- Oxygen saturation <90% (98% is normal); some variability (individual and geographic)
- Acute infection or temperature >100°F
- Persistent drainage or change in drainage from any incision
- Increased swelling, tenderness, and redness around any incision site
- Inability to converse during activity
- Blood pressure (BP) abnormalities
  - Fall in systolic BP with increase in workload; specifically, a decrease of 10 mm Hg or more below any previously recorded BP accompanied by other signs or symptoms
  - Rise in systolic BP above 250 mm Hg or diastolic BP above 115 mm Hg
- Signs of central nervous system involvement (e.g., confusion or delirium, cognitive decline, encephalopathy, seizure, stroke)

Other

- Person indicates need or desire to stop
- Recent myocardial infarction (within 48 hours)

Not all signs and symptoms require immediate cessation of exercise or intervention. The therapist is advised to document any clinical signs or symptoms observed or reported along with any modifications made in the intervention and notify the physician accordingly.

Adapted from Gibbons RJ: ACC/AHA 2002 guideline update for exercise testing. American College of Cardiology Foundation. www.acc.org. Accessed Oct. 1, 2010.

Exercise rehabilitation is an important part of the recovery process. Easy fatigability related to muscular weakness lessens with increased physical activity. Exercise-induced symptoms of angina and light-headedness or syncope disappear immediately after surgery with a successful result.

The exercise capacity of clients soon after MI and bypass surgery is determined by the same parameters as in healthy individuals or for other cardiac problems, including time since MI, age, physical training status, and amount of myocardial dysfunction that occurs with exercise. CNS dysfunction is a common consequence of otherwise uncomplicated CABG surgery that may affect exercise capacity.

An alteration in heart rate variability (HRV) can be transient or may remain for 6 months or more. A high variability in heart rate is a good sign of adaptability, implying that the autonomic nervous system

BOX 9.3 Discharge Instructions after Cardiovascular Surgery

Showers: Permitted 2 days after surgery or hospitalization. Avoid tub baths or soaking in water until incisions are healed; avoid extremely hot water.

Incisions: The incision should be kept dry but can be gently washed with mild soap and warm water (directly over the tapes); lotions, creams, oils, or powders are not permitted until the wound is completely healed unless prescribed by the physician.

Care of surgical leg (for bypass graft involving the leg): Avoid crossing the legs, which impairs circulation; avoid sitting in one position or standing for prolonged periods. Elevate the involved leg when sitting or lying down. Swelling in the grafted leg is common until collateral circulation develops. Swelling should decrease after leg elevation but may recur when standing. Progressive edema must be reported to the physician.

Elastic stockings: Wear for at least 2 weeks after discharge during the daytime and remove at bedtime.

Rest: A balance of rest and exercise is an essential part of the recovery process. Resting between activities and taking short naps are encouraged. Resting may include sitting quietly or reading for 20 to 30 minutes; loss of appetite is common for the first 2 weeks and may contribute to fatigue.

Walking: Walking increases circulation throughout the body and to the heart muscle and is encouraged. Activity must be increased gradually, but frequent walks of short duration are recommended initially. Pacing of activities throughout the day, combined with energy conservation, is important.

Stairs: Climbing stairs is permitted unless the physician indicates otherwise.

Sexual relations: Sexual relations can be resumed when the client feels physically comfortable (usually 2 to 4 weeks after discharge; see also text discussion).

Sternal precautions: See Box 9.1.

Stop any activity immediately if dyspnea, palpitations, chest pain or discomfort, or dizziness or fainting develops. Notify the physician if symptoms do not subside with rest in 20 minutes.

control mechanisms are functioning well. Beneficial effects of exercise training in restoring HRV after coronary angioplasty have been documented.[224]

A program to increase the strength and flexibility of the pectoral and leg muscles is usually recommended. During this time, elastic stockings are usually worn to prevent fluid accumulation at the site of the leg incisions. Special exercises are prescribed to improve chest wall function, facilitate breathing, and prevent adhesive capsulitis, a common finding 6 to 12 weeks after CABG or another open chest procedure.

Data to support the need for early range-of-motion (ROM) exercises to prevent loss associated with surgery are limited. One small study of the effect of shoulder ROM exercises after CABG surgery reported that they do not ameliorate the early loss of ROM associated with surgery, because the loss is a function of the surgical procedure and not lack of ROM challenge.[203] The delay in presentation of adhesive capsulitis suggests that other variables may be present during the time when clients are enrolled in phase I (inpatient) and phase II (outpatient) cardiac rehabilitation programs to account for this development.

Monitoring during Exercise

More than half of all ischemic episodes are not accompanied by angina. Ask any client with identified CAD risk factors or diagnosed CAD to report all unusual sensations, not just episodes of chest pain or discomfort. Exercise testing should be performed before an exercise program is begun, but if this has not been accomplished and baseline measurements are unavailable for use in planning exercise, use pulse oximetry; monitor the heart rate and rhythm, respiratory rate, and blood pressure; and note any accompanying symptoms before, during, and after exercise. This type of monitoring can be modified for each individual and is recommended throughout therapy intervention. Documentation of vital signs can be an excellent way to demonstrate evidence-based outcomes of intervention.

Side effects of cardiovascular medications may not appear until the cardiovascular system is challenged, such as occurs during therapy intervention. Monitoring for drug-related problems is essential, and a basic understanding of how these medications work is helpful (see Table 9.5). Striking a balance between the benefits of cardiovascular medications and acceptable or tolerable side effects can be a challenge, and the therapist and PTA must keep in mind when documenting and reporting drug-related effects that these medications often produce physiologic responses that increase the effectiveness of physical therapy.

Several drugs used in the treatment of CAD are known to alter the heart rate. For example, β-adrenergic blocking agents used in the treatment of angina and hypertension cause a reduction in resting and exercise heart rate. Anyone taking these medications may not be able to achieve a target heart rate above 90 beats/min; therefore using symptoms and rating perceived exertion may be a more appropriate means of monitoring. Avoid increases of more than 20 beats/min over the resting rate for individuals taking these medications.

Conservative limits postoperatively include a maximal heart rate of 130 beats/min, 120 beats/min for medically managed cases, or an increase of 30 beats/min for surgical cases and 20 beats/min for medical cases. A safe rate of exercise will allow the heart rate to return to the resting level within 5 minutes after exercise has been stopped.

Almost all antihypertensive agents, including diuretics that may have a dual action of peripheral dilation and volume depletion, can have a profound effect on postexercise blood pressure. In some healthy people, when exercise is terminated abruptly, precipitous drops in systolic blood pressure can occur because of venous pooling. Some people with CAD have higher levels of systolic blood pressure that exceed peak exercise values; a proper cool down after vigorous exercise is important to prevent such an occurrence.

Side Effects of Medication

As shown in Table 9.5, there is a wide range of commonly prescribed cardiovascular medications with an equally wide variety of potential side effects. The therapist and PTA must make note of medications used by each client and observe for any of the common adverse effects (see Table 9.6).

Of particular note is the potential for muscle pain from statins. Less than 5% of the adult population who take statins develop this problem. A more serious form of this side effect associated with statins (cholesterol-lowering medications) is called *rhabdomyolysis*, the rapid breakdown of skeletal muscle.

Myalgia as a result of taking a statin medication usually occurs within a few weeks of starting the drug. Any unexplained muscle pain, cramps, stiffness, spasm, or weakness in an adult taking a statin should be reported to the physician. This is especially true if there are any predictive risk factors.

Risk factors for this particular effect include age over 80, small body frame or frail health, presence of kidney disease, and polypharmacy. Individuals taking some forms of this medication are especially warned to avoid drinking grapefruit juice while taking statins, because this seems to have an adverse effect.

BOX 9.4 Types of Angina Pectoris

Stable (chronic) angina
- Classic exertional angina

Unstable angina
- Nocturnal angina
- Postinfarction angina
- Chronic crescendo angina
- Resting angina

Variant angina (Prinzmetal's angina)
Microvascular angina (syndrome X)

Angina Pectoris

Definition and Incidence

As blood vessels become obstructed by the formation of atherosclerotic plaque, the blood supply to tissues supplied by these vessels becomes restricted. When the cardiac workload exceeds the oxygen supply to myocardial tissue, ischemia occurs, causing temporary chest pain or discomfort, which is called *angina pectoris*. The exact incidence of angina is unknown, although it is considered common, especially in people age 65 years and older; it occurs more often in men.

Overview

There are several types of anginal pain (Box 9.4). *Chronic stable angina*, classified as classic, exertional angina, occurs at predictable levels of physical or emotional stress and responds promptly to rest or to nitroglycerin. No pain occurs at rest; and the location, duration, intensity, and frequency of chest pain are consistent over time (60 days). *New-onset angina* describes angina that has developed for the first time within the last 2 weeks and is also considered unstable. *Nocturnal angina* may awaken a person from sleep with the same sensation experienced during exertion and is usually caused by increased heart rate associated with dreams or in response to underlying CHF.

Postinfarction angina occurs after MI when residual ischemia triggers an episode of angina. *Preinfarction angina* or *unstable angina*, also known as *progressive angina* or *crescendo angina*, is unpredictable and is characterized by an abrupt change (increase) in the intensity and frequency of symptoms or decreased threshold of stimulus. This angina lasts longer than 15 minutes and is a symptom of worsening cardiac ischemia.

Prinzmetal's, *vasospastic*, or *variant angina* produces symptoms similar to those of typical angina, but it is caused by coronary artery spasm. These spasms periodically squeeze arteries shut and keep the blood from reaching the heart. In this type of angina, coronary arteries are usually clear of plaque or free of physiologic changes that cause obstruction of the vessels. The pattern of Prinzmetal's angina is characterized by early morning occurrence, frequently at the same time each day, and it occurs at rest (i.e., it is unrelated to exertion).

Prinzmetal's angina is more common in women younger than 50; it is often associated with various types of arrhythmias or conduction defects. It is not a benign condition but is less likely to lead to a heart attack than angina caused by atherosclerosis because most heart attacks are caused by the rupture of an atherosclerotic plaque.

Decubitus or *resting angina* is considered atypical; it occurs most often at rest and frequently occurs at the same time every day. This type of anginal chest pain is atypical in that it is paroxysmal

TABLE 9.7   Causes of Myocardial Ischemia

Decreased Oxygen Supply	Increased Oxygen Demand
Vessels	
Atherosclerotic narrowing	Hyperthyroidism
Inadequate collateral circulation	Arteriovenous fistula
Spasm caused by smoking, emotion, or cold	Exercise or exertion
Coronary arteritis	Emotion or excitement
Hypertension	Digestion of large meal
Hypertrophic cardiomyopathy	
Circulatory Factors	
Arrhythmias (↓ blood pressure)	
Aortic stenosis	
Hypotension	
Bleeding	
Blood Factors	
Anemia	
Hypoxemia	
Polycythemia	

From Goodman CC, Snyder TE: Differential diagnosis in physical therapy, ed 4, Philadelphia, 2007, Saunders.

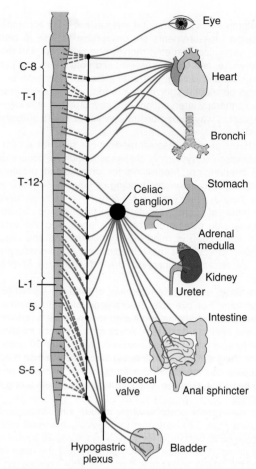

FIG. 9.7 Diagram of the autonomic nervous system. The visceral afferent fibers mediating cardiac pain travel with the sympathetic nerves and enter the spinal cord at multiple levels (C3 to T4). This multisegmental innervation results in a variety of pain patterns associated with myocardial ischemia and infarction.

in nature, not brought on by exercise, and not relieved by rest, but it is reduced when the person sits or stands up.

It is more prevalent among women, particularly those who have undergone hysterectomy. Microvascular angina associated with insulin resistance syndrome affects the microcirculatory system, a network of tiny blood vessels that branch from the large coronary vessels and that provide oxygen to each of the millions of myocardial cells. Why these vessels spasm and cause decreased blood flow remains undetermined; the cause may be a decrease in estrogen during menopause or a specific trigger from within the heart. Long-term survival rates are not reduced in women with this syndrome.

Etiologic and Risk Factors

Any condition that alters the blood (oxygen) supply or demand of the myocardium can cause ischemia (Table 9.7). Increased oxygen needs of the heart, increased cardiac output, or reduced blood flow to the heart can cause angina. CAD accounts for 90% of all cases of angina, although other conditions affecting normal vessels can also cause angina. Disorders of circulation, such as relative hypotension secondary to spinal anesthesia, antihypertensive drugs, or blood loss, can also result in decreased blood return to the heart and subsequent ischemic pain.

Onset of angina may be triggered by physical exertion or exercise, especially involving thoracic or upper extremity muscles or walking rapidly uphill; increase in pulse rate or blood pressure; or vasoconstriction. The threshold for angina is often lower in the morning or after strong emotion; the latter can provoke attacks in the absence of exertion. Angina may also occur less commonly during sexual activity, at rest, or at night during sleep.

Pathogenesis

Angina is a symptom of ischemia usually brought on by an imbalance between cardiac workload and oxygen supply to myocardial tissue usually secondary to CAD. Disruption of a formed plaque with sudden total or near-total arterial occlusion may bring on unstable angina.

Metabolites within the ischemic segment of the myocardium and buildup of lactic acid or abnormal stretching of the myocardium irritate myocardial fibers, resulting in myocardial pain. Afferent sympathetic fibers of the autonomic nervous system enter the spinal cord from levels C3 to T4 (Fig. 9.7), accounting for the varied locations and radiation patterns of anginal pain. The effects of temporary ischemia are reversible; if blood flow is restored, no permanent damage to or necrosis of the heart muscle occurs.

Clinical Manifestations

Angina is characterized by temporary pain or, more often, discomfort that starts suddenly in the chest (substernal or retrosternal) and sometimes radiates to other parts of the body, most commonly to the left shoulder and down the ulnar border of the arm to the fingers. Pain or discomfort may also be referred to any dermatome from C3 to T4, manifesting at the back of the neck, lower jaw, teeth, left upper back, interscapular area, or abdomen occasionally, and possibly down the right arm (Fig. 9.8).

The sensation described is often referred to as squeezing, burning, pressing, heartburn, indigestion, or choking. It is usually mild to moderate (rarely reported as severe); it usually lasts 1 to 3 minutes, sometimes 3 to 5 minutes, but can persist up to 15 to 20 minutes. Symptoms are usually relieved by rest or nitroglycerin; in women, symptoms may be relieved by taking an antacid.

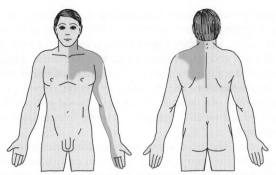

FIG. 9.8 Pain patterns associated with angina. *Left,* Area of substernal discomfort projected to the left shoulder and arm over the distribution of the ulnar nerve. Referred pain may be present only in the left shoulder or in the shoulder and along the arm only to the elbow. *Right,* Occasionally, anginal pain may be referred to the back in the area of the left scapula or the interscapular region. See Fig. 9.12 for the pain pattern associated with myocardial ischemia or infarction experienced by some women (see text for complete description).

Recognizing symptoms of myocardial ischemia in women is more difficult, because the symptoms are less reliable and do not follow the classic pattern described. Many women describe the pain in ways consistent with unstable angina, suggesting that they first become aware of their chest discomfort or have it diagnosed only after it reaches more advanced stages. Some experience a sensation similar to that of inhaling cold air, rather than the more typical shortness of breath. Other women note only weakness and lethargy, and some have observed isolated pain in the midthoracic spine or throbbing and aching in the right biceps muscle.

9.3 Special Implications for the PTA: Angina Pectoris

Identifying Angina

Referred pain from the external oblique abdominal muscle and the pectoral major muscle can cause the sensation referred to as *heartburn* in the anterior chest wall, which mimics angina. When active trigger points are present in the left pectoralis major muscle, the referred pain is easily confused with that from coronary insufficiency. Physical therapy to eliminate the trigger points can aid in the diagnostic process.

Anterior chest wall syndrome with localized tenderness of intercostal muscles, Tietze's syndrome with inflammation of the chondrocostal junctions, intercostal neuritis, and cervical or thoracic spine disease involving the dorsal nerve roots can all produce chest pain that mimics angina. Evaluation of ROM, palpation of soft tissue structures, and analysis of relieving or aggravating factors usually differentiate these conditions from true angina.[85] Likewise, heartburn from indigestion, hiatal hernia, peptic ulcer, esophageal spasm, and gallbladder disease can also cause angina-like symptoms that require a medical evaluation for an accurate medical diagnosis.

The development of unstable angina also requires immediate medical referral and may be reported as the onset of angina at rest, occurrence of typical angina at a significantly lower level of activity than usual, changes in the typical anginal pattern, or changes in blood pressure or heart rate with levels of activity previously well tolerated. Educating the public about reducing delays and getting to an emergency department at the earliest signs of heart attack is essential. Reperfusion therapy within the first 60 to 70 minutes of a heart attack can make a significant difference in outcome.

Nitroglycerin

A person experiencing angina should reduce the pace of, or if necessary stop, all activity and sit down for a few minutes until the symptoms disappear. Exercise can be reinitiated at a reduced intensity, and interval-type training may be required. Some experts suggest waiting several hours before resuming exercise. Anyone experiencing angina regularly with exercise or at a lower exertion than in the past may need a medical evaluation.

Nitroglycerin may be used prophylactically 5 minutes before activities likely to precipitate angina. This is especially true in the intervention or exercise setting for the person with chronic, stable, exertional angina. The use of nitroglycerin must be by physician order and cannot be decided solely by the therapist or PTA and client.

Clients must be reminded that they are not to alter their prescribed drug schedule without consulting their health care provider and that nitrates should be taken as prescribed. Clients should be seated when taking nitroglycerin to avoid syncope and falls. For anginal pain or discomfort not relieved by rest or by up to three nitroglycerin doses in 10 to 15 minutes (i.e., the initial dose followed by a second dose 5 minutes later and a third dose 5 minutes after the second dose), the physician should be contacted. Until the angina is controlled and coronary blood flow reestablished, the client is at risk for myocardial damage from myocardial ischemia.

Nitroglycerin tablets are inactivated by light, heat, air, and moisture, and they should be stored in the refrigerator in an amber container with a tight-fitting cover. Nitroglycerin has a short shelf life and needs to be replaced about every 3 months. A potent nitroglycerin tablet should produce a burning sensation under the tongue when taken sublingually (if it does not, check the expiration date).

Orthostatic Hypotension

Orthostatic hypotension is one of the most common side effects of prophylactic medications for angina. Caution on the part of the PTA is required when exercising or ambulating clients who take these medications. If the person becomes hypotensive, have him or her assume a supine position with legs elevated to increase venous return and to ensure cerebral blood flow.

Extra caution must be taken when placing anyone with orthostatic hypotension and CHF supine with legs elevated, because this may overload an already stressed ventricle. Keeping the head elevated and monitoring carefully are required in this circumstance. Support hose may be recommended, and the person should be reminded to change positions slowly to minimize the effects of orthostatic hypotension. Headache, weakness, increasing pulse, or other unusual signs or symptoms should be reported to the physician. In a home health setting, the home should be evaluated for potentially hazardous conditions. All clients should be encouraged to avoid hazardous activities until their condition has been stabilized by medication, especially in the presence of dizziness.

Monitoring Vital Signs

Exercise testing should be performed before a client begins an exercise program, but if this has not been accomplished and baseline measurements are unavailable for use in planning exercise, monitor the heart rate and blood pressure and note any accompanying symptoms during exercise. Exercise and activity should be performed below the anginal threshold. The PTA must document heart rate and blood pressure when the ischemia began, to establish these parameters. Angina occurring after MI is not considered normal and should be reported to the physician. Exercise testing is recommended before a client resumes an exercise program.

TABLE 9.8 Classification of Blood Pressure for Adults

	Systolic Blood Pressure	Diastolic Blood Pressure
Normal	<120 mm Hg	<80 mm Hg
Prehypertensive	120-139	80-89
Stage 1 hypertension	140-159	90-99
Stage 2 hypertension	≥160	≥100

From The Seventh Report of the Joint National Committee on Prevention, Detection, Evaluation, and Treatment of High Blood Pressure. NIH Publication No. 03-5233, 2003, National Heart, Lung, and Blood Institute (NHLBI). www.nhlbi.nih.gov.
The relationship between blood pressure and risk of coronary vascular disease events is continuous, consistent, and independent of other risk factors. The higher the blood pressure, the greater the chance of heart attack, heart failure, stroke, and kidney disease.
For individuals 40-70 years of age, each 20-mm Hg incremental increase in systolic blood pressure or 10 mm Hg in diastolic blood pressure doubles the risk of coronary vascular disease across the entire blood pressure range from 115/75 to 185/115 mm Hg.

Classification of Blood Pressure for Children and Adolescents

Normal	<90th percentile; 50th percentile is the midpoint of the normal range
Prehypertension	90th-95th percentile or if blood pressure is greater than 120/80 (even if this figure is <90th percentile)
Stage 1 hypertension	95th-99th percentile + 5 mm Hg
Stage 2 hypertension	>99th percentile + 5 mm Hg

From National Heart, Lung, and Blood Institute (NHLBI): Fourth report on the diagnosis, evaluation, and treatment of high blood pressure in children and adolescents, Pediatrics 114:555–576, 2004.

Hypertensive Cardiovascular Disease

Hypertensive cardiovascular disease includes hypertensive vascular disease and hypertensive heart disease.

Hypertension (Hypertensive Vascular Disease)

Definition and overview. Blood pressure is the force exerted against the walls of the arteries and arterioles; diastolic pressure (bottom number) is the pressure in these vessels when the heart is relaxed between beats, and systolic pressure (top number) is the pressure exerted in the arteries when the heart contracts. From age 55 to 60 years, diastolic blood pressure often begins to plateau and may even decline, whereas systolic blood pressure often starts to rise.

Hypertension, or high blood pressure, is defined by the World Health Organization as a persistent elevation of diastolic blood pressure, higher than 90 mm Hg; systolic blood pressure, higher than 140 mm Hg; or both, measured on at least two separate occasions at least 2 weeks apart.

Based on epidemiologic data from the Framingham Heart Study, the development of hypertension is neither inevitable nor beneficial; both systolic pressure and diastolic pressure are important determinants of cardiovascular sequelae.

Hypertension can be classified according to type, cause, and degree of severity. It can also be classified based on risk according to the most recent guidelines (Table 9.8).[53]

Primary (or essential) *hypertension* is also known as idiopathic hypertension and accounts for 90% to 95% of all cases of hypertension. *Secondary hypertension* accounts for only 5% to 10% of cases and results from an identifiable cause. *Malignant hypertension* is a syndrome of markedly elevated blood pressure with organ damage. The elevation of systolic blood pressure independently of change in the diastolic blood pressure is now recognized as a medical condition referred to as *isolated systolic hypertension.*

Incidence. The incidence of hypertension varies considerably among different groups in the American population, but it is estimated that one in four adult Americans (50 million) has high blood pressure. Hypertension is twice as prevalent and more severe among blacks than whites. This phenomenon has been attributed to heredity, greater environmental stress, and greater salt intake or salt sensitivity, although the actual cause is not clear; reduced access to health care increases the prevalence of untreated hypertension.

Blood pressure control rates vary in minority populations and are lowest in Mexican Americans and Native Americans.[55] Socioeconomic factors and lifestyle may be important barriers to blood pressure control in some minority individuals.

Etiologic and risk factors. Primary hypertension has no established cause but is probably related to genetics and other risk factors, such as smoking, obesity, high cholesterol levels, and being of black descent. A familial association with hypertension has been documented, possibly attributable to common genetic background, shared environment, or lifestyle habits.

A variety of specific diseases or problems, such as chronic renal failure, renal artery stenosis, or endocrine disease, can cause *secondary hypertension* (Box 9.5). Small arteries branching from the aorta, called *arterioles,* regulate blood pressure. Any condition that can narrow the opening of these arterioles can increase the blood pressure in the arteries. The risk for cardiovascular disease in adults with hypertension is determined not only by the level of blood pressure but also by the presence or absence of organ damage or factors such as smoking, dyslipidemia, and diabetes.

Risk factors for hypertension may be modifiable or nonmodifiable (Box 9.6). The risk of hypertension increases with age as arteries lose elasticity and become less able to relax. Hypertension occurs slightly more often in men than in women and at an earlier age, but after age 50 years, hypertension begins to develop in more women than men. In all groups the incidence of hypertension increases with age, with a poorer prognosis for people whose hypertension begins at a young age.

White coat hypertension increases the risk of heart disease, because rise in blood pressure occurs in other anxiety-provoking situations as well. Personality traits such as hopelessness and hostility are important factors in cardiovascular disease, including hypertension. Hypertension itself represents a significant risk factor for the development of CAD, stroke, CHF, and renal failure, preceding heart failure in 90% of all cases and increasing in all other associated conditions.

Given the high prevalence of use of nonsteroidal antiinflammatory drugs (NSAIDs) by older adults, especially for conditions such as arthritis, gout, and similar problems,

---

BOX 9.5   Causes of Secondary Hypertension

- Coarctation of the aorta
- Pheochromocytoma (rare catecholamine-secreting tumor)
- Alcohol abuse
- Pregnancy
- Thyrotoxicosis
- Increased intracranial pressure from tumors or trauma
- Collagen disease
- Endocrine disease
  - Acromegaly
  - Cushing's disease
  - Diabetes
  - Hypothyroidism
  - Hyperthyroidism
- Renal disease (e.g., connective tissue diseases, diabetic nephropathy)
- Effects of drugs (e.g., oral contraceptives, corticosteroids, cyclosporine, cocaine)
- Acute stress
  - Surgery
  - Psychogenic hyperventilation
  - Alcohol withdrawal
  - Burns
  - Pancreatitis
  - Sickle cell crisis
- Neurologic disorders
  - Brain tumor
  - Respiratory acidosis
  - Encephalitis
  - Sleep apnea
  - Guillain–Barré syndrome
  - Quadriplegia
  - Lead poisoning

Data from Mann DL, Zipes DP, Libby P, et al, editors: Braunwald's heart disease: a textbook of cardiovascular medicine, ed 10, Philadelphia, 2015, Saunders.

BOX 9.6   Risk Factors of Primary (Essential) Hypertension

Modifiable

- High sodium intake (causes water retention and increases blood volume)
- Obesity (associated with increased intravascular volume)
- Diabetes mellitus
- Hypercholesterolemia and increased serum triglyceride levels
- Smoking (nicotine restricts blood vessels)
- Long-term abuse of alcohol (increases plasma catecholamines)
- Continuous emotional stress (stimulates sympathetic nervous system)
- Personality traits (hostility and sense of hopelessness)
- Sedentary lifestyle
- White coat hypertension (see explanation in text)
- Hormonal status (menopause, especially before age 40 years and without hormone replacement therapy; hysterectomy or oophorectomy)

Nonmodifiable

- Family history of cardiovascular disease
- Age (>55 years)
- Gender (male <55 years; female >55 years)
- Ethnicity (black,[a] Hispanic)

[a]From a pathogenetic point of view, recent research findings have suggested that β-adrenergic receptor downregulation is characteristic of hypertension in whites, whereas heightened vascular α-receptor sensitivity or early vascular hypertrophy may be a feature of hypertension in African Americans.[206] African Americans demonstrate somewhat reduced blood pressure responses to monotherapy with β-blockers, angiotensin-converting enzyme inhibitors, or angiotensin receptor blockers compared with diuretics or calcium channel blockers. These differential responses are largely eliminated by drug combinations.[20,53]

---

the association between this drug use and blood pressure must be observed carefully. Alcohol has been estimated to be responsible for as many as 10% of all cases of hypertension and may be the actual unknown cause of "essential" hypertension.[76]

Blood pressure is linked to salt intake and modulated by the "salt gene" in some people. Those who are salt sensitive may have an increased risk of death.

Inadequate sleep has been identified as a risk factor for hypertension among adults in their fourth to sixth decades who sleep less than 5 hours each night. Short sleep duration is also a risk factor for obesity and diabetes, two conditions commonly linked with hypertension. Men are more likely than women to report getting fewer than 6 hours of sleep, although women are more likely to have trouble falling asleep or getting back to sleep after waking up early.[67,79]

Pathogenesis. Blood pressure is regulated by two factors: blood flow and peripheral vascular resistance. Blood flow is determined by cardiac output. The resistance to flow is primarily determined by the diameter of blood vessels and, to a lesser degree, by the viscosity of blood.

Increased peripheral resistance as a result of the narrowing of the arterioles is the single most common characteristic of hypertension. Constriction of the peripheral arterioles may be controlled by two mechanisms, each with several

components: (1) sympathetic nervous system activity (autonomic regulation) and (2) activation of the renin–angiotensin system.

In the sympathetic nervous system, norepinephrine is released in response to psychogenic stress or baroreceptor activity. The blood vessels constrict, which increases peripheral resistance. At the same time, epinephrine is secreted by the adrenal medulla, resulting in increased force of cardiac contraction, increased cardiac output, and vasoconstriction.

With prolonged hypertension, the elastic tissue in the arterioles is replaced by fibrous collagen tissue. The thickened arteriole wall becomes less distensible, offering even greater resistance to the flow of blood. This process leads to decreased tissue perfusion, especially in the organs of high blood pressure. Atherosclerosis is also accelerated in persons with high blood pressure.

Within the renin–angiotensin system, vasoconstriction results in decreased blood flow to the kidney. Whenever blood flow to the kidney diminishes, renin is secreted and angiotensin is formed, causing vasoconstriction within the renal system and increased total peripheral resistance. Angiotensin also stimulates the secretion of aldosterone, which promotes sodium and water retention by the kidney tubules, causing an increase in intravascular volume. All these factors increase blood pressure.

Clinical manifestations. Hypertension is frequently asymptomatic; this creates a significant health care risk for affected people. When symptoms do occur, they may include headache, vertigo, flushed face, spontaneous nosebleeds, blurred vision, and nocturnal urinary frequency. Elevated blood pressure when measured, especially in the early stages, may be the only sign of hypertension.

Sleep-disordered breathing is also associated with systemic hypertension in middle-aged and older individuals of both genders and different ethnic backgrounds.[162] Progressive hypertension may be characterized by cardiovascular symptoms such as dyspnea, orthopnea, chest pain, and leg edema, or cerebral symptoms such as nausea, vomiting, drowsiness, confusion, and fleeting numbness or tingling in the limbs. It is also well recognized that end-stage renal disease is associated with accelerated and malignant hypertension; hypertension is associated with increased urinary calcium excretion and subsequent bone loss and osteoporosis, especially at the femoral neck.[27]

9.4 Special Implications for the PTA: Hypertension (Hypertensive Vascular Disease)

It is estimated that hypertension remains undiagnosed in nearly half of the 60 million Americans who have it. It is possible that many people in a therapy practice will be hypertensive without knowing it. Cardiac pathology may be unknown, requiring the PTA to remain alert for risk factors that require medical screening. For anyone with identified risk factors, a baseline blood pressure measurement should be taken on two or three separate occasions, and any unusual findings should be reported to the physician. The role of the PTA in screening to identify conditions such as hypertension is important, because an essential early component of intervention for this condition includes exercise.

The potential for osteoporosis and subsequent hip fractures in older adults (especially women) with hypertension points to the importance of osteoporosis screening and prevention in this population. The PTA has an important role in the primary prevention of impairments and functional limitations in people with hypertension. A sudden increase in blood pressure such as occurs with any increase in intraabdominal pressure during exercise or stabilization exercises can be dangerous for already hypertensive persons. The PTA must alert individuals with hypertension to this effect and teach proper breathing techniques during all activities.

Medications

People with CAD taking NSAIDs for pain relief may also be at risk for a myocardial event during times of increased myocardial oxygen demand (e.g., exercise, fever). In addition, older adults taking NSAIDs and antihypertensive agents must be monitored carefully. Regardless of the NSAID chosen, it is important to check blood pressure within the first few weeks after therapy or exercise is initiated and periodically thereafter.

A 2007 statement from the American Heart Association indicates that NSAIDs may cause an increased risk of serious cardiovascular thrombotic events, MI, stroke, heart failure, and hypertension.[21] Individuals with a prior history of cardiovascular disease or with risk factors for cardiovascular disease may be at greater risk. As with all medications, a balance should be considered between the risks and benefits of NSAIDs.

Whenever a health care provider knows that a client has been prescribed antihypertensive medications, appropriate follow-up questions as to whether the client is taking the medication and taking it as prescribed must be addressed. Many people take the medication only when symptoms are perceived and are at risk for the complications described previously.

Obtain as much information as possible about a client's medications so that potential side effects can be anticipated and intervention planned accordingly. Any side effects noted may indicate that a medication adjustment is needed and should be brought to the physician's attention (see Table 9.5).

The following brief description of the impact of various drug classes (all vasodilators) on exercise may assist the therapist and PTA in recommending activities for those who require pharmacologic agents and provide insight into therapeutic decisions for active hypertensive individuals. Antihypertensive medications reduce resting blood pressure levels and may influence blood pressure changes during submaximal and maximal exertion, which affects exercise capacity.

Vasodilators such as nitroglycerin and other nitrates act as prophylactics for angina by dilating the coronary arteries and improving collateral cardiac circulation, increasing oxygen to the heart muscle, and decreasing the blood pressure, which decreases symptoms of angina.

β-Adrenoceptor antagonists (β-blockers) selectively inhibit an increase in heart rate. Clinically, this means that when the person increases his or her activity or exercise level, the normal physiologic response of increased heart rate is blunted. This necessitates a longer warm-up and cool-down period. Sudden changes in position (e.g., supine to standing) should be avoided to prevent dizziness and falls associated with the resulting orthostatic hypotension.

β-Blockers diminish elevations of heart rate, myocardial contractility, and blood pressure. These effects reduce myocardial oxygen requirements during exertion and stress, preventing angina and allowing the person to exercise for longer periods before the onset of angina. The intended action of β-blockers may prevent normal blood pressure and heart rate responses to exercise; therefore using heart rate as an index for monitoring response to exercise is not recommended. Although β-blockers are effective antihypertensives, most of them adversely alter aerobic capacity so that exercise capacity is reduced.

An exercise prescription should be based on exercise stress test results using recommended guidelines.[8] Side effects of β-blockers include bronchospasm, which causes difficulty breathing, and chest tightness, which mimics angina; orthostatic hypotension; syncope; headache; and fatigue and weakness.

Diuretics have been first-line antihypertensive agents for many years, but few studies have observed the effect of diuretic therapy on exercise performance. Existing evidence reveals that peak blood pressures induced by physical activity may not always be controlled with diuretics. Diuretic therapy can result in hypokalemia accompanied by muscular cramps and skeletal muscle fatigue.

Potassium-sparing diuretics may cause hyperkalemia, which can in turn cause ventricular arrhythmias. Exercise tolerance may be reduced with arrhythmias because of a decrease in left ventricular filling time. Prolonged exercise in the heat is not recommended for people taking diuretics because of the cumulative effects of heat, exercise, and diuretics on blood volume and electrolytes. The length of time an individual who is taking a diuretic can safely exercise in the heat varies with the heat index and the physical condition of the person.

Calcium channel antagonists inhibit calcium ion influx across the cell membrane during cardiac depolarization, relax coronary vascular smooth muscle, dilate coronary and peripheral arteries, and increase myocardial oxygen delivery in people with vasospastic angina. This class of vasodilators decreases peripheral vascular resistance at rest and during physical activity, altering exercise tolerance by affecting heart rate and blood pressure during exercise.

During exercise, calcium channel antagonists have been observed to reduce systolic and diastolic pressure at submaximal loads, but higher systolic blood pressures measured during maximal exercise are not lowered. Side effects of calcium antagonists (e.g., drowsiness, dizziness, headache, peripheral edema, tachycardia, bradycardia) may interfere with a client's ability to participate in an exercise program.

Angiotensin-converting enzyme (ACE) inhibitors reduce blood pressure by lowering peripheral vascular resistance and are considered the first line of treatment by many physicians.

Exercise and Blood Pressure

A regular program of aerobic exercise, introduced gradually, facilitates cardiovascular conditioning, may assist in weight reduction, and may provide some benefit in reducing blood pressure. Exercising using primarily the lower extremities can also reduce blood pressure.

Postexercise hypotension in mildly hypertensive individuals has been observed for up to 7 hours after exercise independent of other variables.[175] Diastolic blood pressure reduction seems to be related to the duration of the exercise program. Blood pressure reduction has occurred after just several weeks to 6 months of regular training.[92] On the other hand, blood pressure will return to its previous elevated level if training is discontinued.

Heavy isometric exercises and heavy weightlifting may be harmful, because the blood pressure often rises because of vasovagal reflexes that occur. During fatiguing isometric exercise, the rate and rise of systolic blood pressure appear to be higher in hypertensive individuals, but studies in this area are limited. Generally, antihypertensive drugs have not been found to affect the blood pressure response to isometric exertion. However, the use of isometric exercise to lower blood pressure has not been studied in hypertensive individuals; a fall in resting blood pressure has been observed in normotensive individuals after repetitive isometric contractions equal to 30% of maximal capacity.[242]

Exercise Training Guidelines

The intensity of exercise required to produce health benefits and decrease blood pressure has been confused with the level of exercise necessary to improve physical fitness. Health benefits can be achieved without large gains in fitness. Encouraging people to increase their level of total energy expenditure is the key to increasing activity levels, rather than emphasizing physical fitness. The type, intensity, duration, and frequency of training, as well as progression, should be assessed regularly.

A preexercise evaluation and exercise testing may be prescribed by the physician. This information is helpful in establishing submaximal and maximal blood pressure responses. Monitoring vital signs before, during, and after exercise or activity is essential. Any person with an exaggerated systolic blood pressure response (higher than 250 mm Hg) or failure to reduce diastolic pressure (to less than 90 mm Hg) should be referred to the physician for reevaluation.

Training intensity does not need to be high, and it appears that low-intensity activity three times per week is as effective as high-intensity activity in blood pressure reduction. Training intensity should be based on maximal heart rate using the calculated formulas or measured during a maximal exercise test. After 12 to 16 weeks, if the blood pressure is adequately controlled, the physician may reduce the antihypertensive medication slowly to determine the long-term effect of training on blood pressure.

Monitoring during Exercise

PTAs often treat people who are diagnosed with conditions that are highly correlated with hypertension, such as stroke, obesity, diabetes mellitus, alcoholism, CAD, and pregnancy (see Box 9.5). Monitoring tolerance to exercise by observing for unusual symptoms and measuring blood pressure before, during, and after therapy are important steps in identifying a potential cardiovascular event.

Hypertensive Heart Disease

Definition and overview. The term *hypertensive heart disease* is used when the heart is enlarged as a result of persistently elevated blood pressure (hypertension). Left ventricular hypertrophy and diastolic dysfunction are found in 10% to 30% of the adult population with chronic hypertension, and it may manifest with many of the signs and symptoms of CHF. Both the prevalence and the severity of the disease are greater in blacks than in whites. In all adults, it increases progressively with age.

9.5 Special Implications for the PTA: Hypertensive Heart Disease See 9.2 Special Implications for the PTA: Atherosclerosis (Cardiovascular Disease and Coronary Artery Disease), 9.4 Special Implications for the PTA: Hypertension (Hypertensive Vascular Disease), and 9.7 Special Implications for the PTA: Congestive Heart Failure.

Myocardial Infarction

Definition and Incidence

MI, also known as a "heart attack" or a "coronary," is the development of ischemia with resultant necrosis of myocardial tissue. Any prolonged obstruction depriving the heart muscle of oxygen can cause an MI. It occurs in 1.5 million persons each year and represents the leading cause of death in the adult American population.

Etiologic and Risk Factors

Etiologic and risk factors are the same as for all forms of cardiovascular disease, especially angina pectoris associated with CAD. Eighty percent to 90% of MIs result from coronary thrombus at the site of a preexisting atherosclerotic stenosis. New cases of MI occur in many people with only a borderline risk profile or even lack of known risk factors, suggesting other, unidentified risk factors.

Other causes may include cocaine use, vasculitis, aortic stenosis, or aortic root or coronary artery dissection. Smokers have more than twice as many heart attacks as nonsmokers, and sudden cardiac death occurs two to four times more frequently in smokers. After an infarction, smokers have a poorer chance of recovery than nonsmokers.

It is a well-established fact that heart attacks occur more frequently in the early morning hours. This peak incidence is attributed to an increase in catecholamines with the resultant increased blood pressure, increased workload of the heart, and increased clotting factors in the early morning. Heart attacks also occur in a seasonal pattern, with an increased incidence between Thanksgiving and New Year's Day across all ages, in both genders, and across geographic regions. Whether this can be attributed to mood changes, weather, circadian rhythms, large quantity of food consumed, or some other mechanism remains unknown.

Upper respiratory tract illnesses have been associated with an increased risk of ischemic heart disease and stroke, especially during the flu season in adults 65 years old and older who have not received a flu shot. Studies show a reduction in the risk of hospitalization and mortality for heart disease as well as cerebrovascular disease, pneumonia, and influenza in elderly adults who have received the flu vaccine.[160,161]

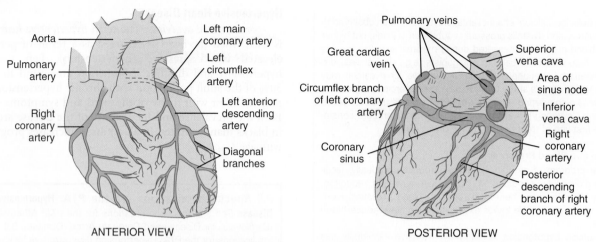

Aorta

Pulmonary artery

Right coronary artery

Left main coronary artery

Left circumflex artery

Left anterior descending artery

Diagonal branches

ANTERIOR VIEW

Pulmonary veins

Great cardiac vein

Circumflex branch of left coronary artery

Coronary sinus

Superior vena cava

Area of sinus node

Inferior vena cava

Right coronary artery

Posterior descending branch of right coronary artery

POSTERIOR VIEW

FIG. 9.9 Areas of myocardium affected by arterial insufficiency of specific coronary arteries. The right and left coronary arteries branch off the aorta just above the aortic valve and normally supply the myocardium with oxygenated blood.

The association between periodontal disease and acute MI is under investigation. There is a definite association between common forms of periodontal disease and cardiovascular disease and stroke, but the causal relations have not been identified.[176]

Researchers have found that bacteria in the mouth spill into the bloodstream and can be found in the walls of major arteries. Recent research showed that intensive periodontal treatment may reverse atherosclerosis by improving elasticity of the arteries, or endothelial function,[223] suggesting that periodontal treatment may reduce cardiovascular risk.

Pathogenesis

The myocardium receives its blood supply from the two large coronary arteries and their branches (Fig. 9.9). One or more of these blood vessels may become occluded by a clot that forms suddenly when an atheromatous plaque ruptures through the sublayers of a blood vessel or when the narrow, roughened inner lining of a sclerosed artery becomes completely filled with thrombus. In most cases, infarcts result from an occlusive thrombus superimposed on an atherosclerotic plaque.

Researchers have found that plaque most likely to rupture (vulnerable plaque) is composed of the soft form of cholesterol and is vulnerable to mechanical forces such as occur with the increase in hormones early in the morning or even the vibration of the heartbeat.

Rupturing plaque does not always result in an MI. It is likely that plaque breaks off frequently without triggering a heart attack, and the large plaques visible on angiograms are often the healed-over and more stable plaques. Although these plaques occlude the coronary vessels, resulting in obstruction, ischemia, and angina, they are not as likely to cause rupture and sudden death as happens with the soft, smaller, and usually undetected plaques.

The most common site involved is the left ventricle, which is the chamber of the heart with the greatest workload. Thrombosis of the anterior descending branch of the left coronary artery is the most common cause of infarction and affects the anterior left ventricle (Fig. 9.10).

Myocardial ischemia or reperfusion injury is accompanied by an inflammatory response. When the myocardium has been completely deprived of oxygen, cells die and the tissue becomes necrotic in an area called the *zone of infarction* (Fig. 9.11). In response to this necrosis, leukocytes aid in removing the dead cells, and fibroblasts form a connective tissue scar within the area of infarction. The remaining heart muscle cells enlarge to compensate for the loss in heart pump function. Usually the formation of fibrous scar tissue is complete within 6 to 8 weeks (Table 9.9).

Immediately surrounding the area of infarction is a less seriously damaged area of injury called the *zone of hypoxic injury*. This zone is able to return to normal, but it may also become necrotic if blood flow is not restored. With adequate collateral circulation, this area may regain its function within 2 to 3 weeks. Adjacent to the zone of hypoxic injury is another reversible zone called the *zone of ischemia*. Ischemic and injured myocardial tissues cause characteristic electrocardiogram (ECG) changes; as the myocardium heals, the ST segment and T waves gradually return to normal, but abnormal Q waves may persist.

Oxygen deprivation is accompanied by electrolyte disturbances, particularly cellular loss of potassium, calcium, and magnesium. Myocardial cells deprived of necessary oxygen and nutrients lose contractility, so the pumping ability of the heart is diminished.

Clinical Manifestations

The most notable symptom of MI is a sudden sensation of pressure, often described as prolonged crushing chest pain, occasionally radiating to the arms, throat, neck, and back (Fig. 9.12). The pain is constant, lasting 30 minutes up to hours, and may be accompanied by pallor, shortness of breath, and profuse perspiration. Angina pectoris pain can be similar, but it is less severe, does not last for hours, and is relieved by cessation of activity, rest, or nitrates.

Symptoms do not always follow the classic pattern, especially in women. Two major symptoms in women are shortness of breath, sometimes occurring in the middle of the night, and chronic, unexplained fatigue. Atypical presentation may include continuous pain in the midthoracic spine or interscapular area, neck and shoulder pain, stomach or abdominal pain,

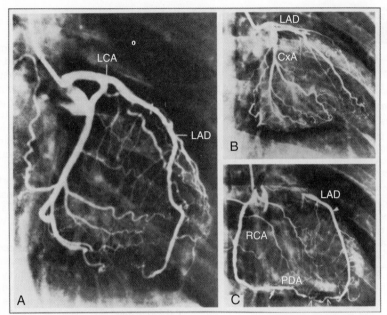

FIG. 9.10 (A) Angiogram of a normal left coronary artery (LCA). (B) Angiogram of a totally obstructed left anterior descending (LAD) coronary artery. (C) Angiogram of the right coronary artery (RCA) and its major branch, the posterior descending artery (PDA) (same heart as in B). The LAD is seen because of collateral vessels connecting the LAD and the RCA system. (From Boucek R, Morales A, Romanelli R, et al: Coronary artery disease: pathologic and clinical assessment, Baltimore, 1984, Williams & Wilkins.)

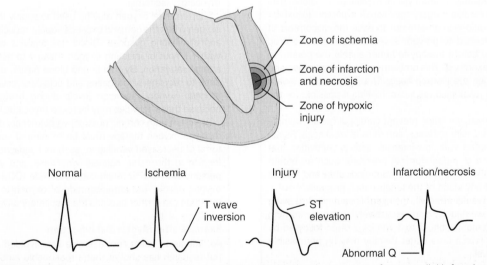

FIG. 9.11 Electrocardiographic alterations associated with the three zones of myocardial infarction.

nausea, unexplained anxiety, or heartburn that is not altered by antacids.

Silent attacks are more common among nonwhites, older adults, all smokers, and adults (men and women) with diabetes, presumably because of reduced sensitivity to pain. Nausea and vomiting may occur because of reflex stimulation of vomiting centers by pain fibers. Fever may develop in the first 24 hours and persist for a week because of inflammatory activity within the myocardium.

Postinfarction complications include arrhythmias, CHF, cardiogenic shock, pericarditis, rupture of the heart, thromboembolism, recurrent infarction, and sudden death. Arrhythmias, affecting more than 90% of individuals, are the most common complication of acute MI and are caused by ischemia, hypoxia, autonomic nervous system imbalances, lactic acidosis, electrolyte imbalances, drug toxicity, or alterations of impulse conduction pathways or conduction defects.

TABLE 9.9 Tissue Changes after Myocardial Infarction

Time after Myocardial Infarction	Tissue Changes
6-12 h	No gross changes; healing process has not begun
18-24 h	Inflammatory response; intercellular enzyme release
2-4 days	Visible necrosis; proteolytic enzymes remove debris; catecholamines, lipolysis, and glycogenolysis elevate plasma glucose and increase free fatty acids to assist depleted myocardium recovery from anaerobic state
4-10 days	Debris cleared; collagen matrix laid down
10-14 days	Weak, fibrotic scar tissue with beginning revascularization; area vulnerable to stress
6 weeks	Scarring usually complete; tough, inelastic scar replaces necrotic myocardium; unable to contract and relax like healthy myocardial tissue

Modified from McCance KL, Huether SE: Pathophysiology: the biologic basis for disease in adults and children, ed 7, St Louis, 2014, Mosby.

9.6 Special Implications for the PTA: Myocardial Infarction

Early Postmyocardial Infarction Considerations

Although the myocardium must rest, bed rest puts the client at risk for development of hypovolemia (low blood volume), hypoxemia (hypoxia), muscle atrophy, and pulmonary embolus (PE). Developing a program of progressive physical activity with adequate pacing and rest periods begins within 24 hours for the acute care client in uncomplicated cases.

Gentle movement exercises, deep breathing, and coughing are usually begun immediately as prophylactic measures. Incisional pain or discomfort from cardiac surgery may cause a person to exhibit rapid, shallow respirations in an attempt to ease the discomfort. If analgesics are prescribed to prevent severe discomfort, the drug can be administered before therapy to better enable the person to carry out breathing exercises. This problem is of limited duration and usually resolves when the incision heals. The PTA must be aware that analgesics also mask pain response, making it possible for the client to overexert.

Early therapeutic exercise helps prevent cardiopulmonary complications, venous stasis, joint stiffness, and muscle weakness. Relaxation is often promoted with low-intensity activity. Activities that increase intrathoracic or intraabdominal pressure, such as breath holding and Valsalva's maneuvers, are contraindicated and should not be performed at any stage of the rehabilitation program.[61]

During the first 6 weeks after MI, the client is cautioned to avoid saunas, hot tubs, whirlpools, and excessively warm swimming pools. Early rehabilitation lasting 2 to 3 weeks is often followed by exercise testing, at which time water therapy may be permissible per physician approval.

Monitoring Vital Signs

The PTA must continually monitor for signs of impending infarction, including generalized or localized pain anywhere over the thorax, upper limbs, and neck; palpitations; dyspnea; light-headedness; syncope; sensation of indigestion; hiccups; and nausea (see Fig. 9.12). Pain medications, such as morphine, used to minimize discomfort initially may also depress the respiratory drive.

The coronary care unit therapist or PTA must monitor corresponding vital signs. The home health PTA must monitor pulse and blood pressure measurements for hypotension because of the side effects precipitated by antihypertensive medications, vasodilators, and other antianginal agents. Initial ambulation and activities at home should be roughly equivalent to levels achieved at the hospital at the time of discharge, depending on the client's physiologic response to the transition from hospital to home.

The client must increase activities gradually to avoid overtaxing the heart as it pumps oxygenated blood to the muscles. The metabolic equivalent system provides one way of measuring the amount of oxygen needed to perform an activity: 1 metabolic equivalent of the task (MET) equals 3.5 mL of oxygen per kilogram of body weight per minute; 1 MET is approximately equivalent to the oxygen uptake a person requires when resting. At 2 METs, the individual is working at twice his or her resting metabolic rate.

Early mobilization activities after acute MI should not exceed 1 to 2 METs (e.g., brushing teeth, eating). In comparison, people who can exercise to 8 or more METs can perform most daily physical activities. Generally 3 to 6 METs is considered the equivalent of moderate exercise. Activities with METs higher than 6 include singles tennis, cycling faster than 10 mph, walking faster than 4 mph, and cross-country skiing.

The MET system may not be as accurate for overweight or obese adults. Research has shown that using the MET system underestimates the energy used for an activity in this population group. Overweight or obese individuals may end up working at a level too high for them. The PTA is advised to use the rate of perceived exertion (RPE) instead.[72]

As activity level increases, the PTA must monitor heart rate, blood pressure, and fatigue, adjusting activity level accordingly. During phase I (acute hospital) care, the heart rate should not rise more than 25% above resting level, and blood pressure must not rise more than 25 mm Hg above resting level.

When systolic blood pressure falls or fails to increase as the intensity of exercise increases, exercise intensity should be immediately reduced. A drop in systolic blood pressure during exercise below the rest value as measured in the standing position is associated with increased risk of lethal arrhythmia in clients with a prior MI or myocardial ischemia.

Supplemental oxygen may be used to supply the myocardium with oxygen when the demand exceeds supply, reducing myocardial stress and eliminating dyspnea. Blood gas analysis is usually performed within 1 hour of initiating oxygen therapy to establish a baseline of arterial saturation. By monitoring blood gases, one can alter oxygen dose to regulate blood gases and acid-base balance. The PTA must monitor oxygen saturation levels during exercise or intervention, because these activities may increase myocardial oxygen demand.

The client with chronic obstructive pulmonary disease (COPD) who receives oxygen therapy must be monitored very closely for symptoms of decreased ventilation, such as headache, giddiness, tinnitus (ringing in the ears), nausea, weakness, and vomiting. Frequently persons with COPD retain carbon dioxide (CO_2), making the use of oxygen deadly. The administration of oxygen to a person with CO_2 retention can further depress the respiratory drive, resulting in death.

Exercise after Myocardial Infarction

As little as 15 years ago, exercise was avoided after a heart attack, but research has shown that a reasonable amount of regular exercise is the best way to strengthen the heart and control blood pressure, cholesterol, diabetes, and weight. Survivors who exercise usually require less medication, are less likely to need future invasive procedures, and are less likely to die of a second heart attack than those who remain sedentary.

Traditionally, isometric exercises have been contraindicated, and resistance training or weightlifting has been excluded from the cardiac client's program. Although weight training is not an isometric (static) exercise, it is similar during maximal lifts (Box 9.7).

A static muscle contraction that involves 70% or more of maximal effort results in a disproportionate increase in heart rate and blood pressure for the absolute level of oxygen uptake, which is potentially harmful for the ischemic heart.[115] For some people, use of a cane or walker is an isometric use of muscles that can increase heart

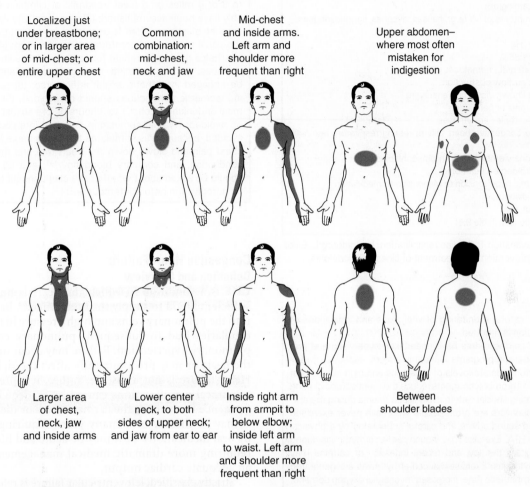

Localized just under breastbone; or in larger area of mid-chest; or entire upper chest

Common combination: mid-chest, neck and jaw

Mid-chest and inside arms. Left arm and shoulder more frequent than right

Upper abdomen– where most often mistaken for indigestion

Larger area of chest, neck, jaw and inside arms

Lower center neck, to both sides of upper neck; and jaw from ear to ear

Inside right arm from armpit to below elbow; inside left arm to waist. Left arm and shoulder more frequent than right

Between shoulder blades

Most common warning signs of heart attack

- Uncomfortable pressure, fullness, squeezing or pain in the center of the chest (prolonged)
- Pain that spreads to the throat, neck, back, jaw, shoulders, or arms
- Chest discomfort with lightheadedness, dizziness, sweating, pallor, nausea, or shortness of breath
- Prolonged symptoms unrelieved by antacids, nitroglycerin, or rest

Atypical, less common warning signs (especially women)

- Unusual chest pain (quality, location, e.g., burning, heaviness; left chest), stomach or abdominal pain
- Continuous midthoracic or interscapular pain
- Continuous neck or shoulder pain
- Isolated right biceps pain
- Pain relieved by antacids; pain unrelieved by rest or nitroglycerin
- Nausea and vomiting; flu-like manifestation without chest pain/discomfort
- Unexplained intense anxiety, weakness, or fatigue
- Breathlessness, dizziness

FIG. 9.12 Early warning signs of a heart attack. Multiple segmental nerve innervation shown in Fig. 9.7 accounts for the varied pain patterns possible. A woman can experience any of the various patterns described but is more likely to develop atypical symptoms of pain as depicted here. (From Goodman CC, Snyder TEK: Differential diagnosis for physical therapists: screening for referral, ed 5, St Louis, 2013.)

BOX 9.7   Contraindications to Exercise after Myocardial Infarction

- Acute myocardial infarction (MI) (<1 or 2 days after an MI without physician approval)
- Unstable angina; easily provoked angina
- New electrocardiogram
- Signs and symptoms of MI (e.g., nausea, dyspnea, light-headedness, chest pain)
- Pao_2 <60 mm Hg
- O_2 saturation <85%
- Hemoglobin <8 g/dL; hematocrit <26%
- Severe aortic outflow obstruction
- Suspected or known dissecting aneurysm
- Acute myocarditis or pericarditis
- Uncontrolled complex arrhythmias
- Active severe congestive heart failure; resting respiratory rate >45 breaths/min
- Recent pulmonary embolism or thrombophlebitis
- Untreated third-degree heart block
- Severe systemic hypertension unresponsive to medication
- Uncontrolled diabetes
- Acute infections
- Digoxin toxicity (see Table 9.5)

Modified from Kavanaugh T: Cardiac rehabilitation. In Goldberg L, Elliot DL: Exercise for prevention and treatment of illness, Philadelphia, 1994, FA Davis.

rate; therefore, careful monitoring of vital signs and indications of perceived exertion is required.

Now, low-risk cardiac clients have undertaken supervised and prescribed weight-training programs without ill effects, especially if regimens incorporate moderate levels of resistance and high numbers of repetitions.[109,212] Thrombolytic agents reduce the client's blood-clotting ability, necessitating special care to avoid tissue trauma during therapy.

Heart attack survivors are often people who have never exercised before and need sound advice and careful supervision by a physical therapist and/or PTA. Exercise may induce cardiac arrhythmias during diuretic and digitalis therapy, and recent ingestion of caffeine may exacerbate arrhythmias. Exercise-induced arrhythmias are generated by enhanced sympathetic tone, increased myocardial oxygen demand, or both. The immediate postexercise period is particularly dangerous because of high catecholamine levels associated with generalized vasodilation. Sudden termination of muscular activity is accompanied by diminished venous return and may lead to a reduction in coronary perfusion while the heart rate is elevated. A careful cool-down period is required, with continued monitoring of vital signs after exercise.

Sexual Activity

People with cardiac disease, both men and women, are prone to sexual dysfunction. The link between cardiovascular disease and erectile dysfunction in men has been the subject of recent studies. Erectile dysfunction is an early predictor of CAD and should be medically evaluated.[188,222] Problems may be caused by medications, anxiety, depression, or limited physical capacity. Hypertensive medications are the most common drugs to cause sexual dysfunction.

Fear of death during sexual intercourse, fear of another infarction caused by sexual activity, and diminished sexual ability caused by illness and aging may be present. The sexual partner may have many similar fears and may want to be included in any information provided about return to sexual function. The relative risk of triggering an MI by sexual activity is less than 1%.[156]

Sexual intercourse with orgasm is physiologically equivalent to activities such as a brisk walk or climbing a flight of stairs. It has been equated to 5 METs of work on an exercise stress test; preorgasmic and postorgasmic phases require about 3.7 METs.

Some general guidelines include the following: (1) when the client can sustain a heart rate of 110 to 120 beats/min with no shortness of breath or anginal pain, he or she can resume sexual activity; (2) sexual activity should be resumed gradually and only after activities such as walking moderate distances (equivalent to 3 or 4 miles on a level treadmill) or climbing stairs comfortably have been accomplished; (3) sexual activity causes the least amount of stress when it occurs in familiar surroundings with the usual partner in a comfortable environment; (4) gradual foreplay helps the heart prepare for coitus, and less strenuous sexual activities, such as cuddling, kissing, touching, and hugging, can be engaged in without sexual intercourse; (5) positions requiring isometric contractions should be avoided; (6) eating a large meal or drinking alcohol 1 to 3 hours before sexual activity should be avoided; (7) anal stimulation and anal intercourse should be avoided, because this stimulates the vagus nerve and may cause chest pain and slows down the heart rate and rhythm, impulse conduction, and coronary blood flow[141]; and (8) the physician should be asked about whether the client should take prophylactic nitroglycerin before intercourse.[119]

Congestive Heart Failure

Definition and Overview

CHF is a condition in which the heart is unable to pump sufficient blood to supply the body's needs. Backup of blood into the pulmonary veins and high pressure in the pulmonary capillaries lead to subsequent pulmonary congestion and pulmonary hypertension. Failure may occur on both sides of the heart or may predominantly affect the right or left side. Heart failure is not a disease; rather, it represents a group of clinical manifestations caused by inadequate pump performance from either the cardiac valves or the myocardium. It may be chronic over many years, requiring management by oral medications, or it may be acute and life-threatening, requiring more dramatic medical management to maintain an adequate cardiac output.

Strictly classified, left ventricular failure is referred to as *congestive heart failure*; acute right ventricular failure, seen almost exclusively in association with massive PE, is labeled *cor pulmonale*. Cor pulmonale is heart disease, but it arises from an underlying pulmonary pathologic condition.

Incidence

CHF is a common complication of ischemic and hypertensive heart disease, occurring most often in the older adult; in its chronic form it is referred to as a *cardiogeriatric syndrome*. Because the heart muscle is damaged during a heart attack, many heart attack survivors develop CHF. In the United States heart failure develops in an estimated 500,000 individuals annually: it is the most common cause for hospitalization in people older than age 65, with an estimated 5 million men and women living with CHF in the United States today. This condition is on the increase as the population ages and more people survive heart attacks.

Etiologic and Risk Factors

Many cardiac conditions predispose individuals to CHF, but hypertension is one of the most prevalent (Table 9.10). People with preexisting heart disease are at greatest risk for the

TABLE 9.10 Etiologic and Risk Factors Associated with Congestive Heart Failure

Etiologic Factors	Risk Factors[a]
Hypertension	Emotional stress
Coronary artery disease	Physical inactivity
Myocardial infarction	Obesity
Valvular heart disease	Diabetes mellitus
Congenital heart disease	Nutritional deficiency (vitamin C
Endocarditis	and thiamin)
Pericarditis	Fever
Myocarditis	Infection
Cardiomyopathy	Anemia
Chronic alcoholism	Thyroid disorders
Atrioventricular malformation	Pregnancy
Thyrotoxicosis (arrhythmia)	Paget disease
Chronic anemia	Pulmonary disease
	Medications (e.g., steroids, NSAIDs)
	Drug toxicity
	Renal disease

[a]Risk factors for new onset or exacerbation of previous congestive heart failure.
NSAIDs, Nonsteroidal antiinflammatory drugs.

development of CHF, because when the heart is stressed, compensatory mechanisms may be inadequate. For example, a faster redistribution of blood volume and increased demand for oxygen by the myocardium occur with increased activity, such as exercise, resulting in heart failure.

CHF occurring during middle age as distinguished from CHF at advanced age includes an increasing proportion of women. Women tend to have more risk factors and concurrent medical problems, such as hypertension, diabetes, or renal insufficiency. In addition, there may be other gender differences contributing to the development of CHF in women, such as differences in myocardial distensibility or hormonal differences as yet undetermined.

Paget disease causes vascular proliferation in the bones. When the disease involves over one-third of the skeleton, a high cardiac output state exists and may tax the compromised heart. Medications such as steroids or NSAIDs and drug toxicity are also risk factors. For the person with chronic, stable heart failure, acute exacerbations may occur, caused by alterations in therapy, client noncompliance with therapy, excessive salt and fluid intake, arrhythmias, excessive activity, PEs, infection, or progression of the underlying disease.

Pathogenesis and Clinical Manifestations

Over the last 15 years, major advances have occurred in our understanding of heart failure. The pathophysiology involves structural changes such as loss of myofilaments, apoptosis (programmed cell death), disturbances in calcium homeostasis, and alteration in receptor density, signal transduction, and collagen synthesis. This cascade of events occurs as a result of a cardiac event (e.g., MI) that develops into a clinical syndrome characterized by impaired cardiac function and circulatory congestion.[75]

CHF is a complex event involving one or both ventricles. This discussion is based on left ventricular failure. When the heart fails to propel blood forward normally, the body uses three neurohormonal compensatory mechanisms; these are effective for a short time but eventually become insufficient to meet the oxygen needs of the body.

First, the failing heart attempts to maintain a normal output of blood by enlarging its pumping chambers so that they can hold a greater volume of blood. This lengthening of the muscle fibers, called *ventricular dilation,* increases the amount of blood ejected from the heart. This compensatory mechanism has limits, because contractility of ventricular muscle fibers ceases to increase when they are stretched beyond a certain point.

During this *first compensatory phase,* the right ventricle continues to pump more blood into the lungs. Congestion occurs in the pulmonary circulation with accumulation of blood in the lungs. The immediate result is shortness of breath (most common symptom), and if the process continues, actual flooding of the air spaces of the lungs occurs, with fluid seeping from the distended blood vessels; this is called *pulmonary congestion* or *pulmonary edema.*

During the *second compensatory phase,* the sympathetic nervous system responds to increase the stimulation of the heart muscle, causing it to pump more often. In response to failing contractility of the myocardial cells, the sympathetic nervous system activates adaptive processes that increase the heart rate and increase its muscle mass to strengthen the force of its contractions. This results in ventricular hypertrophy and a need for more oxygen. Eventually, the coronary arteries cannot meet the oxygen demands of the enlarged myocardium, and the person may experience angina pectoris because of ischemia.

The *third compensatory phase* involves activation of the renin-angiotensin-aldosterone system. With less blood coming from the heart, less blood passes through the kidneys. The kidneys respond by retaining water and sodium in an effort to increase blood volume, which further exacerbates tissue edema. The expanded blood volume increases the load on an already compromised heart. These mechanisms are responsible for the symptoms of diaphoresis, cool skin, tachycardia, cardiac arrhythmias, and oliguria (reduced urine excretion).

When the combined efforts of these three compensatory mechanisms achieve a normal level of cardiac output, the client is said to have compensated CHF. Ultimately, however, the body's efforts to compensate may backfire and produce higher blood volume, higher blood pressure, and more stress on the already weakened heart. The heart's ongoing failure to supply the body with blood compels the body to keep compensating in ways that further burden the heart, and the cycle perpetuates itself. When these mechanisms are no longer effective and the disease progresses to the final stage of impaired heart function, the client has decompensated CHF.

Decompensated CHF ranges from mild congestion with few symptoms to life-threatening fluid overload and total heart failure (Table 9.11). Symptoms usually develop very gradually so that many people do not recognize or report signals of serious disease. The older adult in particular may wrongly associate early symptoms with a lack of fitness or consider them a sign of aging. Confusion and impaired thinking can characterize heart failure in older adults.

Left-sided heart failure. Failure of the left ventricle (Fig. 9.13) prevents the heart from pumping enough blood through the arterial system to meet the body's metabolic needs and causes either pulmonary edema or a disturbance in the respiratory control mechanisms.

TABLE 9.11	Clinical Manifestations of Heart Failure
Left Ventricular Failure	**Right Ventricular Failure**
Progressive dyspnea (exertional first)	Dependent edema (ankle or pretibial first)
Paroxysmal nocturnal dyspnea	Jugular vein distention
Orthopnea	Abdominal pain and distention
Productive spasmodic cough	Weight gain
Pulmonary edema	Right upper quadrant pain (liver congestion)
Extreme breathlessness	
Anxiety (associated with breathlessness)	Cardiac cirrhosis
	Ascites
Frothy pink sputum	Jaundice
Nasal flaring	Anorexia, nausea
Accessory muscle use	Cyanosis (nail beds)
Rales	Psychologic disturbances
Tachypnea	
Diaphoresis	
Cerebral hypoxia	
Irritability	
Restlessness	
Confusion	
Impaired memory	
Sleep disturbances	
Fatigue, exercise intolerance	
Muscular weakness	
Renal changes	

Dyspnea is subjective and does not always correlate with the extent of heart failure; exertional dyspnea occurs in all clients to some degree. The time it takes for dyspnea to subside is an indication of progress or deterioration in a client's status, and it can be measured for documentation. Paroxysmal nocturnal dyspnea resembles the frightening sensation of awakening with suffocation. Once the client is in the upright position, relief from the attack may not occur for 30 minutes or longer. The client often assumes a three-point position, sitting up with both hands on the knees and leaning forward. In severe heart failure, the client may resort to sleeping upright in a chair or recliner. Other sleep disturbances may occur from central sleep apnea present in approximately 40% of all adults with heart failure.

Fatigue and *muscular weakness* are often associated with left ventricular failure, because dyspnea develops along with weight gain and a faster resting heart rate, which decrease the person's ability to exercise. Inadequate cardiac output leads to decreased peripheral blood flow and blood flow to skeletal muscle. The resultant tissue hypoxia and slowed removal of metabolic wastes cause the person to tire easily. Disturbances in sleep and rest patterns may aggravate fatigue; muscle atrophy is common in advanced CHF.

Renal changes can occur in both right- and left-sided heart failure, but they are more evident with left-sided failure. During the day, the client is upright, decreased cardiac output reduces blood flow to the kidneys, and the formation of urine is reduced (oliguria). Sodium and water not excreted in the urine are retained in the vascular system, adding to the blood volume.

Diminished blood supply to the renal system causes the kidney to secrete renin, stimulating production of angiotensin, which causes vasoconstriction that causes an increase in peripheral vascular resistance, increasing blood pressure and cardiac work, and resulting in worse heart failure. Renin secretion also indirectly stimulates the secretion of aldosterone from the adrenal gland. Aldosterone acts on the renal tubules, causing them to increase reabsorption of sodium and water, further increasing fluid volume. At night, urine formation increases with the *recumbent* position as blood flow to the kidney improves. *Nocturia* may interfere with effective sleep patterns, which contributes to fatigue as mentioned.

Right-sided heart failure. Failure of the right ventricle to adequately pump blood to the lungs results in peripheral edema and venous congestion of the organs. Symptoms result from congestion in the heart's right side and throughout the venous system (see Table 9.11).

Dependent edema is one of the early signs of right ventricular failure, although significant CHF can be present in the absence of peripheral edema. In CHF, fluid is retained because the baroreceptors of the body sense a decreased volume of blood as a result of the heart's inability to pump an adequate amount of blood. The receptors subsequently relay a message to the kidneys to retain fluid so that a greater volume of blood can be ejected from the heart to the peripheral tissues.

The retained fluid commonly accumulates in the extracellular spaces of the periphery. The resultant edema is usually symmetric and occurs in the dependent parts of the body in which venous pressure is the highest. In ambulatory persons, edema begins in the feet and ankles and ascends up the lower legs. It is most noticeable at the end of a day and often decreases after a night's rest. In the recumbent person, pitting edema may develop in the presacral area and, as it worsens, progress to the medial thighs and genital area.

Jugular venous distention also results from fluid overload. The jugular veins empty unoxygenated blood directly into the superior vena cava. Because no cardiac valve exists to separate the superior vena cava from the right atrium, the jugular veins give information about activity on the right side of the heart. As fluid is retained and the heart's ability to pump is further compromised, the retained fluid backs up into both the lungs and the venous system, and the jugular veins reveal this. Jugular venous pulsations are examined by inspecting the silhouette of the neck with the person reclining at a 45-degree angle (Fig. 9.14). The right internal jugular vein is recommended because the left internal jugular may be falsely elevated in some people.

As the liver becomes congested with venous blood it becomes enlarged and *abdominal pain* occurs. If this occurs rapidly, stretching of the capsule surrounding the liver causes severe discomfort, and the person may notice either a constant aching or a sharp *right upper quadrant pain*. In chronic CHF, long-standing congestion of the liver with venous blood and anoxia can lead to ascites and jaundice, which are symptoms of liver damage. Anorexia, nausea, and bloating develop secondary to venous congestion of the GI tract. Anorexia and nausea may also result from digitalis toxicity, which is a common problem because digitalis is usually prescribed for CHF.

Cyanosis of the nail beds appears as venous congestion reduces peripheral blood flow. Clients with CHF often feel anxious, frightened, and depressed. Fears may be expressed as frightening nightmares, insomnia, acute anxiety states, depression, or withdrawal from reality.

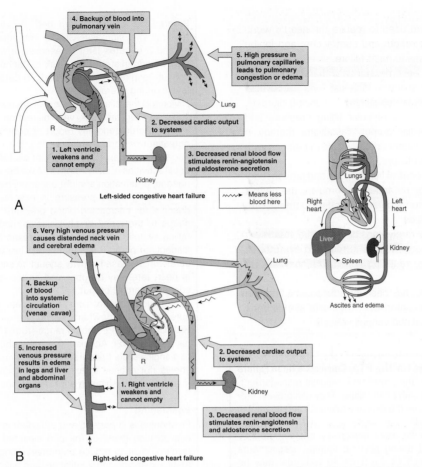

FIG. 9.13 Pathophysiologic mechanisms of congestive heart failure. (A) Left-sided heart failure leads to pulmonary edema (see text description). (B) Right ventricular failure causes peripheral edema that is most prominent in the lower extremities. *Inset,* Integration of the pulmonary and systemic circulation. When the heart contracts normally, it pumps blood simultaneously into both loops, but pump failure causes circulatory or pulmonary problems, depending on the underlying pathologic mechanism. *R,* right; *L,* left. (From Van Meter KC, Hubert RJ: Gould's Pathophysiology for the health professions, ed 5, St Louis, 2014, Saunders; inset from Damjanov I: Pathology for the health-related professions, ed 4, St Louis, 2012, Saunders.)

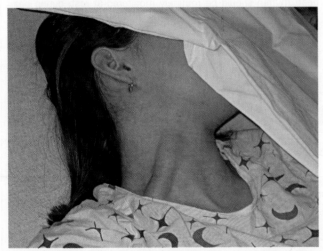

FIG. 9.14 Jugular venous distention occurs bilaterally if there is a cardiac cause such as congestive heart failure; unilateral distention indicates a localized problem. (From Adams JG: Emergency medicine: clinical essentials, ed 2, Philadelphia, 2013, Saunders.)

Medical Management

Prevention and Treatment

Managing heart failure begins with treatment of the underlying cause whenever possible. Nonpharmacologic interventions such as diet and exercise that alter interactions between the heart and the periphery are now accepted therapeutic approaches.

Alterations in lifestyle reduce symptoms and the need for additional medication. There is an urgent need to develop more effective strategies for the prevention and treatment of this increasingly common disorder. Multiple comorbidities in older clients require a multidisciplinary approach to management. Persons with CHF are placed on a sodium-restricted diet, sometimes with limited fluid intake. Emotional and physical rest during the initial phases of intervention is also important in diminishing the workload of the heart.

Pharmacotherapy

Pharmacologic agents are used to reduce the heart's workload, increase muscle strength and contraction, and inhibit neuroendocrine responses to heart failure.

ACE inhibitors have become standard therapy for heart failure because of their ability to increase renal blood flow and decrease renal vascular resistance, enhancing diuresis. ACE inhibitors reduce left ventricular filling pressure and moderately increase cardiac output. Vasodilator therapy in combination with ACE inhibitors prolongs life in persons with moderate to severe heart failure.

Diuretics are used to control fluid buildup and prevent congestion, and digoxin may be added to stimulate the heart's pumping action if symptoms persist despite treatment with ACE inhibitors and diuretics.

The *β-blockers*, once rarely considered in the treatment of CHF, have been shown effective in reducing symptoms, improving clinical status, reducing hospitalizations, and reducing the risk of death.

A new drug, *nesiritide,* has been introduced as a first-line medication for decompensated CHF. It inhibits sympathetic activity and dilates arterial and venous vessels.

9.7 Special Implications for the PTA: Congestive Heart Failure

PTAs have a unique role in the prevention, medical management, and rehabilitation of people with heart failure. They can provide programs that profoundly improve the exercise tolerance and functional status of individuals with CHF.

Medical intervention can be more objectively implemented by using information obtained during physical therapy assessments and interventions. Tests such as the 6-minute walk test may be helpful in predicting peak oxygen consumption and early survival as well as implementing a proper exercise conditioning program for people with advanced heart failure.[46]

Education of physicians and other health care professionals about the role of the physical therapist in defining prescriptive exercise is important. Consideration for the complex pathologic conditions and comorbidities of people in this population is an important contribution to cardiac rehabilitation from the PT's and the PTA's training.

Early Considerations

Clients hospitalized with severe CHF require a therapy program to maintain pulmonary function and prevent complications of bed rest. An important aspect of intervention is functional assessment and physical exercise within the limitations set by the physician.

The PTA should be aware of psychosocial considerations in older adults with CHF. Neuropsychiatric conditions such as Alzheimer's dementia and complications such as delirium are common in older adults with CHF. Persistent alcohol abuse and cigarette smoking often contribute to the onset and progression of heart failure. Major depression, other depressive disorders, anxiety, and social isolation are common and have adverse effects on functional status, quality of life, and prognosis. Working as a team with psychologists and social workers can address these issues effectively.

Monitoring Vital Signs

Aerobic capacity is likely impaired and even more so if the client is deconditioned, adaptive responses to activity may be attenuated or inadequate, activity may exacerbate cardiovascular pump dysfunction, and signs of fatigue and shortness of breath are common. The downward cycle of disease—deconditioning, decreased activity, and disability—necessitates the monitoring of vital signs.[38]

Progressing activities from bed rest to transfers or ambulation requires vital sign assessment immediately after the major activity and 3 minutes later to assess for return to baseline. Oxygen may be administered by mask or cannula; team members should consult respiratory therapy staff to determine appropriate oxygen levels during exercise.

Monitor the client for signs of increasing peripheral edema by assessing jugular neck vein distention, peripheral edema in the legs or sacrum, and any report of right upper quadrant pain. In the outpatient or home health setting, the client is advised to call the nurse or physician if shoes, belt, or pants become too tight to fasten, usual activities of daily living or tasks become difficult, extra sleep is needed, or urination at night becomes more frequent.

Monitoring blood pressure is essential to detect heart failure; observe for decreasing blood pressure and report any change in status to the nurse or physician immediately. Observe for flat or falling systolic blood pressure in response to activity indicative of inadequate pump function (a linear increase of systolic blood pressure with increased activity should be seen). Exaggerated increases in heart rate may be observed as the heart attempts to maintain adequate cardiac output.

Continuous supervision and frequent monitoring of blood pressure are necessary when starting an exercise program for someone with CHF. The RPE should range from 11 to 14 (light to somewhat hard; Table 9.12). Anginal symptoms should not exceed 2 on the 0 to 4 angina scale (moderate to bothersome), and exertional dyspnea should not exceed a rating of mild (some difficulty with activity). Initially, full resuscitation equipment should be available.[31]

Positioning

Positioning is important, and the client is taught to use a high Fowler's position (head of the bed elevated at least 20 inches above level) or chair to reduce pulmonary congestion, facilitate diaphragmatic expansion and ventilation, and ease dyspnea.

The legs are maintained in a dependent position as much as possible to decrease venous return. ROM to decrease venous pooling and monitoring for the development of thrombophlebitis (e.g., unilateral swelling, calf pain, pallor) are required.

Exercise and Congestive Heart Failure

The American College of Sports Medicine's guidelines[10] suggest that CHF clients entering an exercise program should start with moderate-intensity exercise (40% to 60% Vo_{2max}) for a duration of 2 to 6 minutes, followed by 2 minutes of rest. Blood pressure and heart rhythm should be routinely monitored at rest, during peak exercise, and after cool down. The goal is to gradually increase the intensity and duration of exercise. Others advocate starting CHF clients on low to moderate exercise with a shorter duration of exercise initially and a shorter rest period of less than 2 minutes. Recommendations for interval exercise training (following work phases of 30 seconds with recovery phases of 60 seconds) have also been reported.[145,177]

The best guideline is to customize initial exercise intensity for each individual,[238] keeping in mind the individual's goals and expected outcomes. Exercise should be avoided immediately after eating or after taking vasodilator medication. Using an interval training approach is helpful with those individuals who demonstrate marked exercise intolerance.

Symptoms and general fatigue level serve as guidelines to determine frequency, and warm-up and cool-down periods should be longer than normal for observation of possible arrhythmias. Determination of appropriate exercise intensity based on 40% to 60% Vo_{2max} is recommended because the response to exercise is frequently abnormal in people with CHF. Alternately, the initial exercise intensity should be 10 beats below any significant symptoms, including angina, exertional hypotension, arrhythmias, and dyspnea.

TABLE 9.12 Borg Scale of Perceived Exertion[a]

10-Grade Scale	Verbal Rating
0	No exertion at all
0.5	Extremely light
1	Very light
2	Light
3	Moderate
4	Somewhat hard
5	Hard
6	—
7	Very hard
8	—
9	—
10	Very, very hard
—	Maximal exertion

[a]Using a perceived exertion scale is a useful approach to activity prescription. The individual is asked to identify a desirable rating of perceived exertion and uses that level of intensity as a daily guideline for activity. A suggested rating of perceived exertion for most healthy individuals is 3 to 5 (moderate to hard on the 10-grade scale); for the compromised person, a more moderate level of perceived exertion may be recommended by the physician.

Modified from Borg GA: Psychosocial basis of perceived exertion, Med Sci Sports Exerc 472:194–381, 1982.

Rehabilitation personnel must observe for symptoms of cardiac decompensation during exercise, including cough or dyspnea, hypotension, light-headedness, cyanosis, angina, and arrhythmias. Endurance exercise training has been shown to modify neuroendocrine activation in heart failure and may have a long-term beneficial impact.[32]

The PTA should keep in mind that some older CHF clients are unable to increase their exercise intensity or duration despite starting very slowly. These people do not achieve the goal of increased endurance and often leave the program because of increased symptoms and exercise intolerance. Maintaining or even improving functional activities and independence at home may be more appropriate goals for this group.

Medications

Diuretics can produce mild to severe electrolyte imbalance requiring special consideration. A small drop in the serum potassium level can precipitate digoxin poisoning and serious arrhythmias. This situation is a life-threatening condition that occurs in one of every five clients and may have systemic or cardiac manifestations.

Any sign or symptom of digitalis toxicity should be reported to the physician (see Table 9.5). Digitalis toxicity can cause a dip in the ST segment on the ECG; whenever possible, the ECG should be monitored during exercise.

If the serum albumin level is low, digitalis may not be bound to the albumin-binding sites and will be circulating as "free" digoxin. Watch for a low, irregular pulse (less than 60 beats/min); the heart rate normally increases to compensate for CHF, but in the presence of digoxin, heart rate decreases.

NSAIDs, including over-the-counter drugs such as ibuprofen, increase fluid retention independently and significantly blunt the action of diuretics and other cardiovascular drugs, exacerbating preexisting CHF and causing isolated lower extremity edema. The major consideration for exercise in clients taking ACE inhibitors is the possibility of hypotension and accompanying arrhythmias. These problems should be reported to the physician and can be addressed by maintaining proper hydration and by altering dosages and the simultaneous use of other medications.

Orthostatic (Postural) Hypotension

Definition and Overview

The term *orthostatic (postural) hypotension* signifies a decrease of 20 mm Hg or greater in systolic blood pressure or a drop of 10 mm Hg or more in both systolic and diastolic arterial blood pressure with a concomitant pulse increase of 15 beats/min or more on standing from a supine or sitting position.

Orthostatic hypotension may be acute and temporary or chronic. Orthostatic hypotension occurs frequently in older adults and occurs in more than one half of all frail, older adults, contributing significantly to morbidity from syncope, falls, vital organ ischemia, and mortality in older adults with diabetic hypertension. It is highly variable over time but most prevalent in the morning when supine blood pressure is highest and on first arising.

Etiologic Factors

Postural reflexes are slowed as part of the aging process for some, but not all, persons. Normal aging is associated with various changes that may lead to postural hypotension. Cardiac output falls with age; in the older adult with hypertension, it is even lower. These normal changes obviously predispose the aging adult to postural hypotension from any process that further reduces fluid volume or vascular integrity.

In addition, as systolic pressure rises from atherosclerosis, changes further increase the likelihood of postural hypotension. In the older adult with hypertension and cardiovascular disease receiving vasoactive drugs, the circulatory adjustments to maintain blood pressure are disturbed, leaving the person vulnerable to postural hypotension.[117]

Drugs are a major cause of orthostatic hypotension in the aging adult. Many have effects on the autonomic nervous system, both centrally and peripherally, and on fluid balance. Diuretics, calcium channel blockers, nitrates, and L-dopa have hypotensive effects. Antidepressants are a common, overlooked cause of orthostasis, even though this is a known side effect of these medications. A general result of treatment for hypertension may be hypotension. In addition, many older adults with systolic hypertension have postural hypotension that may require management before the hypertension is addressed.

Pathogenesis

Orthostasis is a physiologic stress related to upright posture. When a normal individual stands up, the gravitational changes on the circulation are compensated for by several mechanisms. On standing, the force of gravity causes venous pooling in the lower limbs, a sharp decline in venous return, and reduction in filling pressure of the heart, which increase further on prolonged standing because of shifting of water.

These mechanical events can cause a marked reduction in cardiac output and consequent fall in arterial blood pressure. In healthy people, cardiac output and blood pressure regulation are maintained by powerful compensatory mechanisms involving a rise in heart rate. Blood pressure is maintained by a rise in peripheral resistance. These compensatory mechanisms are initiated by the baroreceptors located in the aortic arch and carotid bifurcation. Orthostatic hypotension results from failure of the arterial baroreflex, most commonly because of disorders of the autonomic nervous system.

In people with autonomic failure or dysreflexia, orthostatic hypotension results from an impaired capacity to increase vascular resistance during standing. This dysfunction leads to increased downward pooling of venous blood and a consequent reduction in stroke volume and cardiac output that exaggerates the orthostatic fall in blood pressure.

Clinical Manifestations

Orthostatic hypotension is often accompanied by dizziness, blurring or loss of vision, and syncope or fainting. There are three main modes of presentation in the older adult: (1) falls or mobility problems, (2) acute or chronic mental confusion, and (3) cardiac symptoms.

A common clinical picture is the person whose legs give way when attempting to stand, usually after prolonged recumbency, after physical exertion, or in a warm environment. These episodes may be accompanied by confusion, pallor, tremor, and unsteadiness. Loss of consciousness may cause frequent falls and additional injuries that can be quite serious. Ischemic neck pain in the suboccipital and paracervical region is often reported by individuals with autonomic failure and orthostatic hypotension.[29]

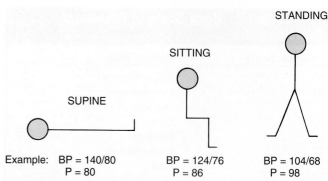

Example: BP = 140/80   BP = 124/76   BP = 104/68
         P = 80   P = 86   P = 98

FIG. 9.15 Assessing postural hypotension. After measuring the blood pressure (BP) and pulse (P) of the person in the supine position, leave the blood pressure cuff in place and assist the person in sitting. Remeasure the blood pressure within 15 to 30 seconds. Assist the person in standing, and measure again. A drop of more than 20 mm Hg systolic and more than 10 mm diastolic accompanied by a 10% to 20% increase in heart rate (pulse) indicates postural hypotension. Sample measurements are given. (From Black JM, Hawks JH: Medical-surgical nursing: clinical management for positive outcomes, ed 8, St Louis, 2009, Saunders.)

9.8 Special Implications for the PTA: Orthostatic Hypotension Many medications used to treat hypertension can result in hypotension, especially when combined with interventions or exercise that results in vasodilation. Of particular concern are heat modalities, such as the whirlpool or Hubbard tank. In addition, moderate to vigorous exercise of large muscle groups can produce significant vasodilation and can result in hypotension. This is particularly true after exercise, when venous return diminishes as exercise abruptly ceases. A cool-down period is essential, and safety measures must be used.[232] Aerobic conditioning is an important part of treatment for orthostatic hypotension resulting from autonomic insufficiency, which is perhaps best accomplished through aquatic exercise therapy.[89]

Stationary standing, as is performed in many activities of daily living, can produce hypotension, especially among those individuals with autonomic failure. With autonomic failure, symptoms of postural hypotension are increased on standing after exercise.

Anyone with orthostatic hypotension, especially persons taking antihypertensive agents, should be instructed to rise slowly from the bed or chair after a long period of recumbency or sitting to avoid loss of balance and prevent falls. Dorsiflexing the feet (ankle pumps), raising the arms overhead with diaphragmatic breathing, and abdominal compression before standing often promote venous return to the heart, accelerate the pulse, and increase blood pressure.

The use of abdominal binders and elastic stockings may also help with venous return. Stockings should not be taken off at night to avoid falls when getting up to go to the bathroom or when getting out of bed in the morning. Elevating the head of the bed 5 to 20 degrees prevents the nocturnal diuresis and supine hypertension caused by nocturnal shifts of interstitial fluid from the legs to the rest of the circulation. Eating small meals may help to avoid postprandial (after eating) hypotension.

The person who becomes hypotensive should assume a supine position with legs elevated to increase venous return and to ensure cerebral blood flow. As previously mentioned, this position must be monitored carefully for anyone with orthostatic hypotension and CHF, possibly necessitating modifying the position to include slight head and upper body elevation. Crossing the legs, which involves contraction of the agonist and antagonist muscles, also has been shown to increase cardiac output, increasing blood pressure.[208]

The physician and supervising PT should be notified if the person remains symptomatic after these measures have been taken. Anyone who is considered borderline hypotensive when tested in the supine position should have blood pressures measured and pulses counted in a sitting position with the legs dangling. If no change occurs when this is done, repeat the measurements with the person standing, if possible. A drop in systolic pressure of 10 to 20 mm Hg or more associated with an increase in pulse rate of more than 15 beats/min suggests depleted intravascular volume (Fig. 9.15).

Myocardial Disease
Myocarditis

Myocarditis is a relatively uncommon acute or chronic inflammatory condition of the muscular walls of the heart (myocardium). It has now been reclassified by the American Heart Association as an acquired (inflammatory) cardiomyopathy.[139]

It is most often a result of bacterial or viral infection, but it also includes those inflammatory processes related to infectious and noninfectious causes of ischemic heart disease. Other possible causes of myocarditis include chest radiation for treatment of malignancy, sarcoidosis, and drugs.

The PTA is most likely to treat the person with systemic lupus erythematosus (SLE) who may have a type of myocarditis called *lupus carditis*. SLE is a multisystem autoimmune disease characterized by a release of autoantibodies into the circulation, with a subsequent inflammatory process that can target the heart and vasculature.

Myocarditis typically evolves through active, healing, and healed stages that are characterized by myocyte necrosis with replacement fibrosis over time. Ventricular tachyarrhythmias develop as a result of the pathologic changes creating an electrically unstable environment.[139]

Clinical evidence of cardiac involvement is found in up to one-half of all people with SLE. Clinical manifestations may include mild continuous chest pain or soreness in the epigastric region or under the sternum, palpitations, fatigue, and dyspnea; onset may follow a viral upper respiratory tract illness in the population at large as well as in persons with SLE. Complications include heart failure, arrhythmias, dilated (congestive) cardiomyopathy, and sudden death.

Myocarditis usually resolves with treatment of the underlying condition or cause; specific antimicrobial therapy is prescribed if an infectious agent can be identified. Viral myocarditis is treated with medications that improve cardiac output and reduce arrhythmias, if present. Management of myocarditis in SLE is usually with corticosteroids, but immunosuppressive agents may be required. Myocarditis that progresses to dilated cardiomyopathy with heart failure is frequently fatal without heart transplantation.

9.9 Special Implications for the PTA: Myocarditis Active myocarditis is considered a contraindication for therapy, because this condition can progress very quickly and stress must be avoided; each case is evaluated by the physician. Athletes in whom myocarditis is suspected or diagnosed should discontinue all sports for 6 months after onset of symptoms. Preparticipation evaluation of cardiac function is essential before resumption of sports activities. An athlete can resume competing when ventricular function and cardiac dimensions return to normal and clinically significant arrhythmias are absent on ambulatory monitoring.[62]

Cardiomyopathy

Definition and overview. Cardiomyopathy is actually part of a group of conditions affecting the heart muscle itself, so that contraction and relaxation of myocardial muscle fibers are impaired. The original definition of *cardiomyopathy* stated that this condition was not caused by other heart or systemic disease, which excluded structural and functional abnormalities caused by valvular disorders, CAD, hypertension, congenital defects, and pulmonary vascular disorders.

The American Heart Association 2006 Expert Consensus Panel proposed the following definition for cardiomyopathy, which reflects the idea that many cardiomyopathies have an underlying cause. Ischemia from CAD is probably the most common.

Cardiomyopathies are a heterogeneous group of diseases of the myocardium associated with mechanical and/or electrical dysfunction that usually (but not invariably) exhibit inappropriate ventricular hypertrophy or dilatation and are caused by a variety of causes that frequently are genetic. Cardiomyopathies either are confined to the heart or are part of generalized systemic disorders, often leading to cardiovascular death or progressive heart failure–related disability.[139]

Cardiomyopathies are classified as *primary* and *secondary*, based on predominant organ involvement. Primary cardiomyopathies are called genetic, mixed (genetic and nongenetic), and acquired. They are confined to the heart muscle.

Generally, congenital or familial types of cardiomyopathies are fairly uncommon individually, but a growing number of different types caused by mutations in genetic encoding have been identified.

Mixed cardiomyopathies include dilated and primary restrictive nonhypertrophied cardiomyopathies. An example of an acquired cardiomyopathy is myocarditis. Considerable overlap can occur among the primary classifications within the same person.

Secondary cardiomyopathies involve myocardial pathology as part of a large number and variety of generalized systemic disorders that affect the heart along with other organs at the same time.

Incidence and risk factors. Cardiomyopathy can affect people of any age and is often seen in young adults in the second and third decades. The actual incidence is unknown, but the disease may be more common than was previously realized.

This increase in incidence may be attributed to two important variables: (1) improved technology, which has allowed for more accurate evaluation of ventricular dimensions and ventricular wall movement and (2) an increased incidence of myocarditis, an important precursor to cardiomyopathy, as a result of a wide variety of pathogens, toxins, and autoimmune reactions.

Delayed-onset cardiotoxic effects of chemotherapeutic agents may appear as chronic cardiomyopathy. Risk factors for the development of this type of cardiomyopathy include increasing doses of chemotherapeutic agents and previous mediastinal radiation.[231]

Dilated cardiomyopathy occurs most often in black men aged 40 to 60 years. About half of the cases of dilated cardiomyopathy are idiopathic, and the remainder result from some known disease process. Risk factors for dilated cardiomyopathy may include obesity, long-term alcohol abuse, systemic hypertension, cigarette smoking, infections, and pregnancy.

Hypertrophic cardiomyopathy appears to be genetically transmitted as an autosomal dominant trait on chromosome 14; currently 11 mutant genes have been linked with hypertrophic cardiomyopathy. It is still the most frequently occurring cardiomyopathy and the most common cause of sudden cardiac death in the young.[139]

Restrictive cardiomyopathy occurs as a result of myocardial fibrosis, hypertrophy, infiltration, or a defect in myocardial relaxation.

Pathogenesis. The exact pathogenesis of cardiomyopathy is unknown; the risk factors mentioned previously seem to lower the threshold for the development of cardiomyopathy.

Regardless of the underlying cause, dilated cardiomyopathy results from extensively damaged myocardial muscle fibers and is characterized by cardiac enlargement. The heart ejects blood less efficiently than normal; thus a large volume of blood remains in the left ventricle after systole, which results in ventricular dilation with enlargement and dilation of all four chambers and eventually leads to CHF (Figs. 9.16 and 9.17).

Clinical manifestations. Generally the symptoms of cardiomyopathy are the same as for heart failure: dyspnea, orthopnea, tachycardia, palpitations, peripheral edema, and distended jugular vein.

Dilated cardiomyopathy is characterized by fatigue and weakness, and chest pain (unlike angina) may occur. Blood pressure is usually normal or low.

Hypertrophic cardiomyopathy is frequently asymptomatic, and sudden death is the presenting sign; hypertrophic cardiomyopathy is the most common cause of sudden death in young competitive athletes. The most common symptom is dyspnea.

Restrictive cardiomyopathy causes clinical manifestations related to decreasing cardiac output. As cardiac output falls and intraventricular pressures rise, signs of CHF appear. The earliest manifestations may include exercise intolerance, fatigue, and shortness of breath followed by other symptoms such as peripheral edema and ascites.

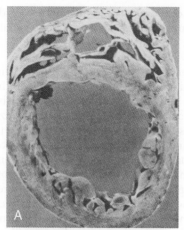

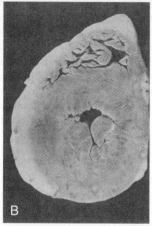

FIG. 9.16 (A) Cross-sectional view of dilated cardiomyopathy. (B) Hypertrophied heart. (From Kinney M: Comprehensive cardiac care, ed 7, St Louis, 1991, Mosby.)

9.10 Special Implications for the PTA: Cardiomyopathy Sudden death can occur, but the incidence is rare. It occurs more often in younger people who have cardiomyopathy, and it may be avoided by eliminating strenuous exercise when a diagnosis has been established. Rest improves cardiac function and reduces heart size.

During the early stages of the disease, many people find it difficult to accept activity restrictions and need encouragement to follow guidelines for activity restriction. Clients should avoid poorly tolerated activities; combine rest with activity; understand that physical stress and emotional stress exacerbate the disease; learn correct breathing techniques, because Valsalva's maneuver should be avoided; and understand that alcohol depresses myocardial contractility and should be eliminated.

The PTA can provide valuable information regarding energy conservation techniques to assist persons with continued independence in activities of daily living and possibly even with improvement of activity tolerance. This is especially true for the person awaiting a cardiac transplant.

The evaluation should include an assessment of current physical activity levels and exercise tolerance and monitoring of heart rate and rhythm, blood pressure, respiratory responses, and any other signs and symptoms of exercise intolerance.[231] A scale that rates perceived exertion (see Table 9.12) is often useful for establishing initial exercise guidelines toward improving endurance.

For the person who has been hospitalized and has not ambulated yet, the therapist will need to assess tolerance to activities in bed before ambulation. During activities, monitor pulse, oxygen saturation, respirations, blood pressure, and color. The heart rate, systolic blood pressure, and respiratory rate normally increase in proportion to the exercise (movement) intensity, whereas the diastolic blood pressure changes minimally (±10 mm Hg).

Improved activity tolerance may be demonstrated by minimal change in pulse or blood pressure during activities with minimal fatigue after the activity. Pulse, respirations, and blood pressure should return to a normal range within 3 minutes of the end of the activity. Discontinue any activity that results in chest pain,

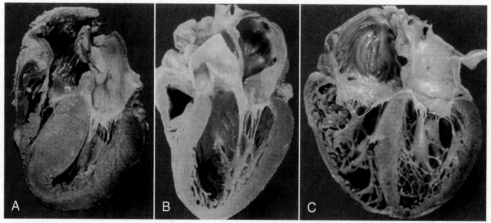

FIG. 9.17 Gross pathologic specimens of the cardiomyopathies. (A) Hypertrophic cardiomyopathy, showing a marked increase in myocardial mass and preferential hypertrophy of the interventricular septum. (B) Normal heart, with normal left ventricular dimensions and thickness. (C) Dilated cardiomyopathy, showing marked increase in chamber size. Atrial enlargement is also evident in both cardiomyopathies (A and C). (From Seidman JG, Seidman C: The genetic basis for cardiomyopathy: from mutation identification to mechanistic paradigms, Cell 104:557, 2001.)

severe dyspnea, cyanosis, dizziness, hypotension, or sustained tachycardia.

Abnormal responses include either blunted or excessive rises in heart rate or systolic blood pressure, excessive increases in diastolic blood pressure or respiratory rate, a fall in systolic blood pressure with increasing activity, or increasing irregularity of the pulse. These signs may be the result of cardiopulmonary toxicity or simply the result of deconditioning. Increasing irregularity in the pulse with pairs or runs of faster beats or more than six isolated irregular beats per minute must be reported to the physician.[231] If the person is taking diuretics, monitor for signs of too-vigorous diuresis (e.g., muscle cramps, orthostatic hypotension). If the person becomes hypotensive, use a supine position with legs elevated to increase venous return and to ensure cerebral blood flow.

Trauma

Nonpenetrating

Any blunt chest trauma, which is especially common in steering wheel impact from an automobile accident, may produce myocardial contusion, resulting in myocardial hemorrhage with little if any myocardial scar once healing is complete. Large contusions may lead to myocardial scars, cardiac rupture, CHF, or formation of aneurysms.

The chest pain of myocardial contusion is similar to that of MI and is often confused with musculoskeletal pain from soft tissue consequences of chest trauma. Myocardial contusion is usually treated similarly to MI, with initial monitoring and subsequent progressive ambulation and cardiac rehabilitation.

Penetrating

Penetrating cardiac injuries are most often caused by external objects, such as bullets or knives, and sometimes from bony fragments secondary to chest injury. Iatrogenic causes of cardiac penetrating injury include perforation of the heart during catheterization and cardiac trauma from cardiopulmonary resuscitation. Complications include arrhythmias, aneurysm formation, death from infection, a form of pericarditis associated with this type of injury, ventricular septal defects, and foreign body embolus.

DISEASE AFFECTING THE CARDIAC NERVOUS SYSTEM

Arrhythmias: Disturbances of Rate or Rhythm

Definition and Overview

The number of times the heart beats (rate) and the heart rhythm are generated and regulated by the sinoatrial (SA) node, which is the internal pacemaker located in the upper right portion of the heart. The signal from the SA node travels through the cardiac conduction system, first through the walls of the atria and then through the walls of the ventricles, causing the atrial (supraventricular) and ventricular chambers of the heart to contract and relax at regular rates necessary to maintain circulation at different levels of activity. An arrhythmia (dysrhythmia) is a disturbance of heart rate or rhythm caused by an abnormal rate of electrical impulse generation by the SA node or the abnormal conduction of impulses.

Arrhythmias can be classified according to their origin as ventricular or supraventricular (atrial), according to the pattern (fibrillation or flutter), or according to the speed or rate at which they occur (tachycardia or bradycardia).

Several types of atrial fibrillation (AF) are now recognized, including the first-detected episode of AF (which may or may not be symptomatic and may self-resolve), recurrent paroxysmal AF (two or more episodes that resolve spontaneously), persistent AF, and permanent AF. Persistent AF is sustained for more than 7 days. It can occur after a first-detected episode of AF or after recurrent paroxysmal AF. Permanent AF, also known as *chronic AF,* occurs when sinus rhythm cannot be sustained after cardioversion (normal heart rhythm returns spontaneously) or when the decision has been made to let AF continue without efforts to restore normal sinus rhythm.[77]

Arrhythmias vary in severity from mild, asymptomatic disturbances that require no intervention to catastrophic ventricular fibrillation, which requires immediate resuscitation. The clinical significance depends on the effect on cardiac output and blood pressure, which is partially influenced by the site of origin.

Etiologic Factors and Incidence

Arrhythmias may be congenital or may result from one of several factors, including hypertrophy of heart muscle fibers secondary to hypertension, previous MI, valvular heart disease, or degeneration of conductive tissue that is necessary to maintain normal heart rhythm (called *sick sinus syndrome*).

Chronic alcohol use and binge drinking have been linked with disturbances in cardiac rhythm, even in individuals without underlying heart disease. *Holiday heart syndrome* is the term used to describe acute arrhythmia (usually supraventricular tachycardia [SVT]) triggered by excessive alcohol intake in an otherwise healthy person. The affected individual experiences intermittent or continuous palpitations, with dyspnea, dizziness, or chest pain often mentioned.

The prevalence of AF doubles with each advancing decade of age beginning at age 50 to 59 years, with a statistically significant increase among men aged 65 to 84 years, although this gap closes with advancing age and remains unexplained.[114,146]

BMI appears to correlate strongly with the risk of AF.[66] With each unit increment of BMI the risk of AF increases 3%. A person who is obese has about a 34% greater risk of AF compared with a person with normal BMI. Moreover, people in the heaviest BMI category have 2.3 times the risk. Improved cardiac care has increased the number of survivors of cardiac incidents who may experience subsequent complications, such as arrhythmias.

Cardiac arrhythmias are very common in the setting of heart failure, with atrial and ventricular arrhythmias often present in the same person. Arrhythmias can occur when a portion of the heart is temporarily deprived of oxygen, disturbing the normal pathway of the heartbeat. Toxic doses of cardioactive drugs, phenylpropanolamine found in some decongestants, alcohol and caffeine consumption, high fevers, and excessive production of thyroid hormone (hyperthyroidism) may also lead to arrhythmias. In many cases, particularly in younger people, there is no known or apparent cause.

Pathogenesis and Clinical Manifestations

Rate. The adult heart beats an average of 60 to 100 times per minute; an arrhythmia is considered to be any significant deviation from the normal range. Whether change in heart rate produces symptoms at rest or on exertion depends on the underlying state of the cardiac muscle and its ability to alter its stroke output to compensate.

Rate arrhythmias are of two basic types: tachycardia and bradycardia. Tachycardia occurs when the heart beats too fast (more than 100 beats/min). Tachycardia develops in the presence of increased sympathetic stimulation, such as occurs with fear, pain, emotion, exertion, or exercise; or with ingestion of artificial stimulants, such as caffeine, nicotine, and amphetamines.

Tachycardia is also found in situations in which the demands for oxygen are increased, such as fever, CHF, infection, anemia, hemorrhage, myocardial injury, and hyperthyroidism. Usually the individual with tachycardia perceives no symptoms, and medical intervention is directed toward the underlying cause.

Bradycardia (less than 50 beats/min) is normal in well-trained athletes, but it is also common in individuals taking β-blockers, those who have had traumatic brain injuries or brain tumors, and those experiencing increased vagal stimulation to the physiologic pacemaker.

Organic disease of the sinus node, especially in older people and those with heart disease, can also cause sinus bradycardia. Bradycardia is usually asymptomatic, but when it is caused by a pathologic condition, the person may experience fatigue, dyspnea, syncope, dizziness, angina, or *diaphoresis* (profuse perspiration). Medical intervention is not usually required unless symptoms interfere with function or are induced by drugs or angina.

Rhythm. Arrhythmias as variations from the normal rhythm of the heart (especially the heartbeat) are detected when they become symptomatic or during monitoring for another cardiac condition. Abnormalities of cardiac rhythm and electrical conduction can be lethal (sudden cardiac death), symptomatic (syncope or near syncope, dizziness, chest pain, dyspnea, and palpitations), or asymptomatic. They are dangerous because they reduce cardiac output so that perfusion of the brain or myocardium is impaired, or they tend to deteriorate into more serious arrhythmias with the same consequences.

The many different types of abnormal cardiac rhythms are usually classified according to their origin, but only the most common ones are included here.

Sinus arrhythmia is an irregularity in rhythm that may be a normal variation in athletes, children, and older people or may be caused by an alteration in vagal stimulation. Sinus arrhythmia may be respiratory (increases and decreases with respiration) or nonrespiratory and associated with infection, drug toxicity, or fever. Treatment for the respiratory type of sinus arrhythmia is not necessary; all other sinus arrhythmias are treated by providing intervention for the underlying cause.

AF is the most common type of SVT or chronic arrhythmia. It is characterized by rapid, involuntary, irregular muscular contractions of the atrial myocardium—quivering or fluttering instead of contracting normally. Consequently, blood remains in the atria after they contract and the ventricles do not fill properly. The heart races, but blood flow may diminish, creating a drop in oxygen levels that results in symptoms of shortness of breath, palpitations, fatigue, and, more rarely, fainting. AF occurs most often

as a secondary arrhythmia associated with rheumatic heart disease, dilated cardiomyopathy, atrial septal defect, hypertension, MVP, recurrent cardiac surgery, and hypertrophic cardiomyopathy.

Secondary AF can also occur in people without cardiac disease but in the presence of a systemic abnormality that predisposes the individual to arrhythmia (e.g., hyperthyroidism, medications, diabetes, obesity, pneumonia, or alcohol intoxication or withdrawal). People with AF are prone to blood clots because blood components that remain in the atria aggregate and attract other components, triggering clot formation. The effect rarely occurs before 72 hours of the first abnormal contraction. AF can result in CHF, cardiac ischemia, and arterial emboli, which can result in an ischemic stroke.

Ventricular fibrillation is an electrical phenomenon that results in involuntary uncoordinated muscular contractions of the ventricular muscle; it is a frequent cause of cardiac arrest. Treatment is directed toward depolarizing the muscle, thus ending the irregular contractions and allowing the heart to resume normal regular contractions.

Heart block is a disorder of the heartbeat caused by an interruption in the passage of impulses through the heart's electrical system. This may occur because the SA node misfires or the impulses it generates are not properly transmitted through the heart's conduction system. Heart blocks are differentiated into three types determined by electrocardiographic testing: first-degree, second-degree, and third-degree (complete) heart block. Causes include CAD, hypertension, myocarditis, and overdose of cardiac medications. Depending on the degree of the heart block, it can cause fatigue, dizziness, or fainting. Heart block can affect people at any age, but this condition primarily affects older people. Mild cases do not require intervention; medication and pacemakers are the two primary forms of management for symptomatic cases.

Sick sinus syndrome, or "brady-tachy syndrome," is a complex cardiac arrhythmia and conduction disturbance that is associated with advanced age, CAD, or drug therapy. Sick sinus syndrome as a result of degeneration of conductive tissue necessary to maintain normal heart rhythm occurs most often among older people. A variety of other heart diseases and other conditions also may result in sinus node dysfunction. Sick sinus syndrome is characterized by bradycardia alone, bradycardia alternating with tachycardia, or bradycardia with atrioventricular block resulting in cerebral manifestations of light-headedness, dizziness, and near or true syncope.

Sinus node dysfunction is suspected in the older adult experiencing episodes of syncope or near syncope, especially in the presence of heart palpitations. An accurate diagnosis is made electrocardiographically, often requiring a 24-hour Holter monitor to document the arrhythmias described. Treatment for the symptomatic person varies according to the specific arrhythmia manifestations and may include antiarrhythmic agents alone or combined with a permanent-demand pacemaker or withdrawal of agents that may be responsible.

Holiday heart syndrome may occur when the heart responds to the increase in catecholamines (epinephrine and norepinephrine) brought on by excessive alcohol intake. Alcohol metabolites may also cause conduction delays.

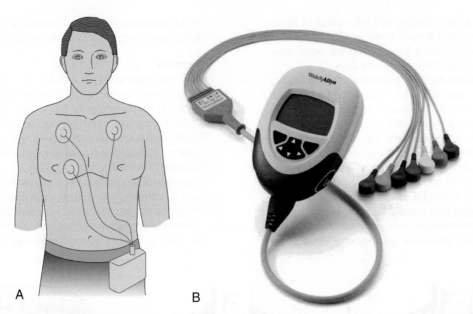

A   B

FIG. 9.18 (A) External cardiac monitoring (a form of telemetry, also called *ambulatory electrocardiography* or *Holter monitoring*) uses a tape recorder that is attached to the skin by electrocardiographic electrodes. It is able to record the heart rhythm over a 24-hour period. Any symptoms experienced while wearing the unit should be recorded by the individual wearing the device. The recording is then analyzed. It may detect changes in heart rhythm or changes in the electrocardiogram that might indicate a lack of blood supply to the heart. (B) Any number of electrodes (up to 12 leads) can be used. The standard three-electrode system in (A) consists of a positive electrode, a negative electrode, and a ground electrode. The unit is small and convenient and can be clipped to the belt or waistband or slipped into a pocket. (B, Courtesy Welch Allyn, Inc., Skaneateles Falls, NY.)

Medical Management

Diagnosis

The ECG is the most common test procedure to document arrhythmias, but if the person is not experiencing symptoms, the heartbeat may look normal. Tape-recorded ambulatory electrocardiography may be used to document arrhythmias. The individual may use continuous monitoring (Fig. 9.18), recording all cardiac cycles over a prescribed period of time, or cardiac event monitoring, recording the ECG just when symptoms are perceived.

Monitoring is especially helpful in recording sporadic arrhythmias that an office or stress test ECG might miss. Monitoring may also be used by persons recovering from MIs, receiving antiarrhythmic medications, or using pacemakers. New pocket-sized devices to allow home monitoring are available; readings may be stored, and the device can be hooked up to the physician's electrocardiograph or diagnostic computer or transmitted over the telephone. For symptoms that occur rarely, an insertable loop recorder can be used. This small device is implanted under the skin in the chest using a local anesthetic.

Treatment

The goal of treatment is to control ventricular rate, prevent thromboembolism, and restore normal sinus rhythm if possible. Normal heart rhythm returns spontaneously (called *cardioversion*) almost immediately in some cases, especially if there is no underlying heart disease. When conversion to normal rate and rhythm does not occur, there are two major approaches to cardioversion: electrical and pharmacologic.

The electrical method uses the a device called a *defibrillator*, is usually more effective, and may require several weeks of anticoagulant therapy (warfarin) to reduce stroke risk. Anyone who has been in AF less than 48 hours but is hemodynamically unstable with serious signs and symptoms related to AF will need immediate electrical cardioversion. Low-voltage electric shocks interrupt the irritable foci of the heart, letting the SA node resume its role as a primary pacemaker.[187]

Pharmacologic treatment may include agents prolonging depolarization and/or other cardiovascular medications (see Table 9.5). If successful, cardioversion restores sinus rhythm, and drug therapy is used to maintain normal heart rate and rhythm. Even with successful electrical cardioversion, long-term antiarrhythmic and anticoagulation drug therapy is used to sustain normal sinus rhythm.

Some tachycardias can be treated with radio wave ablation, a nonsurgical but invasive technique that uses catheterization to thread wires into the heart through which radio waves can be aimed at the heart tissue in which the arrhythmia originates. The catheter-delivered quick bursts of current destroy the specific areas of heart muscle that are generating the abnormal electrical signals causing the arrhythmia. One complication of this technique is the potential destruction of the conducting system (the heart's own internal pacemaker), which necessitates surgical implantation of an artificial pacemaker for some people.

Pacemakers, implants designed to replace the heartbeat by delivering a battery-supplied electrical stimulus through leads attached to electrodes in contact with the heart, may be used in cases of bradycardia, heart block, or refractory tachycardia. Refractory tachycardia is a condition in which the heart is beating very quickly, but only some of those beats are functional; many more beats just echo or make a beat but without contractile force behind the blood flow. Functionally, the heartbeat is actually very slow.

Pacemakers initiate the heartbeat when the heart's intrinsic conduction system fails or is unreliable. In the case of life-threatening arrhythmias that do not respond to other types of intervention, a device called an implantable cardioverter-defibrillator may be implanted (Fig. 9.19). The cardioverter-defibrillator monitors the heart rhythm, and if the heart starts beating abnormally, it generates an electric shock to restore the normal sinus (heart) rhythm.

A more recently developed treatment intervention called *ventricular resynchronization therapy* is gaining recognition for the treatment of intraventricular conduction disturbances associated with CHF. This redesigned pacemaker resynchronizes the right and left ventricles so they pump at the same time, making the heart pump more forcefully instead of pumping faster.

Prognosis

About half of all individuals with AF will spontaneously convert to normal sinus rhythm within 24 to 48 hours; this is less likely to occur in people whose AF has lasted more than 7 days.[243]

Sudden cardiac arrest (sudden death) is responsible for 300,000 deaths annually and is often preceded by fatal heart dysrhythmias in people who have no prior history of heart disease. New data from the Framingham Heart Study indicate that AF is independently associated with a substantially increased risk for death in both men and women, even after adjustment for age and associated factors, such as hypertension, CHF, and stroke.

Defibrillation within the first few minutes of cardiac arrest can save up to 50% of lives; in comparison, an estimated

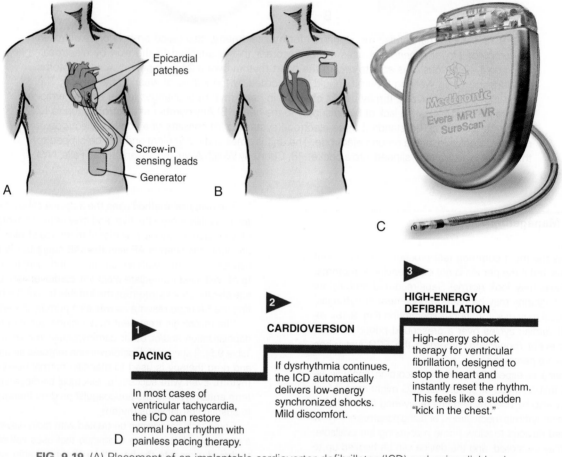

FIG. 9.19 (A) Placement of an implantable cardioverter defibrillator (ICD) and epicardial lead system. The generator is placed in a subcutaneous "pocket" created in the left upper abdominal quadrant. The epicardial screw-in sensing leads monitor the heart rhythm and connect to the generator. If a life-threatening dysrhythmia is sensed, the generator can pace-terminate the dysrhythmia or deliver electrical cardioversion or defibrillation through the epicardial patches. With this system, the leads and patches must be placed during open chest surgery. (B) Transvenous lead system. Open chest surgery is not needed to place this unit. The pacing, cardioversion, and defibrillation functions are all contained in a lead (or leads) inserted into the right atrium and ventricle. New generators are small enough to place in the pectoral region. (C) An example of a dual-chamber ICD (Medtronic Evera MRI SureScan) with tiered therapy and pacing capabilities. (D) Tiered therapy is designed to use increasing levels of intensity to terminate ventricular dysrhythmias. (A, B, and D, From Urden LD, Stacy KM, Lough ME: Critical care nursing: diagnosis and management, ed 6, St Louis, 2009; C, Reproduced with permission of Medtronic, Inc., Northridge, CA.)

5% of sudden cardiac arrest victims in the United States survive without this treatment. Early defibrillation is the key to survival, and toward that end, emergency medical teams are using portable automatic external defibrillator units that use a computer program to sense whether a defibrillatory shock is warranted and will initiate the shock.

The most appropriate and effective drug or drug combination remains unknown, and side effects of long-term rate and rhythm control intervention may prevent long-term use of drug therapy. About 10% of affected individuals continue to have episodes despite treatment, and half of the individuals who are treated have a recurrence within 6 months.

9.11 Special Implications for the PTA: Arrhythmias

Any time a person's pulse is abnormally slow, rapid, or irregular, especially in the presence of known cardiac involvement, documentation and notification of the physician are necessary. Early detection and treatment of AF can be critical in reducing the client's risk of stroke and hemodynamic compromise.

Predisposing factors for arrhythmias include fluid and electrolyte imbalance and drug toxicity. To prevent postoperative cardiac arrhythmias, consult carefully with respiratory therapy personnel to provide adequate oxygen during activities that increase the heart's workload.

Individuals experiencing exercise intolerance because of palpitations, fatigue, and shortness of breath should be assessed further. Keep in mind that people with arrhythmias can be completely asymptomatic. Also, it is possible that clients describing palpitations or similar phenomena may not be experiencing symptoms of arrhythmic heart disease at all.

Palpitations can occur as a result of an overactive thyroid, secondary to caffeine sensitivity, as a side effect of some medications, from decreased estrogen levels, and through the use of drugs such as cocaine. Encourage the client to report any such symptoms to the physician if they have not already been brought to the physician's attention.

PTs and PTAs exercise many people with a history of personal or family heart disease or known risk factors for cardiac disease, potentially necessitating cardiopulmonary resuscitation. Make sure to have advanced cardiac life support equipment available in case of emergency.

Performing an assessment of falls for individuals with cardiac disease, especially for anyone with a personal or family history of arrhythmias, is highly recommended. Screening for syncope, assessing balance and fall risk, and falling prevention programs are important components of a therapist's evaluation. If the individual is also on anticoagulation therapy, he or she should be monitored for signs and symptoms of bleeding; in the acute care setting, the therapist or PTA can monitor the international normalized ratio (INR).

Exercise and Arrhythmias

Exercise often increases arrhythmias because of the increase in activity of the sympathetic nervous system and the increase in circulating catecholamines. Exercise may induce cardiac arrhythmias under several specific conditions, including diuretic and digitalis therapy or recent ingestion of caffeine.

Exercise-induced arrhythmias are generated by enhanced sympathetic tone, increased myocardial oxygen demand, or both. The therapist or PTA can be involved in preparticipation screening of all athletes for conditions that put them at risk for sudden cardiac death. At times, the arrhythmias may disappear with exercise and increased perfusion.

Medications that are effective in controlling arrhythmias at rest may not be effective during exertion or stress. In addition, side effects of antiarrhythmic agents may be more apparent during exercise. For example, decreases in either exercise performance or blood pressure during exercise may occur. Because of their effects on the electrophysiologic characteristics of cardiac cells, these medications have the potential to cause abnormal rhythms. The effect of slowing the impulse through the myocardium may manifest itself during exercise as a partial or complete heart block.

Continued monitoring and observation during the recovery period are also important, because arrhythmias often occur during recovery rather than during peak exercise. If the exercise is stopped abruptly and the individual remains upright, pooling of blood in the lower body occurs. The decreased venous return and subsequent decreased blood flow to the heart may facilitate an irregular rhythm. If exercise is continued at a low intensity during recovery, a sudden decrease in venous return is avoided.

For the client who is wearing or has worn a cardiac monitor, the PTA must obtain the interpretation of the results to determine whether modifications are needed in the person's activities. Anyone with life-threatening arrhythmia should not begin physical therapy activity until intervention for the arrhythmia has been initiated and the condition has been stabilized. Increasing frequency of arrhythmias developing with activity must be evaluated by the physician.[98]

Pacemaker

For the client wearing a pacemaker, the first weeks after surgery may be characterized by fatigue, during which time activity restrictions apply. Most people can drive, but strenuous activities using the arms (e.g., housework, golf, tennis, lifting more than 10 lb) are contraindicated. Once the incision is fully healed and the pacemaker is stable, scar mobilization is permissible. The usual precautions for scar mobilization apply, including mobilizing the tissue in the direction of the scar before using any cross-transverse techniques and mobilizing toward the scar rather than away from the scar to avoid overstretching the healing tissue.

Problems with pacemakers are uncommon, but any unusual deviation from the set heartbeat expected or the development of unusual symptoms, such as dyspnea, dizziness or light-headedness, and syncope or near syncope, must be reported immediately to the physician. It is important that the therapist or PTA understand the underlying problem as well as the type of pacemaker the client is using before monitoring the client's response to an exercise program.

It should be noted that MRIs and prolonged exposure to electromagnetic waves are contraindicated in anyone who is pacemaker dependent. Most exposures to electromagnetic interference are transient and pose no threat to people with pacemakers and implantable cardioverter-defibrillators. Concerns that cellular telephone radiation is linked to pacemaker or implantable cardioverter-defibrillator disruption have not been substantiated or proven clinically important.

The heart rate is limited to the programmed level, and individuals with fixed-rate ventricular synchronous devices require monitoring by blood pressure and perceived exertion scales, with close attention to symptoms of cerebral ischemia. Newer, improved pacemakers produce the cardiac output needed for exercise, making it possible for individuals with pacemakers to be physically active at work and during recreation. Exercise may be limited only by the underlying heart disease and left ventricular function. If the pacemaker recipient has undergone exercise testing safely, aerobic conditioning and endurance training can be initiated, although caution is still advised regarding vigorous upper-body activities.

In some individuals who have survived cardiac arrest and now have a pacemaker, the response to surviving has been compared with posttraumatic stress disorder, which can occur after a person experiences a traumatic event that is outside the realm of usual human experience. Depression, anxiety, difficulty concentrating, negative health beliefs, and increased somatic complaints may be present with or without persistent emotional disability and maladaptation to the event. The therapist or PTA should refer anyone suspected of having persistent depression or anxiety to the physician or mental health professional.

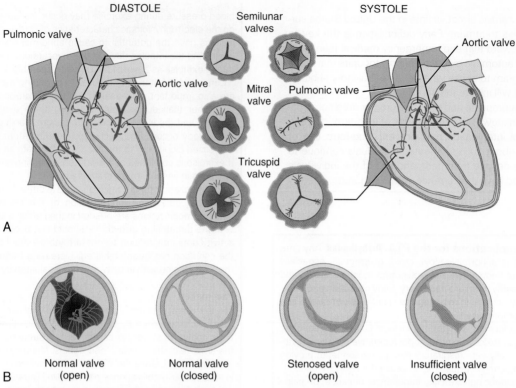

FIG. 9.20 Valves of the heart. (A) The pulmonic, aortic, mitral, and tricuspid valves are shown here as they appear during diastole (ventricular filling) and systole (ventricular contraction). (B) Normal position of the valve leaflets, or cusps, when the valve is open and closed; fully open position of a stenosed valve; closed regurgitant valve showing abnormal opening into which blood can flow back.

DISEASES AFFECTING THE HEART VALVES

Heart problems that occur secondary to impairment of valves may be caused by infections such as endocarditis, congenital deformity, or disease. Valve deformities are classified as functional or anatomic (Fig. 9.20).

Stenosis is a narrowing or constriction that prevents the valve from opening fully and may be caused by scars or abnormal deposits on the leaflets. Valvular stenosis causes obstruction to blood flow, and the chamber behind the narrow valve must produce extra work to sustain cardiac output.

Insufficiency (also referred to as *regurgitation*) occurs when the valve does not close properly and causes blood to flow back into the heart chamber. The heart gradually dilates in response to the increased volume of work. *Prolapse* affects the mitral or tricuspid valve and occurs when enlarged leaflets bulge backward into the atrium.

Valve conditions increase the workload of the heart and require the heart to pump harder to force blood through a stenosed valve or to maintain adequate flow if blood is seeping back. Initially the cardiovascular system compensates for the overload and the person remains asymptomatic, but eventually as stenosis or insufficiency progresses, cardiac muscle dysfunction and accompanying symptoms of heart failure develop.

Over the past 15 years, advances in surgical techniques and a better understanding of timing for surgical intervention have brought tremendous improvement in the clinical outcome of people with valvular heart disease, extending survival rates with less overall morbidity.[45]

Heart transplantation may be necessary when the risk of surgery is prohibitively high in some cases of valvular disease. Continued advances in noninvasive assessment and noninvasive treatment should improve the outlook for anyone with valvular heart disease in the years to come.

Mitral Stenosis
Etiologic Factors and Pathogenesis
Mitral stenosis is a sequela of rheumatic heart disease that primarily affects women. Often a history of rheumatic fever is absent. Because the mitral valve is thickened, it opens in early diastole with a snap that is audible on auscultation and then closes slowly with a resultant murmur.

Clinical Manifestations
In mild cases, left atrial pressure and cardiac output remain normal, and the person is asymptomatic, perhaps until pregnancy or the development of AF, when dyspnea and orthopnea develop. In moderate stenosis, dyspnea and fatigue appear as the left atrial pressure rises and mechanical obstruction of filling of the left ventricle reduces cardiac output.

With severe stenosis, left atrial pressure is high enough to produce pulmonary venous congestion at rest and reduce cardiac output, with resulting dyspnea, fatigue, and right ventricular failure. Lying down at night further increases the pulmonary blood volume, causing orthopnea and paroxysmal nocturnal dyspnea.

Mitral Regurgitation
Etiologic Factors and Pathogenesis
Mitral regurgitation has many possible causes, but involvement of the mitral valve from ischemic heart disease accounts for approximately half of all cases. It is independently associated with female gender, lower BMI, and older age.

During left ventricular systole, the mitral leaflets do not close normally, and blood is ejected into the left atrium as well as through the aortic valve. In acute regurgitation, left atrial pressure rises abruptly, possibly leading to pulmonary edema. When regurgitation is a chronic condition, the left atrium enlarges progressively; the degree of enlargement usually reflects the severity of regurgitation.

Clinical Manifestations
Unfortunately, people with mitral regurgitation lack early warning signs and may remain asymptomatic until severe and often irreversible left ventricular dysfunction occurs. For many years the left ventricular end-diastolic pressure and the cardiac output may be normal at rest, even with considerable increase in left ventricular volume. Eventually, left ventricular overload may lead to left ventricular failure. People with mitral regurgitation experience exertional dyspnea and exercise-induced fatigue. AF may also develop.

Mitral Valve Prolapse
Incidence and Etiologic Factors
MVP has been described as a common disease with frequent complications. There is some dispute about the incidence of MVP. According to data from the Framingham Heart Study, MVP is not as prevalent as previously reported.

The American Heart Association and other sources report that MVP occurs in about 2% to 6% of "normal" adults, especially young women, and is detected most often during pregnancy.[11,46] Other researchers report that MVP is equally common in men and women, although men seem to have a higher incidence of complications.[95]

MVP is characterized by a slight variation in the shape or structure of the mitral (left atrioventricular) valve. The cause remains unknown, although there may be a genetic component. Results of family studies of people with MVP favor an autosomal dominant pattern of transmission for primary MVP with nearly 100% gene expression by females.[65] This condition usually occurs in isolation; however, it can be associated with a number of other conditions, such as Marfan's syndrome, rheumatic fever, endocarditis, myocarditis, atherosclerosis, SLE, muscular dystrophy, acromegaly, adult polycystic kidney disease, and cardiac sarcoidosis.

Pathogenesis
MVP is a pathologic, anatomic, and physiologic abnormality of the mitral valve apparatus affecting mitral valve leaflet motion. Normally, when the lower part of the heart contracts, the mitral valve remains firm and prevents blood from leaking back into the upper chambers. In MVP the slight variation in shape of the mitral valve allows one part of the valve, the leaflet, to billow back into the left atrium during contraction of the ventricle. One or both of the valve leaflets may bulge into the left atrium during ventricular systole. Usually the amount of blood that leaks back into the left atrium is not significant, but in a small number of people, it develops into mitral regurgitation. MVP is the most common cause of isolated mitral regurgitation.

The presence of symptoms linked to neuroendocrine dysfunctions or to the autonomic nervous system has led to the recognition of a pathologic condition known as *mitral valve prolapse syndrome (MVPS)*. Usually diagnosed by chance in asymptomatic individuals during routine tests, MVPS has a high clinical incidence of neuropsychiatric symptoms including anxiety disorder, panic attacks, and depression, as well as symptoms of autonomic dysfunction such as postural hypotension, palpitations, cold hands and feet, shortness of breath, and chest pain.

As the autonomic nervous system is being formed in utero, the mitral valve is also being formed. If there is a slight variation in the structure of the heart valve, there is also a slight variation in the function or balance of the autonomic nervous system.

Clinical Manifestations
More than 50% of all people with MVP are asymptomatic, another 40% experience occasional symptoms that are mildly to moderately uncomfortable, and only 1% experience severe symptoms and lifestyle restrictions. Although the malformation occurs during gestation, it usually remains unnoticed until young adulthood. The person usually becomes aware of symptoms suddenly, and there does not appear to be any correlation between the severity of symptoms and the severity of the prolapse.

The most common triad of symptoms associated with MVP is profound fatigue that cannot be correlated with exercise or stress, palpitations, and dyspnea. Fatigue may not be related to exertion, but deconditioning from prolonged inactivity may develop, further complicating the picture.

The PTA is more likely to see the individual with MVP associated with connective tissue disorders or MVPS with autonomic dysfunction. Frequently occurring musculoskeletal findings in clients with MVPS include joint hypermobility, temporomandibular joint syndrome, pectus excavatum, mild scoliosis, straight thoracic spine, and myalgias.

Other symptoms associated with MVPS may include tremors, swelling of the extremities, sleep disturbances, low back pain, irritable bowel syndrome, excessive perspiration or inability to perspire, rashes, muscular fasciculations, visual changes or disturbances, difficulty in concentrating, memory lapses, and dizziness.

Chest pain or discomfort may occur as a result of autonomic nervous system dysfunction. The autonomic nervous system imbalance results in inadequate relaxation between respirations and eventually causes the chest wall muscles to go into spasm. The chest pain is sharp, lasts several seconds, and is usually felt to the left of the sternum. It is intermittent pain that may occur frequently for a few weeks and then disappear completely, only to return again some weeks later.

MVP or MVPS is a benign condition in the vast majority of people. It is not life-threatening, and only rarely does it result in complications or significantly alter a person's lifestyle. Progressive mitral regurgitation with gradual increase in left atrial and left ventricular size, AF, pulmonary hypertension, and the development of CHF occur in 10% to 15% of people with both murmurs and clicks. Men older than 50 are most often affected.[35]

According to new data available, people with MVP or MVPS are not at greater risk for heart failure, other forms of heart disease, or early death from stroke as was once thought.

Aortic Stenosis
Etiologic Factors and Pathogenesis
Aortic stenosis is a disease of aging that is likely to become more prevalent as the proportion of older people in our population increases. It is most commonly caused by progressive valvular calcification either superimposed on a congenitally bicuspid valve or, in the older adult, involving a previously normal valve after rheumatic fever.

Other risk factors for aortic stenosis are the same as those for heart disease and include obesity, a sedentary lifestyle, smoking, and high cholesterol. Factors affecting the progression of the disease remain uncertain. Over 80% of affected persons are men, and when women are affected, differences are noted that require different postoperative management.[46] Ejection fraction is the amount of blood the ventricle ejects; the normal ejection fraction is about 60% to 75%. A decreased ejection fraction is a hallmark finding of ventricular failure.

Although the deformed valve is not stenotic at birth, it is subjected to abnormal hemodynamic stress, which may lead to thickening and calcification of the leaflets with reduced mobility. The orifice of the aortic valve narrows, causing increased resistance to blood flow from the left ventricle into the aorta.

Outflow obstruction increases pressure within the left ventricle as it tries to eject blood through the narrow opening, causing decreased cardiac output, left ventricular hypertrophy, and pulmonary vascular congestion.

Clinical Manifestations
In adults, aortic stenosis is usually asymptomatic until the sixth (or later) decade. Characteristic sounds may be heard on auscultation, but cardiac output is maintained until the stenosis is severe and left ventricular failure, angina pectoris, or exertional syncope develops. The origin of exertional syncope in aortic stenosis remains controversial; it is perhaps caused by an exercise-induced decrease in total peripheral resistance, which is uncompensated because cardiac output is restricted by the stenotic valve. The most common sign of aortic stenosis is a systolic ejection murmur radiating to the neck. Sudden death may occur, even in previously asymptomatic individuals.

Adults with aortic stenosis who are asymptomatic have a normal life expectancy; they should receive prophylactic antibiotics against infective endocarditis. Once symptoms appear, the prognosis is poor without surgery but excellent with valve replacement even in the older adult, especially in the absence of coexisting illnesses.[45]

Aortic Regurgitation (Insufficiency)
Etiologic Factors and Pathogenesis
In the past, aortic regurgitation occurred secondary to rheumatic fever, but antibiotics have reduced the number of rheumatic fever–related cases. Nonrheumatic causes account for most cases today, including congenitally bicuspid valves, infective endocarditis (valve destruction by bacteria), and hypertension. Aortic regurgitation may also occur secondary to aortic dissection with or without aortic aneurysm, ankylosing spondylitis, Reiter's syndrome, collagen vascular disease, syphilis, and Marfan's syndrome.

When cardiac systole ends, the aortic valve should completely prevent the flow of aortic blood back into the left ventricle. A leakage during diastole is referred to as *aortic regurgitation* or *aortic insufficiency*. When aortic regurgitation develops gradually, the left ventricle compensates by both dilation and enough hypertrophy to maintain a normal wall thickness/cavity ratio, preventing development of symptoms. Eventually the left ventricle fails to stand up under the chronic overload, and symptoms develop.

Clinical Manifestations
Long-standing aortic regurgitation may remain asymptomatic even as the deformity increases, causing enlargement of the left ventricle. The large total stroke volume in aortic regurgitation produces a wide pulse pressure and systolic hypertension, resulting in exertional dyspnea, fatigue, and excessive perspiration with exercise as the most frequent symptoms; paroxysmal nocturnal dyspnea and pulmonary edema may also occur. Angina pectoris or atypical chest pain may be present, but this is uncommon in the absence of CAD.

Tricuspid Stenosis and Regurgitation
Tricuspid stenosis may be congenital or rheumatic in origin and is uncommon. Exercise testing and rehabilitation do not occur until after valve surgery. Surgical repair is more common than valvular replacement for tricuspid valve disease.

9.12 Special Implications for the PTA: Valvular Heart Disease

People with mild valvular malfunction have no symptoms and can usually exercise vigorously and take part in intense sports activities without adverse effects. Although exercise will not improve the mechanical function of a valve, improvement in submaximal cardiac capacity can occur. Exercise is usually stopped for the same reason as it is in healthy adults.

Involvement of more than one valve is not uncommon in people with rheumatic valvular disease and in people who develop valvular regurgitation as a result of ventricular dilation. Usually symptoms and clinical course are determined by the predominant pathologic condition. When two valves are affected equally, symptoms are determined by the most proximally located valve.

Exercise

Exercise testing for most people with valvular disease is of limited value. For example, there is poor correlation between the degree of mitral stenosis and the duration of symptom-limited treadmill exercise. However, exercise echocardiography performed while the individual is on a stationary cycle can be a valuable means for determining left ventricular function in people during exercise.

Prescriptive exercise must be individualized based on the underlying pathologic condition, medical intervention, and condition of the person. General guidelines include exercise a minimum of 3 days per week with alternate days of rest to allow for maximum recuperation. Walking, biking, and swimming are acceptable exercise modalities, but weight training may be considered contraindicated in anyone who is symptomatic with shortness of breath or chest pain or discomfort.

A perceived exertion between light and somewhat hard (RPE of 11 to 14) is the goal, but the individual will usually begin with a much lighter workout and progress over time to this level.[202] Tolerance to symptoms and current exercise habits are important determinants in progressing an exercise program.

Some people with valvular disease avoid physical activity as much as possible and never exercise to the point of developing any symptoms of dyspnea, fatigue, or muscular discomfort. These symptoms develop at light loads in people unaccustomed to any physical activity, regardless of the severity of the valvular disease. Other people force themselves to ignore mild (or even moderate to severe) symptoms to stay on the job or finish a task started.

Fatigue, weakness, and pallor are signs of an inadequate cardiac output for the demands of the exercise. These signs and symptoms are partly subjective, and it is a clinical decision as to how far to allow these people to continue exercising. Chest pain may indicate myocardial ischemia or pulmonary hypertension, or it may be a noncardiac symptom arising from the chest wall.

Follow precautions for angina pectoris. Exercise should be stopped immediately when any signs of reduced cerebral blood flow develop, such as severe facial pallor, confusion, dizziness, heart palpitations, or unsteady gait (see Box 9.5).

Pulmonary edema can be produced by exercising beyond a certain point in people with valvular disease, especially those with mitral stenosis. Pulmonary congestion induced by exercise may cause coughing rather than dyspnea, and exercise should be stopped if coughing becomes significant. Heart failure may occur secondary to chronic, progressive valvular disease. Slight puffiness of the ankles at the end of the day, nocturia, mild nocturnal dyspnea, unexpected weight gain, and more than the usual amount of fatigue can be minor symptoms that are passed over unless specifically sought. Such symptoms must be reported to the physician.

The status of the myocardium is another important variable in exercise impairment relative to valvular heart disease. Severe aortic regurgitation is well tolerated for many years until myocardial weakness occurs. In all forms of heart disease, the healthy myocardium can compensate and maintain the systemic blood flow at or near normal levels for an extended period of time. For the client with valvular disease and myocardial disease or associated CAD, this compensation is not possible, and a lower exercise capacity results.

Stenosis

Valvular stenosis develops or progresses gradually, and because the normal valve orifice is larger than is necessary, stenosis is usually severe before exercise symptoms occur. Stenosis only becomes symptomatic when the condition encroaches on the critical cross-sectional diameter of the opening so that a doubling of the blood flow across the valve quadruples the atrial pressure. The intensity of exertion associated with dyspnea does correlate with the magnitude of atrial pressure, providing a good indicator of the severity of stenosis. However, some people do not complain of dyspnea from lung congestion, only muscular fatigue on exertion as a result of a low cardiac output.

Stress testing may be performed before initiation of an exercise program; with or without those test results, clients should be monitored closely, possibly using the perceived exertion or dyspnea scales mentioned earlier in this chapter. Because of reduced cardiac output, muscle perfusion is reduced and lactate is produced at low workloads. Maximal heart rate may be reduced when dyspnea is the cause of premature termination of exercise. Exercise systolic blood pressure may reach only 130 mm Hg because of low output. Exercise capacity in clients with mitral stenosis can be improved by slowing heart rate and prolonging the diastolic filling period with the use of β-blocking agents.

In the case of symptomatic aortic stenosis, clients are not candidates for exercise programs because of the danger of sudden death. Persons who are asymptomatic must be carefully screened before increasing their physical activity, and for most, exercise intensity should be mild. In people with impaired left ventricular function, cardiac output fails to increase normally with exercise, causing fatigue. Angina with exercise is a common symptom when the aortic stenosis is severe.

Regurgitation

Exercise capacity may be unaffected in cases of mild regurgitation. Mitral regurgitation increases when aortic blood pressure is increased, such as occurs during isometric contractions. Light to moderate rhythmic and repetitive exercise reduces peripheral resistance and is recommended in place of isotonic exercise, which increases the heart rate. Persons with aortic regurgitation caused by weakening of the aortic wall must avoid all strenuous exercise.[63,168]

Prolapse

Most people with MVP can participate in all sports activities, including intense competitive sports. Exercise is a key component in the management of MVP, and although many clients are referred to an exercise physiologist, the PT or PTA may also encounter requests for conditioning and exercise programs. Many times, symptoms of fatigue and dyspnea cause a person to limit physical activity, leading to deconditioning and contributing to a cycle of even more fatigue and shortness of breath.

Caution is advised in the use of weight training for the client with MVP; gradual buildup using light weights and increased repetitions is recommended. Some people with MVPS are prone to exercise-induced arrhythmias, which can (rarely) result in sudden death. Any time tachycardia develops in someone with known MVP, immediate medical referral is necessary.

Postoperative Considerations

Postoperative considerations are the same as for people who have had abdominal or cardiothoracic surgery. After uncomplicated valve ballooning, a return to normal activities is possible within 5 to 7 days. Gradual walking programs can be initiated at home for most people 10 days after surgery, or the client may enroll in a structured cardiac rehabilitation program.

Cardiac rehabilitation postoperatively in people with valvular heart disease is similar to that in post-CABG clients. Care should be taken to avoid high-impact exercises or exercises with a risk of trauma in people who are receiving anticoagulation therapy, to avoid hemarthrosis and bruising.[202]

Exercise outcomes differ after aortic, mitral, and mitral–aortic valve surgery. The degree of improvement in exercise capacity depends on the degree of residual dysfunction, presence or absence of arrhythmia, age of the subject, and effort made to improve exercise capacity. Functional capacity is substantially increased after aortic valve surgery but limited after mitral and mitral–aortic surgery, possibly because of differences in oxygen uptake. As mentioned, for people with mitral stenosis, exercise provides an early warning system, because the onset of dyspnea with strenuous exercise signals the beginning of clinical deterioration.[202]

People with mechanical prosthetic valves receive lifelong anticoagulant therapy and may not tolerate vigorous, weight-bearing activities. Mechanical prostheses have fixed openings that place some limitation, at least theoretically, on cardiac performance during maximal effort.[115] Because stress testing results can be normal, exercise Doppler echocardiography has been used to help prescribe physical activity in clients with prosthetic valves.

Infective Endocarditis

Infective, or bacterial, endocarditis is an infection of the endocardium, the lining inside the heart, including the heart valves; it most commonly damages the mitral valve, followed by the aortic, tricuspid, and pulmonic valves. Bacterial endocarditis may involve normal valves but more often affects valves that have been damaged by a previous pathologic process.

Endocarditis is categorized as either acute or subacute, depending on the clinical course, organisms, and condition of the valves. Endocarditis can occur at any age but rarely occurs in children; half of all clients diagnosed are older than age 60. Older adults may be at greater risk of endocarditis because valvular endocardial disruption is more common, immunity is impaired, and nutrition is poor. Endocarditis is more prevalent among men than women.

Etiologic and Risk Factors

Endocarditis is frequently caused by bacteria normally present in the mouth, respiratory system, or GI tract or as a result of abnormal growths on the closure lines of previously damaged valves.

In addition to those with previous valvular damage, persons with prosthetic heart valves, injection drug users, immunocompromised clients, women who have had a suction abortion or pelvic infection related to intrauterine contraceptive devices, and postcardiac surgical clients are at high risk for developing endocarditis. Congenital heart disease and degenerative heart disease, such as calcific aortic stenosis, may also cause endocarditis.

Hospital-acquired infective endocarditis has become more common as a result of iatrogenic endocardial damage produced by surgery, intracardiac pressure–monitoring catheters, ventriculoatrial shunts, and hyperalimentation lines that reach the right atrium. Portals of entry for microorganisms are also provided by wounds, biopsy sites, pacemakers, intravenous and arterial catheters, indwelling urinary catheters, and intratracheal airways.

Pathogenesis

As an infection, endocarditis causes inflammation of the cardiac endothelium with destruction of the connective tissue. As these blood-borne microorganisms adhere to the endocardial surface, destruction of the connective tissue occurs as a result of the action of bacterial lytic enzymes. The surface endocardium becomes covered with fibrin and platelet thrombi that attract even more thrombogenic material.

The result is the formation of wartlike growths called *vegetations.* These vegetations, consisting of fibrin and platelets, can break off from the valve, embolize, and cause septic infarction in the myocardium, kidney, brain, spleen, abdomen, or extremities. These thromboemboli contain bacteria that not only cause ischemic infarcts but also form new sites of infection, transforming into microabscesses. Bacteria may further invade the valves, causing intravalvular inflammation, destroying portions of the valves, and causing valve deformities.

Clinical Manifestations

Endocarditis can develop insidiously, with symptoms remaining undetected for months, or it can cause symptoms immediately, as in the case of acute bacterial endocarditis. Clinical manifestations can be divided into many groups. It causes varying degrees of valvular dysfunction and may be associated with manifestations involving any number of organ systems, including the lungs, eyes, kidneys, bones, joints, and CNS. The mitral, aortic, tricuspid, and pulmonic valves can be affected; more than one valve can be infected at the same time. Neurologic signs and symptoms are predominant in about one-third of all cases in people over 60 years of age. The classic findings of fever, cardiac murmur, and petechial lesions of the skin, conjunctivae, and oral mucosa are not always present.

Up to 50% of people with infective endocarditis initially have musculoskeletal symptoms, including arthralgia (most common), arthritis, low back pain, and myalgias. Half of these people will have only musculoskeletal symptoms without other manifestations of endocarditis. The early onset of joint pain and myalgia as the first sign of endocarditis is more likely if the person is older and has had a previously diagnosed heart murmur.

Proximal joints are most often affected, especially the shoulder, followed by the knee, hip, wrist, ankle, metatarsophalangeal and metacarpophalangeal joints, and acromioclavicular joints. Most often one or two joints are painful, and symptoms begin suddenly, accompanied by warmth, tenderness, and redness. Symmetric arthralgia in the knees or ankles may lead to a diagnosis of rheumatoid arthritis, but as a rule, morning stiffness is not as prevalent in clients with endocarditis as in those with rheumatoid arthritis or polymyalgia rheumatica.

Bone and joint infections are particularly common in injection drug users. The most common sites of osteoarticular infections are the vertebrae, wrist, and sternoclavicular and sacroiliac joints, often with multiple joint involvement.[191]

Almost one-third of clients with endocarditis have low back pain, which may be the primary symptom reported. Back pain is accompanied by decreased ROM and spinal tenderness. Pain may affect only one side, and it may be limited to the paraspinal muscles. Endocarditis-induced back pain may be very similar to that associated with a herniated lumbar disk, because it radiates to the leg and may be accentuated by raising the leg or by sneezing, coughing, or laughing; however, neurologic deficits are usually absent in persons with endocarditis.

Endocarditis may produce destructive changes in the sacroiliac joint characterized by pain localized over the sacroiliac, probably as a result of seeding of the joint by septic emboli. Widespread diffuse myalgia may occur during periods of fever, but this is not appreciably different from the general myalgia seen in clients with other febrile illnesses. More commonly, myalgia is restricted to the calf or thigh. Bilateral or unilateral leg myalgias occur in approximately 10% to 15% of all persons with endocarditis.

The cause of back pain and leg myalgia associated with endocarditis has not been determined. Rarely, other musculoskeletal symptoms, such as osteomyelitis, tendinitis, hypertrophic osteoarthropathy, bone infarcts, and ischemic bone necrosis, may occur.

9.13 Special Implications for the PTA: Infective Endocarditis Physical exertion beyond normal activities of daily living is usually limited for the person receiving antibiotic therapy for endocarditis and during the following weeks of recovery. The PTA is not likely to treat a person diagnosed during this acute phase of endocarditis. However, because early manifestations of endocarditis may be primarily musculoskeletal or cutaneous in nature, the PTA may be the first to recognize signs and symptoms of a systemic disorder.

Splinter hemorrhages (dark red linear streaks resembling splinters under the nail bed), clubbing, petechiae, purplish red subcutaneous nodes on the finger and toe pads, and lesions on the thenar and hypothenar eminences of the palms, fingers, and sometimes the soles are present in up to 50% of affected individuals.[113]

For any client with known risk factors or a recent history of endocarditis, the PTA must be alert for signs of endocarditis, indications of complications, lack of response to therapy intervention, or signs indicating relapse. Often the client thinks the symptoms are recurrent bouts of the flu.

DISEASE AFFECTING THE PERICARDIUM

The pericardium consists of two layers: the inner visceral layer, which is attached to the epicardium, and an outer parietal layer (see Fig. 9.1). The pericardium stabilizes the heart in its anatomic position despite changes in body position and reduces excess friction between the heart and surrounding structures. It is composed of fibrous tissue that is loose enough to permit moderate changes in cardiac size but that cannot stretch fast enough to accommodate rapid dilation or accumulation of fluid without increasing intracardiac pressure.

The pericardium may be a primary site of disease and is often involved by processes that affect the heart; it may also be affected by diseases of the adjacent tissues. Pericardial diseases are common and have multiple causes. Three conditions primarily affect the pericardium: acute pericarditis, constrictive pericarditis, and pericardial effusion. These three diseases are grouped together for ease of understanding in the following section.

Pericarditis

Definition and Overview

Pericarditis or inflammation of the pericardium, the double-layer membrane surrounding the heart, may be a primary condition or may be secondary to a number of diseases and circumstances (Box 9.8). It may occur as a single acute event, or it may recur and become a chronic condition.

Incidence and Etiologic Factors

The most common types of pericarditis encountered by the PTA will be drug induced or those present in association with autoimmune diseases, after MI, in conjunction with renal failure, after open heart surgery, and after radiation therapy.

Other types encountered less often include viral pericarditis and neoplastic pericarditis. Isolated cases of constrictive pericarditis as a manifestation of chronic graft-versus-host disease after peripheral stem cell transplantation have been reported.[207]

Pathogenesis

Many causes of pericarditis affect both the pericardium and the myocardium with varying degrees of cardiac dysfunction. Constrictive pericarditis is characterized by a fibrotic, thickened, and adherent pericardium that is compressing the heart. The heart becomes restricted in

---

BOX 9.8   Causes of Pericarditis

- Idiopathic (85%)
- Infections
  - Viral (Coxsackie, influenza, Epstein–Barr, hepatitis, and HIV)
  - Bacterial (tuberculosis, *Staphylococcus*, *Streptococcus*, meningococcus, and pneumonia)
  - Parasitic
  - Fungal
- Myocardial injury
  - Myocardial infarction
  - Cardiac trauma: instrumentation; blunt or penetrating pericardium; rib fracture
  - After cardiac surgery
- Hypersensitivity
  - Collagen diseases: rheumatic fever, scleroderma, systemic lupus erythematosus, rheumatoid arthritis
  - Drug reaction
  - Radiation or cobalt therapy
- Metabolic disorders
- Uremia
  - Myxedema
  - Chronic anemia
- Neoplasm
  - Lymphoma, leukemia, lung or breast cancer
- Aortic dissection
- Graft-versus-host disease

---

movement and function (cardiac tamponade). Diastolic filling of the heart is reduced, venous pressures are elevated, cardiac output is decreased, and eventual cardiac failure may result.

When fluid accumulates within the pericardial sac it is referred to as *pericardial effusion.* Blunt chest trauma or any cause of acute pericarditis can lead to pericardial effusion. Rapid distention or excessive fluid accumulation from this condition can also compress the heart and reduce ventricular filling and cardiac output.

Clinical Manifestations

The presentation and course of pericarditis are determined by the underlying cause. For example, pericarditis may occur 2 to 5 days after infarction as a result of an inflammatory reaction to myocardial necrosis, or it may occur within the first year after radiation initiates a fibrinous and fibrotic process in the pericardium. Often there is pleuritic chest pain that is made worse by lying down and by respiratory movements and is relieved by sitting upright or leaning forward. The pain is substernal and may radiate to the neck, shoulders, upper back, upper trapezius, left supraclavicular area, or epigastrium or down the left arm.

Other symptoms may include fever, joint pain, dyspnea, or difficulty swallowing. Auscultation of the lower left sternal border in which the pericardium lies close to the chest wall will produce a pericardial friction rub, which is a high-pitched scratchy sound that may be heard at end expiration. This sound is produced by the friction between the pericardial surfaces that results from inflammation and occurs during heart movement. Symptoms of constrictive pericarditis develop slowly and usually include progressive dyspnea, fatigue, weakness, peripheral edema, and ascites. Constrictive disease can lead to diastolic dysfunction and eventual heart failure.

Medical Management

Treatment

New treatments for pericardial diseases are being developed as a result of modern imaging, new understanding of molecular biology, and immunologic techniques. Comprehensive and systematic implementation of new techniques of pericardiocentesis, pericardial fluid analysis, pericardioscopy, and epicardial and pericardial biopsy, as well as the application of new techniques for pericardial fluid and biopsy analyses, has permitted early specific diagnosis, creating foundations for etiologic intervention in many cases.

Conventional treatment remains twofold, directed toward prevention of long-term complications and the underlying cause. For example, although any underlying infection is treated when possible, symptomatic treatment is provided for idiopathic, viral, or radiation pericarditis; antiinflammatory drugs are given for severe, acute pericarditis or pericarditis associated with connective tissue disorders; chemotherapy is given for neoplastic pericarditis; and dialysis is performed for uremic pericarditis. Analgesics may be prescribed for the pain and fever. Pericardiocentesis (surgical drainage with a needle catheter through a small subxiphoid incision) may be performed if cardiac compression from pericardial effusion does not resolve.

Treatment for constrictive pericarditis is both medical and surgical, including digitalis preparations, diuretics, sodium restriction, and pericardiectomy (surgical excision of the damaged pericardium).

Prognosis

The prognosis in most cases of acute viral pericarditis is excellent when there is no myocardial involvement, because this is frequently a self-limited disease. Without medical intervention, shock and death can occur from decreased cardiac output with cardiac involvement. Constrictive pericarditis is a progressive disease without spontaneous reversal of symptoms. Most people become progressively disabled over time. Surgical removal of the pericardium is associated with a high mortality rate.

9.14 Special Implications for the PTA: Pericarditis Pericardial pain can masquerade as a musculoskeletal problem, manifesting as just upper back, neck, or upper trapezius pain. In such cases, the pain may be diminished by holding the breath or aggravated by swallowing or neck or trunk movements, especially side bending or rotation.

Pain is also aggravated by respiratory movements, such as deep breathing, coughing, and laughing. The PTA must screen for medical disease by assessing aggravating and relieving factors and by asking the client about a history of fever, chills, upper respiratory tract infection (recent cold or flu), weakness, heart disease, or recent MI (heart attack).

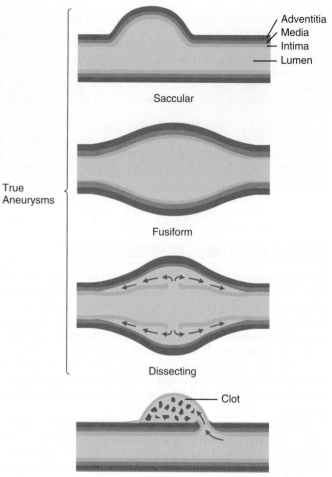

FIG. 9.21 Longitudinal sections showing types of aneurysms. In a true aneurysm, layers of the vessel wall dilate in one of the following ways: saccular, a unilateral outpouching; fusiform, a diffuse dilation involving the entire circumference of the artery wall; or dissecting, a bilateral outpouching in which layers of the vessel wall separate, with creation of a cavity. In a false aneurysm, the wall ruptures, and a blood clot is retained in an outpouching of tissue.

DISEASES AFFECTING THE BLOOD VESSELS

Diseases of blood vessels observed in a therapy setting can include intestinal infarction, aneurysm, PVD, vascular neoplasm, and vascular malformation; only intestinal infarction will not be discussed here.

Aneurysm

Definition and Overview

An aneurysm is an abnormal stretching (dilation) in the wall of an artery, a vein, or the heart with a diameter that is at least 50% greater than normal. When the vessel wall becomes weakened from trauma, congenital vascular disease, infection, or atherosclerosis, a permanent saclike formation develops (Fig. 9.21; see also Fig. 9.23).

Aneurysms are of various types (either arterial or venous) and are named according to the specific site of formation (Fig. 9.22). The most common site for an arterial aneurysm is the aorta, forming a thoracic aneurysm or an abdominal aneurysm.

ANEURYSMS

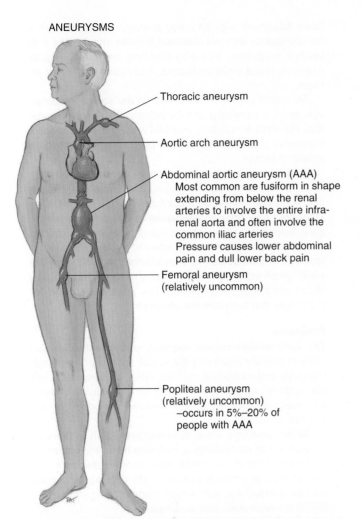

- Thoracic aneurysm

- Aortic arch aneurysm

- Abdominal aortic aneurysm (AAA)
  Most common are fusiform in shape
  extending from below the renal
  arteries to involve the entire infra-
  renal aorta and often involve the
  common iliac arteries
  Pressure causes lower abdominal
  pain and dull lower back pain

- Femoral aneurysm
  (relatively uncommon)

- Popliteal aneurysm
  (relatively uncommon)
  –occurs in 5%–20% of
  people with AAA

FIG. 9.22 Aneurysms are named according to the specific site of formation. Abdominal aortic aneurysms are the most common type; more than 95% of abdominal aortic aneurysms are located below the renal arteries and extend to the umbilicus, causing low back pain. (From Jarvis C: Physical examination and health assessment, ed 7, St. Louis, 2016, Elsevier.)

Thoracic aortic aneurysms located above the diaphragm account for approximately 10% of all aortic aneurysms and occur most frequently in hypertensive men aged 40 to 70 years. Thoracic aortic aneurysms occur less often than other types but tend to be more life-threatening.

Abdominal aortic aneurysms located below the diaphragmatic border occur about four times more often than thoracic aneurysms; this is most likely because the aorta is not supported by skeletal muscle at this location. The incidence of abdominal aortic aneurysm is increasing, probably because of the increasing number of adults over 65 years of age.

Peripheral arterial aneurysms affect the femoral and popliteal arteries.

Incidence and Etiologic Factors

According to the Society for Vascular Surgery, approximately 200,000 people in the United States are diagnosed annually with aortic aneurysm and 15,000 of those aneurysms are severe enough to rupture, causing a medical emergency.[209]

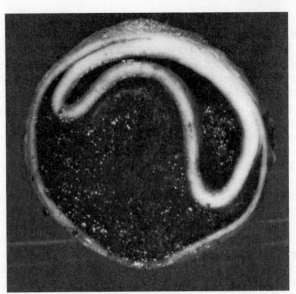

FIG. 9.23 *Dissecting aneurysm.* Cross-section of the aorta with dissecting aneurysm showing true aortic lumen (*above* and *right*) compressed by dissecting column of blood that separates the media and creates a false lumen. (From Kissane JM, ed: Anderson's pathology, ed 9, St Louis, 1990, Mosby.)

Incidence increases with increasing age, usually beginning after age 50 years, presumably as a result of chronic inflammatory cellular changes resulting in atherosclerosis. However, someone without evidence of atherosclerosis can develop an aneurysm, especially in the presence of congenital weakness of the blood vessel walls.

Family members of anyone with an aneurysm have a fourfold increased risk of aneurysm. Aneurysms occur much more often in men than in women, and half of the affected persons are hypertensive.

Atherosclerosis or any injury to the middle or muscular layer of the arterial wall (tunica media) is responsible for most arterial aneurysms. Other, less common causes of aneurysm include trauma (blunt or surgical), Marfan's disease (congenital defects of the arterial wall) and other hereditary abnormalities of connective tissue, and inflammatory diseases and infectious agents.

Pathogenesis

Plaque formation erodes the vessel wall, predisposing the vessel to stretching of the inner and outer layers of the artery and formation of a sac. The stretching of the media produces infarct expansion, a weak and thin layer of necrotic muscle, and fibrous tissue that bulges with each systole.

With time, the aneurysm becomes more fibrotic, but it continues to bulge with each systole, thus acting as a reservoir for some of the stroke volume. In the case of thoracic aortic aneurysms, the shear force of elevated blood pressure causes a tear in the intima with rapid disruption and rupture of the aortic wall. Subsequent hemorrhage causes a lengthwise splitting of the arterial wall, creating a false vessel (Fig. 9.23), and a hematoma may form in either channel.

Clinical Manifestations

Aneurysms may be asymptomatic; when they do occur, manifestations depend largely on the size and position of the aneurysm and its rate of growth. Persistent but vague substernal, back, neck, or jaw pain may occur as enlargement of the aneurysm impinges adjacent structures.

Dissection over the aortic arch and into the descending aorta may be experienced as extreme, sharp pain felt at the base of the neck or along the back into the interscapular areas. When pressure from a large volume of blood is placed on the trachea, esophagus, laryngeal nerve, lung, or superior vena cava, symptoms of dysphagia; hoarseness; edema of the neck, arms, or jaw and distended neck veins; and dyspnea and/or cough may occur, respectively.

Other signs and symptoms may be present in the case of *acute aortic dissection* as a result of compression of branches of the aorta. These include acute MI, reversible ischemic neurologic deficits, stroke, paraplegia, renal failure, intestinal ischemia, and ischemia of the arms and legs.

In the case of an untreated *abdominal aortic aneurysm*, expansion and rupture can occur in one of several places, including the peritoneal cavity, the mesentery, or the retroperitoneum, into the inferior vena cava, or into the duodenum or rectum. *Rupture* refers to a tearing of all three tunicae with bleeding into the thoracic or abdominal cavity. The most common site for an abdominal aortic aneurysm is just below the renal arteries, and it may involve the bifurcation of the aorta (see Fig. 9.22).

Most abdominal aortic aneurysms are asymptomatic, but intermittent or constant pain in the form of mild to severe midabdominal or lower back discomfort is present in some form in 25% to 30% of cases. Groin or flank pain may be experienced because of increasing pressure on other structures.

Early warning signs of an impending rupture may include abdominal heartbeat when lying down or a dull ache (intermittent or constant) in the midabdominal left flank or lower back. Rupture is most likely to occur in aneurysms that are 5 cm or larger, causing intense flank pain with referred pain to the back at the level of the rupture. Pain may radiate to the lower abdomen, groin, or genitalia. Back pain may be the only presenting symptom before rupture occurs.

The most common site for *peripheral arterial aneurysm* is the popliteal space in the lower extremities. Most are caused by atherosclerosis and occur bilaterally in men. Popliteal aneurysm manifests as a pulsating mass, 2 cm or more in diameter, and causes ischemic symptoms in the lower limbs. *Femoral aneurysm* manifests as a pulsating mass in the femoral area on one or both sides.

Medical Management

Diagnosis

Detection of abdominal and peripheral aneurysms often occurs when the physician palpates a pulsating mass during routine examination or when radiographs are taken for other purposes. Radiography, ultrasonography, echocardiography with color Doppler imaging, computed tomography and magnetic resonance imaging, arteriography, and aortography may be used for investigation.

Prevention and Treatment

Annual examination to ensure early identification is recommended for family members of anyone who has previously been diagnosed with an aortic aneurysm. Anyone with a familial risk or signs of diseased arteries should take preventive measures, including smoking cessation, regular exercise, blood pressure control, and cholesterol management.

Treatment is determined based on the size of the bulge, how fast it is expanding, and the individual's clinical presentation. For small aneurysms, watchful waiting is often advised. Preventive pharmacology may be prescribed, depending on individual factors.

Surgical intervention before rupture provides a good prognosis; at 5 cm, the risk of rupture exceeds the risk of repair. A new, less invasive procedure known as *endoluminal stent-graft* may offer an alternative to open abdominal surgery. Guided by angiographic imaging, a catheter is inserted through the femoral or brachial artery to the aneurysm. A balloon within the catheter is then inflated, pushing open the stent, which attaches with tiny hooks to healthy arterial wall above and below the aneurysm. This creates a channel for blood flow that bypasses the aneurysm.

Prognosis

The standard open surgical approach to replace the diseased aorta is steadily improving but is still associated with high morbidity and substantial mortality rates. MI, respiratory failure, renal failure, and stroke are the principal causes of death and morbidity after surgical procedures performed on the thoracic aorta.

At the same time, the endoluminal stent-graft comes with its own set of complications, including fever, breakdown or migration of the device, leaks, and unknown durability. Further studies to improve treatment are ongoing. Aneurysm rupture is associated with a high mortality; frequently aneurysms are discovered only at autopsy.

9.15 Special Implications for the PTA: Aneurysm Anyone with complications associated with an aneurysm is also at risk for pulmonary complications.

Because the prevalence of all diseases of the aorta increases with age and because the population in the United States is aging, it is expected that aortic aneurysm will be encountered with increasing frequency. Knowledge of the natural history, familial history, and clinical features of this disorder may alert the PTA to the need for medical intervention.

For the person who has had a surgically repaired aneurysm, activities are restricted and are only gradually reintroduced. The PTA may be involved in bedside exercises and early mobility, which are especially important to prevent thromboembolism as a result of venous stasis during prolonged bed rest and immobility.

Because of the invasiveness of open abdominal surgery, anyone undergoing this procedure is at high risk for pulmonary complications. Incisional pain and the use of abdominal musculature in coughing discourage the person from full inspirations as well as effective forceful huffing or coughing. The acute care PTA will use clinical techniques to assist with cough with pillows or towel rolls at the incisional site and forceful huffing.[99]

Proper lifting techniques should be reviewed before discharge, even though the client will not be able to provide a return demonstration. Activities that require pushing, pulling, straining, or lifting more than 10 lb are restricted for 6 to 10 weeks postoperatively.

Anterior or abdominal soft tissue mobilization for persons with back pain who have postoperative abdominal scars may require indirect techniques. This precaution is especially true for the person with a previous abdominal aneurysm, the person with a known nonoperative aneurysm (less than 5 cm), or the person with a family history of aneurysm or an undiagnosed aneurysm.

The PTA must always palpate the abdomen for a pulsating mass before performing anterior or abdominal therapy. It is possible to palpate the width of the pulse beginning at the abdominal midline and progressing laterally. The pulse should be characterized by a uniform width on either side of the abdominal midline until the umbilicus is reached, at which point the aortic bifurcation results in expansion of the pulse width. Throbbing pain that increases with exertion should alert the PTA to the need to monitor vital signs and palpate pulses.

Peripheral Vascular Disease

Although PVD is usually thought to refer to diseases of the blood vessels supplying the extremities, it actually encompasses pathologic conditions of blood vessels supplying the extremities and the major abdominal organs, and is most often apparent in the intestines and kidneys.

PVD is organized based on the underlying pathologic finding. Although the terms *peripheral arterial disease* (PAD) and *peripheral vascular disease* are often used interchangeably, PVD is a broader, more encompassing grouping of disorders of both the arterial and venous blood vessels, whereas PAD refers only to arterial blood vessels. PVD typically affects the legs more often than the arms, but upper extremity involvement is not uncommon.

Approximately 8 million Americans over age 60 years are affected by PVD, with 20% of those people over age 70 years. Arterial occlusive forms of PVD are most common as a result of atherosclerosis. Intermittent claudication is the classic symptom of PAD. Intermittent claudication associated with PAD is predictable and nearly always develops after the same amount of exertion, generally occurs in the calves and less commonly in the thighs and buttocks,[49] and usually improves rapidly with rest.

Data from the Framingham Heart Study and other population studies indicate that incidence of intermittent claudication sharply increases in late middle age and is somewhat higher in men than in women. The true prevalence of PAD is at least five times higher than expected based on the reported prevalence of intermittent claudication.[59] Specific symptoms of the various forms of PVD depend on the underlying pathologic condition, the blood vessels involved, and the location of the affected blood vessels.

Inflammatory Disorders

Inflammatory conditions of the blood vessels are often discussed as immunologic conditions, because inflammation and damage to large and small vessels result in end-stage organ damage. Vasculitis is the most commonly encountered inflammatory blood vessel disease in a therapy practice.

Vasculitis is actually a group of disorders that share a common pathogenesis of inflammation of the blood vessels involving arteries, veins, or nerves, resulting in narrowing or occlusion of the lumen or formation of aneurysms that can rupture. Vascular inflammation is a central feature of many rheumatic diseases, especially rheumatoid arthritis and scleroderma.

Vasculitis. Vasculitis can involve blood vessels of any size, type, or location and can affect any organ system, including the nervous system; classification is usually according to the size of the predominant vessels involved. Vasculitis may be acute or chronic with varying degrees of involvement. The distribution of lesions may be irregular and segmental rather than continuous.

Neurologic manifestations of vasculitis can occur in conjunction with any of the vasculitides listed, affecting the peripheral nervous system or the CNS. The primary target organ involvement is usually muscle and nerve, skin, testicle, kidney, and, less often, the CNS.

Immune (antibody–antigen) complexes to each disorder are deposited in the blood vessels, resulting in varying symptoms depending on the organs affected.

Phagocytosis of the immune complexes takes place, and release of free radicals and proteolytic enzymes disrupts cell membranes and damages blood vessel walls. The resulting damage to endothelial cells results in thickening of the vessel wall, occlusion, and ischemia of the affected nerves with axonal degeneration and the resultant neuropathy.

Thromboangiitis obliterans (Buerger's disease)

Overview and pathogenesis. Thromboangiitis obliterans, also referred to as *Buerger's disease,* is a vasculitis affecting the peripheral blood vessels (both arteries and veins), primarily in the extremities. The cause is not known, but it is most often found in men younger than age 40 who smoke heavily, although the incidence in women is increasing. There has been some suggestion that unrecognized cocaine use may masquerade as Buerger's disease.[137]

The pathogenesis of thromboangiitis obliterans is unknown; general inflammatory concepts apply. The inflammatory lesions of the peripheral blood vessels are accompanied by thrombus formation and vasospasm occluding and eventually obliterating (destroying) small and medium-sized vessels of the feet and hands.

Clinical manifestations. Clinical manifestations of pain and tenderness of the affected part are caused by occlusion of the arteries, reduced blood flow, and subsequent reduced oxygenation. The symptoms are episodic and segmental, meaning that the symptoms come and go intermittently over time and appear in different asymmetric anatomic locations. The plantar, tibial, and digital vessels are most commonly affected in the lower leg and foot. Intermittent claudication centered in the arch of the foot or the palm of the hand is often the first symptom.

When the hands are affected, the digital, palmar, and ulnar arteries are most commonly involved. Pain at rest occurs, with persistent ischemia of one or more digits. Other symptoms include edema; cold sensitivity; rubor (redness of the skin from dilated capillaries under the skin); cyanosis; and thin, shiny, hairless skin from chronic ischemia. Paresthesias, diminished or absent posterior tibial and dorsalis pedis pulses, painful ischemic ulceration, and eventual gangrene may develop. Inflammatory superficial thrombophlebitis is common.

Medical Management

Diagnosis, Treatment, and Prognosis

Arteriography may be used in the diagnosis, but definitive diagnosis of thromboangiitis obliterans is determined by histologic examination of the blood vessels in a leg amputated because of gangrene. Given the new findings that cocaine use may cause presenting symptoms very much like those of Buerger's disease, laboratory screening for drug use may be appropriate in some cases.[137]

Intervention should begin with cessation of smoking and avoidance of any environmental or secondhand smoke inhalation. All other treatment techniques are aimed at improving circulation to the foot or hand, including pharmacologic intervention and physical or occupational therapy.

Thromboangiitis is not life-threatening, but it can result in progressive disability from pain and loss of function secondary to amputation. Cessation of smoking is the key determinant in prognosis.

9.16 Special Implications for the PTA: Inflammatory Disorders Peripheral neuropathy is a well-known and frequently early manifestation of many vasculitic syndromes. The pattern of neuropathic involvement depends on the extent and temporal progression of the vasculitic process that produces ischemia. A severe, burning dysesthetic pain in the involved area is present in 70% to 80% of all cases.

Other symptoms may include paresthesias and sensory deficit; severe proximal muscle weakness and muscular atrophy can occur secondary to the neuropathy. In the early phase, one nerve is affected and causes symptoms in one extremity, but other nerves can become involved as the disorder progresses.

The PTA should watch for anyone with neuropathy who exhibits constitutional symptoms, such as fever, arthralgia, or skin involvement. This may herald a possible vasculitic syndrome and requires medical referral for accurate diagnosis. Early recognition of vasculitis can help prevent a poor outcome. With no treatment or with a poor outcome to intervention, CNS involvement can occur late in the course of vasculitis.

When corticosteroids are used, the PTA must be aware of the need for osteoporosis prevention and attend to the other potential side effects from the chronic use of these medications.

Alternative methods of pain control may be offered in a rehabilitation setting, such as biofeedback, transcutaneous electrical nerve stimulation, and physiologic modulation.

Vasculitis (Inflammatory Disease of Arteries and Veins)

The PTA's role in management of vasculitis may be primarily for relief of painful muscular and joint symptoms when present and in the prevention of functional loss in the case of neuropathies. For the client with thromboangiitis obliterans (Buerger's disease), exercise must be graded to avoid claudication, and the client must be instructed in a home program for preventive skin care. Gangrene can occur as a result of prolonged ischemia from vessel obliteration; clients are typically treated for wound care and postoperatively after amputation.

Often a client with some other primary orthopedic or neurologic diagnosis has also been medically diagnosed with vasculitis.

Arteritis. Early recognition and referral can prevent the serious complications associated with arteritis. Older adults who experience sudden or unexplained headaches, lingering flulike symptoms such as muscle aches (myalgia) and fatigue, persistent fever, unexplained weight loss, jaw pain when eating, or visual disturbances must be referred to their physicians. This is especially true for anyone with a previous diagnosis of polymyalgia rheumatica.

The use of corticosteroids can result in side effects such as osteoporosis and bone fractures, weight gain, diabetes, and high blood pressure. The client must be advised regarding an osteoporosis prevention program and how to handle an increase in appetite. Remaining physically active and exercising are key components for both these issues.

Arterial Occlusive Diseases

Occlusive diseases of the blood vessels are a common cause of disability and usually occur as a result of atherosclerosis. Other causes of arterial occlusion include trauma, thrombus or embolism, vasculitis, vasomotor disorders such as Raynaud's disease or phenomenon and reflex sympathetic dystrophy (now called *complex regional pain syndrome*), arterial punctures, polycythemia, and chronic mechanical irritation of the subclavian artery resulting from compression by a cervical rib. For each individual case, see the discussion of the underlying cause of the occlusion to understand etiologic and risk factors and pathogenesis.

Atherosclerotic occlusive disease can also affect other vessels throughout the body and not just the cardiac blood vessels.

Occlusive cerebrovascular disease as a result of atherosclerosis accounts for many episodes of weakness, dizziness, blurred vision, or sudden cerebrovascular accident or stroke. Extracranial arterial ischemia accounts for over half of these types of strokes.

Arterial thrombosis and embolism. Occlusive diseases may be complicated by arterial thrombosis and embolism (Fig. 9.24). Chronic, incomplete arterial obstruction usually results in the development of collateral vessels before complete occlusion threatens circulation to the extremity. Arterial embolism is generally a complication of ischemic or rheumatic heart disease, with or without MI.

Signs and symptoms of pain, numbness, coldness, tingling or changes in sensation, skin changes (pallor and mottling), weakness, and muscle spasm occur in the extremity distal to the block (Fig. 9.25). Treatment may include immediate or delayed embolectomy, anticoagulation therapy, and protection of the limb.

Arteriosclerosis obliterans (peripheral arterial disease)

Definition and overview. Arteriosclerosis obliterans, defined as arteriosclerosis in which proliferation of the intima has caused complete obliteration of the lumen of the artery, is also known as *peripheral arterial disease*. It is the most common arterial occlusive disease and accounts for about 95% of cases. It is a progressive disease that causes ischemic ulcers of the legs and feet and is most often seen in older clients, associated with diabetes mellitus.

Etiologic and risk factors. Atherosclerosis as the underlying cause of occlusive disease, with its known etiologic and associated risk factors, is discussed earlier in the chapter. PAD correlates most strongly with cigarette

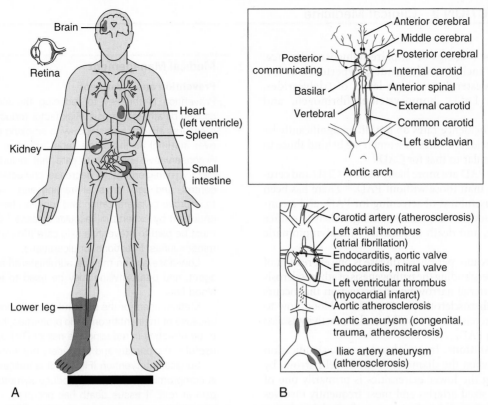

Brain

Retina

Heart
(left ventricle)

Spleen

Kidney

Small
intestine

Lower leg

Anterior cerebral
Middle cerebral
Posterior cerebral
Internal carotid
Anterior spinal
External carotid
Common carotid
Left subclavian

Posterior
communicating

Basilar

Vertebral

Aortic arch

Carotid artery (atherosclerosis)
Left atrial thrombus
(atrial fibrillation)
Endocarditis, aortic valve
Endocarditis, mitral valve
Left ventricular thrombus
(myocardial infarct)
Aortic atherosclerosis
Aortic aneurysm (congenital,
trauma, atherosclerosis)
Iliac artery aneurysm
(atherosclerosis)

A   B

FIG. 9.24 (A) Common sites of infarction from arterial emboli. (B) Sources of arterial emboli.

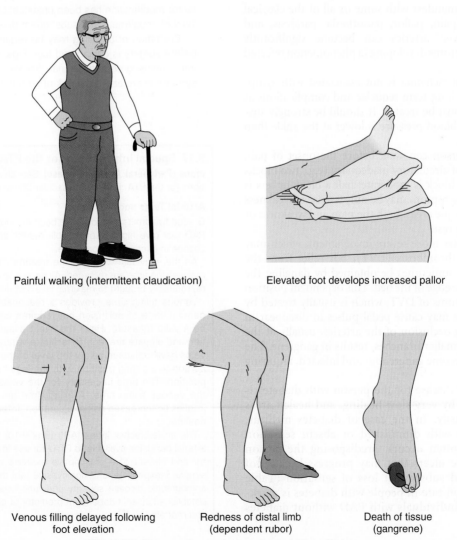

Painful walking (intermittent claudication)

Elevated foot develops increased pallor

Venous filling delayed following
foot elevation

Redness of distal limb
(dependent rubor)

Death of tissue
(gangrene)

FIG. 9.25 Signs and symptoms of arterial insufficiency.

smoking and either diabetes or impaired glucose tolerance. Other risk factors include male gender; hypertension; low levels of HDL cholesterol; and high levels of triglycerides, apolipoprotein B, Lp(a), homocysteine, fibrinogen, and blood viscosity.

Prevalence and incidence rates do not differ significantly by gender, although incidence rates in women lag behind those in men in a pattern similar to that for CAD.[153]

Individuals with PAD are more likely to have CHD and cerebrovascular disease than those without PAD.[59] There has been a debate as to the usefulness of screening for PAD, and a conclusion has been made that targeted screening is likely to reduce heart attack, stroke, and death in patients with asymptomatic PAD.[24]

Pathogenesis. Because peripheral disease is one expression of atherosclerosis, understanding the pathogenesis of atherosclerosis is important. The arterial narrowing or obstruction that occurs as a result of the atherosclerotic process reduces blood flow to the limbs during exercise or at rest. Muscular reactivity is also adversely affected in PAD.

Clinical manifestations. In peripheral vessels, claudication symptoms appear when the diameter of the vessel narrows by 50%. PAD affecting the lower extremities is primarily one of large and medium-sized arteries and most frequently involves branch points and bifurcations. Symptoms of arterial occlusive disease usually occur distal to the narrowing or obstruction. Acute ischemia may manifest with some or all of the classical symptoms, such as pain, pallor, paresthesia, paralysis, and pulselessness. However, arteries can become significantly blocked without symptoms developing (a phenomenon referred to as *silent ischemia*).

Even though silent ischemia is not associated with symptoms, it has the same long-term sequelae and complications as overt ischemia and must be treated. It should be strongly suspected when systolic blood pressure is lower at the ankle than at the arm.

The distance a person can walk before the onset of pain indicates the degree of circulatory inadequacy (e.g., two blocks or more is mild; one block is moderate; half a block or less is severe). The primary symptom may be only a sense of weakness or tiredness in these same areas; both the pain and weakness or fatigue are relieved by rest.

Pain at rest indicates more severe involvement, which may mimic deep venous thrombosis (DVT), but relief from the occlusive disease can sometimes be obtained by dangling the uncovered leg over the edge of the bed. This dependent position would increase symptoms of DVT, which is usually treated by leg elevation. Exercise may cause pedal pulses to disappear in some people. Sudden occlusion of the arteries, usually at the level of one of these smaller branches, results in gangrene. The necrotic tissue may become gangrenous and infected, requiring surgical intervention.

Occlusive arterial disease for the person with diabetes is further complicated by very slow healing, and healed areas may break down easily. In the case of diabetes mellitus, diabetic neuropathy with diminished or absent sensation of the toes or feet often occurs, predisposing the person to injury or pressure ulcers that may progress because of poor blood flow and subsequent loss of sensation (Table 9.13). The amputation rate in people with diabetes is markedly higher than in individuals with PAD without diabetes mellitus.

Medical Management

Prevention and Treatment

Prevention is the key to reducing the incidence of PVD caused by atherosclerosis. Risk factor reduction and lifestyle measures are the first steps, with smoking cessation (or not ever starting) as the single most effective prevention tool. A conservative approach to care that includes a program of dietary management to decrease cholesterol and fat, pain control, and daily physical training and exercise[48] therapy to improve collateralization and function has been uniformly endorsed by experts in vascular disease.[7] Careful attention must be paid to preventive skin care (Box 9.9) to avoid even minor injuries, infections, or ulcerations.

Low-dose aspirin may be administered as an antiplatelet agent, and pentoxifylline may be used to improve capillary blood flow.

Statins, used for the prevention of cardiovascular disease because of their antithrombotic properties, have been shown to be effective in reducing the risk of DVT and may become useful in the primary and secondary prevention of DVT.[179]

Surgical intervention (Fig. 9.26) is indicated if blood flow is compromised enough to produce symptoms of ischemic pain at rest, if tissue death has occurred, or if claudication interferes with essential activities or work.[49] This decision is usually made after exercise therapy combined with risk factor modification has been unsuccessful in preventing this level of impairment and subsequent disability.

Cessation of smoking may be required by the physician before surgery is considered (see Figs. 9.3 and 9.5). People with multisegmented arterial disease with more involved symptoms are at greater risk of amputation.

9.17 Special Implications for the PTA: Arteriosclerosis Obliterans (Peripheral Arterial Disease) See also 9.22 Special Implications for the PTA: Peripheral Vascular Disease.

Arterial Tests and Measures

Graded treadmill protocols have been developed to test people with PAD that give highly reproducible results and are able to evaluate change in exercise performance.

As the individual walks on the treadmill, time to pain and maximal walking time are recorded. All people limited by claudication are reproducibly brought to maximal levels of discomfort.[10]

Venous filling time provides a reasonable assessment of the general state of perfusion but requires patent venous valves to be a valid measure. Have the client assume a recumbent position and elevate the legs to facilitate venous drainage. When the veins have collapsed below the level of the skin, quickly bring the person to a sitting position with the legs hanging in a dependent position. The time necessary for the veins to fill to skin level is the venous filling time. A filling time greater than 25 seconds implies an increased risk of ulceration, infection, and poor wound healing.

The ankle/brachial index (ABI) (Box 9.10) is another measure of arterial perfusion available to PTAs for use in documenting the need for and benefit of a prescriptive exercise program. The ABI is a simple, inexpensive, and noninvasive tool that correlates well with angiographic disease severity and functional symptoms. It is well established as an independent predictor of cardiovascular morbidity and mortality.[149,194]

TABLE 9.13   Comparison of Arterial, Venous, and Neuropathic Ulcers

	Arterial Ulcer	Venous Ulcer	Neuropathic (Diabetic) Ulcer
Etiology[a]	Arteriosclerosis obliterans Atheroembolism Large- or medium-vessel atherosclerosis Raynaud's disease Diabetes mellitus Collagen disease Vasculitis	Valvular incompetence History of DVT Venous insufficiency accompanied by hypertension Peripheral incompetence; varicose veins	Diabetes mellitus; combination of arterial disease and peripheral neuropathy Repetitive unrecognized trauma
Location	Anywhere on leg or dorsum of foot or toes Bone prominences (anterior tibial) Lateral malleolus	Medial aspect of distal one-third of lower extremity Behind medial malleolus	Same areas in which arterial ulcers appear, especially toes Areas in which peripheral neuropathy occurs (pressure points on plantar aspect of foot, toes, and heels)
Clinical manifestations	Painful, especially with legs elevated Pulses poor quality or absent Intermittent claudication (exertional calf pain) Rest pain or nocturnal aching of foot or forefoot relieved by dependent dangling position Integumentary (trophic) changes Hair loss Thin, shiny skin Ischemia: pale, white skin color Areas of sluggish blood flow: red-purple mottling Hypersensitivity to palpation History of minor nonhealing trauma	Can be very painful; venous insufficiency can cause aching pain; more comfortable with legs elevated Normal arterial pulses Eczema or stasis dermatitis Edema Venous periwound (dark pigmentation) is called *hemosiderin staining*; leakage of hemosiderin is caused by blood that cannot return because of vascular incompetence	Classic symmetric ascending stocking-glove distribution of sensory loss (begins in feet and ascends to knees, then symptoms begin in the hands) May not be painful because of loss of sensation (e.g., neuropathic ulcers are painless or insensate when palpated) Some people experience unpleasant sensations (tingling or hypersensitivity to normally painless stimuli) Loss of vibratory sense and light touch Pulses may be present or diminished (arteries become calcified) Neuropathic foot is warm and dry Loss of vascular tone increases arteriovenous shunting and impairs blood flow necessary for wound healing; sepsis common Altered biomechanics and weight bearing
Wound appearance	Minimal exudate with dry necrosis Blanched wound base and periwound tissue	Superficial Highly exudative Red wound base Irregular edges	Round, craterlike with elevated rim; diabetes hastens changes described in figure at left (arterial ulcer) Minimal drainage Frequently deep High infection rate

[a]Ulceration may also occur as a result of lymphatic disorders, skin cancer, metabolic abnormalities, and vasculitis.
Images from Bryant R, Nix D: *Acute and chronic wounds: current management concepts,* ed 5, St Louis, 2016, Elsevier; neuropathic ulcer courtesy of J. Lebretton and V. Driver.
DVT, Deep vein thrombosis.

BOX 9.9   Guidelines for Skin Care and Protection

Temperature Protection

- Nicotine causes vasoconstriction of the small vessels in the hands and feet; avoid all tobacco products.
- Recognize and avoid other triggers that cause vasoconstriction (e.g., emotional distress, caffeine, cold or cough remedies that contain a decongestant).
- Wear layers of clothing made of natural fibers, such as cotton, to draw moisture away from the skin; in cold weather, wear a hat and scarf because heat is lost through the scalp. Silk is a good insulator; consider it for socks and long underwear.
- Wear thick mittens, which are warmer than gloves, and socks purchased from an outdoor clothing or ski shop designed to wick moisture away while retaining body heat.
- Avoid air conditioning; wear warmer clothes, layer light clothing, or wear a sweater or jacket in air conditioning; be careful when going into an air-conditioned environment after being out in the heat and vice versa.
- Test water temperature before bathing or showering or have a member of the family test first; use another portion of the body to test if insensitivity exists in hand or foot.
- Use a heating pad, a hot water bottle, or an electric blanket to warm the sheets of your bed before getting into bed, but *do not* apply these directly to the skin and do not sleep with any electric device left on; if necessary wear light socks and mittens or gloves to bed. Do not soak hands or feet in hot water.
- Keep household temperatures at a constant, even, and comfortable level.
- Keep protective covering available at all times, even in the summer.
- Avoid contact with extremes of temperature, such as oven, dishwasher (hot dishes), refrigerator, or freezer; wear thick oven mitts whenever reaching into the oven. Keep mittens or warm gloves by the refrigerator and freezer to prevent symptoms when reaching into it.
- Wear rubber gloves whenever cleaning, washing dishes, or rinsing or peeling vegetables under water.
- Avoid holding ice, ice-cold fruit, hot or cold drinks, or frozen foods; wear protective gloves whenever making contact with any of these items.

Skin Care

- Take care of your skin, and give your hands and feet extra care and protection; examine hands and feet daily; at the first sign of bruising, skin changes (e.g., cracking, calluses, blisters, redness), swelling, infection, or ulcer, immediately contact a member of your health care team (e.g., nurse, physical therapist, physician). If vision is impaired, have a family member or health care professional inspect your hands and feet.
- Circulation problems tend to create dry skin and delay healing; keep your skin clean and well moisturized; wash with a mild, creamy, or moisturizing liquid soap or gel; clean carefully between fingers and toes; *do not* soak them.
- Avoid perfumed lotions, and do not put lotion on sores or between toes.
- Observe carefully for any activities that might put pressure on your fingertips, such as using a manual typewriter, playing a musical instrument (e.g., guitar, piano), and doing crafts or needlework.

- Do not go barefoot indoors or outdoors; this includes getting up at night; avoid wearing open-toed shoes, pointy-toed shoes, high heels, or sandals; always wear absorbent socks or socks that wick perspiration away from skin; avoid nylon material (including pantyhose material); avoid stockings with seams or with mends; change socks or stockings daily.
- Make sure shoes provide good support without being too tight, avoid shoes that cause excessive foot perspiration, and alternate shoes throughout the week (i.e., do not wear the same shoes every day). Do not wear shoes without socks or stockings.
- Avoid hot tubs and prolonged baths; dry carefully between toes; water temperature should be 90°F to 95°F.
- Use heel protectors, sheepskin, and other protective devices whenever recommended.

Other Tips

- For Raynaud's disease or phenomenon, avoid situations that precipitate excitement, anxiety, or feelings of fear; teach yourself how to recognize early signs of these emotions and use relaxation techniques to reduce stress.
- For Raynaud's disease or phenomenon, when you have an attack, gently rewarm fingers or toes as soon as possible; place your hands under your armpits, wiggle fingers or toes, or move or walk around to improve circulation; if possible, run warm (*not* hot) water over the affected body part until normal color returns.
- Do not use razor blades; use electric razors.
- Avoid medications and substances (e.g., nicotine; caffeine in chocolate, tea, coffee, and soft drinks) that can cause blood vessels to narrow; discuss all medications with your physician.
- Maintain good circulation; do not stay in one position for more than 30 minutes; use breathing and stretching exercises whenever confined to a desk, chair, car, or bed for more than 30 minutes.
- Do not wear constricting or tight clothing, especially tight socks; avoid elastic around wrists or ankles.
- Do not wear jewelry, such as watches or bracelets, to bed at night.
- Leave a night light on in dark areas; turn on lights in dark areas and hallways.
- Do not sit with legs crossed because this can cause pressure on the nerves and blood vessels.
- Avoid sunburn.
- Do not scratch insect bites; do not scratch areas of itchy skin.
- Do not do bathroom surgery on corns or calluses; do not use chemical agents for the removal of corns or calluses; see your physician.

Care of Nails

- Use clippers, not scissors; *do not* use razor blades; cut toenails straight across, but file fingernails in a rounded fashion to the tips of your fingers.
- Take care of your nails; use cuticle softener or moisturizing cream or lotion around cuticles; push the cuticles back very gently with a cotton swab soaked in cuticle remover; *do not* push cuticles back with a sharp object and *do not* cut the cuticles with scissors or nail clippers.
- Use lamb's wool between overlapping toes.

Blood pressures are measured both in the arm (brachial blood pressure) and in the ankle, with the client in a supine position for both measurements. The ankle blood pressure may be auscultated using the dorsalis pedis pulse or posterior tibialis artery with the cuff placed above the ankle. The systolic ankle pressure is divided by the brachial systolic pressure.

With increasing degrees of arterial narrowing, there is a progressive fall in systolic blood pressure distal to the sites of involvement. If both pressures are measured with the person in the supine position and the vessels are unobstructed, the ratio of ankle to brachial pressures should be 1.0.[193]

If flow to the lower extremity is decreased, the ratio will be less than 1.0. Based on two large population-based studies, the

reference standard of ABI less than 0.90 at rest or less than 0.85 after exercise in adults older than 55 indicates PAD.[73,189] ABI measurements may be of limited value in anyone with diabetes, because calcification of the tibial and peroneal arteries may render them noncompressible.[7]

ABI can be measured before and after exercise to assess the dynamics of intermittent claudication. This can be accomplished by leaving the ankle pressure cuffs in place during the exercise. Once the walk is completed or pain develops, the person rapidly assumes a supine position and the ankle pressures are measured.

At modest workloads, the healthy adult can maintain ankle systolic pressures at normal levels. If the exercise is strenuous, there may be a transient fall in systolic pressure that rapidly returns to

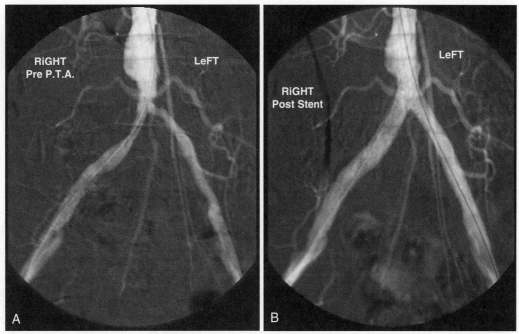

FIG. 9.26 Percutaneous transluminal angioplasty (PTA) may be used in peripheral vascular disease. (A) Significant narrowing of the aortic bifurcation and both common iliac arteries. The narrowing in both iliac arteries was successfully treated by angioplasty, and bilateral stents were inserted to maintain patency. (B) The client had bilateral calf claudication, which was relieved by this procedure. (From Forbes CD, Jackson WF: Color atlas and text of clinical medicine, ed 3, London, 2003, Mosby.)

BOX 9.10 Ankle/Brachial Index[a]

≥1.1	Suspicious for arterial calcification; blood vessels do not compress (e.g., diabetes)
1.0	Adequate blood supply; compression acceptable
<1.0	Inadequate blood supply; impaired wound healing; requires medical evaluation; prescriptive exercise beneficial
0.5-0.9	Indicates arterial occlusion; prescriptive exercise may be beneficial; delayed wound healing; light compression acceptable
<0.5	Severe arterial occlusive disease; may require surgical revascularization procedure; wound healing unlikely; rarely compress

[a]Values vary slightly from institution to institution and geographically from one area of the United States to another. Consider these values a general guideline, and check the standard used at your current facility or location.

baseline levels. If a person walks to the point of claudication, ankle systolic pressure falls precipitously, often to unrecordable levels, and will not return to baseline levels for several minutes. Generally if ankle pressure falls by more than 20% of the baseline value and requires more than 3 minutes to recovery, the test result is considered abnormal.[7,171]

Prescriptive Exercise

In prescribing an exercise program for someone with claudication secondary to occlusive disease, exercise tolerance must be determined. A training heart rate should be based on the exercise tolerance test, because persons with PVD frequently have CAD as well. Frequently symptoms of claudication occur before training heart rate is reached, but the heart rate should be monitored and should not exceed the training heart rate, even in the absence of symptoms. Anginal chest pain is a red flag to decrease intensity.

A progressive conditioning program, including walking for fixed periods, is essential, even if the initial length of walking time is only 1 minute. Exercise can protect against atherothrombotic events by improving ambulatory function; increasing cells that line the blood vessels capable of blood vessel repair,[201] endothelial-dependent dilation, and calf blood flow[36]; and favorably altering cardiovascular risk factor profile, an important element in the management of PAD.[107]

The greatest improvement occurs with intermittent exercise to near-maximal pain progressing to a long-term program of structured walking for at least 30 minutes three times weekly.[81] The most effective program begins with brisk treadmill walking at a pace that is comfortable for the individual until claudication begins, followed by immediate rest and continued walking when the pain subsides.

The PTA can direct the client to progress quickly to levels of exercise at maximal tolerable pain to obtain optimal symptomatic benefit over time. This pattern is repeated starting with intervals as short as 1 to 5 minutes, alternating with rest periods of sufficient duration to eliminate pain (usually 2 to 10 minutes). Without complicating factors, the individual is usually able to complete at least a 30- to 45-minute walk without pain or rest breaks within 6 to 8 weeks.

Claudication is influenced by the speed, incline, and surface of the walk, which should be modified whenever possible to improve exercise tolerance. Supervised exercise and social support are recommended to improve both physical function and quality of life in people with PAD and intermittent claudication.[192]

Altered gait pattern has been documented with PAD,[80] with less time spent in the swing phase of the gait cycle and more time in double stance. This ambulatory pattern favors greater gait stability at the expense of greater walking speed and can be improved with exercise rehabilitation. People with intermittent claudication associated with PAD are also functionally limited by dorsiflexion weakness, impairing their ability to perform tasks requiring distal lower extremity strength.[196]

After exercise, numbness in the foot as well as pain in the calf may occur. The foot may be cold and pale, which is an indication that the circulation has been diverted to the arteriolar bed of the leg muscles.

The main factor limiting success of exercise therapy is lack of client motivation. For this reason, the most successful programs combine regular, supervised outpatient sessions with home exercise programs; regularity rather than intensity should be stressed.

Precautions

When arterial thrombosis or embolism is suspected, the affected limb must be protected by proper positioning below the horizontal plane, and protective skin care must be provided. Heat or cold application and massage are contraindicated, and family members must also be notified of these restrictions. The home health PTA must be alert to the possibility of hot water bottles, heating pads, electric blankets, and hot foot soaks being used by the client without physician approval. This precaution is especially true for people with diabetes-associated peripheral neuropathies and for people with paraplegia.

Encourage the person with vascular disease to prevent becoming chilled by keeping the thermostat at home set at 70°F to 72°F (21.1°C to 22.2°C) and to avoid prolonged exposure to cold outdoors.

In addition, many people with PVD and diabetes mellitus have peripheral sensory neuropathy and are at greater risk for skin breakdown on the foot from weight-bearing activities such as walking or running (see Box 9.9). These individuals should participate in alternate forms of exercise even though these exercises may not improve walking ability as much as a structured walking program.[154]

Venous Diseases

Venous disease can be acute or chronic; acute venous disease includes thrombophlebitis, and chronic venous disease includes varicose vein formation and chronic venous insufficiency (CVI).

Venous thrombosis and pulmonary embolus[219]

Definition and overview. Venous thrombosis is a partial occlusion or complete occlusion of a vein by a thrombus (clot) with secondary inflammatory reaction in the wall of the vein. A venous thrombus is an intravascular collection of platelets, erythrocytes, leukocytes, and fibrin, with the potential to produce significant morbidity and mortality.[220]

There are two types of venous thrombosis: superficial (Fig. 9.27) and deep. Superficial venous thrombosis of the upper extremity can occur, although it is much less common and is usually seen in people with a systemic illness in the presence of an indwelling central venous catheter, malignancy, or, less often, hemodialysis.[138]

In the lower extremities, superficial venous thrombus is usually the result of varicose veins, is self-limiting, and is not a serious condition. Calf vein thrombosis is usually clinically silent and benign without complications, although silent calf vein thromboses can extend into more proximal veins.[17] Proximal DVTs are much more likely to become PEs.[220]

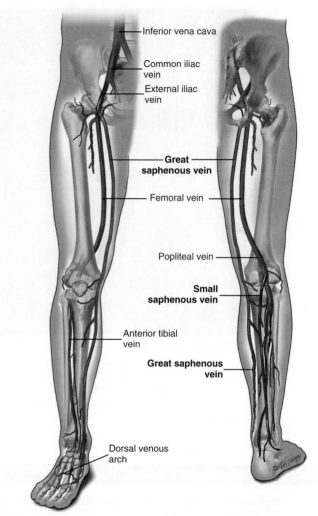

FIG. 9.27 Veins in the leg. The legs have three types of veins: deep veins (femoral and popliteal) coursing alongside the deep arteries to conduct most of the venous return from the legs; superficial veins, the great and small saphenous veins; and perforators (not pictured), the connecting veins that join the two sets and route blood from the superficial into the deep veins. The great saphenous vein starts at the medial side of the dorsum of the foot and ascends in front of the medial malleolus, crossing the tibia obliquely and ascending along the medial side of the thigh. The small saphenous vein starts on the lateral side of the dorsum of the foot and ascends behind the lateral malleolus and up the back of the leg in which it joins the popliteal vein. (From Jarvis C: Physical examination and health assessment, ed 7, St. Louis, 2016, Elsevier. ©Pat Thomas, 2011.)

Incidence and etiologic and risk factors. DVT is the third most common cardiovascular disease after acute coronary artery episodes and cerebrovascular accidents, affecting up to 2 million Americans annually.[158]

High-risk surgical candidates have a history of recent venous thromboembolism or have undergone extensive pelvic or abdominal surgery for advanced malignancy, CABG, renal transplantation, splenectomy, or major orthopedic surgery to the lower limbs.

Approximately 30% to 60% of all people undergoing major general surgical procedures or having common pathologies such as cerebrovascular accidents develop

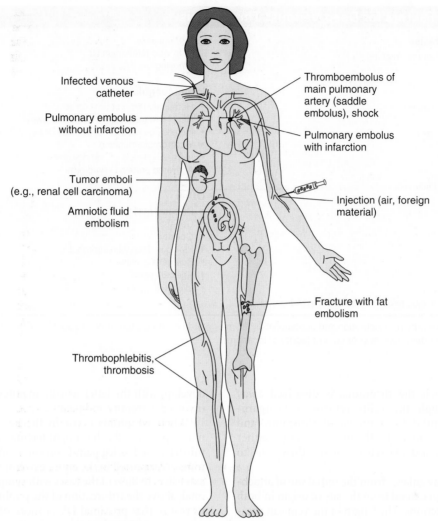

FIG. 9.28 Sources and effects of venous emboli.

Infected venous catheter

Pulmonary embolus without infarction

Tumor emboli (e.g., renal cell carcinoma)

Amniotic fluid embolism

Thrombophlebitis, thrombosis

Thromboembolus of main pulmonary artery (saddle embolus), shock

Pulmonary embolus with infarction

Injection (air, foreign material)

Fracture with fat embolism

clinical manifestations of DVT up to 4 weeks after the operation or incident[6,240] (Fig. 9.28).

Fat embolism syndrome from fat thromboembolic phenomena is a well-known consequence of femoral total hip replacement arthroplasty. Intravasation of fat into the bloodstream during prosthetic implantation has been linked with postoperative confusion and cognitive decline. The risk of fat embolism syndrome is four times greater with simultaneous bilateral total knee or total hip replacements.[120,125,184] Changes have been made in the arthroplasty surgical technique that may result in a reduced incidence of this complication.

Brain microemboli from cardiac surgery with subsequent neurologic dysfunction have also been reported. The major source of the microemboli is lipid droplets of the patient's fat that drip into the blood in the surgical field. The lipid-laden blood is aspirated and returned to the patient via the cardiopulmonary bypass apparatus.[214]

Substantial evidence indicates that the pathologic processes of venous (and arterial) thromboembolism involve both genetic and lifestyle influences. Scientific progress over the past decade has revealed a growing number of genetic factors present in more than 1% of the population that increase the relative risk

of venous thrombosis twofold to sevenfold. Several of these factors have been demonstrated to interact adversely with lifestyle influences, such as oral contraceptives and smoking.

Thrombus formation is usually attributed to venous stasis, hypercoagulability, or injury to the venous wall, although other risk factors may be present (Box 9.11). It is commonly held that at least two of these three conditions must be present for thrombi to form. What were previously considered to be idiopathic causes of thrombosis now have been identified as abnormalities associated with thrombophilia.

Pathogenesis. Any trauma to the endothelium of the vein wall exposes subendothelial tissues to platelets and clotting factors in the venous blood, initiating thrombosis. Platelets adhering to the vein wall attract the deposition of fibrin, leukocytes, and erythrocytes, forming a thrombus that may remain attached to the vessel wall. There are two types of thrombus: (1) mural thrombus, in which the thrombus is attached to the wall of the vein but does not occlude the vessel lumen, and (2) occlusive thrombus, which begins by attachment to the vessel wall and progresses to completely occlude the vessel lumen.

Both mural and occlusive thrombi may undergo one of the following forms of evolution or resolution: (1) lysis

---

BOX 9.11   Risk Factors for Deep Venous[a] Thrombosis

Immobility (Venous Stasis)
- Prolonged bed rest (e.g., burns, fracture)
- Prolonged air travel
- Neurologic disorder (e.g., spinal cord injury, stroke)
- Cardiac failure
- Absence of ankle muscle pump

Trauma (Venous Damage)
- Varicose veins
- Smoking
- Surgery
- Local trauma (e.g., direct injury)
- Intravenous injections
- Fracture or dislocation
- Childbirth and delivery
- Sclerosing agents

Lifestyle
- Hormonal status
  - Oral contraceptive use
  - Hormonal medications (e.g., tamoxifen, doxorubicin [Adriamycin])

- Pregnancy
- In vitro fertilization (?)
- Smoking

Hypercoagulation
- Hereditary thrombotic disorders
- Neoplasm (especially viscera and ovary)
- Increasing levels of coagulation factors (VIII and XI)
- Prothrombin mutation
- Increasing levels of homocysteine
- Activated protein C syndrome

Other
- Diabetes mellitus
- Genetic
- Obesity
- Previous deep vein thrombosis
- Buerger's disease
- Age >60 years
- Idiopathic cause

[a]Values vary slightly from institution to institution and geographically from one area of the United States to another. Consider these values a general guideline, and check the standard used at your current facility or location.

---

or dissolution, in which the thrombus is dissolved away and blood flow through the veins returns; (2) organization, with the potential for removal of thrombus and vein; (3) extension, in which the thrombus enlarges either proximally or distally; and (4) release of the thrombus to form a PE.

A *mural thrombus* may enlarge from the initial site of attachment, however. Clots can extend from the site of origin in both proximal and distal directions. The length of the vein can measure more than 1 m.

An *occlusive thrombus* may undergo restoration of the central venous canal. Although blood flow is restored through the vein, the valves do not recover function, resulting in backflow of blood and other secondary functional and anatomic problems.

Most occlusive thrombi heal by removal of the clot and the nonfunctional vein. Adherence of the thrombus to the vein often leads to phagocytic cell removal of both the clot and the vein followed by deposition of scar tissue (often leading to venous insufficiency under these circumstances, a condition sometimes referred to as *postthrombotic syndrome*).

Finally, the thrombus may break off and become free floating as an *embolism*. The embolus travels through the progressively enlarging venous vessels and through the right side of the heart to the progressively narrowing pulmonary artery in which it may become lodged and occlude pulmonary circulation (PE).[220] If a thrombus occludes a major vein, the venous pressure and volume rise distally. However, if a thrombus occludes a deep small vein (e.g., tibial, popliteal), collateral vessels develop and relieve the increased venous pressure and volume. This is why the majority of PEs come from proximal DVTs.

Clinical manifestations. In the early stages, approximately half of the people with DVT are asymptomatic in the affected extremity. The lower extremities are affected more often (more than 90%) but upper extremity venous thrombi can also

develop, with the latter usually manifesting with edema of the involved extremity and pain.

When symptoms occur in the lower extremity, the client may report a dull ache, a tight feeling, or pain in the calf, often misdiagnosed as leg pain from some other cause. When symptoms are reported in the entire extremity, the condition is more extensive. In 80% of the cases with symptoms, the DVT is proximal, above the trifurcation of the popliteal vein. It is important to realize that proximal DVTs more often lead to severe consequences of DVT and that at the time of diagnosis more than 50% of affected individuals already have PEs.[16]

Signs are often absent; when present but taken alone, they may be variable and unreliable. Signs and symptoms include leg or calf swelling, pain or tenderness, dilation of superficial veins, and pitting edema. The skin of the leg and ankle on the affected side may be relatively warmer than on the unaffected side. If venous obstruction is severe, the skin may be cyanotic.

Any of these symptoms can occur without DVT, possibly associated with other vascular, inflammatory, musculoskeletal, or lymphatic conditions that produce signs and symptoms similar to those of DVT.[220]

PEs, most often from the large, deep veins of the pelvis and legs, are the most devastating complication of DVT and can occur without apparent warning. Signs and symptoms of PE are dependent on the size and location of the PE[101,183] and may include the following[85]:

- Possible sudden death
- Pleuritic chest pain
- Diffuse chest discomfort
- Tachypnea
- Tachycardia
- Hemoptysis
- Anxiety, restlessness, apprehension
- Dyspnea
- Persistent cough

Upper Extremity Venous Thrombosis. In the case of upper extremity superficial venous thrombosis, dull pain and local tenderness in the region of the involved vein may be accompanied by signs of superficial induration and redness. Upper extremity superficial venous thrombosis is self-limiting and does not cause PE, because the blood flow to deeper veins is through small perforating venous channels. Iatrogenic superficial venous thrombosis is often secondary to prolonged intravenous catheter use.

Medical Management

Diagnosis

Use of the clinical decision rule (CDR) of Wells and colleagues in anyone with suspected DVT clusters signs, symptoms, and risk factors and classifies the person's likelihood of having DVT as low, moderate, or high (Table 9.14).[235-237] The CDR has been shown to be a reliable and valid tool for clinical assessment for predicting the risk of DVT in the lower extremity.[18,19,122] The CDR has been specifically shown to be valid with orthopedic outpatients.[182] A recent investigation revealed that physical therapists and PTAs often underestimate the likelihood of DVT in high-risk individuals and frequently do not refer to a physician when they should.[183]

Moderate- to high-risk individuals receive Doppler duplex ultrasonography as a rapid screening procedure to detect thrombosis.

It is recognized that often other calf muscle strain or contusion may be difficult to differentiate from venous thrombosis; further diagnostic testing may be required to determine the correct diagnosis. Although Homans' sign was once used for differential diagnosis of acute DVT, it is no longer considered a sensitive or specific test for ruling DVT in or out.

Prevention

Primary prevention of DVT is important through the use of early mobilization for low-risk individuals and prophylactic use of anticoagulants (see Table 9.5) in people considered at moderate to high risk for DVT. Although such interventions reduce the risk of DVT, it must be understood that even people receiving anticoagulant therapy may still develop DVTs. The highest incidence of DVT occurs with abdominal, thoracic, pelvic, hip, or knee surgical procedures; neurologic or other conditions leading to paresis or paralysis; and prolonged immobilization, cancer, and CHF.

Routine use of knee elastic stockings in all postoperative clients has been adopted in most hospitals, and many facilities use pneumatic pressure devices with on-off cycles applied for the first few hours after major surgery to mimic the calf pump. Once the person is able, ankle pumping is added, because this has been shown effective in increasing average peak venous velocity (flow) from the lower extremity with dorsiflexion of the ankle by over 200%, reducing DVT while the person is immobilized.[241]

Treatment

The goals of DVT management are to prevent progression to PE, limit extension of the thrombus, limit damage to the vein, and prevent another clot from forming. Current therapy is to administer low molecular weight heparin (LMWH) followed by long-term oral anticoagulation (warfarin). Anticoagulation

TABLE 9.14 **Wells' Clinical Decision Rule for Deep Venous Thrombosis**	
Clinical Presentation	**Score**
Active cancer (within 6 months of diagnosis or receipt of palliative care)	1
Paralysis, paresis, or recent immobilization of lower extremity	1
Bedridden for more than 3 days or major surgery in the last 4 weeks	1
Localized tenderness in the center of the posterior calf, the popliteal space, or along the femoral vein in the anterior thigh or groin	1
Entire lower extremity swelling	1
Unilateral calf swelling (more than 3 mm larger than uninvolved side)	1
Unilateral pitting edema	1
Collateral superficial veins (nonvaricose)	1
An alternative diagnosis that is as likely as (or more likely than) DVT (e.g., cellulitis, postoperative swelling, calf strain)	−2
Total Points	
Key	
−2 to 0: Low probability of DVT (3%)	
1 or 2: Moderate probability of DVT (17%)	
3 or more: High probability of DVT (75%)	

DVT, Deep venous thrombosis. Medical consultation is advised in the presence of low probability; medical referral is required with moderate or high score.
From Wells PS, Anderson DR, Bormanis J, et al: Value of assessment of pretest probability of deep-vein thrombosis in clinical management, Lancet 350:1795–1798, 1997.

therapy for acute DVT prevents enlargement of the thrombus and allows for further attachment of the thrombus to the vessel wall, reducing the likelihood of PE.[220]

Today, routine practice is to authorize ambulation in all cases of DVT after adequate anticoagulation by LMWH or heparin has been administered if local symptoms and general condition permit. The concern in an acute care or rehabilitation setting is the increased risk of PE in clients who are aggressively mobilized too soon after a diagnosis of a DVT and before adequate anticoagulation has been administered. Bed rest (up to 24 hours) may be advised before a person with acute DVT is returned to ambulation and physical therapy.

Elastic stockings must be worn whenever the person is ambulating or in the upright position. The standard of care for DVT is moving toward the following protocol: inject with LMWH and discharge to home with additional doses the client can use to inject at home over the next week while taking warfarin and return for follow-up in 1 week with evaluation of INR. Clients are advised to remain active but avoid any straining maneuvers.

For cases of massive DVT, thrombolysis, thrombectomy, and embolectomy are being used with increasing skill and improved outcomes.

Prognosis

DVTs that are not diagnosed can lead to life-threatening consequences, such as PE. With appropriate intervention and in the absence of complications, a return to normal health and activity can be expected within 1 to 3 weeks for the person with a calf DVT and within 6 weeks for the person with thigh or pelvic DVT.

Prognosis depends on the size of the vessel involved, the presence of collateral circulation, and the underlying cause of the thrombosis. Recurrence occurs in 5% of DVT cases and 1% of PE cases and may be related to risk factors listed in Box 9.11 or too short a time on anticoagulants.

It remains unknown whether anticoagulant therapy should be extended for longer periods, if lower intensity should be recommended during this extension, or if the benefits of extended anticoagulant therapy outweigh the risk of bleeding complications.

A potential long-term complication of DVT is venous stasis or insufficiency when permanent damage to the vein has occurred. Of people who have had DVT treated with anticoagulants, 25% to 30% will develop some form of postthrombotic syndrome in the first 10 years after DVT.

9.18 Special Implications for the PTA: Venous Thrombosis and Pulmonary Embolism

Risk Assessment

Populations at risk (see Box 9.11), especially postoperative, postpartum, and immobilized clients, should be identified by the medical staff and observed carefully. Risk factor assessment scales for use in a therapy practice are available.

The person at risk for DVT secondary to fracture and subsequent immobility involving a lower extremity cast should be carefully evaluated when the cast is removed. Normally, calf muscle atrophy is easily observed when the cast is removed. Normal calf size (less than 1-cm difference between left and right) without atrophy on cast removal may signal swelling associated with DVT.

For the client with diagnosed thrombophlebitis, the PTA should monitor and report any signs of PE, such as chest pain, hemoptysis, cough, diaphoresis, dyspnea, and apprehension. Clients with a history of DVT may develop CVI even years later and therefore must be monitored periodically for life.

Anyone receiving anticoagulant therapy must be monitored for manifestations of bleeding, as evidenced by blood in the urine, in the stool, or along the gums or teeth; subcutaneous bruising; or back, pelvic, or flank pain. The presence of any of these signs or symptoms must be reported to the physician immediately.

The risk for bleeding is increased with alcohol use, especially if there is concomitant liver disease, because alcohol also can potentiate warfarin. Many herbs have natural anticoagulant effects that can potentiate the effect of warfarin, and others can counteract its effect. Ginkgo biloba, garlic, dong quai, dan shen, and ginseng should not be used or taken at the same time as warfarin. Anyone using these products should be encouraged to discuss medication dosage with the prescribing physician. Eating large quantities of vitamin K–rich foods can also interfere with the drug's anticoagulant effects, necessitating careful monitoring of food intake in patients who are on warfarin.

Bleeding under the skin and easy bruising in response to the slightest trauma can occur when platelet production is altered. This condition necessitates extreme care in the therapy setting, especially for any intervention requiring soft tissue mobilization, manual therapy, or the use of any equipment, including any modalities and weight-training devices.

Prevention and Intervention

Prevention is the key to treatment of thrombophlebitis, both preventing thrombus formation and preventing thrombi from becoming emboli. Preventive therapy can be tailored to the individual's level of risk and may include active and passive ROM exercise, early ambulation for brief but regular periods whenever possible, coughing and deep-breathing exercises, and proper positioning.

The person at risk must be taught the importance of avoiding one position for prolonged periods and avoiding pillows under the legs postoperatively to facilitate venous return. At the same time, elevation of the legs just above the level of the heart aids blood flow by gravitational force and prevents venous stasis as a contributing factor to the formation of new thrombi.

Placing the foot of the bed in Trendelenburg's position (6-inch elevation with slight knee bend to prevent popliteal pressure) decreases venous pressure and helps relieve pain and edema. Prolonged sitting in a chair in the early postoperative period should be avoided.

After thrombosis of a deep calf vein, elastic support hose should be worn for at least 6 to 8 weeks or longer if risk is moderate or high. Helping the client find easier ways to put the hose on and explaining the purpose may increase compliance in using the hose consistently and correctly.

Support pantyhose may be an acceptable alternative for some people who have trouble putting on the compressive stockings or who live in very hot climates. The hypothesis for the use of compressive or elastic stockings is that the compressive force applied by the stocking causes the vessel wall to become applied to the thrombus, keeping the thrombus in its location and preventing movement inside the blood vessel. Without the external compressive force of the stocking, once the person stands, increased hydrostatic pressure causes venous distention and permits the thrombus to become free floating inside the vessel.[220]

Varicose veins

Definition and incidence. Varicose veins are an abnormal dilation of veins, usually the saphenous veins of the lower extremities, leading to tortuosity (twisting and turning) of the vessel, incompetence of the valves, and a propensity to thrombosis. Women are affected with leg varicosities more often than men (secondary to pregnancy) until age 70 years, when the gender difference disappears. Forty-one percent of women aged 40 to 50 years and 72% of women aged 60 to 70 years have varicose veins.[94]

This condition most often develops from age 30 to 50 years for all persons. A separate but similar condition called *spider veins* or *telangiectasia* (broken capillaries) results in fine-lined networks of red, blue, or purple veins, usually on the thighs, calves, and ankles. The veins may form patterns resembling a sunburst, a spider web, or a tree with branches but can also appear as short, unconnected, or parallel lines.

Etiologic and risk factors. Varicose veins may be an inherited trait, but it is unclear whether the valvular incompetence is secondary to defective valves in the saphenous veins or to a fundamental weakness of the walls of the vein leading to dilation of the vessel.

Periods of high venous pressure associated with heavy lifting or prolonged sitting or standing are risk factors. Hormonal changes often contribute to the development of this condition by relaxing the vein walls.

Other risk factors include pressure associated with pregnancy or obesity, heart failure, hemorrhoids, constipation, esophageal

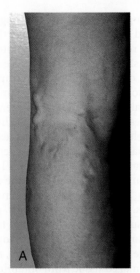
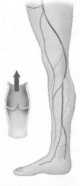
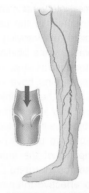

NORMAL VEINS
Functional valves aid
in flow of venous blood
back to heart

VARICOSE VEINS
Failure of valves and
pooling of blood in
superficial veins

FIG. 9.29 (A) The appearance of superficial varicose veins. (B) Diagrams of normal and varicose veins. (From Leonard PC: Building a medical vocabulary: with Spanish translations, ed 9, St Louis, 2015, Saunders.)

varices, and hepatic cirrhosis. Risk factors for spider veins are similar but also include local injury.

Pathogenesis. Blood returning to the heart from the legs must flow upward through the veins, against the pull of gravity. This blood is milked upward, principally by the massaging action of the muscles against the veins. To prevent the blood from flowing backward, the veins contain one-way valves located at intervals, which operate in pairs by closing to stop the reverse movement of the blood.

The vessels most commonly affected by varicosities are located just beneath the skin superficial to the deep fascia and function without the kind of support deep veins of the legs receive from surrounding muscles. As the one-way valves become incompetent or the veins become more elastic, the veins engorge with stagnant blood and become pooled. Any condition accompanied by pressure changes places a strain on these veins, and the lack of pumping action of the lower leg muscles causes blood to pool.

The weight of the blood continually pressing downward against the closed venous valves causes the veins to distend and eventually lose their elasticity. When several valves lose their ability to function properly, the blood collects in the veins, causing the veins to become swollen and distended. During pregnancy, the uterus may press against the veins coming from the lower extremities and prevent the free flow of returning blood. More force is required to push the blood through the veins, and the increased back-pressure can result in varicose veins.

Clinical manifestations. The clinical picture is not directly correlated with the severity of the varicosities; extensive varicose veins may be asymptomatic, but minimal varicosities may result in multiple symptoms. The development of varicose veins is usually gradual; the most common symptom reported is a dull, aching heaviness, tension, or feeling of fatigue brought on by periods of standing. Cramps of the lower legs may occur, especially at night, and elevation of the legs often provides relief. Itching from an associated dermatitis may also occur above the ankle.

The most visible sign of varicosities is the dilated, tortuous, elongated veins beneath the skin, which are usually readily visible when the person is standing (Fig. 9.29). Varicosities of long duration may be accompanied by secondary tissue changes, such as a brownish pigmentation of the skin and a thinning of the skin above the ankle. Swelling may also occur around the ankles.

Untreated, the veins become thick and hard to the touch; impaired circulation and skin changes may lead to ulcers of the lower legs, especially around the ankles (see Table 9.13). One of the most important distinctions between varicose veins and spider veins is that in some cases varicose veins can result in thromboses (blood clots) and phlebitis (inflammation of the vein) or venous insufficiency ulcers. Spider veins are merely a cosmetic issue with no adverse effects.

Medical Management

Diagnosis
The physician must distinguish between the symptoms of arteriosclerotic PVD, such as intermittent claudication and coldness of the feet, and symptoms of venous disease, because occlusive arterial disease usually contraindicates the operative management of varicosities below the knee. When the two conditions coexist, the reduced blood flow caused by the atherosclerosis may even improve the varicosities by reducing blood flow through the veins.

Visual inspection and palpation identify varicose veins of the legs, and Doppler ultrasonography or the duplex scanner is useful in detecting the location of incompetent valves.

Treatment
Treatment of mild varicose veins is conservative, consisting of periodic daily rest periods with feet elevated slightly above the heart. Client education as to the importance of promoting circulation is stressed, including instructions to make frequent changes in posture, practice a daily exercise program, and use properly fitting elastic stockings appropriately.

When varicosities have progressed past the stage at which conservative care is helpful, surgical intervention and compression sclerotherapy may be considered. In the past, surgical treatment of varicose veins consisted of removing the varicosities and the incompetent perforating veins (ligation and stripping), a procedure sometimes referred to as *stripping the veins.*

Other procedures for varicose veins have been developed, including radiofrequency, sclerotherapy (injections of a hardening, or sclerosing, solution; over several months' time the injected veins atrophy and blood is channeled into other veins), and laser therapy (noninvasive use of near-infrared wavelengths). Ligation and stripping of the greater saphenous vein prevent its use as a source for future CABGs, motivating researchers to develop effective intervention techniques that salvage large veins.

Prognosis
Good results with relief of symptoms are usually possible in the majority of cases. Early conservative care for varicose veins during initial stages may help prevent the condition from worsening, but advanced disease may not be prevented from recurring, even with surgical intervention or sclerotherapy. Although surgery for varicose veins can improve appearance, it may not reduce the physical discomfort, suggesting that most lower limb symptoms may have a nonvenous cause.

9.19 Special Implications for the PTA: Varicose Veins The PTA can be very instrumental in developing prescriptive exercise and preventive measures for anyone at risk for, or already diagnosed with, varicose veins. Because excessive sitting or standing contributes to this condition, the PTA can individualize a program to help the person avoid static postures and use quick stretch or movement breaks coordinated with deep-breathing exercises.

Over-the-counter pantyhose should be replaced with special compressive hose that do not constrict the area behind the knee, the upper leg, the waist, or the groin. These should be worn as much as possible during the daytime hours (including during exercise for some people) but may be removed at night. After exercise and at the end of the day, instruct the individual to elevate the legs in a supported position above the level of the heart for 10 to 15 minutes.

Encourage the person to practice good breathing techniques during this time. Aerobic exercise, strength training, or resistive exercises are encouraged, but high-impact activities, such as jogging or step aerobics, should be avoided. Brisk walking, cycling, cross-country skiing or Nordic track, rowing, and swimming are all good alternatives to high-impact activities.

Chronic venous insufficiency

Definition and incidence. CVI, also known as *postphlebitic syndrome* and *venous stasis,* is defined as inadequate venous return over a long period of time. This condition follows most severe cases of DVT, although it is possible to develop CVI without prior episodes of DVT. CVI may also occur as a result of leg trauma, varicose veins, and neoplastic obstruction of the pelvic veins. The long-term sequelae of CVI may be chronic leg ulcers, accounting for the majority of vascular ulceration; incidence is expected to continue rising with the aging of America.[158]

Etiologic factors and pathogenesis. CVI occurs when damaged or destroyed valves in the veins result in decreased venous return, increasing venous pressure and producing venous stasis. Without adequate valve function and in the absence of the calf muscle pump, blood flows in the veins bidirectionally, causing high ambulatory venous pressures in the calf veins (venous hypertension). Superficial veins and capillaries dilate in response to the venous hypertension. Red blood cells, proteins, and fluids leak out of the capillaries into interstitial spaces, producing edema and the reddish brown pigmentation characteristic of CVI.

Chronic pooling of blood in the veins of the lower extremities prevents adequate cellular oxygenation and removal of waste products. Any trauma, especially pressure, further lowers the oxygen supply by reducing blood flow into the area. Cell death occurs, and necrotic tissue develops into venous stasis ulcers. The cycle of reduced oxygenation, necrosis, and ulceration prevents damaged tissue from obtaining necessary nutrients, causing delayed healing and persistent ulceration. Poor circulation impairs immune and inflammatory responses, leaving venous stasis ulcers susceptible to infection.

Other contributing factors may include poor nutrition, immobility, and local trauma (past or present). A previous history of burns requiring skin grafts predisposes the individual to venous insufficiency. The area of the graft usually lacks superficial veins, properly functioning capillaries, or both, resulting in blood pooling in these areas. As a result, previously burned areas and skin grafts in the lower extremity are susceptible to vascular ulceration.

Clinical manifestations. CVI is characterized by progressive edema of the leg; thickening, coarsening, and brownish pigmentation of skin around the ankles; and venous stasis ulceration (see Table 9.13). Venous insufficiency ulcers constitute approximately 80% of all lower extremity ulcers, occurring most often above the medial malleolus in which venous hypertension is greatest.

These ulcers characteristically are shallow wounds with a white creamy to fibrous slough over a base of good granulation tissue. They can be very painful, with a moderate to large amount of drainage. The wounds typically have irregular borders and are partial to full thickness, often with signs of reepithelialization (e.g., pink or red granulation base). Frequently, moderate to severe edema is present in the limb; in long-standing cases, this edema becomes hardened to a dense, woody texture. The skin of the involved extremity is usually thin, shiny, dry, and cyanotic. Dermatitis and cellulitis may develop later in this condition.

9.20 Special Implications for the PTA: Chronic Venous Insufficiency The PTA can be very instrumental in providing clients with venous insufficiency with education and prevention to avoid complications that can occur with vascular ulceration and chronic wounds. Formulating an exercise prescription; collaborating with a nutritionist; and understanding the underlying cause, hemodynamics, comorbidities, and principles of tissue repair are essential in developing a plan of care.

Compression therapy is the gold standard for treatment of venous insufficiency, especially when venous leg ulcers are present. The goal is to promote venous return from peripheral veins to central circulation. The PTA may also use layered gradient compression wraps. The presence of CHF is considered a precaution for the use of external compression and requires close collaboration between the physician and the therapist and PTA.

Before initiation of compression therapy the ABI should be measured. Compression may not be tolerated and/or may have to be modified if arterial circulation is compromised. Arterial obstruction in the presence of venous insufficiency may not be readily recognized.

Assessing ABI is also warranted if wounds associated with CVI do not demonstrate healing within 2 weeks of beginning wound care. ABIs can be higher than 1.0 in individuals with diabetes because the vessels do not compress due to arterial calcification.[7]

Assessment of the legs should be performed frequently to observe for insufficiency (stasis) ulcers, skin changes, impaired growth of nails, and discrepancy in size of extremities, including observations and measurements for edema.

In the home health setting, the client or family should be instructed to contact a member of the medical team if any edema or change in the condition of the extremity occurs. When a stasis ulcer of any size is detected, treatment is initiated. A wound care specialist (usually a PT or a nurse) is a vital part of the health care team in the management of stasis ulcers.

Whirlpool beyond an initial one or two treatments is contraindicated, because the increased blood volume and dependent position (underlying causes of wound) can make the edema worse. When pulsatile debridement devices are unavailable, limited hydrotherapy (maximal temperature 80°F [26.7°C]) may be indicated to remove loose debris, and antiseptics may be indicated to moisten dried exudate or to facilitate debridement.

The client should be advised to avoid prolonged standing and sitting; crossing the legs; sitting too high for feet to touch the floor or too deep, causing pressure against the popliteal space; and wearing tight clothing or support hose or stockings that extend above the knee, which act as a tourniquet at the popliteal fossa. Elastic stockings are recommended, but they must be worn properly to avoid bunching behind the knee or uneven compression in the popliteal fossa.

Vasomotor disorders
Raynaud's disease and Raynaud's phenomenon
Definition and Overview. Intermittent episodes of small artery or arteriole constriction of the extremities causing temporary pallor and cyanosis of the digits and changes in skin temperature are called *Raynaud's phenomenon*. These episodes occur in response to cold temperature or strong emotion, such as anxiety or excitement. When this condition is a primary vasospastic disorder it is called (idiopathic) *Raynaud's disease.* If the disorder is secondary to another disease or underlying cause, the term *Raynaud's phenomenon* is used.

Incidence and Etiologic Factors
Raynaud's Disease. Eighty percent of persons with Raynaud's disease are women aged 20 to 49 years. The exact cause of Raynaud's disease remains unknown, but it appears to be caused by hypersensitivity of digital arteries to cold, release of serotonin, and genetic susceptibility to vasospasm. It is usually experienced as more annoying than medically serious.

Raynaud's Phenomenon. Epidemiologists estimate that Raynaud's phenomenon is a problem for 10% to 20% of the general population; it affects women 20 times more frequently than men, usually from ages 15 to 40 years. Risk factors for Raynaud's phenomenon are different between men and women. The Framingham Offspring Study reports that age and smoking are associated with Raynaud's phenomenon in men only, whereas an association with marital status and alcohol use was observed in women only. These findings suggest that different mechanisms influence the expression of Raynaud's phenomenon in men and women.[74]

Raynaud's phenomenon as a condition secondary to another disease is often associated with Buerger's disease or connective tissue disorders. Raynaud's phenomenon can be a sign of occult (hidden) neoplasm, which should especially be suspected when it presents unilaterally.

Raynaud's phenomenon may also occur with change in temperature, such as occurs when going from a warm outside environment to an air-conditioned room. In addition, it may be associated with occlusive arterial diseases and neurogenic lesions, such as thoracic outlet syndrome, or with the effects of long-term exposure to cold (occupational or frostbite), trauma, or use of vibrating equipment such as jackhammers. Injuries to the small vessels of the hands may produce Raynaud's phenomenon. The trauma can be a result of repetitive stress that comes from using crutches for extended periods, typing on a computer keyboard, or even playing the piano.

Because nicotine causes small blood vessels to constrict, smoking can trigger attacks in persons who are predisposed to this phenomenon.

Pathogenesis and Clinical Manifestations. Scientists theorize that Raynaud's phenomenon is associated with a disturbance in the control of vascular reflexes. Although the causes differ for Raynaud's disease and Raynaud's phenomenon, the clinical manifestations are the same, based on a pathogenesis of arterial vasospasm in the skin.

It begins with the release of chemical messengers, which cause blood vessels to constrict and remain constricted. The flow of oxygenated blood to these areas is reduced, and the skin becomes pale and cold. The blood in the constricted vessels, which has released its oxygen to the tissues surrounding the vessels, pools in the tissues, producing a bluish or purplish color.

In most cases, the skin color progresses from blue to white to red. First, ischemia from vasospastic attacks causes cyanosis, numbness, and the sensation of cold in the digits (thumbs usually remain unaffected). The affected tissues become numb or painful. For unknown reasons, the flow of chemical that triggered the process eventually stops. The vessels relax, and blood flow is restored. The skin becomes white (characterized by pallor) and then red (characterized by rubor) as the vasospasm subsides and the capillaries become engorged with oxygenated blood. Oxygen-rich blood returns to the area, and as it does, the skin becomes warm and flushed. The person may experience throbbing, paresthesia, and slight swelling as this occurs.

Sensory changes, such as numbness, stiffness, diminished sensation, and aching pain, often accompany vasomotor manifestations. Initially no abnormal findings are present between attacks, but over time, frequent, prolonged episodes of vasospasm causing ischemia interfere with cellular metabolism, causing the skin of the fingertips to thicken and the fingernails to become brittle.

In severe, chronic Raynaud's phenomenon, the underlying condition may have produced scars in the vessels, reducing the

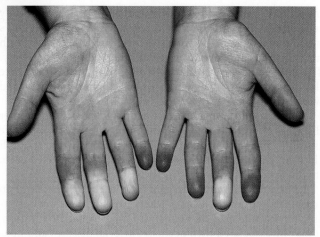

FIG. 9.30 Raynaud's disease or phenomenon. White color (pallor) from arteriospasm and resulting deficit in blood supply may initially involve only one or two fingers. Cold and numbness or pain may accompany the pallor or cyanosis stage. Subsequent episodes may involve the entire finger and may include all the fingers. Toes are affected in 40% of cases. (From Hallett JW, Mills JL, Earnshaw J, et al: Comprehensive vascular and endovascular surgery, ed 2, Philadelphia, 2009, Mosby.)

vessel diameter and therefore blood flow. When attacks occur, they are often more severe, resulting in prolonged loss of blood to fingers and toes, which can produce painful skin ulcers; rarely, gangrene may develop. Episodes of Raynaud's disease are often bilateral, progressing distally to proximally along the digits. Raynaud's phenomenon may be unilateral, involving only one or two fingers, but this clinical presentation warrants a physician's differential diagnosis because it can be associated with cancer (Fig. 9.30).

9.21 Special Implications for the PTA: Vasomotor Disorders

Raynaud's Disease and Phenomenon

Prevention of episodes of Raynaud's is important. The affected individual must be encouraged to keep warm, avoid air conditioning, and dress warmly in the winter.

Aquatic therapy is often helpful in diminishing symptoms, but again, the individual must be careful when moving from place to place with extreme temperature changes. The use of antihypertensives for Raynaud's can result in postural hypotension; the physician should be notified of these findings to alter the dosage.

Physical or occupational therapy is often prescribed and should include client education about managing symptoms through protective skin care and cold protection (see Box 9.9), biofeedback, stress management and relaxation techniques, whirlpool or other gentle heat modalities, and exercise. Large-movement arm circles in a windmill fashion can restore circulation in some people. The individual will have to experiment with the speed at which to move the arms; some people benefit from slow, gentle movement, whereas others find greater success with fast rotations.

9.22 Special Implications for the PTA: Peripheral Vascular Disease

Even though Special Implications for the PTA boxes for each individual disease making PVD have been presented, a brief overview or summary of PVD as a whole seems warranted and a reminder that because of the prevalence of atherosclerotic disease in anyone with PVD, heart rate and blood pressure should be monitored during the evaluative process and during initial interventions. This is especially important in those with diabetes mellitus and anyone who has undergone an amputation, which implies severe disease.

Notably, people with PAD may exhibit precipitous rises in blood pressure during exercise because of the atherosclerotic process present and the diminished vascular bed.[231] Examination of the pedal pulses should be part of the physical examination for all clients older than age 55, and measurement of the ABI is recommended for those who have diminished or nonpalpable pedal pulses but who do not have diabetes.[7]

For the client with back pain, buttock pain, or leg pain of unknown or previously undiagnosed cause, screening for medical disease, including assessment of risk factors, past medical history, and special tests and measurements (e.g., bicycle test, palpation of pulses), is essential.[85,88]

PVD can be confusing, with the wide range of diseases affecting veins and arteries, the causes of which are sometimes occlusive, sometimes inflammatory, and, occasionally, as in the case of Buerger's disease, both occlusive and inflammatory. The basic point to keep in mind is how arterial disease differs (significantly) from venous disease in clinical presentation, pathogenesis, and management.

Focusing on the underlying etiologic factors is the key to choosing the most appropriate and effective intervention.

During the acute phase of arterial ischemia rehabilitation, intervention and movement are minimized, heat and massage are contraindicated, and the person is instructed in the use of positions that will increase blood flow to the tissues involved.

Chronic arterial disease can be treated by physical therapy by concentrating on improving collateral circulation and increasing vasodilation. The role of exercise in PAD has been well documented.[34] It has been suggested that supervised exercise may be more beneficial than unsupervised exercise.[131]

In venous disorders, the tissues are oxygenated but the blood is not moving, and stasis occurs. With venous occlusion, the skin is discolored rather than pale, edema is prominent, and pain is most marked at the site of occlusion, although extreme edema can render all the skin of the limb quite tender.

The goal of therapy is to create compressive pumping forces to move fluid volume and reduce edema. For this reason, heat or cold, compressive stockings, massage, and activity (e.g., ankle pumps, heel slides, quad sets, ambulation) are part of the treatment protocol.

Modifying cardiovascular risk factors, improving exercise duration and decreasing claudication, preventing joint contractures and muscle atrophy, preventing skin ulcerations, promoting healing of any pressure ulcers, and improving quality of life are part of the therapy plan of care. In the case of lower extremity amputation, the use of unweighted ambulation to reduce the physiologic demands of walking during early rehabilitation has been reported.[155]

For people with vascular ulcers, improving the arterial supply or venous return will lessen pain, increase mobility, and allow ulcers to heal. Whenever ulcers are present, understanding the type of ulcer and the underlying cause will point to the best intervention.

Lymphatic Vessels

The lymphatic system is part of the circulatory system that collects excess tissue fluid and plasma that has leaked out of capillaries into the interstitial space and returns it to the bloodstream.

Disorders of the lymphatic system may result from inflammation of a lymphatic vessel (lymphangitis), inflammation of one or more lymph nodes (lymphadenitis), an increased amount of lymph (lymphedema), or enlargement of the lymph nodes (lymphadenopathy). There are also three forms of lymph vascular insufficiency that can occur.

9.23 Special Implications for the PTA: The Cardiac Client and Surgery

Noncardiac Surgery

Therapy for people with cardiovascular disease undergoing orthopedic surgery or neurosurgery is altered only by the need for more deliberate and careful monitoring of the person's response to activity and exercise.

Postoperative rehabilitation may take longer because of the underlying cardiac condition and any complications that may arise as a result of cardiovascular compromise. Careful observation for DVT must be ongoing during the first 1 to 3 weeks postoperatively.

Physical therapy initiated in the intensive care unit focuses on restoring mobility, increasing strength, and improving balance and reflexes; heel slides, ankle pumps, and bedside standing are included in the early postoperative protocol. Airway clearance techniques and breathing exercises are essential to prevent atelectasis, especially in the case of implantation of an artificial heart, because of the location of the device. Frequent, slow, rhythmic reaching, turning, bending, and stretching of the trunk and all extremities many times throughout the day help alleviate the surgical pain–tension cycle and facilitate pulmonary function.

Cardiac Surgery

Progressive ambulation can be initiated as soon as the client can transfer. In the case of open heart surgery, *sternal precautions* are standard postoperative orders (see Box 9.1); preventing separation of the sternum may require handheld assistance in place of assistive devices initially. It is important to know whether the chest has been closed; the skin may be closed, but the chest may not be.

Upper extremity precautions are determined by the physician according to the surgery that was performed and the status of the incision. When the chest is closed, shoulder flexion and abduction can proceed until the point of movement at the chest wall or rib cage. This rotation can cause a torque, and further motion must be limited at that point.

When the client can ambulate 1000 feet, the treadmill (1 mile/hour) or exercise cycle (0.5 RPE) can be used (see Table 9.12), usually around the fourth postoperative day if there are no complications. Whether to use the treadmill or bicycle is generally an individual decision made by the client based on personal preference; presence of orthopedic problems must be taken into consideration. Resistive elastic or small weights and aerobic training are introduced 4 to 6 weeks postoperatively. Pushing or pulling activities and lifting more than 10 lb are contraindicated in the first 4 to 6 weeks.

Chest (and in women, breast) discomfort, shortness of breath, upper quadrant myalgia (chest, arms, neck, and upper back), palpitations, low activity tolerance, mood swings, and localized swelling in the case of grafts taken from the leg are all commonly reported in the early days and weeks after cardiac surgery.

Exercise

The use of lower extremity–derived aerobic exercise to improve hemodynamics, normalize heart rate, improve oxygen uptake and delivery, and decrease diastolic blood pressure has been well documented and discussed earlier in this chapter. Many of these individuals have not exercised in years and remain deconditioned or fearful of exercise.

The PTA must firmly encourage active participation in a program of physical activity and exercise for anyone who has given up and chosen to remain sedentary. Exercise tolerance must be monitored closely during the early weeks after surgery. The PTA is encouraged to use perceived exertion scales (see Table 9.12), monitor changes in diastolic pressure, and rely on measurements of oxygen uptake to set exercise limits.

Psychosocial Considerations

Psychologic and emotional recovery from cardiac surgery is not always addressed or discussed. Recent research has documented that cardiac surgery is often accompanied by significant cognitive decline, especially memory loss and decline in task planning ability and psychomotor speed.

Additional research is needed to determine whether the observed cognitive decline is related to the surgery itself, normal aging in a population with cardiovascular risk factors, or a combination of these and other factors.[198-200]

Depression is commonly reported after CABG and after cardiac surgery in general. The majority of people who are depressed after cardiac surgery were depressed before surgery. There does not appear to be any correlation between depressed mood and cognitive decline after cardiac surgery, which suggests that depression alone cannot account for the cognitive decline.

Because cardiac surgery is increasingly performed in older adults with more comorbidities, identifying people at risk for adverse neurocognitive outcomes will be helpful in protecting them by modification of the surgical procedure or by more effective medical therapy.[142,198-200]

Cardiogenic Shock

Shock is acute, severe circulatory failure associated with a variety of precipitating conditions. Regardless of the cause, shock is associated with marked reduction of blood flow to vital organs, eventually leading to cellular damage and death.

Clinical manifestations of shock may include tachycardia, increased respiratory rate, and distended neck veins. In early septic shock (vascular shock caused by infection), there is hyperdynamic change with increased circulation, so the skin is warm and flushed and the pulse is bounding rather than weak.

In the second phase of shock (late septic shock), hypoperfusion (reduced blood flow) occurs with cold skin and weak pulses, hypotension (systolic blood pressure of 90 mm Hg or less), mottled extremities with weak or absent peripheral pulses, and collapsed neck veins. This phase is usually irreversible; the client is unresponsive, and cardiovascular collapse eventually occurs.

Treatment is directed toward both the manifestations of shock and its cause.

9.24 Special Implications for the PTA: Cardiogenic Shock

PTA in an acute care or home health setting may be working with a client who is demonstrating signs and symptoms of impending shock. Careful monitoring of vital signs and clinical observations will alert the PTA to the need for medical intervention. The client in question may demonstrate normal mental status or may become restless, agitated, and confused.

For the acute care therapist or PTA, people hospitalized with shock are critically ill and are usually unresponsive. Cardiopulmonary and musculoskeletal function as well as prevention of further complications will be the focus of the therapist. Treatment for the immobile person in shock, which is directed toward positioning, skin care, and pulmonary function, must be short in duration but effective, to avoid fatiguing the person.

The Cardiac Client and Pregnancy

Normal physiologic changes during pregnancy can exacerbate symptoms of underlying cardiac disease, even in previously asymptomatic individuals. The most common cardiovascular complications of pregnancy are peripartum cardiomyopathy, aortic dissection, and pregnancy-related hypertension.

Peripartum cardiomyopathy or cardiomyopathy of pregnancy is discussed briefly earlier in the chapter. Pregnancy predisposes to aortic dissection, possibly because of the accompanying connective tissue changes. Dissection usually occurs near term or shortly postpartum in the arteries or the aorta, and special implications are the same as for aneurysm.

Cardiac Complications of Cancer and Cancer Treatment[151]

Many treatments for cancers are also known to be cardiotoxic. People with cancer experience all the usual cardiac problems that occur in the general population in addition to complications of cancer and its therapy. Tumor masses can cause compression of the heart and great vessels, resulting in pericardial effusions and tamponade. Certain tumors can cause arrhythmias and may secrete mediators that are directly toxic to the heart. Pericardial effusions and tamponade can follow surgery, radiation, or chemotherapy.

Cardiac toxicity may occur after chest irradiation, especially when combined with the administration of many chemotherapeutic agents. Chest radiation for any type of cancer exposes the heart (and lungs) to varying degrees and doses of radiation. Previous mediastinal radiation and increasing cumulative doses of chemotherapy or irradiation are known risk factors for the development of cardiotoxicity.

Pericardial effusion is the most common manifestation of radiation heart disease, but coronary arteries are known to become fibrotic and undergo luminal narrowing, resulting in hypertension, angina, and MI.

Chemotherapy agents may prompt acute and chronic heart failure[173] or coronary spasm leading to angina, MI, arrhythmias, or sudden death.

The most common manifestations of cardiotoxicity are cardiac arrhythmias or acute or chronic pericarditis. Other cardiac problems that may develop include blood pressure changes, thrombosis, ECG changes, myocardial fibrosis with a resultant restrictive cardiomyopathy, conduction disturbances, CHF, accelerated and radiation-induced CAD, and valvular dysfunction. These may occur during or shortly after treatment or within days or weeks after treatment; or they may not be apparent until months and sometimes years after completion of chemotherapy.[169]

Although only a small percentage of persons develop serious problems or obvious symptoms of cardiotoxicity, many people have functional limitations that are not clinically apparent because they are physically inactive.

9.25 Special Implications for the PTA: Cardiac Complications of Cancer Treatment Any client referred to therapy who has completed oncologic treatment should be assessed for potential cardiac (and pulmonary) dysfunction, including questions about previous and current activity levels, evaluation of exercise tolerance or endurance, monitoring of heart rate and rhythm, blood pressure, and respiratory responses. Any symptoms of exercise intolerance must be noted.

Clients may be asymptomatic, with the only manifestation being changes on the ECG. Ideally, the oncology and cardiac team will recommend continuous cardiac monitoring with baseline and regular ECG and echocardiographic studies and measurement of serum electrolytes and cardiac enzymes for those individuals with risk factors or a history of cardiotoxicity.

REFERENCES/SUGGESTED READINGS

To enhance this text and add value for the reader, references and suggested readings are included on the companion Evolve site that accompanies this textbook. The reader can view the source and access it online whenever possible.

10

The Hematologic System

CHAPTER OBJECTIVES

1. Review basic components of blood, and the physiology of the hematologic system.
2. Describe signs and symptoms of common hematologic conditions.
3. Recognize the interaction between physical therapy interventions and hematologic conditions.

OUTLINE

VOCAB BUILDERS

Anaphylaxis	Ferritin	Proliferative
Anastomoses	Ionizing radiation	Recombinant
Autologous	Koilonychia	Spherocytosis
Disseminated	Leukopenia	Strongyloidiasis
Ecchymoses	Normovolemic	Thyrotoxicosis
Epistaxis	Palliation	Transient
Erythematous	Perfusion	Urticaria
Extravasation	Petechiae	Viscosity

Hematology is the branch of science that studies the form and structure of blood and blood-forming tissues. Two major components of blood are examined: plasma and formed elements (erythrocytes, or red blood cells [RBCs]; leukocytes, or white blood cells [WBCs]; and platelets, or thrombocytes).

Delivery of these formed elements throughout the body tissues is necessary for cellular metabolism, defense against injury and invading microorganisms, and acid–base balance. The formation and development of blood cells, which usually take place in the red bone marrow, are controlled by hormones (specifically erythropoietin) and feedback mechanisms that maintain an ideal number of cells.

The hematologic system is integrated with the lymphatic and immune systems. The lymph nodes are part of the lymphatic system but also part of the hematopoietic (blood-forming) system and the lymphoid system, which consists of organs and tissues of the immune system.

Lymph fluid passes through these nodes, or valves, which are located in the lymph channels at 1- to 2-cm intervals. As the fluid passes through the nodes, it is purified of harmful bacteria and viruses. Networks of the lymphatic system are situated in several areas of the body and may be considered primary (thymus and bone marrow) or secondary (spleen, lymph nodes, tonsils, and Peyer's patches of the small intestine).

All the lymphoid organs link the hematologic and immune systems in that they are sites of residence, proliferation, differentiation, or function of lymphocytes and mononuclear phagocytes (mononuclear phagocyte system: macrophage and monocyte cells capable of ingesting microorganisms and other antigens).

Lymphocytes are any of the nonphagocytic leukocytes (WBCs) found in the blood, lymph, and lymphoid tissues that make up the body's immunologically competent cells. They are divided into two classes: B and T lymphocytes (see the section on leukocytosis in this chapter). For example, in the hematologic system, the lymphocytes of the spleen produce approximately one-third of the antibody available to the immune system.

SIGNS AND SYMPTOMS OF HEMATOLOGIC DISORDERS

Disruption of the hematologic system results in circulatory disorders as well as signs and symptoms noted in the hematologic tissues themselves. The circulatory disorders can be characterized by edema and congestion, infarction, thrombosis and embolism, lymphedema, bleeding and bruising, and hypotension and shock (Box 10.1).

Edema is the accumulation of excessive fluid within the interstitial tissues or within body cavities. *Congestion* is the

> ### BOX 10.1 Most Common Signs and Symptoms of Hematologic Disorders
>
> - Edema
>   - Lymphedema
>   - Cerebral edema
>   - Inflammatory edema
>   - Peripheral dependent edema
>   - Pulmonary edema
> - Lymphadenopathy
> - Congestion
> - Infarction (brain, heart, gastrointestinal tract, kidney, spleen)
> - Thrombosis
> - Splenomegaly
> - Embolism
> - Bleeding and bruising
> - Shock
>   - Rapid, weak pulse (late phase)
>   - Hypotension (systolic blood pressure less than 90 mm Hg)
>   - Cool, moist skin (late phase)
>   - Pallor
>   - Weak or absent peripheral pulses

accumulation of excessive blood within the blood vessels of an organ or tissue. The forms of lymphedema include cerebral edema, inflammatory edema, peripheral dependent edema, and pulmonary edema. Congestion may be localized, as with a venous thrombosis, or generalized, as with heart failure (e.g., congestive heart failure [CHF]), which results in congestion in the lungs, lower extremities, and abdominal viscera.

Infarction is a localized region of necrosis caused by reduction of arterial *perfusion* below a level required for cell viability. Such a situation occurs as a result of arterial obstruction due to atherosclerosis, arterial thrombosis, or embolism, when oxygen supply fails to meet the oxygen requirements of organs with end arteries, such as the gastrointestinal (GI) tract, the heart, and, less often, the kidneys and spleen. Cerebral cortical neurons (cerebral infarction) and myocardial cells (myocardial infarction) are most vulnerable to ischemia, although protective collateral blood flow develops in the heart through *anastomoses*.

A *thrombus* is a solid mass of clotted blood within an intact blood vessel or chamber of the heart. An *embolus* is a mass of solid, liquid, or gas that moves within a blood vessel to lodge at a site distant from its place of origin. Most emboli are thromboemboli, although other possible origins of emboli include fragments of cholesterol separating from sclerotic plaque deposits, fatty droplets commonly developed from bone fractures, and nitrogen bubbles that develop as a result of decompression sickness. Thrombosis (development of a thrombus or clot) results from pathologic activation of the hemostatic mechanisms involving platelets, coagulation factors, and blood vessel walls. Endothelial injury, alteration in blood flow (stasis and turbulence), and hypercoagulability of the blood (e.g., protein abnormalities either primary or associated with cancers) promote thrombosis and thromboembolism.

Lymphedema, or chronic swelling of an area from accumulation of interstitial fluid (edema), occurs in hematolymphatic disorders secondary to obstruction of lymphatic vessels or lymph nodes. Obstruction may be of an inflammatory or mechanical nature from trauma, regional lymph node resection or irradiation, or extensive involvement of regional nodes by malignant disease.

Women who have been treated surgically for breast cancer with lymph node dissection, mastectomy, and/or radiation therapy are at double the risk of developing lymphedema of the arm and/or chest wall. When the obstruction that slows the lymph fluid exceeds the pumping capacity of the system, the fluid accumulates in the tissues in the extremity, causing edema in one or more limbs. This accumulation of fluid may become a source for bacterial growth, leading to infection, fibrosis, and possible loss of functional limb use.

Bleeding and bruising can occur from trauma of various types and are normal consequences of injury. However, when bleeding and bruising are elicited with minor trauma (e.g., brushing teeth) or bleeding continues longer than normal, there is more concern for a disorder of the blood. These symptoms are often a result of platelet abnormalities (function or quantity) such as idiopathic thrombocytopenic purpura, thrombotic thrombocytopenic purpura, or von Willebrand's disease.

Purpura is a hemorrhagic condition that occurs when not enough normal platelets are available to plug damaged vessels or prevent leakage from even minor injury to normal capillaries. Purpura is characterized by movement of blood into the surrounding tissue *(extravasation),* under the skin, and through the mucous membranes, producing spontaneous *ecchymoses* (bruises) and *petechiae* (small, red patches) on the skin. When accompanied by a decrease in the circulating platelets, it is called *thrombocytopenic purpura.* In the acute form, bleeding can occur from any of the body orifices, such as hematuria, nosebleed, vaginal bleeding, and bleeding gums.

Shock occurs when the circulatory system (heart as well as arteries) is unable to maintain adequate pressure in order to perfuse organs. Common clinical signs include tachycardia, tachypnea, cool extremities, decreased pulses, decreased urine output, and an altered mental status. Hypotension is typically present but may be initially absent. The end result is hypoxia to end organ tissues, particularly the kidneys, brain, and heart.

Diagnosis as to the cause of shock should include an evaluation of the heart and the peripheral arteries (systemic vascular resistance). Myocardial infarction and heart failure are problems that make it difficult for the heart to pump an adequate amount of blood to the body. Decreased blood volume (hypovolemia) from hemorrhaging or severe volume depletion (e.g., nausea, vomiting, and diarrhea) also reduces the body's ability to perfuse tissue.

Disorders that cause a decrease in the arterial pressure include sepsis (infection from any source), liver failure, severe pancreatitis, *anaphylaxis,* and *thyrotoxicosis.* The three most common classes of shock therefore are cardiogenic (heart related), hypovolemic, and causes related to reduced systemic vascular resistance, although many overlap (Table 10.1).

TABLE 10.1	Etiologic Factors of Shock
Category of Shock	**Causes**
Hypovolemic	Hemorrhage (loss of blood, shock)
	Vomiting
	Diarrhea
	Dehydration secondary to decreased fluid intake, diabetes mellitus (diuresis during diabetic ketoacidosis or severe hyperglycemia), diabetes insipidus, inadequate rehydration of long-distance runner
	Addison's disease
	Burns
Cardiogenic	Arrhythmias
	Acute valvular dysfunction
	Acute myocardial infarction
	Severe congestive heart failure
	Cardiomyopathy
	Obstructive valvular disease (aortic or mitral stenosis)
	Cardiac tumor (atrial myxoma)
Reduced systemic vascular resistance	Bacteremia; overwhelming infections
	Spinal cord injury
	Pain
	Trauma
	Vasodilator drugs
	Burns
	Thyrotoxicosis
	Pancreatitis
	Anaphylaxis
	Liver failure

Lymphadenopathy is the abnormal enlargement of a lymph node(s). Lymph nodes filter lymph as it returns to the heart. Infectious organisms (e.g., Epstein–Barr virus [EBV] and tuberculosis) and autoimmune disorders (e.g., rheumatoid arthritis [RA] and systemic lupus erythematosus [SLE]) can cause an inflammatory expansion and enlargement of lymph nodes. Malignant diseases such as lymphoma, chronic lymphocytic leukemia, and Hodgkin's lymphoma can also cause enlarged lymph nodes.

Lymph nodes are typically "rubbery" in feel, unattached to surrounding tissue (mobile), and small (usually less than 1 cm in diameter). Inflammatory nodes may be tender to the touch, warm, and enlarged but usually remain mobile and soft. Although malignant nodes are often not tender or mobile, they are firm and enlarged. Most cases of lymphadenopathy are not malignancy related, although all instances of abnormal adenopathy should be investigated.

Enlargement of the spleen, or *splenomegaly,* is present in many hematologic diseases. The spleen is normally involved in removing old or deformed erythrocytes, producing antibodies, and removing antibody-laden bacteria or cells. When the spleen exceeds normal function in one of these areas, it becomes enlarged. For example, if a client has hereditary *spherocytosis* and forms abnormally shaped erythrocytes, the spleen attempts to remove all these cells, thereby increasing in size to accomplish this task.

Splenomegaly is often noted in people with infectious mononucleosis or malignancies such as Hodgkin's lymphoma (where the spleen is infiltrated by disease). If the bone marrow is unable to produce cells (because of an infiltrative process), the spleen often assumes that role and becomes enlarged (extramedullary hematopoiesis).

10.1 Special Implications for the PTA: **Hematologic Disorders** Hematologic conditions alter the oxygen-carrying capacity of the blood and the constituents, structure, consistency, and flow of the blood. These changes can contribute to hypocoagulopathy or hypercoagulopathy, increased work of the heart and breathing, impaired tissue perfusion, and increased risk of thrombus.

Hematologic abnormalities require that the results of the client's blood analysis and clotting factors be monitored so that therapy intervention can be modified to minimize risk.[48]

Platelet disorders require special consideration by the clinician during exercise. Decreased platelets are associated with the risk of life-threatening hemorrhage, and physical therapy intervention must be tailored to the individual's platelet levels. For example, platelet levels between 40,000 and 60,000 µL face an increased risk of postsurgical or traumatic bleed. Low-load resistance exercise is permitted with 1- to 2-lb weights. Safe exercise includes walking, stationary bicycling with light resistance, and minimal activities of daily living.

For clients with platelet levels in the 20,000 to 40,000 range, low-intensity exercise with no weights or resistance up to 2 lb is permitted but with no resistance during stationary biking. Activity and exercise restriction is even more stringent when platelet levels are below 20,000. Below 10,000, spontaneous central nervous system (CNS), GI, and/or respiratory tract bleeding may occur.[210] In all cases, clients are monitored carefully for any signs of bleeding. Guidelines vary from one geographic region to another and even from center to center within a single geographic location.

Splenomegaly

Because splenomegaly is often associated with conditions characterized by rapid destruction of blood cells, it is important to follow the usual precautions for anyone with poor clotting abilities (e.g., see 10.4 Special Implications for the PTA: The Anemias in this chapter).

The client must be taught proper breathing techniques in conjunction with ways to avoid activities or positions that could traumatize the abdominal region or increase intracranial, intrathoracic, or intraabdominal pressure.

The person with a small or absent spleen is more susceptible to streptococcal infection, which calls for prevention techniques such as good handwashing.

Exercise and Sports

Exercise training can induce blood volume expansion immediately (plasma volume) and over a period (erythrocyte volume) and is associated with healing, improved quality of life, and improved exercise capabilities in cases of anemia from hemorrhage, trauma, renal disease, and chronic diseases. The reestablishment of erythropoiesis through exercise and effects of exercise on blood volume in other groups remain unknown but are a potential area for further investigation and consideration in the clinical setting.[66,171]

Improvements in athletic performance with exogenous erythropoietin (referred to as "blood doping") have been documented as improvements in running time and maximal oxygen uptake. However, these effects are not without risk for increased blood *viscosity* and thrombosis, with potentially fatal results. Until a definitive test is developed for detection of exogenous erythropoietin, the clinician must remain aware of this potential problem.[178,179]

Monitoring Vital Signs

Clients in whom shock develops may exhibit orthostatic changes in vital signs. A drop in systolic blood pressure of 10 to 20 mm Hg or more, associated with an increase in pulse rate of more than 15 beats/minute, may indicate a depleted intravascular volume.

The clinician is unlikely to see a client with acute hypovolemia; hypovolemia is more likely the result of dehydration, as in the case of the long-distance runner or the client with severe diarrhea or slow GI tract bleeding. The aging population is especially vulnerable to development of unknown slow intestinal bleeding, especially with the use of aspirin or nonsteroidal antiinflammatory drugs (NSAIDs).

Clients with peripheral neuropathies or clients taking medications such as certain antihypertensive drugs may be *normovolemic* and experience an orthostatic fall in blood pressure but without associated increase in pulse rate. If any doubt exists, the client should be placed in the supine position with legs elevated to maximize cerebral blood flow. The Trendelenburg position, in which the head is lower than the rest of the body, is no longer used because of the increased difficulty of breathing in this position.

AGING AND THE HEMATOPOIETIC SYSTEM

Although blood composition changes little with age, the percentage of the marrow space occupied by hematopoietic (blood-forming) tissue declines progressively. The percentage of bone marrow fat is equal to the person's age, reaching a plateau at approximately age 50 years.

Other changes include decreased total serum iron, total iron-binding capacity, and intestinal iron absorption but with increased total body and bone marrow iron; increased fragility of plasma membranes; a rise in fibrinogen and increased platelet adhesiveness; red cell rigidity; and early activation of the coagulation system. Platelet morphology (form and structure) does not appear to change with age, but platelet count and function have been found to vary from normal to increased or decreased.

The cumulative effect of these changes appears in the form of disturbed blood flow in older subjects, leading to the development or aggravation of various circulatory disorders, especially hypertension, stroke, and diabetes. In addition, correlations found between hematologic changes and changes in behavioral patterns and some cognitive functions suggest that hematologic changes contribute to other changes associated with aging as well.[5]

Age-related changes in the peripheral blood include slightly decreased hemoglobin and hematocrit, although levels remain within the normal adult range. Low hemoglobin levels noted in aging adults can be caused by iron deficiency (usually via blood loss such as ulcer, telangiectasia, colon polyps, or cancer) or can be associated with a long-standing condition such as rheumatologic conditions often seen in a therapy practice (referred to as *anemia of chronic disease*). Vitamin B_{12}, which is required to produce blood cells, and the subsequent development of anemia (resulting from a B_{12} deficiency) with its hematologic, neurologic, and GI manifestations, are discussed later in this chapter.

Aging is also associated with a decreased number of lymph nodes and diminished size of remaining nodes, decreased function of lymphocytes, and decline in cellular immunity caused by altered T-cell function. The effect of aging on quantity, form, and structure of lymphocytes is not well documented.

BLOOD TRANSFUSIONS

Advances in treating hematologic/immunologic disorders through blood transfusions and bone marrow transplantation have provided new success in long-term treatment and a cure for some previously fatal disorders. Modern blood banking and transfusion medicine have developed techniques to administer only the blood component needed by the client, such as packed RBCs for anemia or cryoprecipitate for bleeding disorders.

Clients in a therapy setting who have undergone numerous surgical procedures (e.g., traumatic injuries) or elective orthopedic or cardiac procedures may also receive *autologous* blood transfusions (i.e., reinfusion of a person's own blood) when significant blood loss may be a complication and a transfusion may be anticipated.

The development of *recombinant* human erythropoietin (rHuEpo, EPO, or Epogen), with its ability to stimulate erythropoiesis and elevate RBCs, has reduced the need for blood transfusion in a variety of clinical situations (e.g., chronic renal disease, hematologic malignancies, cancer-related anemia, and surgical procedures, especially joint arthroplasty and cardiac procedures).

Reaction to Blood and Blood Products

Febrile, Nonhemolytic Reaction

Because blood products are most often donated from another person, reactions may occur. The most common transfusion-related reaction is a febrile, nonhemolytic reaction (occurring in 0.5% to 1% of erythrocyte transfusions and 30% of platelet transfusions). The condition is characterized by an increase in temperature by more than 1° F during or soon after the transfusion. These reactions are a result of either donor leukocyte cytokines or alloantibodies of the recipient directed against the leukocytes of the donor.

Treatment includes stopping the transfusion, checking the blood for a direct hemolytic process (in the laboratory), and administering antipyretics or corticosteroids. Symptoms are usually *transient*, and the removal of donor leukocytes from the blood (leukocyte reduction) can reduce the risk of another similar reaction (Box 10.2).

Transfusion-Related Acute Lung Injury

Transfusion-related acute lung injury occurs in as many as 1 in every 2000 transfusions.[114] This reaction may present with mild shortness of breath or appear clinically similar to adult respiratory distress syndrome. With appropriate respiratory intervention, most people recover without permanent pulmonary damage.[160] Other complications may include transmission of disease (human immunodeficiency virus [HIV], hepatitis, cytomegalovirus), iron overload, air embolism, hypotension in clients taking angiotensin-converting enzyme inhibitors,[122] and circulatory overload when blood is administered rapidly in large amounts.

Acute Hemolytic Transfusion Reaction

Less common (only 1 in every 25,000 transfusions) but more severe is the acute hemolytic transfusion reaction. This is due to ABO incompatibility: typically a mistake is made by giving the wrong blood to a person or blood is mislabeled. Symptoms begin soon after the transfusion is begun (see Box 10.2). Erythrocytes are destroyed intravascularly with resultant red plasma and red urine.

The mortality rate is high, ranging from 17% to 60%. The transfusion is immediately terminated and the client given cardiovascular support. Renal failure, *disseminated* intravascular coagulation, and severe hypotension may occur.

BOX 10.2   Signs and Symptoms of Reactions to Blood and Blood Products

Febrile, Nonhemolytic Transfusion Reaction
- Fever, chills
- Headache
- Nausea, vomiting
- Hypertension
- Tachycardia

Transfusion-Related Acute Lung Injury
- Pulmonary edema
- Acute respiratory distress
- Severe hypoxia

Acute Hemolytic Transfusion Reaction
- Fever, chills
- Nausea, vomiting
- Flank and abdominal pain
- Headache
- Dyspnea
- Hypotension
- Tachycardia
- Red urine

Delayed Hemolytic Transfusion Reaction
- Unexplained drop in hemoglobin—anemia
- Increased bilirubin level—jaundice
- Increased lactate dehydrogenase (LDH) level

Allergic Reactions
- Hives, rash
- Wheezing
- Mucosal edema

Anaphylaxis
- Abrupt hypotension
- Edema of the larynx
- Difficulty breathing
- Nausea
- Abdominal pain
- Diarrhea
- Shock
- Respiratory arrest

Septic Reactions
- Fever, chills
- Hypotension
- Headache
- Back, chest, abdominal pain
- Shortness of breath

Circulatory Overload
- Red face
- Shortness of breath
- Tachycardia
- Orthopnea
- Hypertension
- Headache
- Seizures

Delayed Hemolytic Transfusion

Delayed hemolytic transfusion reactions occur when the donated erythrocytes are quickly removed from the circulatory system because of an alloantibody. There are often asymptomatic reactions that are noted only because there was not a rise in the hemoglobin following the transfusion.

Allergic Reaction

If the client reacts to the donated plasma an allergic reaction may occur, with associated *urticaria* (hives), rash, mucosal edema, wheezing, and other respiratory symptoms. These types of reactions are more typical with fresh frozen plasma and platelet transfusions and seen in about 1% to 3% of all transfusions. Antihistamines and/or corticosteroids aid in treating the symptoms, and premedication before the next transfusion may help reduce or prevent subsequent reactions.

Anaphylaxis

True anaphylaxis is rare (approximately 1 in 20,000 to 50,000 transfusions) and may occur with or without allergic reactions. Symptoms include acute onset of hypotension and edema of the larynx with associated difficulty breathing. Nausea, abdominal pain, and diarrhea may accompany the reaction. This reaction can be severe and fatal and is associated with shock, respiratory failure, and vascular collapse. The earlier the symptoms occur, the more severe the reaction. Treatment consists of immediately discontinuing the transfusion, administering epinephrine and corticosteroids, and providing cardiovascular and respiratory support.

Septic Reactions

Rarely, septic reactions can occur secondary to bacterial contamination of blood products, principally platelets (they are not stored at cold temperatures). In March 2004, all blood banks began to routinely screen platelets for bacterial contamination, with a subsequent reduction in septic reactions. Symptoms of such reactions include fever/chills; hypotension; headache; back, chest, and abdominal pain; and shortness of breath. Culture of the product and appropriate antibiotics and cardiovascular support are the mainstays of treatment.

Transfusion as a source for hepatitis (B and C) has been reduced since the initiation of donor screening for the hepatitis antibody. People with hemophilia who received coagulation factor concentrates before 1984 have been at highest risk among transfusion recipients because of exposures to pooled blood products prepared from thousands of donors. The availability of nonhuman plasma factors has virtually eliminated the transmission of viruses among people with hemophilia.

The risk of HIV infection by transfusion is low overall, calculated at 1 in 1 million transfusions. The risk of HIV transmission by blood transfusion has been continually reduced through the elimination of high-risk individuals from blood donor pools and the use of more sensitive screening. Acquired immune deficiency syndrome (AIDS) has developed in a small percentage of people receiving transfusion of RBCs, platelets, or commercial coagulation factor concentrates. AIDS has also been reported in infants after neonatal exchange, but the majority of pediatric cases were associated with maternal transmission from mothers with HIV.

Bloodless Medicine

Bloodless medicine and surgery is the use of technologic and pharmaceutical techniques to minimize blood loss and avoid the use of allogenic blood transfusions. Bloodless medicine and surgery programs began over the past 20 years to meet the needs of Jehovah's Witnesses, whose beliefs do not allow blood transfusions.

In recent years, the number of bloodless medicine programs has increased as a result of a growing number of individuals seeking this type of treatment to avoid potential exposure to bloodborne pathogens or because of a family history of transfusion reactions.[175]

As bloodless programs have grown, researchers have found other advantages to avoiding blood transfusions. The length of time banked blood spends in storage can affect the hemoglobin molecule's ability to release the oxygen it is carrying, potentially decreasing its oxygen-carrying capacity. Furthermore, cold storage of blood can negatively affect an RBC's elasticity, potentially leading to its early destruction.[147,175]

Candidates for Bloodless Procedures

The first step in ensuring successful use of bloodless techniques is a thorough history, including a history of any personal or family history of bleeding abnormalities.[76,147] Any history of bleeding abnormalities requires further evaluation.

Preoperative blood work is needed to detect anemia because individuals with low preoperative hemoglobin levels are more likely to need a transfusion.[77] Bloodless techniques can still be used if a low hemoglobin level is increased by giving recombinant human erythropoietin and iron.[147,184]

Bloodless Techniques

There are a variety of techniques that are used during surgical procedures to avoid the need for a blood transfusion. *Minimally invasive surgery* can significantly reduce blood loss, as does meticulous surgical technique. Technologic advances such as the gamma knife, harmonic scalpel, and argon beams have also improved the surgeon's ability to achieve hemostasis during procedures by coagulating vessels while causing less tissue damage.[76]

Another technique, acute *normovolemic hemodilution,* which removes a quantity of a person's blood and replaces it with intravenous crystalloid and colloid solution to maintain volume, can also be used.

With acute normovolemic hemodilution, fluid loss during a procedure is mainly the crystalloid/colloid solution, which limits loss of RBCs while preserving clotting factors. At the conclusion of the surgical procedure, the withdrawn blood is returned to the patient. Because this process is completed through a closed circuit, it is acceptable to most Jehovah's Witnesses.[176,184]

Cell salvage techniques can be used in the intraoperative and postoperative phases to retransfuse lost blood. These techniques have been associated with infection and hemolysis but are believed to be safe as part of an overall blood loss management program.[176]

Steps should be taken postoperatively to minimize blood loss by close observation for bleeding with immediate steps being taken to regain hemostasis (halt bleeding). Additionally, postoperative phlebotomy should be kept to a minimum and the blood drawn using microsampling techniques.[76,176] Use of recombinant human erythropoietin and iron should be continued as needed during the postoperative phase.

Finally, clinician acceptance of low hemoglobin levels is essential in bloodless medicine and surgery. Research has shown that the body can tolerate lower hemoglobin levels than would be thought acceptable without compromising oxygen delivery. Hemoglobin levels alone should not be used as the deciding factor for a blood transfusion. The individual's condition and comorbidities should also be taken into account.[175]

The advances in bloodless medicine and surgery have led to use of these techniques in many surgical procedures, including the Whipple procedure, joint replacements, and coronary artery bypass.[147]

10.2 Special Implications for the PTA: Blood Transfusions Most blood transfusion reactions occur during the actual transfusion and are not of consequence to the clinician, but when autologous transfusion is unavailable or inappropriate, the clinician must be alert for any signs of adverse reaction. Among the most common transfusion reactions are febrile, nonhemolytic transfusion reactions and delayed hemolytic transfusion reactions. Clinical symptoms from these reactions are typically mild and can usually be prevented on subsequent transfusions.

One of the most severe, but uncommon, reactions is the acute hemolytic transfusion reaction. This is due to antigen–antibody reactions resulting from blood type incompatibility, with clumping of cells, hemolysis, and release of cellular elements into the serum. Signs and symptoms indicating such a reaction are listed in Box 10.2.

Occasionally, a client may develop an allergic reaction observed as dyspnea or urticaria; the latter may be brought to the clinician's attention after local modality intervention. The clinician may also be the first to recognize early signs of hepatitis (jaundice), especially changes in sclerae or skin color or reported changes in urine (dark or tea colored) and stools (light colored or white).

Bloodless Medicine

Clinicians who work where bloodless techniques are used must have an awareness of the impact of lower hemoglobin levels on a person's ability to participate in therapy, especially exercise. Clinicians should review blood work before each therapy session, looking specifically at hemoglobin levels. Routine vital signs and pulse oximetry need to be monitored throughout the therapy sessions.

Finally, patients/clients need to be observed closely to monitor how they are tolerating sitting, standing, and therapeutic activities. Although no studies have yet documented the relationship between hemoglobin levels and safe activity levels in therapy, patients participating in the Englewood Hospital and Medical Center (Englewood, NJ) bloodless medicine program have tolerated therapeutic activities with hemoglobin levels in the 7 to 9 g/dL range.

DISORDERS OF IRON ABSORPTION

Hereditary Hemochromatosis

Hemochromatosis is an autosomal recessive hereditary disorder characterized by excessive iron absorption by the small intestine. Most inherited forms of the disease are caused by abnormalities of the *HFE* gene located on chromosome 6. Although the exact mechanism of this gene is unknown, two hypotheses exist that may explain the pathology of the disease.

Pathogenesis

The *crypt hypothesis* suggests that the abnormal protein product of *HFE* is unable to interact with transferrin and leads to a decrease in absorption of iron by the intestinal crypt cells. This then triggers an inappropriate increase in iron absorbed by the intestinal villus cells.

The second hypothesis relates to hepcidin, a recently discovered peptide hormone produced by the liver that appears to be the master regulator of iron homeostasis in human beings and other mammals. Hepcidin levels increase when iron plasma is high but is not produced when iron plasma is low. Hepcidin inhibits the release of iron by macrophages, but in its absence macrophages can release needed iron.

The product of *HFE* most likely plays a role in regulating the production of hepcidin, thus an abnormal gene product would alter iron metabolism, leading to increased absorption despite already high iron plasma levels.[153]

Most likely these two hypotheses are interrelated. Abnormalities of the hemochromatosis gene occur in 1 in every 200 people of Northern European descent, although not all people with the gene will develop the disease. Hemochromatosis is present at birth but remains asymptomatic until the development of iron overloading and onset of symptoms between ages 40 and 60 years (sometimes as early as age 30 years). The prevalence is equal among men and women, but men experience symptoms 5 to 10 times more often than do women (menstruation and pregnancy help to slow progression of the disorder).

Clinical Manifestations

The body typically absorbs iron at a rate equal to body requirements. But in hemochromatosis, there is an uncoupling between absorption and body needs. Excess iron is slowly deposited in cells, particularly in the liver, pancreas, heart, and, to a lesser extent, other endocrine glands (e.g., the pituitary gland).

Early signs and symptoms can include weakness, chronic fatigue, myalgias, joint pain, abdominal pain, hepatomegaly, elevated hemoglobin, and elevated liver enzymes. Continued iron overload leads to tissue damage. The liver is the most commonly affected organ, and clients may present with hepatomegaly without liver enzyme abnormalities. If the disease progresses without treatment, cirrhosis with liver failure may ensue.

Other complications of untreated hemochromatosis include diabetes mellitus, cardiac myopathy (with associated CHF) and arrhythmias, "bronzing" of the skin (from iron deposition in the dermis and increase of melanin), destructive arthritis, and impotence (men) or decreased libido (women) and sterility.

10.3 Special Implications for the PTA: Hemochromatosis Arthropathy occurs in 40% to 60% of individuals with hemochromatosis and can be the first manifestation of the disease.[92] The arthropathy associated with hemochromatosis is not reversible and often continues to progress even with effective medical intervention.

Osteoarthritic manifestations are diverse, with minimal joint inflammation at first. The affected individual may report twinges of pain on flexing the small joints of the hand, especially the second and third metacarpophalangeal joints. Involvement of these joints often helps to distinguish hemochromatosis-related arthropathy from osteoarthritis.

Acute joint presentation can occur with progression that involves the large joints, including the hips, knees, and shoulders, accompanied by destruction to the joint, severe impairment, and resulting disability. Hemochromatosis may be associated with calcium pyrophosphate dihydrate deposition disease. This presents as an acute inflammatory arthritis.[181]

Therapeutic intervention is essential in providing flexibility, strength, and proper alignment to promote function, prevent falls, and prevent the loss of independence in activities of daily living. The clinician can be very helpful in evaluating the need for assistive devices, orthotics, and splints toward these goals.

DISORDERS OF ERYTHROCYTES

The Anemias

Definition

Anemia is a reduction in the oxygen-carrying capacity of the blood from an abnormality in the quantity or quality of erythrocytes (RBCs). The World Health Organization (WHO) has defined anemia in terms of the level of hemoglobin: less than 14 g/100 mL for men and less than 12 g/100 mL for women. Different ranges exist for men and women, infants and growing children, and different metabolic and physiologic states.

These normal values must be evaluated on an individual basis; normal levels may be inadequate if tissue oxygen delivery is impaired by pulmonary insufficiency, cardiac disorders, or an increase in hemoglobin oxygen affinity, whereas low levels may be appropriate if tissue oxygen requirements are decreased, as in the case of hypothyroidism.

Overview

Anemia is not a disease but rather a symptom of many other disorders, such as dietary deficiency (anemia due to folate or vitamin B_{12} deficiency); acute or chronic blood loss (iron deficiency); congenital defects of hemoglobin (sickle cell diseases); exposure to industrial poisons; diseases of the bone marrow; chronic inflammatory, infectious, or neoplastic disease; or any other disorder that upsets the balance between blood loss through bleeding or destruction of blood cells and production of blood cells.

Many types and causes of anemia exist; not all are discussed in this text. The most common anemias observed in a therapy setting fall into five broad disease-related categories: (1) iron deficiency associated with chronic GI blood loss secondary to NSAID use, (2) chronic diseases or inflammatory diseases, such as RA or SLE, (3) nutritional conditions (e.g., malabsorption syndrome leading to vitamin B_{12}, folate, or iron deficiency; alcohol abuse leading to folate deficiency), (4) infectious diseases such as tuberculosis or AIDS, and (5) neoplastic disease (bone marrow failure). Anemia with neoplasia may be a complication of chemotherapy (e.g., with cisplatin, carboplatin, or taxol administration), as a consequence of radiation to the pelvis, or caused by bone marrow infiltration.

Anemias are classified according to etiologic factors (Box 10.3) or morphology (form/structure) (Box 10.4). Descriptions of anemias based on erythrocyte morphology refer to the size and hemoglobin content of the RBC. In some anemias, variations occur in size (e.g., anisocytosis) or shape (e.g., poikilocytosis) of erythrocytes.

Etiologic Factors and Pathogenesis

Anemia results from (1) excessive blood loss, (2) increased destruction of erythrocytes, or (3) decreased production of erythrocytes. Anemia is the most common hematologic abnormality; only the anemias most commonly observed in rehabilitation or therapy settings are discussed here, using the three etiologic categories from Box 10.3 as a guideline.

The underlying pathogenesis can be multifactorial and depends on the condition causing the anemia. A number of physiologic compensatory responses to anemia occur, depending on the rapidity of onset and duration of anemia and the condition of the individual. In acute-onset anemia with severe loss of intravascular volume, peripheral vasoconstriction and central vasodilation occur to preserve blood flow to the vital organs.

BOX 10.3   Causes of Anemia

Excessive Blood Loss (Hemorrhage)
- Trauma, wound
- Gastrointestinal cancers
- Angiectasia
- Bleeding peptic ulcer
- Excessive menstruation
- Bleeding hemorrhoids
- Varices, diverticulosis

Destruction of Erythrocytes (Hemolytic)
- Mechanical (e.g., microangiopathic hemolytic anemia, damage by a mechanical heart valve)
- Autoimmune hemolytic anemia (AIHA)
- Hemoglobinopathies (e.g., sickle cell disease)
- Enzyme defects (e.g., glucose-6-phosphate dehydrogenase deficiency)
- Parasites (e.g., malaria)
- Hypersplenism
- Cell membrane abnormalities (e.g., hereditary spherocytosis)
- Thalassemias

Decreased Production of Erythrocytes
- Chronic diseases (e.g., rheumatoid arthritis, tuberculosis, cancer)
- Nutritional deficiency (e.g., iron, vitamin B_{12}, alcohol abuse, folic acid deficiency)
- Cellular maturational defects (e.g., thalassemias, cytotoxic or antineoplastic drugs)
- Decreased bone marrow stimulation (e.g., hypothyroidism, decreased erythropoietin production)
- Bone marrow failure (e.g., leukemia, aplasia)
- Bone marrow replacement (myelophthisis, neoplasm)
- Myelodysplastic syndromes (sideroblastic anemia)

BOX 10.4   Anemia Classified by Morphology

- Normocytic (normal size)
- Macrocytic (abnormally large)
- Microcytic (abnormally small)
- Normochromic (normal amounts of hemoglobin [Hb])
- Hyperchromic (high concentration of Hb)
- Hypochromic (low concentration of Hb)
- Anisocytosis (various sizes)
- Poikilocytosis (various shapes)

If the anemia persists, small-vessel vasodilation will provide increased blood flow to ensure better tissue oxygenation. These vascular compensations result in decreased systemic vascular resistance, increased cardiac output, and tachycardia, resulting in a higher rate of delivery of oxygen-bearing erythrocytes to the tissues. Other compensatory mechanisms include an increase in plasma volume to maintain total blood volume and enhance tissue perfusion and stimulation of erythropoietin production to increase new erythrocyte production.

Excessive blood loss. Excessive blood loss, such as occurs with GI bleeding in the client with a history of aspirin or NSAID use, is a cause of anemia seen in a therapy practice. Slow, chronic GI blood loss from medication or any GI disorder (e.g., peptic and duodenal ulcers, gastritis, GI cancers, hemorrhoids, diverticulosis, ulcerative colitis, and colon polyps) can result in iron-deficiency anemia.

Destruction of erythrocytes. Destruction of erythrocytes (hemolysis) can occur as a result of congenital RBC membrane abnormalities, lack of necessary enzymes needed for normal metabolism, autoimmune processes, or infection. All but the autoimmune processes are discussed elsewhere in this chapter.

Autoimmune hemolytic anemia (AIHA) is caused by an autoantibody that attaches to the RBC, leading to its destruction. The most common form of AIHA is warm antibody mediated, an immunoglobulin (Ig) G autoantibody that binds to erythrocytes at body temperature. Macrophages are attracted to the attached autoantibody and release enzymes that begin to destroy the cell membrane. The resultant spherical cells are removed by the spleen.

Cold agglutinin disease is another autoimmune hemolytic process caused by IgM autoantibodies that bind to erythrocytes at temperatures less than 37° C and trigger complement fixation and clumping of erythrocytes. These complement-laden erythrocytes may be destroyed intravascularly or removed by the liver. Hemolytic anemia can be idiopathic or a result of collagen vascular diseases (e.g., SLE), lymphoproliferative diseases (e.g., chronic lymphocytic leukemia or lymphoma), or other malignancies. Medications such as dapsone, penicillin, quinidine, quinine, and methyldopa can also cause AIHA.

Decreased production of erythrocytes. Anemias resulting in the underproduction of RBCs usually stem from either a lack of erythropoietin (as seen in kidney disease) or an inability of the bone marrow to respond to erythropoietin. Hyporesponsiveness of the bone marrow may be a result of a nutrient deficiency or a chronic disease such as RA, SLE, tuberculosis, or cancer.

Nutritional deficiency as a cause of anemia can occur at any age. Iron, vitamin B_{12}, and folate are among the most important vitamins and minerals in the production of hemoglobin and the formation of erythrocytes. Iron is necessary for DNA synthesis, oxygen transport, and respiration. Iron deficiency can occur secondary to blood loss (RBCs are the principal site of iron storage), malabsorption, normal growth, and pregnancy. Menstruating women, pregnant women, growing children, lower socioeconomic groups, and older adults (as a result of economic constraints, lack of interest in food preparation, and poor dentition) are the most common groups to develop iron-deficiency anemia.

Vitamin B_{12} (cobalamin) is required for DNA synthesis. Deficiency of the vitamin may infrequently occur because of a lack in the diet (the body is very efficient at retaining cobalamin) but most often develops because of an absence of intrinsic factor (IF).

After cobalamin is ingested it normally combines with R binders in the stomach and then binds to IF in the small intestine. IF is produced by gastric parietal cells and is required for cobalamin absorption in the terminal small bowel. Without IF, cobalamin is not absorbed.

Pernicious anemia is an anemia due to a loss of IF. Antibodies against the membrane of gastric parietal cells cause an atrophy of these cells, resulting in a lack of IF production. Destruction of IF production sites may also occur with gastrectomy.

Other causes of vitamin B_{12} deficiency include bacterial overgrowth in the lumen of the intestine (competes for vitamin B_{12}), surgical resection of the ileum (eliminates the site of vitamin B_{12} absorption), severe Crohn's disease, and, more rarely, dietary deficiency (e.g., strict vegetarian diet) and tapeworm infection. Crohn's disease can cause sufficient destruction of the ileum to retard vitamin B_{12} absorption.

Folic acid deficiency is a common cause of decreased production of erythrocytes. Folic acid deficiency has many causes, but it usually results from inadequate dietary intake, chronic alcoholism, malabsorption syndromes, anorexia, and consumption of overcooked food. In anemia due to folic acid deficiency associated with alcoholism, not only is the diet poor in folate but alcohol inhibits the enzyme needed to absorb folate.

The common occurrence of folic acid deficiency during the growth spurts of childhood and adolescence and during the third trimester of pregnancy is explained by the increased demands for folate required for DNA synthesis in these circumstances. Pregnant women need six times the normal amount of folic acid to meet the needs of the developing fetus. Long-term use of anticonvulsants (e.g., primidone, diphenylhydantoin, phenobarbital), antimetabolites administered for cancer and leukemia, and certain oral contraceptives may interfere with folate absorption.

Anemia of chronic disease is very common in the therapy setting. It is characterized by a modest reduction in hemoglobin (9 to 11 g/dL), the presence of inflammation (secondary to a disease), and decreased responsiveness of the bone marrow to erythropoietin. Many diseases associated with inflammation have accompanying elevated levels of cytokines and interferons. The production of hepcidin, a protein synthesized by the liver, is induced by the presence of interferon 6 (IF-6); hepcidin both inhibits the absorption of iron from the gut and the release of iron from macrophages for bone marrow use. Clients with an underlying chronic illness usually do not need iron, and anemia of chronic disease does not respond to iron.

Bone marrow disorders constitute another source of anemia caused by decreased production of erythrocytes in a therapy practice. Aplastic anemia, marrow replacement with fibrotic tissue or tumor, acute leukemia, and infiltrative disease (e.g., lymphoma, myeloma, and carcinoma) fall into this etiologic category.

Anemias of radiation-induced bone marrow failure occur because the bone marrow stem cells are destroyed and mitosis (cell division) is inhibited, preventing the synthesis of RBCs. Antimetabolites used in cancer therapy also cause bone marrow failure by blocking the synthesis of purines or nucleic acids required for synthesis of DNA within the cell. Aplastic anemia may result from either damage to the stem cells or immune-mediated destruction of the stem cells.

Clinical Manifestations

Mild anemia often causes only minimal and usually vague symptoms such as fatigue until hemoglobin concentration and hematocrit fall below half of normal. As the anemia progresses, general signs and symptoms caused by the inability of anemic blood to supply the body tissues with enough oxygen may include weakness, dyspnea on exertion, easy fatigue, pallor or yellowing of skin (especially the palms of the hands, fingernails, mucosa, and conjunctiva), tachycardia, increased angina in preexisting coronary artery disease, leg ulcers (sickle cell), and, occasionally, *koilonychia* (Fig. 10.1).

Pallor in dark-skinned people may be observed by the absence of the underlying red tones that normally give brown or black skin its luster. The brown-skinned individual demonstrates pallor with a more yellowish-brown color, and the black-skinned person appears ashen or gray.

Neuropsychiatric complications such as dementia, ataxia, psychosis, and peripheral neuropathies can develop in cases of B_{12} deficiency. These abnormalities are caused by lesions in the spinal column, the cerebrum, and peripheral nerves. The lack of cobalamin initially leads to demyelination of the nerves followed by axonal degeneration. Axonal death may result if cobalamin deficiency persists.

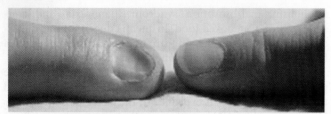

FIG. 10.1 Normal nail *(right)* compared with nail referred to as koilonychia and sometimes called spoon-shaped nails or spoon nails *(left)*. They are thin, depressed nails with lateral edges turned up and are concave from side to side. They may be idiopathic, congenital, or a hereditary trait and are occasionally due to iron-deficiency anemia. (From Swartz MH: Textbook of physical diagnosis, ed 6, Philadelphia, 2014, Saunders.)

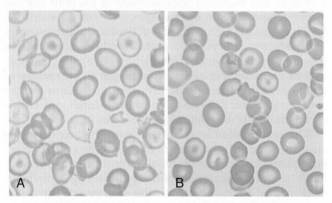

Thalassemia major   Thalassemia minor

FIG. 10.2 Thalassemia is a hemolytic hemoglobinopathy anemia characterized by microcytic, short-lived RBCs caused by deficient synthesis of Hb polypeptide chains. Classification of type depends on the chain involved (α-thalassemia, β-thalassemia). β-thalassemia occurs in two forms: thalassemia major and thalassemia minor. Characteristic bull's-eye or target cells are shown here in both forms. (From Damjanov I, Linder J: Pathology: a color atlas, St. Louis, 2000, Mosby.)

Reversal of symptoms may be possible if treatment is initiated before permanent damage to the nerves. The findings typically consist of a symmetric sensory neuropathy that begins in the feet and lower legs, although rarely it may involve the upper extremities, especially fine motor coordination of the hands. This upper extremity neuropathy may clinically manifest as problems with deteriorating handwriting.

Affected individuals may also describe moderate pain or paresthesias of the extremities, especially the feet. Individuals may interpret the neuropathy as difficulty with locomotion when, in fact, they are experiencing the loss of proprioception. The affected individual may need to hold on to the wall, countertops, or furniture at home because of difficulties maintaining balance. An associated positive Romberg's sign may be present. Loss of motor function is a late manifestation of B_{12} deficiency.

Although a symmetrical neuropathy is the usual pattern, B_{12} deficiency occasionally presents as a unilateral neuropathy and/or bilateral but asymmetrical neuropathy. CNS manifestations range from mild cognitive changes to dementia to frank psychosis. Clients may present with personality changes and/or inappropriate behavior.

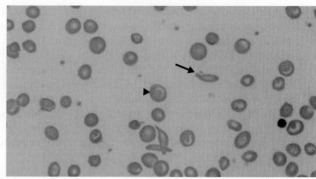

FIG. 10.3 Target *(arrowhead)* and sickle *(arrow)* cells typical of sickle cell anemia. (From Currie G, Douglas G: The flesh and bones of medicine, Edinburgh, Mosby, 2011.)

Complications depend on the specific type of anemia; severe anemia can cause heart failure and hypoxic damage to the liver and kidney with all the signs and symptoms associated with either of those conditions. Anemia in the presence of a coronary obstruction precipitates cardiac ischemia.

Medical Management

Diagnosis

Anemia in the early stages often goes unnoticed because symptoms may not be recognized until hemoglobin concentration is reduced to half of normal. Once symptoms become pronounced or noted on routine laboratory tests, the diagnosis is most often made by blood tests.

The RBC indexes indicate if the RBCs are normal (normocytic), larger than normal (macrocytic, as seen with B_{12} and folate deficiency), or smaller than normal (microcytic, as seen with thalassemias and iron deficiency). The peripheral smear may reveal structural characteristics, which give clues to the underlying cause of the anemia. For example, target cells (bull's-eye erythrocytes) are often associated with thalassemia (Fig. 10.2) and microspherocytes can be seen in warm antibody–induced hemolysis, whereas sickled erythrocytes are noted with sickle cell disease (Fig. 10.3).

Personal and family history may point to congenital anemia, and a physical examination may elicit signs of primary hematologic diseases such as lymphadenopathy, hepatosplenomegaly, skin and mucosal changes, stool positive for blood, or bone tenderness.

Following these initial tests, more specific laboratory tests can be done to verify the diagnosis. These may include a complete blood cell count (CBC), an iron profile, serum *ferritin*, reticulocyte count, haptoglobin, B_{12} level, folate level, and lactate dehydrogenase.

Treatment

Treatment of anemia is directed toward alleviating or controlling the causes, relieving the symptoms, and preventing complications. It is critical that the underlying cause of anemia is determined so that appropriate treatment can be given. For example, endoscopy to identify the source of GI blood loss for a client with a long-term history of NSAID use would indicate the need to stop taking the medication and prescribe the use of proton pump inhibitors.

Treating the underlying cause can include the replacement of deficient vitamins and minerals (e.g., vitamin B_{12}, folate, or iron) or corticosteroids for warm-antibody AIHA. The anemia of cold agglutinin disease is typically mild, requiring only a warm environment, whereas bone marrow transplantation may be required for malignancies. Immunosuppressive therapy with antithymocyte globulin and cyclosporine is the initial treatment for clients with aplastic anemia, and individuals with kidney disease are given erythropoietin or darbepoetin.

Prognosis

The prognosis for anemia depends on the etiologic factors and potential treatment for the underlying cause. For example, the prognosis is good for anemia related to nutritional deficiency but poor for lymphoproliferative diseases. Likewise, treatment is aimed at correcting the underlying pathogenesis.

Untreated or misdiagnosed B_{12} deficiency can be progressive, resulting in irreversible neurologic damage. Anemia in the older adult (age 85 years or older) is associated with an increased risk of death. Although anemia was once considered a normal consequence of aging, it is now recognized as a sign of other disease in the older adult (e.g., hip fracture, RA, erosive gastritis, peptic ulcer, malnutrition, cirrhosis, ulcerative colitis) requiring further assessment.[95]

10.4 Special Implications for the PTA: The Anemias

Exercise and Anemia

The impact of anemia on functional recovery in the acute care or rehabilitation setting and the theoretical risk of increased morbidity and mortality during prescribed therapeutic exercise have not been thoroughly investigated. Further study is indicated to examine the implications for anemia on functional recovery and cardiopulmonary complications during rehabilitation.[53]

The following guidelines should be used until proven protocols are developed. Exercise for any anemic person should be approved by the physician. Diminished exercise tolerance may be expected in anyone with anemia along with easy fatigability, depending on the cause of the anemia. Increased physical activity increases the demand for oxygen, which may not be adequately available in the circulating blood. Pacing and training that distribute the intensity of the workload over time can be used to promote physiologic recovery.[48] For the sedentary aging adult, decreased activity can mask exercise intolerance; observe carefully for any changes in mental status.

The prevalence of iron-deficiency anemia is likely to be higher in athletic populations and groups, especially in younger female athletes, than in sedentary individuals. In anemic individuals, iron deficiency decreases athletic performance and impairs immune function, leading to other physiologic dysfunction.

Although it is likely that blood losses secondary to exercise, such as foot-strike hemolysis or iron loss through sweat, may contribute to anemia, nonathletic causes must also be considered. Dietary choices explain much of a negative iron balance, but the GI and genitourinary systems must be evaluated for blood loss.[179]

Evidence also exists for increased rates of RBC iron and whole-body iron turnover. The young female athlete may want to speak with medical or dietary consultants about the use of low-dose iron supplements during training.[18,213]

Research has shown that people with chronic renal failure who have severe anemia are able to exercise but must do so at a lower intensity than the normal population. The maximum oxygen consumption (VO_{2max}) for the anemic client is at least 20% less than that for the normal population. Exercise testing and prescribed exercise(s) in anemic clients must be initiated with extreme caution and should proceed gradually to tolerance and/or perceived exertion levels.[61,148]

Precautions

Knowing the underlying cause of the anemia may be helpful in identifying red flag symptoms indicating the need for alteration of the program or medical referral. For example, GI blood loss associated with NSAID use may worsen suddenly, precipitating a crisis in a therapy setting.

It is not uncommon for clients to present with both anemia and cardiovascular disease, precipitating angina. New studies show that the amount of oxygen-carrying hemoglobin (Hb) circulating in the blood of older women is an independent risk factor for mobility problems. Hb perceived as mildly low and even low-normal (12 g/dL) in women at least 70 years old increases the likelihood of difficulty performing daily tasks by 1.5 times.[35,36]

The clinician may identify older adults who have a difficult time with general mobility, such as walking more than one block, climbing a flight of stairs, or doing housework. When they have difficulty, they become more sedentary, resulting in a decline in independence. The condition of mildly low Hb is no longer considered clinically benign because mortality risk has been shown to be lower with higher Hb levels.[37] It may be appropriate to request assessment of Hb levels and/or communicate with the physician about the potential harm of low-normal Hb levels.

Bleeding under the skin and easy bruising in response to the slightest trauma often occur when platelet production is altered (thrombocytopenia) secondary to hypoplastic or aplastic anemia. This condition necessitates extreme care in the therapy setting, especially any intervention requiring manual therapy or the use of any equipment, including modalities and weight-training devices. Splenomegaly associated with some types of anemia requires precautions in performing soft tissue techniques in the left upper quadrant, especially up and under the rib cage; indirect techniques away from the spleen are indicated.

Decreased oxygen delivery to the skin results in impaired healing and loss of elasticity as well as delaying wound healing and healing of other musculoskeletal injuries. If the anemia is caused by vitamin B_{12} deficiency (e.g., pernicious anemia, pregnancy, hyperthyroidism), the nervous system is affected.

Alteration of the structure and function of the peripheral nerves, spinal cord (myelin degeneration), and brain may occur. Paresthesias, especially numbness mimicking carpal tunnel syndrome; gait disturbances; extreme weakness; spasticity; and abnormal reflexes can result. Permanent neurologic damage unresponsive to vitamin B_{12} therapy can occur in extreme cases when intervention has been delayed.

Monitoring Vital Signs

Tachycardia may be the first change observed when monitoring vital signs, usually accompanied by a sense of fatigue, generalized weakness, loss of stamina, and exertional dyspnea. Systolic blood pressure may not be affected, but diastolic pressure may be lower than normal, with an associated increase in the resting pulse rate.

Resting cardiac output is usually normal in people with anemia, but cardiac output increases with exercise more than in nonanemic people. As the anemia becomes more severe, resting cardiac output increases and exercise tolerance progressively decreases until dyspnea, tachycardia, and palpitations occur at rest.

DISORDERS OF LEUKOCYTES

Alterations in blood leukocyte (WBC) concentration and in the relative proportions of the several leukocyte types are recognized as measures of the reaction of the body to infection, inflammation, tissue damage, or degeneration. In many instances, these alterations give useful indications of the nature of the pathologic process and may be seen in association not only with acute infections but also with many chronic ailments treated by the clinician.

Leukocytes may be classified in three main groups: granulocytes (basophils, eosinophils, neutrophils), monocytes, and lymphocytes. *Granulocytes* (granular leukocytes) contain lysing agents within their granules that are capable of digesting various foreign materials. The main type of granulocyte is the neutrophil, also called the *polymorphonuclear leukocyte*; these are usually not found in normal "healthy" tissue and are referred to as the first line of hematologic defense against invading pathogens.

Granulocytes are also involved in the pathophysiology of organ damage in ischemia/reperfusion, trauma, sepsis, or organ transplantation. Basophils and eosinophils are involved with allergic reactions and respond to parasitic and fungal infections.

Monocytes are the largest circulating blood cells and represent an immature cell until it leaves the blood and travels to the tissues. Once migrated, monocytes form macrophages when activated by foreign substances such as bacteria. Monocytes/macrophages participate in inflammation by synthesizing numerous mediators and eliminating various pathogens.

Lymphocytes are further divided into B and T cells. B lymphocytes are responsible for the humoral portion of the immune system and are known to secrete antibodies that react with antigens and initiate complement-mediated destruction or phagocytosis of foreign pathogens, particularly bacteria. T lymphocytes are in control of cell-mediated immunity and are able to recognize and destroy cells altered by viruses.

These cells are also responsible for coordinating the immune response through the release of lymphokines and inflammatory modulators, creating a cell-to-cell communication with B cells and monocytes. The exact role or function of leukocytes during inflammatory processes remains the subject of considerable investigation.

Leukocytosis
Definition and Etiology
Leukocytosis, defined as an increase in the number of leukocytes in the blood, may occur as a result of a variety of causes (Box 10.5) and may also occur as a normal protective response to physiologic stressors such as strenuous exercise, emotional changes, temperature changes, anesthesia, surgery, pregnancy, some drugs, toxins, and hormones.

Leukocytosis develops within 1 or 2 hours after the onset of acute hemorrhage and is greater when the bleeding occurs internally (e.g., into the peritoneal cavity, pleural space, or joint cavity, or as a result of a skull fracture with associated intracranial bleed or subarachnoid hemorrhage) than when the bleeding is external.

Leukocytosis is a common finding in and characterizes many infectious diseases recognized by a count of more than 10,000 WBCs/mm^3. An elevated WBC count (greater than 50,000/mm^3, with the majority of cells being neutrophils and neutrophil precursors) in response to a serious underlying process is referred to as a leukemoid reaction (see Box 10.5).

Leukocytosis frequently results from an increase in circulating neutrophils (neutrophilia) recruited in large numbers

---

BOX 10.5 Causes of Leukocytosis

- Acute hemorrhage
- Infection (viral, bacterial, or fungal)
- Malignancies (leukemia, lymphoma, non–small cell lung cancer, multiple myeloma)
- Myeloproliferative disorders
- Glucocorticosteroid therapy
- Trauma (e.g., burns)
- Tissue necrosis (e.g., infarction)
- Inflammation (autoimmune-mediated, such as myositis or vasculitis)

---

in the course of infections and in the presence of some rapidly growing neoplasms (e.g., leukemia, non–small cell lung cancer, renal cell carcinoma, and gastric carcinoma). The counts may be especially high in tumors with significant necrosis. Some tumors can also release hormone-like substances that cause leukocytosis.

Clinical Manifestations
Clinical signs and symptoms of leukocytosis are usually associated with symptoms of the conditions listed in Box 10.5 and may include fever, headache, shortness of breath, symptoms of localized or systemic infection, and symptoms of inflammation or trauma to tissue.

Medical Management

Diagnosis, Treatment, and Prognosis
Major leukocyte functions are accomplished in the tissues so that the leukocytes in the blood are in transit from the site of production or storage to the tissues, even in normal people. Variations in the blood concentrations of each leukocyte type may be of brief duration and easily missed or may persist for days or weeks. Laboratory tests for detecting leukocyte abnormalities include total leukocyte count, leukocyte differential cell count, peripheral blood morphology, and bone marrow morphology.

Treatment is directed toward the underlying cause of the change in leukocytes and control of any infections. Prognosis depends on the etiology of the leukocytosis.

10.5 Special Implications for the PTA: Leukocytes It is important for the clinician to be aware of the client's most recent leukocyte (WBC) count before and during episodes of care if that person is immunosuppressed. At that time, the client is extremely susceptible to opportunistic infections and severe complications.

The importance of good handwashing and hygiene practices cannot be overemphasized when treating immunocompromised clients. Some centers recommend that people with a WBC count of less than 1000/mm^3 or a neutrophil count of less than 500/mm^3 wear a protective mask. Clinicians should ensure that these people are provided with equipment that has been disinfected according to standard precautions.

Leukopenia
Definition and Etiology
Leukopenia, or reduction of the number of leukocytes in the blood below 5000/mL, can be caused by a variety of factors such as HIV (or other viral infection such as hepatitis), alcohol and nutritional deficiencies, drug-induced condition, and connective tissue disorders (e.g., SLE). It can occur in many forms of bone marrow failure, such as that following

antineoplastic chemotherapy or radiation therapy or in overwhelming infections.

People with leukemia, lymphoma, myeloma, and Hodgkin's lymphoma have serious underlying WBC abnormalities that contribute to the risk of infection associated with leukopenia. Unlike leukocytosis, leukopenia is never beneficial. As the leukocyte count decreases, the risk for various infections increases.

The risk of infection from leukopenia after bone marrow radiation has been reduced with continued improvements in medical treatment. The use of naturally occurring glycoproteins to help collect blood stem cells administered after chemotherapy reduces the duration of blood cell reduction and prevents the serious problems encountered in the past.

These glycoproteins are hematopoietic growth factors called colony-stimulating factors (CSFs) or, more specifically, granulocyte colony-stimulating factor (GCSF), or filgrastim (Neupogen). Growth factors move the stem cells from the bone marrow into the peripheral blood and can result in a temporary tenfold to hundredfold increase in the numbers of circulating stem cells at the time of bone marrow recovery. Filgrastim not only increases the number but also the function of granulocytes.

Clinical Manifestations

Leukopenia may be asymptomatic (and detected by routine tests) or associated with clinical signs and symptoms consistent with infection, such as sore throat, cough, high fever, chills, sweating, ulcerations of mucous membranes (e.g., mouth, rectum, vagina), frequent or painful urination, or persistent infections.

Medical Management

Diagnosis and Treatment

As with leukocytosis, diagnosis is by laboratory testing for leukocyte abnormalities. Treatment is directed toward elimination of the cause of the reduced leukocytes and control of any infections. Pharmacologic therapy includes the use of antibiotics, antifungal agents, and CSF drugs such as filgrastim (Neupogen). This drug markedly assists in decreasing the incidence of infection in people who have received bone marrow–depressing antineoplastic agents.

Basophilia

Basophils are a subtype of leukocytes involved in inflammatory and allergic reactions. Their granules contain heparin (an anticoagulant but without significant systemic effects), histamine (the cause of most of the systemic symptoms), chondroitin sulfate, platelet-activating factor, and other proteins.

The antibody IgE is the most common stimulator of basophilic degranulation. IgE may be secreted in response to the body's detection of a foreign particle (such as insect venom or some drugs). The histamine and other proteins released by the basophil lead to a local inflammatory and allergic response. This response varies from person to person. Some clients may have reactions that are not modulated and develop anaphylaxis, asthma, urticaria, and allergic rhinitis. Basophilia is primarily associated with myeloproliferative disorders, particularly chronic myeloid leukemia.

The remaining categories (e.g., basophilia/basopenia, eosinophilia/eosinopenia, neutrophilia/neutropenia) are all types of leukocytosis or leukopenia. The specific type is determined when the leukocyte differential (WBC count) determines the percentage of each type of granular and nongranular leukocyte.

Eosinophilia

Following their maturation and release from the bone marrow into the circulation, eosinophils soon migrate into tissue. These tissues are in areas that have contact with the external environment, such as the skin, GI tract, genital tract, and lungs. Eosinophils can be recruited to areas of inflammation by various antibodies and interleukins and stimulated to release chemokines, growth factors, cytokines, peroxidase, and other modulating proteins.

Chemokines are any of a group of low-molecular-weight cytokines (e.g., interleukins) identified on the basis of their ability to induce chemotaxis (cell movement) or chemokinesis (cell activity due to the presence of a chemical substance) in leukocytes in inflammation. Chemokines function as regulators of the immune system and may play roles in the circulatory system and CNS.

Eosinophils, however, are not central participants in defending the body against most infections but do play key roles in fighting parasitic infections, such as hookworm or *strongyloidiasis*. Eosinophils are also involved in allergic reactions such as asthma, cutaneous reactions, and other hypersensitivity states.

Eosinophilia is an elevation in the number of eosinophils in the blood (with an eosinophil count greater than 500/μL). It is seen most often in allergic reactions to drugs (aspirin, sulfonamides, penicillins), in hay fever, eczema, collagen vascular diseases (RA, eosinophilic fasciitis, periarteritis nodosa), and malignancies (Hodgkin's lymphoma; mycosis fungoides; chronic myeloid leukemia; and cancer of the stomach, pancreas, and lung).

Idiopathic hypereosinophilia syndrome (counts from 50,000 to 100,000/μL), eosinophilic leukemia, and Loeffler's syndrome are uncommon illnesses but are associated with dramatic eosinophilia. Increased levels of eosinophils were also identified during outbreaks of *eosinophilia myalgia syndrome*, a connective tissue disease induced by the ingestion of contaminated L-tryptophan supplements, sometimes taken for insomnia or back pain.[47]

Neutrophilia

Granulocytes assist in initiating the inflammatory response, and they defend the body against infectious agents by phagocytosing bacteria and other infectious substances. Generally the neutrophils (the most plentiful of the granulocytes) are the first phagocytic cells to reach an infected area, followed by monocytes; neutrophils and monocytes work together to phagocytose all foreign material present.

Granulocytosis (an excess of granulocytes in the blood) or *neutrophilia* (increased number of neutrophils in the blood) are terms used to describe the early stages of infection or inflammation. The capacity of corticosteroids or alcohol to diminish the accumulation of neutrophils in inflamed areas may be due to their ability to reduce cell adherence.

The many potential causes of neutrophilia include inflammation or tissue necrosis (e.g., after surgery from tissue damage, severe burns, myocardial infarction, pneumonitis, rheumatic fever, RA); acute infection (e.g., *Staphylococcus, Streptococcus, Pneumococcus*); drug- or chemical-induced causes (e.g., epinephrine, steroids, heparin, histamine); metabolic causes (e.g., acidosis associated with diabetes, gout, thyroid storm, eclampsia); and neoplasms of the liver, GI tract, or bone marrow. Physiologic neutrophilia may also occur as a result of exercise, extreme heat/cold, third-trimester pregnancy, and emotional distress.

Neutropenia

Neutropenia is the condition associated with a reduction in circulating neutrophils (less than 2500/µL). Causes are either acquired or congenital. Acquired neutropenias are typically a result of toxicity to neutrophil precursors in the bone marrow. This may be due to drugs (e.g., NSAIDs, sulfonamides, penicillins, anticonvulsants) or infectious agents (e.g., hepatitis B, cytomegalovirus, EBV, HIV). Other drugs can cause an autoimmune-related peripheral destruction of neutrophils, leading to neutropenia.

Other causes of neutropenia include carcinoma of the lung, breast, prostate, and stomach and malignant hematopoietic disorders that can occupy enough of the bone marrow to cause global marrow failure with resultant pancytopenias (all cell lines are decreased in number). Congenital causes usually come to attention early in life and are much less common than acquired causes.

The longer an individual exists without neutrophils, the higher the risk for significant infection. Drug-induced neutropenia generally resolves in 10 to 12 days, whereas administration of GCSF may shorten the time to resolution.

Lymphocytosis/Lymphocytopenia

Lymphocytosis occurs most commonly in acute viral infections, especially those caused by EBV. Other causes include endocrine disorders (e.g., thyrotoxicosis, adrenal insufficiency) and malignancies (e.g., acute and chronic lymphocytic leukemia).

Lymphocytopenia may be acquired or congenital. Acquired lymphocytopenias can be attributed to abnormalities of lymphocyte production associated with neoplasms and immune deficiencies and destruction of lymphocytes by drugs, viruses, or radiation.

Other causes include corticosteroid therapy, severe systemic illnesses (e.g., miliary tuberculosis), SLE, sarcoidosis, or severe right-sided heart failure. Lymphocytopenia can be a major problem for individuals with AIDS, increasing their susceptibility to viral illnesses, malignancies, and fungal infections.

Monocytosis

Monocytosis, an increase in monocytes, is most often seen in chronic infections such as tuberculosis and subacute endocarditis and other inflammatory processes, such as SLE and RA. Monocytosis is present in more than 50% of people with collagen vascular disease.

Clients with sarcoidosis or other granulomatous processes may also have elevated monocytes. Monocytosis also exists as a normal physiologic response in newborns (first 2 weeks of life). Although not common, monocytes can go through a transformation, becoming leukemia, or an elevation of normal monocytes can be seen in malignancies such as Hodgkin's and non-Hodgkin's lymphoma. Monocytosis can be indicative of bone marrow recovery following a drug-induced loss of granulocytes.

NEOPLASTIC DISEASES OF THE BLOOD AND LYMPH SYSTEMS

Hematologic malignancies include diseases in any hematologic tissue (e.g., bone marrow, spleen, thymus) that arise from changes in stem cells or clonal (genetically identical cells) proliferation of abnormal cells. The primary hematologic disorders that result from stem cell abnormalities include the myeloproliferative disorders (e.g., polycythemia vera, essential thrombocythemia, chronic myeloid leukemia, and myelofibrosis with myeloid metaplasia) and acute myeloid leukemia. Myelofibrosis is the replacement of hematopoietic bone marrow with fibrous tissue such as fibroblasts and collagen.

Multiple myeloma and plasma cell diseases arise from clonal proliferation of abnormal plasma cells. Lymphoid malignancies are also a clonal proliferation of malignant cells and can be categorized according to the malignant cell type: B-cell, T-cell/natural killer cell, and Hodgkin's lymphoma. For ease of discussion, the leukemias are presented together.

Bone Marrow and Stem Cell Transplantation

Bone marrow transplantation is often a treatment choice for many of the neoplastic diseases of the blood and lymph systems.

The Leukemias

Leukemia is a malignant neoplasm of the blood-forming cells that replaces the normal bone marrow with a malignant clone (genetically identical cell) of lymphocytic or myelogenous cells. The disease may be acute or chronic based on its natural course; acute leukemias have a rapid clinical course, resulting in death in a few months without treatment, whereas chronic leukemias have a more prolonged course. The four major types of leukemia are acute or chronic lymphocytic and acute or chronic myeloid leukemia (Table 10.2).

When leukemia is classified according to its morphology (i.e., the predominant cell type and level of maturity), the following descriptors are used: *lympho-,* for leukemias involving the lymphoid or lymphatic system; *myelo-,* for leukemias of myeloid or bone marrow origin involving hematopoietic stem cells; -*blastic,* for leukemia involving large, immature (functionless) cells; and -*cytic,* for leukemia involving mature, smaller cells. If classified immunologically, T-cell/natural killer cell and B-cell leukemias are described.

Acute leukemia is an accumulation of neoplastic, immature lymphoid or myeloid cells in the bone marrow and peripheral blood. It is defined as more than 30% blasts in the bone marrow (the WHO classification accepts 20% as the definition of leukemia).

Chronic leukemia is a neoplastic accumulation of mature lymphoid or myeloid elements of the blood that usually progresses more slowly than an acute leukemic process and permits the production of greater numbers of more mature, functional cells. With rapid proliferation of leukemic cells, the bone marrow becomes overcrowded with abnormal cells, which then spill over into the peripheral circulation. Crowding of the bone marrow by leukemic cells inhibits normal blood cell production.

The three main symptoms that occur as a consequence of this infiltration and replacement process are (1) *anemia* and reduced tissue oxygenation from decreased erythrocytes, (2) *infection* from neutropenia as leukemic cells are functionally unable to defend

TABLE 10.2 Overview of Leukemia

	ALL	CLL	AML	CML
Incidence (% of all leukemias)	20%	25%	40%	15%–20%
Adults	30%	100% (common)	80% (most common)	95%–100%
Children	65%–70% (most common)	NA	20%	2%
Age	Peak, 3–7 years 65 + (older adults)	50+ years	Mean, 63 years; incidence increases with age from 45–80+ years	Average, 66 years (mostly adults)
Etiologic factors	Unknown; chromosomal abnormalities; Down syndrome (high incidence)	Chromosomal abnormalities; slow accumulation of CLL lymphocytes	Benzene; alkylating agents; radiation; myeloproliferative disorders; chromosome abnormalities	Philadelphia chromosome; radiation exposure
Prognosis	Adults: 40% Children: 80% survival	Poor cytogenetics: median, 8 years; good cytogenetics: median, 25 years	Adults: Median survival, 10–14 years	Moderately progressive with new treatment; current survival rate unknown

ALL, Acute lymphoblastic leukemia; *AML*, acute myelogenous leukemia; *CLL*, chronic lymphocytic leukemia; *CML*, chronic myeloid leukemia.

the body against pathogens, and (3) *bleeding tendencies* from decreased platelet production (thrombocytopenia) (Fig. 10.4).

Leukemia is not limited to the bone marrow and peripheral blood. Abnormalities in the CNS or other organ systems can result from the infiltration and replacement of any tissue of the body with nonfunctional leukemic cells or metabolic complications related to leukemia.

Leukemia is a complex disease that requires careful identification of the subtype for appropriate treatment. Molecular probes can be used to establish a morphologic diagnosis of the type of leukemia, which then determines treatment and prognosis. These analyses are sufficiently sensitive to detect one leukemic cell among 100,000 or even in 1 million normal cells. Because of this extreme sensitivity, molecular markers have generally been used to determine the presence or absence of a few leukemic cells remaining after intensive therapy, so-called *residual disease.*

During the past 25 years, death rates for leukemia have been falling significantly (57% decline) for children and more modestly for adults younger than age 65 years. These declines in mortality reflect the advances made in the biologic and pathologic understanding of leukemia, technologic advances in medical care, and subsequent treatment that is more specifically targeted at the molecular level.

The aim of treatment is to bring about complete remission, or no evidence of the disease, with return to normal blood and marrow cells without relapse. For leukemia, a complete remission that lasts 5 years after treatment often indicates a cure. Future clinical and laboratory investigation will likely lead to the development of new, even more effective treatments specifically for different subsets of leukemia. The development of new chemotherapeutic and biologic agents combined with refined dose and schedule and stem cell transplantation has already contributed to the clinical success of treatment.

Acute Leukemia

Acute leukemia is a rapidly progressive malignant disease that results in the accumulation of immature, functionless cells called *blast cells* in the bone marrow and blood that block the development of normal cell development.

The two major forms of acute leukemia are *acute lymphoblastic leukemia* (ALL) and *acute myelogenous leukemia* (AML).

Lymphocytic leukemia involves the lymphocytes and lymphoid organs, and myelogenous leukemia involves hematopoietic stem cells that differentiate into myeloid cells (monocytes, granulocytes, erythrocytes, and platelets).

Acute Myelogenous Leukemia

Incidence and risk factors. AML is the most common leukemia in adults, constituting 80% of adult acute leukemias, whereas only 20% of AML patients are children. AML remains a rare disease, with about 12,000 cases per year.[15]

The incidence of AML increases with each decade of life, with the median age at onset of 63 years.[120] People older than age 70 years have a twelvefold increase of developing AML. Most cases of AML develop for unknown reasons, whereas some cases occur following treatment for another cancer (chemotherapy or radiation induced) or from a preexisting myelodysplastic syndrome.

Two types of chemotherapy treatment–related AML are described. The first typically occurs 5 to 7 years following exposure to an alkylating agent and is often heralded by a dysplastic phase. The other appears shortly after exposure to a topoisomerase II inhibitor (1 to 3 years) and lacks a dysplastic phase. Abnormalities in chromosome 7 are often seen in treatment-related AML and carry a worse prognosis than those cases that are idiopathic.[169]

Other risk factors for AML include previous radiation exposure and chemical/occupational exposure (e.g., benzene, herbicides, pesticides, cigarette smoking). Persons with uncommon genetic disorders, such as Down syndrome or Fanconi syndrome, also have a higher incidence of developing acute leukemia than the general population.

Pathogenesis. AML is a heterogeneous group (not all the same) of neoplastic myeloid cells. Myeloid stem cells have the capability of differentiating into granulocytes, monocytes, erythrocytes, and platelets; neoplastic changes can occur along any line, resulting in many subtypes of AML.

Current techniques allow for cytogenetic analyses that can reveal specific chromosomal abnormalities where portions of a chromosome translocate (move) and fuse with another gene, creating a fusion gene. It is these abnormalities that lead to the development of leukemia, either allowing the cell to divide without regulation or failing to undergo programmed cell death (apoptosis).

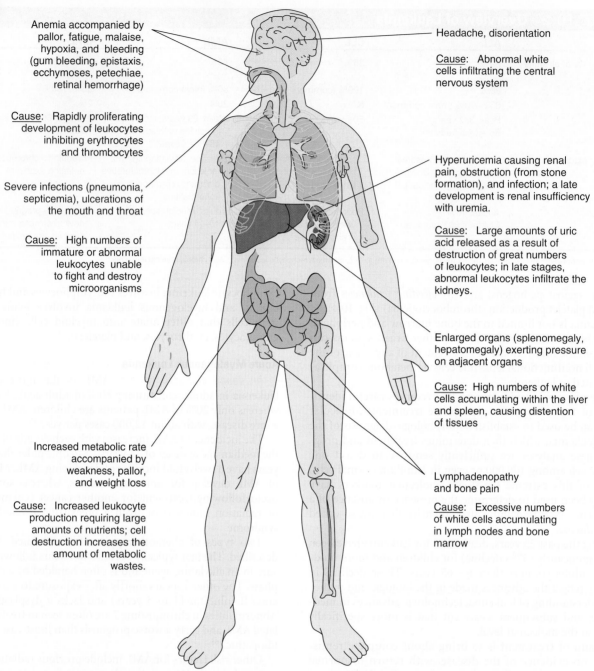

Anemia accompanied by pallor, fatigue, malaise, hypoxia, and bleeding (gum bleeding, epistaxis, ecchymoses, petechiae, retinal hemorrhage)

<u>Cause</u>: Rapidly proliferating development of leukocytes inhibiting erythrocytes and thrombocytes

Severe infections (pneumonia, septicemia), ulcerations of the mouth and throat

<u>Cause</u>: High numbers of immature or abnormal leukocytes unable to fight and destroy microorganisms

Increased metabolic rate accompanied by weakness, pallor, and weight loss

<u>Cause</u>: Increased leukocyte production requiring large amounts of nutrients; cell destruction increases the amount of metabolic wastes.

Headache, disorientation

<u>Cause</u>: Abnormal white cells infiltrating the central nervous system

Hyperuricemia causing renal pain, obstruction (from stone formation), and infection; a late development is renal insufficiency with uremia.

<u>Cause</u>: Large amounts of uric acid released as a result of destruction of great numbers of leukocytes; in late stages, abnormal leukocytes infiltrate the kidneys.

Enlarged organs (splenomegaly, hepatomegaly) exerting pressure on adjacent organs

<u>Cause</u>: High numbers of white cells accumulating within the liver and spleen, causing distention of tissues

Lymphadenopathy and bone pain

<u>Cause</u>: Excessive numbers of white cells accumulating in lymph nodes and bone marrow

FIG. 10.4 Pathologic basis for the clinical manifestations of leukemia. (Modified from Black JM, Matassarin-Jacobs E, editors: Luckmann and Sorensen's medical-surgical nursing, ed 4, Philadelphia, 1993, Saunders.)

Clinical manifestations. Initial clinical indications of AML are related to pancytopenia (reduction in all cell lines), reflecting leukemic cell replacement of bone marrow. Clients often have infections because of a lack of neutrophils or bleeding secondary to platelet deficiency (thrombocytopenia).

Spontaneous bleeding or bleeding with minor trauma often occurs in the skin and mucosal surfaces, manifested as gingival bleeding, *epistaxis,* midcycle menstrual bleeding, or heavy bleeding associated with menstruation (see Fig. 10.4). Petechiae (small, purplish spots caused by intradermal bleeding) are common clinical manifestations of thrombocytopenia particularly noted on the extremities after prolonged standing or minor trauma.

Fatigue, loss of energy, and shortness of breath with physical exertion are common as a result of anemia. Leukemia cells may infiltrate the skin (known as leukemia cutis), seen most often in the acute monocytic or myelomonocytic subtypes of AML. Leukemia cutis may present as multiple purplish papules or as a diffuse rash (Fig. 10.5).

Modest splenomegaly is seen in 50% of clients with AML, whereas lymphadenopathy is uncommon. Expanded leukemic marrow may cause discomfort in the bones, especially the sternum, ribs, and tibia. In the older adult, the disease can present insidiously with progressive weakness, pallor, a change in sense of well-being, and delirium.

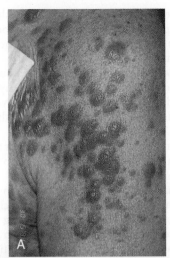

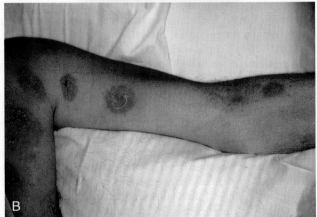

FIG. 10.5 (A) Leukemia cutis in an individual with monoblastic leukemia. (B) Another example of leukemia cutis in the form of *erythematous* nodular tumors. (A, From Hoffman R: Hematology: basic principles and practice, ed 4, Philadelphia, 2005, Churchill Livingstone. B, From Noble J: Textbook of primary care medicine, ed 3, St, Louis, 2001, Mosby.)

CNS involvement is uncommon, occurring in only 1% to 2% of adults presenting with AML.[31] These people present with symptoms similar to meningitis (e.g., headache, stiff neck, and fever). Some clients may develop cerebral bleeding or meningitis due to pancytopenia. In a small number of cases, AML may be more subtle, presenting at first with progressive fatigue and normal blood counts.

Treatment. The diagnosis of acute leukemia is a medical emergency, especially if the WBC count is high (greater than 100,000/mL), placing the person at risk for cerebral hemorrhage caused by leukostasis (obstruction of and damage to blood vessels plugged with rigid, large blasts).

Treatment decisions are based on the subtype of AML. Most induction (initial) treatment protocols use aggressive combination chemotherapy in order to eradicate the neoplastic cells and restore normal hematopoiesis. Supportive care, including fluids, blood product replacement, and prompt treatment of infection with broad-spectrum antibiotics, is frequently needed during the 3- to 4-week hospitalization required for bone marrow recovery. Significant complications occur during this period, with a death rate of 5% to 10%.[15]

Induction chemotherapy is followed by consolidation chemotherapy, which is intended to maintain a complete remission. Consolidation treatment is administered in a cyclic fashion over 2 to 4 months.

The discovery of mutations and translocations that may be causing leukemia has led to the development of targeted therapeutic agents. One example is tretinoin. It is used against acute promyelocytic leukemia and targets the t(15;17) translocation. Experimental drugs are in clinical trials for persons with *FLT3* mutations, and other agents will be designed in hopes of targeting the genetic abnormalities without affecting normal cells.

Prognosis. If left untreated, all leukemias are fatal. With induction treatment, approximately 80% of clients younger than 60 years achieve remission. The rate of remission decreases as age increases to over 60 years.

According to the WHO classification, persons with AML with favorable cytogenetics (good prognosis) have a 60% 5-year survival rate, whereas those with a poor prognosis have only a 10% 5-year survival rate. Clients with an intermediate prognosis (the majority of AML cases) have a 40% 5-year survival rate.

Improvement in outcomes for people with a poor prognosis is a major goal of clinical research. Because this group rarely remains in remission after consolidation therapy, current protocols include allogeneic, unrelated-donor or cord-blood transplantation following induction (e.g., transplant done in first remission). Consolidation therapy is offered to those people with good prognostic cytogenetics. Autologous transplantation and consolidation therapy are the options for clients with normal cytogenetics but an intermediate risk for recurrence.

Acute Lymphoblastic Leukemia

Incidence and risk factors. In contrast to AML, ALL is diagnosed more frequently in children. Of the 4000 cases of ALL identified each year, two-thirds occur in children, whereas only one-third are diagnosed in adults.[162] Yet of the 1500 annual deaths, almost two-thirds occur in adults.

Like AML, most ALL cases develop for unknown reasons. A few risk factors have been identified, including significant exposure to radiation and infection with HTLV-1 (human T-cell lymphoma/leukemia virus). Persons with genetic disorders such as Down syndrome also have an increased risk.

Questions have been raised as to whether electromagnetic fields, such as those generated in high-voltage power lines, increase the risk of developing ALL. Currently, large studies are ongoing, with initial data suggestive of no increased risk or a very slight increased risk. Answers should be available at the conclusion of these studies. Burkitt's lymphoma can form a type of ALL that responds poorly to treatment.

Pathogenesis. Abnormal cytogenetics or translocations and mutations are frequently seen in ALL cases. These genetic changes lead to abnormal cell growth and division or inability of the cells to decrease their growth and die (scheduled cell death or apoptosis). These various abnormalities are associated with poor or good prognosis. For instance, leukemic cells with more than 50 chromosomes (hyperdiploidy) and the translocation t(12;21) have a good prognosis. More than 50% of children with ALL have this defect, whereas only 10% of adults have it. Leukemic cells with fewer than 45 chromosomes are difficult to treat and carry a poor prognosis. Translocations t(4;11) (50% of infant cases) and t(9;22) (50% of adults older than age 50 years) also have a poor prognosis.[162]

Clinical manifestations. ALL exhibits clinical signs and symptoms resulting from an abnormal bone marrow that is unable to engage in normal hematopoiesis. Fever and frequent infections indicate a lack of normal neutrophils, whereas easy bleeding and bruising are indicative of thrombocytopenia. Clients are often tired as a result of anemia.

ALL is more likely than AML to have leukemic cells spread to extramedullary sites. The CNS is frequently involved, causing headache, weakness, seizures, vomiting, difficulty with balance, and blurred vision.[9] Testicles in males and ovaries in females commonly harbor leukemic cells and are difficult to reach with chemotherapy agents.

Bone and joint pain from leukemic infiltration or hemorrhage into a joint may be the initial symptoms (more common finding in children than adults). Involvement of the synovium may lead to symptoms suggestive of a rheumatic disease, especially in children.

Hepatosplenomegaly and lymphadenopathy (particularly in the mediastinum) are frequently encountered along with an enlarged thymus. If thymic swelling is significant, the client may exhibit difficulty breathing or upper extremity swelling from increased pressure on the bronchus or superior vena cava (superior vena cava syndrome), which requires immediate attention.

Chronic Leukemia

Chronic leukemia is a malignant disease of the bone marrow and blood that progresses slowly and permits numbers of more mature, functional cells to be made. Chronic leukemia has two major groups: chronic myeloid leukemia (CML) and chronic lymphocytic leukemia (CLL), each with several subtypes.

These are entirely different diseases and are presented separately. CML is also known as chronic myelogenous leukemia or chronic myelocytic leukemia. Other less common forms include prolymphocytic leukemia (terminal transformation of CLL) and hairy cell leukemia (accounting for only 1% to 2% of adult leukemias).

Chronic Myeloid Leukemia

Incidence and etiologic factors. CML is a neoplasm of the hematopoietic stem cell. The genetic abnormalities created in the stem cell are the result of acquired injury to the DNA and passed on to all related cell lines, resulting in increases in myeloid cells and clonal anomalies in erythroid cells and platelets. This leads to abnormal cells in peripheral blood and marked hyperplasia in the bone marrow.

CML accounts for 15% of all leukemias, with approximately 4600 cases diagnosed per year. This type of leukemia occurs mostly in adults, with only 2% developing in children. Although the exact etiologic factors are unknown, the incidence of CML is increased in people with severe radiation exposure. No chemical or other environmental risk factors are known to cause CML.

CML was the first form of leukemia with a known genetic predisposition (Philadelphia chromosome [Ph]; named after the city in which researchers first observed the chromosome). The specific genetic anomaly is a translocation that fuses the long arm of chromosome 22 to chromosome 9. Detached pieces of chromosome 9 adhere to the broken end

of chromosome 22 and vice versa. This translocation occurs only in the stem cell and in the various blood cells derived from that stem cell. The chromosomes of the cells in other tissues are normal.

Pathogenesis. CML originates in the hematopoietic stem cell (i.e., this cell has the ability to develop into any one of several blood cells) and involves overproduction of myeloid cells. The genetic defect detected in CML cells is called the Philadelphia chromosome. This translocation [t(9;22)] was the first consistent chromosomal anomaly identified in a cancer and is now detected in all cases of CML and known to be the cause of CML.

The abnormal chromosome develops from the accidental translocation and fusion of the *BRC* gene on chromosome 22 and the *ABL* gene on chromosome 9, creating a unique gene (*BRC-ABL*). The *BRC-ABL* gene encodes for an abnormal protein product that acts as a tyrosine kinase, resulting in a dysregulated proliferation signal.

Tyrosine kinase is an enzyme that is necessary for normal cell growth. In normal cells, the enzyme turns on and off as it should, but in people with CML this enzyme appears to be in the permanent "switched on" state, eliminating the normal checks and balances on proliferation.

Unlike AML, CML permits the development of mature WBCs that generally can function normally. This important distinction from acute leukemia accounts for the less severe early course of the disease.[165]

Clinical manifestations. Presenting signs and symptoms are often quite nonspecific. The most typical symptoms at presentation are fatigue, anorexia, and weight loss, although approximately 40% of affected individuals are asymptomatic. Sweats, malaise, and shortness of breath during physical activity are also reported.

Splenomegaly is present in 50% of all cases, with thrombocytosis being very common. Discomfort on the left side of the abdomen from the enlarged spleen is not uncommon.

The natural history of CML is a progression (over years) from a *proliferative* phase (chronic phase), into an accelerated phase (more symptoms but not acute leukemia), to an aggressive acute leukemia (blast crisis) that can be rapidly fatal within months.

Chronic Lymphocytic Leukemia

Incidence and etiologic and risk factors. CLL is a common type of adult leukemia, accounting for 25% to 30% of all leukemias, with almost 10,000 cases per year.[97] The incidence of CLL increases with advancing age; 90% are older than age 50 years, and men are affected more often than women. CLL may occur in as many as 3% of people older than age 70 years.

The cause of CLL is also unknown but a few environmental factors have been implicated, such as farming pesticides and the chemical warfare herbicide Agent Orange, although conclusive evidence is lacking. Some groups of people may have a genetic predisposition, including persons with a first-degree family member with CLL.[209]

Pathogenesis. The cell type responsible for more than 95% of the cases of CLL is the B cell (T-cell CLL is uncommon). When a normal B cell is stimulated by an antigen, it enters a proliferative phase, creating clones able to fight infection. It is during this stage that a cell may develop a mutation and predispose it to become cancerous. A mutation allowing the cell to continue to proliferate places that cell at an advantage but the human host at a disadvantage. With continuous exposure to this antigen and the aid of stromal cells, cytokines, and chemokines, cells would be stimulated to proliferate and avoid apoptosis (programmed cell death), potentially leading to cancer.

CLL cells may develop from this type of cell because most initial CLL cells lack major cytogenetic abnormalities (translocations are uncommon). As the mutated B cell continues to divide, more mutations develop, creating a heterogenous group of abnormal cells. Different mutations appear to affect the course of the disease.

Mutations in the immunoglobulin-forming genes can proffer a prolonged, milder course of disease or a more aggressive, symptomatic illness. For example, clients with no or few *V* gene mutations or multiple CD38 + or ZAP-70 + mutations followed an aggressive, often fatal course, whereas cancerous clones with few CD38 + or ZAP-70 + mutations resulted in a more indolent course.[38] ZAP-70 + is a protein normally found in T lymphocytes and is responsible for transferring signals inside the cell.

There are few unifying mutations except the deletion of 13q14.3, which is present in more than half of all people with CLL.[130] The frequency of this mutation suggests that the genes in this region offer the clonal cells an advantage over other cells. Other mutations are noted to be in genes that control apoptosis or confer chemotherapy resistance, resulting in a poor prognosis.

Clinical manifestations. In the early stages of the disease, most clients remain asymptomatic or complain of vague, nonspecific symptoms such as fatigue or enlarged lymph nodes. Depending on the mutations present in the abnormal clone, clients may experience a prolonged, indolent course with few symptoms.

Those people with more aggressive CLL develop pancytopenia (with accompanying symptoms of infections, hemorrhage, and significant fatigue) and decreased immunoglobulin levels (also resulting in infections). With progression of the disease, clients may develop lymphadenopathy, splenomegaly, hepatomegaly, weight loss, bone pain, and bone marrow infiltration. Approximately 10% to 25% of clients develop the complication of AIHA,[150] and immune thrombocytopenia occurs in 2% of cases.[24]

10.6 Special Implications for the PTA: Leukemia Like all cancers, medical innovations in the treatment of leukemia are increasing the patient's lifespan while increasing the likelihood of treatment side effects. Strengthening and energy-enhancing programs during cancer treatment may reduce the disabling fatigue and other effects of chemotherapy and radiation therapy.

Precautions

The period after chemically induced remission is critical for each client, who is now highly susceptible to spontaneous hemorrhage and defenseless against invading organisms. The usual precautions for thrombocytopenia, neutropenia, and infection control must be adhered to strictly. The importance of strict handwashing technique cannot be overemphasized. The clinician should be alert to any sign of infection and report any potential site of infection, such as mucosal ulceration, skin abrasion, or a tear (even a hangnail). Precautions are as for anemia, outlined earlier in this chapter.

Anticipating potential side effects of medications used in the treatment of leukemia can help the clinician better understand client reactions during the episode of care. Drug-induced mood changes, ranging from feelings of well-being and euphoria to depression and irritability, may occur; depression and irritability may also be associated with the cancer. Exercise intensity and duration and activity modifications are necessary for clients with anemia.

Clients with a history of prolonged corticosteroid use should be assessed for muscle weakness and avascular necrosis of the hips and shoulders.

Joint Involvement

Arthralgias or arthritis occurs in approximately 12% of adults with chronic leukemia, 13% of adults with acute leukemia, and up to 60% of children with ALL. Articular symptoms are the result of leukemic infiltrates of the synovium, periosteum, or periarticular bone or of secondary gout or hemarthrosis. Asymmetrical involvement of the large joints is most commonly observed. Pain that is disproportionate to the physical findings may occur, and joint symptoms are often transient.

Children with Leukemia

Because of increasing survival rates for children with ALL and the extensive side effects of the treatments, the clinician must pay attention to specific measures of cognition, function, activity, and participation when planning an appropriate intervention program. All components are needed in a comprehensive program.[126]

Short- and long-term impairments can affect any or all of these components. Decreased Hb levels, osteonecrosis, joint range of motion (ROM), strength, gross and fine motor performance, fitness, and attendance or absence from school are all factors to consider.[126]

Long-term effects of treatment and CNS prophylaxis can include peripheral neuropathies, neuropsychologic disorders, problems with balance, decreased muscle strength, and obesity. CNS prophylaxis includes intrathecal chemotherapy (injection of drugs into the spinal fluid) and cranial irradiation. Cranial irradiation and obesity are significant predictors of impaired balance.[207]

Preschool children with immature nervous systems may be more sensitive to the neurotoxicity of radiation and chemotherapy, placing them at a greater risk for CNS damage than children with fully developed neurologic systems.[131] Learning difficulties, cognitive deficits, attention problems, and lack of participation in physical activities can be sequelae of medical treatment.[207]

Personal factors such as a family's cultural belief system may influence how children and their parents perceive rehabilitation and specific interventions. Health-related quality of life and goals may be driven by family and cultural values that are not necessarily what the clinician perceives as in the best interest of the child's function and fitness.

The clinician should try to match the program with the family's cultural expectations, ability to participate, and emotional and financial resources. Expecting from the family only what they can succeed at and providing support and education where they are needed to help the family grow and care for their child with medical needs will create the best therapeutic environment for the child to thrive in.

Malignant Lymphomas

Lymphoma is a general term for cancers that develop in the lymphatic system. Lymphomas are divided into two groups: Hodgkin's lymphoma (HL; also known as Hodgkin's disease) and non-Hodgkin's lymphoma (NHL). With the extensive progression in cytogenetic research that has occurred over the past 5 years, this distinction is beginning to blur.

It is becoming more useful to categorize lymphomas according to their clinical behavior—indolent or aggressive—and their chromosome features. Currently HL is distinguished from other lymphomas by the presence of a characteristic type of cell known as the Reed–Sternberg cell. All other types of lymphoma are called NHL.

Hodgkin's Lymphoma

Definition and overview. HL is lymphoid neoplasm with the primary histologic finding of giant Reed–Sternberg cells in the lymph nodes. These cells are part of the tissue macrophage system and have twin nuclei and nucleoli that give them the appearance of owl eyes (Fig. 10.6).

Although this malignancy originates in the lymphoid system and primarily involves the lymph nodes, it can spread to other sites such as the spleen, liver, bone marrow, and lungs. There are two subtypes of HL: classic HL (further divided into the categories of nodular sclerosing HL, mixed-cellularity HL [MCHL], lymphocyte-rich classic HL, and lymphocyte-depleted HL) and nodular lymphocyte-predominant HL (LPHL). LPHL is uncommon and represents only 4% to 5% of HL cases.

Incidence and risk factors. Classic HL can occur in both children and adults, but peaks at two different ages: between the ages of 25 and 30 years and after the age of 55 years. Children younger than 5 years rarely develop this disease, whereas only 10% of HL cases occur in children 16 years old and younger. LPHL typically has only one peak incidence around the fourth decade. Approximately 7800 cases of HL are diagnosed in the United States each year (typically men more than women).[97]

Although the exact cause of HL remains under investigation, certain risk factors have been identified (Table 10.3). One factor that has been related to HL is previous infection with EBV. The DNA of this virus has been found in the Reed–Sternberg cells of about 50% of clients with classic HL (about 90% in developing countries).

Pathogenesis. HL is a B-cell–type malignancy with clonal expansion of a malignant B cell. The reason for the transformation from a normal B cell to a malignant cell is still under investigation, but significant progress has been made. Recent evidence suggests that an infection or inflammation may be involved. As just discussed, genes from EBV are found in half of all HL cases in the industrialized world.

Products from these genes (*LMP1*, *LMP2*, and *EBNA1*) have the ability to mimic transmembrane receptors and activate the transcription factor NF-κB (which is normally inhibited). NF-κB plays a key role in the proliferation and survival of the malignant clones through its function of regulating dozens of genes within the cell. The products of these genes include cytokines and chemokines.

Many cytokines, particularly interleukins, are involved in producing an environment where the Reed–Sternberg cells thrive. For example, some interleukins attract inflammatory cells (eosinophils, monocytes, and mast cells), which aid in the survival of the cell. In the laboratory, if these inflammatory cells are not surrounding the Reed–Sternberg cells, they do not survive.

Other interleukins expressed by the Reed–Sternberg cells inhibit the activation of T cells, which normally destroy abnormal cells. This inhibition creates an area of local immunosuppression and allows the Reed–Sternberg cell to evade detection. Some interleukins act as growth factors, encouraging proliferation, metastasis, and angiogenesis. Another protein induced by NF-κB, termed c-FLIP, is incorporated into a complex that signals cell death but is not functional in that capacity, thereby evading apoptosis and making the cell immortal.[105]

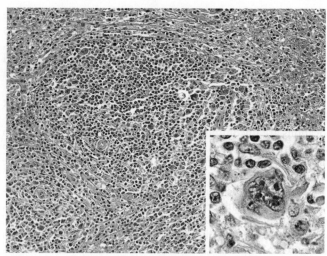

FIG. 10.6 Reed–Sternberg cell. Named for Dorothy M. Reed, American pathologist (1874–1964) and Karl Sternberg, Austrian pathologist (1872–1935). This is one example of the large, abnormal, multinucleated reticuloendothelial cells in the lymphatic system found in Hodgkin's lymphoma (HL). The number and proportion of Reed–Sternberg cells identified are the basis for the histopathologic classification of HL. (From Jaffe ES, Arber DA, Campo E, et al. (eds): Hematopathology, ed 2, Philadelphia, 2017, Elsevier.)

TABLE 10.3   Risk Factors for Malignant Lymphomas

NHL	HL
Age (increased risk with increasing age)	Familial
Sex (males more than females)	
Environmental Contaminants	
Herbicides and pesticides (?)	
Benzene (?)	
Polychlorinated biphenyls (PCBs) (?)	
Radiation	
Viral Infection	
EBV, mononucleosis virus	EBV, mononucleosis virus
Human T-lymphotrophic virus type I (HTLV-1)	
HIV	
Congenital Immunodeficiency Syndromes	
Hepatitis C (?)	
Immunocompromise/immunodeficiency	
Chronic disease or illness; autoimmune diseases	Chronic disease or illness; autoimmune diseases
Immunosuppressants	Immunosuppressants
Cancer treatment with alkylating or cytotoxic agents	Cancer treatment with alkylating or cytotoxic agents
Inherited immune deficiencies (e.g., collagen vascular disease)	SLE
HIV	HIV
AIDS	AIDS
Helicobacter pylori bacteria (gastric lymphoma)	Ulcerative colitis
Methotrexate	Drug abuse
Obesity (women)	Obesity (men)

EBV, Epstein–Barr virus; *HL,* Hodgkin's lymphoma; *NHL,* non-Hodgkin's lymphoma; *SLE,* systemic lupus erythematosus.

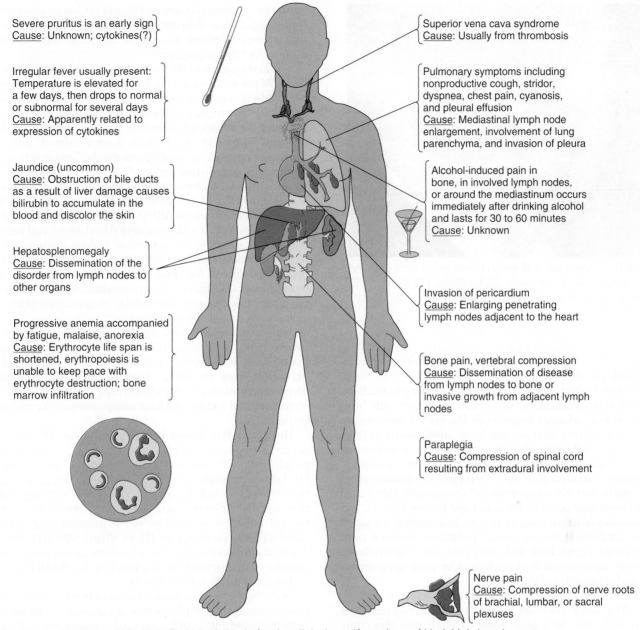

Severe pruritus is an early sign
Cause: Unknown; cytokines(?)

Irregular fever usually present:
Temperature is elevated for
a few days, then drops to normal
or subnormal for several days
Cause: Apparently related to
expression of cytokines

Jaundice (uncommon)
Cause: Obstruction of bile ducts
as a result of liver damage causes
bilirubin to accumulate in the
blood and discolor the skin

Hepatosplenomegaly
Cause: Dissemination of the
disorder from lymph nodes to
other organs

Progressive anemia accompanied
by fatigue, malaise, anorexia
Cause: Erythrocyte life span is
shortened, erythropoiesis is
unable to keep pace with
erythrocyte destruction; bone
marrow infiltration

Superior vena cava syndrome
Cause: Usually from thrombosis

Pulmonary symptoms including
nonproductive cough, stridor,
dyspnea, chest pain, cyanosis,
and pleural effusion
Cause: Mediastinal lymph node
enlargement, involvement of lung
parenchyma, and invasion of pleura

Alcohol-induced pain in
bone, in involved lymph nodes,
or around the mediastinum occurs
immediately after drinking alcohol
and lasts for 30 to 60 minutes
Cause: Unknown

Invasion of pericardium
Cause: Enlarging penetrating
lymph nodes adjacent to the heart

Bone pain, vertebral compression
Cause: Dissemination of disease
from lymph nodes to bone or
invasive growth from adjacent lymph
nodes

Paraplegia
Cause: Compression of spinal cord
resulting from extradural involvement

Nerve pain
Cause: Compression of nerve roots
of brachial, lumbar, or sacral
plexuses

FIG. 10.7 Pathologic basis for the clinical manifestations of Hodgkin's lymphoma.

Reed–Sternberg cells also express receptors for receiving signals from inflammatory cells, creating "cross-talking" between the malignant cells and surrounding inflammatory cells, which may contribute to the ability of the Reed–Sternberg cells to metastasize.

Clinical manifestations. See Fig. 10.7.

Classic HL and LPHL present with different clinical manifestations and progression of disease. Because of these distinctions, these two subgroups are discussed separately.

Classic Hodgkin's lymphoma. Classic HL begins in a group of lymph nodes and spreads contiguously to other lymph node chains. The cervical, axillary, and paraaortic lymph nodes and mediastinum are the most common initial locations for involvement (Fig. 10.8). These lymph nodes are usually nontender and firm.[55]

Nodular sclerosing HL typically presents with supradiaphragmatic lymph node involvement, whereas MCHL often exhibits smaller involved lymph nodes in a subdiaphragmatic location or involves organs. Clients who have disease below the diaphragm, MCHL, or "B" symptoms are more likely to develop splenic involvement. Splenic involvement is seen in 30% to 40% of people with HL, but detection is often difficult. An enlarged spleen does not necessarily indicate involvement, whereas a normal-size spleen does not rule out involvement. HL in the liver is rare and seen only with splenic involvement.[55]

Bone marrow involvement occurs in less than 10% of newly diagnosed cases. If lymph nodes become large and bulky, they can lead to further symptoms, such as tracheal or bronchial compression (with accompanying shortness of breath) or obstruction of the GI tract. Lymph nodes may grow and enlarge and finally perforate the lymph node capsule, continuing to grow and invade into adjacent tissue

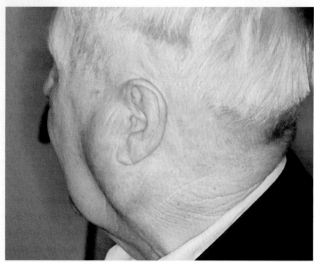

FIG. 10.8 Enlarged cervical lymph nodes associated with Hodgkin's lymphoma. (From Sapp JP, Eversole, LR, Wysocki GP: Contemporary oral and maxillofacial pathology, ed 2, St. Louis, 2004, Mosby.)

or organs. This can occur in the lung, pericardium, pleura, chest wall, gut, or bone.[55]

Effusions (collections of fluid) may also develop in the lung, heart, or abdominal cavity. Tumor can spread not only from lymph node to adjacent lymph node but via the bloodstream to lung, liver, bone marrow, and bone. Involvement in these areas is often indicative of extensive disease. As bone marrow is replaced, infections, anemia, and thrombocytopenia result.[55]

Primary involvement of the CNS is rare, and dissemination of disease to the CNS is uncommon.[21] Occasionally spinal cord involvement may occur in the dorsal and lumbar regions, and compression of nerve roots of the brachial, lumbar, or sacral plexus can cause nerve root pain. Epidural involvement (also uncommon) causes back and neck pain with hyperreflexia. Extremity involvement is characterized by pain, nerve irritation, and obliteration of the pulse.

Twenty-five percent of people present with "B" symptoms. The fever associated with HL is intermittent and occurs with drenching night sweats. Clients may also complain of fatigue, pruritus (itching), and pain associated with drinking alcohol.

Lymphocyte-predominant Hodgkin's lymphoma. LPHL typically presents with one-node involvement rather than groups of involved lymph nodes. This occurs in peripheral lymph nodes such as the cervical, axillary, or inguinal lymph node chains. Unlike classic HL, LPHL does not follow an orderly pattern of spread, but can be found in lymph nodes distant from the original node of disease. LPHL infrequently involves the bone marrow, spleen, or thymus. "B" symptoms rarely occur. LPHL has an indolent clinical course with long disease-free intervals. Relapse is common but responds well to treatment.[154]

Special problems

Pregnancy and Hodgkin's lymphoma. Because the mean age at diagnosis of HL is 32 years, it is not uncommon for women to develop HL while pregnant. Diagnostic staging can be accomplished safely with magnetic resonance imaging (MRI) because it does not use *ionizing radiation*[140]; it has no adverse

impact on the natural course of HL; and HL has no effect on the course of gestation, delivery, or the incidence of prematurity or spontaneous abortions. The risk of metastatic involvement of the fetus by HL is negligible.[66]

The management of HL during pregnancy must be individualized. Many women have been successfully treated while pregnant without adverse effects on the fetus.[67] In cases of disease onset early in pregnancy, the recommendation may be made to consider a therapeutic abortion. Women presenting in later pregnancy are often able to have therapy delayed until after delivery or can undergo modified or standard combination chemotherapy and radiation therapy.[66]

Antiretroviral treatment and prophylaxis for opportunistic infection may also be administered for HIV-positive women.[108] With the increased use of ABVD therapy (doxorubicin [Adriamycin], bleomycin, vinblastine, and dacarbazine) and reduced reliance on radiation therapy, most women do not have to receive radiation. However, with appropriate shielding, the estimated fetal dose of radiation can be reduced by 50% or more in most cases if required.[79] In nonpregnant women, to further reduce any risk, it is advisable to delay pregnancy for 12 months after completion of radiation therapy.[67]

Long-term semen banking is available for men whose future fertility may be compromised by suppression of spermatogenesis secondary to administration of chemotherapy or radiotherapy treatment. Banking of a single ejaculate before chemotherapy or radiotherapy treatment may preserve potential fertility without compromising the oncology treatment.[91]

Hodgkin's lymphoma in AIDS. Although HL does not occur as frequently in HIV-positive clients as does NHL, people with HIV are still at increased risk of developing HL (about eightfold to tenfold increase). When it occurs, the histology is usually MCHL associated with aggressive, disseminated disease and systemic symptoms. Since the introduction of highly active antiretroviral therapy (HAART), the incidence of HL in clients with HIV has not changed significantly, but there has been an improvement in mortality rate, particularly as a result of the HAART therapy and reduced AIDS-related deaths.[72]

Once the diagnosis is made, staging of the disease is accomplished through a complete physical examination; blood tests (sedimentation rate); and computed tomographic (CT) scan of the chest, abdomen, and pelvis (Fig. 10.9). Often a bone marrow biopsy or aspirate is needed to determine the extent of the disease. Because systemic chemotherapy is used, extensive staging is no longer required, including exploratory laparotomy or splenectomy (which can be more dangerous than helpful).

The stage of the neoplasm depends on the number of nodes involved, the location of the nodes, the presence of "B" symptoms (fever, weight loss, night sweats), the sedimentation rate, and size of nodes. Staging is by the Ann Arbor system or the modified version called the Cotswolds classification, denoting stages I to IV (Box 10.6), which helps determine treatment.

Three prognostic groups have also been proposed: early favorable, early unfavorable, and advanced disease. Advanced disease is further divided according to the presence of seven risk factors: advanced disease plus zero to three risk factors is staged as advanced disease with favorable prognosis, and advanced disease with greater than three risk factors is termed advanced disease with unfavorable prognosis.[83]

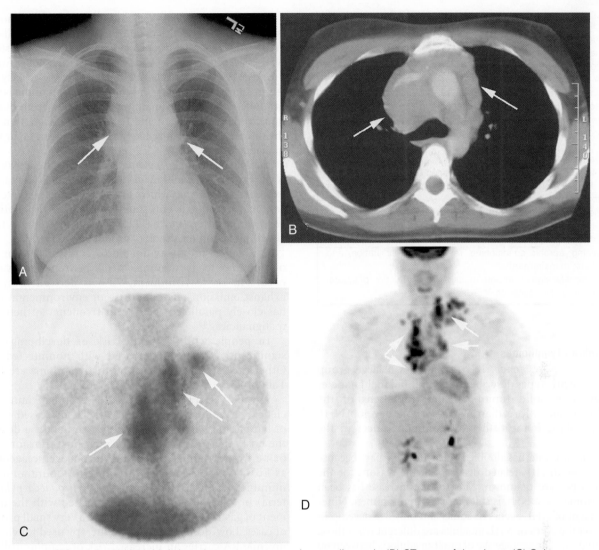

FIG. 10.9 (A) Hodgkin's lymphoma as seen on chest radiograph. (B) CT scan of the chest. (C) Gallium scan of the head, neck, and chest. (D) PET scan. The arrows indicate sites of diseases. Note that PET and CT scans provide more detailed information compared with chest radiograph and gallium scan. (From Goldman L: Goldman-Cecil medicine, ed 25, Philadelphia, 2016, Saunders.)

BOX 10.6 Ann Arbor Staging Classification for Hodgkin's Lymphoma[a]

Stage I:	Involvement of a single lymph node, group of nodes, or a single extralymphatic site I_E (e.g., spleen, thymus, Waldeyer's tonsillar ring) except liver and bone marrow
Stage II:	Involvement of two or more lymph node regions on the same side of the diaphragm or an extralymphatic site and its regional lymph nodes with or without other lymph nodes on the same side of the diaphragm
Stage III:	Involvement of lymph node regions or structures on both sides of the diaphragm; may include spleen or localized extranodal disease
Stage IV:	Widespread extralymphatic involvement (liver, bone marrow, lung, skin)

[a]Stages can be further classified by A to indicate absence or B to indicate presence of systemic symptoms. Systemic symptoms usually occur in Stages III and IV.

10.7 Special Implications for the PTA: Hodgkin's Lymphoma The clinician may palpate enlarged, painless lymph nodes during a cervical, spine, shoulder, or hip examination. Lymph nodes are evaluated on the basis of size, consistency, mobility, and tenderness. Lymph nodes up to 2 cm in diameter that are soft in consistency, freely and easily moveable, tender to palpation, and transient are considered within normal limits but must be followed carefully.

Lymph nodes greater than 2 cm in diameter that are firm in consistency, nontender to palpation, fixed, and hard are considered suspicious and require evaluation. Enlarged lymph nodes associated with infection are more likely to be tender than slow-growing nodes associated with cancer.

Changes in size, shape, tenderness, and consistency should raise a red flag. The physician should be notified of these findings and the client advised to have the lymph nodes evaluated by the physician; immediate medical referral is necessary in someone with a history of cancer.

The clinician's role in lymphoma addresses (1) quality-of-life issues, including emotional and spiritual needs; (2) impairments, functional limitations, and disabilities; and (3) physical conditioning and deconditioning.

A few of the identified signs and symptoms of impairment common with this group of people are generalized weakness, decreased endurance, impaired mobility, altered kinesthetic awareness and balance (including unstable gait); respiratory impairment; involvement of the lymphatic system (lymphedema); and pain.

Requirements for infection control and treatment subsequent to the cytotoxic effects on the CNS are outlined previously in the section on the leukemias. Additionally, side effects of radiation and/or chemotherapy must be considered.

Depending on the results of the client's established plan of care, intervention strategies may include client and family education, pain management, mobility and gait training, therapeutic exercise, balance training, aerobic conditioning, respiratory rehabilitation, and lymphedema management.

Monitoring vital signs is important, as is daily evaluation of laboratory values (e.g., Hb, platelets, WBCs, hematocrit).[17]

Non-Hodgkin's Lymphomas

Overview and incidence. NHL comprises a large group (about 30 specific types described) of lymphoid malignancies that present as solid tumors arising from cells of the lymphatic system. More than 67,000 people develop NHL per year, making it the fifth most common cancer in the United States.

The incidence rate has doubled since 1970, in part because of the increase in HIV-related disease, but the reasons for the remaining cases are unknown. Most of the increase has been noted in women, but NHL is still more common in men. Ninety-five percent of NHL occurs in adults and only 5% develop in children, yet the types of NHL in adults are different from those seen in children. The average age of onset in adults is between 60 and 70 years.

The lymph nodes are usually involved first, and any extranodal lymphoid tissue, particularly the spleen, thymus, and GI tract, may also be involved. The bone marrow is commonly infiltrated by lymphoma cells, but this is rarely the primary site of a lymphoma.

Lymphomas are classified according to the Revised European/American Lymphoma/WHO system, which relies on the histochemical, genetic, and cytologic features. Lymphomas are classified as either B cell or T cell. B-cell lymphomas are more common than T-cell lymphomas.

The clinical course for each of the NHLs, even subtypes, is variable. The most common lymphoma is diffuse large B-cell lymphoma (DLBCL), which is 33% of all NHLs. It is an aggressive, fast-growing tumor. Studies have demonstrated three subtypes with different response rates and prognosis.

Burkitt's lymphoma is a highly aggressive B-cell tumor requiring intensive treatment; only 1% to 2% of lymphomas are classified as Burkitt's. *Follicular lymphoma* is slow growing and clinically indolent (slow growing, painless, continually relapsing). Follicular lymphomas constitute about 14% of lymphomas. Follicular lymphoma, although indolent, may transform to a more rapidly progressive form, DLBCL.

Mantle cell lymphoma makes up only 2% of lymphomas but is typically widespread at diagnosis. Although these cells grow at an intermediate rate, the prognosis is poor. Clinical staging of NHL is according to the Ann Arbor system, ranging from stage I to stage IV. Compared with HL, NHLs are more likely to present in an extranodal site, and the progression of the NHL does not follow the orderly anatomic progression from one lymph node to the next. Stage I and II NHLs are uncommon because the disease is much more likely to be disseminated at the time of diagnosis.

Etiologic and risk factors. Studies in the 1990s linked NHL to two widespread environmental contaminants: exposure to *benzene*, which originates from cigarette smoke, gasoline, automobile emissions, and industrial pollution, and *polychlorinated biphenyls* (PCBs) found throughout the food chain (highest in meats, dairy products, and fish).[82]

One large study was unable to confirm the connection of benzene to lymphoma.[205] Of benzene exposure that occurs in the environment, 70% is derived from vehicle exhaust emissions. The increase of environmental benzene has closely paralleled the rise in frequency of hematologic malignancies.[143]

In people with HIV, the risk of developing NHL is significantly elevated compared with noninfected people. Other predisposing risk factors for lymphoma are listed in Table 10.3.[152]

A wide variety of primary and secondary immunodeficiencies have been associated with an increased incidence of lymphomas. This phenomenon may reflect a decrease in the host's surveillance mechanism against transformed cells or be from prolonged exposure to oncogenic agents, such as EBV, as a consequence of failure to mount an adequate immune response. The presence of *Helicobacter pylori* (bacteria) in the stomach lining is associated with the development of gastric lymphoma, but this is a very small proportion of cases. Low-dose methotrexate therapy used for classic and juvenile RA carries an increased risk of lymphoproliferative disease.[23,46]

Pathogenesis. Although the exact cause of NHL is unknown, studies using techniques of molecular biology have provided some clues to the pathogenesis. The malignant lymphomas develop from the malignant transformation of a single lymphocyte that is arrested at a specific stage of B- or T-lymphoid cell differentiation and begins to multiply, eventually crowding out healthy cells and creating tumors, which enlarge lymph nodes.

Because immunosuppressed people have a greater incidence of the disease, an immune mechanism is suspected. Unlike in HL, T-cell function is minimally affected (30%), but B-cell abnormalities are more common in NHL (70%). In children, virtually all malignant lymphomas are high-grade, aggressive neoplasms.

Clinical manifestations. The NHLs are variable in clinical presentation and course, varying from indolent disease to rapidly progressive disease. Lymphadenopathy is the first symptom of NHL, with painless enlargement of isolated or generalized lymph nodes of the cervical, axillary, supraclavicular, inguinal, and femoral (pelvic) chains. This development may occur slowly and progressively or rapidly depending on lymphoma type.

Extranodal sites of involvement may include the nasopharynx, GI tract, bone (accompanied by bone pain), thyroid, testes, and soft tissue. Abdominal lymphoma may cause abdominal pain and fullness, GI obstruction or bleeding, ascites, back pain, and leg swelling.

Lymph node enlargement in the chest can lead to compression of the trachea or bronchus, causing shortness of breath and coughing. Development of the superior vena cava (SVC) syndrome can occur secondary to compression of the SVC by enlarged nodes; this causes edema of the upper extremities and face. SVC syndrome is life threatening and requires immediate attention.

NHL presenting as polyarthritis has been reported, and Sjögren's syndrome is associated with malignant lymphomas.[63,197] Constitutional symptoms include fever, night sweats, pallor, fatigue, and weight loss; when present, these systemic B symptoms typically predict a poor prognosis.

Primary CNS lymphoma is an NHL restricted to the nervous system. Presenting symptoms may include headache, confusion, seizures, extremity weakness/numbness, personality changes, difficulty speaking, and lethargy. Before the spread of HIV, this type of lymphoma was rare.

HIV and NHL. NHL is more common in clients with HIV than is HL and is an AIDS-defining illness. Typically lymphomas that occur in clients with HIV are aggressive, fast-growing tumors. The two major subtypes of lymphomas are CNS and systemic lymphomas (with or without CNS involvement).

Two rare lymphomas seen more frequently in people with HIV are primary effusion lymphoma and plasmablastic lymphoma of the oral cavity, but the most common types are DLBCL and Burkitt's lymphoma. Tumor is frequently diffusely spread at the time of diagnosis, with extranodal involvement common.

As discussed earlier, many illnesses that are accompanied by a reduced immune system demonstrate an increased incidence of NHL. Before aggressive HIV therapy (i.e., HAART), lymphomas in persons with HIV were associated with a very poor prognosis.

Currently the use of HAART has significantly reduced the risk of developing NHL and also improved tolerance for chemotherapy once diagnosed with NHL. This reduction is based on higher CD4 counts and improving the immune system. It appears that if HAART therapy is not effective, people with AIDS still have the same increased risk of developing NHL.[117] The improved immune status derived from HAART has increased treatment options for HIV-related lymphoma. Clients are now treated with the intent to cure, receiving chemotherapy, immune modulators, and bone marrow transplantation.

10.8 Special Implications for the PTA: Non-Hodgkin's Lymphoma See 10.7 Special Implications for the PTA: Hodgkin's Lymphoma in this chapter.

Although uncommon, the association between the use of methotrexate in RA and the development of lymphoma has been reported.[23,46] Any time an individual receiving methotrexate for RA complains of back pain accompanied by constitutional symptoms and/or GI symptoms and/or the clinician palpates enlarged lymph nodes at any of the nodal sites, a medical referral is warranted.

Multiple Myeloma

Definition and overview. Multiple myeloma (MM) is a primary malignant neoplasm of plasma cells arising in the bone marrow. This tumor initially affects the bones and bone marrow of the vertebrae, ribs, skull, pelvis, and femur. Progression of the disease causes damage to the kidney, leads to recurrent infections, and often affects the nervous system. The extent, clinical course, complications, and sensitivity to treatment vary widely among affected people.

Incidence and etiologic factors. The incidence of MM has doubled in the past 2 decades, with an annual incidence of approximately 16,570 cases in the United States and 11,310 deaths from MM in the United States in 2006.[10,97] Because more people are living longer, much of this increase is due to the occurrence of MM in people older than age 85.

MM occurs less often than the most common cancers (e.g., breast, lung, or colon), but its incidence is double that of HL. This disease can develop at any age but is most commonly seen in older people. The median age of diagnosis is 69 years for men and 71 years for women; only 5% of clients with MM are younger than 40 years.

African American men are affected twice as often as Caucasian men,[164] and MM is slightly more common in men than in women. Risk factors and the cause of MM are unknown, but exposure to ionizing radiation may be linked. Certain occupational hazards found in the petroleum, leather, lumber, and agricultural industries may be linked as well.

Pathogenesis. MM is a malignancy that increases the rate of cell division of plasma cells produced in bone marrow. In the normal development of plasma cells, a hematopoietic stem cell in the bone marrow gives rise to an immature B lymphocyte. This cell then enters the bloodstream and travels to lymphoid tissue. Here it is activated by an antigen-presenting cell and exposed to an antigen, becoming a centroblast.

Centroblasts undergo a maturation process that requires gene rearrangements and switching its Ig isotype from IgM to IgG or IgA. Centroblasts become centrocytes, which then differentiate into plasmablasts or memory B cells. Plasmablasts then migrate back to the bone marrow and terminally differentiate into plasma cells, which no longer divide.

Although it is unknown which cell is the progenitor to the malignant clonal plasma cells, research suggests that it involves the memory B cell or plasmablast—cells that have already been exposed to antigen and undergone gene rearrangements. It is during these times of rearrangement in the gene's coding for the immunoglobulin that breaks naturally occur and mutations can occur, leading to MM.

Although this process takes place in lymph tissue (where MM is not typically involved), these cells leave and acquire adhesion molecules, allowing them to attach to the bone marrow stromal cells (structure cells of the bone marrow). It is also these adhesion molecules that attract malignant plasma cells together, forming plasmacytomas or masses of plasma cells.

Similar to other cancers, these clonal cells require the aid of surrounding cells for survival and proliferation. Stromal cells, once a myeloma cell attaches, release cytokines and inflammatory proteins such as IL-6 and IL-1, and tumor necrosis factor (TNF). These proteins then induce the stromal cells to express a surface protein that binds osteoclast precursor cells, inducing them to mature and differentiate. Osteoclasts then break down bone.

This process can be inhibited by osteoprotegerin (OPG), which is secreted by many cell types, but myeloma cells are able to internalize and break down OPG. This leads to an imbalanced situation in the bones, with increased osteoclast activity and reduced OPG. What is unknown is why osteoblasts (bone-building cells) undergo apoptosis (programmed cell death). These areas of bone destruction can be seen on plain radiographs, CT, or MRI.

These clonal plasma cells also release high concentrations of immunoglobulins known as M-protein. Monoclonal immunoglobulins in the urine are termed Bence Jones protein. These proteins contribute to renal dysfunction and suppress normal immunoglobulin synthesis.

This decreased level of normal antibodies leaves people with MM unable to adequately respond to infections. Bleeding problems are seen in 15% to 30% of clients with MM. Although thrombocytopenia is uncommon in the early stages of the disease (IL-6 may stimulate megakaryocytes), acquired coagulopathies or platelet dysfunction can occur. Anemia is common because of low levels of erythropoietin and increased levels of cytokines that decrease the production of erythrocytes.

Clinical manifestations. The onset of MM is usually gradual and insidious. Common presenting features include fatigue, bone pain, and recurrent infections. Fatigue is a frequent problem due to anemia and elevated levels of cytokines.

Infections are common, particularly gram-negative organisms (60% of infections). MM in older adults (older than 75 years) is the same as that reported in younger people except for a higher rate of infection in the older population.[167] These malignant plasma cells can also form large masses known as plasmacytomas, which can grow in bones and soft tissues.

Musculoskeletal. Most people with MM develop bone pain (more than two-thirds present with it) and other bone-related problems as bone marrow expands and bone is destroyed. The initial symptom is usually bone pain, particularly at the sites containing red marrow (ribs, pelvis, spine, clavicles, skull, and humeri). Bone loss, the major clinical manifestation of MM, often leads to pathologic fractures, spinal cord compression, osteolysis-induced hypercalcemia, and bone pain.

Initially the bone pain may be mild and intermittent or may develop suddenly as a severe pain in the back, rib, leg, or arm, which is often the result of an abrupt movement or effort that has caused a spontaneous (pathologic) bone fracture. The pain is often radicular and sharp to one or both sides and is aggravated by movement. Symptoms associated with bone pain usually subside within days to weeks after initiation of systemic chemotherapy, but if the disease progresses more areas of bone destruction develop.

Bone destruction leads to hypercalcemia, seen in 30% to 40% of people with MM, which can be life threatening. Symptoms of hypercalcemia may include confusion, increased urination, loss of appetite, abdominal pain, constipation, and vomiting.

Muscular weakness and wasting affect nearly half of all individuals with cancer and contribute to the cause of cancer-related fatigue. Muscle wasting occurs as a result of disuse, pathology, anemia, nutritional imbalances, or decreased rates of muscle protein synthesis.[6]

Renal. Renal impairment is a common complication of MM, occurring in 50% of all cases at some stage in the disease process. The pathogenesis is multifactorial, but myeloma of the kidney and hypercalcemia account for two of the major causes.

The large amount of monoclonal light chains secreted by the malignant plasma cells can form large casts in the tubules of the kidneys, causing dilation and atrophy, which leads to the inability of the nephron to function and interstitial nephritis. Hypercalcemia occurs from increased bone destruction and absorption of calcium into the blood. In an effort to rid the body of the excess calcium, the kidneys increase the output of urine, which can lead to serious dehydration and result in further kidney damage if intake of fluids is inadequate.

Calcium can also be deposited in the kidney, creating another source of interstitial nephritis. Hypercalcemia is a common presenting feature but is less common after adequate chemotherapy. Recurrent urinary tract infections are also common and detrimental to the kidneys.

Many medications are nephrotoxic, including some antibiotics, radiographic dyes, and chemotherapy agents. NSAIDs can reduce blood flow to the kidneys, causing further damage. Because of the many factors that can cause injury to the kidneys, nephrotoxic medications should be avoided or used with caution in clients with MM because renal dysfunction and renal failure can occur.

Neurologic. Neurologic complications of MM stem from bone loss or tumor invasion or are protein related. Collapse of the bone with subsequent compression of the nerves can occur as bone is destroyed in the vertebrae. Clients may complain of back pain, numbness, tingling, or loss of strength.

Large plasmacytomas (particularly in the spinal canal or skull) can compress nerves, leading to spinal cord or cranial nerve compressions. Spinal cord compression is usually observed early or in the late relapse phase of the disease. Presenting symptoms include back pain with radiating numbness/tingling, muscle weakness or paralysis of the lower extremities, and loss of bowel or bladder control.

Spinal cord compression is a medical emergency requiring immediate attention. High concentrations of protein are also neuropathic. Amyloidosis (deposits of insoluble fragments of a protein) develops in approximately 10% of people with MM (up to 35% have asymptomatic amyloidosis). These deposits cause tissues to become waxy and immobile and may affect nerves, muscles, and ligaments, especially the carpal tunnel area of the wrist. Carpal tunnel syndrome with pain, numbness, or tingling of the hands and fingers may develop. The association between MM and RA, Sjögren's syndrome, and other autoimmune diseases has been established, but it is not clear why this occurs.

10.9 Special Implications for the PTA: Multiple Myeloma MM can have severe and devastating effects on the musculoskeletal system. Fatigue and skeletal muscle wasting can result in a weak and debilitated individual who is at risk for falls and subsequent musculoskeletal injuries. Bone pathology with fracture can also be very painful and disabling, affecting function and quality of life. The clinician may be instrumental in early detection and referral to minimize detrimental secondary effects.[100]

Multiple Myeloma and Exercise

Clinicians can assist individuals with MM to manage both the disease and treatment-related symptoms, improve overall quality of life, and prevent further complications associated with decreased activity and exercise.

The clinician may play an important role in various stages of the progression of this disease, including prevention and management of skeletal muscle wasting, cancer-related fatigue, and pathologic fractures.[100] Individualized exercise programs for patients receiving aggressive treatment for MM may be effective for decreasing fatigue and mood disturbance and for improving sleep.[41]

Symptoms such as fatigue can be so overwhelming at times that some people have even said that they would rather just die than continue suffering the extremes of fatigue and malaise.[44] The National Comprehensive Cancer Network continues to recommend exercise in their updated clinical practice guidelines for the management of cancer-related fatigue.[135,136]

The guidelines suggest referral to physical therapy for fitness assessment and exercise recommendations with emphasis on getting clients to gradually increase their activity level to avoid sustaining an injury or becoming discouraged. Short, low-intensity exercise programs may be helpful at first. The key is to get the individual to implement and maintain the program.

Individuals with MM have a number of intrinsic and extrinsic factors that can challenge their ability to engage in an exercise program. Intrinsic factors include a belief that exercise will help, a commitment to one's health, creation of personal goals, and a plan to reach them. Extrinsic factors include a good support system and adequate medical care (e.g., prophylactic epoetin alfa used to treat anemia).[42]

The clinician's ability to implement fall assessments and prevention programs can be a life-saving intervention for the individual at risk for pathologic fractures. Exercise interventions to improve function and decrease muscle wasting and cancer-related fatigue during and after cancer treatment for MM have been shown effective. Suggested exercise protocols for MM are available.[189]

Complications

Specific examination and evaluation can provide early recognition of complications such as hypercalcemia and spinal cord compression. Any symptoms of hypercalcemia (see Clinical Manifestations in this section) must be reported to the physician; the client should seek immediate medical care because this condition can be life threatening. (For the client with amyloidosis, anemia, or renal failure, see the Special Implications for the PTA for each of these conditions.) Adequate hydration and mobility help minimize the development of hypercalcemia.

The client with MM who develops signs of cord compression must be referred to the physician. Emergency MRI is required to locate the area of cord compression. A laminectomy may be required when spinal cord compression occurs, but immediate radiation and high-dose glucocorticoid therapy usually relieve the compression, avoiding the need for surgical intervention.

Spinal instability may be a problem. Orthopedic stabilizing orthoses such as thoracic, lumbar, or sacral orthosis (TLSO or back braces) may help with pain management and reduce the risk of further trauma but are often poorly tolerated; newer lightweight supports with hook-and-loop fasteners may be more useful. Vertebroplasty and kyphoplasty procedures may help improve spinal stability; cement injected into the collapsed vertebrae reinforces the bone. In the case of kyphoplasty, vertebral height is restored.[69]

Weight Bearing

There is little clinical evidence to guide the clinician in choosing a safe amount of weight bearing through cancer-lysed metastatic bone during exercise, transfers, ambulation, or other activities of daily living skills.[100] Some general guidelines based on radiographic findings have been suggested for individuals with bone metastases[73]:

>50% (cortical metastatic involvement)	Non–weight bearing with crutches or walking; touch down permitted
25%–50%	Partial weight bearing; avoid twisting or stretching
0%–25%	Full weight bearing; avoid lifting or straining

These recommendations must be used with caution, taking into consideration the client's age, general health, overall level of fitness, and level of pain. Through careful assessment, the clinician guides the client in maintaining mobility as much as possible while preventing fracture. Continual monitoring of symptoms to detect developing or new fracture is imperative. The affected individual must be taught what to look for and when to seek medical attention if signs and symptoms of new fracture appear.

Supportive and Palliative Care

In preterminal and terminal stages, attention to supportive therapy and *palliation* are integral and can make a great impact on the quality of life of the individual and his or her family. The role of the clinician increases in late stages when immobility and renal failure complicate the clinical picture.[161]

Myeloproliferative Disorders

Myeloproliferative disorders are a group of diseases that originate from a hematopoietic stem cell that has undergone a transformation. This transformation allows the cells to mature and function, yet there is uncontrolled production. Myeloproliferative disorders also share other characteristics, including a hypercellular bone marrow, tendency toward thrombosis and hemorrhage, and an increased risk of evolving into acute leukemia over time.[29]

The four main myeloproliferative diseases are CML, polycythemia vera, essential thrombocythemia, and idiopathic myelofibrosis. Although all of these disorders can exhibit elevations in all cell lines, each disease has a main cell line that is affected.

Polycythemia vera is an uncontrolled production of erythrocytes. Essential thrombocythemia is characterized by an elevated platelet count. Excessive fibrosis of the marrow is a dominant feature of idiopathic myelofibrosis. Myelofibrosis and other more rare diseases are not covered in this text. CML is discussed with the leukemias.

Polycythemia Vera

Definition, overview, and etiologic factors. Polycythemia (rubra) vera (PV) is a myeloproliferative disorder of bone marrow stem cells affecting the production of erythrocytes. The diagnosis of polycythemia means an elevated RBC mass that may be primary or secondary.

Secondary polycythemia is typically acquired as a result of decreased oxygen availability to the tissues (e.g., smoking, high altitudes, and chronic heart and lung disorders); the body attempts to compensate for the reduced oxygen by producing more erythrocytes. However, PV is a primary cause of polycythemia and results from a genetic abnormality that allows erythrocytes to mature and function but in an uncontrolled fashion.

The incidence of PV is approximately two to three cases per 100,000.[12] PV develops following a transformation of a hematopoietic stem cell. The etiologic factors of PV are attributed to benzene and other occupational exposures, including radiation. It typically occurs in older people between age 50 and 60 years (people with PV younger than 30 years is rare), with a slightly higher incidence in men than in women.

Pathogenesis. Recently, specific mutations have been discovered that tie many of the myeloproliferative disorders together. One was a change in Janus kinase 2 (JAK2), reported in 2005. This protein normally initiates intracellular signals after a cell membrane receptor binds erythropoietin, thrombopoietin, IL-3, GCSF, or granulocyte-macrophage CSF.[29]

Once JAK2 is activated, a cascade of signals is sent that leads to the production of cells. In up to 95% of clients with PV, there is a mutation in the *JAK2* gene. Valine is replaced for phenylalanine at position 617 (V617F). This region normally exerts a negative effect in that it controls signals and the production of cells. But with this mutation cellular production occurs despite the lack of binding cytokines (cells become cytokine independent), leading to many of the problems seen in myeloproliferative disorders, including PV.

Other genetic abnormalities are also described, and several genetic modifications are most likely required for cellular transformation. There is also an increased risk of PV evolving into AML over time. Although the mechanisms are not understood, clients without the JAK2 mutation can develop AML, demonstrating that other mutations may be the source.

Clinical manifestations. Symptoms are related to hyperviscosity, hypervolemia, and hypermetabolism. The increased concentration of erythrocytes may cause hypertension or neurologic symptoms such as headache, blurred vision, a feeling of fullness in the head, disturbances of sensation in the hands and feet, and vertigo.

Blockage of the capillaries supplying the digits of either the hands or feet may cause a peripheral vascular neuropathy with decreased sensation, burning numbness, or tingling. This same small blood vessel occlusion can also contribute to the development of cyanosis and clubbing of the digits. If untreated, the worst-case scenario may include gangrene, requiring amputation.

The client may demonstrate increased skin coloration (e.g., ruddy complexion of face, hands, feet, ears, and mucous membranes), and splenomegaly is common. Dyspnea may develop secondary to hypervolemia. Abnormal interactions among erythrocytes, leukocytes, platelets, and the endothelium lead to thrombosis (e.g., splenic infarctions and Budd–Chiari syndrome, which is a thrombosis of the hepatic vein) or bleeding (e.g., easy bruising, GI bleeding, and epistaxis).

Gout and uric acid stones may develop because of hypermetabolism. Intolerable pruritus (itching), especially after bathing in warm water, may be prominent. The symptoms of PV are often insidious in onset and characterized by vague complaints such as irritability, general malaise and fatigue, backache, and weight loss. Diagnosis may not be made until a secondary complication, such as stroke or thrombosis, occurs.

Prognosis. The prognosis for PV is good, and median survival is 15 years with appropriate treatment. Without proper treatment, the mortality rate (18 months from the time of symptomatic onset) is 50%. The risk for stroke, myocardial infarction, and thromboembolism is high for people with this condition; thrombosis or hemorrhage is the major cause of death. Late in the course of this disease, bone marrow may be replaced with fibrous tissue (myelofibrosis) or transform into AML.

10.10 Special Implications for the PTA: Polycythemia Vera Thrombosis occurs more often in clients with PV, which requires the clinician to be alert to any possible signs of Budd–Chiari syndrome (abdominal pain, ascites, and liver function abnormalities) and deep vein thrombosis or stroke (e.g., weakness, numbness, inability to speak, visual changes, headache.

GI bleeding, bruising, and epistaxis are also common. Watch for other complications such as dyspnea and splenomegaly. If the person has symptomatic splenomegaly, follow precautions for soft tissue techniques required in the left upper quadrant, especially up and under the rib cage. These procedures must be secondary or indirect techniques away from the spleen.

DISORDERS OF HEMOSTASIS

Hemostasis is the arrest of bleeding after blood vessel injury and involves the interaction among the blood vessel wall, the platelets, and the plasma coagulation proteins. Normal hemostasis is divided into two separate and independent processes: primary and secondary.

Primary hemostasis involves the formation of a platelet plug at the site of vascular injury. When a vessel is disrupted, collagen fibrils and von Willebrand's factor (vWF) in the subendothelial matrix of the blood vessel become exposed to blood. The vWF (which is usually coiled when inactive) in the plasma and the subendothelium becomes uncoiled and binds the collagen fibrils to the platelets via special receptors on the platelets. This ultimately leads to the formation of a platelet plug.

Secondary hemostasis is triggered when vascular damage exposes tissue factor. Tissue factor is found in places not normally exposed to blood flow, where the presence of blood is pathologic. It is present in significant amounts in the brain, subendothelium, smooth muscle, and epithelium. Tissue factor is not found in skeletal muscle or synovium, the usual locations for spontaneous bleeding in people with hemophilia.

Tissue factor then binds the clotting factor VII, which in turn activates factor X and IX. This eventually leads to the formation of thrombin, which cleaves fibrinogen into fibrin, creating a fibrin clot at the site of injury.

Normal primary hemostasis requires normal number and function of platelets and vWF. Persons who have abnormalities in primary hemostasis have defects in either the number or function of platelets or a deficiency or dysfunction of vWF.

A decrease in the number of platelets, called *thrombocytopenia*, can prevent hemostasis. An exceptionally high number of platelets, called thrombocytosis, may cause bleeding, thrombosis, or both (see section on essential thrombocythemia). Persons with a deficiency or dysfunction in vWF have von Willebrand's disease (vWD).

Bleeding caused by platelet disorders or vWD is characterized by mucosal or skin bleeding. Normal secondary hemostasis necessitates the presence of clotting factors. Defects in secondary hemostasis result from clotting factor deficiencies or dysfunction, such as those seen in hemophilia A and B. Persons with abnormalities in secondary hemostasis tend to have more serious bleeding such as deep muscle hematomas and spontaneous hemarthrosis.

von Willebrand's Disease
Definition and Overview
von Willebrand's disease (vWD) is the most common inherited bleeding disorder and is caused by a lack or dysfunction of vWF. The prevalence of this illness may be as high as 1% to 2% of the population (based on population screening studies), yet studies that used only data from clients referred for bleeding disorders found only 30 to 100 cases per 1 million, which is similar to hemophilia A.[166]

vWF is a large molecule made of multiple glycoproteins (dimers). It is produced by megakaryocytes, which secrete vWF into the blood plasma, and also by vascular endothelial cells, which release it into the subendothelial matrix. The function of vWF is to bind collagen fibrils and platelets in areas of vascular injury to create a platelet plug. It also stabilizes factor VIII and prevents it from being inactivated and cleared from the plasma during times of bleeding.

vWD is classified into three main subtypes: types 1, 2, and 3. Type 1 is the most common subtype and accounts for 60% to 80% of clients with vWD. Persons with this subtype have 5% to 30%

of the normal amount of vWF, leading to mild to moderate symptoms. Type 1 is inherited through an autosomal dominant fashion.

Type 2 is less common and seen in only 10% to 30% of vWD cases. It is caused by a dysfunction in vWF rather than a reduction in quantity of vWF. Because the severity of the abnormality can vary, this subtype is further divided into types 2A, 2B, 2M, and 2N. This subtype is also inherited in an autosomal dominant manner.

The rarest of vWD subtypes is type 3, which makes up only 1% to 5% of cases. Persons affected with this form have less than 1% of the normal plasma levels of vWF (levels may be undetectable) and very low levels of the clotting factor VIII. Because these clients are lacking both vWF and factor VIII, their symptoms are more severe and resemble hemophilia A. Inheritance is autosomal recessive.

Pathogenesis

vWF is produced from a gene located on chromosome 12. Many factors are involved in determining inheritance of the disease, yet often only one mutation on one chromosome leads to minor bleeding problems, whereas abnormalities on both genes (homozygous) have more serious problems.

vWD occurs as a result of a qualitative lack of vWF or because of an abnormally functioning vWF (although vWF is produced, a mutation causes a malformation in the function of the proteins). Significant investigation has been placed into the discovery of the genetic abnormalities associated with vWD, and more than 250 mutations of multiple types have been documented.[102]

Clinical Manifestations

Symptoms experienced by clients with vWD vary depending on the subtype and severity of the abnormality. Clients with type 1 experience bleeding consistent with a primary hemostasis defect. This most frequently involves mucosal and skin bleeding such as petechiae and prolonged oozing of blood after trauma or surgery.

Other common problems include epistaxis, gum bleeding, and GI bleeding. Symptoms associated with type 2 depend on the severity of the mutation and the quantity of functional vWF. It is estimated that 10% to 20% of women with menorrhagia (excessive menstruation) have vWD. Menorrhagia is a common presenting symptom yet is frequently overlooked and undiagnosed because gynecologists only rarely (less than 1%) perform tests to confirm or exclude a bleeding disorder.[32,49,57]

Type 3 clients present not only with symptoms of mucosal and skin bleeding but also more frequent and severe symptoms including hemarthrosis and muscular hematomas (similar to hemophilia A).

Hemophilia
Overview

Hemophilia is a bleeding disorder inherited as a sex-linked autosomal recessive trait. The two primary types of hemophilia are *hemophilia A,* or classic hemophilia, and *hemophilia B,* or Christmas disease. Hemophilia A results from a lack of the clotting factor VIII and constitutes 80% of all cases of hemophilia. Hemophilia B is less common, affecting about 15% of all people with hemophilia, and is caused by a deficiency of factor IX. Other less-common deficiencies, such as deficiencies of clotting factors I, II, V, VII, X, or XIII, are rare and are not fully discussed in this text. Unless otherwise noted, hemophilia refers to both hemophilia A and B in this text.

Factors VIII and IX are required in secondary hemostasis (in contrast to vWF, which is needed in primary hemostasis). These clotting factors are activated and result in the production of thrombin, which cleaves fibrinogen to fibrin, creating a stable clot.

The level of severity of the disease depends on the defect in the clotting factor gene and is classified according to the percentage of clotting factor present in plasma (determined through blood tests): mild (6% to 30%), moderate (1% to 5%), and severe (less than 1%). Normal concentrations of coagulation factors are between 50% and 150%.

For people with *mild* hemophilia (25% of all cases), spontaneous hemorrhages (bleeding that occurs with no apparent cause) are rare, and joint and deep muscle bleeding are uncommon. Surgical, dental, or other injury or trauma precipitates symptoms that must be treated the same as for severe hemophilia.

For those people with *moderate* hemophilia (15% of all people with hemophilia), spontaneous hemorrhage is not usually a problem, but major bleeding episodes can occur after minor trauma. People with *severe* hemophilia comprise 60% of people with hemophilia and may bleed spontaneously or with only slight trauma, particularly into the joints and deep muscle.

Incidence

Hemophilia A and B are the most common inherited clotting factor deficiencies,[22] with 17,000 people affected by hemophilia A or B (approximately 10,500 with hemophilia A and 3200 with hemophilia B).[32] Hemophilia primarily affects males without bias for race or socioeconomic group.

Etiologic Factors

The gene responsible for codes for factors VIII and IX are located on the X chromosome, making hemophilia a gender-linked recessive disorder. Because females normally carry two X chromosomes, they only develop hemophilia if both genes are affected, if the normal X gene is inactivated, or if they only have one X chromosome (i.e., Turner's syndrome), making hemophilia rare in females.

Males, on the other hand, only inherit one X chromosome and therefore develop hemophilia because they lack another normal X chromosome to provide these clotting factors (such as most females do). Thus females are the carriers of the abnormality, whereas males present with the disease (Fig. 10.10).

Every carrier has a one in four chance of having a child with hemophilia. Men with the mutation will pass this on to their daughters (making them carriers), yet their sons will only inherit a normal Y chromosome and not develop hemophilia. Although in two thirds of the cases of hemophilia a known family history is evident, this disorder can occur in families (approximately one third) without a previous history of blood-clotting disorders because of spontaneous genetic mutation. The remaining rare clotting factor deficiencies are inherited in an autosomal recessive manner.

Pathogenesis

At least 10 proteins called *clotting factors* in the blood must work in a precise order to make a blood clot. Hemophilia A is due to a deficiency of the protein clotting factor VIII (antihemophilic factor), whereas hemophilia B is a lack of factor IX. These clotting factors are produced by the liver and released into the blood. Factor VIII, once in the plasma, combines with vWF (as previously discussed). Factors VIII and IX are necessary for the formation of thrombin, which converts fibrinogen into fibrin, generating a clot. Clients with these factor deficiencies are unable to produce thrombin and clot.

The genetic pattern of hemophilia is quite different from that of disorders such as sickle cell disease, in which every affected

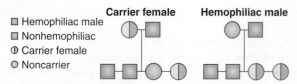

FIG. 10.10 Inheritance patterns in hemophilia for all family members. A woman is definitely a carrier if she is (1) the biologic daughter of a man with hemophilia, (2) the biologic mother of more than one son with hemophilia, or (3) the biologic mother of one hemophilic son with at least one other blood relative with hemophilia. A woman may or may not be a carrier if she is (1) the biologic mother of one son with hemophilia; (2) the sister of a male with hemophilia; (3) an aunt, cousin, or niece of an affected male related through maternal ties; or (4) the biologic grandmother of one grandson with hemophilia. (From Beare PG, Myers JL: Adult health nursing, ed 3, St. Louis, 1998, Mosby.)

individual has the identical genetic defect. The presence of such variable defects in the same gene accounts for the differences in severity of hemophilia.

Many different genetic lesions cause factor VIII deficiency, such as gene deletions, with all or part of the gene missing, or missense and nonsense mutations, which cause the clotting factor to be made incorrectly or not at all. Not all mutations are inherited; 25% to 30% of cases are due to new mutations. Hundreds of different mutations have been discovered. Most of these mutations are nucleotide substitutions (missense) or small deletions, whereas one common mutation noted in more than 40% of people with severe hemophilia A is a partial inversion. An Internet database is available that documents the mutations in the factor VIII gene.[129]

Although uncommon, a woman who is a carrier of hemophilia can have very low levels of factors VIII or IX. This is due to the fact that in every cell of the body either the normal X chromosome or the affected X chromosome is randomly inactivated (turned off) in a process called *lyonization*. If the majority of the inactivated chromosomes are the normal X, then the levels of clotting factors may be very low, and such carriers may experience excessive bleeding.

Clinical Manifestations

Clinically, hemophilia A and hemophilia B present with the same symptoms and can only be distinguished by specific factor assay tests. Unlike most clients with vWD, those with hemophilia manifest delayed joint and deep muscle bleeding.

Occurrences of bleeding are noted during the newborn period in infants who have hemophilia. The most common instances include immunizations, heel sticks, blood draws, and circumcision. If a child is born to a known carrier, circumcision should not be performed until appropriate tests are completed. As the child grows, bleeding problems will continue to be manifested.

Hematoma formation may result from injections or after firm holding (such as occurs when a child is held under the arms or by the elbow and lifted), excessive bruising from minor trauma, delayed hemorrhage (hours to days after injury) after a minor injury, persistent bleeding after tooth loss, and recurrent bleeding into muscles and joints.

Bruising, bleeding from the mouth or frenulum, intracranial bleeding, hematomas of the head, and hemarthrosis (bleeding into the joints) can occur during early ambulation. By age 3 to 4 years, 90% of children with severe hemophilia have had an episode of persistent bleeding not seen in mild cases.

Clients with severe hemophilia often display episodes of spontaneous bleeding (into the joints, muscles, and internal organs) along with severe bleeding with trauma or surgery. Those persons affected with mild to moderate hemophilia do not commonly have spontaneous bleeding but exhibit excessive bleeding with trauma and surgery.

Women with hemophilia. Women with hemophilia experience excessive uterine bleeding during their menstrual cycle, with possible oozing from the ovary after ovulation midcycle. Heavy menstrual flow is often the symptom that initiates a coagulation evaluation or more often is reported but not adequately diagnosed.

Cases have occurred in which a female carrier of the hemophilia gene has abnormal bleeding when the level of clotting factor is low enough to cause significant problems with coagulation, especially after trauma or surgery. Abnormal bleeding from bruising, dental extractions, abortion or miscarriage, complications of pregnancy (e.g., placenta not delivered completely, episiotomy or tearing, prolonged postpartum hemorrhage), nosebleeds, and minor trauma (such as cuts with prolonged oozing) may be overlooked because of the misconception that hemophilia does not occur in women.

Joint. Bleeding into the joint spaces (hemarthrosis) is one of the most common clinical manifestations of hemophilia, significantly affecting synovial joints. The knee is the most frequently affected joint followed by the ankle, elbow, hip, shoulder, and wrist. Bleeding in the synovial joints of the feet, hands, temporomandibular joint, and spine is less common.

Joints with at least four bleeds in 6 months are called target joints, and in children with severe hemophilia, this can occur during toddlerhood. According to the Centers for Disease Control and Prevention, target joints may occur in as many as 37% of people with hemophilia. When blood is introduced into the joint, the joint becomes distended, causing swelling, pain, warmth, and stiffness.

The synovial membrane responds by producing an increased number of synovial villi and undergoing vascular hyperplasia in an attempt to reabsorb the blood. Blood is an irritant to the synovium, which releases enzymes that break down RBCs and the cell byproducts (e.g., iron). This process causes the synovium to become hypertrophied, with formation of finger-like projections of tissue extending onto the articular surface.

The mechanical trauma of normal weight-bearing motion may then impinge and further injure the inflamed synovium. Iron in the form of hemosiderin is deposited in the synovium, which impairs the production of synovial fluid. A vicious cycle is established as the synovium attempts to cleanse the joint of blood and debris, becoming more hypertrophic and susceptible to still further bleeding.[11] Erosive damage of the cartilage follows these changes in the synovium with narrowing of the joint space (Fig. 10.11), erosions at the joint margins, and subchondral cyst formation. Collapse of the joint, joint sclerosis, and eventual spontaneous ankylosis may occur.

In later stages of joint degeneration, chronic pain, severe loss of motion, muscle atrophy, crepitus, and joint deformities occur. Despite advances in medical management, target joints can progress to advanced arthropathy. This is most commonly seen in people with severe hemophilia. The articular cartilage softens, turns brown (due to hemosiderin), and becomes pitted and fragmented. The inflamed synovium is thick and highly vascularized and can grow over the joint surfaces, becoming pannus.

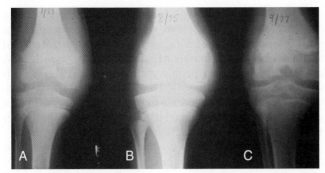

FIG. 10.11 Stages of hemophilic arthropathy according to the Arnold–Hilgartner scale. (A) Stage I (1973). (B) Stage III (1975). (C) Stage IV (1977). (Courtesy Mountain States Regional Hemophilia Center, Colorado State Treatment Program, Denver.)

Eventually, lesions in the deeper layers of cartilage result in subchondral bone breakdown and the formation of subchondral cysts. Osteophyte formation occurs along the edges of the joint (Box 10.7 and Table 10.4). With the destruction of the cartilage, little to no joint space is left. This bone-on-bone contact can lead to significant pain, limitation of motion, joint malalignment, muscle atrophy, functional impairment, and disability.

At this point joint bleeds are rare. For the child, recurrent bleeds into the same joint can lead to growth abnormalities. The epiphyses, where bone growth takes place, are stimulated to grow in the presence of hyperemia caused by bleeding. Postural asymmetries may develop (e.g., leg length differences, angulatory deformities, bony enlargement at the affected joint).[11]

Classification of hemophilic arthropathy. Several different classification scales are used to identify progression of hemophilic arthropathy. The Arnold–Hilgartner and Pettersson score classification scales have been in use for many years. With the Arnold–Hilgartner scale, the arthropathy is divided into stages that are assumed to be progressive. With the Pettersson score, a number of specific findings are evaluated and the additive sum of the assigned points is calculated (see Table 10.4).

In addition, some MRI information is now being used for classification. With improvements in hemophilia care, evaluation of subtle joint changes not readily apparent with conventional radiography has become increasingly important. MRI can visualize effusion, hemarthrosis, synovial hypertrophy and/or hemosiderin deposition, subchondral cysts and/or surface erosions, and loss of cartilage (Fig. 10.12).

Different MRI methods for joint scoring use either a progressive or additive scoring strategy. Using proposed MRI scoring methods, imaging specialists can detect and monitor early joint changes, assess therapeutic outcomes, and further define the pathophysiology of hemophilic joint disease. An in-depth discussion of these techniques is available for readers interested in the specifics.[121]

Muscle. Muscle hemorrhages can be more insidious and massive than joint bleeding, and although they can occur anywhere, muscle hemorrhages most often involve the flexor muscle groups (e.g., iliopsoas, gastrocnemius, forearm flexors). Intramuscular hemorrhage that is visible in superficial areas such as the calf or forearm will also result in pain and limitation of motion of the affected part. Less obvious intramuscular hemorrhage

---

BOX 10.7   Arnold–Hilgartner Hemophilic Arthropathy Stages

Staging scheme to classify joint changes seen on radiographs:

0:	Normal joint
I:	No skeletal abnormalities; soft tissue swelling
II:	Osteoporosis and overgrowth of epiphysis; no erosions; no narrowing of cartilage space
III:	Early subchondral bone cysts, squaring of the patella; intercondylar notch of distal femur and humerus widened; cartilage space remains preserved
IV:	Finding of stage III more advanced; cartilage space narrowed significantly; cartilage destruction
V:	End stage; fibrous joint contracture, loss of joint cartilage space, marked enlargement of the epiphyses, and substantial disorganization of the joints

Data from Arnold WD, Hilgartner MW: Hemophilic arthropathy, J Bone Joint Surg Am 59:287–305, 1977.

TABLE 10.4   Pettersson Classification of Hemophilic Arthropathy

Type of Change	Finding	Score[a]
Osteoporosis	Absent	0
	Present	1
Enlarged epiphysis	Absent	0
	Present	1
Irregular subchondral surface	Absent	0
	Slight	1
	Pronounced	2
Narrowing of joint space	Absent	0
	<50%	1
	>50%	2
Subchondral cyst formation	Absent	0
	1 Cyst	1
	>1 Cyst	2
Erosions at joint margins	Absent	0
	Present	1
Incongruence between joint surfaces	Absent	0
	Slight	1
	Pronounced	2
Joint deformity (angulation and/or displacement between articulating bones)	Absent	0
	Slight	1
	Pronounced	2

[a]Possible total joint score is 0–13 points.
This classification is a joint scoring system based on radiographic findings used to classify and monitor joint changes and damage.
Modified from Anderson A, Holtzman TS, Masley J: Physical therapy in bleeding disorders, New York, 2000, National Hemophilia Foundation.

---

such as occurs in the iliopsoas may result in groin pain, pain on extension of the hip, and reflexive flexion of the hip and thigh.

Other signs and symptoms may include warmth, swelling, palpable hematoma, and neurologic signs such as numbness and tingling. A large iliopsoas hemorrhage can cause displacement of the kidney and ureter and can compress the neurovascular bundle, including the femoral nerve with subsequent weakness; decreased sensation over the thigh and knee in the L2, L3, and L4 distribution; decreased or absent knee reflexes; temperature changes; and even permanent impairment. Iliopsoas bleeds are considered a medical emergency requiring immediate referral to a physician.

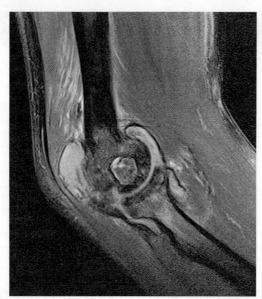

FIG. 10.12 MRI demonstrates subchondral cysts, synovial hyperplasia and synovitis, and chondral changes in this elbow of a 21-year-old man with hemophilia A. (From Adams JE, Reding MT: Hemophilic arthropathy of the elbow. Hand Clinics 27(2):151-163, 2011.)

Nervous system. In general, compression of peripheral nerves and blood vessels by hematoma may result in severe pain, anesthesia of the innervated part, loss of perfusion, permanent nerve damage, and even paralysis. The femoral, ulnar, and median nerves are most commonly affected.

CNS hemorrhage may include intracranial hemorrhage and, rarely, intraspinal hemorrhage. Intracranial hemorrhages (ICHs), or head bleeds inside the skull, in a newborn can occur regardless of the severity of hemophilia and may have long-term consequences such as paralysis, seizures, cerebral palsy, and other neurologic deficits.

Although signs and symptoms of ICH may be dramatic (e.g., seizures, paralysis, apnea, unequal pupils, excessive vomiting, or tense and bulging fontanelles), they are often vague (e.g., crankiness or irritability, lethargy, feeding difficulty), leading to a delay in diagnosis. The lifetime risk of ICH is about 2% to 8% although many are asymptomatic and unreported.[109] ICH in clients with hemophilia carries a mortality rate of up to 30% when it occurs, making it one of the most common causes of death after HIV.

Inhibitors. With the production of safer factor concentrates, the development of antibody inhibitors (antibodies that destroy the infused factor) poses the most serious complication to hemophilia treatment. Inhibitors occur infrequently, approximately two cases per 1000 person-years, but can be serious, causing complications in 20% to 33% of persons who develop an inhibitor.[65,103]

The risk of developing an inhibitor does not remain the same during the lifetime of a person with hemophilia, and the appearance of antibodies can be transient or low titers. Factors that increase the risk for developing inhibitors are still under investigation, including significant exposure to factor VIII concentrates (continuous infusion)[177] or the type of factor VIII product used. Clients with high titers of inhibitors, which decrease therapy efficacy, may receive factor IX concentrates or undergo immune tolerance therapy (frequent infusions of factor VIII).

Transmissible diseases. Individuals (primarily those with severe hemophilia) who were treated before current purification techniques for factor concentrates (before 1986) may have been exposed to hepatitis B or C and/or HIV. Approximately 50% of people with hemophilia during this period became infected with HIV. No other at-risk group had such a high prevalence. Currently, about 10% to 15% of people with hemophilia have HIV, but since 1986 no further HIV transmission has occurred.

Transmission of hepatitis is equally serious, and about 70% to 90% of people with hemophilia who received clotting factor before the mid-1980s test positive for hepatitis C.[134] Current improved methods of viral inactivation of factor concentrates through pasteurization and solvent treatment and monoclonal and recombinant technology have resulted in safer products.

Improved screening methods to identify donors with hepatitis have also reduced the risk of hepatitis transmission. As of 1997, there have been no reports of hepatitis A, B, or C transmission through clotting factor treated with these improved processes.[89] Up to one-third of individuals with a bleeding disorder and hepatitis C were coinfected with HIV, and everyone who was infected with HIV also contracted hepatitis C.[138]

The transmission of hepatitis A and parvovirus B19 has also been reduced in plasma-derived products, but hepatitis A can now be prevented by immunization with a vaccine. All newborns with hemophilia now receive the hepatitis B vaccination series, but older clients often have hepatitis B along with its long-term sequelae.

Effective treatment of hemophilia is based on an accurate diagnosis of the deficient clotting factor and its level in the blood. Diagnosis is not always straightforward, as a variety of factors can confound the test results (e.g., blood type; factor levels can be elevated by stress, hyperthyroidism, and pregnancy, yet decreased in hypothyroidism).

Currently no known cure or prenatal treatment for hemophilia exists. Until a medical cure is developed, primary goals for intervention in the case of bleeding episodes are to stop any bleeding that is occurring as quickly as possible and to infuse the missing factors until the bleeding stops.

Treatment for severe forms of hemophilia is recommended to take place in specialized hemophilia treatment centers across the United States and its territories. In these centers the specialized care required can be provided through a multidisciplinary team approach with appropriately trained and experienced health care providers. Treatment at a hemophilia treatment center has been shown to minimize disability, morbidity, and mortality rates.[32,182]

Physical therapy intervention (see 10.11 Special Implications for the PTA: Hemophilia in this chapter) has been effective in reducing the number of bleeding episodes through protective strengthening of the musculature surrounding affected joints, muscle reeducation, gait training, and client education. Physical therapy is used during episodes of acute hemorrhage to control pain and additional bleeding and to maintain positioning and prevent further deformity.

Gene therapy is still in experimental stages but appears very promising. When successful, gene therapy will deliver a normal (unaffected) copy of a gene into a target cell that contains a defective gene. Human trials are underway for hemophilia A and B using a variety of different delivery techniques. In fact, hemophilia is considered a model disease for treatment with gene therapy because it is caused by a single malfunctioning gene, and only a small increase in clotting factor could provide a great benefit.[124]

Prognosis

Years ago, most men with hemophilia died in their youth. Currently, the majority of deaths in persons with hemophilia are viral related (hepatitis B and C, HIV), yet with improved diagnosis and significantly improved treatment (including safety), they have a greater life expectancy.[158]

Tremendous improvement has been made in carrier detection and prenatal diagnosis to provide early treatment and prevent complications. Gene therapy for hemophilia A and B, now in clinical trials, holds promise of a cure. Additionally, home infusion therapy provides immediate treatment with clotting factor for joint and muscle bleeds recognized early. Early treatment has significantly reduced the morbidity formerly associated with hemophilia.

10.11 Special Implications for the PTA: Hemophilia Physical therapy intervention for individuals with hemophilia has undergone a drastic change. Two decades ago, everyone in the hemophilia community had joint disease in varying degrees of severity. Today treatment protocols are more aggressive, with more frequent infusions given at younger ages, resulting in less joint damage.[40]

Many children with hemophilia are growing up without having a single joint bleed. The focus has shifted from rehabilitation to prevention; PTs and PTAs are important health care professionals in helping these individuals lead normal, active lives.[40] Only a brief discussion of treatment for the adult or child with hemophilia can be included in this text. For more detailed information regarding intervention and treatment, the reader is referred to other more specific references.[11,26,84,137]

Hemophilia and Exercise

A regular exercise program—including appropriate sports activities, resistance training, cardiovascular/aerobic training, and therapeutic strengthening and stretching exercises for affected extremities—is an important part of the comprehensive care of the individual with hemophilia. The clinician can help individuals with hemophilia identify, seek out, and enjoy physical activity, exercise, and sport participation that provide benefits that outweigh the risks.[84]

Exercise not only promotes physical wellness in the form of improved work capacity, it protects joints, enhances joint function, and is beneficial for decreasing the frequency of bleeds and has been shown to temporarily increase the levels of circulating clotting factor in individuals with a factor VIII deficiency.[139] Immobilization of joints can lead to deterioration of muscles, which in turn leads to joint instability and repeated bleeding and premature development of arthropathy.[133,188]

Growing evidence suggests that exercise, coupled with a healthy diet, may boost the immune system of people with hemophilia who also have HIV and/or are living with hepatitis C.[202] The clinician can be instrumental in helping the person with hemophilia individualize an exercise or sports activity plan with specific but realistic goals and a schedule with alternating exercises (cross-training).

Although many factors related to joint bleeding are fixed, one risk factor that can be modified by the clinician is the body mass index. Clients with more severe disease develop joint problems earlier with accompanying ROM problems. An increased body mass index also increases the risk of limited joint ROM and may be a modifiable risk factor in clients with hemophilia.[183]

An overall therapy program includes client education early on for family, client, school personnel, and coaches for prevention, conditioning, and wellness. Specific guidelines are available including all age levels from infants, toddlers, and preschoolers to adults, including sports safety information and the categorization of sports and activities by risk.[11,137]

For older children and adolescents, selecting a sport with a good chance of success and adequate preparation (e.g., stretching and flexibility, conditioning including strength and weight training, endurance including an aerobic component, and possibly infusion before participation) for the sport is crucial.

Although it is obvious that some bleeding may result from participation in a sport, fewer bleeding episodes occur when children engage in physical activities on a regular basis than when they are sedentary. When a particular sport or activity is often followed by bleeding, then that activity should be reevaluated. A joint that requires multiple infusions to stop bleeding, remains symptomatic, or has persistent synovitis is not likely to withstand the stresses of a sport that relies on that joint.[137]

As orthopedic problems occur, a problem-oriented program is developed specific to the pathology. Generally, a therapy program includes exercises to strengthen muscles and improve coordination; methods to prevent and reduce deformity; methods to influence abnormal muscle tone and pathologic patterns of movement; techniques to decrease pain; functional training related to everyday activities; special techniques such as manual traction and mobilization; massage; and physiotechnical modalities such as cold, heat (including ultrasound), and electric modalities.

Aquatic therapy is an excellent modality, especially for chronic arthropathy. The buoyancy of the water allows for ease of active movements across joints without the compressive force induced by gravity, thus decreasing pain. Water's density creates a resistive force to allow muscle strengthening, and the hydrostatic pressure can help reduce swelling.[11]

Guidelines to Strength Training

In the past, people with bleeding disorders were told to avoid strenuous exercise and any kind of weight training to avoid the risk of bleeding episodes. Today we know that a well-planned exercise program can be extremely beneficial to all individuals with a bleeding disorder. Weight training is still approached with caution as overly strenuous free-weight lifting can still cause microtears in the muscles and intramuscular bleeds.[7,128]

Strength training, also known as resistance training, builds muscle, increases strength, stabilizes joints, improves circulation, and potentially reduces the risk of injury and spontaneous bleeding episodes. It is not body building, power lifting, or competitive weightlifting; these activities should be avoided.

The importance of warm-up and cool-down periods should be emphasized. Little or no weight is used until the individual can complete 10 to 15 repetitions with proper form. Weight or resistance can be gradually increased by 5% to 10% when the first phase of 10 to 15 repetitions is easy. The client should be reminded never to attempt to lift maximal weight.[7,8]

As with all strength training, it is best to utilize full pain-free ROM slowly and with good breathing throughout the cycle of contraction and relaxation. Maintain adequate hydration at all times. Adolescents must especially be reminded that pain is a red flag to stop and seek help. Most injuries result from improper form and performing the exercise too fast. Any time an individual of any age with hemophilia experiences joint trauma or injury, strength training may have to be discontinued and gradually reintroduced after healing occurs.[7]

Maintaining Joint Range of Motion

The clinician and client must be alert to recognize any signs of early (first 24 to 48 hours) bleeding episodes (Table 10.5). Providing immediate factor replacement to stop the bleeding and following the RICE principle (Table 10.6) to promote comfort and healing are two goals for treating an acute joint (hemarthrosis) or muscle bleed (intramuscular hemorrhage).

The joint ROM can be measured during this acute episode in the pain-free range but should not be strength tested. Elastic wraps, splints, slings, and/or assistive devices may be necessary and a tolerance and/or weaning schedule established.[11] Static or dynamic night splints may be used to apply a low-load stretch to a muscle shortened because of an underlying condition such as synovitis or articular contracture.

A static splint made of plaster, synthetic casting materials, or thermoplastic splinting materials holds the joint in a single position. The material is molded to the extremity, then hardens, and straps are applied to keep it in place. A static splint does not bend or straighten the joint. It must be remolded or remade as the individual gains ROM.[99]

A dynamic splint applies a small amount of pressure (1 to 2 lb) to stretch a joint over a long period. The individual can still bend and straighten the joint and the clinician can adjust the amount of load applied as needed. There is less irritation and fewer bleeds with the dynamic splint.

Repeated bleeds in the same area can cause a muscle to shorten, limiting joint ROM. Individuals with inhibitors or limited access to treatment are at increased risk for this type of problem. Night splints may be a good option for people who have muscle contractures that are not responding to other treatment interventions. The desired effect can be obtained in 6 to 8 weeks for individuals who do not have an inhibitor. For those clients with inhibitors, night splinting can take much longer (6 months to 1 year).[99] Serial casting may be a better choice for clients with longstanding problems; either splinting or casting should be used before resorting to surgery.[74,168]

The clinician must maintain awareness for possible leg length discrepancy secondary to various arthropathies. Even minor discrepancies can affect standing posture and gait mechanics and contribute to low-back pain and other lower quadrant impairments. Shoe lifts in conjunction with appropriate prophylactic therapy and exercise can be effective.[81,98]

Specific Exercise Guidelines

Initiation of exercise after a bleed must be delayed, and rehabilitation progress is typically slower for individuals with factor VIII and factor IX deficiency who develop factor inhibitors. Prognosis for full return of function is diminished in such cases. In all cases of joint bleed, the use of heat is contraindicated; if used, hydrotherapy or aquatic intervention must be performed in comfortable but not hot temperatures to avoid blood vessel dilation.[210]

Isometric muscle exercise should be initiated when active bleeding stops to prevent muscular atrophy. This exercise is especially critical with recurrent knee hemarthroses to prevent the visible atrophy of the quadriceps femoris muscle. As pain and edema diminish, the client should begin gentle active ROM exercises followed by slowly progressing strengthening exercises when the joint is pain free through its full range. In the case of an iliopsoas bleed, when ambulation is resumed, crutches and toe-touch weight bearing are initiated. Active movement should be performed in a pain-free range and progressed very slowly.[11]

As the strengthening program is progressed, strengthening aids such as elastic bands or tubing and cuff weights can be used for all muscles before transitioning to weight equipment. Preadolescents should avoid using high–weight lifting machines.

Postbleed exercise should also take into consideration any damage that may have occurred to the joint, such as ligamentous or capsular stretching. Closed chain and other exercises to restore proprioception should be incorporated into the rehabilitation program.[11]

As a prophylactic measure, clients with severe hemophilia generally need to infuse with clotting factor when participating in a strengthening program. With careful supervision and progression of the exercise program, the individual can progress to aerobic activities.

In some individuals, increased stress levels result in increased frequency of spontaneous bleeding. Biofeedback may be considered especially helpful for these clients who experience spontaneous bleeding during emotional upsets and periods of depression. Biofeedback can also be used for muscle retraining or relaxation techniques to control muscle spasm and ROM.

The Older Adult with Hemophilia

Life expectancy has increased dramatically with modern treatment for hemophilia. Although today's treatments have reduced the number and severity of joint bleeds, middle-aged and older adults with hemophilia did not have the benefit of powdered concentrates and prompt home care.

As children they were hospitalized and/or bed bound with casts, packed in ice while whole blood was administered slowly by intravenous drip. It took days for their levels to go up. Before factor replacement it could take weeks to get a joint bleed under control. The consequence of this type of treatment was contracted joints and severe arthritis.[28]

Today's older adult still may not have quick and easy access to factor replacement. Mobility impairments can make it difficult, if not impossible, to get to a hemophilia treatment center. Loss of fine motor control or the onset of tremors makes self-care at home equally problematic. Adults with hemophilia are not spared from other health care concerns such as diabetes, heart disease, stroke, or cancer. The management of comorbidities may be complicated even more by the bleeding disorder.

The clinician can begin education about long-term planning with middle-aged clients. Introducing the idea of home modifications to improve accessibility should begin early. The importance of staying active cannot be overemphasized. All older adults find that recovery time and rehabilitation take longer as they advance through the decades. Resuming normal activities after injury, surgery, or health conditions that set them back is extremely important.[28]

It is also important to keep educating young clients who are noncompliant with their treatment and ignore recommendations. These individuals likely will have problems in the future similar to those experienced by today's older adult population, who did not have the benefit of modern treatment interventions.

The same is true for young adults during the college years or transitioning from living at home with adult supervision during high school to living on their own independently. For many people with bleeding disorders, this is the first time they will assume "ownership" of their disease.[128] Maintaining physical fitness at every stage of life is a key part of management for hemophilia.

Orthopedic/Surgical Interventions

Whereas factor replacement can be used to control bleeding associated with surgery, any operative procedure is complicated for individuals who develop inhibitors. Sometimes a joint becomes a chronic problem even with optimal infusion therapy and aggressive hemophilia care. In such cases, orthopedic or surgical intervention may be indicated to alleviate pain and deformity and to restore the joint to a more functional state. This may include prescription for an orthosis or a splint or serial casting to increase ROM. Joint replacement (arthroplasty) is now a treatment option as well.

Synovectomy (removal of the joint synovium) is recommended to stop a target joint from its cycle of bleeding. This procedure is not usually done to improve ROM or to decrease pain but rather to prevent further damage to the joint caused by bleeding. Arthroscopic synovectomy is best performed before joint degeneration has progressed beyond stage II on the Arnold–Hilgartner scale (see Box 10.7).

One option is injection of a radioactive isotope (referred to as *isotopic synovectomy* or *synoviorthesis*, usually[33] P in the United States) that causes scarring to the synovium to arrest bleeding. This procedure has unique advantages and disadvantages and may be more appropriate for one type of client than another.[59,60]

Arthroplasty (joint replacement) is indicated when a joint shows end-stage damage and has become extremely painful. Client age, ROM, and level of pain and function are determinants as to the timing of this procedure. Knees, hips, and shoulders are most commonly helped through arthroplasty, with restoration of pain-free joint movement.

The benefits of a 6-week preoperative physical therapy program (prehabilitation) combined with 6 weeks of postoperative rehabilitation have been demonstrated. An individually tailored and supervised program to increase ROM and muscle strength enables rapid mobilization and recovery of function while minimizing the risk of bleeding.[187]

Long-term results of joint replacement are still under investigation. Mechanical survival of the implant is reported as good or excellent for 80% of knees, but the incidence of late infection (months to years later) resulting in implant failure remains high (16%).[141,180]

Arthrodesis (joint fusion) may be performed in a joint with advanced, painful arthropathy untreatable by arthroplasty. Joint fusion can relieve or eliminate pain to provide improved quality of life, but it also causes permanent loss of joint motion. Arthrodesis can be a very effective way to provide the individual a more stable base for weight-bearing activities.

Osteotomy (removal of a section of bone) may be done to correct angular deformities in a joint and may be considered before arthroplasty to reduce the stresses placed on a joint caused by poor alignment. Other less common interventions may include excision of a hemophilia pseudotumor or removal of cysts or exostoses.

The Person with Hemophilia and HIV

It is important for anyone with both hemophilia and HIV to maintain optimal care of their musculoskeletal systems during and between bleeding episodes. It is especially important in the presence of chronic arthropathy and HIV or AIDS to maintain joint function through nonsurgical means, especially exercise.

Surgery may be contraindicated if the risk of infection is too great (e.g., when the CD4 cell count is less than 200). Activities such as tai chi and yoga provide stretching, strengthening (including weight bearing), and a mild aerobic component. Aquatics or swimming must be approached with caution because of the potential for transmission of *Cryptosporidiosis* oocysts, which cause infection in immunocompromised individuals.[11]

TABLE 10.5 Clinical Signs and Symptoms of Hemophilia Bleeding Episodes

Acute hemarthrosis	Aura, tingling, or prickling sensation
	Stiffening into the position of comfort (usually flexion)
	Decreased range of motion
	Pain/tenderness
	Swelling
	Protective muscle spasm
	Increased warmth around joint
Muscle hemorrhage	Gradually intensifying pain
	Protective spasm of muscle
	Limitation of movement at the surrounding joints
	Muscle assumes a position of comfort (usually shortened)
	Loss of sensation
Gastrointestinal involvement	Abdominal pain and distention
	Melena (blood in stool)
	Hematemesis (vomiting blood)
	Fever
	Low abdominal/groin pain from bleeding into wall of large intestine or iliopsoas muscle
	Hip flexion contracture from spasm of the iliopsoas muscle secondary to retroperitoneal hemorrhage
Central nervous system involvement	Impaired judgment
	Decreased visual and spatial awareness
	Short-term memory deficits
	Inappropriate behavior
	Motor deficits: spasticity, ataxia, abnormal gait, apraxia, decreased balance, loss of coordination

Modified from Goodman CC, Snyder TE: Differential diagnosis for the physical therapist: screening for referral, ed 5, St. Louis, 2013, Saunders.

Thrombocytopenia

Thrombocytopenia, a decrease in the platelet count below $150,000/mm^3$ of blood, is caused by inadequate platelet

TABLE 10.6 Management of Joint and Muscle Bleeds

Joint: Acute Stage	Joint: Subacute Stage	Muscle
Factor replacement	Factor replacement (if indicated)	Factor replacement
RICE	Progressive movement and exercises	RICE
Pain-free movement	Wean splints and slings	Appropriate weight-bearing status; bed rest for iliopsoas bleed
Pain medication	Progressive weight bearing	Progressive movement

RICE, Rest, ice, compression (applying pressure to the area for at least 10 to 15 minutes), and elevation (immobilizing and elevating the body part above the heart while applying ice). Modified from Anderson A, Holtzman TS, Masley J: Physical therapy in bleeding disorders, New York, 2000, National Hemophilia Foundation.

BOX 10.8 Causes of Thrombocytopenia

Increased Platelet Destruction
- Immune thrombocytopenic purpura
- Drug induced, immune related (e.g., heparin, sulfa drugs)
- Thrombotic microangiopathy (also called thrombotic thrombocytopenic purpura)
- Disseminated intravascular coagulation
- Vasculitis
- Bypass during heart surgery
- Mechanical heart valve
- Splenic sequestration
- von Willebrand's disease

Decreased Platelet Production
- Bone marrow infiltration (metastatic neoplasms, leukemia, lymphoma, myeloma)
- Bacterial infections (mycobacteria)
- Viral infections (HIV, cytomegalovirus, hepatitis C)
- Nutritional deficiencies (folate, B_{12})
- Aplastic anemia
- Myelofibrosis
- Drug induced, not immune related (e.g., alcohol, chemotherapy agents, chloramphenicol)

production from the bone marrow, increased platelet destruction outside the bone marrow, or splenic sequestration (entrapment of blood and enlargement in the spleen). Thrombocytopenia is a common complication of leukemia or metastatic cancer (bone marrow infiltration) and aggressive cancer chemotherapy (cytotoxic agents). Thrombocytopenia may also be a presenting symptom of aplastic anemia (bone marrow failure); other causes are listed in Box 10.8.

Mucosal bleeding is the most common event and occurs by simply blowing the nose or brushing the teeth. Other sites of mucosal bleeding may include the uterus, GI tract, urinary tract, respiratory tract, and brain (intracranial hemorrhaging [ICH]). Symptoms include epistaxis (frequent and difficult to stop), petechiae and/or purpura in the skin (especially the legs) and oropharynx, easy bruising, melena, hematuria, excessive menstrual bleeding, and gingival bleeding.

Diagnosis requires laboratory examination of blood and perhaps bone marrow (if clinically indicated) to confirm the diagnosis. Treatment depends on the precipitating cause (e.g., treatment of underlying leukemia or cessation of cytotoxic drugs until platelet count elevates).

Other treatment methods for immune-related thrombocytopenia (e.g., immune thrombocytopenic purpura) may include use of corticosteroids (e.g., prednisone); intravenous immune globulin and $Rh_o(D)$; splenectomy; monoclonal antibody agents (e.g., rituximab); and plasmapheresis, a procedure that removes blood from the body, separates the portion containing the antiplatelet antibodies, and then returns the cleansed blood to the body. Newer drugs, thrombopoietic agents, are being tested to provide medications with fewer adverse events.[25]

Transfusions with platelets are avoided in clients with immune thrombocytopenic purpura unless severe bleeding occurs. However, clients with a secondary cause for thrombocytopenia (e.g., acute leukemia treatment and severe complications of chemotherapy agents that cause thrombocytopenia) may require platelet transfusions for bleeding and/or counts less than 15,000/mm^3.

The prognosis is variable depending on the underlying cause; it is poor when associated with leukemia or aplastic anemia but good with conditions amenable to treatment.

10.12 Special Implications for the PTA: Thrombocytopenia Thrombocytopenia can cause bleeding into the muscles or joints, and the clinician may encounter the severe consequences of this condition. The clinician must be alert for obvious skin or mucous membrane symptoms of thrombocytopenia such as severe bruising, external hematomas, and the presence of petechiae.

Such signs usually indicate a platelet level below 150,000/mm^3. Instruct the client to watch for signs of thrombocytopenia and when noted to immediately apply ice and pressure to any external bleeding site. They should avoid aspirin and aspirin-containing compounds without a physician's approval because of the risk of increased bleeding.

Strenuous exercise or any exercise that involves straining or bearing down could precipitate a hemorrhage, particularly of the eyes or brain. Exercise prescription is highly individualized and should take into account intensity, duration, and frequency appropriate for the individual's condition, age, and previous activity level.

Blood pressure cuffs and similar devices must be used with caution. When used, elastic support stockings must be thigh high, never knee high. Mechanical compression with a pneumatic pump and soft tissue mobilization are contraindicated unless approved by the physician. Practice good handwashing and observe carefully for any signs of infection. (See also Special Implications for the PTA 10.4: The Anemias in this chapter.)

Effects of Aspirin and Other Nonsteroidal Antiinflammatory Drugs on Platelet Function

Acquired disorders of platelet function can occur through the use of aspirin and other NSAIDs that inactivate platelet cyclooxygenase. This key enzyme is required for the production of thromboxane A_2, a potent inducer of platelet aggregation and constrictor of arterial smooth muscle.

A single dose of aspirin can suppress normal platelet aggregation for 48 hours or longer (up to 1 week) until newly formed platelets have been released. Platelets are anucleated, and once aspirin irreversibly inhibits cyclooxygenase, the platelet is unable to synthesize new enzyme and remains inactive for the rest of its life span.

NSAIDs have less potent antiplatelet effects than aspirin because they reversibly inhibit cyclooxygenase. Symptoms from this phenomenon are mild and may consist of easy bruising and bleeding, usually confined to the skin. The use of aspirin or NSAIDs is usually contraindicated before any surgical procedure. Prolonged oozing may occur following dental procedures or surgery.

Hemoglobinopathies

Several diseases are a result of an abnormality in the formation of Hb. Because Hb is essential for life, anomalies in the shape, size, content, or oxygen-carrying capacity can lead to severe problems. Sickle cell disease and thalassemia are two hemoglobinopathies with potential for serious complications and are discussed further.

Hereditary spherocytosis, hereditary elliptocytosis, hereditary stomatocytosis, and pyropoikilocytosis are rare diseases that occur because of defects in the erythrocyte membrane that cause premature clearance of RBCs (hemolysis). Glucose-6-phosphate dehydrogenase deficiency also leads to hemolysis. Discussions of these diseases can be found elsewhere.

Sickle Cell Disease

Overview and incidence. *Sickle cell disease* (SCD) is an autosomal recessive disorder characterized by the presence of an abnormal form of Hb (Hb S) within the erythrocytes. This irregular form of Hb is the result of a single mutation in the β-Hb chain where the amino acid glutamic acid at position 6 is substituted with valine.

The presence of Hb S can cause RBCs to change from their usual biconcave disk shape to a crescent or sickle shape once the oxygen is released (deoxygenated). SCD occurs when two sickle cell genes are inherited (one from each parent) or one sickle cell gene and another abnormal Hb is inherited, so that almost all of the Hb is abnormal.

Homozygous Hb S occurs when an individual inherits two sickle cell genes. *Heterozygous Hb SC* is the result of inheriting one sickle cell gene and one gene for another abnormal type of Hb called C. Persons with this type of abnormality have fewer complications than those with homozygous Hb S, but they exhibit more ophthalmologic and orthopedic complications.

Heterozygous *Hb S β-thalassemia* is the result of inheriting one sickle cell gene and one gene for a type of thalassemia, another inherited anemia. β-Thalassemias are caused by genetic mutations that abolish or reduce production of the beta globin subunit of Hb.[151]

The sickle cell trait refers to people who carry only one *Hg S* gene and is discussed at the end of this section. Hb F, or fetal Hb, is found in infants. Although most infants switch to making α- and β-Hb, some continue to make Hb F, termed hereditary persistence of fetal Hb. People who inherit one sickle gene and the hereditary persistence of fetal Hb abnormalities make $\alpha_2\gamma_2$ Hb and do not develop the severe symptoms of SCD.

Approximately three out of every 1000 black newborns and between 50,000 and 70,000 individuals in the United States have a sickle cell syndrome; the number in Africa is correspondingly higher.[132] It is a worldwide health problem, affecting many races, countries, and ethnic groups, and is the most common inherited hematologic disorder. The WHO estimates that each year more than 300,000 babies are born worldwide with this inherited blood disorder.[206]

About one in 400 African American newborns in the United States has sickle cell anemia, and one in 12 African Americans (8%) carries the sickle cell trait.[204] The disease is particularly common among people whose ancestors come from sub-Saharan Africa, India, Saudi Arabia, and Mediterranean countries.[206]

Etiologic factors. The cause of SCD and its worldwide incidence is the result of several factors. The sickle cell trait may have developed as a single genetic mutation that provided a selective advantage against severe forms of falciparum malaria.

Anyone who carries the inherited trait for SCD but does not have the actual illness is protected against this form of malaria. In countries with malaria, children born with sickle cell trait survived and then passed the gene for SCD to their offspring. As populations migrated (including the slave trade), the sickle cell trait and sickle cell anemia moved throughout the world.

Several theories purport to explain the origination of SCD, but its actual origin is unknown. Four separate haplotypes are known; each is related to the severity of illness and each is associated with a different geographic location, including different locations in Africa, eastern Saudi Arabia, and India.

Risk factors. Because SCD is inherited as an autosomal recessive trait, both parents of an offspring must have the sickle Hb gene. When both parents have sickle cell trait, they have a 25% chance with each pregnancy of having a child with sickle cell anemia. If one parent has sickle cell trait and the other has a β-thalassemic disorder, they are at the same risk for having a child with a sickle β-thalassemia syndrome.

In couples in which one individual has sickle cell trait and one has Hb C trait, the chance of having a child with Hb SC disease is also 25% with each pregnancy. If one parent has sickle cell anemia and the other has the sickle cell trait, the risk of having a child with sickle cell anemia is 50% (Fig. 10.13).

Individuals with sickle cell trait can receive nondirective genetic counseling (given objective information without personal bias and without provision of specific recommendations) after Hb electrophoresis and other measurements have been performed on each prospective parent.

Risk factors likely to induce symptoms or episodes (*episode* is now the preferred term over *crisis;* however, clinicians may find that some affected individuals prefer the term *crisis*) are factors that cause physiologic stress, resulting in sickling of the erythrocytes. Stress from viral or bacterial infection, hypoxia, dehydration, extreme temperatures (hot or cold), alcohol consumption, or fatigue may precipitate an episode.

Additionally, episodes may be precipitated by the presence of acidosis; exposure to low oxygen tensions as a result of strenuous physical exertion, climbing to high altitudes, flying in nonpressurized planes, or undergoing anesthesia without receiving adequate oxygenation; pregnancy; trauma; and fever. Any of these factors may increase the body's need for oxygen, increasing the percentage of erythrocytes that deoxygenate, thereby precipitating an episode.

Pathogenesis. The sickle cell defect occurs in Hb, the oxygen-carrying constituent of erythrocytes. Hb contains four chains of amino acids, the compounds that make up proteins. Two of the amino acid chains are known as α-*globin chains,* and two are called β-*globin chains.*

In normal Hb, the amino acid in the sixth position on the β-globin chains is glutamic acid. In people with SCD, the sixth position is occupied by another amino acid, valine (Fig. 10.14). DNA recombinant technology has identified the genetic locus for the β-globin on chromosome 11.

This single-point mutation of valine for glutamic acid results in a loss of two negative charges that causes surface abnormalities. The sickle Hb transports oxygen normally, but after releasing oxygen, Hb molecules that contain the β-globin chain defect stick to one another instead of remaining separate and polymerize (change molecular arrangement), forming long, rigid rods or tubules inside RBCs.

The higher the concentration of deoxygenated sickle Hb molecules and the lower the blood pH, the faster the polymerization occurs.[156] The rods cause the normally smooth, doughnut-shaped RBCs to take on a sickle or curved shape and to lose their vital ability to deform and squeeze through tiny blood vessels (Fig. 10.15).

This sickling is reversible for a time because the cells are reoxygenated in the lungs, but eventually the change becomes irreversible. The erythrocyte membrane becomes damaged in the process of sickling and unsickling and the cells are removed (hemolyzed).

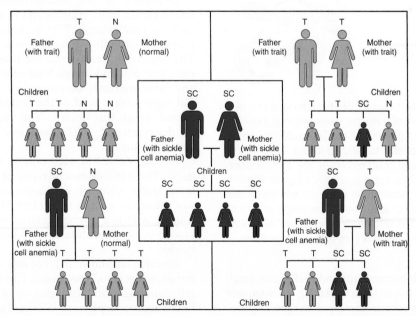

FIG. 10.13 Statistical probabilities of inheriting sickle cell anemia. (From O'Toole MT: Miller-Keane encyclopedia and dictionary of medicine, nursing, and allied health, rev ed 7, Philadelphia, 2005, Saunders.)

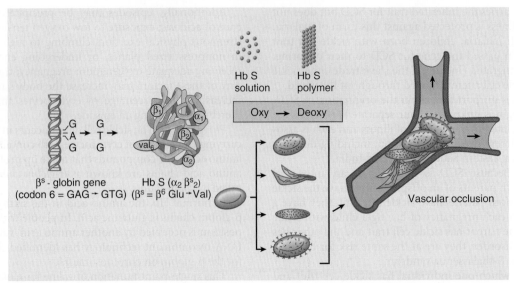

FIG. 10.14 Schematic view of the pathophysiologic characteristics of SCD. The double-stranded DNA molecule on the left represents a β-globin gene in which a GAG→GTG substitution in the sixth codon has created the sickle cell gene. Valine is substituted for glutamic acid as the sixth amino acid, creating a mutant Hb tetramer (Hb S). A tetramer is a protein with four subunits (tetrameric). Hb S loses solubility and polymerizes when deprived of oxygen. Upon deoxygenation, most sickle cells lose deformability. Some cells sickle; a fraction becomes dehydrated, irreversibly sickled, and poorly deformable; a few become highly adherent. Vasoocclusion (*right*) is initiated by adherent cells sticking to the vascular endothelium, thereby creating a nidus that traps rigid cells and facilitates linking together in a chain formation, a process called polymerization. (From Goldman L: Cecil textbook of medicine, ed 22, Philadelphia, 2004, Saunders.)

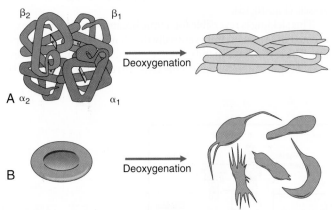

FIG. 10.15 (A) The molecular structure of Hb contains a pair of α polypeptide chains and a pair of α chains, each wrapped around a heme group (an iron atom in a porphyrin ring). The quaternary structure of the Hb molecule enables it to carry up to four molecules of oxygen. In the folded β-globin chain molecule, the sixth position contacts the α-globin chain. The amino acid substitution at the sixth position of the β-globin chain occurring in sickle cell anemia causes the Hb to aggregate into long chains, altering the shape of the cell (Hb S). (B) The change of the RBC from a biconcave disk to an elongated or crescent (sickle) shape occurs with deoxygenation.

The sickled cells, which become stiff and sticky, clog small blood vessels, depriving tissue from receiving an adequate blood supply. Tissues experience increased oxygen requirements under stress, causing more Hb to release its oxygen, which leads to increased numbers of deoxygenated and polymerized cells.

Deoxygenation of sickle cells induces potassium (followed by water) efflux, which increases cell density and the tendency of Hb S to polymerize. The sickle cell also has a chemical on the cell surface that binds to blood vessel walls, leading to endothelial cell activation. As a result, these sickle-shaped, rigid, sticky blood cells cannot pass through the capillaries and thus they block the flow of blood.[151]

Occlusion of the microcirculation increases hypoxia, which causes more erythrocytes to sickle, and thus a vicious cycle is precipitated. This accumulation of sickled erythrocytes obstructing blood vessels produces tissue injury. The organs at greatest risk are those with sluggish circulation, low pH, and a high level of oxygen extraction (spleen and bone marrow) or those with a limited terminal arterial supply (eye, head of the femur). No tissue or organ is spared from this injury. The higher the concentration of deoxygenated cells, the more severe (clinically) the complications.

Average sickle RBCs last only 10 to 20 days (normal is 120 days). The RBCs cannot be replaced fast enough, and anemia is the result. Although significant injury occurs in the microvasculature as a result of sickling, the most severe complication of SCD is a cerebral infarct, which occurs in the large blood vessels, where blood is moving rapidly and the diameter is wide.

Research has shown that not only are the Hb cells abnormal but so are the blood vessel walls. This is likely a product of sickle cells adhering to and damaging endothelium, which leads to an inflammatory response of WBCs, cytokines, chemoattractants, and procoagulants. Over time, smooth muscle cells migrate into the wall, where they proliferate and narrow the lumen of the vessel.[155]

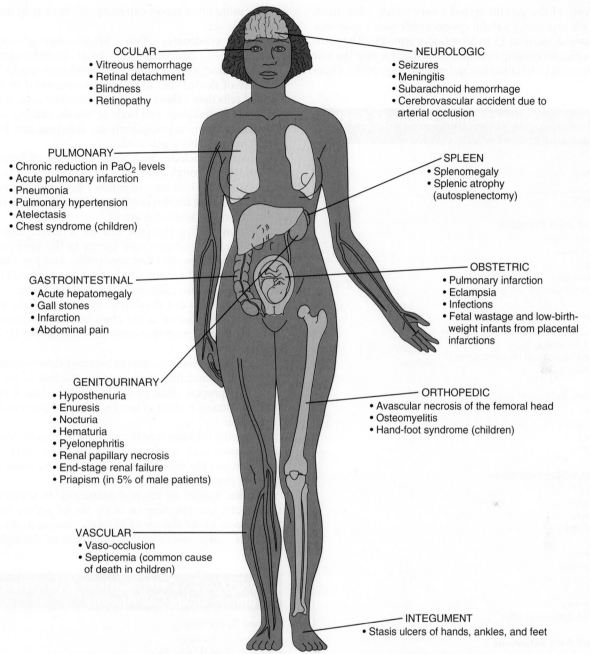

OCULAR
- Vitreous hemorrhage
- Retinal detachment
- Blindness
- Retinopathy

NEUROLOGIC
- Seizures
- Meningitis
- Subarachnoid hemorrhage
- Cerebrovascular accident due to arterial occlusion

PULMONARY
- Chronic reduction in PaO_2 levels
- Acute pulmonary infarction
- Pneumonia
- Pulmonary hypertension
- Atelectasis
- Chest syndrome (children)

SPLEEN
- Splenomegaly
- Splenic atrophy (autosplenectomy)

GASTROINTESTINAL
- Acute hepatomegaly
- Gall stones
- Infarction
- Abdominal pain

OBSTETRIC
- Pulmonary infarction
- Eclampsia
- Infections
- Fetal wastage and low-birth-weight infants from placental infarctions

GENITOURINARY
- Hyposthenuria
- Enuresis
- Nocturia
- Hematuria
- Pyelonephritis
- Renal papillary necrosis
- End-stage renal failure
- Priapism (in 5% of male patients)

ORTHOPEDIC
- Avascular necrosis of the femoral head
- Osteomyelitis
- Hand-foot syndrome (children)

VASCULAR
- Vaso-occlusion
- Septicemia (common cause of death in children)

INTEGUMENT
- Stasis ulcers of hands, ankles, and feet

FIG. 10.16 Clinical manifestations and possible complications associated with SCD. These findings are a consequence of infarctions, anemia, hemolysis, and recurrent infections.

Significantly narrowed or stenotic arteries can further collect sickled cells, thereby occluding the lumen and resulting in stroke. Further complicating stroke and pulmonary hypertension is the lack of nitric oxide production. Normally, when hypoxia is present, nitric oxide is produced to cause local vasodilatation, inhibit endothelial damage, and prevent proliferation of vascular smooth muscle.[195] But the hemolysis of erythrocytes and release of Hb inhibits the production of nitric oxide, thus blocking the beneficial effects of nitric oxide.

Clinical manifestations. Sickled erythrocytes cause hemolytic anemia and tend to occlude the microvasculature, resulting in both acute and chronic tissue injury. Intravascular sickling and hemolysis can begin by 6 to 8 weeks of age, but clinical manifestations do not usually appear until the infant is at least 6 months old, at which time the postnatal decrease in Hb F, which inhibits sickling, and increased production of Hb S lead to the increased concentration of Hb S.

Acute clinical manifestations of sickling, called *crises* or *episodes*, usually fall into one of four categories: vasoocclusive or thrombotic, aplastic, sequestration or, rarely, hyperhemolytic (Fig. 10.16).

Pain caused by the blockage of sickled RBCs (thrombosis) is the most common symptom of SCD, occurring unpredictably in any organ, bone, or joint of the body, wherever and whenever a blood clot develops. The symptoms and frequency, duration, and intensity of the painful episodes vary widely (Box 10.9). Some people experience painful episodes only once a year; others may have as many as 15 to 20 episodes annually. The vaso-occlusive episodes causing ischemic tissue damage may last 5 or 6 days, requiring hospitalization and subsiding gradually. Older clients more often report extremity and back pain during vascular episodes.

Chest syndrome. Two life-threatening thrombotic complications associated with SCD include acute chest syndrome and stroke. Acute chest syndrome results from the inability of sickled cells to become reoxygenated in the lungs. Sickled cells then adhere to lung endothelium cells, resulting in further inflammation, and occlude vessels, causing infarction. The most common precipitants are infection and fat emboli (from infarcted bone marrow).

Symptoms include chest pain, shortness of breath, fever, wheezing, and cough (Box 10.10). Chest radiographs typically demonstrate an infiltrate, sometimes days after the symptoms began. Prognosis for this complication is poor and is one of the most common causes of death.[156]

Pulmonary hypertension can be a severe consequence of repeated microthrombotic events in the lung even without a history of acute chest syndrome. Autopsy studies suggest that more than one-third of people with SCD develop this complication (although the real incidence is probably higher). This can develop in clients who have not had a significant number of acute chest syndrome crises because of the continual microthrombosis that may not be clinically evident.

These small vessels eventually become thickened and blocked by thrombin and fibrous tissue with the loss of the vascular bed. This process often proceeds without clinical symptoms until the person is short of breath, at which time the damage is irreversible.

Currently the most sensitive method of detecting pulmonary hypertension early is echocardiography. Pulmonary hypertension increases the risk of sudden death and is a common cause of death in people with SCD.

Stroke. Stroke, or cerebral infarction, is another serious thrombotic complication of SCD. Stroke occurs in 11% of SCD clients under the age of 20 years, causing death or severe disability. Large vessels can become stenotic through chronic

---

BOX 10.9   Clinical Manifestations of Sickle Cell Anemia

Pain
- Abdominal
- Chest
- Headache

Bone and Joint Episodes
- Low-grade fever
- Extremity pain
- Back pain
- Periosteal pain
- Joint pain, especially shoulder and hip

Vascular Complications
- Cerebrovascular accidents
- Chronic leg ulcers
- Avascular necrosis of the femoral head
- Bone infarcts

Pulmonary Episodes
- Hypoxia
- Chest pain
- Dyspnea
- Tachypnea

Neurologic Manifestations
- Seizures
- Hemiplegia
- Dizziness
- Drowsiness
- Coma
- Stiff neck
- Paresthesias
- Cranial nerve palsies
- Blindness
- Nystagmus
- Transient ischemic attacks

Hand-and-Foot Syndrome
- Fever
- Pain
- Dactylitis

Splenic Sequestration Episodes
- Liver and spleen enlargement, tenderness
- Hypovolemia

Renal Complications
- Enuresis
- Nocturia
- Hematuria
- Pyelonephritis
- Renal papillary necrosis
- End-stage renal failure (older adult population)

Modified from Goodman CC, Snyder TE: Differential diagnosis for physical therapists: screening for referral, ed 5, St. Louis, 2013, Saunders.

BOX 10.10   Complications Associated with Pediatric Sickle Cell Anemia

Chest Syndrome
- Severe chest pain
- Fever of ≥38.8° C (≥102° F)
- Very congested
- Cough
- Dyspnea
- Tachypnea
- Sternal or costal retractions
- Wheezing

Stroke
- Seizures
- Unusual or strange behavior
- Inability to move an arm and/or a leg
- Ataxia or unsteady gait (do not assume these are guarding responses to pain)
- Stutter or slurred speech
- Distal muscular weakness in the hands, feet, or legs
- Changes in vision
- Severe, unrelieved headaches
- Severe vomiting

injury to the endothelium. Once the diameter of an affected artery is significantly narrowed, acute occluding of the vessel can occur (by a clot made of sickle and normal cells, WBCs, platelets, and thrombin), causing a cerebral infarct.[155]

Local production of nitric oxide is typically stimulated by hypoxia to cause a beneficial vasodilatation, but free Hb (from sickle cells breaking apart) inhibits nitric oxide production, resulting in no valuable vasodilatation and further complicating strokes.

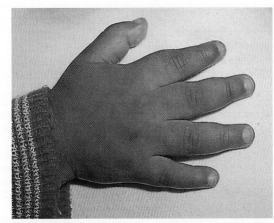

FIG. 10.17 Dactylitis. Painful swelling of the hands or feet can occur when a clot forms in the hands or feet. This problem, known as hand-and-foot syndrome, occurs most often in children affected by SCD. (From Lissauer T, Clayden G: Illustrated textbook of paediatrics, ed 4, Edinburgh, 2012, Mosby.)

Symptoms are similar to strokes in people without SCD, including paralysis, weakness, speech difficulties, seizures, and tingling/numbness of extremities. Infarcts can occur in the microvasculature as well. MRI and magnetic resonance angiography of the head and neck may show more extensive changes than are seen clinically, suggesting that silent strokes are not uncommon.

Additionally, many cognitive effects from these microvasculature strokes result in learning problems. Children demonstrate problems with memory, attention, visual–motor performance, and academic or social skills; neuromotor delays; mild hearing loss and auditory processing disorders; and failed speech and language screening.[4,88,107,185]

Other complications. For most people with SCD, the incidence of complications can be reduced by simple protective measures such as prophylactic administration of penicillin in childhood, avoidance of excessive heat or cold and dehydration, and contact as early as possible with a specialist center. These precautions are most effective if susceptible infants are identified at birth.

Other thrombotic complications include *hand-and-foot syndrome* (dactylitis), which occurs when a microinfarction (clot) occludes the blood vessels that supply the metacarpal and metatarsal bones, causing ischemia; it may be an infant's first problem caused by SCD.

It presents with low-grade fever and symmetric, painful, diffuse, nonpitting edema in the hands and feet, extending to the fingers and toes (Fig. 10.17). This is a fairly common phenomenon seen almost exclusively in the young infant and child. Despite radiographic changes and swelling, the syndrome is almost always self-limiting, and bones usually heal without permanent deformity (Fig. 10.18).

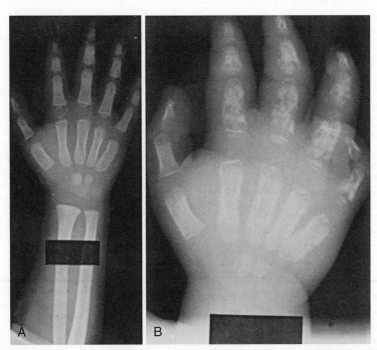

FIG. 10.18 Radiographs of an infant with sickle cell anemia and acute dactylitis. (A) The bones appear normal at the onset of the episode. (B) Destructive changes and periosteal reaction are evident 2 weeks later. (From Kliegman RM, Stanton BMD, St. Geme J, et al. (eds): Nelson textbook of pediatrics, ed 20, Philadelphia, 2016, Elsevier.)

Medical Management

Prevention

Sickle cell anemia can be prevented. Couples at risk of having affected children can be identified by inexpensive and reliable blood tests; chorionic villus sampling from 9 weeks of gestation can be performed for prenatal diagnosis.

Adoption of such measures goes hand in hand with health education. However, prenatal diagnosis can raise ethical questions that differ from one culture to another. Experience has clearly shown that genetic counseling, coupled with the offer of prenatal diagnosis, can lead to a large-scale reduction in births of affected children.

The risk of having affected children can be detected before marriage or pregnancy; however, to do so requires a carrier screening program. There is extensive experience with such programs in low- and high-income countries. For example, in the case of thalassemia prevention, unmarried people in Montreal (Canada) and the Maldives are offered screening. Premarital screening is a national policy in Cyprus and the Islamic Republic of Iran, and prereproductive screening is emphasized in Greece and Italy.

The WHO recommends these approaches be practiced in conformity with the three core principles of medical genetics: the autonomy of the individual or the couple, their right to adequate and complete information, and the highest standards of confidentiality.[206]

Diagnosis

It is required in every state that all infants be screened for SCD regardless of race or ethnic background (universal screening). This recommendation is based on several factors: (1) one out of every 200 Hispanic and 400 white children in Texas carries the sickle cell trait; (2) although SCD is more prevalent in certain racial and ethnic groups, it is not possible to define accurately an individual's heritage by physical appearance or surname; and (3) prophylactic penicillin and pneumococcal vaccination reduce both morbidity and mortality from pneumococcal infections in infants with sickle cell anemia and sickle thalassemia.

Screening targeted to specific racial and ethnic groups will therefore miss some affected infants, subjecting them to an increased risk of early mortality. Universal screening is the best, most reliable, and most cost-effective screening method to identify affected infants.[149] The cord blood of newborns is tested in the United States.

The diagnosis of sickle cell trait or any of the other sickle syndromes depends on the demonstration of sickling under reduced oxygen tension.

Stroke is a relatively infrequent complication in the young infant; the median age for occurrence of stroke in children is 7 years. Splenic sequestration (entrapment of blood and enlargement in the spleen) can occur in children younger than 6 years with homozygous Hb S and at any age with other types of SCD. Circulatory collapse and death can occur in less than 30 minutes.

Any signs of weakness, abdominal pain, fatigue, dyspnea, tachycardia accompanied by pallor, and hypotension require emergency medical attention. Client and family education should emphasize the importance of regularly scheduled medical evaluations for anyone receiving hydroxyurea. The risk of developing an undetected toxicity that can result in severe bone marrow depression must be explained. Outward signs of drug complications are rarely evident.

Neurodevelopment

SCD is a blood disorder; however, the CNS is one of the organs frequently affected by the disease.[87,173] Brain disease can begin early in life and often leads to neurocognitive dysfunction.

Approximately one-fourth to one-third of children with SCD have some form of CNS effects from the disease, which typically manifest as deficits in specific cognitive domains and academic difficulties.

The impact of the disease on families shares many features similar to other neurodevelopmental disorders, but social-environmental factors related to low socioeconomic status; worry and concerns about social stigma; and recurrent, unpredictable medical complications can be sources of relatively higher stress in SCD.

Greater public awareness of the neurocognitive effects of SCD and their impact on child outcomes is a critical step toward improved treatment, adaptation to illness, and quality of life.

Exercise

Multiple factors contribute to exercise intolerance in individuals with sickle cell anemia, but little information exists regarding the safety of maximal cardiopulmonary exercise testing or the mechanisms of exercise limitation in these clients.

For example, low peak VO_2, low anaerobic threshold, gas exchange abnormalities, and high ventilatory reserve comprise a pattern consistent with exercise limitation due to pulmonary vascular disease in this population group. Low peak VO_2, low anaerobic threshold, no gas exchange abnormalities, and a high heart rate reserve reflect peripheral vascular disease and/or myopathy. Low peak VO_2, low anaerobic threshold, no gas exchange abnormalities, and a low heart rate reserve are best explained by anemia.[27] These kinds of cardiopulmonary factors must be considered when prescribing exercise for this population.[146]

During a sickle cell episode, the clinician may be involved in nonpharmacologic pain control or management. Precautions include avoiding stressors that can precipitate an episode, such as overexertion, dehydration, smoking, and exposure to cold or the use of cryotherapy for painful, swollen joints. (See 10.1 Special Implications for the PTA: Hematologic Disorders in this chapter.)

Should a person with SCD experience an isolated musculoskeletal injury (e.g., sprained ankle) in the absence of any sickle cell episodes, careful application of ice can be undertaken.

Pain Management

People with SCD suffer both physically and psychosocially. They may describe feelings of helplessness against the disease and fear a premature death. Frequent hospitalizations and consequent job absences often result in stressful financial constraints.

Depression is a common finding in this group of people. A program offering holistic treatment focuses on pharmacologic and nonpharmacologic strategies, offering the client multiple self-management options. The sickle cell pain can be successfully managed using whirlpool therapy at a slightly warmer temperature (102° F to 104° F), facilitating muscle relaxation through active movement in the water.

10.13 Special Implications for the PTA: Sickle Cell Disease It is important for the clinician to recognize signs of complications, especially signs of acute chest syndrome, stroke, and neurodevelopmental impairment (see Box 10.10). Providing client education is also an important role. Clients should be taught about risks and risk prevention, including the importance of physical activity and/or mobility, prevention of pulmonary complications using breathing and incentive spirometry, and the importance of remaining well hydrated.

The clinician should teach the client alternative methods of pain control, such as the appropriate application of mild heat to painful areas or the use of visualization or relaxation techniques. Combined use of medications, psychologic support, relaxation techniques, biofeedback, and imagery is a useful intervention to lessen the effects of painful episodes.[85] Cognitive-behavioral therapy can be helpful in the management of sickle pain because of the high level of psychologic stress among people with SCD experience.[193]

Joint effusions in SCD can occur secondary to long bone infarctions with extension of swelling and septic arthritis. Clients with SCD may also have coexistent rheumatic or collagen vascular disease or osteoarthritis, necessitating careful evaluation to determine the presence of marked inflammation or fever before initiating intervention procedures.

Teaching joint protection is important and may include assistive devices, equipment, and technology and pain-free strengthening exercises. Persistent thigh, buttock, or groin pain in anyone with known SCD may be an indication of aseptic necrosis of the femoral head. Blood supply to the hip is only adequate, even in healthy people, so the associated microvascular obstruction can leave the hip especially vulnerable to ischemia and necrosis. Up to 50% of sickle cell cases develop this condition.

Total hip replacement may be indicated in cases in which severe structural damage occurs; sickle cell–related surgical complications most commonly include excessive intraoperative blood loss, postoperative hemorrhage, wound abscess, pulmonary complications, and transfusion reactions.[196]

Tolerance, Dependence, and Addiction

It is helpful if the client, family, and clinician understand the differences among tolerance, dependence, and addiction as they relate to the individual with SCD receiving or needing narcotic medications. Tolerance and dependence are both involuntary and predictable physiologic changes that develop with repeated administration of narcotics; these terms do not indicate that the person is addicted.

Tolerance occurs when, after repeated administration of a narcotic, larger doses are needed to obtain the same effect. *Dependence* has occurred if withdrawal symptoms emerge when the narcotic is stopped abruptly. In either case, this means that once the medication is no longer needed, the dosage will have to be tapered down to avoid withdrawal symptoms.

Addiction, although also based on physiologic changes associated with drug use, has a psychologic and behavioral component characterized by continuous craving for the substance. Addicted people will use a drug to relieve psychologic symptoms even after the physical pain is gone.

The chronic use of narcotics for pain relief may lead to addictive use in vulnerable individuals, but even if someone is addicted, the pain should still be treated and narcotics should not be withheld if they are the drugs of choice for the pain condition. Ironically, undertreating the pain because of fear of fostering addiction actually encourages a pattern of drug-seeking and drug-hoarding behaviors.[78]

REFERENCES/SUGGESTED READINGS

To enhance this text and add value for the reader, references and suggested readings are included on the companion Evolve site that accompanies this textbook. The reader can view the source and access it online whenever possible.

11

The Respiratory System

1. Understand the common signs, symptoms, and prognoses in pulmonary diseases.
2. Review infectious pulmonary conditions.
3. Understand the nature and prognoses of obstructive conditions.
4. Understand the interlink between cardiac and pulmonary conditions.

OUTLINE

VOCAB BUILDERS

Acini
Ameliorate
Asbestos
Auscultation
Aspergillus
Atopy
Bifurcation
Blebs
Bullae
Cavitation
Clubbing
Compliance
CPAP
Cytotoxic
Empyema
Exacerbation

Extrapulmonary
FEV
Fractionation
FVC
Genotoxicity
Granulomas
Hypercoagulable
Iatrogenic
Infiltrate
Insidious
Inspissated
Leukotriene
Methacholine
Morphologically
Mucolytic
Mycoplasmal

Narcolepsy
Palliative
Paraseptal
Percussion
Percutaneous
Perfusion
Pleurisy
Prophylaxis
Remodeling
Sequelae
Spirometry
Sympathomimetic
Viscosity
WOB

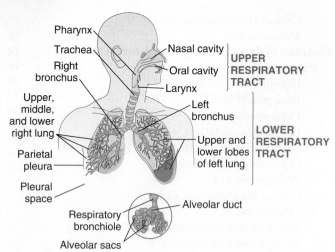

FIG. 11.1 Structures of the upper and lower respiratory tracts. The upper respiratory tract consists of the nasal cavity, pharynx, and larynx; the lower respiratory tract includes the trachea, bronchi, and lungs. The circle shows the acinus, the terminal respiratory unit, which consists of the respiratory bronchioles, alveolar ducts, and alveolar sacs. This is the portion of the lungs where oxygen and carbon dioxide are exchanged.

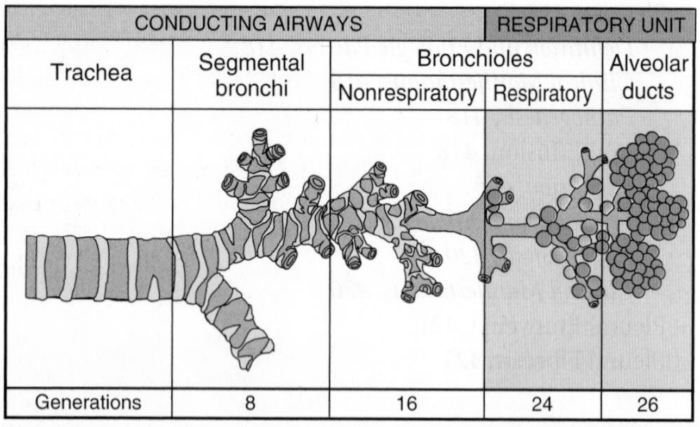

TABLE 11.1	**Causes of Hypoxemia**
Mechanism	**Common Clinical Cause**
Ventilation–perfusion mismatch	Asthma Chronic bronchitis Pneumonia
Decreased oxygen content	High altitude Low oxygen content Enclosed breathing space (suffocation)
Hypoventilation	Lack of neurologic stimulation of the respiratory center Oversedation Drug overdose Neurologic damage COPD
Alveolocapillary diffusion abnormality	Emphysema Fibrosis Edema
Pulmonary shunting	ARDS Hyaline membrane disease (ARDS in newborn) Atelectasis

ARDS, Acute respiratory distress syndrome; *COPD,* chronic obstructive pulmonary disease.
Modified from McCance KL, Huether SE, editors: Pathophysiology: the biologic basis for disease in adults and children, ed 7, St. Louis, 2014, Mosby.

CONDUCTING AIRWAYS				RESPIRATORY UNIT
Trachea	Segmental bronchi	Bronchioles		Alveolar ducts
		Nonrespiratory	Respiratory	
Generations	8	16	24	26

FIG. 11.2 Structures of the lower airway. The first 16 generations of the airways branching in human lungs are purely conducting; transitional airways lead into the final respiratory zone consisting of alveoli, where gas exchange takes place.

OVERVIEW

Anatomically, the respiratory system can be divided into three main portions: the upper airway, the lower airway, and the terminal alveoli (Fig. 11.1). The upper airway consists of the nasal cavities, sinuses, pharynx, tonsils, and larynx. The lower airway consists of the conducting airways, including the trachea, bronchi, and bronchioles (Fig. 11.2). The alveoli, or air sacs, at the end of the conducting airways in the lower respiratory tract are the primary lobules, sometimes called the *acini,* of the lung.

Physiologically, lung function is composed of ventilation and respiration. *Ventilation* is the ability to move the air in and out of the lungs via a pressure gradient. *Respiration* is the gas exchange that supplies oxygen to the blood and body tissues and removes carbon dioxide. Pathology or impairment of the airways, lungs, chest wall, and diaphragm will affect ventilation. Pathology of the lungs and cardiovascular system, as well as peripheral tissues, will affect respiration.

Major Sequelae of Pulmonary Disease or Injury

Hypoxemia is the most common condition caused by pulmonary disease or injury. *Hypoxemia,* deficient oxygenation of arterial blood, may lead to *hypoxia,* a broad term meaning diminished availability of oxygen to the body tissues; *hypercapnia* is the presence of abnormally large amounts of carbon dioxide in the blood, which correspond with abnormally low amounts of oxygen in the blood. Prolonged hypoxia will cause tissue damage or death. Hypoxemia is caused by respiratory alterations (Table 11.1) or cardiovascular compromise, whereas hypoxia may occur anywhere in the body as a result of alterations of other systems and may not be related to changes in the pulmonary system.

Signs and symptoms of hypoxemia vary, depending on the level of oxygenation in the blood (Table 11.2). Exercise testing may be performed to determine the degree of oxygen desaturation and/or hypoxemia that occurs on exertion. This testing requires analysis of arterial blood samples drawn with the subject at rest and at peak exercise. Continuous noninvasive measurement of arterial oxyhemoglobin saturation is usually determined by pulse oximetry.

Oxygen Transport Deficits in Systemic Disease

Although this chapter focuses on primary pulmonary impairment, pathologic conditions of every major organ system can have secondary effects on pulmonary function and on the oxygen transport pathway (which includes the cardiovascular system). Such effects are of considerable clinical significance given that they can be life threatening and that therapy interventions usually put additional demands on the oxygen transport system. The resulting secondary effect may include a large range of pulmonary impairments such as altered ventilation, *perfusion,* and ventilation–perfusion matching; reduced lung volumes, capacities, and flow rates; atelectasis; reduced surfactant production and distribution; impaired mucociliary transport; secretion accumulation;

TABLE 11.2   Signs and Symptoms of Hypoxemia

Pao₂ (mm Hg)	Signs and Symptoms
80–100	Normal
60–80	Moderate tachycardia, possible onset of respiratory distress, dyspnea on exertion
50–60	Malaise Light-headedness Nausea Vertigo Impaired judgment Incoordination Restlessness
35–50	Marked confusion Cardiac arrhythmias Labored respiration
25–35	Cardiac arrest Decreased renal blood flow Decreased urine output Lactic acidosis Lethargy Loss of consciousness
<25	Decreased minute ventilation[a] secondary to depression of the respiratory center

[a]The total volume of air inhaled or exhaled in 1 minute.
Pao₂, Partial pressure of arterial oxygen.
Modified from Frownfelter DL, Dean E: Principles and practice of cardiopulmonary physical therapy, ed 4, St. Louis, 2006, Mosby.

BOX 11.1   Most Common Signs and Symptoms of Pulmonary Disease

- Cough
- Dyspnea
- Abnormal sputum
- Chest pain
- Hemoptysis
- Cyanosis
- Digital clubbing
- Altered breathing patterns

pulmonary aspiration; impaired lymphatic drainage; pulmonary edema; impaired coughing; and respiratory muscle weakness or fatigue.[85]

Signs and Symptoms of Pulmonary Disease

Pulmonary disease is often classified as acute or chronic, obstructive or restrictive, or infectious or noninfectious and is associated with many common signs and symptoms. The most common of these are cough and dyspnea. Others include chest pain, abnormal sputum, hemoptysis, cyanosis, digital clubbing, and altered breathing patterns (Box 11.1 and Table 11.3).

Cough

As a physiologic response, cough occurs frequently in healthy people, but a persistent dry cough may be caused by a tumor, congestion, or hypersensitive airways (allergies). A productive cough with purulent sputum may indicate infection, whereas a productive cough with nonpurulent sputum is nonspecific and indicates airway irritation. Hemoptysis (coughing and spitting blood) indicates a pathologic condition—infection, inflammation, abscess, tumor, or infarction.

Dyspnea

Dyspnea is defined as the subjective feeling of shortness of breath (SOB). It usually indicates hypoxemia but can be associated with emotional states, particularly fear and anxiety. Dyspnea is usually caused by diffuse and extensive rather than focal pulmonary disease, pulmonary embolism (PE) being the exception. Factors contributing to the sensation of dyspnea include increased work of breathing (*WOB*), respiratory muscle fatigue, increased systemic metabolic demands, and decreased respiratory reserve capacity. Dyspnea that occurs when the person is lying down is called *orthopnea* and is caused by redistribution of body water. Fluid shift leads to increased fluid in the lung, which interferes with gas exchange and leads to orthopnea. In the supine and prone positions, the abdominal contents also exert pressure on the diaphragm and can cause dyspnea by increasing the WOB and often limiting vital capacity.

Chest Pain

Pulmonary pain patterns are usually localized in the substernal or chest region over involved lung fields, including the anterior aspect of the chest, side, or back. However, pulmonary pain can radiate to the neck, upper trapezius, costal margins, thoracic area of the back, scapulae, or shoulder. Shoulder pain caused by pulmonary involvement may radiate along the medial aspect of the arm, mimicking other neuromuscular causes of neck or shoulder pain. Musculoskeletal causes of chest (wall) pain must be differentiated from pain of cardiac, pulmonary, epigastric, and breast origins.

Extensive disease may occur in the lung without occurrence of pain until the process extends to the parietal pleura (Fig. 11.3). Pleural irritation then results in sharp, localized pain that is aggravated by any respiratory movement. Clients usually note that the pain is alleviated by autosplinting—that is, lying on the affected side, which diminishes the movement of that side of the chest.[296,309]

Cyanosis

The presence of cyanosis, a bluish color of the skin and mucous membranes, depends on the oxygen saturation of arterial blood and the total amount of circulating hemoglobin. It is further differentiated as central or peripheral. Central cyanosis is best observed as a bluish discoloration in the oral mucous membranes, lips, and conjunctivae (i.e., the warmer, more central areas) and is most often associated with cardiac right-to-left shunts and pulmonary disease. Peripheral cyanosis is associated with decreased perfusion to the extremities, nail beds, and nose (i.e., the cooler, exposed areas) and is commonly caused by cold external temperature, anxiety, heart failure, or shock.

Clinically detectable cyanosis depends not only on oxygen saturation but also on the total amount of circulating hemoglobin that is bound to oxygen. For example, a child with severe anemia may not be cyanotic because all available hemoglobin is fully saturated with oxygen. However, a child with polycythemia may demonstrate signs of cyanosis because the overproduction of red blood cells (RBCs) results in increased amounts of hemoglobin that are not fully saturated with oxygen. In some instances, however, such as in carbon monoxide poisoning, hemoglobin is bound with a substance other than oxygen. Cyanosis is not present because the hemoglobin is fully bound; but because the hemoglobin is not bound to oxygen, there is inadequate tissue oxygenation, and tissue death may occur.

TABLE 11.3   Descriptions of Altered Breathing Patterns and Sounds

Breathing Pattern or Sound	Description
Apneustic	Gasping inspiration followed by short expiration
Biot's respiration (ataxia)	An irregular pattern of deep and shallow breaths; fast, deep breaths interspersed with abrupt pauses in breathing
Cheyne–Stokes respiration	Repeated cycle of deep breathing followed by shallow breaths or cessation of breathing
Crackles, rales	Discontinuous, low-pitched sounds predominantly heard during inspiration that indicate secretions in the peripheral airways[13]
Hyperventilation	Abnormally prolonged and deep breathing
Hypoventilation	Reduction in the amount of air entering the pulmonary alveoli, which causes an increase in the arterial CO_2 level
Kussmaul's respiration	A distressing dyspnea characterized by increased respiratory rate (>20/min), increased depth of respiration, panting, and labored respiration typical of air hunger
Lateral–costal breathing	Chest becomes flattened anteriorly with excessive flaring of the lower ribs (supine position); minimal to no upper chest expansion or accessory muscle involvement with outward flaring of the lower rib cage instead; the person breathes into the lateral plane of respiration (gravity eliminated) because the weakened diaphragm and intercostal muscles cannot effectively oppose the force of gravity in the anterior plane; used to focus expansion in areas of the chest wall that have decreased expansion (e.g., spinal cord injury with atelectasis or pneumonia, asymmetric chest expansion with scoliosis)[a]
Paradoxical breathing (sometimes referred to as *reverse breathing*)	All or part of the chest wall falls in during inspiration; may be abdominal expansion during exhalation; can lead to a flattened anterior chest wall or pectus excavatum
Stridor	A shrill, harsh sound heard during inspiration in the presence of laryngeal obstruction
Wheezing	High-pitched, continuous whistling sound, usually with expiration and related to bronchospasm or other constriction of the airways

[a]Data from Massery M: Personal communication, 2001.

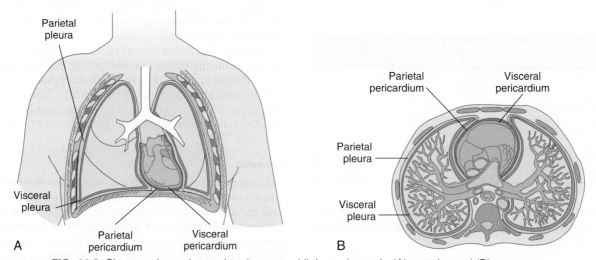

FIG. 11.3 Chest cavity and associated structural linings shown in (A) anterior and (B) cross-sectional views. For instructional purposes the layers are depicted larger than actually found in the human body.

Arterial saturation in central cyanosis is usually decreased, whereas arterial saturation may be normal in peripheral cyanosis. In the case of peripheral cyanosis, vasoconstriction with decreased blood supply and perfusion rather than unsaturated blood is the underlying cause of symptoms.

Clubbing

Thickening and widening of the terminal phalanges of the fingers and toes result in a painless clublike appearance recognized by the loss of the angle between the nail and the nail bed (Fig. 11.4). Conditions that chronically interfere with tissue perfusion and nutrition may cause *clubbing*. These include cystic fibrosis (CF), chronic obstructive pulmonary disease (COPD), lung cancer, bronchiectasis, pulmonary fibrosis, congenital heart disease, and lung abscess. Although 75% to 85% of clubbing is caused by pulmonary disease and resultant hypoxia (diminished availability of blood to the body tissues), clubbing does not always indicate lung disease. It is sometimes present in heart disease, peripheral vascular disease, and disorders of the liver and gastrointestinal tract.

Altered Breathing Patterns

Changes in the rate, depth, regularity, and effort of breathing occur in response to any condition affecting the pulmonary

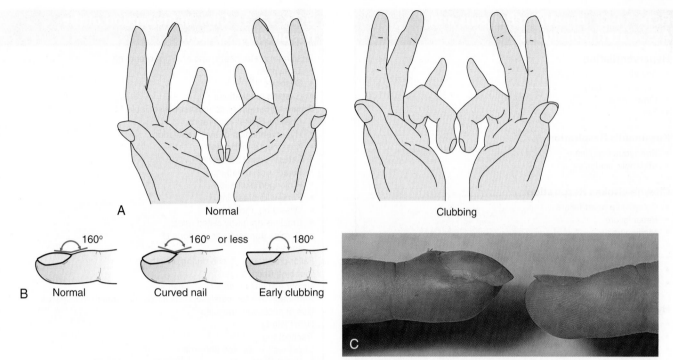

FIG. 11.4 (A) Assessment of clubbing by the Schamroth method. The client places the fingernails of opposite fingers together and holds them up to a light. If a diamond shape can be seen between the nails, there is no clubbing. (B) The profile of the index finger is examined, and the angle of the nail base is noted; it should be about 160 degrees. The nail base is firm to palpation. Curved nails are a variation of normal with a convex profile and may look like clubbed nails, but the angle between the nail base and the nail is 160 degrees or less. In early clubbing, the angle straightens out to 180 degrees and the nail base feels spongy to palpation. (C) Photograph of advanced clubbing of the finger *(left)* compared with normal finger *(right)*.

system (see Table 11.3). Breathing patterns can vary, depending on the neuromuscular or neurologic disease or trauma (Box 11.2).

In a large cross-section of people and clinical disorders, hypoventilation is one of the most common changes in breathing patterns observed. Anything that can cause hypoxemia (e.g., fever, malnutrition, metabolic disturbance, loss of blood or blood flow, or reduced availability of oxygen) reduces energy supplies and results in respiratory muscle dysfunction and altered breathing patterns.

Breathing pattern abnormalities seen with head trauma, brain abscess, diaphragmatic paralysis of chest wall muscles and thorax (e.g., generalized myopathy or neuropathy), heat stroke, spinal meningitis, and encephalitis can include *apneustic breathing, ataxic breathing,* or *Cheyne–Stokes respiration* (CSR) (see Table 11.3).

Spinal cord injuries above C3 result in loss of phrenic nerve innervation, necessitating ventilator support and a tracheostomy. *Ventilatory support* is used to refer to a variety of interventions, including mechanical ventilation via endotracheal intubation, noninvasive ventilatory support with continuous positive airway pressure (*CPAP*), positive end-expiratory pressure (PEEP), and bilevel positive airway pressure (BiPAP).

Clients with generalized weakness, as in Guillain–Barré syndrome, some myopathies or neuropathies, or incomplete spinal cord injuries, may show a tendency toward a specific breathing pattern called *lateral–costal breathing* (see Table 11.3).

11.1 Special Implications for the PTA: Signs and Symptoms of Pulmonary Disease Monitoring cardiopulmonary status is important because many of the interventions provided by a physical therapist assistant (PTA) elicit an exercise stimulus and stress the oxygen transport system. Because impairment can result from diseases other than cardiopulmonary conditions, PTAs in all settings need knowledge in anticipating and detecting pulmonary dysfunction in the absence of primary pulmonary disease.[85,107]

Recognizing abnormal responses to interventions is important in identifying the client who needs additional intervention or who needs to be referred to another health care professional. Clinical observation of the client as he or she breathes is important (Box 11.3) and can alert the PTA to respiratory pathologic conditions. Techniques to improve ventilation can enhance motor performance and improve a client's functional level.[107,149] The reader is referred to more specific texts for information about intervention techniques.

The PTA involved in performing airway clearance techniques and pulmonary rehabilitation must recognize precautions for and contraindications to therapy interventions in the medical client (Table 11.4).

AGING AND THE PULMONARY SYSTEM

Aging affects not only the physiologic functions of the lungs (ventilation and respiration) but also the ability of the respiratory system to defend itself. More than any other organ, the lung is susceptible to infectious processes and environmental and occupational pollutants (see the section on environmental

BOX 11.2   Breathing Patterns and Associated Conditions

Hyperventilation

- Anxiety
- Acute head injury
- Hypoxemia
- Fever

Kussmaul's Respiration

- Strenuous exercise
- Metabolic acidosis

Cheyne–Stokes Respiration

- Congestive heart failure
- Renal failure
- Meningitis
- Drug overdose
- Increased intracranial pressure
- Infants (normal)
- Older people during sleep (normal)

Hypoventilation

- Fibromyalgia syndrome
- Chronic fatigue syndrome
- Sleep disorder
- Muscle fatigue
- Muscle weakness
- Malnutrition
- Neuromuscular disease
  - Guillain–Barré syndrome
  - Myasthenia gravis
  - Poliomyelitis
  - Amyotrophic lateral sclerosis (ALS)
- Pickwickian or obesity hypoventilation syndrome
- Severe kyphoscoliosis

Apneustic

- Midpons lesion
- Basilar artery infarct

Biot's Respiration (Ataxia)

- Exercise
- Shock
- Cerebral hypoxia
- Heat stroke
- Spinal meningitis
- Head injury
- Brain abscess
- Encephalitis

BOX 11.3   Clinical Inspection of the Respiratory System

Respiratory rate, depth, and effort of breathing
- Tachypnea
- Dyspnea
- Gasping respirations

Breathing pattern or sounds (see also Table 11.3)
- Cheyne–Stokes respiration
- Hyperventilation or hypoventilation
- Kussmaul's respiration
- Lateral–costal breathing
- Paradoxical breathing
- Prolonged expiration
- Pursed-lip breathing
- Wheezing, rhonchi
- Crackles (formerly called *rales*)
- Gurgles (formerly called *rhonchi*)

Cyanosis

Pallor or redness of skin during activity

Clubbing (toes, fingers)

Nicotine stains on fingers and hands

Retraction of intercostal, supraclavicular, or suprasternal spaces

Use of accessory muscles

Nasal flaring

Tracheal tug

Chest wall shape and deformity
- Barrel chest
- Pectus excavatum
- Pectus carinatum
- Kyphosis
- Scoliosis

Cough

Sputum: frothy; red-tinged, green, or yellow

---

and occupational diseases in this chapter). These factors, combined with the normal aging process, contribute to the decline of lung function.

Age-related alterations in the respiratory system are based on structural changes that lead to functional impairment of gas exchange.[314,360] Chest wall compliance decreases with aging because of changes in joints of the ribs and spine, as well as alterations in collagen. This increased stiffness affects the volume of air moved and the WOB. Elastic recoil also is decreased by intermolecular collagen crosslinks. Alveolar walls flatten, surface area is reduced, and the small airways more readily collapse and trap air, reducing the capacity for gas exchange.[107,167] Thus diminished gas exchange is primarily a result of increased physiologic dead space.

Many changes that occur with aging affect the lower airway, but in the upper airway the movement of the cilia slows and becomes less effective in sweeping away mucus and debris. This reduced ciliary action combined with the other changes noted predisposes the older client to increased respiratory infections.

Reduction in respiratory muscle strength and endurance and subsequent increase in WOB requiring greater muscle oxygen consumption at any workload are observed with increasing age.[41,107] Respiratory muscle strength is measured by maximum inspiratory pressure and maximum expiratory pressure. These measurements have been correlated with spirometry, nutritional status, and grip strength. Loss of respiratory muscle strength can lead to dyspnea and ultimately to ventilatory pump failure.

Normal ventilation of older adults is comparable to that of younger people. For older adults, tidal volumes are smaller and rate is higher. There is a significant blunting of response to hypoxia and hypercapnia from both the respiratory and cardiovascular systems, particularly at rest. The hypercapnia response during exercise is greater in older adults, contributing to more dyspnea for a given workload even in the absence of oxygen desaturation or metabolic acidosis. Most adults attain maximal lung function (as measured by forced expiratory volume [FEV]) during their early twenties, but with increasing age, especially after age 55 years, there is an overall decrease in the functional ability of the lungs to move air in and out. This decline peaks by age 75 years, falling to about 70% of our maximum. Aging reduces the reserve capacity of virtually all pulmonary functions regardless of lifestyle, although a sedentary lifestyle accelerates the decline in functional capacity.[188]

TABLE 11.4 Considerations for and Contraindications to Airway Clearance Techniques in the Medical Client

Considerations	Contraindications
Hemoptysis	Untreated tension pneumothorax; treat when chest tube has been inserted and client's condition is stable
Fragile ribs (e.g., metastatic bone cancer, osteoporosis, flail chest, rib fractures, osteomyelitis of the ribs)	
Burns, open wounds, skin infections in thoracic area	Unstable cardiovascular system
	Hypotension
Pulmonary edema, congestive heart failure	Uncontrolled hypertension
Large pleural effusion	Acute myocardial infarction
Pulmonary embolism (controversial)[a]	Arrhythmias
	Conditions prone to hemorrhages (platelet count <20,000/mm³: must have physician's approval)
Symptomatic aneurysm or decrease in circulation of the main blood vessels	Unstabilized head and neck injury
Platelet count of 20,000–50,000/mm³	Intracranial pressure >20 mm Hg
Postoperative status	
Neurosurgery (positioning may cause increased intracranial pressure; can begin gentle breathing exercises)	
Esophageal anastamosis (gastric juices may affect suture line)	
Orthopedic clients who are limited in positioning	
Recent spinal fusion	
Surgical complications (e.g., pericardial sac tear)	
Recent skin grafts or flaps	
Resected tumors (avoid tumor area)	
Recently placed pacemaker	
Older or nervous clients who become agitated or upset with therapy	
Acute spinal injury or recent spinal surgery such as laminectomy (precaution: log-roll and position with care to maintain vertebral alignment)	

[a]A question remains whether there may be a recurrence (repeat emboli in the medically unstable client, i.e., one whose blood level of anticoagulants is not yet adequate to prevent a possible second embolus from dislodging) with movement in positioning the client for airway clearance techniques. However, allowing the client to lie still can contribute to the development of further venous stasis.

All of these changes contribute to the increased WOB, meaning that the older adult works harder for the same air exchange as the younger person. These changes are influenced by lifestyle and environmental factors, respiratory disease, and body size. The effects of age are not nearly as influential as the effects of smoking in causing a premature decline in lung function and in limiting the ability to exercise.

Pulmonary complications during anesthesia and the postoperative period are significantly increased in older adults with preexisting diseases. Loss of an effective cough reflex contributes to an increased susceptibility to pneumonia and postoperative atelectasis in the older population. Other contributing factors to the loss of an effective cough reflex include conditions more common in older age such as reduced consciousness, use of sedatives, impaired esophageal motility, dysphagia, and neurologic diseases.

11.2 Special Implications for the PTA: Aging and the Pulmonary System The PTA practicing in a geriatric setting needs to be knowledgeable about the normal consequences of aging to be able to identify the origin of and differences between impairments of aging and pathology. The ability to measure and discriminate between the process of aging and the *sequelae* of pathologic conditions (including consideration of the impact of comorbidities) is essential in the management of impairment and prevention of functional decline. Descriptions of the normal progressive decline of the respiratory system and the physiologic effects of pathologic conditions (both acute and chronic) as these conditions relate to the aging adult are available.[41,107,244]

Pulmonary Capacity and Exercise

Although ventilatory and respiratory functions of older adults undergo a process of change related to aging that begins in early adulthood, it does not appear that healthy older people are limited by these changes in exercise capacity for activities that require moderate levels of oxygen consumption (VO_2). On the other hand, clients with obstructive lung disease have a significant loss of vital capacity and may experience SOB at relatively low exercise intensities. In fact, the older person with obstructive lung disease may self-limit exercise because of dyspnea as opposed to exercise limitation by reduced cardiovascular capacity.

Exercise capacity or exercise tolerance does decrease in the older adult as the Pao_2 (measure of oxygen in arterial blood) decreases. Daily physical activity can be assessed using the following categories: sedentary; sedentary with some daily activity; active through occupation or recreational activity; and trained athlete. A higher level of habitual physical activity is one factor favorably influencing oxygen delivery.

The ability to deliver oxygen to the tissues is called *maximal* VO_2 (VO_{2max}) and reflects the functioning of the oxygen transport pathway. Age-associated reductions in cardiac output may compromise the ventilation–perfusion balance, and the Pao_2 (and thus oxygen delivery) may be reduced even more.

Regular exercise can substantially slow the decline in VO_{2max} delivery caused by cardiovascular deconditioning related to age or lowered levels of habitual physical activity. Decreased respiratory muscle strength and endurance occurring with age can be enhanced with exercise, although much of the improved ventilatory efficiency has been attributed to peripheral changes (decreased carbon dioxide production and blood lactate).[343] In other words, peripheral conditioning improves function but does not make changes in the lung parenchyma.

INFECTIOUS AND INFLAMMATORY DISEASES

Pneumonia

Incidence

Pneumonia is a commonly encountered disease, with more than 4 million cases diagnosed each year. The combined cost of pneumonia and influenza to the U.S. economy was $37.5 billion in 2004.[268] It is a leading cause of death in the United States, claiming the lives of approximately 65,000 Americans annually. Approximately 30% of pneumonias are bacterial—especially prevalent in the older adult. Viral pneumonia, accounting for nearly one-half of all cases, is not usually life threatening except in the immunocompromised person. The remaining 20% of all cases are caused by mycoplasma.

Definition and Etiologic Factors

Pneumonia is an inflammation affecting the parenchyma of the lungs and can be caused by (1) a bacterial, viral, fungal, or *mycoplasmal* infection (organisms that have both viral and bacterial characteristics); (2) inhalation of toxic or caustic chemicals, smoke, dusts, or gases; or (3) aspiration of food, fluids, or vomitus.

It may be primary or secondary, and it often follows influenza. The common feature of all types of pneumonia is an inflammatory pulmonary response to the offending organism or agent. This response may involve one or both lungs at the level of the lobe (lobar pneumonia) or more distally at the bronchioles and alveoli (bronchopneumonia).

The major routes of infection are airborne pathogens, circulation, sinus or contiguous infection, and aspiration. Nosocomial (hospital-acquired) infections have twice the mortality and morbidity of non–hospital-acquired infections.[54]

Risk Factors

Infectious agents responsible for pneumonia are typically present in the upper respiratory tract and cause no harm unless resistance is lowered by some other factor. Many host conditions promote the growth of pathogenic organisms, but cigarette smoking (more than 20 cigarettes per day) is highly correlated with community-acquired pneumonia (CAP).[10] Pneumonia is also a frequent complication of acute respiratory infections such as influenza and sinusitis.

Other risk factors include chronic bronchitis, poorly controlled diabetes mellitus, uremia, dehydration, malnutrition, and prior existing critical illnesses such as chronic renal failure, chronic lung disease, or acquired immunodeficiency syndrome (AIDS). In addition, the stress of hospitalization, confinement to an extended care facility or intensive care unit, surgery, tracheal intubation, treatment with antineoplastic chemotherapy or immunosuppressive drugs, and urinary incontinence promote rapid colonization of pathogenic organisms.

Infants, older adults, people with profound disabilities or who are bedridden, and persons with altered consciousness (e.g., caused by alcoholic stupor, head injury, seizure disorder, drug overdose, or general anesthesia) are most vulnerable. Inactivity and immobility cause pooling of normal secretions in the airways, which creates an environment promoting bacterial growth. People with severe periodontal disease, those who have difficulty swallowing, those who have an inability to take oral medications, and those whose cough reflexes are impaired by drugs, alcohol, or neuromuscular disease are at increased risk for the development of pneumonia as a result of aspiration.

Pathogenesis

Although a common disease, pneumonia is relatively rare in healthy people because of the effectiveness of the respiratory host defense system and the fact that healthy lungs are generally kept sterile below the first major bronchial divisions. In the compromised person, the normal release of biochemical mediators by alveolar macrophages as part of the inflammatory response does not eliminate invading pathogens. The multiplying microorganisms release damaging toxins, stimulating full-scale inflammatory and immune responses with damaging side effects.

Inflammation and edema cause the acini and terminal bronchioles to fill with infectious debris and exudate so that air cannot enter the alveoli and gas exchange is impaired, leading to ventilation–perfusion abnormalities and dyspnea. With the appearance of an inflammatory response, clinical illness usually occurs.

Resolution of the infection with eventual healing occurs with successful containment of the pathogenic microorganisms. However, little is known about the actual processes that halt the acute inflammatory reaction in pneumonia and initiate recovery.

Aspiration pneumonia. The risk of aspiration pneumonia arises when anatomic defense mechanisms are impaired such as occurs with seizures; a depressed central nervous system (CNS) inhibiting the cough reflex; recurrent gastroesophageal reflux; neuromuscular disorders, especially with suck–swallow dysfunction; anatomic abnormalities (laryngeal cleft or tracheoesophageal fistula); and debilitating illnesses. Chronic aspiration often causes recurrent bouts of acute febrile pneumonia. Although any region may be affected, the right side—especially the right upper lobe in the supine person—is commonly affected because of the anatomic configuration of the right main-stem bronchus.

Fungal pneumonia. Pneumonia caused by fungi may manifest with mild symptoms, although some people become very ill. The three most common types, *histoplasmosis, coccidioidomycosis,* and *blastomycosis,* are generally specific to a limited geographic area. Other fungal lung infections primarily affect people with compromised immune systems. Diagnosis is made by culturing sputum samples.

Viral pneumonia. Viral pneumonia is usually mild and self-limiting, often bilateral and panlobular but confined to the septa rather than the intraalveolar spaces as is more likely with bacterial pneumonia. Viral pneumonia can be a primary infection creating an ideal environment for a secondary bacterial infection, or it can be a complication of another viral illness such as measles or chickenpox. The virus destroys ciliated epithelial cells and invades goblet cells and bronchial mucous glands. Bronchial walls become edematous and infiltrated with leukocytes. The destroyed bronchial epithelium sloughs throughout the respiratory tract, preventing mucociliary clearance.

Bacterial pneumonia. Destruction of the respiratory epithelium by infection with the influenza virus may be one mechanism whereby influenza predisposes people to bacterial pneumonia. The lung parenchyma, especially the alveoli in the lower lobes, is the most common site of bacterial pneumonia.

The infection is usually limited to one or two lobes.

***Pneumocystis carinii* pneumonia.** *Pneumocystis carinii* pneumonia (PCP) is a progressive, often fatal pneumonia with an unknown origin of organism. It is possibly acquired from the environment, from infected humans, or from animals, fungi, or protozoa. Previously the majority of people with AIDS developed PCP during the course of their illness, but this is much less common now with pharmacologic *prophylaxis.* PCP has been shown to be the first indicator of conversion from human immunodeficiency virus (HIV) infection to the designation of AIDS. In a retrospective 10-year analysis of people with PCP, 6 out of 18 patients were HIV positive.[158] Other people at risk for the development of PCP include anyone who is immunosuppressed for organ transplantation, by chemotherapy for lymphoma or leukemia, by steroid therapy, or by malnutrition.

Clinical Manifestations

Most cases of bacterial pneumonia are preceded by an upper respiratory infection (URI), frequently viral. Signs and symptoms of pneumonia include sudden and sharp pleuritic chest pain aggravated by chest movement and accompanied by a hacking, productive cough with rust-colored or green purulent sputum. Other symptoms include dyspnea, tachypnea accompanied by decreased chest excursion on the affected side, cyanosis, headache, fatigue, fever and chills, and generalized aches and myalgias that may extend to the thighs and calves. Older adults with bronchopneumonia have fewer symptoms than younger people, and 25%

remain afebrile because of the changes in temperature regulation as part of the normal aging process. Associated changes in gas exchange (hypoxia and hypercapnia) may result in altered mental status (e.g., confusion) or loss of balance, which may lead to falls.

Most cases of pneumonia are relatively mild and resolve within 1 to 2 weeks, although symptoms may linger for 3 to 4 weeks total (more typical of viral or mycoplasmal pneumonia). If the infection develops slowly with a fever so low as to be unnoticeable, the person may have what is referred to as "walking pneumonia." This form tends to last longer than any other form of pneumonia. Complications of pneumonia can include pleural effusion (fluid around the lung), *empyema* (pus in the pleural cavity), and, more rarely, lung abscess.

Medical Management

Diagnosis

The clinical presentations of pneumonias caused by different pathogenic microorganisms overlap considerably, requiring microscopic examination of respiratory secretions in making a differential diagnosis. A blood culture may help identify the bacteria, but bacterial counts are positive in only approximately 10% of bacterial pneumonias; 90% of bacterial pneumonias do not show a positive bacterial count.

The U.S. Food and Drug Administration (FDA) has approved a simple, quick urine test (urinary antigen testing) for detecting *Streptococcus pneumoniae* that provides results in 15 minutes. Immediate test results allow specific treatment to begin right away, thus controlling antibiotic overuse and antibiotic resistance by using cost-effective targeted antibiotics. Results of the urine test should be confirmed with a culture. Research continues to develop new diagnostic techniques to determine the microbiologic cause of pneumonia.

Other diagnostic procedures may include chest x-ray studies and computed tomography (CT) scans. These will show *infiltrates* that may involve a single lobe (lobar pneumonia from staphylococci), or may be more diffuse, as in the case of bronchopneumonia (usually streptococci). *Percussion* and *auscultation* of the chest may reveal signs of lung consolidation such as dullness, inspiratory crackles, or bronchial breath sounds.

Treatment

The primary treatment for bacterial and mycoplasmal forms of pneumonia is antibiotic therapy along with rest and fluids. Treatment with specific antibiotics is based on the history; whether the pneumonia was acquired in the community, hospital, or extended care facility; and on the medical status and overall condition of the client (e.g., otherwise healthy or debilitated). Airway clearance techniques (ACTs) (also known as *chest physical therapy, pulmonary physical therapy,* and *pulmonary hygiene*) may aid in clearing purulent sputum. ACTs can include but are not limited to percussion and vibration complemented by postural drainage; deep breathing and cough assisted techniques; and the use of mechanical devices (e.g., the Vest, Acapella, Flutter).

Fungal pneumonia is treated with antifungal drugs. Viral pneumonia is treated symptomatically unless secondary bacterial pneumonia develops. Hospitalization may be required for the immunocompromised client.

A vaccine is recommended for everyone age 65 years or older; for people with chronic disorders of the lungs, heart, liver, or kidneys; for individuals with poorly controlled diabetes mellitus; and for those with a compromised immune system or confined to a long-term care facility. Immunization can provide protection from pneumococcal disease for a period of 3 to 5 years in over 80% of vaccinated persons. A pneumococcal conjugate vaccine that is effective against invasive pneumococcal disease—and to a lesser degree against otitis media and pneumonia—has been licensed in the United States for routine use in infants and in high-risk children.[243,304]

The pneumonia vaccine has been successful in reducing incidence of penicillin-resistant *S. pneumoniae* by 81% in infants and 49% in the elderly from 1999 to 2004. Because pneumonia is a common complication of the flu, the U.S. Centers for Disease Control and Prevention (CDC) recommends annual flu vaccinations as well.

Prognosis

CAP remains a common and serious clinical problem despite the availability of potent antibiotics and aggressive supportive measures. Hospital-acquired pneumonia (HAP) has an even higher mortality rate. Pneumonia ranks seventh among the causes of death in the United States and currently accounts for almost 40% of hospital deaths; 90% of those fatalities occur in people over age 65 years, largely a result of coexisting medical problems that weaken the immune system.

Highly effective prevention and treatment methods can improve survival and reduce the likelihood of developing pneumonia, but one-half of older adults do not get vaccinations that could cut the death rate in half. *Healthy People 2020* objective 1-9c is to reduce hospitalization for immunization-preventable pneumonia to 8 per 10,000 in persons age 65 years or older.

11.3 Special Implications for the PTA: Pneumonia The Centers for Disease Control and Prevention (CDC) recommends adherence to standard precautions for clients with pneumonia. At the very least, careful handwashing by all personnel involved is essential for reducing the transmission of infectious agents. Adequate hydration and pulmonary hygiene, including deep breathing, coughing, and airway clearance techniques, should be instituted in all clients hospitalized with pneumonia. Ventilatory support and supplemental oxygen may be needed to maintain adequate gas exchange in severely compromised clients.

Preventive measures are important and include early ambulation in postoperative clients and postpartal women unless contraindicated. Proper positioning to prevent aspiration during the postoperative period and for all people who are immobilized or who have a poor gag reflex is important.

Occasionally a lower lobe infection can irritate the diaphragmatic surface so that pain referred to the shoulder is the presenting symptom. For the client with a known diagnosis of pneumonia, the breathing pattern and the position assumed in bed can indicate the client's discomfort, reveal tachypnea, and demonstrate splinting of the chest to minimize pleuritic pain (i.e., lying on the affected side reduces the pleural rubbing that often causes discomfort).

Lobes affected by pneumonia will remain vulnerable to further infection for some time, especially in the bedridden, debilitated, or neuromuscularly compromised population. Airway clearance techniques are not usually helpful in adults with uncomplicated pneumonias. However, the client, family, or caretakers should be instructed in breathing exercises and a positional rotation program with frequent positional changes to prevent secretions from accumulating in dependent positions and to optimize ventilation–perfusion matching.

Pulmonary Tuberculosis

Definition

Tuberculosis (TB), historically known as *consumption,* is an infectious, inflammatory systemic disease that affects the lungs and may disseminate to involve lymph nodes and other organs. TB is caused by infection with *Mycobacterium tuberculosis* and is characterized by granulomas, caseous (resembling cheese) necrosis, and subsequent cavity formation typically in the lungs. Latent infection is defined as harboring *M. tuberculosis* without evidence of active infection; active infection is based on the presence of clinical and laboratory findings.

Overview

TB may be primary or secondary. The first or primary infection with the tubercle bacillus is usually asymptomatic and almost always (99%) remains quiet after the development of a hypersensitivity to the microorganism. The primary infection usually involves the middle or lower lung area with lesions in the lung parenchyma. These lesions quickly spread to the bronchopulmonary lymph nodes, where they gain access to the bloodstream. This predisposes the person to the subsequent development of chronic pulmonary and *extrapulmonary* TB at a later time.

Secondary TB develops as a result of reinfection by the tubercle bacillus. This is the most common form of clinical TB. Reactivated TB usually causes abnormalities in the upper lobes of one or both lungs. In the United States, development of secondary TB is almost always the result of reinfection that occurs when the primary lesion becomes active as a result of debilitation or lowered resistance.

Incidence

Despite improved methods of detection and treatment, TB remains a global health problem with the highest rates in Southeast Asia, sub-Saharan Africa, and Eastern Europe (new cases 200 to 400 per 100,000).[62] Before the development of anti-TB drugs in the late 1940s, TB was the leading cause of death in the United States. Drug therapy, along with improvements in public health and general living standards, resulted in a marked decline in incidence. However, recent influxes of immigrants from developing nations, rising homeless populations, prolonged life spans, and the emergence of HIV led to an increase in reported cases in the mid-1980s, reversing a 40-year period of decline.

Overall, from 1985 to 1992 there was a 20% increase in new TB cases in the United States. Now, after years of rising TB infection rates, the United States has started to see a decrease in the annual number of cases (current incidence is 4.8 cases per 100,000 U.S.–born individuals) by 3.8%, and the incidence among foreign-born persons has not risen.[71,170] Cases of multidrug-resistant TB have continued to rise annually, and there remains a huge reservoir of individuals who are infected.

Multidrug-resistant TB has emerged as a major infectious disease problem throughout the world. The infected individual begins taking the prescribed medication, feels better, and discontinues taking the drugs, which are normally required to be taken 6 to 9 months. The disease flares up months later and is now resistant to the medications, and the infected person passes it along as a new drug-resistant strain characterized by mutations in existing genes.[106] The factors contributing to the rise in multidrug-resistant TB are the increased incidence of TB in populations without easy access to anti-TB medications (e.g., homeless people and economically disadvantaged people), the deterioration of the public health infrastructure, interruptions in the drug supply, and inadequate training of health care providers regarding the epidemiology of TB and the AIDS pandemic.

Risk Factors

Although TB can affect anyone, certain segments of the population have an increased risk of contracting the disease, particularly those with HIV infection and people age 65 or older. The latter constitute nearly one-half of the newly diagnosed cases of TB in the United States and most cases of reactivation of dormant mycobacteria.

Other groups at risk include (1) economically disadvantaged or homeless people living in overcrowded conditions, frequently ethnic groups such as Hispanics, Native Americans, and Asian/Pacific Islanders; (2) immigrants from Southeast Asia, Africa (high HIV incidence), Eastern Europe, Mexico, and Latin America; (3) persons dependent on injection drugs, alcohol, or other drugs associated with malnutrition, debilitation, and poor health; (4) infants and children under the age of 5; (5) current or past prison inmates; (6) persons with diabetes mellitus; (7) persons with end-stage renal disease; and (8) others who are immunocompromised (not only those who are HIV infected but also those who are malnourished, organ transplant recipients, and anyone receiving cancer chemotherapy or prolonged corticosteroid therapy).

The Institute of Medicine (IOM) estimates that more than one-half of all TB cases in the United States are attributable to foreign-born residents. The IOM has published a report calling for TB screening of all U.S. immigrants to prevent a predicted resurgence of the disease in the United States.[162]

Limited access to health care because of socioeconomic status or illegal alien status and sociocultural differences contribute to delays in seeking care and influence adherence to treatment, contributing to the rise in TB among foreign-born residents, especially along the U.S.–Mexican border.[238]

Environmental factors that enhance transmission include contact between susceptible persons and an infectious person in relatively small, enclosed spaces (e.g., evidence of limited transmission during extended airline, train, or bus travel has been documented)[182]; inadequate ventilation that results in insufficient dilution or removal of infectious droplet nuclei (e.g., older buildings such as hospitals, prisons, government buildings, universities); and recirculation of air containing infectious droplet nuclei. Adequate ventilation is the most important measure to reduce the infectiousness of the environment. Mycobacteria are susceptible to ultraviolet irradiation (i.e., sunshine), so outdoor transmission of infection rarely occurs.

Etiologic Factors

The causative agent is the tubercle bacillus (Fig. 11.5), commonly transmitted in the United States by inhalation of infected airborne particles, known as *droplet nuclei,* which are produced when the infected persons sneeze, laugh, speak, sing, or cough.

Casual contact or brief exposure to a few bacilli will not result in transmission of sufficient bacilli to infect a person. Rather, prolonged exposure in an enclosed space is required for transmission. Genetic factors determining susceptibility and resistance to the infection are suspected but have not been proven.

The tubercle bacillus is capable of surviving for months in sputum that is not exposed to sunlight. Within the body it becomes encapsulated and can lie dormant for decades and then become reactivated years after an initial infection. This is

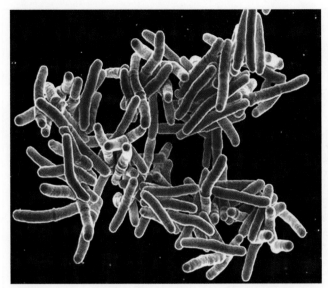

FIG. 11.5 Tuberculosis (TB) bacteria. (Courtesy National Institute of Allergy and Infectious Diseases [NIAID].)

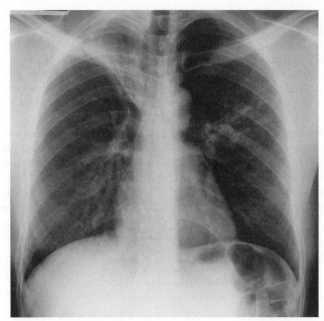

FIG. 11.6 Segmental consolidation in tuberculous bronchopneumonia. The right upper lobe is grossly collapsed, scarred, and bronchiectatic. It had remained stable for many years until segmental nodular and linear consolidation appeared in the left middle zone, signaling reactivation. The segmental lesion was thought to be secondary to aspiration of bacteria from the right upper lobe.

how secondary TB infection can occur at any time the person's resistance is lowered (e.g., alcoholism, immunosuppression, silicosis, advancing age, or cancer).

The older people of today were children when transmission of tubercle bacilli occurred more often. Now reactivation of the disease is developing in their later years because an increasing portion of older adults who were previously not infected are acquiring new infections in extended care facilities.

Pathogenesis

After a susceptible person has inhaled droplet nuclei containing *M. tuberculosis* and bacilli have become established in the alveoli of the lungs, epithelial cells surround and encapsulate the multiplying bacilli in an attempt to wall off the invading organisms, thus forming a typical tubercle.

Two to 10 weeks after initial human infection with the bacilli, immunity usually limits further multiplication and spread of the TB bacilli. Although the TB bacilli are walled off inside a tubercle, the bacilli are not necessarily destroyed; they can remain alive but dormant inside the structure.

No one yet knows how the TB bacterium does its damage. The organisms grow for 2 to 12 weeks until they reach a number sufficient to elicit a cellular immune response that can be detected by a reaction to the tuberculin skin test.

The organisms tend to be localized or focused at sites of infection. In persons with intact immunity, granulomas are formed that limit multiplication and spread of the organism, rendering the infection inactive, or *latent*. The tubercles stay intact as long as the immune system is maintained.

For the majority of individuals with an intact immune system, latent infection is clinically and radiographically undetected; a positive tuberculin (protein purified derivative [PPD]) skin test result is the only indication that infection has taken place. Individuals with latent TB infection (LTBI) but not active disease are not infectious and cannot transmit the organism. When residual lesions are visible on a chest radiograph, these sites remain potential lesions for reactivation.

If, however, the infection is not controlled by the immune defenses, the person develops symptoms of progressive primary

TB. The granulomas become necrotic in the center and eventually produce fibrosis and calcification of the tissues.

Tubercle bacilli can spread to other parts of the body by way of the lymphatics to the lymph nodes and then through the bloodstream to more distant sites. This produces a condition called *miliary* (evenly distributed small nodules) *TB*, most common in people 50 years old or older and in very young children with unstable or underdeveloped immune systems.

Once TB has entered the circulatory system, bacilli are carried to all areas of the body and may lodge in any organ, especially the lymph system, the spine and weight-bearing joints, the urogenital system, and the meninges. Untreated, these tiny lesions spread and produce large areas of infection (e.g., TB pneumonia, tubercular meningitis). The same pharmacologic treatment is used for extrapulmonary and pulmonary TB, though the duration may be extended for some neurologic or skeletal infections.[126]

Clinical Manifestations

Most symptoms associated with TB do not appear in the early, most curable stage of the disease, although a skin test administered would be positive. Often symptoms are delayed until 1 year or more after initial exposure to the bacilli. Symptoms suggestive of TB include productive cough of more than 3 weeks' duration accompanied by weight loss, fever, night sweats, fatigue, malaise, and anorexia. Rales may be heard in the area of lung involvement, as well as bronchial breath sounds, if there is lung consolidation.

Complications associated with TB can include bronchopleural fistulae, esophagopleural fistulae, pleurisy with effusion, tuberculous pneumonia or laryngitis, and sudden lung atelectasis, indicating that a deep tuberculous cavity in the lung has perforated or created an opening into the pleural cavity, allowing air and infected material to flow to it (Fig. 11.6).

Extrapulmonary involvement (e.g., abdominal, pericardial, genitourinary, lymph node, CNS, or skeletal TB) increases in frequency in the presence of declining immunocompetency. Extrapulmonary TB occurs alone (i.e., without pulmonary involvement) in one-third of HIV-infected persons and in another one-third of HIV-infected persons with pulmonary involvement.[12] Tuberculous involvement of the brain and spinal cord is a common neurologic disorder in developing countries and has recently shown resurgence when associated with HIV. In tuberculous meningitis the process is located primarily at the base of the brain, and symptoms include those related to cranial nerve involvement, as well as headache, decreased level of consciousness, and neck stiffness. Tuberculous meningitis is associated with high morbidity and mortality. Tuberculous spondylitis (Pott's disease) is a rare complication of extrapulmonary TB.

Medical Management

Prevention

Preventing the transmission of TB is essential and can be done by using such simple measures as covering the mouth and nose with a tissue when coughing and sneezing, reducing the number of organisms excreted into the air. However, preventive and therapeutic interventions must address not only the bacillus but also the financial, nutritional, and employment status of those people at risk.

Adequate room ventilation and preventing overcrowding in homeless shelters and prisons are well-known preventive measures.

The term *preventive drug therapy* has been changed to *treatment of LTBI*. The failure of vaccination with bacille to control the global TB epidemic and the spread of multidrug resistance has resulted in renewed research efforts to develop a better vaccine. New vaccines could be soon available, and live vaccines are currently being tested.[217]

Diagnosis

Diagnostic measures for identifying TB currently include history, physical examination, tuberculin skin test, chest radiograph, and microscopic examination and culture of sputum. The tuberculin skin test determines whether the body's immune response has been activated by the presence of the bacillus. The skin and other tissues become sensitized to the protein part of the tubercle bacilli. A positive reaction causes a swelling or hardness at the site of infection and develops 3 to 10 weeks after the initial infection. A positive skin test reaction indicates the presence of a TB infection but does not show whether the infection is dormant or is causing a clinical illness. Other diagnostic methods, such as sputum analysis, bronchoscopy, or biopsy, may be indicated in some cases.

Because of the dormant properties of the tubercle bacillus, anyone infected with TB should have periodic TB testing performed. In the case of someone with known TB, the skin test will always be positive, requiring periodic screening with chest x-ray studies. Previously an annual examination was recommended, but currently screening is based on symptomatic presentation (if asymptomatic, testing is not required) and job exposure (e.g., health care workers treating persons with active TB, AIDS, or HIV infection are at increased risk of exposure).

11.4 Special Implications for the PTA: Pulmonary Tuberculosis

Health care workers should be alert at all times to the need for preventing TB transmission when cough-inducing procedures are being performed, but especially in cases of known TB or human immunodeficiency virus (HIV) infection. Isolation measures for anyone who may be dispersing *Mycobacterium tuberculosis* must be taken both in the acute care setting and in outpatient areas. Inpatient rooms must be posted with airborne and acid-fast bacilli (AFB) precautions.

If there is a high degree of suspicion or proved TB, clients should be cared for in negative-pressure isolation rooms while undergoing assessment and/or treatment. Procedures that may generate infectious aerosols should be carried out in similarly ventilated rooms. Precautions must be followed by all health care personnel having contact with clients diagnosed with TB (Box 11.4).

PTAs may be asked to assist individuals with a weak cough to generate a stronger one, either to improve ventilation or sometimes to obtain a sputum sample without performance of the more invasive bronchoscopy. In such cases, the PTA should always check to see if the person has ever been diagnosed with pulmonary TB or had a recent TB test. When in doubt, the PTA should practice self-protective measures such as wearing a high-efficiency particulate air (HEPA) respirator or a protective mask. Training in the use of the mask and the proper sizing for the PTA are important.

People with TB typically have poor nutritional status and progressive weight loss that may have secondary effects on the musculoskeletal system such as postural defects and trigger point irritability. The effects of isolation result in disuse atrophy and cardiopulmonary and physical deconditioning, including progressive dyspnea.

Chest expansion may be decreased because of diffuse fibrotic changes in progressive disease. Tracheal deviation may be present if there is a significant loss of volume in the upper lobes. Postural adaptations may have developed in late stages of the disease because of poor breathing patterns.[112] Other areas of treatment should include correcting overall posture, gait pattern, muscle strength, balance, and functional mobility.

Finding the balance between exercise and clinical limitations is challenging, and there is little evidence that exercise is effective in people with active TB. Exercise training for patients with post-TB lung disorders has been shown to be effective in improving oxygen uptake, dyspnea, functional outcomes, and timed walking distance.[14,358]

Side effects of the medication can lead to peripheral neuritis that may be brought to the attention of the PTA. This and any other complication, such as hepatitis, hemoptysis, optic neuritis, or purpura, should be reported to the physician.

Extrapulmonary TB is much less common than pulmonary TB but occurs in 50% of individuals with concurrent HIV. Musculoskeletal and nervous system lesions are prevalent in extrapulmonary TB cases. Treatment of Pott's disease follows the same chemotherapy regimen, with prompt response. Immobilization and avoidance of weight bearing may be required to relieve pain, with attention to maintaining strength and range of motion.

Treatment for the Health Care Worker

For the health care worker who is exposed to TB and develops active disease, treatment will yield a "cure" if the appropriate pharmacologic intervention is followed for the full course prescribed, usually a minimum of 6 months. A cure simply means the active TB will not likely recur, but the person can be reexposed and reinfected. Treatment failure (not taking enough medication or for long enough duration) is a more likely outcome than reinfection or redisease because treatment compliance (i.e., noncompliance) is a much bigger problem.

A person with active disease who misses 2 weeks of treatment must restart the entire course and risks the development of drug-resistant infection. After 2 weeks on effective medication, more than

85% of people with positive sputum cultures convert to a noninfectious status. Although the individual is no longer considered infectious, a minimum of 6 months is required before the disease is considered cured.

If the health care worker is exposed and infected but does not develop active disease (approximately 90% of all cases), there is a 10% lifetime risk that active disease can develop; one-half of that risk is present in the first 2 years. That 10% risk can be reduced to approximately a 1% risk if a single prophylactic medication is taken properly for 6 months.

In such cases, the individual is considered a "TB reactor" and will always test positive on skin tests for TB. These individuals will require TB clearance in order to work in health care settings, schools, or similar settings. Clearance is provided via medical documentation of treatment and a letter from the attending physician.

The TB bacterium must be inhaled and cannot be transmitted by physical contact with extrapulmonary sites unless the organism is expelled, aerosolized, and then inhaled. Although unusual, this type of situation may be encountered during wound care involving the integument and should be approached with appropriate standard precautions.

Lung Abscess

Definition

Described as a localized accumulation of purulent exudate within the lung, an abscess usually develops as a complication of pneumonia, especially aspiration and staphylococcal pneumonia. This can occur when bacteria are aspirated from the oropharynx along with foreign material or vomitus, or it can occur from septic embolus from a heart valve. Septic pulmonary emboli from staphylococcal endocarditis of the tricuspid or pulmonary valves are most often a complication of the use of illicit injection drugs. An abscess may also form when a neoplasm becomes necrotic and contains purulent material that does not drain from the area because of partial or complete obstruction.

Risk Factors

Aspiration associated with alcoholism is the single most common condition predisposing to lung abscess. Other predisposed persons include those with altered levels of consciousness because of drug or alcohol use as mentioned, seizures, general anesthesia, lung cancer, or CNS disease; impaired gag reflex as a result of esophageal disease or neurologic disorders; poor dentition and periodontal care; and tracheal or nasogastric tubes, which disrupt the mechanical defenses of the airways.

Pathogenesis and Clinical Manifestations

As with all abscesses, a lung abscess is a natural defense mechanism in which the body attempts to localize an infection and wall off the microorganisms so these cannot spread throughout the body. As the microorganisms destroy the local parenchymal tissue (including alveoli, airways, and blood vessels), an inflammatory process causes alveoli to fill with fluid, pus, and microorganisms (consolidation). Death and decay of consolidated tissue may progress proximally until the abscess drains into the bronchus, spreading the infection to other parts of the lung and forming cavities (*cavitation*).

Clinical signs and symptoms of abscess formation almost always include a productive cough of foul-smelling sputum and persistent fever. Other characteristic features include chills,

---

BOX 11.4   Guidelines for Therapists for Preventing Transmission of Tuberculosis

All tuberculosis (TB) control recommendations for inpatient facilities apply to hospices and home health services and outpatient settings.

All facilities should have a supervisor in charge of infection control *compliance*.

All new employees (and student therapists) should be screened with the two-step tuberculin skin test or blood assay *Mycobacterium tuberculosis* test (BAMT).

Doors to airborne infection isolation (AII) rooms must be kept closed.

Clients infected with TB must cover mouth and nose with tissues when coughing, sneezing, or laughing.

Cough-inducing procedures should not be performed on TB clients unless absolutely necessary; such procedures should be performed using local exhaust in a HEPA-filtered booth or individual TB isolation room. After completion of treatment, such persons should remain in the booth or enclosure until the cough has subsided.

Clients must wear a mask when leaving the room.

Anyone entering the room must wear a protective mask, or HEPA respirator, properly.

Therapists must be adequately trained in the use and disposal of masks and should use a PR, which is a special mask,[a] whenever the client is undergoing cough-inducement or aerosol-generating procedures.

The therapist must check the condition of both the face piece and face seal each time the PR is worn.

Gloves are worn when touching infective material.

Disinfect the stethoscope between treatment sessions.

Staff and employees attending clients in all settings must be tested for TB: every 6 months for high-risk therapists, and other personnel annually.

Handwashing is required before and after contact with the client.

Isolation precautions must be continued until a clinical and bacteriologic response to medical treatment has been demonstrated.

Environmental surfaces (e.g., walls, crutches, bed rails, and walkers) are not associated with transmission of infections; only routine cleaning of such items is required.

Therapists with current pulmonary or laryngeal TB should be excluded from work until adequate treatment is instituted, cough is resolved, and sputum is free of bacilli on three consecutive smears.

Home health personnel can reinforce client education about the importance of taking medications as prescribed.

HEPA, High-efficiency particulate air; *PR,* particulate respirator.
[a]There are several types of face masks designated as particulate respirators; all National Institute for Occupational Safety and Health (NIOSH)–certified respirators are acceptable protection for health care workers against *M. tuberculosis.* The respiratory protection standard set by the Occupational Safety and Health Administration (OSHA) requires a NIOSH-certified respirator; when such a respirator is used, the law requires that a training and fit-test program be present.
From Jensen PA, Lambert LA, Iademarco MF, et al.: Guidelines for preventing the transmission of *Mycobacterium tuberculosis* in healthcare settings, MMWR Recomm Rep 54:1–141, 2005.

---

dyspnea, pleuritic chest pain, cyanosis, and clubbing of fingernails, which can develop over a short period of time. Cavitation causes severe cough with copious amounts of purulent sputum and sometimes hemoptysis.

Pneumonitis

Pneumonitis is an acute inflammation of lung tissue. It is usually caused by infections and is discussed in this chapter (see section on environmental and occupational diseases) under its most common presentation as hypersensitivity pneumonitis. Other causes of pneumonitis include lupus pneumonitis associated with systemic lupus erythematosus (SLE), aspiration pneumonitis associated with inspiration of acidic gastric fluid, obstructive pneumonitis associated with lung cancer, and interstitial pneumonitis associated with AIDS. Consolidation with impaired gas exchange may occur in the involved lung tissue, but with successful inactivation of the infecting agent, resolution occurs with restoration of normal lung structure.

Acute Bronchitis

Acute bronchitis is an inflammation of the trachea and bronchi (tracheobronchial tree) that is of short duration (1 to 3 weeks) and self-limiting with few pulmonary signs. It may result from chemical irritation, such as from smoke, fumes, or gas, or it may occur with viral infections such as influenza, measles, chickenpox, or whooping cough.

Symptoms of acute bronchitis include the early symptoms of a URI or a common cold that progress to fever; a dry, irritating cough caused by transient hyperresponsiveness; sore throat; possible laryngitis; and chest pain from the effort of coughing. Later, the cough becomes more productive of purulent sputum, followed by wheezing. There may be constitutional symptoms, including moderate fever with accompanying chills, back pain, muscle pain and soreness, and headache.

Clients with viral bronchitis have a nonproductive cough that is aggravated by cold, dry, or dusty air. Bacterial bronchitis (common in clients with COPD) causes retrosternal (behind the sternum) pain that is aggravated by coughing.

Acute bronchitis should be differentiated from chronic bronchitis, pneumonia, whooping cough, rhinosinus conditions, and gastrointestinal reflux disease before treatment begins.[46] Treatment is conservative and symptomatic with cough suppressants, rest, humidity, good nutrition, and hydration.

Seasonal vaccination of people with recurrent bouts of bronchitis reduces the number and severity of *exacerbations* over the winter months.[104] Bronchodilators are not indicated, and the use of antibiotics for acute bronchitis is not recommended.[46,342]

Prognosis is usually good with treatment, and although acute bronchitis is usually mild, it can become complicated in people with chronic lung or heart disease and in older adults because they are more susceptible to secondary infections. Pneumonia is a critical complication.

OBSTRUCTIVE DISEASES

Chronic Obstructive Pulmonary Disease
Definition

COPD, also called *chronic obstructive lung disease,* refers to chronic airflow limitation that is not fully reversible. Asthma, chronic bronchitis, obstructive bronchiolitis,[322] and emphysema are all forms of pathology that manifest as COPD. Although these diseases share a common obstructive component and can occur independently, they most commonly coexist, requiring differing treatment and having different prognoses.

Incidence and Risk Factors

COPD is second only to heart disease as a cause of disability in adults younger than 65 years of age. It is the fourth leading cause of death in the United States, predicted to be the third leading cause of death by 2020. Nearly 12 million people in the United States were diagnosed with COPD in 2000, but the prevalence is much

higher (nearly 24 million adults have documented lung impairment). There were approximately 119,000 deaths from COPD in 2000. The estimated cost of COPD was $32.1 billion in 2002.

COPD is almost always caused by exposure to environmental irritants, especially smoking, which is the most common cause of COPD; this condition rarely occurs in nonsmokers. As with all chronic diseases, the prevalence of COPD is strongly associated with age, and the condition usually manifests at age 55 to 60 years. More men are affected than women, but the incidence in women is increasing with the concomitant increase in smoking by women. Because smoking is the major cause of both emphysema and chronic bronchitis, these two conditions often occur together.

Morbidity and mortality rates for COPD increase with the effects of repeated or chronic exposure to irritating gases, dusts, or allergens; chronic irritation; and pollution in urban environments. Other contributing factors include chronic respiratory infections (e.g., sinusitis), periodontal disease,[295] the aging process, heredity, and genetic predisposition.

Pathogenesis and Clinical Manifestations

The pathogenesis and clinical manifestations of each component of COPD are discussed separately in their respective sections. A broad overview of COPD is shown in Fig. 11.7. The person with COPD often develops a characteristic look with shoulders raised and muscles tensed from SOB and the increased WOB (Fig. 11.8).

Medical Management

At least two sets of guidelines for diagnosis and management of COPD are available.[125] One set of guidelines was developed by the Global Initiative for Chronic Obstructive Lung Disease (GOLD), a joint project of the National Heart, Lung, and Blood Institute and the World Health Organization (WHO). Guidelines were also developed jointly by the American Thoracic Society and European Respiratory Society. These groups have set standards and made recommendations for management and future research of COPD.

Diagnosis

Physical examination and air-flow limitation on pulmonary function testing are assessment tools for determining the presence and extent of COPD. A simple and inexpensive portable spirometer permits such testing in the outpatient setting, but it may also be conducted in a respiratory laboratory with a computerized spirometer; the results should not be used interchangeably.

Spirometry is the most basic and frequently performed test of pulmonary (lung) function. The spirometer measures how much air the lungs can hold and how well the respiratory system is able to move air into and out of the lungs. Because spirometry is based on a maximal forced exhalation, the accuracy of its results are highly dependent on the person's understanding, cooperation, and best efforts. Spirometry differs from peak flow readings in that spirometry records the entire forced breathing capacity against time, and peak flow records the largest breathing flow that can be sustained.

The spirometer measures the expired air-flow rate and volume in a specific time period. More than a 10% difference measured before and after activity or before and after medication (a bronchodilator) is considered diagnostic for a reactive airway disease component of COPD. Predicted values based on age, height, gender, and body weight are compared with actual values to determine the numeric (%) comparison (Table 11.5).[60]

Spirometry results are expressed as a percentage and are considered abnormal if they are less than 80% of the normal predicted value. An abnormal result usually indicates the presence of some degree of obstructive lung disease. Forced expiratory volume in 1 second (FEV_1) values (percentage of predicted) can be used to classify the obstruction, which may occur as mild to very severe.

History, clinical examination, x-ray studies, and laboratory findings usually enable the physician to distinguish COPD from other obstructive pulmonary disorders, such as bronchiectasis, adult CF, and central airway obstruction. High-resolution CT scan is used to diagnose and quantify emphysema. Most cases of emphysema involve a history of cigarette smoking, chronic cough and sputum production, and dyspnea.

Laboratory analysis may include blood gas measurements and blood pH to determine the presence of hypoxemia or hypercapnia (excess carbon dioxide in blood) and acid–base balance, sputum culture, or presence of immunoglobulin E (IgE) antibodies against specific allergens.

Treatment

The successful management of COPD requires a multifaceted approach that includes smoking cessation, pharmacologic management, airway clearance as needed, exercise (aerobic, strength, flexibility, posture, and breathing), control of complications, avoidance of irritants, psychologic support, and dietary management.

The main goals for the client with COPD are to improve oxygenation and decrease carbon dioxide retention. These are accomplished by:

1. Reducing airway edema secondary to inflammation and bronchospasm (asthma) through the use of bronchodilator medication
2. Facilitating the elimination of bronchial secretions
3. Preventing and treating respiratory infection
4. Increasing exercise tolerance
5. Controlling complications
6. Avoiding airway irritants and allergens
7. Relieving anxiety and treating depression, which often accompany COPD
8. Exercising to improve muscle oxidative capacity

Common classifications of medications used in the treatment of COPD include oral or inhaled bronchodilators, antiinflammatory agents, antibiotics, mucolytic expectorants, mast cell membrane stabilizers, and antihistamines. These medications may have side effects that will affect the person's response to physical therapy treatments (Table 11.6). Combining bronchodilators improves effectiveness in reducing exacerbations and improves lung function.[94] Systemic corticosteroids are of some help in acute exacerbations of COPD but have some side effects, including hyperglycemia,[353] and do not produce any long-term benefits.[250]

The benefits of pneumococcal vaccine have been proved (decreased mortality and hospitalization), and vaccination is recommended for all people with COPD. Annual prophylactic vaccination against influenza is also recommended.

Narcotics, tranquilizers, and sedatives are used with caution because these depress the respiratory center. Pharmacologic research includes investigation of multiple mediator antagonists, antiinflammatories with better delivery of the medication and lower side effects, induced repair of alveolar tissue, and effects of drug combinations.[94,100]

Long-term oxygen treatment (LTOT) reduces morbidity and extends life in clients with hypoxemia.[76] People with PaO_2 of 55 to 59 mm Hg or less (determined by arterial blood gases [ABGs]) with signs of tissue hypoxemia (see Table 11.2) are considered for long-term oxygen therapy. Oxygen therapy is also considered for those who desaturate during sleep or exercise. The National Heart, Lung, and Blood Institute in collaboration with the Centers for Medicare and Medicaid Services has identified areas of future research to improve care and/or reduce cost of care.[76]

Surgical treatment for COPD remains controversial, but lung-volume reduction surgery (LVRS), which is bilateral pneumectomy or removal of large bullae that compress the lung and add to dead space, has been shown to reduce the lung volume, relieve thoracic distention, improve respiratory mechanics, and reduce morbidity.[61,150] LVRS may be an alternative treatment to lung transplantation for selected individuals with end-stage COPD.

Lung transplantation, both single and double, is appropriate for clients with COPD when FEV_1 is less than 24% predicted and/or the partial pressure of arterial carbon dioxide ($PaCO_2$) is equal to or greater than 55 mm Hg. Pulmonary rehabilitation is considered important in selecting surgical candidates and preparing them for surgery.[279] Survival rates are approximately 80% at year 1, 50% at year 5, and 35% at year 10.[56,219]

Prognosis

The prognosis for individuals with chronic bronchitis and emphysema is poor because these are chronic, progressive, and debilitating diseases. The death rate from COPD has increased 22% in the last decade, especially among older men, and the mortality rate 10 years after diagnosis is greater than 50%. COPD is largely preventable, and many believe that early recognition of small airway obstruction with appropriate treatment and cessation of smoking may prevent relentless progression of this disease. Early treatment of airway infections and vaccination against influenza and pneumococcal disease have an effect on morbidity and mortality of individuals with COPD.

There is no cure for COPD, but smoking cessation and oxygen therapy have been shown to increase the survival rate. Pulmonary rehabilitation has also been shown to improve quality of life, decrease hospitalizations, and decrease incidence of COPD exacerbations.[42,301]

11.5 Special Implications for the PTA: Chronic Obstructive Pulmonary Disease

Pulmonary Rehabilitation

The pulmonary rehabilitation program model contains many intervention components beyond just airway clearance techniques and exercise, including (but not limited to) smoking cessation, nutrition and weight control, psychosocial support, and lifestyle modification, as well as optimal medical care.[107] Treatment of chronic obstructive pulmonary disease (COPD) includes breathing exercises, postural drainage, physical training, a program to improve posture, and strengthening of respiratory musculature. For the motivated child with asthma, breathing exercises and controlled breathing are of value in preventing overinflation, improving the strength of respiratory muscles and the efficiency of the cough, and reducing the work of breathing (WOB).

People with COPD often adopt a sedentary lifestyle owing to their decreased ability to tolerate activity. This leads to progressive deconditioning, which will lead to progressive deterioration in limb and respiratory muscle function that could adversely affect exercise capacity.

Although there is little evidence that rehabilitation efforts can result in improved pulmonary function or arterial blood gases (ABGs), there is strong and growing evidence that programs that include exercise retraining can result in significant benefits such as reduced hospitalizations, increased exercise tolerance, reduced dyspnea, improved skills in using inspiratory muscle training devices, increased independent activities of daily living (ADL) skills, and increased sense of well-being and quality of life.[279]

Exercise

Exercise limitation is a common and disturbing manifestation of COPD caused by multiple interrelated anatomic and physiologic disturbances. Exercise tolerance can be improved despite the presence of fixed structural abnormalities in the lung. Only a weak correlation between degree of airway obstruction and exercise tolerance has been shown, suggesting that factors other than lung function impairment (e.g., deconditioning and peripheral muscle dysfunction) play a predominant role in limiting exercise capacity in people with COPD. In fact, inspiratory capacity is a more powerful predictor of exercise tolerance than forced expiratory volume in 1 second (FEV_1) or forced vital capacity *(FVC)*.[233]

Muscle weakness in stable COPD does not affect all muscles equally. For example, proximal upper limb muscle strength may be impaired more than distal upper limb muscle strength, peripheral muscle may be limited mainly by endurance capacity, and the diaphragm muscle may be altered structurally (e.g., changes in muscle length and configuration affecting the mechanical force and action) and limited in strength capacity. These alterations in different muscle types require individual assessment and exercise prescription.[132,133]

Clients with COPD must be encouraged to remain active, with specific attention directed toward activities they enjoy. Training in pacing and energy conservation allows even those with limited exercise tolerance to increase their daily activities. Exercise testing that is individualized to the specific client's needs and goals is used to determine the person's baseline and for prescribing a training regimen. Medications and oxygen may be used or timed to determine the effect of these interventions. Oximetry, heart rate, respiratory rate, and blood pressure are routinely monitored, and blood gases or expired gases may be used to assess response to testing. Respiratory muscle strength testing is measured as maximum inspiratory and expiratory pressures.[107]

Strengthening the muscles of respiration is done by teaching the person with COPD to take slow, deep breaths and to use pursed-lip breathing. Pursed-lip breathing helps slow the respiratory rate and prevent airway collapse during exhalation. The client is instructed to inhale through the nose and exhale with the lips pursed in a whistling or kissing position. Each inhalation should take about 4 seconds and each exhalation about 6 seconds.

Effective coughing techniques using diaphragmatic breathing help to mobilize secretions. Ventilatory muscle training should be included for anyone who continues to experience exercise limitation and breathlessness despite medical therapy and general exercise reconditioning. Respiratory muscle training improves exercise tolerance, dyspnea, and quality of life.[189]

People with chronic airflow obstruction report disabling dyspnea when performing seemingly trivial tasks (e.g., activity with unsupported arms). Some muscles of the upper torso and shoulder girdle share both a respiratory and a positional function for the arms, resulting in functional limitations in many clients with lung disease during unsupported upper extremity activities.

Simple arm elevation results in significant increases in metabolic and ventilatory requirements in clients with long-term airflow limitations. Pulmonary rehabilitation that includes upper extremity training (progressive resistance exercises [PREs]) reduces metabolic and ventilatory requirements for arm elevation. This type of program may allow clients with COPD to perform sustained upper extremity activities with less dyspnea.[115]

Lower extremity training should be included routinely in the exercise prescription. The choice of type and intensity of training should be based primarily on the individual's baseline functional status, symptoms, needs, and long-term goals. Progressively increased walking is the most common form of exercise for COPD. Swimming is a preferred exercise option for clients with bronchial asthma (see next discussion). PTAs working with these clients should encourage them to maintain hydration by drinking fluids (including before, during, and after exercise) to prevent mucous plugs from hardening and to take medications as prescribed. When tolerated, high-intensity (continuous or interval), short-term training may lead to greater improvements in quality of life and aerobic fitness than low-intensity training of longer duration, but it is not absolutely necessary to achieve gains in exercise endurance.[42,110]

Exercise tolerance may improve after exercise training (including weight training)[67] because of gains in aerobic fitness or peripheral muscle strength,[211] enhanced mechanical skill and efficiency of exercise, and improvements in respiratory muscle function, breathing pattern, or lung hyperinflation. Exercise improves muscle oxidative capacity and recovery in individuals with COPD.[274]

Exercise training can also reduce anxiety, fear, and dyspnea previously associated with exercise in the deconditioned person. Exercises for flexibility, posture, and motor control can improve mechanical and kinetic efficiency and thus can reduce oxygen demand during daily activities and exercise.

Gains made in exercise tolerance, peripheral and respiratory muscle strength, and quality of life can last up to 2 years after a limited duration (6- to 12-week) rehabilitation program.[42,329] The optimal duration for an exercise program remains unknown; a 7-week course provides greater benefits than a 4-week course in terms of improvements in health status. Further studies in this area are needed.[134]

Three training sessions per week improve exercise performance and health status, whereas a program consisting of two sessions per week for 8 weeks may not be effective in people with moderate COPD.[281] Maximally intense exercise sustained over 45 minutes daily, 5 days per week for 6 weeks has been reported more effective in endurance training than exercise of a moderate intensity.[119] Information about other considerations for exercise training in chronic lung disease is available.[2,129,177,348]

Monitoring Vital Signs

Using a pulse oximeter can help the PTA and client observe for a decrease in oxygen saturation before hypoxemia occurs. Oxygen saturation is generally kept at 90% or above by adjusting supplemental oxygen levels, adjusting activity level, and practicing physiologic modulation or physiologic quieting.[160] Some people with COPD retain carbon dioxide and have a depressed hypoxic drive, requiring low oxygen levels to stimulate the respiratory drive. In such cases the upward adjustment of supplemental oxygen levels must be monitored very carefully; increasing total oxygen administered via nasal cannula higher than 1 to 2 L requires careful monitoring of the respiratory system (e.g., respiratory rate and breathing pattern), documentation, and consultation with other members of the pulmonary rehabilitation team.

Blood pressure and pulse should be observed at rest and in response to exercise, especially in anyone with COPD and cardiac arrhythmias. Most people with COPD who have mild arrhythmias at rest do not tend to have increased arrhythmias during exercise. Arrhythmias may disappear with exercise and increased perfusion.

Breath sounds are changed because the loss of interstitial elasticity and the presence of interalveolar septa lead to air trapping with increased volume of air in the lungs. Air pockets are poor transmitters of vibrations; thus vocal fremitus (the client whispers "99, 99, 99"), breath sounds, and the whispered and spoken voice are impaired or absent on auscultation.

This absence of the vesicular quality of lung sounds is distinctive and may be heard before radiographic evidence of COPD. On the other hand, when there is fluid in the lung or lungs, consolidation, or collapse (e.g., atelectasis), whispered words are heard perfectly and clearly. This is the earliest sign of atelectasis.

A peak flowmeter, a home monitoring device to measure fast expiratory flow (a reflection of bronchorestriction), can be used to determine how compromised a client with asthma or reactive airways may be compared with the normal values for that person. This may be a useful measure in determining response to therapy intervention and documenting measurable outcomes.

Exercise and Medication

The majority of pulmonary medications are used to promote bronchodilation and improve alveolar ventilation and oxygenation and are delivered as an aerosol spray through a device called a *metered-dose inhaler* (MDI). Older adults sometimes have difficulty using an inhaler because of arthritis or other medical problems that impair hand–breath coordination.

Proper technique is important to ensure delivery of the medication to the desired location (Box 11.5).[43] When medications are properly used, their effects should improve an individual's ability to exercise and more effectively obtain the benefits of training. However, the many side effects of pulmonary medications may interfere with normal adaptations to habitual exercise so that exercise tolerance and conditioning may not occur.[57]

For example, corticosteroids mask or impede the beneficial effects of exercise. Anyone with pulmonary disease taking corticosteroids for a prolonged period may develop steroid myopathy and muscular atrophy not only in the peripheral skeletal muscles but also in the muscle fibers of the diaphragm. Animal studies also suggest that severe undernutrition causes a decrease in muscle energy status, which contributes to diaphragmatic fatigue.[186] Recent studies have shown promise for use of anabolic steroids and L-carnitine supplements in combating muscle changes in COPD.[38,75]

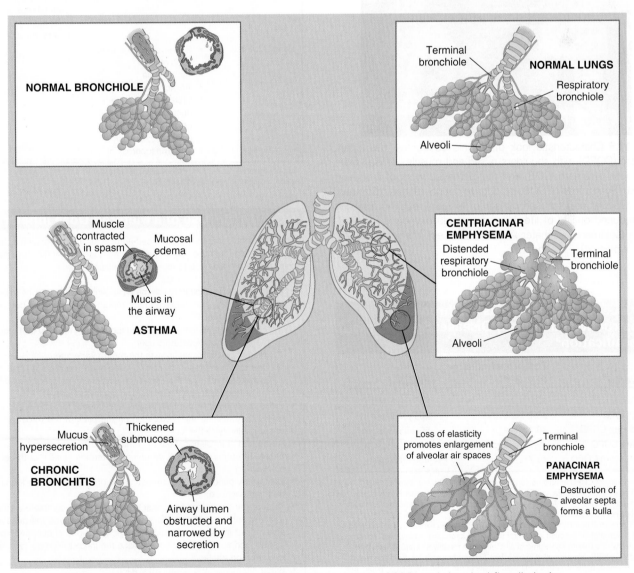

FIG. 11.7 What happens in chronic obstructive lung disease (COPD) and chronic airflow limitation.

Chronic Bronchitis
Definition and Overview

Chronic bronchitis is clinically defined as a condition of productive cough lasting for at least 3 months (usually the winter months) per year for 2 consecutive years. If obstructive lung disease characterized by a decreased FEV_1/FVC ratio less than 75% is combined with chronic cough, chronic bronchitis is diagnosed. Initially, only the larger bronchi are involved, but eventually all airways become obstructed, especially during expiration.

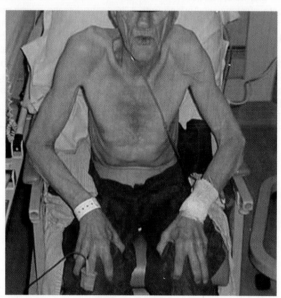

FIG. 11.8 Characteristic look of chronic obstructive pulmonary disease (COPD) with shoulders raised and muscles tensed from shortness of breath (SOB) and the increased work of breathing (WOB). Symptoms of SOB, productive cough, fatigue, dizziness, and muscular pain (caused by lack of oxygen) result in disability and reduced quality of life. Use of portable oxygen is required. (From Goldman L, Schafer AI: Goldman-Cecil medicine, ed 25, Philadelphia, 2016, Saunders.)

TABLE 11.5   Diagnosis of Chronic Obstructive Pulmonary Disease: Spirometric Classification[a]

Severity	Postbronchodilator FEV$_1$/FVC	FEV$_1$ %
At risk	>0.7	≥80 predicted
Mild COPD	≤0.7	≥80 predicted
Moderate COPD	≤0.7	50–80 predicted
Severe COPD	≤0.7	30–50 predicted
Very severe COPD	≤0.7	<30 predicted

[a]The diagnosis of COPD should be considered in anyone who has chronic cough, sputum production, dyspnea, or history of risk factors for COPD. Spirometry is required in making the diagnosis: air-flow limitation that is not reversible is indicated by a post-bronchodilator FEV$_1$/FVC ratio of ≤0.7.

COPD, Chronic obstructive pulmonary disease; *FEV$_1$,* forced expiratory volume in one second (volume of air expelled in the first second of forced expiration); *FVC,* forced vital capacity (the maximum volume of air that can be forcibly and rapidly exhaled). Data from Celli BR, MacNee W; ATS/ERS Task Force: Standards for the diagnosis and treatment of patients with COPD: a summary of the ATS/ERS position paper, Eur Respir J 23:932, 2004.

Risk Factors and Pathogenesis

Chronic bronchitis is characterized by inflammation and scarring of the bronchial lining. This inflammation obstructs air flow to and from the lungs and increases mucus production. Irritants such as cigarette smoke, long-term dust inhalation, or air pollution cause mucus hypersecretion and hypertrophy (increased number and size) of mucus-producing glands in the large bronchi.

The swollen mucous membrane and thick sputum obstruct the airways, causing wheezing and a subsequent cough as the

TABLE 11-6   Common Side Effects of Pulmonary Medications Used to Treat Pulmonary Diseases

	Emphysema, Chronic Bronchitis, Asthma	Cystic Fibrosis
Acute treatment	• Tachycardia • Dizziness • Tremor • Confusion • GI distress	• GI distress • Tachycardia • Tremor • Collagenous tissue destruction (skin, skeletal muscle, cartilage, ligaments, bones)
Long-term use	• GI distress (ibuprofen, antibiotics) • Tachycardia • Tremor • Collagenous tissue destruction (skin, skeletal muscle, cartilage, ligaments, bones) • Immunosuppression	

Courtesy Susan A. Queen, PT, PhD, Associate Professor Emeritus, University of New Mexico, Division of Physical Therapy, 2016.

BOX 11.5   Use of a Metered-Dose Inhaler

The PTA should watch the client self-administer the medication at least one time. Schedule the use of the metered-dose inhaler (MDI) 15 to 20 minutes before exercise to maximize ventilation.

- Shake the unit 5 to 10 times.
- Exhale to normal expiratory volume while slightly tilting your head back.
- Place the inhaler mouthpiece in the mouth in one of three positions (client preference):
  1. In the mouth with the tongue and teeth out of the way (not recommended for corticosteroid use)
  2. Resting on the lower lip with the mouth wide open
  3. One to 1½ inches in front of a wide-open mouth; a 4- to 6-inch spacer that fits over the end of the inhaler can be used to maintain the correct distance while avoiding spraying the eyes
- Press the inhaler and inhale slowly and deeply for 3 to 5 seconds to avoid depositing the medication on the back of the throat and to ensure delivery to the lungs.
- At the end of inhalation, hold the breath for 10 seconds.
- Exhale through pursed lips; when using steroids, rinse mouth before swallowing.
- Wait a few minutes before repeating the procedure if more than one puff is prescribed.
- To determine whether an inhaler is empty, keep a completely empty (marked) inhaler on hand. Place the empty inhaler and the questionable inhaler in a bowl (or sink) of water. If the one in question floats just as high as the empty one, replace the inhaler. Number of doses is written on the label.
- Rinse the inhaler and spacer after each use.

person tries to clear the airways. In addition, impaired ciliary function reduces mucus clearance and increases client susceptibility to infection. Infection results in even more mucus production with bronchial wall inflammation and thickening. As airways collapse, air is trapped in the distal portion of the lung, causing reduced alveolar ventilation, hypoxia, and acidosis. This downward spiral continues because the client now has an abnormal ventilation–perfusion (V/Q) ratio and resultant decreased Pao$_2$.

Clinical Manifestations

The symptoms of chronic bronchitis are persistent cough and sputum production (worse in the morning and evening than at midday). The increased secretion from the bronchial mucosa and obstruction of the respiratory passages interfere with the flow of air to and from the lungs. The result is SOB, prolonged expiration, persistent coughing with expectoration, and recurrent infection. Infection may be accompanied by fever and malaise.

Over time, reduced chest expansion, wheezing, cyanosis, and decreased exercise tolerance develop. In addition, the obstruction results in decreased alveolar ventilation and increased Paco$_2$. Hypoxemia (deficient oxygenation of the blood) leads to polycythemia (overproduction of erythrocytes) and cyanosis. If not reversed, pulmonary hypertension (PH) leads to cor pulmonale. Severe disability or death is the final clinical picture.

Emphysema
Definition and Overview
Emphysema is defined as a pathologic accumulation of air in tissues, particularly in the lungs, and is found in most people with COPD. There are different types of emphysema (see Fig. 11.7).
1. *Centriacinar emphysema* occurs most often in smokers and consists of the following two forms:
    a. Centrilobular emphysema, the most common type, produces destruction in the bronchioles, usually in the upper lung regions. Inflammation develops in the bronchioles, but usually the alveolar sac (distal to the respiratory bronchioles) remains intact.
    b. Panlobular emphysema destroys the air spaces of the entire acinus and most commonly involves the lower lung.
2. *Paraseptal* (panacinar) emphysema destroys the alveoli in the lower lobes of the lungs, resulting in isolated blebs along the lung periphery. Paraseptal emphysema is believed to be the likely cause of spontaneous pneumothorax.

Etiologic Factors
Cigarette smoking is the major etiologic factor in the development of emphysema and has been shown to increase the numbers of alveolar macrophages and neutrophils in the lung. However, other factors, such as heredity, must determine susceptibility to emphysema because fewer than 10% to 15% of people who smoke develop clinical evidence of airway obstruction.

In many cases emphysema occurs as a result of prolonged respiratory difficulties, such as chronic bronchitis that has caused partial obstruction of the smaller divisions of the bronchi. Emphysema can also occur without serious preceding respiratory problems as in the case of a defect in the elastic tissue of the lungs or in older persons whose lungs have lost their natural elasticity.

A number of clients with early onset of COPD have an inherited deficiency of (low levels or absent) AAT, a protective protein. AAT is made in the liver but circulates in the blood to protect the tissues in the body, including the lungs. Epidemiologists report approximately 100,000 people with this disorder; 20 million more may be undiagnosed asymptomatic carriers. AAT deficiency is suspected in smokers who develop emphysema before age 40 years and in nonsmokers who develop emphysema. Symptoms may not develop until affected individuals are in their seventies. Progressive liver (cirrhosis) and lung disease (panlobular emphysema) occur when AAT is absent.[316]

Pathogenesis
Emphysema is a disorder in which destruction of elastin protein in the lung that normally maintains the strength of the alveolar walls leads to permanent enlargement of the acini.

Eventually the loss of elasticity in the lung tissue causes narrowing or collapse of the bronchioles so that inspired air becomes trapped in the lungs, making breathing difficult, especially during the expiratory phase. Obstruction results from changes in lung tissues, rather than from mucus production and swelling as in chronic bronchitis (which is why steroids are usually not helpful in this condition).

The permanent overdistention of the air spaces with destruction of the walls (septa) between the alveoli is accompanied by partial airway collapse and loss of elastic recoil. Pockets of air form between the alveolar spaces (*blebs*) and within the lung parenchyma (*bullae*). This process leads to increased ventilatory dead space, or areas that do not participate in gas or blood exchange (Fig. 11.9).

The WOB is increased as a result of ventilatory drive from hypoxemia and hypercapnia, increased effort during exhalation (normally passive recoil), and flattening of the diaphragm caused by hyperinflation. As the disease progresses, increasing dyspnea and pulmonary infection develop. Respiratory muscle atrophy can lead to deterioration of lung function and increased WOB.[322] PH develops from capillary loss and vessel intimal thickening, and this eventually leads to cor pulmonale (right-sided congestive heart failure).

In centrilobular emphysema the destruction of the lung is uneven and originates around the airways. The membranous bronchioles are thicker, narrower, and more reactive than in panlobular emphysema. Lung compliance is low or normal and does not relate to the extent of the emphysema (i.e., not to the losses of elastic recoil), but rather the decrease in airflow is related mainly to the degree of airway abnormality.

In contrast, panlobular emphysema is characterized by even destruction of the lung, and the small airways appear less narrowed and less inflamed than in centrilobular emphysema. Lung compliance is increased and is related to the extent of the emphysema; the decrease in airflow is primarily associated with the loss of elastic recoil rather than with the abnormalities in the airways.[72]

Clinical Manifestations
At first, symptoms may be apparent only during physical exertion. Eventually marked exertional dyspnea progresses to dyspnea at rest. This occurs as a result of the irreversible destruction reducing elasticity of the lungs and increasing the effort to exhale trapped air. Cough is uncommon, with little sputum production. The client is often thin, has tachypnea with prolonged expiration, and must use accessory

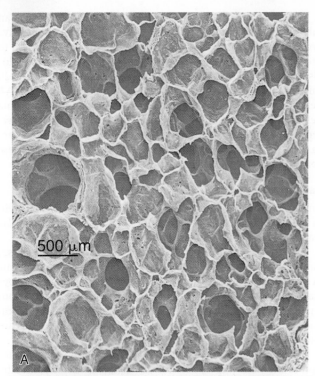

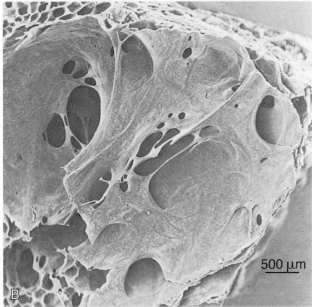

FIG. 11.9 Effects of emphysema seen in these scanning electron micrographs of lung tissue. (A) Normal lung with many small alveoli. (B) Lung tissue affected by emphysema. Notice that the alveoli have merged into larger air spaces, reducing the surface area for gas exchange. (From Patton KT, Thibodeau GA: Structure and function of the body, ed 15, St. Louis, 2016, Elsevier.)

muscles for ventilation. To increase lung capacity and use of accessory muscles, the client often leans forward with arms braced on the knees supporting the shoulders and chest. The combined effects of trapped air and alveolar distention change the size and shape of the client's chest, causing a barrel chest and increased expiratory effort. The normal arterial oxygen levels and dyspnea give clients a classic appearance (Fig. 11.10).

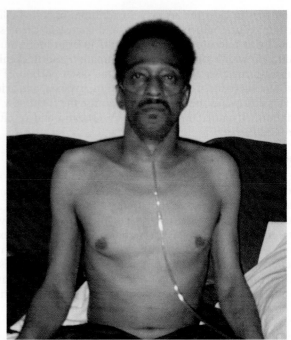

FIG. 11.10 The person with emphysema manifests classic findings. Use of respiratory accessory (intercostal, neck, shoulder) muscles and cachectic appearance (wasting caused by ill health) reflect two factors: (1) shortness of breath (SOB), the most disturbing symptom, and (2) the tremendous increased work of breathing (WOB) necessary to increase ventilation and maintain normal arterial blood gases (ABGs). (From Linton AD: Introduction to medical-surgical nursing, ed 5, St. Louis, 2012, Saunders.)

Persons with emphysema have three times the rate of anxiety as the general public. This anxiety is associated with dyspnea or fear of dyspnea. Antianxiety medications, particularly selective serotonin reuptake inhibitors (SSRIs), and cognitive behavioral therapy have been shown to be helpful, although more research is needed.[48]

Medical Management

Diagnosis and Treatment

Diagnosis is made on the basis of history (usually cigarette smoking), physical examination, chest film, and pulmonary function tests. The most important factor in the treatment of emphysema is cessation of smoking. Human lungs benefit no matter when someone quits smoking; quitting smoking is the most effective way of preventing lung function decline caused by emphysema (and chronic bronchitis).

Different breathing techniques can assist with controlling dyspnea. Pursed-lip breathing causes resistance to outflow at the lips, which in turn maintains intrabronchial pressure and improves the mixture of gases in the lungs. This type of breathing should be encouraged to help the client get rid of the stale air trapped in the lungs. However, this type of breathing pattern has been found to be ineffective for some people; methods to examine diaphragmatic movement and the potential for success with diaphragmatic breathing are available.[57] Pulmonary rehabilitation and supplemental oxygen are critical aspects of management of COPD and emphysema.[61]

TABLE 11.7 Types of Asthma

Classification	Triggers
Extrinsic	Immunoglobulin E (IgE)–mediated external allergens
	Foods; sulfite additives (wines)
	Indoor and outdoor pollutants, including ozone, smoke, exhaust
	Pollen, dust, molds
	Animal dander, feathers
Intrinsic	Unknown; secondary to respiratory infections
Adult-onset	Unknown
Exercise-induced	Alteration in airway temperature and humidity; mediator release
Aspirin-sensitive (associated with nasal polyps)	Aspirin and other nonsteroidal antiinflammatory drugs
Allergic bronchopulmonary aspergillosis	Hypersensitivity to *Aspergillus* species
Occupational	Metal salts (platinum, chrome, nickel)
	Antibiotic powder (penicillin, sulfathiazole, tetracycline)
	Toluene diisocyanate (TDI)
	Flour
	Wood dusts
	Cotton dust (byssinosis)
	Animal proteins
	Smoke inhalation (firefighters)
	Latex-induced
	Emotional stress

Prognosis

Prognosis for individuals with emphysema associated with symptomatic AAT deficiency (AATD) is poor, with a high incidence of transplantation for liver and lung disease and with many on a transplant waiting list.[317] LVRS (surgically removing damaged areas of the lung) may help improve breathing and ventilation. Studies have not been able to predict who can benefit the most from this treatment approach.

Asthma

Definition and Overview

Asthma is defined as a reversible obstructive lung disease characterized by inflammation and increased smooth muscle reaction of the airways to various stimuli. It is a chronic condition with acute exacerbations and characterized as a complex disorder involving biochemical, autonomic, immunologic, infectious, endocrine, and psychologic factors in varying degrees in different individuals. This condition can be divided into two main types according to causative factors: extrinsic (allergic) and intrinsic (nonallergic), but other recognized categories include adult-onset, exercise-induced, aspirin-sensitive, *Aspergillus*-hypersensitive, and occupational asthma (Table 11.7).

Incidence

Asthma, as one component of COPD, is the most common chronic disease in adults (11.9% incidence) and children (7% to 9% incidence), and the prevalence, morbidity, and mortality of asthma are increasing in the United States. Puerto Ricans have the highest incidence, followed by non-Hispanic blacks and Native Americans. Explanations include increased accuracy of medical diagnosis and increased chart documentation among physicians, as well as increased prevalence as a result of an increase in average life expectancy. Adults with asthma are 12 times more likely to develop COPD,[138] and there are more than 4500 deaths from asthma each year in the United States.

Risk Factors

The environment, including air pollution and exposure to other environmental toxins (including pesticides),[118,156] homes that are airtight, exposure to pets, and windowless offices may also be risk factors contributing to the significant rise in incidence. The *hygiene hypothesis* blames lack of exposure to stimulants or overexposure to cleaning agents.[215,291] Large families, early exposure to pets, early infections, and attending daycare may protect against allergic sensitization.[332]

Asthma can occur at any age, although it is more likely to occur for the first time before the age of 5. Antibiotic exposure during infancy appears to be a risk factor for developing childhood asthma. In childhood, asthma is three times more common and more severe in boys; however, after puberty the incidence in the genders is equal, although monthly variations in asthma episodes seem to correlate with estrogen levels for women.[90]

Children with lower birth weight (less than 5.5 lb at birth) and prematurity (more than 3 weeks premature) are more susceptible to the effects of ozone (air pollution) compared with children who are born at full term or full weight.[241] It is estimated that asthma goes unrecognized as an adverse factor affecting performance in 1 in 10 adolescent athletes.

Asthma is found most often in urban, industrialized settings; in colder climates; and among the urban disadvantaged population (areas of poverty). Asthma is more prevalent and more severe among black children, but this may not be a result of race or low income per se but rather of demographic location because all children living in an urban setting are at increased risk for asthma.[85]

Overcrowded living conditions with repeated exposure to cigarette smoke, dust, cockroaches, and mold and where a gas stove or oven is used for heat may be contributing factors.[196] Alcoholic drinks, particularly wines, appear to be important triggers for asthmatic responses. Sensitivity to the sulfite additives and salicylates present in wine seems likely to play an important role in these reactions.[333]

There is a relationship between obesity and asthma. Data from the Nurses Health Study II show that obesity increases women's risk of developing adult-onset asthma, possibly as a result of estrogen stored in lipids. The higher the body mass index (BMI), the greater the risk of developing asthma.[59] One study demonstrated reduced respiratory function in 32% of obese children and only 3% of children with a normal BMI.[331]

Etiologic Factors

Asthma occurs in families, which indicates that it is an inherited disorder. Asthma is influenced by two genetic tendencies: one associated with the capacity to develop allergies (*atopy*), and the other with the tendency to develop hyperresponsiveness of the airways independent of atopy. Eighty percent of individuals with asthma report allergic rhinitis. Studies have shown that stimulation of the nasal mucosa causes bronchi to react.[262] Environmental factors interact with inherited factors to cause attacks of bronchospasm. Asthma can develop when predisposed persons are infected by viruses or exposed to allergens or pollutants.

Extrinsic asthma, also known as atopic or allergic asthma, is the result of an allergy to specific triggers; usually the offending allergens are foods or environmental antigens suspended in the air in the form of pollen, dust, molds, smoke, automobile exhaust, and animal dander. More than one-half of the cases of asthma in children and young adults are of this type.

Intrinsic asthma, or nonallergic asthma, has no known allergic cause or trigger, has an adult onset (usually over 40 years of age), and is most often secondary to chronic or recurrent infections of the bronchi, sinuses, or tonsils and adenoids. This type of asthma may develop from a hypersensitivity to the bacteria or, more commonly, viruses causing the infection. Other factors precipitating intrinsic asthma include drugs (aspirin and β-adrenergic antagonists), environmental irritants (occupational chemicals and air pollution), cold dry air, exercise, and emotional stress.

Occupational asthma is defined as variable narrowing of airways, causally related to exposure in the working environment to specific airborne dusts, gases, acids, molds, dyes, vapors, or fumes. Many of these substances are very common and not ordinarily considered hazardous. Only a small proportion of exposed workers develop occupational asthma, but it has received considerable attention recently as the most frequent occupational lung disease worldwide.

New substances and processes involving new chemicals have increased dramatically in the last two decades, and there is little information about "safe" levels of exposure that protect all workers.[24] High-risk occupations for asthma include farmers, animal handlers, and agricultural workers; painters; plastics and rubber workers; cleaners and homemakers (especially if cooking is done with a gas stove); textile workers; metal workers; and bakers, millers, and other food processors. Exposure to biologic dusts and gases and fumes can cause a 30% to 50% increased risk of asthma.

Pathogenesis

The airways are the site of an inflammatory response consisting of cellular infiltration, epithelial disruption, mucosal edema, and mucous plugging (Fig. 11.11). The release of inflammatory mediators produces bronchial smooth muscle spasm; vascular congestion; increased vascular permeability; edema formation; production of thick, tenacious mucus; and impaired mucociliary function.

Several mediators also cause thickening of airway walls and increased contractile response of bronchial smooth muscles. These changes in the bronchial musculature, combined with the epithelial cell damage caused by eosinophil infiltration, result in the airway hyperresponsiveness characteristic of asthma.

Once the airway is in spasm and airways are swollen, mucous plugs the airway, trapping distal air. V/Q mismatch, hypoxemia, obstructed expiratory flow, and increased workload of breathing follow. Most attacks of asthmatic bronchospasm are short lived, with freedom from symptoms between episodes, although airway inflammation is present even in people who are asymptomatic.

Excessive airway narrowing occurs when the smooth muscle shortens (not necessarily to an abnormal degree). The relationship between the mechanical and contractile properties of smooth muscle and lung volume and how these interact to

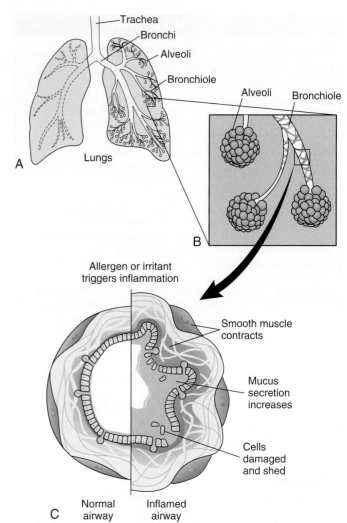

FIG. 11.11 Bronchiole response in asthma. (A) Air is distributed throughout the lungs via small airways called *bronchioles.* (B) Healthy bronchioles accommodate a constant flow of air when open and relaxed. (C) In asthma, exposure to an allergen or irritant triggers inflammation, causing constriction of the smooth muscle surrounding the bronchus (bronchospasm). The airway tissue swells; this edema of the mucous membrane further narrows airways, with production of excess mucus also interfering with breathing.

determine smooth muscle length are the subject of new research. The relative importance of smooth muscle area and mechanical properties, altered airway structure, and airway inflammation in asthma has not yet been determined.[166]

Clinical Manifestations

Clinical signs and symptoms of asthma differ in presentation (Box 11.6), degree (Table 11.8), and frequency among clients, and although current symptoms are the most important concern of affected people, they reflect the current level of asthma control more than underlying disease severity.[256]

During full remission, clients are asymptomatic and pulmonary function test findings are normal. Over time, repeated attacks cause airway *remodeling,* chronic air trapping, proliferation of submucosal glands, and hypertrophied smooth muscle. This may progress to irreversible changes and COPD.

BOX 11.6 Clinical Manifestations of Bronchial Asthma

Cough
- Hacking, paroxysmal, exhausting, irritative, involuntary, nonproductive
- Becomes rattling and productive of frothy, clear, gelatinous sputum
- Main or only symptom
- Tickle in the back of the throat accompanied by a cough

Respiratory-Related Signs
- Shortness of breath; may occur at rest
- Prolonged expiratory phase
- Audible wheeze on inspiration and expiration or on expiration only; never on inspiration only
- Often appears pale
- May have a malar flush and red ears
- Lips deep dark red color
- May progress to cyanosis of nail beds, around mouth and lips
- Restlessness
- Apprehension
- Anxious facial expression
- Itching around nose, eyes, throat, chin, scalp
- Sweating may be prominent as attack progresses
- May sit upright with shoulders in a hunched-over position, hands on the bed or chair, and arms braced (older children)
- Speaks with short, panting broken phrases

Chest
- Coarse, loud breath sounds (may become quiet or silent if severe)
- Prolonged expiration
- Generalized inspiratory and expiratory wheezing; increasingly high pitched
- Loss of breath sounds with severe cases

With Repeated Episodes
- Barrel chest
- Elevated shoulders
- Use of accessory muscles of respiration
- Skin retraction (clavicles, ribs, sternum)
- Facial appearance: flattened malar bones, circles beneath the eyes, narrow nose, prominent upper teeth, nostrils flaring

Modified from Hockenberry MJ, Wilson D: Wong's essentials of pediatric nursing, ed 9, St. Louis, 2013, Mosby.

TABLE 11.8 Stages of Asthma

Stage	Symptoms
Mild	Symptoms reverse with cessation of activity; daytime symptoms ≤2 times/wk; nighttime symptoms ≤2 times/mo; inhaled medication as needed (not usually daily)
Moderate	Audible wheezing
	Use of accessory muscles of respiration
	Leaning forward to catch breath
	Daily (but not continual) daytime symptoms requiring short-acting inhalant and long-term treatment
	Episodes ≥2 times/wk; nighttime symptoms ≥4 times/mo
Severe	Blue lips and fingernails
	Tachypnea (30–40 breaths/min) despite cessation of activity
	Cyanosis-induced seizures
	Skin and rib retraction
	Activity limited; frequent daytime and nighttime episodes, sometimes continual

An acute attack that cannot be altered with routine care is called *status asthmaticus*. This is a medical emergency requiring more vigorous pharmacologic and support measures. Despite appropriate treatment, this condition can be fatal.

When air is trapped, a severe paradoxical pulse develops as venous return is obstructed; blood pressure drops over 10 mm Hg during inspiration. Pneumothorax occasionally develops. If status asthmaticus continues, hypoxemia worsens and acidosis begins. If the condition is untreated or not reversed, respiratory or cardiac arrest will occur.

Medical Management

Prevention
Heavier emphasis on teaching self-management and especially prevention for anyone with asthma is recommended by the American Academy of Allergy, Asthma, and Immunology. An excellent daily asthma management plan is available.[11]

Diagnosis
Pulse oximetry, pulmonary function studies, bronchial challenge test with *methacholine*, skin prick tests, ABG analysis, serum IgE and blood eosinophil counts, induced sputum cell counts, exhaled nitric oxide (marker for eosinophilic inflammation),[326] questionnaires, and chest films may be used in assessing for both the presence and the severity of asthma. The methacholine challenge test is a valuable diagnostic measure. There are strong correlations with this test and some symptoms.[359] Inexpensive but reliable spirometer testing can be used to obtain evidence of the bronchial hyperreactivity associated with asthma.

Diagnosis may be delayed in older clients who have other illnesses that cause similar symptoms or who attribute their breathlessness to the effects of aging and respond to the onset of asthma by limiting their activities to avoid eliciting symptoms. The diagnosis of occupational asthma is usually based on history of a temporal association between exposure and the onset of symptoms and objective evidence that these symptoms are related to airflow limitation. Sputum induction and analysis may be helpful in confirming occupational asthma.[120]

At the beginning of an attack, there is a sensation of chest constriction, inspiratory and expiratory wheezing, nonproductive coughing, prolonged expiration, tachycardia, and tachypnea. Secondary bronchospasm is marked by recurrent attacks of dyspnea, with wheezing caused by the spasmodic constriction of the bronchi. Other symptoms may include fatigue, a tickle in the back of the throat accompanied by a cough in an attempt to clear the airways, and nostril flaring (advanced).

The person usually assumes a classic sitting or squatting position to reduce venous return, leaning forward so as to use all the accessory muscles of respiration. The skin is usually pale and moist with perspiration, but in a severe attack there may be cyanosis of the lips and nail beds. In the early stages of the attack coughing may be dry, but as the attack progresses, the cough becomes more productive of a thick, tenacious mucoid sputum. The nocturnal worsening of asthma is a common feature of this disease and may affect daytime alertness, even in children.[88] Rhinitis, chronic cough, snoring, and apnea may be responsible for sleep disturbance.

Treatment

Identifying specific allergens for each individual and avoidance of asthma triggers, combined with the use of two classes of medications (bronchodilators and antiinflammatory agents; see Table 11.6), has been recommended in the management of asthma. In the past, asthma was thought to be caused by spasms of the muscles surrounding the airways between the trachea and lungs and therefore was treated first with bronchodilator drugs to widen the constricted airways and ease symptoms. It is now clear that asthma attacks are actually episodic flare-ups of chronic inflammation in the lining of the airways necessitating the use of inhaled antiinflammatories to suppress the underlying inflammation and allow the airways to heal.

Most people require bronchodilator therapy to control symptoms by activating β-agonist receptors on smooth muscle cells in the respiratory tract, thereby relaxing the bronchial muscle and opening the airways; those with mild symptoms may use metered-dose inhaler (MDI) devices to administer *sympathomimetic* bronchodilators on an as-needed basis.

People who experience moderate to severe asthma may require daily administration of antiinflammatory agents, such as corticosteroids, to prevent asthma attacks. Corticosteroids dampen the entire immune system response. Antiinflammatory drugs have a preventive action by interrupting the development of bronchial inflammation. They may also modify or terminate ongoing inflammatory reactions in the airways.

It is important that people with asthma know the difference between medications that must be taken daily to prevent asthma symptoms and medications that relieve symptoms once they have begun. Low-dose corticosteroid inhalants are recommended to reduce the risk of side effects (e.g., psychiatric problems, reduced growth in children, ocular effects, death, osteoporosis, or alopecia and hirsutism) from prolonged use.[89,319] *Leukotriene*-receptor antagonists inhibit inflammation and have been shown to be safe and effective in adults with asthma and allergic rhinitis.[337]

Low dietary intake and blood levels of vitamins C and E, selenium, and flavonoids are seen in people with asthma.[237,263,302] Although some researchers suggest that antioxidant nutrients (especially obtained from food sources such as fruits and vegetables) appear helpful in asthma treatment,[225,235,248,263] others report that people with asthma may have a diminished capacity to restore the antioxidant defenses, making the use of supplemental antioxidants questionable in this population.[266]

Many complementary treatments have been used to *ameliorate* asthma symptoms, although there has been minimal research to validate most of these claims. There is minimal but growing evidence to support the use of acupuncture.[206] Spinal manipulation and other forms of manual therapy have been deemed to be ineffective in the treatment of asthma.[97,154] In one study of 65 people, yoga was found to have no effect on asthma.[293] Complementary treatments are still being studied for benefits and adverse effects.[34]

Prognosis

The outlook for clients with bronchial asthma is excellent despite the recent increase in the death rate. Childhood asthma may disappear, but only about one-quarter of the children with asthma become symptom free when their airways reach adult size. Factors that predict adult asthma include gender (males are more likely to outgrow asthma), smoking, allergy to dust mites, degree of airway hyperresponsiveness, and early age of onset.[298,325] Adults with asthma are 12 times more likely to develop COPD, but studies indicate that the majority of people with asthma do not experience a decline in pulmonary mechanics or appear to be at risk of reduced life expectancy.[138,227]

Attention to general health measures and use of pharmacologic agents permit control of symptoms in nearly all cases. The risk of lung cancer is two times greater in people with asthma compared with those who do not have a history of asthma.[53]

Status asthmaticus can result in respiratory or cardiac arrest and possible death (see previous discussion). If ventilation becomes necessary, prognosis for recovery can be poor (see discussion of effects of exercise for more information).

11.6 Special Implications for the PTA: Asthma Many people with asthma do not even know they have the disease. Some think they simply have chronic bronchitis, colds, or allergies. Anyone who reports coughing or a feeling of tightness in the chest when others smoke nearby and especially anyone who gasps for breath after exercise should be referred to a physician for evaluation of these symptoms.

Exercise-Induced Asthma

Exercise-induced bronchospasm (EIB), or exercise-induced asthma (EIA), is not a unique syndrome but rather an example of the airway hyperreactivity common to all persons with asthma. EIA is an acute, reversible, usually self-terminating airway obstruction that develops 5 to 15 minutes after strenuous exercise when the person no longer breathes through the nose, warming and humidifying the air, but opens the mouth. Breathing cold, dry air through the mouth degranulates mast cells, which release bronchoconstrictive mediators inducing EIB. EIB or EIA lasts 15 to 60 minutes after the onset.

Because PTAs recommend and observe exercise, they may be the first to recognize symptoms of undiagnosed asthma. Coughing is the most common symptom of EIA, but other symptoms include chest tightness, wheezing, and shortness of breath (SOB). The affected (but undiagnosed) individual may comment, "I am more out of shape than I thought." This should be a red flag for the PTA to consider the possibility of asthma and need for medical diagnosis and intervention.

If an asthma attack should occur during therapy, first assess the severity of the attack. Place the person in high Fowler's position (an inclined position in which the head of the bed is raised to promote dependent drainage) and encourage diaphragmatic and pursed-lip breathing. If the client has an inhaler available, provide whatever assistance is necessary for that person to self-administer the medication. Help the person relax while assessing the person's response to the medication.

Usually the episode subsides spontaneously in 30 to 60 minutes. The severity of an attack increases as the exercise becomes increasingly strenuous. The problem is rare in activities that require only short bursts of energy (e.g., baseball, sprints, gymnastics, or skiing) compared with those that involve endurance exercise (e.g., soccer, basketball, distance running, or biking).

Swimming, even long-distance swimming, is well tolerated by people with EIA, partly because they are breathing air fully saturated with moisture, but the type of breathing required may also play a role. Exhaling underwater, which is essentially pursed-lip breathing, is beneficial because it prolongs each expiration and increases the end-expiratory pressure within the respiratory tree.

Effect of Exercise

There are many barriers to exercise for people with asthma, including lack of motivation, time constraints, weather conditions, and belief that exercise is not good for this condition.[212] To prevent secondary complication of a sedentary lifestyle and because obesity can contribute to the inflammatory process associated with asthma, exercise and education about exercise should be part of any treatment program.

There is strong evidence to support physical training for cardiovascular training in this population.[275] There is inadequate evidence for a positive effect of breathing exercises and inspiratory muscle training in individuals who have asthma.[153,276]

Exercise and Medication

Bronchospasm can occur during exercise (especially in EIA) if the person with asthma has a low blood oxygen level before exercise. For this reason, it is helpful to take bronchodilators by metered-dose inhaler (MDI) 20 to 30 minutes before exercise, performing mild stretching and warm-up exercises during that time period to avoid bronchospasm with higher workload exercise. Increased exercise should be accompanied by good bronchodilator coverage to promote bronchodilation and improve alveolar ventilation and oxygenation. Exercise guidelines for adults with asthma can be modified from recommendations for children with asthma (Table 11.9).

Many clients have found that using their inhalers in this way before exercise permits them to exercise without onset of symptoms. Proper administration of an MDI is essential (see Box 11.5). The first dose induces dilation of the larger, central bronchial tubes, relaxing smooth muscles in the airways; the second dose dilates the bronchioles (smaller airways).

Metabolism of certain drugs administered can be altered by exercise, tobacco, marijuana, or phenobarbital (all of which increase drug metabolism). Cimetidine (Tagamet), erythromycin, or the presence of a viral infection may decrease drug metabolism.

The physician must be informed if a client develops signs of asthma or any bronchial reactivity during exercise. Medication dosage can then be altered to maintain optimal physical performance. Excessive use of inhaled β-adrenergic agents (using three or more full canisters monthly) requires physician referral for further evaluation.

Common manifestations of drug-induced (theophylline) toxicity include nausea, vomiting, tremors, anxiety, tachycardia and arrhythmias, and hypotension. The use of nonsteroidal antiinflammatory drugs (NSAIDs), including aspirin, in older people with asthma should be avoided if possible because the drug interactions can cause increased bronchospasm in susceptible individuals.

Some athletes do not achieve the control needed for the performance demands of competition. The effectiveness of short-acting medications and medications in general for asthma varies widely among people with asthma while exercising. The preventive benefits of each medication dose may wane after a new drug has been taken for several weeks. Any athlete with asthma who cannot perform at the levels desired or expected because of asthma symptoms should be advised to review medications and medication use with the physician.

Medication and Bone Density

Long-term use of inhaled corticosteroids in the management of moderate to severe asthma is associated with decreased bone mineral density (BMD) and associated increased risk of fractures and a high occurrence of asymptomatic vertebral fractures, particularly in high-risk postmenopausal women (i.e., those not receiving hormone replacement therapy).[15,286,350] African American children may be afforded some protection from osteoporosis as compared with Caucasian children using high-dose inhaled corticosteroids.[135]

The PTA can be very instrumental in providing education for the prevention and intervention for the treatment of osteopenia and osteoporosis.

Monitoring Vital Signs

Monitoring vital signs can alert the PTA to important changes in bronchopulmonary function. Developing or increasing tachypnea may indicate worsening asthma or drug toxicity. Other signs of toxicity, such as diarrhea, headache, and vomiting, may be misinterpreted as influenza. Hypertensive blood pressure readings may indicate asthma-related hypoxemia.

Auscultate the lungs frequently, noting breath sounds including the degree of wheezing and the quality of air movement. In this way, any change in respiratory status will be more readily perceived.

If the client does not have a productive cough in the presence of rhonchi (dry rattling in the bronchial tube), teach effective coughing techniques.

Status Asthmaticus

Therapy can augment the medical management of the client with status asthmaticus. In coordination with the individual's medications, the PTA helps to remove secretions; promotes relaxed, more efficient breathing; reduces hypoxemia; and teaches the client to coordinate relaxed breathing with general body movement.

Caution needs to be observed to avoid stimuli that bring on bronchospasm and deterioration (e.g., aggressive percussion, forced expiration maneuvers, aggressive bag ventilation, or manual hyperinflation with an intubated individual). Certain body positions may have to be avoided because of client intolerance or exacerbation of symptoms in those positions.[85]

Immediate medical care is recommended for anyone with asthma who is struggling to breathe with no improvement in 15 to 20 minutes after initial treatment with medications or who is hunched over and unable to straighten up or resume activity after medication administration. The presence of blue or gray lips or nail beds is another indication of the need for immediate medical attention.

TABLE 11.9 Exercise Guidelines for Children with Asthma

Recommendation	Benefit
General exercise, school-based physical education	Maintains motor control, flexibility, strength, cardiovascular fitness; prevents or reverses side effects of medication (e.g., corticosteroids)
	Raises threshold for strenuous exercise before mouth breathing and EIB occur
Low-impact exercise (aerobics, weight training, stationary bike)	Permits exercise without increased bronchospasm
Warm-up before aerobic activity	Helps control airway reactivity; gradually desensitizes mast cells, reducing release of bronchoconstrictive mediators
Exercise in a trigger-free environment (i.e., avoid cold, pollution, or increased pollen outdoors; exercise indoors; avoid tobacco smoke; swimming program is ideal)	Prevents bronchospasm; controls symptoms
Take prescribed medication properly before exercise or activity producing bronchospasm	Prevents bronchospasm
Monitor FEV₁/FVC ratio before, during, and after physical activity[a]	Determines whether shortness of breath is caused by intensity of exercise or diminished air flow from bronchospasm
Decrease of 10% requires slowing activity	
Drop of 15%–20% from initial measurement necessitates cessation of exercise	

[a]Peak flowmeters can be used to obtain this information. Determine the child's normal range of lung function by having the child blow in the meter in the morning and evening for 1 wk. The average level measured varies from person to person and is influenced by gender and height. Testing should establish a peak flow protocol against which lung function can be compared to determine whether deterioration has occurred.

EIB, Exercise-induced bronchospasm; *FEV₁/FVC,* ratio of forced expiratory volume in 1 sec to forced vital capacity.

Bronchiectasis

Definition

Bronchiectasis is a progressive form of obstructive lung disease characterized by irreversible destruction and dilation of airways generally associated with chronic bacterial infections. Clinically, it is considered an extreme form of bronchitis and no longer considered part of COPD. Abnormal and permanent dilation of the bronchi and bronchioles develops when the supporting structures (bronchial walls) are weakened by chronic inflammatory changes associated with secondary infection.

Incidence and Etiologic and Risk Factors

The incidence of bronchiectasis is low in the United States because of improved control of bronchopulmonary infections. However, any condition producing a narrowing of the lumen of the bronchioles may create bronchiectasis, including TB, adenoviral infections, and pneumonia. Bronchiectasis also develops in people with immunodeficiencies involving humoral immunity, recurrent aspiration, and abnormal mucociliary clearance (immotile cilia syndromes).

CF causes about one-half of all cases of bronchiectasis. Sinusitis, dextrocardia (heart located on right side of chest), Kartagener's syndrome (alterations in ciliary activity), defective development of bronchial cartilage (Williams–Campbell syndrome), and endobronchial tumor predispose a person to bronchiectasis.

Pathogenesis

Although bronchiectasis has been viewed as a progressive disease of destruction and dilation of the medium and large airways, there is now evidence of the importance of the small airways in the pathogenesis of this condition. Chronic inflammation of the bronchial wall by mononuclear cells is common to all types of bronchiectasis. Abnormal bronchial dilation characteristic of bronchiectasis is accompanied by accumulation of wet secretions that plug the airway and cause bronchospasm, producing even more mucus. A vicious cycle of bacteria-provoked inflammatory lung damage occurs with irreversible destruction or fragmentation of the bronchial wall and resultant fibrosis further obstructing and obliterating the bronchial lumen (Fig. 11.12). In response to these changes, large anastomoses develop between the bronchial and pulmonary blood vessels to increase the blood flow through the bronchial circulation. V/Q mismatch causes hypoxia and hypercapnia.

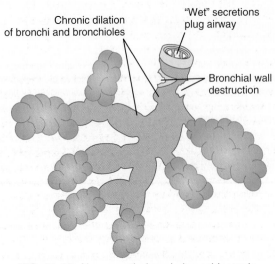

Chronic dilation of bronchi and bronchioles

"Wet" secretions plug airway

Bronchial wall destruction

FIG. 11.12 Airway pathology in bronchiectasis.

Clinical Manifestations

The most immediate symptom of bronchiectasis is persistent coughing, with large amounts of purulent sputum production (worse in the morning). Rhinosinusitis, dyspnea, and fatigue are also strongly related to bronchiectasis. For those without other significant disease, most report chronic childhood respiratory problems.[184]

Weight loss, anemia, and other systemic manifestations, such as low-grade fever, hemoptysis, and weakness, are also common. Clubbing may occur, and the breath and sputum may become foul-smelling with advanced disease. Heart failure may occur as a result of the vascular fibrosis. There is a known correlation between bronchiectasis and rheumatoid arthritis, but the exact mechanism remains unknown.

Medical Management

Diagnosis

Imaging studies (e.g., high-resolution CT scan) have become increasingly accurate in depicting the features of early bronchiectasis, as have radiographic studies and laboratory tests.

Treatment

The goals of treatment are removal of secretions and prevention of infection. The principal treatment involves ACTs, bronchodilators, and antibiotics selected on the basis of sputum smears and cultures. A recent study demonstrated that use of inhaled corticosteroids improved quality of life for people with steady-state bronchiectasis.[220] Hydration is important, and supplemental oxygen may be administered. Surgical resection is reserved for the few clients with localized bronchiectasis and adequate pulmonary function who fail to respond to conservative management or for the person with massive hemoptysis. Long-term care is the same as for any person with COPD.

Prognosis

The morbidity and mortality associated with bronchiectasis have declined markedly in industrialized nations, but prevalence remains high in Pacific and Asian countries. The overall prognosis is often poor, and although bronchiectasis is usually localized to a lung lobe or segment, persistent, nonresolving infection may cause the disorder to spread to other parts of the same lung. Complications of bronchiectasis include recurrent pneumonia, lung abscesses, metastatic infections in other organs (e.g., brain abscess), and cardiac and respiratory failure. Good pulmonary hygiene and avoidance of infectious complications in the involved areas may reverse some cases of bronchiectasis.

11.7 Special Implications for the PTA: Bronchiectasis The effects of bronchopulmonary airway clearance techniques (also referred to as *hygiene physical therapy, chest therapy, chest physical therapy*) to improve pulmonary function in bronchiectasis remain inconclusive because of insufficient research.[173,174] The beneficial effects of airway clearance techniques to mobilize secretions and improve pulmonary clearance (e.g., sputum production or radioaerosol clearance) in the treatment of bronchiectasis have been documented in one small study.[174]

In many settings, postural drainage and percussion for the person with bronchiectasis are administered routinely on the basis of diagnosis rather than specific clinical criteria. Further research to clarify outcomes of airway clearance techniques is necessary and may provide the PTA with clinical goals other than secretion mobilization.

Inspiratory muscle training appears to have an effect on exercise endurance, but insufficient evidence exists to support other types of physical training.[45] However, a recent randomized controlled study demonstrated improvement in exercise tolerance with pulmonary rehabilitation.[44]

The selection of techniques to include in an airway clearance regimen varies among institutions as well as among practitioners and may include positioning, postural drainage, and chest percussion of involved lobes performed several times per day. Family members can be instructed in how to provide this care at home.

Directed coughing and breathing exercises to promote good ventilation and removal of secretions should follow positional or percussive therapy. The best times to do this are in the early morning and several hours after eating the final meal; performing these techniques just before bedtime may result in increased coughing and prevent the person from sleeping. An excellent review of the use of airway clearance techniques in the acute care setting is available.[107]

Bronchiolitis

Definition and Overview

Bronchiolitis refers to several *morphologically* distinct pathologic conditions that involve the small airways. Acute bronchiolitis is a commonly occurring, diffuse, and often severe inflammation of the lower airways (bronchioles) caused by a viral infection in children under 2 years of age. Acute adult onset is related to asthma, aspiration, or bronchiectasis.

Bronchiolitis was once classified as a type of chronic interstitial pneumonia and referred to as *small airways disease;* progress in pathology has provided more specific cause-directed diagnoses that reflect the individual reaction patterns observed. Constrictive bronchiolitis, diffuse panbronchiolitis, and airway-centered fibrosis are also forms of bronchiolitis.

Bronchiolitis obliterans in the adult is now considered acute or chronic with identification of these special forms (e.g., obliterative, eosinophilic bronchiolitis in asthma, necrotizing bronchiolitis in viral infection, or toxic fume bronchiolitis after exposure to noxious gases and the development of chemical pneumonitis).[270,338] Bronchiolitis obliterans is the most important clinical complication in heart–lung and lung transplant recipients and may represent a form of allograft rejection; it is a rare complication of allogeneic (human-to-human) bone marrow transplantation. Circulating fibroblast precursors from bone marrow may be implicated in transplant recipients with bronchiolitis.[50]

Bronchiolitis obliterans may occur in association with rheumatoid arthritis, polymyositis, and dermatomyositis. Penicillamine therapy has been implicated as a possible cause of bronchiolitis obliterans in clients with rheumatoid arthritis.

Sleep-Disordered Breathing

Definition

Sleep-disordered breathing is a collection of syndromes characterized by breathing abnormalities during sleep that result in intermittently disrupted gas exchange and in sleep interruption. Sleep-disordered breathing includes CSR, hypoventilation syndromes with and without chronic lung disease, heavy snoring with daytime sleepiness (upper airway resistance syndrome), and sleep apnea. The most common and only condition discussed here, sleep apnea syndrome, is defined as significant daytime symptoms (e.g., sleepiness) in conjunction with evidence of sleep-related upper airway obstruction and sleep disturbance.[32]

There are three types of sleep apnea: central, obstructive, and mixed.

- *Central sleep apnea* is caused by altered chemosensitivity and cerebral respiratory control. The brain fails to send the appropriate signals to the respiratory muscles to initiate breathing, resulting in no diaphragmatic movement and no airflow. This is seen in infants younger than 40 weeks' conceptual age and in people with neurologic disorders (e.g., tumors, brain infarcts, diffuse encephalopathies).
- *Obstructive sleep apnea* (OSA), the most commonly diagnosed form of sleep apnea, is characterized by respiratory effort without airflow because of upper airway obstruction. This form manifests with repetitive episodes of apnea during sleep and results in extreme daytime sleepiness.
- *Mixed sleep apnea* is central apnea that is immediately followed by an obstructive event.

Incidence

Depending on geographic area, prevalence of OSA ranges from 2% to 58% in men and 10% to 37% in women.[273] Gender differences in upper airway collapse have not been observed, although there appears to be a relationship to testosterone levels.[289,362,363] Forty percent of obese people have OSA, and 70% of people with sleep apnea are obese. OSA in children without neurologic impairment is most commonly caused by adenotonsillar hypertrophy, although obesity is positively correlated with this disorder in children also.[17] Children with Down syndrome are particularly vulnerable to OSA and should be tested at age 3 to 4 years.[305]

Etiologic and Risk Factors

OSA is a result of partial or complete pharyngeal collapse during sleep, leading to either reduction (hypopnea) or cessation (apnea) of breathing. Both conditions can lead to substantial hypoxia and hypercapnia, with arousal from sleep required to reestablish airway patency and a resumption of ventilation. This cycle of recurrent pharyngeal collapse with subsequent arousal from sleep leads to the primary symptoms of daytime somnolence.

The main cause of sleep apnea in adults is upper body obesity, especially a large neck circumference. A neck circumference greater than 16 inches for a woman or greater than 17 inches in a man correlates with an increased risk of this disorder.[335] Enlarged tonsils or adenoids are the primary cause of sleep apnea in children.[277]

People with anatomically narrowed upper airways, such as occur in micrognathia, macroglossia (large tongue), and adenoid, uvula, elongated soft palate, or tonsillar hypertrophy, are predisposed to the development of OSA. Fat deposits or swelling in any or all of these tissues causes further obstruction.

Other risk factors include increasing age, genetic factors (sleep-disordered breathing clusters in families), neurologic disorders, smoking, and cardiopulmonary dysfunctions such as hypertension, moderate to severe heart failure (including cor pulmonale), calcification of carotid arteries, chronic bronchitis, or cardiac dysrhythmia. Drinking alcohol or taking sedatives before sleeping may precipitate or worsen the condition.

Clinical Manifestations

The frequent interruptions of deep, restorative sleep often lead to daytime (including morning) sluggishness and headaches, daytime fatigue, excessive daytime sleepiness, cognitive impairment, weight gain, and sexual impotence. Bed partners usually report loud cyclic snoring with periods of silence (breath cessation), restlessness, frequent episodes of waking up gasping, and often thrashing movements of the extremities during sleep.

Neurocognitive effects may include personality changes; irritability, hyperactivity, and depression; judgment impairment or poor school performance; domestic, work-related, or automobile accidents; memory loss; and difficulty concentrating.

Neurocognitive effects of apnea may also cause a mood disorder leading to an erroneous diagnosis of dysthymia; treatment with standard antidepressant medications may exacerbate the condition.[178] Anyone with acquired or congenital neurologic disorders, such as tetraplegia, stroke, and Down syndrome, is susceptible to sleep disorders.[305,315]

Fragmented sleep with its repetitive cycles of snoring, airway collapse, and arousal may cause hypertension in some people. Sleep-disordered breathing may be a risk factor for cardiovascular involvement, including angina pectoris, acute myocardial infarction, cardiac arrhythmias, and ischemic stroke.[51,52,264] The exact mechanisms for this are yet unknown, but there is an association with inflammation and prothrombotic factors, as well as CNS effects.[180] Risk of stroke is independent of other risk factors, including obesity and hypertension.[354]

Medical Management

Diagnosis

Diagnosis may be made using sleep monitoring devices, radiologic imaging, laboratory assays, questionnaires, and clinical signs and symptoms, but the most reliable test to confirm the diagnosis is overnight polysomnography (i.e., monitoring the subject during sleep for periods of apnea and lowered blood oxygen saturation).

The physician must differentiate sleep apnea syndrome from seizure disorder, *narcolepsy*, or psychiatric depression. A hemoglobin level is obtained, and thyroid function tests are performed. Diagnostic criteria for children have not been standardized, although it is recognized that they should be different from adult criteria.[277] The primary symptom in children is hyperactivity, not daytime somnolence.

Treatment

Obstructive and mixed types of sleep apnea syndrome can be treated. Because many clients with sleep apnea are overweight, weight loss is recommended. Weight loss may be curative, but only a small percentage of people maintain their weight loss, and symptoms return with weight gain. Therefore alternative interventions have been developed, and the most common treatment for OSA is CPAP used during sleep. CPAP provides positive pressure from a CPAP machine that pumps open the airway and prevents it from obstructing. This treatment technique may not be tolerated by some people, and adherence to its use is only about 40%.[204] Adherence level is demonstrated in the first 2 weeks, but there may be increased compliance after 2 years because the perceived benefits outweigh the barriers such as noise and discomfort.[114,318]

One study has evaluated adherence and effectiveness of CPAP in children. CPAP was effective in improving oxygen saturation, and the average nightly use was 5.3 hours (a time markedly overestimated by parents).[214]

In adults, use of CPAP is more effective than no treatment and treatment with oral appliances in reducing apnea, decreasing blood pressure, and improving quality of life.[116] Guidelines for use of CPAP have been published.[192] Oral appliances may be inserted into the mouth at bedtime and used to hold the jaw forward, thus preventing pharyngeal occlusion. Such devices are regulated by the FDA. There is evidence that oral appliances reduce sleepiness and disordered breathing when compared with control but that CPAP is more effective overall. It is recommended that oral appliances be used for mild sleep disorders or when the person does not tolerate CPAP.[200]

Surgery is recommended if an airway obstruction can be determined as the cause of the sleep apnea. Neurogenic causes of sleep apnea are more difficult to control. There is insufficient evidence to draw any conclusions about the effectiveness of medication. Medication has been directed at improving tone in the upper airway, increasing ventilatory drive, reducing rapid eye movement (REM) sleep, and reducing airway resistance or surface tension.[307] Alcohol and hypnotic medications should be avoided. In children, performance of tonsillectomy and adenoidectomy has been shown be effective in a majority of cases.[277,303]

Prognosis

Evidence indicates that OSA may be associated with increased long-term cardiovascular and neurophysiologic morbidity. Cardiac and vascular morbidity may include systemic hypertension, cardiac arrhythmias, PH, cor pulmonale, left ventricular dysfunction, stroke, and sudden death. Recognition and appropriate treatment of OSA and related disorders will often significantly enhance the client's quality of life, overall health, productivity, and safety on the highway and job.

11.8 Special Implications for the PTA: Sleep-Disordered Breathing: Apnea There has been very little research on the effects of pulmonary rehabilitation in persons with sleep apnea. Two studies demonstrated positive responses to exercise training, although exercise alone was not an adequate intervention.[252] One small study showed that physical activity level was better correlated with subjective measures of well-being than severity of apnea disorder.[155]

Pulmonary rehabilitation may be an effective adjunct intervention to improve quality of life and cardiovascular fitness and to assist with weight loss. Because of the possible cardiovascular complications associated with clients who have obstructive sleep apnea (OSA), vital signs should be monitored before, during, and after submaximal or maximal exercise. The client should not be left in the supine position for prolonged periods of time, even while awake.

There are some reports of sleep apnea in association with cervical lesions (e.g., osteophytes caused by diffuse idiopathic skeletal hyperostosis [DISH]),[208] as well as after anterior cervical spine fusion.[139] Individuals with rheumatoid arthritis complicated with temporomandibular joint destruction and cervical involvement can also develop OSA.[258] Physical therapy may be explored in developing treatment protocols when the musculoskeletal structures of the mandible contribute to the problem.

Restrictive Lung Disease

Overview

Restrictive lung disorders are a major category of pulmonary problems, including any condition that reduces the lung volume and decreases compliance. Examples include but are not limited to pulmonary fibrosis, systemic sclerosis (SS) lung diseases, and chest wall trauma or lung injury, which are all discussed here. There are many causes of restrictive lung diseases that are covered in other sections of this chapter or book. More than 100 identified interstitial lung diseases (ILDs) can cause restrictive lung disease.

Extrapulmonary causes may include neurologic or neuromuscular disorders (e.g., head or spinal cord injury, amyotrophic lateral sclerosis [ALS], myasthenia gravis, Guillain–Barré syndrome, muscular dystrophy, or poliomyelitis), musculoskeletal disorders (e.g., ankylosing spondylitis, kyphosis or scoliosis, or chest wall injury or deformity), postsurgical conditions, particularly involving the abdomen or thorax, and obesity.

Clinical Manifestations

Clinical presentation varies according to the cause of the restrictive disorder. Generally, clients with restrictive lung disease exhibit a rapid, shallow respiratory pattern. Chronic tachypnea (fast rate) occurs in an effort to overcome the effects of reduced lung volume and compliance. Pulmonary function tests are characterized by a decrease in total lung capacity.

Exertional dyspnea progresses to dyspnea at rest because of the loss of inspiratory reserves. As the disease progresses, respiratory muscle fatigue may occur, leading to inadequate alveolar ventilation and carbon dioxide retention. Hypoxemia is a common finding, especially in the later stages of restrictive disease.

Medical Management

Treatment and Prognosis

The management of restrictive lung disease is based in part on the underlying cause. Treatment goals are oriented toward adequate oxygenation, maintaining an airway, and obtaining maximal function. For example, persons with spinal deformities may be helped with corrective surgery, and obese persons may experience improved breathing after weight loss.

Corticosteroids may help control inflammation and reduce further impairment, but previously damaged alveolocapillary units cannot be regenerated or replaced. Some clients with end-stage disease may be candidates for lung transplantation. Most restrictive lung diseases are not reversible, and the disease progresses to include PH, cor pulmonale, severe hypoxia, and eventual ventilatory or cardiac failure.

11.9 Special Implications for the PTA: Restrictive Lung Disease Exercise testing (6-minute walk tests or other submaximal exercise evaluation) plays an important role in determining the extent of the disease and assessing outcomes. Many residual effects of pulmonary pathology are neuromuscular in nature and can be addressed by appropriate physical therapy.[221]

A primary problem for clients with restrictive lung disease secondary to generalized weakness and neuromuscular disease is ineffective cough. Airway clearance techniques to facilitate cough and effectively dislodge secretions to the central airways may be exhausting for the client. Rest periods must be incorporated in the treatment.

A person with restrictive lung disease will be more adversely affected by the restriction of lung function in the recumbent position, emphasizing the importance of routine positioning for immobile clients and active or active-assisted movements whenever possible. Extrapulmonary causes of restriction are most amenable to physical therapy intervention. Consider manual therapy for improving chest wall compliance with injury or after surgery, as well as flexibility exercises.

Pulmonary Fibrosis

Definition and Overview

Pulmonary fibrosis (also known as *interstitial lung disease*) is a general term that refers to a variety of disorders in which ongoing epithelial damage or chronic inflammation of lung tissue leads to progressive scarring (fibrosis) of the lungs, predominantly fibroblasts and small blood vessels that progressively remove and replace normal tissue.[251]

Etiologic and Risk Factors

Two-thirds of cases of pulmonary fibrosis are idiopathic pulmonary fibrosis (IPF), in which the cause is unknown. In the remaining one-third, fibrosis in the lung is caused by healing scar tissue after active disease, such as TB, SS, or acute respiratory distress syndrome (ARDS), or after inhalation of harmful particles such as moldy hay, metal dust, coal dust, or *asbestos*.

Other risk factors include some infections and connective tissue diseases, such as rheumatoid arthritis or SLE; certain drugs, particularly some chemotherapy agents; and in rare cases, genetic or familial predisposition.

Thoracic radiation (e.g., postmastectomy irradiation of the chest wall and regional lymphatics in clients with breast cancer) may result in pericarditis and pneumonitis, which can progress to pulmonary fibrosis weeks, or even months, after radiation treatments have ended. In addition, some chemotherapies can cause pulmonary fibrosis.[257]

Pathogenesis and Clinical Manifestations

Fibrosis irreversibly distorts and shrinks the lung lobe at the alveolar level and causes a marked loss of lung compliance. The lung becomes stiff and difficult to ventilate with decreased diffusing capacity of the alveolocapillary membrane, causing hypoxemia. There does not appear to be an inflammatory process but rather abnormal wound healing in response to multiple, microscopic sites of ongoing alveolar epithelial injury and fibrosis.[251,300] The course of pulmonary fibrosis varies, with early symptoms such as SOB and a dry cough potentially progressing to further complications.

Medical Management

Diagnosis

Definitive diagnosis of IPF is with surgical biopsy. Clinical assessment, pulmonary function tests, and radiographic studies support the pathologic findings.

Treatment and Prognosis

Although past treatment for IPF has included corticosteroids, there is insufficient evidence to support their use. Because of the more recent hypothesis that repeated lung injury is the cause, antiinflammatory treatment is not warranted. Other types of pulmonary fibrosis may respond to corticosteroids.[278]

The clinical course of people with pulmonary fibrosis and rheumatoid arthritis is chronic and progressive. Response to treatment is unpredictable, and the overall prognosis is poor, with median survival time less than 4 years.[122]

11.10 Special Implications for the PTA: Pulmonary Fibrosis One of the most common late effects of chest irradiation is pulmonary fibrosis, which may not occur for months to years after radiation to the thorax. The total dose of radiation and the size of the treatment portal determine the severity of this condition. The changes in pulmonary function are usually a progressive decline in lung volumes and a decrease in lung compliance and diffusing capacity. As doses increase, the frequency of pulmonary fibrosis increases, but with improved dosage *fractionation*, most people die from the cancer before these complications develop.

Early identification of idiopathic pulmonary fibrosis (IPF) may improve morbidity. Identifying and referring anyone who has unusual SOB or progressive decrease in exercise tolerance may help with early diagnosis. Physical therapy intervention depends on clinical presentation following the appropriate preferred practice pattern or patterns and may focus on peripheral conditioning and motor control for more efficient oxygen usage.

Systemic Sclerosis Lung Disease
Definition
SS, or scleroderma, is an autoimmune disease of connective tissue characterized by excessive collagen deposition in the skin and internal organs, particularly the kidneys and lungs.

Incidence, Pathogenesis and Clinical Manifestations
Clinically, more than one-half of all people with SS die of pulmonary disease.[313] The presence of pulmonary arterial hypertension is a major prognostic factor in mortality. The lungs, as a result of a rich vascular supply and abundant connective tissue, are a frequent target organ (second to the esophagus in visceral involvement). Skin changes generally precede visceral alterations, and lung involvement rarely causes symptoms at first, but pulmonary symptoms develop after an average of 7 years.[30]

Three pathways produce organ damage with SS.
- First, inflammation is caused by T cells and cytokines, resulting in alveolitis before fibrosis.
- Second, severe thickening and obstruction of vessels occurs, resulting in PH and renal failure.
- Third, cutaneous fibrosis occurs.[312] Immunosuppressive therapy may delay onset of symptoms by up to 4 years.[30]

Recent studies have determined that the balance between fibrotic and inflammatory mediators may be important to developing pathology.[148] As a result, initial symptoms of dyspnea on exertion and nonproductive cough develop. As fibroblast proliferation and collagen deposition progress, fibrosis of the alveolar wall occurs and the capillaries are obliterated. Traditional tests, such as pulmonary function tests and chest radiographs, are insensitive and not predictive of outcome. Clinically, the client demonstrates more severe dyspnea and has a greater risk of deterioration in pulmonary function.

Medical Management
Treatment
Successful treatment of SS pulmonary disease remains an area for further development. Pharmacologic treatment using low-dose prednisone is recommended because of the possible association of high-dose corticosteroids with renal failure in clients with SS.

Investigations conclude that lung transplantation is a viable option for carefully selected individuals with scleroderma-related lung disease; survival rates are equivalent to those of lung transplant recipients with other disorders.[222]

Prognosis
SS lung disease is unpredictable and may have a mild, prolonged course, but as the pulmonary fibrosis advances and causes PH, cor pulmonale characterized by peripheral edema may develop, progressing rapidly to respiratory failure and death. Lung disease is the most frequent cause of death from SS. Morbidity and mortality in adults over 75 years of age are worse than in younger adults, in part related to late diagnosis.[87]

11.11 Special Implications for the PTA: Systemic Sclerosis Lung Disease The effectiveness of a pulmonary rehabilitation program with systemic sclerosis lung disease remains unknown and warrants research investigation. Therapy implications and interventions should be based on general principles regarding pulmonary involvement and specific clinical presentation.

Chest Wall Trauma or Lung Injury
Chest or thoracic trauma ranges from superficial wounds such as contusions and abrasions to flail chest to life-threatening tension pneumothorax (which is discussed later in this chapter). A flail chest consists of fractures of two or more adjacent ribs on the same side, and possibly the sternum, with each bone fractured into two or more segments. The fractured rib segments are detached (free floating) from the rest of the chest wall. The integrity of the thorax is compromised, and the inspiratory force of the diaphragm causes inward (paradoxical) movement of the fractured ribs. The number of rib fractures is directly correlated with lung-related complications, and the presence of six or more rib fractures significantly increases mortality from nonpulmonary causes.[103]

Early identification of rib fractures or a flail chest improves outcomes, particularly in children, in whom chest trauma is the second leading cause of death.[294] Complex soft tissue injury can occur in the absence of chest wall fractures.[3] Cough-induced rib fractures occur primarily in women and can occur in persons with normal bone density.[142] These fractures are typically lateral, in the middle ribs, and do not cause flail chest.

Clinical Manifestations
It is common for a fractured rib end to tear the pleura and lung surface, thereby producing hemopneumothorax. This causes the lung to collapse from the loss of negative pressure. Fractured ribs can also lacerate abdominal organs, the brachial plexus, and blood vessels.

In flail chest, the paradoxical chest motion impairs movement of gas in and out of the lungs (Fig. 11.13), promotes

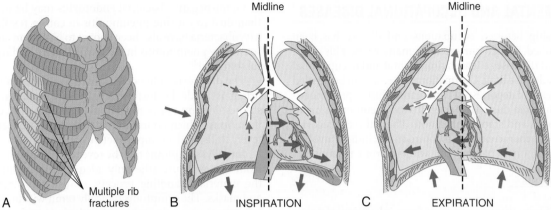

FIG. 11.13 Flail chest. Arrows indicate air movement or structural movement. (A) Flail chest consists of fractured rib segments that are detached (free floating) from the rest of the chest wall. (B) On inspiration, the flail segment of ribs is sucked inward. The affected lung and mediastinal structures shift to the unaffected side. This compromises the amount of inspired air in the unaffected lung. (C) On expiration, the flail segment of ribs bellows outward. The affected lung and mediastinal structures shift to the affected side with the diaphragm elevated on that side (not shown). Some air within the lungs is shunted back and forth between the lungs instead of passing through the upper airway.

atelectasis, and impairs pulmonary drainage. Other clinical manifestations of flail chest include excruciating pain, severe dyspnea, hypoventilation, cyanosis, and hypoxemia, leading to respiratory failure without the appropriate intervention.

Medical Management

Diagnosis and Treatment

In a retrospective study of 492 adults, the combination of pain with palpation and hypoxia predicted 100% of all significant acute intrathoracic injuries seen on radiographs.[284] Because blunt trauma may also involve significant soft tissue injury, multidetector CT is recommended to more accurately determine the extent of injury.[236]

Initial treatment follows the ABCs of emergency treatment (airway, breathing, and circulation) to treat the pneumothorax, thereby enabling the person to breathe deeply and to effectively clear secretions. A chest tube removes both air and blood in the pleural cavity after chest trauma and regains the negative pressure in the pleural space so the lungs can remain inflated. The tube is usually positioned in the sixth intercostal space in the posterior axillary line. CPAP or PEEP via a machine may be used to enhance or maintain lung expansion.[25]

Treatment may also require internal fixation by controlled mechanical ventilation until the chest wall has stabilized, which may take 14 to 21 days or more. Ventilators are able to monitor pressure, flow, and volume so treatment can be prescribed and modified for each person.[35]

Whenever pulmonary function is adequate, intubation is avoided to help reduce infection, the most common complication associated with morbidity and mortality in clients with blunt chest trauma. Pharmacologic treatment may include muscle relaxants or musculoskeletal paralyzing agents (e.g., pancuronium bromide) to reduce the risk of separation of the healing costochondral junctions.

Older adults are more likely to have comorbid conditions and less likely to tolerate traumatic respiratory compromise.

Older adults have a significantly higher rate of chest injuries sustained in motor vehicle accidents.[198] Age and its effects on the body are the strongest predictor of outcome with flail chest, and increasing age is associated with increased complications and mortality.[8]

11.12 Special Implications for the PTA: Chest Wall Trauma or Lung Injury Transcutaneous electrical nerve stimulation (TENS) units have been shown to be more effective than nonsteroidal antiinflammatory drugs (NSAIDs) for controlling pain associated with rib fractures and chest wall trauma.[255] This is important because pain can further compromise pulmonary function.[179]

Once the person's condition has been stabilized, PTAs are likely to come into contact during the recovery period. Manual techniques for secretion removal are used with precaution.

Airway clearance techniques may have a role in facilitating chest tube drainage but must be used carefully in the presence of any rib fractures. Percussion and vibration techniques are contraindicated directly over fractures but can be used over other lung segments. Rib or chest taping and ultrasound over the site of the fracture should not be used. Once the fractures have healed and are stable, rib mobilization and soft tissue mobilization for the intercostals may be necessary to restore normal respiratory movements.

It should be noted that airway clearance techniques can cause rib fractures owing to repeated internal pressure and force of coughing, and that infants are particularly vulnerable to rib fractures.[63] Frequent turning and position changes, as well as deep-breathing and coughing exercises, are important. A semi-Fowler's position may help with lung reexpansion necessary to prevent atelectasis. In the case of flail chest from injury, simultaneous cardiac damage may have occurred, necessitating the same care as for a person who has suffered a myocardial infarction.

Sternal fractures associated with clinically silent myocardial contusion are best visualized on chest computed tomography (CT) scans, but scapular fractures are often overlooked when only supine chest radiographs are performed. The PTA may recognize a suspicious clinical presentation (e.g., loss of scapular–humeral motion, symptoms out of proportion to the injury, or development of previously undocumented large hematomas) suggesting the need for more definitive medical diagnosis. In the case of scapular or humeral fractures, once the fracture has healed the PTA may become more involved in restoration of movement and strength.

ENVIRONMENTAL AND OCCUPATIONAL DISEASES

The relationship between occupations and disease has been observed, studied, and documented for many years. This chapter defines and discusses a few environmental and occupational diseases related to the lung. Occupational diseases can be divided into three major categories: (1) inorganic dusts (pneumoconioses); (2) organic dusts (hypersensitivity pneumonitis); and (3) fumes, gases, and smoke inhalation. These three categories have pathologic characteristics in common, including involvement of the pulmonary parenchyma with a fibrotic response.

Pneumoconiosis
Overview
Any group of lung diseases resulting from inhalation of particles of industrial substances, particularly inorganic dusts such as those from iron ore or coal, with permanent deposition of substantial amounts of such particles in the lung, is included in the generic term of *pneumoconiosis* (dusty lungs). Clinically common pneumoconioses include coal worker's pneumoconiosis (also known as *black lung disease*), silicosis, and asbestosis. Other types of pneumoconiosis include talc pneumoconiosis, beryllium lung disease (berylliosis), aluminum pneumoconiosis, cadmium worker's disease, and siderosis (inhalation of iron or other metallic particles). Farmers in dry climate regions exposed to respirable dust (inorganic agricultural dusts) during farming activities (e.g., plowing and tilling) and toxic gases (e.g., from animal confinement) may develop chronic bronchitis, hypersensitivity pneumonitis, and pulmonary fibrosis.

11.13 Special Implications for the PTA: Pneumoconioses New materials are being introduced into the workplace at a faster rate than their potential toxicities can be evaluated despite the fact that many have a pathologic effect on the pulmonary system. The possibility of occupational lung disease should be considered whenever a working or retired person has unexplained respiratory illness.

Steam inhalation and airway clearance techniques, such as controlled coughing and segmental bronchial drainage with chest percussion and vibration, help clear secretions. Exercise tolerance must be increased slowly over a long period beginning with increasing regular activities of daily living. Daily activities should be planned carefully to conserve energy, to decrease the work of breathing, and to afford frequent rest periods.

Graded progression from increasing tolerance for daily activities to a conditioning program may precede or replace an aggressive exercise program. In severe cases, oxygen may be necessary for any increase in activity level or exercise and the person may not progress beyond self-care skills.

Hypersensitivity Pneumonitis

Exposure to organic dusts may result in hypersensitivity pneumonitis, also called *extrinsic allergic alveolitis*. The alveoli and distal airways are most often involved as a result of inhalation of organic dusts and active chemicals. Most of the diseases are named according to the specific antigen or occupation and involve organic materials such as molds (e.g., mushroom compost, moldy hay, sugar cane, or logs left unprotected from moisture), fungal spores (e.g., stagnant water in air conditioners and central heating units), plant fibers or wood dust (particularly redwood and maple and cotton), cork dust, coffee beans, bird feathers, and hydroxyurea (*cytotoxic* agent).

Gram-negative bacterial endotoxins may be more to blame than dust in causing pneumonitis in cotton textile workers.[340] Mycobacteria have also been shown to be responsible for hypersensitivity pneumonitis in industrial metal grinding and in "hot tub lung."[7,143]

The diagnosis of hypersensitivity pneumonitis of an organic origin is made by history of exposure, pulmonary function studies, inflammatory mediators in sputum, and clinical manifestations, which commonly include abrupt onset of dyspnea, fever, chills, and a nonproductive cough.

Initially, symptoms may be reversed by removing the worker from the exposure (the only adequate treatment), modifying the materials-handling process, or using protective clothing and masks. The symptoms typically remit within 24 to 48 hours but return on reexposure and with time, and in some people they may become chronic.

Hypersensitivity pneumonitis may manifest as acute, subacute, or chronic pulmonary disease depending on the frequency and intensity of exposure to the antigen. The prognosis is poor with repeated exposure to these organic dusts, resulting in nonreversible interstitial fibrosis and other adverse respiratory effects.

Noxious Gases, Fumes, and Smoke Inhalation

Exposure to toxic gases and fumes is an increasing problem in modern industrial society. Any time oxygen in the air is replaced by another toxic or nontoxic agent, asphyxia (deficient blood oxygen and increased carbon dioxide in blood and tissues) occurs. Such is the case when products manufactured from synthetic compounds are heated at high temperatures, releasing fumes. For example, workers who use heating elements to seal meat in plastic wrappers and workers involved in the manufacture of plastics and packaging materials made of polyvinyl chlorides are exposed to these fumes. Workers exposed to the artificial butter flavoring for popcorn, diacetyl, have developed significant respiratory obstruction.[191]

The most common mechanism of injury is local irritation, the specific type and extent depending on the type and concentration of gas and the duration of exposure. For example, highly soluble gases, such as ammonia, rapidly injure the mucous membranes of the eye and upper airway, causing an intense burning pain in the eyes, nose, and throat. Insoluble gases such as nitrogen dioxide, encountered by farmers, cause diffuse lung injury.

Metal fume fever is a systemic response to inhalation of certain metal dusts and fumes such as zinc oxide, which is used in galvanizing iron, the manufacture of brass, and chrome and copper plating. Symptoms include fever and chills, cough, dyspnea, thirst, metallic taste, salivation, myalgias, headache, and malaise. Welding fumes create exposure to multiple hazardous agents and cause varied respiratory and systemic pathology.[232] *Polymer fume fever*, associated with heating of polymers, may cause similar symptoms. With brief exposures, the symptoms associated with these two syndromes are self-limiting, but prolonged exposure results in chronic cough, hemoptysis, and impairment of pulmonary function associated with a wide range of lung pathologic conditions.

Chemical pneumonitis can result from exposure to toxic fumes. The acute reaction may produce diffuse lung injury characterized by air space disease typical of pulmonary edema. In its chronic form, bronchiolitis obliterans develops.

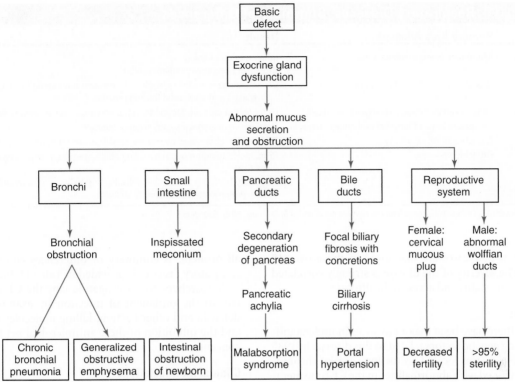

FIG. 11.14 Various effects of exocrine gland dysfunction in cystic fibrosis. (Adapted from Hockenberry MJ, Wilson D: Wong's essentials of pediatric nursing, ed 9, St. Louis, 2013, Mosby.)

Smoke inhalation injury produces direct mucosal injury secondary to hot gases, tissue anoxia caused by combustion products, and asphyxia as oxygen is consumed by fire. Thermal injury seen in the upper airway is characterized by edema and obstruction. Incomplete combustion of industrial compounds produces ammonia, acrolein, sulfur dioxide, and other substances in today's fires.

Environmental tobacco smoke (ETS), or exposure to secondhand smoke among nonsmokers, is widespread. Home and workplace environments are major sources of exposure. A total of 15 million children are estimated to be exposed to secondhand smoke in their homes annually. ETS increases the risk of heart disease and respiratory infections in children, increases the risk of lung cancer by a factor of 2 to 3, and is responsible for an estimated 3000 cancer deaths of adult nonsmokers and 2300 deaths from sudden infant death syndrome (SIDS) annually.[268]

Infants born to women exposed to ETS during pregnancy have an increased chance of decreased birth weight and intrauterine growth retardation.[147] Prenatal exposure to mainstream smoke from the mother and even to ETS from the mother has been shown to change fetal lung development and cause airflow obstruction, promote airway hyperresponsiveness and early development of asthma and allergy, and double the odds of future attention deficit hyperactivity disorder.[164,195]

Newborns, infants, and children under the age of 2 are at high risk for cardiovascular effects if they are exposed to household ETS. Endothelial cells of the blood vessels damaged as a result of exposure to passive smoking can be measured during the first decade of life. ETS over a period of more than 10 years changes the intima/media ratio by enhancing the thickness of the vessel wall. Other effects of involuntary smoking among children may include middle ear disease, upper and lower respiratory infections, and asthma.[165,324]

ETS is associated with rhinitis symptoms of runny nose and nasal congestion in some people and is associated with decreased flow in the airways, bronchial hyperresponsiveness, and increased respiratory infections.[124] Other symptoms following exposure to secondhand tobacco smoke may include headache, chest discomfort or tightness, and cough. See also the section on lung cancer in this chapter.

CONGENITAL DISORDERS

Cystic Fibrosis

Definition and Overview

CF is an inherited disorder of ion transport (sodium and chloride) in the exocrine glands that affects the hepatic, digestive, male reproductive, and respiratory systems (Fig. 11.14). The basic genetic defect predisposes to chronic bacterial airway infections, and almost all persons develop obstructive lung disease associated with chronic infection that leads to progressive loss of pulmonary function.

Incidence

CF is the most common inherited genetic disease in the white population, affecting approximately 30,000 children and young adults (equal gender distribution) in the United States. More than 1000 new cases are diagnosed each year. The disease is inherited as an autosomal recessive trait, meaning that both parents must be carriers so that the child inherits a defective gene from each one. In the United States 5% of the population, or 12 million people, carry a single copy of the CF gene. Each time two carriers conceive a child, there is a 25% chance (1:4) that the child will have CF, a 50% (1:2) chance that the child will be a carrier, and a 25% chance that the child will be a noncarrier.

TABLE 11.10	**Respiratory Diseases: Summary of Differences**	
Disease	**Primary Area Affected**	**Result**
Acute bronchitis	Membrane lining bronchial tubes	Inflammation of lining Bronchial dilation with inflammation
Bronchiectasis	Bronchial tubes (bronchi or air passages)	Causative agent invades alveoli with resultant outpouring from lung capillaries into air spaces and continued healing process
Pneumonia	Alveoli (air sacs)	
Chronic bronchitis	Larger bronchi initially; all airways eventually	Increased mucus production (number and size) causing airway obstruction
Emphysema	Air spaces beyond terminal bronchioles (alveoli)	Breakdown of alveolar walls; spaces enlarged
Asthma	Bronchioles (small airways)	Bronchioles obstructed by muscle spasm, swelling of mucosa, thick secretions
Cystic fibrosis	Bronchioles	Bronchioles become obstructed and obliterated; later larger airways become involved Mucous plugs cling to airways walls, leading to bronchitis, bronchiectasis, atelectasis, pneumonia, or pulmonary abscess

From Goodman CC, Snyder TE: Differential diagnosis for the physical therapist, ed 5, St. Louis, 2013, Saunders.

Ten percent of new cases are diagnosed in those over 18 years of age.[79] The severity of the disease is strongly correlated with socioeconomic status and access to health care.[297]

Etiologic Factors

In recent years, there have been major advances in understanding the underlying genetic factors related to this disease. In 1985 and 1989 the CF gene was located on the long arm of chromosome 7 and was cloned with abnormalities in the CF transmembrane conductance regulator (CFTR) protein being attributed to CF.

In healthy people, this CFTR protein provides a channel by which chloride (a component of salt) can pass in and out of the plasma membrane of many epithelial cells, including those of the kidney, gut, and conducting airways. Clients with CF have a defective gene that normally enables cells to form or regulate that channel.

Over 300 mutations in the CF gene affecting the CFTR protein have been described, but not all of the mutations have been identified, so mass screening cannot yet identify individuals carrying the gene for CF who would otherwise test negative. New tests are being developed to more reliably detect for mutations.[176]

Inflammation plays a role in lung damage associated with CF unrelated to the genetic defect.[84] The role of polymorphism (individual variation) of a gene that regulates protection from lung injury (by producing a substance called *glutathione*) has strong association with the severity of CF lung disease.[229]

Pathogenesis

Much about the complex pathogenesis of CF is still unknown, but it does appear that this impermeability of epithelial cells to chloride results in (1) dehydrated and increased *viscosity* of mucous gland secretions, primarily in the lungs, pancreas, intestine, and sweat glands; (2) elevation of sweat electrolytes (sodium chloride); and (3) pancreatic enzyme insufficiency. The dehydration resulting in thick, viscous mucous gland secretions causes the mechanical obstruction responsible for the multiple clinical manifestations of CF.

Bronchial and bronchiolar obstruction by the abnormal mucus predisposes the lung to infection and causes patchy atelectasis with hyperinflation. The disease progresses from mucous plugging and inflammation of small airways (bronchiolitis) to bronchitis, followed by bronchiectasis, pneumonia, fibrosis, and the formation of large cystic dilations that involve

all bronchi. A summary of differences among these various respiratory diseases is provided in Table 11.10.

Researchers are investigating why the CF lung is so receptive to the onslaught of infection by examining the role of defensin and other bacteria-killing molecules in the CF airway and the inhibition of these antimicrobial peptides by high salt concentrations.

Clinical Manifestations

The consistent finding of abnormally high sodium and chloride concentrations in the sweat is a unique characteristic of CF. Parents frequently observe that their infants taste salty when they kiss them. Almost all clinical manifestations of CF are a result of overproduction of extremely viscous mucus and deficiency of pancreatic enzymes.

A complete list of clinical manifestations by organ and in order of progression is given in Box 11.7. Recurrent pneumothorax, hemoptysis, PH, and cor pulmonale are serious and life-threatening complications of severe and diffuse CF pulmonary disease.

Pancreas. Approximately 90% of clients have pancreatic insufficiency with thick secretions blocking the pancreatic ducts and causing dilation of the small lobes of the pancreas, degeneration, and eventual progressive fibrosis throughout. The blockage also prevents essential pancreatic enzymes from reaching the duodenum, thus impairing digestion and absorption of nutrients. Clinically, this process results in bulky, frothy (undigested fats because of a lack of amylase and tryptase enzymes), and foul-smelling stools (decomposition of proteins producing compounds such as hydrogen sulfide and ammonia).

As the life expectancy for people with CF has improved, the incidence of glucose intolerance and CF-related diabetes has increased. Hyperglycemia may adversely influence nutritional status and weight, pulmonary function, and development of late microvascular complications.[349]

Gastrointestinal. The earliest manifestation of CF, *meconium ileus* (sometimes referred to as *distal intestinal obstruction syndrome*), is present in approximately 10% to 15% of newborns with CF. The small intestine is blocked with thick, puttylike tenacious meconium. Prolapse of the rectum is the most common gastrointestinal complication associated with CF, occurring most often in infancy and childhood. Children of all ages with CF are susceptible to intestinal obstruction from thickened, dried, or impacted stools (*inspissated* meconium). Advances in investigative techniques have led to increasing

BOX 11.7   Clinical Manifestations of Cystic Fibrosis

Early Stages
- Persistent coughing
- Sputum production
- Persistent wheezing
- Recurrent pulmonary infection
- Excessive appetite, poor weight gain
- Salty skin and sweat
- Bulky, foul-smelling stools

Pulmonary
Initial
- Wheezy respirations
- Dry, nonproductive cough

Progressive Involvement
- Increased dyspnea
- Decreased exercise tolerance
- Paroxysmal cough
- Tachypnea
- Obstructive emphysema
- Patchy areas of atelectasis
- Nasal polyps, chronic sinusitis

Advanced Stage
- Barrel chest
- Kyphosis
- Pectus carinatum
- Cyanosis
- Clubbing (fingers and toes)
- Recurrent bronchitis
- Recurrent bronchopneumonia
- Pneumothorax
- Hemoptysis
- Right-sided heart failure secondary to pulmonary hypertension

Gastrointestinal
- Voracious appetite (early)
- Anorexia (late)
- Weight loss

- Failure to thrive or grow; protein-calorie malnutrition
- Distended abdomen
- Thin extremities
- Sallow (yellowish) skin
- Acute gastroesophageal reflux (GERD)
- Intussusception

Distal Intestinal Obstruction Syndrome (Meconium Ileus)
- Abdominal distention
- Colicky, abdominal pain
- Vomiting
- Failure to pass stools (constipation)
- Rapid development of dehydration
- Anemia

Liver
- Cirrhosis
- Portal hypertension

Pancreatic
- Large, bulky, loose, frothy, foul-smelling stools (pancreatic enzyme insufficiency)
- Fat-soluble vitamin deficiency (vitamins A, D, E, K)
- Recurrent pancreatitis
- Iron deficiency anemia
- Malnutrition
- Diabetes mellitus

Genitourinary
- Male urogenital abnormalities
- Delay in sexual development
- Sterility (most males); infertility (some females)

Musculoskeletal
- Marked tissue wasting, muscle atrophy
- Myalgia
- Osteoarthropathy (adult)
- Rheumatoid arthritis (adult)
- Osteopenia, osteoporosis (adult)

reports of Crohn's disease and ischemic bowel disease in persons with CF. Poor nutrition and weight loss are common as a result of malabsorption, inadequate oral intake, early satiety, and increased usage of calories.

Pulmonary. Chronic cough and purulent sputum production are symptomatic of lung involvement. The child is unable to expectorate the mucus because of its increased viscosity. This retained mucus provides an excellent medium for bacterial growth, placing the individual at increased risk for infection. Reduced oxygen–carbon dioxide exchange causes variable degrees of hypoxia, clubbing (see Fig. 11.4), cyanosis, hypercapnia, and resultant acidosis. Chronic pulmonary infection and hyperinflation lead to secondary manifestations of barrel chest, pectus carinatum, and kyphosis.

The most common complication of CF is an exacerbation of pulmonary disease requiring medical and physical therapy intervention. Early warning signs (Box 11.8) must be recognized and treatment initiated (referred to as a "tune-up"), preferably at home but sometimes in the hospital. Respiratory failure is a frequent complication of severe pulmonary disease in persons with CF and is the most common cause of CF-related deaths.

BOX 11.8   Signs and Symptoms of Pulmonary Exacerbation in Cystic Fibrosis

- Increased cough
- Increased sputum production and/or a change in appearance of sputum
- Fever
- Weight loss
- School or work absenteeism (because of illness)
- Increased respiratory rate and/or WOB
- New findings on chest examination (e.g., wheezing, crackles)
- Decreased exercise tolerance
- Decrease in FEV_1 of 10% or more from baseline value within past 3 months
- Decrease in hemoglobin saturation of 10% or more from baseline value within past 3 months
- New finding(s) on chest radiograph

FEV_1, Forced expiratory volume in 1 second, *WOB*, work of breathing. From Cystic Fibrosis Foundation: Clinical practice guidelines for cystic fibrosis, Bethesda, MD, 1997, Cystic Fibrosis Foundation.

Liver. Liver involvement in CF is much less frequent than both pulmonary and pancreatic diseases, which are present in 80% to 90% of individuals with CF. Liver disease affects only one-third of the CF population; however, because of the decreasing mortality from extrahepatic causes, its recognition and management are becoming a relevant clinical issue.[69]

Recent observations suggest that clinical expression of liver disease in CF may be influenced by genetic modifiers; their identification is an important issue because it may allow recognition of people at risk for the development of liver disease at the time of diagnosis of CF and early institution of prophylactic strategies.[69]

Genitourinary. Genitourinary manifestations are primarily related to reproduction; infertility, once thought to be universal in men and common in women, may be treated successfully with new techniques for in vitro fertilization. The vas deferens may be absent bilaterally, or if present it is obstructed so that although sperm production is normal, blockage or fibrosis of the vas deferens prevents release of the sperm into the semen (azoospermia). Women experience decreased fertility because thick mucus in the cervical canal prevents conception. As the disease progresses, there is also an increased incidence of amenorrhea.

Musculoskeletal. Muscle pain is reported and may be alleviated with proper nutrition and exercise, although this is based on anecdotal information and has not been verified in studies. Decreased bone mineral density (BMD) and bone mineral content are common at all ages in CF, attributed to multifactorial causes (e.g., nutrition, exposure to glucocorticoid therapy, gonadal dysfunction, age, body mass, or activity). Spinal consequences of bone loss include excessive kyphosis and neck and back pain. Lung transplant is also associated with increased osteoporosis from long-term immunosuppression.

Hypertrophic pulmonary osteoarthropathy occurs with increasing frequency with increasing age and severity of disease in 2% to 7% of affected individuals. This condition is accompanied by clubbing of the fingers and toes; arthritis; painful periosteal new bone formation (especially over the tibia); and swelling of the wrists, elbows, knees, or ankles. The periostitis is observed radiographically in the diaphysis of the tubular bones and may be a single layer or a solid cloaking of the bone.

Separately—and usually without association with other manifestations of CF—attacks of episodic arthritis accompanied by severe joint pain, stiffness, rash, and fever may occur intermittently but repeatedly. Also related to CF are rheumatoid arthritis, spondyloarthropathies, sarcoidosis, and amyloidosis, which are caused by coexistent conditions and drug reactions.[40]

Medical Management

Diagnosis

Now that the gene responsible for CF has been identified, prenatal diagnosis and screening of carriers are possible as part of genetic counseling. The tests detect only mutations already observed but account for 70% (those with the DF508 mutation) of all CF carriers. In 2004 the CDC issued a recommendation that all newborns be screened for CF, and currently 18 states and the District of Columbia do routine screening. Prepregnancy genetic testing that involves DNA analysis of oocytes is available for couples at risk for having children with CF.

About one-half of all children with CF have presenting symptoms in infancy that include failure to thrive, respiratory compromise, or both. The age at presentation can vary, and some people are not diagnosed until adulthood. CF is traditionally diagnosed using the sweat test; a positive test occurs when the sodium chloride concentration is greater than 60 mEq/L for anyone younger than 20 years (reference value: 40 mEq/L) and above 80 mEq/L for those over 20 years.[311]

Pulmonary function tests are performed in affected individuals from the age of 6 and up to measure and monitor lung function over time. These tests are used to classify the severity of baseline lung disease. Almost all measures are based on the flow of air into and out of the lungs in a given period of time.

Treatment

A multidisciplinary approach must be taken in treating CF, with the goal of promoting a normal life for the individual. The treatment of CF depends on the stage of the disease and which organs are involved. Medical management is oriented toward alleviating symptoms and includes the use of antibiotics, aggressive pulmonary therapy with drugs (*mucolytics*) to thin mucus secretions, ACTs, supplemental oxygen, and adequate hydration and enhanced nutrition with pancreatic enzymes administered before or with meals.

Pharmacotherapy

Drug therapy for CF has been primarily directed at prophylaxis and treatment of infections with antibiotics, targeting inflammation, and supplementing digestive enzymes and vitamins. Pharmacotherapy to date has included broad-spectrum antimicrobials to protect the respiratory epithelium from damage and aerosolized antibiotics (e.g., tobramycin) that deliver a more concentrated dose directly to the site of infection. Common side effects of medications used to treat CF are found in Table 11.6. The PTA will need to be aware of how these physical symptoms will require a change in the treatment approach according to the patient's activity tolerance.

Transplantation

Double-lung or heart-lung transplants have been used with children and adults with advanced pulmonary vascular disease and who are severely disabled by dyspnea and hypoxia. In the United States the United Network for Organ Sharing has addressed perceived inequities in organ distribution by allocating organs by illness severity rather than time on the waiting list. A lung allocation score ranks severity for patients 12 years of age and older for transplantation based on variables including lung function, oxygen and ventilatory needs, diabetes, weight, and physical performance.[201]

Liver transplantation should be offered to anyone with CF and progressive liver failure and/or with life-threatening sequelae of portal hypertension, who also have mild pulmonary involvement that is expected to support long-term survival.[69]

Long-term survival after transplant has yet to be determined, but improved quality of life has been achieved. The new lungs do not acquire the CF ion-transport abnormalities but are subject to the usual posttransplant complications. CF problems in other organ systems persist and may be worsened by some of the immunosuppressive regimens.[357] CNS complications occur more frequently in

CF transplant recipients than in other lung transplant recipients.[128] Criteria for lung transplant have been published, and early referral and continuous monitoring are required because decline as a result of the long waiting period can be expected.[121]

Prognosis

Using its innovative CF patient registry, which tracks information on approximately 23,000 clients who receive care through the CF Foundation's Care Center Network, researchers have analyzed the numbers and continue to assess trends in the health status of registered individuals. When CF was first distinguished from celiac disease in 1938, life expectancy with CF was approximately 6 months.[84] Data show that the prognosis has steadily improved over the past 20 years with a gradual increase in longevity; in 2008, the median predicted age of survival had risen to 37.4 years.[247]

More than 50% of children with CF live into adulthood. The new median age of survival is based on 2013 data that include date of birth, date of death, gender, and date of diagnosis.[81a] A detailed CF Foundation Annual Patient Registry Data Report is available.

11.14 Special Implications for the PTA: Cystic Fibrosis

Airway Clearance Techniques

The PTA must always be aware that anyone with CF is susceptible to infections, in particular with *Burkholderia cepacia.* Care must be taken to avoid transmission via equipment, other patients, or oneself. Handwashing is essential, and high-alcohol hand rubs may be more effective.[123] The PTA will be involved with airway clearance techniques carried out several times per day or as often as the person is able to tolerate them without undue fatigue. Airway clearance techniques should not be performed before or immediately after meals to prevent regurgitation and/or vomiting. Treatment must be scheduled to avoid mealtimes.

Aerosol therapy to deliver medication to the lower respiratory tract should be administered just before airway clearance techniques to maximize the effectiveness of both treatments. Breathing exercises, improved posture, mobilization of the thorax through active exercise, and manual therapy are part of promoting good breathing patterns and improving inspiratory muscle endurance. Specifics of airway clearance techniques for this population are beyond the scope of this text; the reader is referred to more detailed materials available.[77,78,80,107]

The many difficulties surrounding percussion and postural drainage (e.g., is associated with poor compliance, is time consuming, and requires the assistance of a trained individual) have resulted in the development of alternative airway clearance techniques that can be accomplished without the assistance of another caregiver.

Each of these techniques (e.g., autogenic drainage, active cycle breathing, positive expiratory pressure [PEP], Flutter valve, Acapella, and Quake) requires a certain level of compliance, motivation, understanding, neuromuscular function, and breath control. Autogenic drainage, active cycle breathing, and PEP help the individual to move the mucus up to the larger airways where it can be coughed out more easily. Autogenic drainage comprises a series of sequential breathing exercises designed to clear the small, medium, and large airways in that order. The PARI PEP S device maintains pressure in the lungs, keeping the airways open and allowing air to get behind the mucus

(Fig. 11.15). This device has been shown to be effective in increased sputum production, improved lung function, and improved oxygenation.[83]

The Flutter valve is similar to the PEP device but uses a stainless steel ball that vibrates, alternately opening and closing the device's air hole, pulsing air back into the airways (Fig. 11.16). Current practice is to use one of the devices (PEP or Flutter valve) followed by autogenic breathing techniques. The total treatment time is about 15 minutes, and treatment can be carried out independently by some children and most adolescents and adults with mild to moderate disease who can follow the directions and control their breathing.

Preliminary studies on the Flutter device suggest that Flutter valve therapy is an acceptable alternative to postural drainage and percussion and may be more effective than postural drainage in prolonging the ability to raise secretions. Sputum production increased significantly 30 minutes after the end of treatment, and 1 hour after the end of treatment, it was significantly greater than the amount produced after postural drainage.[23,130] In a comparison study lasting 1 year, PEP was superior to the Flutter in maintaining pulmonary function, reducing hospitalizations, and reducing antibiotic use.[228]

A high-frequency chest wall oscillation vest can provide mucus clearance for individuals who lack the ability to perform the simpler techniques and is especially helpful with children (although the cost may seem prohibitive, it is less than a single hospitalization for a pulmonary exacerbation). The device consists of an inflatable vest (the Vest) attached to an air pulse generator (Fig. 11.17). The generator, a compressor-like device, rapidly inflates and deflates the vest, gently compressing and releasing the chest wall to create airflow within the lungs. This device treats all lobes simultaneously for the duration of the time it is activated. This process moves mucus toward the larger airways where it can be cleared by coughing.

The effectiveness of this mechanized device has been supported by the limited research published to date. Results from the Vest are becoming quite well documented, demonstrating decreased hospitalizations and slower rate of FEV_1 decline.[194] The Vest Airway Clearance System website (http://www.thevest.com/research/bibliography.asp) has an extensive bibliography. Future research should determine optimal compression frequencies and wave forms.[194,234] The Vest is comparable to PEP in effectiveness, but arterial oxygen saturation may drop during its use, so this must be monitored during exacerbations.[83]

Nutrition

Malnutrition and deterioration of lung function are closely interrelated and interdependent in the person with CF. Each affects the other, leading to a spiral decline in both. The occurrence of malnutrition during childhood seems to be associated with impaired growth and repair of the airway walls. In children, when growth in body length occurs, good nutrition is associated with better lung function. When adequate nutrition is combined with physical training and aerobic exercise, improved body weight, respiratory muscle function, lung function, and exercise tolerance occur, with increases in both respiratory and other muscle mass.[146]

Exercise

Increasingly, exercise and sport are being advanced as core components of treatment for individuals with CF of all ages. A large portfolio of exercise literature has already established that supervised exercise programs enhance fitness (and thereby improve survival), increase sputum clearance, delay the onset of dyspnea, delay declines in pulmonary function, prevent decrease in bone density,[345] enhance cellular immune response,[36] and increase feelings of well-being, thereby potentially improving self-image, self-confidence, and quality of life for the person with CF. Both short- and long-term aerobic and anaerobic training have positive effects on exercise capacity, strength, and lung function.[44] Even unsupervised programs produce a training effect and pulmonary benefits.[239] Inspiratory muscle training alone in individuals with CF has shown improved lung function and increased work capacity, as well as improved psychosocial status.[86,96]

The PTA can be very instrumental in providing client and family education about the importance of combining good nutrition and exercise and activity. The PTA helps each individual develop an exercise routine that includes strengthening, stretching, aerobic, and endurance components, with special attention to breathing exercises to aerate all areas of the lungs. Weight loss with exercise is of special concern in this population, especially for the individual with CF and diabetes mellitus.

Energy expenditure is higher than usual for individuals with CF and diabetes during periods of recovery from mild exercise or activity because of increased work of breathing (WOB) consistent with higher ventilatory requirements.[341] This requires careful collaboration among the client and family, therapy team, and nutritionist. In addition, systemic inflammatory response to exercise may be greater for individuals with CF, potentially exacerbating the disease.[163]

As longevity increases with CF, quality-of-life issues are more important; thus these issues, such as posture, arthropathies, and neuromuscular control, are becoming more important for the PTA.[92,223] When treating anyone with CF who has sustained trauma, a multisystem approach is critical for optimal outcomes in physical therapy.[322]

Individuals with CF who are awaiting a transplant must remain as active as possible; whenever possible, the PTA should design a safe but effective exercise program. If significant oxygen desaturation or severe breathlessness limits activity, then exercise on a treadmill, stationary bike, or even a stationary device for seated pedaling is recommended, with supplemental oxygen supplied at sufficient flow to match minute ventilatory requirements.[345]

Studies of exercise performance in lung transplant recipients with end-stage CF report that exercise performance improves after transplantation but remains well below normal.[254] In a study of 12 individuals 8 to 95 months after lung transplant, the diaphragm and abdominal muscle strength was preserved relative to healthy controls, but quadriceps strength was significantly diminished and affected exercise performance. Corticosteroid use partly contributed to this strength deficit.[267]

Transition to Adult Care

CF centers and other centers providing lifelong care for clients with CF have realized the need for a transition phase between pediatric and adult care and the provision of counseling for parents and the young adult with CF to assist them with this marked change in approach to the young adult's care.

The PTA can and should have an integral role in preparing families and clients for various phases in care from pediatrics to adolescent care to a more independent model of adult care. Materials and resources are available to help get such a program started and established if one does not exist in your current facility.[31,65,226,356]

Many families receive care for their child for years at a pediatric center and develop lifelong relationships with health care agencies and staff. Every effort should be made to accomplish a smooth transition for the client and the family, because the move from the well-established pediatric facility to a new facility or medical team can be a stressful transition for all.

Families in rural settings or who travel distances to benefit from centralized services in CF clinics or centers have some unique needs that should be addressed as well. For example, maintaining a complete medical record in more than one facility is not always possible. Without a good systems coordinator, gaps in the medical record from one clinic to another become all too common.

Transition to adult care should be a planned process over time. Every effort should be made to avoid an abrupt transfer. The pediatric team has the responsibility to "set the stage" for the transition. The process can be started early with expectations for an eventual adult transition reinforced in intervals. Written information about the transition, setting an actual time frame, and planning each step in the process are important.[226]

Three guiding principles are suggested, regardless of the format chosen for transition. First, there must be an adult team that is both interested and able to provide care. Second, there needs to be a very well planned, coordinated approach to the transition. Third, there must be excellent communication and interaction between the pediatric and adult teams.[226] Transition programs should be flexible enough to meet the needs of a wide range of young people, health conditions, and circumstances. The actual transfer of care should be individualized to meet the specific needs of young people and their families.[285] Family involvement, including parents, guardians, and/or partner and the client, is essential to the success of any transition phase. The omission of any key people from the transition team can result in frustration, feelings of abandonment, and miscommunication, which could ultimately lead to compromised care for the individual with CF.

Adults with Cystic Fibrosis

As individuals with CF survive longer into adulthood, the unique needs of this population group are being considered. Health care in the adult setting encourages independence and increased self-reliance.[357] Achieving an ideal nutritional status is an integral part of management of people with CF, but how these requirements change as the individual ages remains unknown. Emphasis is continually placed on dietary intake and weight; the effects of this on eating behavior and self-perceptions are under investigation.[1,330,347]

Other concerns include the effects of long-term use of pancreatic enzymes, osteoporosis associated with late-stage CF and its complications of increased fracture rates and severe kyphosis,[18,19,145] the effects of hormonal changes in relation to the menstrual cycle on lung function,[172] psychosocial–spiritual issues,[151] and infertility issues.[159]

The origin of bone disease in CF is multifactorial and not completely understood. However, glucocorticoid therapy, delayed pubertal maturation, malabsorption of vitamin D, poor nutritional status, inactivity, and hypogonadism are all potential contributing factors.[81] Decreases in bone mineral density resulting from these factors can lead to osteoporosis, fragility fractures, and possible exclusion from lung transplant candidacy.[81] An in-depth discussion of bone health and disease in CF is available.[81]

Stress urinary incontinence has also been shown to affect many girls and women with CF, probably caused by the forceful and prolonged coughing bouts characteristic of the disease.[70,231] Interventions aimed at improving pelvic floor muscle strength and coordination may be appropriate for these individuals.

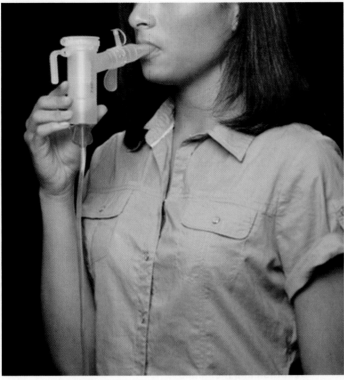
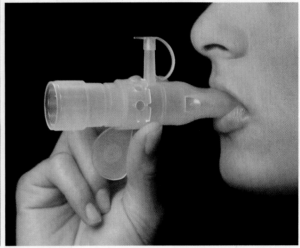

FIG. 11.15 PARI PEP S. The positive expiratory pressure (PEP) device maintains pressure in the lungs, keeping the airways open and allowing air to get behind the mucus to improve airway clearance, lung volume capacity, and oxygenation. (Courtesy PARI Respiratory Equipment, Inc., Midlothian, VA.)

PARENCHYMAL DISORDERS

Atelectasis

Definition

Atelectasis is the collapse of normally expanded and aerated lung tissue at any structural level (e.g., lung parenchyma, alveoli, pleura, chest wall, bronchi) involving all or part of the lung. Most cases are categorized as obstructive–absorptive or compressive atelectasis.

Etiologic Factors and Pathogenesis

The primary cause of atelectasis is obstruction of the bronchus serving the affected area. If a bronchus is obstructed (e.g., by tumors, mucus, or foreign material), atelectasis occurs as air in the alveoli is slowly absorbed into the bloodstream with subsequent collapse of the alveoli. Atelectasis can also develop when there is interference with the natural forces that promote lung expansion (e.g., hypoventilation associated with decreased motion or decreased pulmonary expansion such as occurs with paralysis, pleural disease, diaphragmatic disease, severe scoliosis, or masses in the thorax). Failure to breathe deeply postoperatively (e.g., because of muscular guarding and splinting from pain or discomfort with an upper abdominal, chest, or sternal incision), oversedation, immobility, coma, or neuromuscular disease can also interfere with the natural forces that promote lung expansion, leading to atelectasis.

Insufficient pulmonary surfactant, such as occurs in respiratory distress syndrome, inhalation of anesthesia, high concentrations of oxygen, lung contusion, aspiration of gastric contents

or smoke inhalation, or increased elastic recoil as a result of interstitial fibrosis (e.g., silicosis, asbestosis, radiation pneumonitis), can also interfere with lung distention. When atelectasis is caused by inhalation of concentrated oxygen or anesthetic agents, quick absorption of these gases into the bloodstream can lead to collapse of alveoli in dependent portions of the lung.

Although atelectasis is usually caused by bronchial obstruction, direct compression can also cause it. The compressive type is caused by air (pneumothorax), blood (hemothorax), or fluid (hydrothorax) filling the pleural space. Abdominal distention that presses on a portion of the lung can also collapse alveoli, causing atelectasis.

Clinical Manifestations

When sudden obstruction of the bronchus occurs, there may be dyspnea, tachypnea, cyanosis, elevation of temperature, drop in blood pressure, substernal retractions, or shock. In the chronic form of atelectasis, the client may be asymptomatic with gradual onset of dyspnea and weakness.

Medical Management

Diagnosis

Atelectasis should be suspected in penetrating or other chest injuries. X-ray examination may show a shadow in the area of collapse. If an entire lobe is collapsed, the radiograph will show the trachea, heart, and mediastinum deviated toward the collapsed area, with the diaphragm

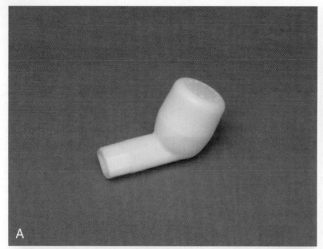

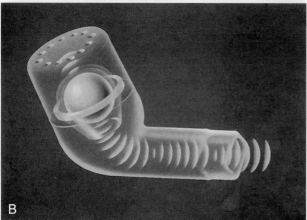

FIG. 11.16 The Flutter mucus clearance device. (A) The Flutter device provides positive expiratory pressure therapy for patients with mucus-producing respiratory conditions, including chronic obstructive pulmonary disease (COPD). (B) The Flutter device shown in this schematic uses a stainless steel ball that vibrates, alternately opening and closing the device's air hole, producing vibrations of the airway, loosening and upward movement of the mucus and, ideally, airway clearance. (Courtesy Aptalis Pharma US, Inc., an Allergan affiliate.)

elevated on that side. Chest auscultation and physical assessment add to the clinical diagnostic picture. Blood gas measurements may show decreased oxygen saturation.

Treatment and Prognosis

Once atelectasis has occurred, treatment is directed toward removing the cause whenever possible. Suctioning or bronchoscopy may be employed to remove airway obstruction. ACTs are helpful to remove secretions and promote segmental inflation after the obstruction has been removed.

Surfactant has been used to resolve atelectasis in infants with respiratory distress syndrome, meconium aspiration, and other pathologies.[101] Antibiotics are used to combat infection accompanying secondary atelectasis. Re-expansion of the lung is often possible, but the final prognosis depends on the underlying cause. Chronic atelectasis may require surgical removal of the affected segment or lobe of lung.

11.15 Special Implications for the PTA: Atelectasis Atelectasis is usually a postoperative complication of thoracic or high abdominal surgery, and left lower lobe atelectasis can occur after cardiac surgery. Within a few hours after surgery, atelectasis becomes increasingly resistant to reinflation. This complication is exacerbated in people receiving narcotics.

Diminished respiratory movement as a result of postoperative pain is often addressed by the PTA. Frequent, gentle position changes, deep breathing, coughing, and early ambulation help promote drainage of all lung segments. Deep breathing and effective coughing enhance lung expansion and prevent airway obstruction. Deep breathing is beneficial because it promotes the ciliary clearance of secretions, stabilizes the alveoli by redistributing surfactant, and permits collateral ventilation of the alveoli.

With deep breathing, air passes from well-ventilated alveoli to obstructed alveoli, minimizing the tendency for collapse and facilitating removal of the obstruction. To minimize postoperative pain during deep-breathing and coughing exercises, teach the client to splint the incision. This can be done by holding a pillow firmly over the incision or simply placing hands over the incision when taking a deep breath.

There is evidence that vigorous airway clearance techniques are as effective in resolving atelectasis from mucous plugs as bronchoscopy.[190] Bronchoscopy has the adverse effect of temporarily lowering oxygen saturation and further irritating lung tissue.

Pulmonary Edema

Definition and Incidence

Pulmonary edema or pulmonary congestion occurs when excessive fluid in the lungs leaks into the alveolar spaces, the interstitial tissue, or both. This decreases the space available for gas exchange. Normally the lung is kept dry by lymphatic drainage and a balance among capillary pressures and capillary permeability.

Pulmonary edema is a common complication of many disease processes. It occurs at any age but with increasing incidence in older people with left-sided heart failure.

Etiologic and Risk Factors

Most cases of pulmonary edema are caused by the following:

- Cardiac conditions: left ventricular failure, acute hypertension, or mitral valve disease
- Noncardiac conditions: kidney or liver disorders prone to the development of sodium and water retention, IV narcotics, increased intracerebral pressure, brain injury, high altitude, diving and submersion, sepsis, medications, inhalation of smoke or toxins (e.g., ammonia), blood transfusion reactions, shock, and disseminated intravascular coagulation[111]

Other risk factors include hyperaldosteronism, Cushing's syndrome, use of glucocorticoids, and use of hypotonic fluids to irrigate nasogastric tubes. Pulmonary edema itself is a major predisposing factor in the development of pneumonia that complicates heart failure and ARDS.

Clinical Manifestations

Clinical manifestations of pulmonary edema occur in stages. During the initial stage, clients may be asymptomatic or they may complain of restlessness and anxiety and the feeling that they are developing a common cold. Other signs include a persistent cough, slight dyspnea, diaphoresis, and intolerance to exercise. As fluid continues to fill the pulmonary interstitial spaces, the dyspnea becomes more acute, respirations increase in rate, and there is audible wheezing. If the edema is severe, the cough becomes productive of frothy sputum tinged with blood, giving it a pinkish hue. If the condition persists, the person becomes hypoxic and less responsive and may lose consciousness.

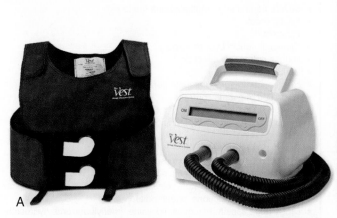
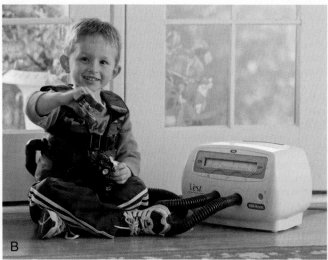

FIG. 11.17 (A) The Vest Airway Clearance System used to self-administer high-velocity oscillations. The vest can accommodate a child as young as 2 years old and is worn 30 minutes twice each day. (B) It has multiple programming options for treatment flexibility. Any position can be assumed, and a child can do everything himself. This device promotes compliance and is accompanied by reduced use of medications and infections. (Courtesy Hill-Rom Services PTE Ltd., St. Paul, MN.)

Medical Management

Prevention

Prevention is a key component with persons at increased risk for the development of pulmonary edema. Preventive measures may be as simple as lowering salt intake or monitoring and changing medications to maintain proper homeostasis of fluid balances. Specific pharmacologic treatment includes the use of digoxin and diuretics.

Diagnosis

Pulmonary edema is usually recognized by its characteristic clinical presentation. Cardiogenic pulmonary edema is differentiated from pulmonary edema of noncardiac causes by the history and physical examination; an underlying cardiac abnormality can usually be detected clinically or by the electrocardiogram (ECG), chest film, or echocardiogram. A chest film may show increased vascular pattern; increased opacity of the lung, especially at the bases; and pleural effusion.

There are no specific laboratory tests diagnostic of pulmonary edema; when the condition progresses enough to cause liver involvement the physician may observe the hepatojugular reflex (positional or palpatory pressure on the liver results in distention of the jugular vein). Auscultation reveals distinct abnormal breath sounds with crackles or rales. Blood gas measurements indicate the degree of functional impairment, and sputum cultures may indicate accompanying infection.

Treatment

Once pulmonary edema has been diagnosed, treatment is aimed at enhancing gas exchange, reducing fluid overload, and strengthening and slowing the heartbeat. Oxygen by mask or through ventilatory support is used along with diuretics, diet, and fluid restriction to remove excess alveolar fluid.

Morphine may be used to relieve anxiety and reduce the effort of breathing for people who do not have narcotic-induced pulmonary edema. Other pharmacologic-based treatment may be used to help dilate the bronchi, strengthen contractions of the heart, and increase cardiac output.

Prognosis

The prognosis depends on the underlying condition. The presence of pulmonary edema is a medical emergency requiring immediate intervention to prevent further respiratory distress and death. It is often reversible with clinical management.

11.16 Special Implications for the PTA: Pulmonary Edema Signs and symptoms of pulmonary edema that may come to the PTA's attention include engorged neck and hand veins (because of peripheral vascular fluid overload), pitting edema of the extremities, adventitious breath sounds, and paroxysmal nocturnal dyspnea (very common with this condition). One of the first signs of dyspnea may be increased difficulty breathing when lying down that is relieved by sitting up (orthopnea).

Any liver involvement requires precautions when performing any soft tissue mobilization techniques to the anterior part of the abdomen, including the diaphragm. Indirect techniques or mobilization away from the liver is recommended.

When working with a client already diagnosed with pulmonary edema, the sitting (high Fowler's) position is preferred, with legs dangling over the side of the bed or plinth. This facilitates respiration and reduces venous return. Monitor for decreased respiratory drive (less than 12 breaths/min is significant), which should be documented and reported immediately. If oxygen is being administered, the PTA monitors the oxyhemoglobin saturation levels and titrates oxygen accordingly. It may be necessary to increase oxygen levels before exercise, but respiratory rate and breathing pattern must be monitored.

Pulmonary edema can become life-threatening within minutes, requiring immediate action by the PTA to get medical assistance for this person. The client may be taking nitroglycerin sublingually, which will increase vasodilation and decrease ventricular preload. Monitor blood pressure closely and observe for signs of hypotension because nitroglycerin can drop blood pressure dangerously. The PTA should consult with nursing or respiratory staff for any special considerations for each individual client.

If pulmonary edema is left untreated, gradual exercise intolerance usually occurs as the dyspnea progresses. The client may comment about weight gain or difficulty fastening clothes. Check for peripheral edema in the immobile or bedridden client. In this group of people, edema can occur in the sacral hollow rather than in the feet and legs because the sacrum is the lowest place on the trunk. Care must be taken to prevent pressure ulcers in this area.

> **BOX 11.9** **Causes of Acute (Adult) Respiratory Distress Syndrome**
>
> - Severe trauma (e.g., multiple bone fractures)
> - Septic shock
> - Pancreatitis
> - Cardiopulmonary bypass surgery
> - Diffuse pulmonary infection
> - Burns
> - High concentrations of supplemental oxygen
> - Aspiration of gastric contents
> - Massive blood transfusions
> - Embolism: fat, thrombus, amniotic fluid, venous air
> - Near drowning
> - Radiation therapy
> - Inhalation of smoke or toxic fumes
> - Thrombotic thrombocytopenic purpura
> - Indirect: chemical mediators released in response to systemic disorders (e.g., viral infections, pneumonia)
> - Drugs (e.g., aspirin, narcotics, lidocaine, phenylbutazone, hydrochlorothiazide, most chemotherapeutic and cytotoxic agents)
>
> Listed in order of decreasing frequency.

Acute Respiratory Distress Syndrome

Definition

ARDS is a form of acute respiratory failure after a systemic or pulmonary insult. It is also called *adult respiratory distress syndrome, shock lung, wet lung, stiff lung, hyaline membrane disease (adult* or *newborn), posttraumatic lung,* or *diffuse alveolar damage* (DAD). It is often a fatal complication of serious illness (e.g., sepsis), trauma, or major surgery.

Incidence, Etiology, and Risk Factors

ARDS has been identified only within the last 40 years, affecting a reported 150,000 people per year in the United States. This figure has been challenged, and part of the reason for the uncertainty of numbers is the lack of uniform definitions for ARDS and the diversity of diseases underlying ARDS. The incidence has increased as improvements in intensive care have allowed more people to survive the catastrophic illnesses that precede ARDS. People of any age can be affected, but most often young adults with traumatic injuries develop ARDS.

ARDS occurs as a result of injury to the lung by a variety of unrelated causes; the most common are listed in Box 11.9.

Pathogenesis

Alveolocapillary units, alveolar spaces, alveolar walls, and lungs are the site of initial damage (thus the name *diffuse alveolar damage*). Although the mechanism of lung injury varies with the cause, damage to capillary cells and alveolar cells is common in ARDS regardless of cause. Cell death plays a role in this syndrome.[218] This results in pulmonary edema and alveolar collapse, which impairs respiration (gas exchange).

Pulmonary edema decreases lung compliance and impairs gas exchange. The loss of surfactant (because of cell death) leads to atelectasis and further impairment in lung compliance and results in hypoxia and hypercapnia. These are only the pulmonary manifestations of what is now recognized as a more systemic process called *multiple organ dysfunction syndrome* (MODS), formerly called *multiple organ failure* (MOF).

Clinical Manifestations

The clinical presentation is relatively uniform regardless of cause and occurs within 12 to 48 hours of the initiating event. The earliest sign of ARDS is usually an increased respiratory rate characterized by shallow, rapid breathing. Pulmonary edema, atelectasis, and decreased lung compliance cause dyspnea, hyperventilation, and the changes observed on chest radiographs (Fig. 11.18).

As breathing becomes increasingly difficult, the individual may gasp for air and exhibit intercostal, clavicular, or sternal retractions and cyanosis. Unless the underlying disease is reversed rapidly, especially in the presence of sepsis (toxins in the blood), the condition quickly progresses to full-blown MODS, involving the kidneys, liver, gut, CNS, and cardiovascular system.

Medical Management

Diagnosis

Because ARDS is a collection of symptoms rather than a specific disease, differential diagnosis is through a process of diagnostic elimination. Cardiogenic pulmonary edema and bacterial pneumonia must be ruled out because there are specific treatments for those disorders. By definition, respiratory failure in the proper clinical setting (history and physical findings) constitutes ARDS. Physical examination, blood gas analysis to assess the severity of hypoxemia, microbiologic cultures to identify or exclude infection, and radiographs may be part of the diagnostic process.

Treatment

Specific treatment is administered for any underlying conditions (e.g., sepsis or pneumonia). Otherwise treatment is supportive and aimed toward prevention of complications. Supportive therapy to maintain adequate blood oxygen levels may include administration of humidified oxygen by a tight-fitting face mask, allowing for CPAP. Traditional ventilator management of ARDS emphasized normalization of blood gases and promoted high rates of further lung damage. It is now known that overdistention and cyclic inflation of injured lung can exacerbate lung injury and promote systemic inflammation. Mechanical ventilation with PEEP can minimize these effects, but evidence for protective ventilation is still lacking.[117,240]

Sedation to reduce anxiety and restlessness during ventilation is required in some cases. If tachypnea, restlessness, or respirations out of phase with the ventilator (bucking) cannot be managed by sedation, pharmacologic paralysis may be induced. Other pharmacologic agents have been ineffective in altering morbidity or mortality.[5,165]

11.17 Special Implications for the PTA: Acute (Adult) Respiratory Distress Syndrome

Acute respiratory distress syndrome (ARDS) requires careful monitoring and supportive care. Timely physical therapy interventions improve gas exchange and reverse pathologic progression, thereby curtailing or avoiding artificial ventilation.[351]

Assess the client's respiratory status frequently, and observe for retractions on inspiration, the use of accessory muscles of respiration, and developing or worsening dyspnea. On auscultation, listen for adventitious breath sounds (rales or rhonchi) or diminished breath sounds, and report any clear, frothy sputum that may indicate pulmonary edema.

Closely monitor heart rate and blood pressure. Watch for arrhythmias, which may result from hypoxemia, acid–base disturbances, or electrolyte imbalance. Empty condensation from the tubing of the ventilator to ensure maximal oxygen delivery during therapy.

Critical illness polyneuropathy is a neurologic complication of ARDS, multiple organ dysfunction syndrome, and other trauma. PTAs should be alert for signs of motor or sensory changes in clients with ARDS.[6]

V/Q mismatch is common in ARDS and can be altered by position changes that can facilitate lung expansion and redistribute fluid in the lungs. Oxygenation in clients with ARDS may sometimes be improved by turning them from the supine to the prone position, dramatically reducing pulmonary dead space and improving aeration.[99] This change takes the weight off (and improves ventilation in) the posterior regions of the lungs while promoting perfusion in the anterior aspects. The net result is improved oxygenation, expansion of atelectatic alveoli, and increased functional residual lung capacity. Caregivers may be reluctant to use the prone position. The PTA can be very instrumental in providing education on proper technique and rationale.

The client should be turned as far as possible on the abdomen; a 270-degree turn can improve oxygenation in some individuals, but ideally the full prone position is optimal. The person can be turned almost fully prone and supported with two or three pillows to help protect the airway, permit visualization, and allow suctioning as necessary. The better the person responds to the prone position, the longer that position can be maintained, although tolerance may build up with repeated use of the position. It is the repeated change from supine to prone positioning that redistributes pulmonary fluid and improves aeration and oxygenation overall.

Before turning, identify all invasive lines and bring them above the person's waist and over the head; lines inserted in the groin area can be moved over to the side that will remain nondependent. Taking these precautions will reduce the chances that the lines will get kinked or dislodged. One person should be in charge of the person's airway during the turning, supporting the client's head and watching the intravenous lines. Any side-port line of a pulmonary artery catheter must be monitored especially carefully because it is closest to the client and more likely to kink. When the turn is completed, the same clinician turns the client's head to one side, making sure the airway is visible and open. Extra pillows or foam or gel pads may be needed to make room for the airway and increase comfort level. The dependent shoulder should be positioned with the elbow directly to the side and the hand facing up toward the head to prevent dislocation. A pad around the mouth to absorb bronchial secretions will decrease the potential for eye contamination.

The prone position promotes secretion removal by propelling secretions toward the upper airways. It also makes it easy to perform back care and help maintain sacral and heel skin integrity. Disadvantages include the potential for facial skin irritation (especially on the forehead), loss of important vascular accesses, and difficulty performing

cardiopulmonary resuscitation if required. Blood pressure may drop after the turn but should stabilize within a few minutes; unstable blood pressure will necessitate returning the person to the supine position. Other indicators of poor position tolerance include a decline in SaO_2, SvO_2, or the tidal volume over time.[91,99]

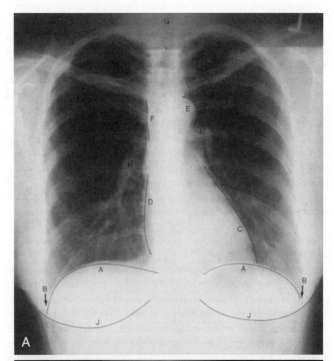

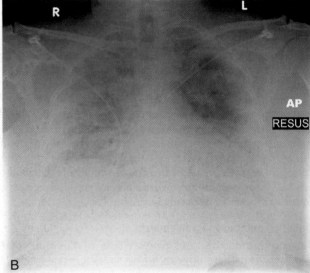

FIG. 11.18 (A) Normal chest film taken from a posteroanterior (PA) view. The backward L in the upper right corner is placed on the film to indicate the left side of the chest. Some anatomic structures can be seen on the x-ray study and are outlined: A, diaphragm; B, costophrenic angle; C, left ventricle, D, right atrium; E, aortic arch; F, superior vena cava; G, trachea; H, right bronchus; I, left bronchus; J, breast shadows. (B) This chest film shows massive consolidation from pulmonary edema associated with acute (adult) respiratory distress syndrome (ARDS). (A, From Black JM, Hawks, JH: Medical-surgical nursing, ed 8, St. Louis, 2009, Saunders. B, From Garden OJ, Bradbury AW, Forsythe JLR, et al., editors: Principles and practice of surgery, Edinburgh, 2012, Churchill Livingstone.)

Postoperative Respiratory Failure

Postoperative respiratory failure can result in the same pathophysiologic and clinical manifestations as ARDS but without the severe progression to MODS (see previous discussion of ARDS). Risk factors include surgical procedures of the thorax or abdomen, limited cardiac reserve, chronic renal failure, chronic hepatic disease, infection, period of hypotension during surgery, sepsis, and smoking, especially in the presence of preexisting lung disease. In the pediatric population, a difficult respiratory course may result in necrotizing enterocolitis, a postoperative gastrointestinal complication related to ischemia of the bowel.

The most common postoperative pulmonary problems include atelectasis, pneumonia, pulmonary edema, and pulmonary emboli (see these diagnoses elsewhere in the chapter for more detail). Prevention of any of these problems involves frequent turning, deep breathing, humidified air to loosen secretions, antibiotics for infection as appropriate, supplemental oxygen for hypoxemia, and early ambulation.

If respiratory failure develops, mechanical ventilation may be required, and treatment is very similar to that for ARDS.

Sarcoidosis

Definition

Sarcoidosis is a systemic disease of unknown cause involving any organ that is characterized by granulomatous inflammation present diffusely throughout the body. Technically this condition could be included earlier in this chapter in the section on infectious and inflammatory diseases, but without a better sense of the underlying cause, it remains here under diseases that affect the lung parenchyma. The *granulomas* consist of a collection of macrophages surrounded by lymphocytes taking a nodular form. In fact, granulomatous inflammation of the lung is present in 90% of clients with sarcoidosis. Secondary sites include the skin, eyes, liver, spleen, heart, and small bones in the hands and feet.

Incidence

Sarcoidosis occurs predominantly in the third and fourth decades (between the ages of 20 and 40 years) and has a slightly higher incidence in women than in men. It is present worldwide with some interesting differences in prevalence among ethnic groups. It is more prevalent in African Americans and Puerto Ricans.[197a] Socioeconomic, environmental, and genetic factors appear to influence the occurrence.[74]

Etiologic Factors and Pathogenesis

The etiologic factors and pathogenesis of sarcoidosis are unknown, but there appears to be an exaggerated cellular immune response on the part of the helper T lymphocytes to a foreign antigen whose identity remains unclear. Increasing evidence points to a triggering agent that may be genetic, infectious (bacterial or viral), immunologic, or toxic. Abnormalities of immune function—as well as autoantibody production, including rheumatoid factor and antinuclear antibodies—are seen in sarcoidosis and in connective tissue diseases, suggesting a common immunopathogenetic mechanism.

Granuloma formation may regress with therapy or as a result of the disease's natural course but may also progress to fibrosis and restrictive lung disease.

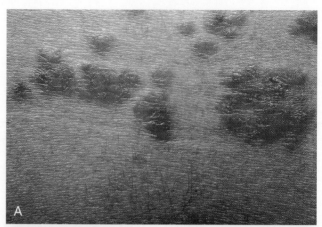
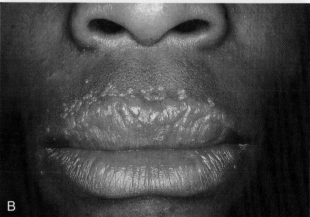

FIG. 11.19 Sarcoidosis. (A) Cutaneous sarcoidosis usually consists of papules and plaques with a typical reddish brown color. (B) Lesions often favor the lips and perioral region. (From Bolognia JL, Jorizzo JL, Schaffer JV: Dermatology, ed 3, London, 2012, Saunders.)

Clinical Manifestations

Sarcoidosis can affect any organ, including bones, joints, muscles, and vessels. Lungs and thoracic lymph nodes are most often involved, with acute or *insidious* respiratory problems sometimes accompanied by symptoms affecting the skin, eyes, or other organs. The diverse manifestations of this disorder lend support to the hypothesis that sarcoidosis has more than one cause. The clinical impact of sarcoidosis is directly related to the extent of granulomatous inflammation and its effect on the function of vital organs.

Pulmonary sarcoidosis has a variable natural course from an asymptomatic state to a progressive life-threatening condition. Signs and symptoms may develop over a period of a few weeks to a few months and include dyspnea, cough, fever, malaise, weight loss, skin lesions (Fig. 11.19), and erythema nodosum (multiple tender, nonulcerating nodules). This condition may also be entirely asymptomatic, manifesting with abnormal findings on routine chest radiographs. Respiratory symptoms of dry cough and dyspnea without constitutional symptoms (symptoms of systemic illness, including fatigue, weakness, malaise, weight loss, sweating, and fever) occur in over one-half of all people with sarcoidosis, and up to 15% develop progressive fibrosis. Chest pain, hemoptysis, or pneumothorax may be present.

Sarcoidosis may manifest with extrapulmonary symptoms referable to bone marrow, skin, eyes, cranial nerves or peripheral nerves (neurosarcoidosis), liver, or heart

BOX 11.10 Clinical Manifestations of Sarcoidosis

Pulmonary

- Asymptomatic with abnormal chest film
- Gradually progressive cough and shortness of breath
- Pulmonary fibrosis with pulmonary insufficiency
- Laryngeal and endobronchial obstruction

Extrapulmonary

- Löfgren's syndrome: fever, arthralgias, bilateral hilar adenopathy, erythema nodosum
- Heerfordt's syndrome (uveoparotid fever): fever, swelling of parotid gland and uveal tracts, seventh cranial nerve palsy
- Erythema nodosum
- Peripheral lymphadenopathy or splenomegaly
- Lymphoma
- *Eyes:* excessive tearing, swelling, uveitis, iritis, glaucoma, cataracts
- *Skin:* nodules or skin plaques (see Fig. 11.19); skin cancer
- *Central nervous system:* cranial nerve palsies, subacute meningitis, diabetes insipidus
- *Joints:* polyarticular and monarticular arthritis
- *Bones:* punched-out cystic lesions in phalangeal and metacarpal bones
- *Heart:* paroxysmal arrhythmias, conduction disturbances, congestive heart failure, sudden death
- *Kidney:* hypercalcemia with nephrocalcinosis or nephrolithiasis
- *Liver:* granulomatous hepatitis, liver cancer

(Box 11.10). Neurosarcoidosis is an uncommon but severe and sometimes life-threatening manifestation of sarcoidosis occurring in 5% to 15% of cases. Sarcoidosis appears to be associated with a significantly increased risk of cancer in affected organs (e.g., skin, liver, lymphoma, or lung). Chronic inflammation is the mediator of this risk.[20]

Medical Management

Diagnosis

There is no specific test other than history for sarcoidosis, so diagnosis is based on clinical examination, radiographic, CT, pulmonary function and laboratory test findings, and biopsy of easily accessible granulomas (e.g., skin lesions, salivary gland, or palpable lymph nodes). When lung involvement is suspected, further testing may be required, and new imaging techniques improve detection. Other granulomatous diseases (e.g., TB, berylliosis, lymphoma, carcinoma, or fungal disease) must be ruled out.

Treatment

Pulmonary treatment may not be required, especially in clients who are asymptomatic. Short-term (less than 6 months) use of inhaled steroids may improve symptoms, especially in people who mainly have a cough. The long-term use of corticosteroids is the treatment of choice for those clients who have impaired lung function with pulmonary granulomas. Corticosteroids are quite effective in reducing the acute granulomatous inflammation as seen on radiographs, but their efficacy in improving lung function and altering the long-term prognosis is unproven. Oral steroids may be beneficial for stage 2 and 3 disease.[253,260]

11.18 Special Implications for the PTA: Sarcoidosis

There is a distinct arthritic component associated with sarcoidosis, variously reported in 10% to 35% of people who develop extrapulmonary involvement. The knees or ankles are the most common sites of acute arthritis. Distribution of joint involvement is usually polyarticular and symmetric, and the arthritis is commonly self-limiting after several weeks or months. Occasionally the arthritis is recurrent or chronic, but even then, joint destruction and deformity are rare. Treatment of arthritis in sarcoidosis is usually as for any other form of arthritis. The arthritic symptoms may develop early as the first manifestation of the disease or late in the disease.

PTAs should be alert to any presenting signs or symptoms of increased disease activity associated with sarcoidosis because medical vigilance with attention to new symptoms is important in the management of sarcoidosis. This disease manifests in many and diverse patterns, but observe especially for exertional dyspnea that progresses to dyspnea at rest, chest pain, joint swelling, or increased fatigue and malaise, reducing the client's functional level or ability to participate in therapy. Muscle involvement and bone involvement are frequently underdiagnosed. Symptoms of muscle weakness, aches, tenderness, and fatigue, often accompanied by neurogenic atrophy, may indicate sarcoid myositis.[26]

Cranial nerve palsies (especially facial palsy), multiple mononeuropathy, and less commonly, symmetric polyneuropathy may all occur. Improvement of neurologic function may occur with the use of corticosteroids.

For clients receiving steroid therapy, increased side effects of the medication should be reported to the physician. For example, long-term use of steroids lowers resistance to infection, may induce diabetes and myopathy, and is associated with weight gain, loss of potassium in the urine, and gastric irritation.

Lung Cancer

Overview

Lung cancer, a malignancy of the epithelium of the respiratory tract, is the most frequent cause of cancer death in the United States. The term *lung cancer*, also known as *bronchogenic carcinoma*, excludes other pulmonary tumors such as sarcomas, lymphomas, blastomas, hematomas, and mesotheliomas.

Types of Lung Cancer

At least a dozen different types of tumors are included under the broad heading of lung cancer. Clinically, lung cancers are classified as follows:

- Small cell lung cancer (SCLC), or 20% of all lung cancers
- Non–SCLC (NSCLC), or 80% of all lung cancers

Within these two broad categories, there are four major types of primary malignant lung tumors:

- SCLC includes small cell carcinoma or oat cell carcinoma
- NSCLC includes:
  - Squamous cell carcinoma
  - Adenocarcinoma
  - Large cell carcinoma

The characteristics of these four lung cancers are summarized in Table 11.11.

Adenocarcinoma, the most common form of lung cancer in the United States, tends to arise in the periphery, usually in the upper lobes at different levels of the bronchial tree. An individual tumor may reflect the cell structure of any part of the respiratory mucosa from the large bronchi to the smallest bronchioles. Because of this, *adenocarcinoma* refers to a heterogeneous group of neoplasms that have in common the formation of glandlike structures. Adenocarcinoma is further subdivided

TABLE 11.11   Characteristics of Lung Cancer

Tumor type	Incidence	Growth Rate	Metastasis	Treatment
Small Cell Lung Cancer (SCLC)				
Small cell (oat cell)	20%–25%	Very rapid	Very early; to mediastinum or distal area of lung	Combination chemotherapy; surgical resectability is poor
Non–Small Cell Lung Cancer (NSCLC)				
Squamous cell (epidermal)	17% (greater in men)	Slow	Localized metastasis not common or occurs late, usually to hilar lymph nodes, adrenals, liver	Surgically resectability is good if stage I or II. Chemotherapy and radiation therapy for all stages are under continued investigation
Adenocarcinoma	35%–40%[a]	Slow to moderate	Early; metastasis throughout lung and brain or to other organs	Surgical resectability is good if localized stage I or II. Chemotherapy or chemoradiation and surgery may be combined for stage III
Large cell (anaplastic)	10%–15%	Rapid	Early and widespread metastasis to kidney, liver, adrenals	Surgical respectability is poor if involvement is widespread; better prognosis if stage I or II. Chemotherapy of limited use, radiation therapy is palliative

[a]A major histologic change has occurred over the last three decades as the most common cell type has shifted from squamous cell to adenocarcinoma. This shift appears to be the result of physiochemical changes in the late 20th-century smoke (e.g., increased levels of tobacco-specific nitrosamines).
From Statistical data from the U.S. Department of Health Services, Publication No. 96–691, Washington, DC, 1996.
From Austin JHM, Stellman SD, Pearson GDN: Screening for lung cancer, N Engl J Med 344:935–936, 2001.

into four categories: acinar, papillary, bronchioloalveolar, and solid carcinoma. Increasing incidence of adenocarcinoma cell–type lung cancer is currently attributed to changes in smoking patterns (e.g., deeper and more intense inhalation) in response to reduced tar and nicotine in cigarettes. Presumably, the excess volume inhaled to satisfy addictive needs for nicotine delivers increased amounts of carcinogens and toxins to the peripheral areas of the lungs.[314]

Large cell carcinomas are so poorly differentiated that they cannot be classified with the other three categories and require special diagnostic testing procedures to differentiate from other pathologic lung conditions.

Incidence

Lung cancer remains the leading cause of cancer death in the United States (estimated 167,050 deaths in 2006) and one of the world's leading causes of preventable death.[170] More people die of lung cancer than of colon, breast, and prostate cancer combined. In 1987 lung cancer overtook breast cancer to become the most common cause of death from cancer among women in the United States.

Among men and women, both incidence and mortality have slowed with the decline in cigarette smoking. Smoking among adolescents peaked in 1996 and has been on the decline, yet a survey in 2002 showed that 9.8% of middle school students and 22.5% of high school students reported that they currently smoke cigarettes.[216] Deaths from lung cancer increase at ages 35 to 44 years, with a sharp increase at ages 45 to 55 years. Incidence continues to increase up until age 74 years, after which the incidence levels off and decreases among the very old. There are differences in mortality rates for racial and ethnic groups.

Black males have the highest death rate, and Asian/Pacific Islanders, American Indian/Alaska natives, and Hispanic males have the lowest death rate. Among women, blacks and whites have the highest mortality, whereas Asian/Pacific Islander and Hispanic females have the lowest death rate from lung cancer.[169] Women taking hormone replacement therapy have an earlier onset of and greater mortality from lung cancer.[113]

Risk Factors

Contributions to lung cancer include environment (smoking, secondhand smoke, occupational exposure, or air pollution), nutrition, and genetic factors.[185] Age, family history, and medical history, especially of lung disease, also influence the occurrence, morbidity, and mortality.

Cigarette smoking. Cigarette smoking (more than 20 cigarettes per day) remains the greatest risk factor for lung cancer; 85% to 90% of all lung cancers occur in smokers, although, remarkably, fewer than 20% of cigarette smokers develop lung cancer. The relative risk of lung cancer increases with the number of cigarettes smoked per day and the number of years of smoking history. The people at highest risk began smoking in their teens, inhale deeply, and smoke at least one-half pack per day.

Smoking is a major cause of cancers of the oropharynx and bladder among women. Evidence is also strong that women who smoke have increased risks for liver, colorectal, and cervical cancer and cancers of the pancreas and kidney. There is also an increased risk for stroke, death from ruptured abdominal aortic aneurysm, and peripheral vascular disease among smokers compared with nonsmokers.[147]

Former smokers have about one-half the risk of current smokers of dying from lung cancer. Compared with current smokers, the risk for lung and bronchus cancer among former smokers declines as the duration of abstinence lengthens, but it takes over 20 years to reach the risk level of people who never smoked.[185] These statistics support the fact that lung cancer is the most preventable of all cancers. The elimination of cigarette smoking would virtually eliminate SCLC. Smoking cessation also appears to slow the rate of progression of carotid atherosclerosis and other vascular disease.

There are approximately 50 known carcinogens and promoting substances found in tobacco smoke; the major causal agents of lung cancer are the polynuclear aromatic hydrocarbons and tobacco-specific *N*-nitrosamines (nicotine). Tobacco smoking also results in increased exposure to ethylene oxide, aromatic amines, and other agents that cause damage to DNA.[265] For this reason, the risk of lung cancer is increased in a smoker who is also exposed to other carcinogenic agents, such as radioactive isotopes, polycyclic aromatic hydrocarbons and arsenicals, vinyl chloride, metallurgic ores, and mustard gas.

Marijuana. Marijuana contains many of the same organic and inorganic compounds that are carcinogens, cocarcinogens, or tumor promoters found in tobacco smoke. Marijuana produces inflammation, edema, and cell injury in the tracheobronchial mucosa of smokers and contributes to oxidative stress, which is a precursor for DNA mutations.[320] Cannabinoids have been shown to inhibit certain breast, lung, and brain cancers,[187] although other studies have shown an increase in head, neck, and lung cancers.[144] Unfortunately, most studies do not examine the magnitude of exposure and concurrent tobacco use.

The risk of marijuana smoking does not appear to approach that of smoking tobacco, and any increased risk may be associated with the route of delivery (the heat and particulate irritation of smoking) rather than the drug itself. Further studies are needed.

Environmental tobacco smoke. In 1992, the U.S. Environmental Protection Agency (EPA) declared secondhand smoke or ETS to be a group A human carcinogen. ETS increases the relative risk of lung cancer about 1.5-fold, and there are 3000 lung cancer deaths each year from ETS.[97] This exposure increases the risk for the children and partners of smokers and becomes an occupational hazard in individuals working in bars, restaurants, or other places that are not smoke free.

Occupational exposure. Studies on whether occupational factors increase the risk of cancer development in the nonsmoker are limited in number but confirm that certain occupational exposures are associated with an increased risk of lung cancer in both male and female nonsmokers.[269] The inhalation of asbestos fibers is associated with higher cancer risks for both smokers and nonsmokers, although the rate is considerably higher for smokers.

The rate of lung cancer in people who live in urban areas is 2.3 times greater than that of those living in rural areas, possibly implicating air pollution as a risk factor in lung cancer. The exact role of air pollution is still unknown, but carcinogens with known *genotoxicity* continue to be released into outdoor air from industrial sources, power plants, and motor vehicles; epidemiologic research provides evidence for an association between air pollution and lung cancer.[68,336]

Indoor exposure to radon, which is a colorless, odorless gas that is a product of uranium and radium produced from the decomposition of rocks and soil, is a known carcinogen and the second leading cause of lung cancer. Concentrations vary geographically (more in the northern United States), and radon gas levels are highest in basements, nearest the soil.[108] Other sources of radon exposure include radioactive waste and underground mines; exposure to tobacco smoke multiplies the risk of concurrent exposure to radon.

Other occupational or environmental risk factors associated with lung cancer include diesel exhaust, benzopyrenes, silica, formaldehyde, copper, chromium, cadmium, arsenic, alkylating compounds, sulfur dioxide, and ionizing radiation.

Previous lung disease. The presence of other lung diseases, such as pulmonary fibrosis, scleroderma, and sarcoidosis, may increase the risk of developing lung cancer. COPD or fibrosis of the lungs inhibits the clearance of carcinogens from the lungs, thereby increasing the risk of alteration of DNA with resultant malignant cell growth.

Nutrition. Other risk factors may include low consumption of fruits and vegetables, reduced physical activity, increased dietary fat (especially diets high in saturated or animal fat and cholesterol), and high alcohol intake. A recent prospective study demonstrated positive effects of fruit consumption, but not of vegetables.[131]

Studies have shown no beneficial effect of vitamin E, beta-carotene, or retinol, and several studies have determined that beta-carotene supplementation in smokers increases the risk for lung cancer. The mechanism for this carcinogenic action remains unknown.[290]

Genetic susceptibility. Several published studies suggest that lung cancer can aggregate in some families, and it has been hypothesized that the defect in the body's ability to defend against the carcinogens in tobacco smoke may be inherited.[352] A first-degree smoking relative of an individual with lung cancer has an increased risk of developing lung cancer. This predilection may be the result of a genetic predisposition, but the trait (lung cancer) may be expressed only in the presence of its major predisposing factor (i.e., tobacco). Carcinogenic chemicals may induce genomic instability either directly or indirectly through inflammatory processes in the lung epithelial cells.

Pathogenesis

As mentioned, there is a clear relationship between cigarette smoking and the development of SCLC. The effects of smoking include structural, functional, malignant, and toxic changes. DNA-mutating agents in cigarettes produce alterations in both oncogenes and tumor suppressor genes, as well as genes that detoxify and assist with DNA repair. Normal polymorphism (variations in genes) also plays a role in the development of or resistance to cancer.

Small cell lung cancer. When the cells become so dense that there is almost no cytoplasm present and the cells are compressed into an ovoid mass, the tumor is called *small cell carcinoma* or *oat cell carcinoma*. SCLC develops most often in the bronchial submucosa, the layer of tissue beneath the epithelium, and tends to be located centrally, most often near the hilum of the lung. These tumors can produce hormones that stimulate their own growth and the rapid growth of neighboring cells, causing bronchial obstruction and pneumonia with early intralymphatic invasion. Lymphatic and distant metastases are usually present at the time of diagnosis.

Non–small cell lung cancer. Squamous cell carcinomas arise in the central portion of the lung near the hilum, projecting into the major or segmental bronchi. Although these tumors tend to grow rapidly, they often remain located within the thoracic cavity, making curative treatment more likely compared with other NSCLC types. These tumors may be difficult to differentiate from TB or an abscess because they often undergo central cavitation (formation of a cavity or hollow space).

Clinical Manifestations

Symptoms of early stage localized lung cancer do not differ much from pulmonary symptoms associated with chronic smoking (e.g., cough, dyspnea, and sputum production), so the person does not seek medical attention. Women with lung cancer have lower incidence or severity of COPD, so symptoms may be fewer and diagnosis delayed.[202] Symptoms may depend on the location within the pulmonary system, whether centrally located, peripheral, or in the apices of the lungs. Systemic symptoms, such as anorexia, fatigue, weakness, and weight loss, are common, especially with advanced disease (metastases) and associated with poor prognosis.[29]

Bone pain associated with bone metastasis is common; other symptoms resulting from metastases depend on the site of involvement (e.g., hepatomegaly and jaundice with liver metastasis and seizures, headaches, confusion, or focal neurologic signs with brain metastasis). Other signs and symptoms of disease include recurring bronchitis or pneumonia; productive cough with hemoptysis; wheezing; poorly defined persistent chest pain; difficulty swallowing or hoarseness; orthopnea; nerve involvement (phrenic, laryngeal, brachial plexus, or sympathetic ganglion); and vascular (superior vena cava [SVC]), cardiac, and esophageal compression as a result of local tumor invasion.[29,109,271]

Small cell lung cancer. Signs and symptoms of SCLC depend on the size and location of the tumor and the presence and extent of metastases. Because SCLCs most commonly arise in the central endobronchial location in people who are almost exclusively long-term smokers, typical symptoms are a result of obstructed air flow and consist of persistent, new, or changing cough, dyspnea, stridor, wheezing, hemoptysis, and chest pain.[49]

Intercostal retractions on inspiration and bulging intercostal spaces on expiration indicate obstruction. As obstruction increases, bronchopulmonary infection (obstructive pneumonitis) often occurs distal to the obstruction. Centrally located tumors cause chest pain with perivascular nerve or peribronchial involvement that can refer pain to the shoulder, scapula, upper back, or arm.

Non–small cell lung cancer. The less common peripheral pulmonary tumors (large cell) often do not produce signs or symptoms until disease progression produces localized, sharp, and severe pleural pain increased on inspiration, limiting lung expansion; cough and dyspnea are present. Pleural effusion may develop and limit lung expansion even more.

Tumors in the apex of the lung, called *Pancoast's tumors,* occur both in squamous cell and adenocarcinomatous cancers. Symptoms do not occur until the tumors invade the brachial plexus (see 11.19 Special Implications for the PTA: Lung Cancer). Destruction of the first and second ribs can occur. Paralysis, elevation of the hemidiaphragm, and dyspnea secondary to phrenic nerve involvement can also occur.

Other manifestations may include digital clubbing, skin changes, joint swelling associated with hypertrophic pulmonary osteoarthropathy (see previous discussion of this condition in the section on CF), decreased or absent breath sounds on auscultation, or pleural rub (inflammatory response to invading tumor).

Metastasis

The rich supply of blood vessels and lymphatics in the lungs allows the disease to metastasize rapidly.[48] Lung cancers spread by direct extension, lymphatic invasion, and bloodborne metastases. Tumors spread by direct invasion in the bronchus of origin; others may invade the bronchial wall and circle and obstruct the airway. Intrapulmonary spread may lead to compression of lung structures other than airways such as blood or lymph vessels, alveoli, and nerves.

Direct extension through the pleura can result in spread over the surface of the lung, chest wall, or diaphragm. Carcinomas of the lung of all types metastasize most frequently to the regional lymph nodes, particularly the hilar and mediastinal nodes. Supraclavicular, cervical, and abdominal channels may also be invaded. Tumors originating in the lower lobes tend to spread through the lymph channels.

Lung cancer generally has a widespread pattern of hematogenous metastases. This is caused by the invasion of the pulmonary vascular system. After tumor cells enter the pulmonary venous system, they can be carried through the heart and disseminated systemically. Tumor emboli can become lodged in areas of organ systems where vessels become too narrow for their passage or where blood flow is reduced.

The most frequent site of extranodal metastases is the adrenal gland. Lung cancer can also metastasize to the brain, bone, and liver before manifesting symptomatically. Brain metastases constitute nearly one-third of all observed recurrences in people with resected NSCLC of the adenocarcinoma type. Metastases to the brain usually result in CNS symptoms of confusion, gait disturbances, headaches, or personality changes.

Tumor spread intrathoracically to the mediastinum and beyond can produce SVC syndrome with swelling of the face, neck, and arms. SVC syndrome is usually a sign of advanced disease. If left untreated, SVC syndrome results in cerebral edema and possible death. Increased intracranial pressure, headaches, dizziness, visual disturbances, and alteration in mental status are signs of progressive compression. Cardiac metastasis can occur and results in arrhythmias, congestive heart failure, and pericardial tamponade.

As a form of secondary malignancy, the lungs are the most frequent site of metastases from other types of cancer. Any tumor cell dislodged from a primary neoplasm can find its way into the circulation or lymphatics, which are filtered by the lungs. Carcinomas of the kidney, breast, pancreas, colon, and uterus are especially likely to metastasize to the lungs.

Medical Management

Prevention

Prevention is the key to eliminating or at least reducing the need for treatment of lung cancer. Targeted state and federal antitobacco programs have contributed to significant drops in cigarette consumption.

Healthy People 2010 set a goal of reducing the lung cancer mortality rate from 57.6 per 100,000 population (1998 figure) to 44.9 per 100,000 population, representing a 22% improvement. This goal has been retained in the draft of *Healthy People 2020. Healthy People 2010* outlined a systematic approach to health improvement that includes methods for lung cancer prevention through prevention of tobacco use and tobacco addiction in all age, ethnic, and socioeconomic groups. (*Healthy People 2010* and *Healthy People 2020* are available online at http://www.healthypeople.gov/).

Other strategies for lung cancer prevention have included chemoprevention (i.e., administration of agents—usually drugs but also nutraceuticals or nutritional supplements—before the diagnosis of invasive cancer to absorb free oxygen radicals and to block or reverse carcinogenesis), adoption of a diet high in fruits and vegetables, and reduction of ETS.

Although significantly lower levels of vitamin C and E are found in people with lung cancer, a review of eight prospective studies show no reduction in cancer risk from diet or vitamin supplements.[4,66] Reduction or prevention of occupational exposure may be achieved through a combination of approaches, including toxicologic testing of new compounds before they are marketed, application of industrial hygiene techniques, industry regulation, and epidemiologic surveillance.

Diagnosis

Many lung cancers are detected on routine chest film in clients undergoing evaluation for unrelated medical conditions without pulmonary symptoms, although 90% of the people with lung cancer are symptomatic at diagnosis. Unfortunately, chest radiography is not sensitive enough to show tumors when they are small and operable, and routine screening is not supported by the evidence.

A chest scan called *low-dose spiral CT* (LDCT) detects tumors too small to be seen on radiographs. There are some concerns with the LDCT (e.g., cost, false-positive findings, unnecessary biopsies of small benign tumors), although the availability of this type of diagnostic procedure may bring about annual screening for lung cancer for those at risk. However, mass screening for lung cancer with CT is not currently advocated because to date no randomized population trial has demonstrated a significant reduction in lung carcinoma mortality as a result of any screening intervention.[22,213]

Treatment

Current treatment with new agents used in combination—as well as when combined with radiation and hormones—has led to an improved response rate in the treatment of some lung cancers.[55] Chemotherapy approaches are numerous and address different targets. Newer agents that inhibit epidermal growth factor receptors are showing promise alone and in combination with other drugs.[327]

Small Cell Lung Cancer

The cornerstone treatment for SCLC is chemotherapy, which is the cornerstone of treatment for all stages of this disease, resulting in high response rates (65% to 85%).[181] Surgical resection for the treatment of SCLC is not usually considered but when used seems most effective for clients in the early stages of SCLC. For clients with more advanced disease, surgery causes unnecessary risk and stress with no valid benefits. Laser therapy is a surgical treatment used when the tumor mass is causing nonresectable bronchial obstructions and when accessible by bronchoscope.

SCLC is quite sensitive to radiation therapy, which, in conjunction with chemotherapy, is now routinely administered to those with limited disease.[33] Individuals with extensive disease usually receive combination chemotherapy initially. Other treatment options depend on the clinical manifestations and client needs (e.g., radiation therapy may be administered to the brain, bone, spine, or other sites of metastasis). In the future, tumor growth may be halted by replacement or substitution of mutated tumor suppressor gene functions or biochemical modulation of oncogene products. New forms of immunotherapy may also be targeted specifically toward mutant oncogenes in cancer cells.

Non–Small Cell Lung Cancer

Options for *palliative* treatment of late obstructing NSCLC by photodynamic therapy, brachytherapy, electrocautery, cryotherapy, and laser therapy are currently being used as primary treatment of early disease with some success.[224] Surgical resection by lobectomy or pneumonectomy for treatment of stage I carcinoma is recommended with curative intent.[213,308] Postoperative radiation is considered harmful and is not recommended, particularly in early stage NSCLC.[272] Concurrent chemoradiation reduces risk of death at 2 years by 14% compared with sequential chemoradiotherapy, and a 7% reduction compared with radiation alone.[288]

Surgery is usually not warranted for stage III NSCLC. Combinations of treatments appear to help, but optimal treatment techniques and dose are controversial and primarily directed to increasing survival time.[173,282] Approach to stage IV disease is palliative and depends on location and extent of disease and clinical manifestations. For example, clients who develop spinal cord compromise secondary to metastatic disease can be palliated effectively with short-course external-beam radiotherapy.

SVC obstruction can also be ameliorated by chemotherapy and radiotherapy as well as the placement of stents.[287] Short-term radiotherapy can also reduce some lung symptoms.[207] Chemotherapy has also been useful in improving palliation and increasing survival in stage IV disease.[310]

Prognosis

The curability of lung cancer remains poor usually because by the time lung cancer is detected, invasion and metastasis have already occurred. The prognosis is influenced by the stage of the disease at presentation, the cell type, the treatment that can be given, and the status of the client at the time of diagnosis (e.g., people who are ambulatory respond to treatment better than those who are confined to bed more than 50% of the time).

Other factors associated with poor prognosis include weight loss of more than 10% of body weight in 6 months and generalized weakness. Overall 5-year survival rate among older blacks with NSCLC is significantly lower compared with whites, largely explained by lower rates of surgical treatment.[21] Although women appear to be more susceptible to lung cancer, they have higher survival rates.[109]

Currently, with treatment, only 14% of people with lung cancer survive beyond 5 years after diagnosis, but if caught early, lung cancer can be cured up to 70% of the time. Survival without treatment is rarely possible, and most untreated persons die within 1 year of diagnosis, with a median survival of less than 6 months. Curative treatment requires effective control of the primary tumor before metastasis occurs. Chemotherapy is usually combined with surgery or irradiation for more advanced tumors.

Other factors thought to confer poor prognosis include male gender, age older than 70 years, prior chemotherapy, elevated serum lactic dehydrogenase levels, low serum sodium, and elevated alkaline phosphatase levels.

11.19 Special Implications for the PTA: Lung Cancer

The effective management of short- and long-term side effects from lung cancer and its treatment is essential for rehabilitation. The American College of Chest Physicians has developed recommendations for improving quality of life in end-of-life care.[137] Increasing the PTA's knowledge of psychosocial–spiritual effects in these cases assists the PTA in planning appropriate intervention programs and promoting the optimal use of resources. If clients and their families can overcome treatment barriers, they will be more motivated toward achieving increased and sustained independence and quality of life.

The PTA can be very helpful in teaching clients with lung cancer nonpharmacologic means of pain relief and energy conservation techniques while providing an optimal rest schedule and activity program in accordance with the degree of pulmonary involvement. Effective breathing and coughing techniques should be taught and reinforced.

Cigarette smoking should be discouraged. Numerous surveys have shown that the majority of current smokers demonstrate a desire to stop smoking and that intervention through smoking-cessation programs can be successful. The Agency for Health Care Policy and Research (AHCPR), which is now called the Agency for Healthcare Research and Quality (AHRQ), has recommended specific guidelines with intervention strategies to assist health care providers in giving smokers consistent and effective smoking cessation guidelines. Every therapy and rehabilitation department should have information available about local smoking-cessation programs and a listing of local physicians willing to help anyone who expresses a desire to cease smoking.

Metastasis

Metastatic spread of pulmonary tumors to the long bones and to the vertebral column, especially the thoracic vertebrae, is common, occurring in as many as 50% of all cases. Local metastases by direct extension may involve the chest wall and may even erode the first and second ribs and associated vertebrae, causing bone pain and paravertebral pain associated with involvement of sympathetic nerve ganglia. Subsequently, chest, shoulder, arm, or back pain can be the presenting symptom but usually with accompanying pulmonary symptoms.

The client may not associate the musculoskeletal symptoms with the pulmonary symptoms, so the therapy team must always remember to screen for medical disease. Cases of patients with lung cancer and shoulder pain for which no local cause could be found have been reported, and in each case, radiotherapy to the ipsilateral mediastinum eliminated symptoms. Pain referred from intrathoracic involvement of the phrenic nerve was the suspected underlying pain generator.[183]

Any time a mechanical cause is not found or the client fails to progress or improve in therapy, he or she should be reevaluated by the physical therapist, and referring physician contact is recommended. Spinal cord compression from extradural metastases of lung cancer usually occurs from direct extension of vertebral metastases. Back pain is often the first sign and may occur as progressive back pain 6 months before the diagnosis is made. The pain may be constant and aggravated by Valsalva maneuver, sneezing or coughing, movement, and lying down, and may be diminished by sitting up. Weakness, sensory loss, and a positive Babinski's reflex may be observed.

Radiation is usually the treatment of choice for epidural metastases from lung cancer. Neurosurgical intervention may be indicated if the area of compression has been previously irradiated to maximal tolerance. Surgical decompression may also be indicated if neurologic deterioration occurs during the initiation of radiation therapy. The treatment field extends two vertebral bodies above and below the level of blockage. Corticosteroids are prescribed to reduce swelling and inflammation around the cord.[48]

Apical (Pancoast's) tumors do not usually cause symptoms while confined to the pulmonary parenchyma, but once they extend into the surrounding structures, the brachial plexus (C8 to T1) may become involved, manifesting as a form of thoracic outlet syndrome. This nerve involvement produces sharp pleuritic pain in the axilla, shoulder (radiating in an ulnar nerve distribution down the arm), and subscapular area of the affected side, with atrophy and weakness of the upper extremity muscles. Invasion of the cervical sympathetic plexus may cause *Horner's syndrome* with unilateral miosis, ptosis, and absence of sweating on the affected side of the face and neck.

Treatment for these two conditions may combine surgery with radiation. Local anesthetics administered through an axillary catheter placed in the brachial plexus for intractable neuropathic pain have also been reported; this approach is reversible and may be preferable to destructive procedures, such as cordotomy. Therapy intervention for the thoracic outlet syndrome is an important part of the palliative treatment for this condition.

Trigger points of the serratus anterior muscle also mimic the distribution of pain caused by C8 nerve root compression and must be ruled out by palpation, lack of neurologic deficits, and possible elimination with appropriate trigger point therapy. Pancoast's tumors may also masquerade as subacromial bursitis.

Paraneoplastic Syndrome

Paraneoplastic syndromes occur in 10% to 20% of lung cancer clients. These usually result from hormones secreted by the tumor that act on target organs and produce a variety of symptoms, most commonly hypercalcemia, digital clubbing, osteoarthropathies, or rheumatologic disorders such as polymyositis, lupus, and dermatomyositis.

Chemotherapy and Radiation Treatment

Clients undergoing chemotherapy, radiation therapy, or a combination of both must, along with their families, work closely with members of the multidisciplinary health team to obtain the information and emotional support they need. It is important that PTAs have knowledge of side effects associated with different antineoplastic interventions and anticipate toxicities.

For example, side effects of chemotherapy, including nausea and vomiting, require careful scheduling of therapy to optimize treatment success. Some chemotherapy is neurotoxic, and the PTA should watch for peripheral neuropathies. In the presence of cancer pain, pain medication should be timed to allow maximal comfort during therapy (e.g., approximately 30 to 60 minutes before therapy).

Loss of appetite with accompanying weight loss may result in muscle weakness and decreased physical endurance requiring more frequent rest periods. The PTA may be able to assist the client with reduced functional status exhibiting other symptoms, such as dyspnea and fatigue, by teaching diaphragmatic breathing techniques, use of relaxation techniques for overused respiratory accessory muscles, and positioning for easing the work of breathing (WOB) (e.g., sitting upright and leaning forward slightly with elbows resting on knees).

Energy conservation should be addressed by teaching the client to schedule strenuous activities at times of the day when energy levels are the highest, alternating strenuous tasks with easier ones, using frequent rest breaks, planning activities to minimize the use of stairs or walking long distances, and reducing workload (encourage the client to perform elective tasks, especially household chores, less often and in the sitting position whenever possible).

Monitoring platelet, hematocrit, and hemoglobin levels can help guide the PTA and client in establishing activity level. Vital signs should be monitored before and after periods of increased activity; heart and lung sounds and oxygen saturation should be monitored during activity. Observe for signs of extreme fatigue, chest pain, or diaphoresis.

Other concerns addressed by the PTA may include regaining strength and endurance after chemotherapy or radiation therapy, mobility training for those clients with gait and balance disturbances, instruction for sleeping postures and bed mobility for clients with bone pain from metastasis, and in late-stage cancer, prevention or treatment of contractures or skin breakdown. Helping the client recognize short- and long-term side effects associated with treatment before these effects become life threatening is essential.

DISORDERS OF THE PULMONARY VASCULATURE

Pulmonary Embolism and Infarction

Definition and Incidence

PE is the lodging of a blood clot in a pulmonary artery with subsequent obstruction of blood supply to the lung parenchyma. Although a blood clot is the most common cause of occlusion, air, fat, bone marrow (e.g., fracture), foreign IV material, vegetations on heart valves that develop with endocarditis, amniotic fluid, and tumor cells (tumor emboli) can also embolize and occlude the pulmonary vessels.

PE is common, and in the United States the incidence is estimated at approximately 600,000 cases and 50,000 to 200,000 deaths annually.[193] It is the most common cause of sudden death in the hospitalized population. The overall incidence of PE appears to be declining, probably because of better treatment of established deep vein thrombosis (DVT) and increased use of thromboprophylaxis.

Etiologic and Risk Factors

The most common cause of PE is a DVT originating in the proximal deep venous system primarily of the lower extremity, but 20% come from the upper extremity. Before the introduction of routine prophylaxis with heparin (now low-molecular-weight heparin [LMWH]) or warfarin sodium (Coumadin), the incidence of DVT after hip fracture, total hip replacement, or other surgeries involving the abdomen, pelvis, prostate, hip, or knee was extremely high.

Three major physiologic risk factors linked with PE are as follows:

1. Blood stasis (e.g., immobilization or bed rest for any reason, including prolonged trips and air travel, spinal cord injury, burn patients, pneumonia, obstetric and gynecologic clients, fracture care with casting or pinning, and older or obese people)
2. Endothelial injury (local trauma) secondary to surgical procedures (as late as 1 month postoperatively), trauma, or fractures of the legs or pelvis
3. *Hypercoagulable* states (e.g., oral contraceptive use, cancer, and hereditary thrombotic disorders)

Major clinical risk factors for PE (DVT) include immobility; abdominal or pelvic surgery; hip or knee replacement; late pregnancy; cesarean section; lower limb fractures; malignancy of pelvis or abdomen; and previous PE. Minor risk factors include congenital heart disease, congestive heart failure, hypertension, superficial venous thrombosis, indwelling catheter, COPD, oral contraceptive use, hormone replacement therapy, neurologic disability, long distance travel, obesity, and smoking.[193]

Pathogenesis

In DVT, clots form in the popliteal or iliofemoral arteries (50%), deep calf veins (5%), or subclavian vein (up to 20%). Part or all of the clot may embolize, traveling through the venous system, the right side of the heart, and into the lungs. Each embolus is a mass of fresh or organizing thrombus composed of alternating bands of red cells, fibrin strands, and leukocytes with a rim of fibroblasts at the periphery Any level of the pulmonary artery, from the main trunk to the distal branches, is a site for emboli to lodge. This causes an area of blockage and ischemic necrosis to the area perfused by that vessel.

PE ranges from peripheral and clinically insignificant to massive embolism causing sudden death. PE may lead to ventilation-perfusion (V/Q) mismatch, which leads to hypoxia. PE and DVT should be considered part of the same pathologic process, and in fact, studies showed that a large percentage of people with DVT but no symptoms of PE also had evidence of PE on lung scanning. Conversely, people with PE often have abnormalities on ultrasonographic studies of leg veins.[127]

In addition to the loss of capillary beds, pulmonary emboli cause increased pulmonary vascular resistance, PH, and right ventricular failure (in severe cases).

Clinical Manifestations

Clients may be asymptomatic in the presence of small thromboemboli or may sustain cardiac arrest, depending on the size and location of the embolus and the individual's preexisting cardiopulmonary status. Common symptoms in people with PE include dyspnea (84%), pleuritic chest pain (74%), apprehension (59%), and cough (53%). Common signs include tachypnea greater than 16 breaths/min (92%), rales (58%), accentuated S2 (53%), tachycardia (44%), and fever (43%). Other signs and symptoms may include hemoptysis, diaphoresis, S3 or S4 gallop, lower extremity edema, cardiac murmur, and cyanosis.[193]

A DVT may manifest up to 2 weeks postoperatively as tenderness, leg pain, swelling (a difference in leg circumference of 1.4 cm in men and 1.2 cm in women is significant), and warmth. One exception to this presentation is the person who has been immobilized for a prolonged period in a cast. Immobilization causes muscle atrophy in the involved leg, so equal leg circumference should be a clinical red flag for medical evaluation.

A positive Homans' sign (deep calf pain on slow dorsiflexion of the foot or gentle squeezing of the affected calf) is not specific for this condition and should not be relied on because it also occurs with Achilles tendinitis and gastrocnemius and plantar muscle injury. Only one-half of the people with DVT experience pain with this test in the presence of a thrombus. Other signs of DVT may include subcutaneous venous distention, discoloration, swelling, warmth, a palpable cord (superficial thrombus), and pain on placement of a blood pressure cuff around the calf (considerable pain with the cuff inflated to 160 to 180 mm Hg).

Medical Management

Diagnosis

PE is difficult to diagnose because the signs and symptoms are nonspecific. PE may mimic (and even coexist with) pneumonia, congestive heart failure, pericarditis, myocardial infarction, pneumothorax, anxiety, and even rib fractures. The physician must also differentiate conditions that can mimic thromboembolism to the calf, such as cellulitis, muscle strain or rupture, lymphangitis, and rupture of a Baker cyst. Circumstances such as the sudden onset of chest pain or dyspnea in hospitalized, postsurgical, or trauma patients are highly suggestive of PE.

Clinical screening and assessment of need for further testing are conducted using Wells, Wicki, or Charlotte criteria and nonimaging laboratory tests (especially D-dimer, which is a byproduct of fibrin crosslinks). Negative clinical assessment and D-dimer test results may limit the need for further testing.[230]

Using combinations of additional tests to rule out or rule in PE to make the diagnosis is optimal. V/Q scans can rule out PE if findings are normal in the presence of normal x-ray findings and with no other cardiopulmonary disease.[193]

Alveolar dead space evaluation in combination with D-dimer has been found to create a false-negative response of less than 1%. Echocardiogram can detect PE in 80% of cases. Conventional angiogram has potential for serious side effects and has poor reliability. Spiral CT scan has become the initial diagnostic tool and is useful to exclude PE.[152] The major disadvantage of spiral CT is its inability to visualize beyond fourth-order branches of the pulmonary artery so that small distal emboli are not seen. Compression ultrasonography is used for the detection of DVT, but a negative result should not rule out DVT.

Prevention and Treatment

The management of DVT and PE has changed dramatically in the last few years. Given the mortality of PE and the difficulties involved in its clinical diagnosis, prevention of DVT and PE is crucial. Primary prevention of DVT through the prophylactic use of anticoagulants is important for persons undergoing total hip replacement, major knee surgery, abdominal or pelvic surgery, prostate surgery, and neurosurgery. In fact, anyone hospitalized should be evaluated for risk of PE and placed on prophylaxis as appropriate.

LMWH (anticoagulant now replacing unfractionated heparin) is the most common agent for prophylaxis because it prolongs the clotting time and allows the body time to resolve the existing clot, thereby preventing further development of the thrombus; it does not reduce the immediate embolic risk or enhance clot lysis. LMWHs have fewer major bleeding complications and do not require laboratory monitoring of coagulation tests to adjust medications. The U.S. FDA has approved outpatient treatment of DVT with the LMWH enoxaparin as a bridge to warfarin. Warfarin (Coumadin), an oral anticoagulant, is used simultaneously with heparin or during the transition from IV to oral anticoagulant, with a targeted activated partial thromboplastin time of 1.5 to 2.5 times the baseline value and an international normalized ratio of 2 to 3.

Prophylaxis and treatment with these medications for PE and DVT are different. Direct thrombin inhibitors fondaparinux, idraparinux, and ximelagatran have been shown to be at least as effective as LMWH and well tolerated.[242]

Thrombolytic therapy (a controversial, expensive treatment used with massive embolism) to lyse pulmonary thromboemboli in situ is accomplished through the use of thrombolytic agents such as streptokinase, urokinase, recombinant tissue plasminogen activator, and newer agents such as reteplase, saruplase, and recombinant staphylokinase. These drugs enhance fibrinolysis by activating plasminogen, generating plasmin.

Plasmin directly lyses thrombi both in the pulmonary artery and in the venous circulation and has a secondary anticoagulant effect. Successfully used, PE thrombolysis reverses right-sided heart failure rapidly and safely. There is limited evidence that thrombolytics are better than heparin for PE[93] but moderate evidence that they are effective in reducing postthrombotic syndrome and maintaining vessel patency.[344]

Surgical implantation of a filter in the vena cava (known as *inferior vena cava* [IVC] *filters* or *Greenfield filters*) may be used to prevent PE in anyone who cannot tolerate anticoagulation therapy by filtering the blood and preventing clots from moving past the screen. There is an increased risk of caval occlusion and dependent edema as a result of obstruction of the filter with this procedure. As temporary measures, the filters are helpful, but permanent filters have not improved survival rates.[242] Other procedures used in the case of massive DVT or hemodynamically unstable PE may include thrombectomy and embolectomy performed surgically in an angiography laboratory or suite.

Mechanical compression or use of sequential compression devices (SCDs) reduces the risk of DVT by two-thirds alone and by 50% when used with anticoagulants. A risk reduction for PE by two-fifths has also been seen.[283]

Prognosis

PE is the primary cause of death for as many as 100,000 people each year (perhaps double that amount) and a contributory factor in another 100,000 deaths annually. About 10% of victims die within the first hour, but prognosis for survivors (depending on underlying disease and on proper diagnosis and treatment) is generally favorable. Clients with PE who have cancer, congestive heart failure, or chronic lung disease have a higher risk of dying within 1 year than do clients with an isolated PE.

Small emboli resolve without serious morbidity, but large or multiple emboli (especially in the presence of severe underlying cardiac or pulmonary disease) have a poorer prognosis. PE may recur despite LMWH therapy, most commonly in people with massive PE or in whom anticoagulant therapy has been inadequate. PE is the leading cause of pregnancy-related mortality in the United States.

11.20 Special Implications for the PTA: Pulmonary Embolism and Infarction A careful review of the client's medical history may alert the therapy team to the presence of predisposing factors for the development of a deep vein thrombosis (DVT) or pulmonary embolism (PE). Frequent changing of position, exercise, the use of graduated-compression stockings, devices that provide intermittent pneumatic compression, and early ambulation are necessary to prevent thrombosis and embolism; sudden and extreme movements should be avoided. All postsurgical patients should be taught to do ankle pumps hourly. Under no circumstances should the legs be massaged to relieve muscle cramps, especially when the pain is located in the calf and the person has not been up and about.

Restrictive clothing, crossing the legs, and prolonged sitting or standing should be avoided. Elevating the legs, bending the bed at the knees, or propping pillows under the knees can produce venous stasis and should be done with caution to avoid severe flexion of the hips, which will slow blood flow and increase the risk of new thrombi.

Paget–Schroetter syndrome is a DVT of the upper extremity primarily caused by weight lifting and results in compression and subsequent stenosis of the subclavian vein. PTAs should be aware of this syndrome because early detection can prevent PE and other complications.[47]

After the diagnosis of a PE (especially associated with cardiovascular surgeries and total hip replacements), treatment with anticoagulation continues for those at high risk of recurrence. Anyone taking anticoagulants should be monitored carefully for signs of bleeding such as bloody stool, blood in urine, vaginal bleeding, bloody gums or nose, or large ecchymoses. If the person mentions any of these symptoms to the PTA, the client should be instructed to contact the physician immediately.

Medications should not be changed without the physician's approval; the use of additional medications, especially over-the-counter preparations for colds, headaches, rheumatic pain, and so on, must be approved by the physician.

Pulmonary Hypertension
Definition and Incidence

PH is high blood pressure in the pulmonary arteries defined as a rise in pulmonary artery pressure of 5 to 10 mm Hg above normal (normal is 15 to 18 mm Hg). There is no definitive set of values used to diagnose PH, but the National Institutes of Health (NIH) requires a resting mean artery pressure of more than 25 mm Hg at rest and 30 mm Hg during exercise.

WHO established a classification of pulmonary hypertensive diseases in 1998. The classification includes five major categories:
1. Pulmonary artery hypertension (PAH)
2. Pulmonary venous hypertension
3. PAH associated with disorders of the respiratory system or hypoxemia
4. PAH caused by chronic thrombotic or embolic disease
5. PAH caused by disorders directly affecting the pulmonary vasculature

There are several subcategories for each major category.[306]

Primary PH (PPH) is rare—that is, one or two cases per 1 million in the United States. PAH in neonates occurs in 1.9/1000 births from a variety of conditions.[136] PPH occurs most commonly in young and middle-aged women (pregnant women have the highest mortality). It may have no known cause (idiopathic), although familial disease (defects in the bone morphogenetic protein receptor type II gene and transforming growth factor–β [TGF-β]) has been found[323] to account for approximately 10% of cases. An epidemic of PAH was caused by the appetite suppressant aminorex fumarate, which was sold from 1965 to 1968. This drug produced the same vascular lesions as those seen in PPH and was the stimulus for new research.[102]

Pathogenesis

PPH is characterized by diffuse narrowing of the pulmonary arterioles caused by hypertrophy of smooth muscle in the vessel walls and formation of fibrous lesions in and around the vessels. The underlying cause of these changes is unknown, but looking beyond simple pulmonary vasoconstriction, it is now recognized that defects in endothelial function, pulmonary vascular smooth muscle cells, and platelets may all be involved in the pathogenesis and progression of PPH.

Defects in ion channel activity in smooth muscle cells in the pulmonary artery also may contribute to vasoconstriction and vascular proliferation.[161] These changes create increased resistance to the right side of the heart, which can eventually cause heart failure (cor pulmonale).

Secondary PH is caused by any respiratory or cardiovascular disorder that increases the volume or pressure of blood entering the pulmonary arteries; narrows, obstructs, or destroys the pulmonary arteries; or increases the pressure of blood leaving the heart (pulmonary veins).

Increased volume or pressure overloads the pulmonary circulation, whereas narrowing or obstruction elevates the blood pressure by increasing resistance to flow within the lungs. For example, COPD destroys alveoli and associated capillary beds, thus increasing pressure through the remaining vasculature. Left-sided heart failure causes blood to "back up," and thus resistance is increased.

With persistent PAH, the result is right ventricular hypertrophy and eventual cor pulmonale.

Clinical Manifestations

The most common symptoms of primary or secondary PH are atypical cardiorespiratory symptoms such as fatigue, weakness, chest discomfort or pain, syncope, peripheral edema, abdominal distention, and unexplained SOB that begin with exercise and later occur with minimal activity or at rest.[27] Signs and symptoms of secondary PH are difficult to recognize in the early stages when the symptoms of the underlying disease are more prominent.

11.21 Special Implications for the PTA: Pulmonary Hypertension Impairment of exercise performance is associated with pulmonary hypertension (PH) because pulmonary vascular resistance and pulmonary artery pressure increase dramatically with exercise. There may be impaired heart rate kinetics during exercise with corresponding impaired cardiac output response and slow recovery of the heart.[280] For these reasons, clients with PH must be closely monitored when participating in activities or therapy that causes increased physical stress.

Maintenance of adequate systemic blood pressure is essential, and the PTA must be familiar with the medications used and potential side effects, especially if blood pressure is altered pharmacologically. A drop in blood pressure can indicate heart failure. Inhaled N_2O and prostacyclin, which are endogenous vasodilators, increase oxygen consumption at the same workload during exercise, thereby improving exercise capacity. N_2O use is diminishing as a result of its toxicity and cost.[205]

Secondary PH may occur in clients with connective tissue diseases, such as scleroderma, because the disease affects the vasculature of several organs, including the lungs (pulmonary fibrosis) and kidneys. The arterioles usually demonstrate intimal proliferation with progressive luminal occlusion. The development of hypertension often indicates the onset of an accelerated scleroderma renal crisis. Medical treatment is toward control of the blood pressure.

Cor Pulmonale
Definition and Incidence

Cor pulmonale, also called *pulmonary heart disease,* is the enlargement of the right ventricle secondary to PH that occurs in diseases of the thorax, lung, and pulmonary circulation. It is a term that describes the pathologic effects of lung dysfunction as it affects the right side of the heart. Right-sided heart dysfunction secondary to left-sided heart failure, vascular dysfunction, or congenital heart disease is excluded in the definition of cor pulmonale.

Chronic cor pulmonale occurs most frequently in adult male smokers, although the incidence in women is increasing as heavy smoking in females becomes more prevalent. The actual prevalence of cor pulmonale is difficult to determine because cor pulmonale does not occur in all cases of chronic lung disease and because routine physical examination and laboratory tests are relatively insensitive to the presence of PH. It has been estimated that cor pulmonale accounts for 5% to 10% of organic heart disease.

Etiologic and Risk Factors

Pulmonary vascular diseases and respiratory diseases (e.g., emphysema, chronic bronchitis) are the primary causes of cor pulmonale. Emphysema and chronic bronchitis cause over 50% of cases of cor pulmonale in the United States. When a PE has been sufficiently massive to obstruct 60% to 75% of the pulmonary circulation, acute cor pulmonale can occur. Cor pulmonale is frequently the cause of death in COPD.[346]

Cor pulmonale can also develop under conditions of sustained elevations in intrathoracic pressure associated with mechanical ventilation (and PEEP). The intrathoracic vessels narrow, leading to reduced cardiac output and possible cor pulmonale. Chronic widespread vasculitis—such as occurs in association with the collagen vascular disorders (e.g., rheumatoid arthritis, SLE, dermatomyositis, polymyositis, Sjögren's syndrome, CREST [*c*alcinosis cutis, *R*aynaud's phenomenon, *e*sophageal dysfunction, *s*clerodactyly, and *t*elangiectasis] syndrome accompanying scleroderma)—can also cause chronic cor pulmonale. Occasionally, widespread radiation pneumonitis can be the underlying cause of cor pulmonale.

Other (uncommon) causes include pneumoconiosis, pulmonary fibrosis, kyphoscoliosis, pickwickian syndrome, lymphangitic infiltration from metastatic carcinoma, and obliterative pulmonary capillary changes that cause vasoconstriction and later hypertension. The feature common to all these conditions that predisposes to cor pulmonale is hypoxia, which leads to vasoconstriction.[346]

Pathogenesis

Sustained elevation in pulmonary arterial hypertension can be mediated through persistent vasoconstriction, abnormal vascular structural remodeling, or vessel obliteration (see discussion of PH in this chapter). Cor pulmonale develops as these factors increase pulmonary vessel pressure and overload in the right ventricle. Normally the ventricle is a thin-walled (heart) muscle able to meet an increase in volume and pressure, but long-term pressure overload from hypertension causes the tissue to hypertrophy.

In the case of acute cor pulmonale caused by emboli from DVT, the thrombus breaks loose and lodges at or near the *bifurcation* of the main pulmonary artery. Whether caused by vascular abnormalities or embolic obstruction, there is a marked fall in pressure necessary to drive blood through the compromised vascular bed because the right ventricle is compromised.

Clinical Manifestations

Evidence of cor pulmonale may be obscured by primary respiratory disease and may appear only during exercise testing. The heart appears normal at rest, but with exercise, cardiac output falls and the ECG shows right ventricular hypertrophy. The predominant symptoms are related to the pulmonary disorder and include chronic productive cough, exertional dyspnea, wheezing respirations, easy fatigability, and weakness.

With a large pulmonary embolus, sudden severe, central chest pain can occur as a result of acute dilation of the root of the pulmonary artery and secondary to ischemia. The person may collapse, often with loss of consciousness, and death may occur within minutes if the thrombus is large and does not dislodge. If the thrombus is small or moves more peripherally in response to pounding on the chest or chest compression during resuscitation, acute cor pulmonale develops rather than sudden death.

Low cardiac output causes pallor, sweating, hypotension, anxiety, impaired consciousness, and a rapid pulse of small amplitude. The specific signs associated with cor pulmonale include exercise-induced peripheral cyanosis, clubbing (see Fig. 11.4), distended neck veins, and bilateral dependent edema. Hypoxia can cause pulmonary vasoconstriction and worsen symptoms.

Medical Management

Diagnosis

Diagnosis is made on the basis of physical examination, radiologic studies, and ECG or echocardiogram, sometimes both. Echocardiogram can be performed at bedside and can effectively and efficiently detect right ventricular enlargement, as well as excessive right ventricular afterload.[168] Pulmonary function tests usually confirm the underlying lung disease. Laboratory findings may include polycythemia present in cor pulmonale secondary to COPD. ECG and chest film may not be diagnostic in the early stages of cor pulmonale.

Treatment

The primary goal of medical treatment is to reduce the workload of the right ventricle. This is accomplished by lowering pulmonary artery pressure, as in the treatment of PH (see discussion of PH in this chapter). Oxygen administration, salt and fluid restriction, and diuretics are essential, as well as treatment of the underlying chronic pulmonary disease, while at the same time relieving the hypoxemia, hypercapnia, or acidosis. There is no specific surgical treatment available for most causes of chronic cor pulmonale. Heart–lung transplantation for clients with PPH is valuable in late-stage disease.

Prognosis

Because cor pulmonale generally occurs late during the course of COPD and other irreversible disease, the prognosis is poor. Once congestive signs appear, the average life expectancy is 2 to 5 years, but survival is significantly longer when uncomplicated emphysema is the cause. Although cor pulmonale can be caused by obstructive and restrictive lung diseases, restrictive lung diseases are associated with a lower life expectancy once they reach the stage of cor pulmonale.

11.22 Special Implications for the PTA: Cor Pulmonale Because pulmonary infection exacerbates chronic obstructive pulmonary disease (COPD) and cor pulmonale, all health care workers must practice careful handwashing and follow standard precautions. Early signs of infection (e.g., increased sputum production, change in sputum color, chest pain or chest tightness, or fever) must be reported to the physician immediately. Watch for signs of respiratory failure such as change in pulse rate; deep, labored respirations; and increased fatigue produced by exertion.

People who are bedridden must be repositioned frequently to prevent atelectasis (and skin breakdown). Breathing exercises should be carried out frequently throughout the day. Diaphragmatic and pursed-lip breathing exercises should be reviewed for anyone with COPD and used with appropriate individuals.[58]

Teach the client (or family member) how to detect edema in the lower extremities, especially the ankles, by pressing the skin over the shins for 1 to 2 seconds and looking for a lasting finger impression. Watch for signs of digitalis toxicity such as complaints of anorexia, nausea, vomiting, or yellow halos around visual images.

DISORDERS OF THE PLEURAL SPACE

Pneumothorax

Definition

Pneumothorax is an accumulation of air or gas in the pleural cavity caused by a defect in the visceral pleura or chest wall. The result is collapse of the lung on the affected side. Pneumothorax is classified as spontaneous or traumatic. Primary spontaneous pneumothorax (PSP) develops with no underlying lung pathology. Secondary spontaneous pneumothorax (SSP) is typically a result of blebs or bullae that occur in COPD, CF, or other lung disorders. Traumatic pneumothoraces are iatrogenic or noniatrogenic[28] (Fig. 11.20).

Incidence and Risk Factors

Spontaneous pneumothorax may affect up to 20,000 people per year in the United States. Although pneumothorax can develop at any age, spontaneous pneumothorax is especially common in tall, slender boys and men aged 20 to 40 years. Smoking appears to increase the risk of PSP in men by as much as a factor of 20 in a dose-dependent manner (i.e., chances increase as number of cigarettes smoked increases).[292]

The most common causes of iatrogenic pneumothorax are transthoracic needle lung biopsy, subclavian vein catheterization, thoracentesis, transbronchial lung biopsy, and positive pressure ventilation. Surgical procedures that involve the chest wall and abdomen also can precipitate pneumothorax.

Pathogenesis

When air enters the pleural cavity the lung collapses and a separation between the visceral and parietal pleurae (see Fig. 11.3) occurs, destroying the negative pressure of the pleural space. This disruption in the normal equilibrium between the forces of elastic recoil and the chest wall causes the lung to recoil by collapsing toward the hilum. Depending on the individual's overall lung function, a loss of 40% may be present before symptoms appear.[292] The result is SOB and mediastinal shift toward the unaffected side, compressing the opposite lung. The causative pleural defect may be in the lung and visceral pleura (lung lining) or the parietal pleura (chest wall lining).

Spontaneous pneumothorax occurs when there is an opening on the surface of the lung allowing leakage of air from the airways or lung parenchyma into the pleural cavity. Most often this happens when an emphysematous bleb (blisterlike formation) or bulla (larger vesicle) or other weakened area on the lung ruptures. The majority of people with spontaneous pneumothorax have subpleural bullae that are most likely induced by the degradation of elastic fibers in the lung caused by the smoking-related influx of neutrophils and macrophages. Spontaneous pneumothorax can occur during sleep, at rest, or during exercise and can progress to become a tension pneumothorax. Other causes of this type of pneumothorax include TB, sarcoidosis, lung abscess, ARDS, and PCP.

Traumatic pneumothorax is a secondary pneumothorax with the entry of air directly through the chest wall or from laceration of the lung caused by penetrating or nonpenetrating chest trauma, such as a rib fracture or stab or bullet wound that tears the pleura.

Hemopneumothorax, in which both air and blood escape into the pleural space, can occur after chest trauma.

Open pneumothorax is a type of traumatic pneumothorax that occurs when air pressure in the pleural space equals barometric pressure because air that is drawn into the pleural space during inspiration (through the damaged chest wall and parietal pleura or through the parietal pleura and damaged visceral pleura) is forced back out during expiration. This can rapidly lead to hypoventilation and hypoxia.

Iatrogenic pneumothorax develops as a result of direct puncture or laceration of the visceral pleura during attempts at central line placement, *percutaneous* lung aspiration, thoracentesis, or closed pleural biopsy. Direct alveolar distention can occur with anesthesia, CPR, or mechanical ventilation with PEEP.

Tension pneumothorax can result from any type of pneumothorax and is life threatening. In tension pneumothorax, the site of pleural rupture acts as a one-way valve, permitting air to enter on inspiration but preventing its escape by closing up during expiration. Under these conditions, continuously increasing air pressure in the pleural cavity may cause progressive collapse of the lung tissue. Air pressure in the pleural space pushes against the already recoiled lung, causing compression atelectasis, and against the mediastinum, compressing and displacing the heart and great vessels. Venous return and cardiac output decrease.[354]

Clinical Manifestations

Dyspnea is the first and primary symptom of pneumothorax, but other symptoms may include a sudden sharp pleural chest pain, fall in blood pressure, weak and rapid pulse, and cessation of normal respiratory movements on the affected side of the chest.

If the pneumothorax is large or if there is a tension pneumothorax, it may push the mediastinum toward the unaffected lung, causing the chest to appear asymmetric and the trachea to move to the contralateral side. The pain may be referred to the ipsilateral shoulder (corresponding shoulder on the same side as the pneumothorax), across the chest, or over the abdomen.

Clinical manifestations of tension pneumothorax include severe hypoxemia, dyspnea, and hypotension (low blood pressure) in addition to the other signs and symptoms of pneumothorax already mentioned. Increased intrathoracic pressure from a tension pneumothorax may result in neck vein distention. Untreated tension pneumothorax may quickly produce life-threatening shock and bradycardia.

Medical Management

Diagnosis and Treatment

Diagnosis is made by chest film at inspiration. CT scan has been shown to be more sensitive in the person with chest trauma.[236] There are no specific laboratory tests, but blood gas measurements indicate the degree of respiratory impairment. The presence of dyspnea, tachycardia, decrease or loss of breath sounds, percussive hyperresonance, decreased fremitus, asymmetric chest wall movement, and subcutaneous emphysema (swelling and crepitus with palpation) will assist in the diagnosis.

Depending on the size of the pneumothorax, no specific treatment is required for PSP less than 20% beyond rest and the administration of oxygen to relieve dyspnea.[334] However, recurrences are frequent and associated with increased mortality in SSP.

Thoracoscopic procedures of pleurodesis (pleural abrasion, talc poudrage, and pleurectomy) are recommended to prevent further recurrence in SSP. Placement of a chest tube is standard procedure for traumatic pneumothoraces.[28] Surgical repair is sometimes warranted, particularly with major trauma.

Pneumothorax is an unwanted sequela to respiratory distress syndrome in premature infants. The use of prophylactic surfactant significantly reduces the incidence of pneumothorax in this population.[311]

It is not a good idea to travel by airplane (because of air pressure changes) or to have pulmonary function tests performed (e.g., in CF) for at least 2 weeks after a pneumothorax has healed. Encouraging smoking cessation is essential.

Prognosis

There is a low mortality rate with idiopathic pneumothorax, but a corresponding 15% mortality rate for pneumothorax associated with underlying lung disease. From 30% to 50% of affected persons experience a recurrence, and after one recurrence, subsequent episodes are much more likely. The physiologic events associated with tension pneumothorax are life-threatening, requiring immediate treatment.

11.23 Special Implications for the PTA: Pneumothorax When getting someone up for the first time, monitor vital signs, especially blood pressure and pulse, and request emergency medical help immediately anytime someone with a suggestive history demonstrates sudden shoulder or chest pain, altered breathing pattern, or drop of blood pressure accompanied by weak and fast pulse, pallor, dyspnea, or extreme anxiety.

In the case of trauma (e.g., motor vehicle accident, assault, or traumatic falls) the presence of undiagnosed nondisplaced rib fractures or rib fragments must be considered when getting a person up for the first time. The client's movements and the action of parasternal intercostal muscles can displace the rib, causing puncture of the lung or penetrating aortic injury.

Anyone with a history of SSP should also be monitored closely during treatment because of the chance for recurrence and complications. See also in this chapter 11.12 Special Implications for the PTA: Chest Wall Trauma or Lung Injury.

Pleurisy
Definition and Etiologic Factors
Pleurisy (pleuritis) is an inflammation of the pleura caused by viral or bacterial infection, injury (e.g., rib fracture), or tumor (particularly malignant pleural mesothelioma). It may be a complication of lung disease, particularly of pneumonia, but also of TB, lung abscesses, influenza, SLE, rheumatoid arthritis, or pulmonary infarction.

Clinical Manifestations

The symptoms develop suddenly, usually with a sharp, sticking chest pain that is worse on inspiration, coughing, sneezing, or movement associated with deep inspiration. Other symptoms may include cough, fever, chills, and rapid shallow breathing (tachypnea). The visceral pleurae is insensitive; pain results from inflammation of the parietal pleurae. Because the latter is innervated by the intercostal nerves, chest pain is usually felt over the site of the pleuritis, but pain may be referred to the lower chest wall, abdomen, neck, upper trapezius muscle, and shoulder. On auscultation, a pleural rub can be heard (sound caused by the rubbing together of the visceral and costal pleurae).

Pathogenesis

There are two types of pleurisy: wet and dry. The membranous pleura that encases each lung is composed of two close-fitting layers; between these layers is a lubricating fluid. If the fluid content remains unchanged by the disease, the pleurisy is said to be dry. If the fluid increases abnormally, it is a wet pleurisy, or pleurisy with effusion (Fig. 11.21). Inflammation of the part of the pleura that covers the diaphragm is called *diaphragmatic pleurisy* and occurs secondary to pneumonia.

When the central portion of the diaphragmatic pleura is irritated, sharp pain may be referred to the neck, upper trapezius, or shoulder. Stimulation of the peripheral portions of the diaphragmatic pleura results in sharp pain felt along the costal margins, which can be referred to the lumbar region by the lower thoracic somatic nerves (Fig. 11.22).

Wet pleurisy is less likely to cause pain because there usually is no chafing. The fluid may interfere with breathing by compressing the lung. If the excess fluid of wet pleurisy becomes infected with formation of pus, the condition is known as *purulent pleurisy* or *empyema*. Pleurisy causes pleurae to become reddened and covered with an exudate of lymph, fibrin, and cellular elements and may lead to pleural effusion. In dry pleurisy, the two layers of membrane may become congested and swollen and rub against each other, which is painful. Although only the outer layer causes pain (the inner layer has no pain nerves), the pain may be severe enough to require the use of a strong analgesic.

Medical Management

Treatment is usually with aspirin and time or, if the pleurisy is severe and unresponsive, NSAIDs. Antibiotics may be prescribed for a specific infection. Sclerosing therapy for chronic or recurrent pleurisy may be recommended.

11.24 Special Implications for the PTA: Pleurisy Bed rest is an important part of the care plan for the client with pleurisy. Therapy in the acute care setting should be coordinated to provide as much uninterrupted rest as possible. Breathing and coughing exercises are important but often avoided because of the pain these respiratory movements cause. To minimize discomfort, have the patient use a splinted technique of applying firm pressure with hands or a pillow to the site of the pain during deep breathing and coughing.

Pleural Effusion
Definition
Pleural effusion is the collection of fluid in the pleural space (between the membrane encasing the lung and the membrane lining the thoracic cavity) where there is normally only a small amount of fluid to prevent friction as the lung expands and deflates (see Fig. 11.21). Pleural fluid normally seeps continually into the pleural space from the capillaries lining the parietal pleura and is then reabsorbed by the visceral pleural capillaries and lymphatics.

Incidence and Etiologic Factors

The causes of pleural effusion are best considered in terms of the underlying pathophysiology:

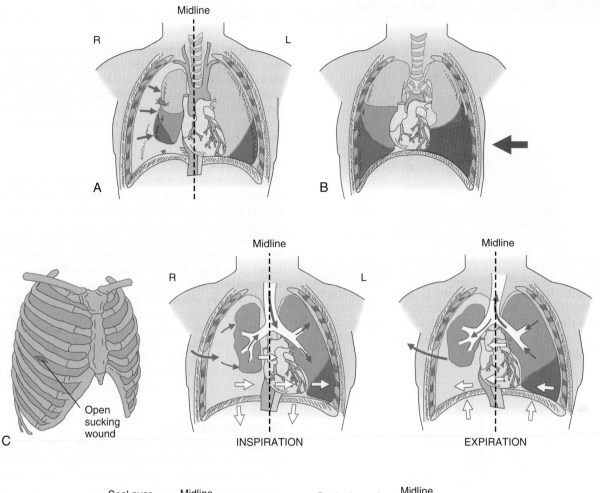

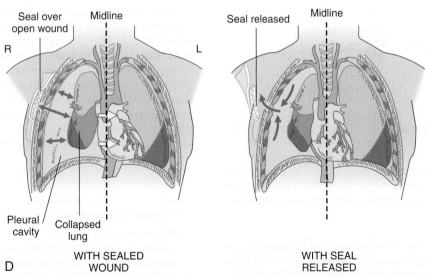

FIG. 11.20 (A) Pneumothorax. Lung collapses as air gathers in the pleural space between the parietal and visceral pleurae. (B) Massive hemothorax, blood in the pleural space *(arrow)* below the left lung, causing collapse of lung tissue. (C) Open pneumothorax (sucking chest wound). Air movement *(solid arrows)* and structural movement *(open arrows)*. A chest wall wound connects the pleural space with atmospheric air. During inspiration, atmospheric air is sucked into the pleural space through the chest wall wound. Positive pressure in the pleural space collapses the lung on the affected side and pushes the mediastinal contents toward the unaffected side. This reduces the volume of air in the unaffected side considerably. During expiration, air escapes through the chest wall wound, lessening positive pressure in the affected side and allowing the mediastinal contents to swing back toward the affected side. Movement of mediastinal structure from side to side is called mediastinal flutter. (D) Tension pneumothorax. If an open pneumothorax is covered (e.g., with a dressing), it forms a seal and tension pneumothorax with a mediastinal shift develops. A tear in lung structure continues to allow air into the pleural space. As positive pressure builds in the pleural space, the affected lung collapses, and the mediastinal contents shift to the unaffected side. Tension pneumothorax is corrected by removing the seal (i.e., dressing), allowing air trapped in the pleural space to escape.

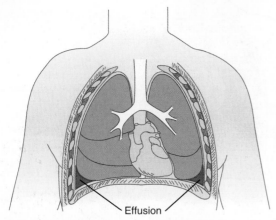

FIG. 11.21 Pleural effusion, a collection of fluid in the pleural space between the membrane encasing the lung and the membrane lining the thoracic cavity, as seen on upright x-ray examination. Pleurisy (pleuritis) is an inflammation of the visceral and parietal pleurae. When there is an abnormal increase in the lubricating fluid between these two layers, it is called *pleurisy with effusion.*

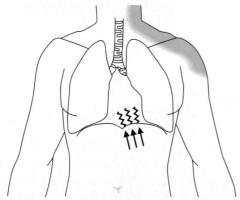

FIG. 11.22 Diaphragmatic pleurisy. Irritation of the peritoneal (outside) or pleural (inside) surface of the central area of the diaphragm refers sharp pain to the neck, supraclavicular fossa, and upper trapezius muscle. The pain pattern is ipsilateral to the area of irritation. Irritation to the peripheral portion of the diaphragm refers sharp pain to the costal margins and lumbar region (not shown).

1. Transudates caused by abnormalities of hydrostatic or osmotic pressure (e.g., congestive heart failure, cirrhosis with ascites, nephrotic syndrome, or peritoneal dialysis)
2. Exudates resulting from increased permeability or trauma (e.g., infection, primary or secondary malignancy, PE, trauma including surgical trauma [e.g., cardiotomy])

An exudate is a fluid with a high content of protein and cellular debris that has escaped from blood vessels and has been deposited in tissues or on tissue surfaces, usually as a result of inflammation. A transudate is a fluid substance that has passed through a membrane or has been forced out from a tissue; in contrast to an exudate, a transudate is characterized by high fluidity and a low content of protein, cells, or solid matter derived from cells.

Any condition that interferes with either the secretion or drainage of this fluid will lead to pleural effusion. Pleural effusion is common with heart failure and lymphatic obstruction caused by neoplasm. Less common causes include drug-induced effusion, pancreatitis, collagen vascular diseases (SLE or rheumatoid arthritis), intraabdominal abscess, or esophageal perforation. A person of any age can be affected, but it is more common in the older adult because of the increased incidence of heart failure and cancer.

Pathogenesis

The most common mechanism of pleural effusion is migration of fluids and other blood components through the walls of intact capillaries bordering the pleura. When stimulated by biochemical mediators of inflammation, junctions in the capillary endothelium separate slightly, enabling leukocytes and plasma proteins to migrate out into affected tissues. Rupture of a blood vessel or leakage of blood from an injured vessel causes a form of pleural effusion called *hemothorax* (see Fig. 11.21).

Malignancy effusion is usually a local effect of the tumor such as lymphatic obstruction or bronchial obstruction with pneumonia or atelectasis. Lymphatic blockage from any cause can result in drainage of the contents of lymphatic vessels into the pleural space. It can also be a result of systemic effects of tumor elsewhere, but in either case, malignant cells in the pleural effusion of a person with lung cancer indicate an inoperable situation.

Clinical Manifestations

Clinical manifestations of pleural effusion will depend on the amount of fluid present and the degree of lung compression. A small amount of effusion may be discovered only by chest x-ray examination. Large effusions cause clinical manifestations related to their volume and the rate at which they accumulate in the pleural space causing restriction of lung expansion. Clients usually have dyspnea on exertion that becomes progressive. They may develop nonspecific chest discomfort; sometimes the chest pain is pleuritic, which is a sharp, stabbing pain exacerbated by coughing or breathing and changes in position. Other symptoms characteristic of the underlying cause of pleural effusion may be the primary clinical picture (e.g., weight loss and fever with TB or cancer or signs of heart failure).

Medical Management

Diagnosis

Examination of the pleural fluid via transthoracic aspiration biopsy (surgical puncture and drainage of the thoracic cavity) includes analysis of pH; specific gravity; protein; stains and cultures for bacteria, TB, and fungi; eosinophilia count; and glucose concentration to aid in the differential diagnosis.[299]

Some markers, such as neutrophil-derived enzymes, may be indicators for necessity of chest tubes for drainage. Chest pain must be differentiated from pain of pericardial or musculoskeletal origin. Chest radiographs and physical examination with possible CT scan are necessary components of the diagnostic process.

Treatment

Treatment may not be required when the individual is asymptomatic; if the client is only mildly symptomatic, transthoracic aspiration may be all that is necessary. In the case of an underlying disease process (e.g., congestive heart failure or renal pathologic findings associated with transudates), treatment is aimed toward that condition.

Drainage of the fluid for exudate-caused effusion provides symptomatic improvement but does not significantly alter lung volumes or gas exchange. Removal of fluid associated with malignancy is considered only if the individual is symptomatic and could benefit from aspiration. Repeated aspiration is avoided because significant protein loss can occur and the fluid reaccumulates in 1 to 3 days.

Some (exudate) pleural effusions resolve with antibiotic therapy. Recurrent (exudate) pleural effusions may be treated by pleurectomy (surgically stripping the parietal pleura away from the visceral pleura) and pleurodesis (sclerosing substance introduced into the pleural space to create an inflammatory response that scleroses tissues together). Both of these procedures have negative effects that must be taken into consideration.

Prognosis

Prognosis depends on the underlying disease; in cancer, recurrent pleural effusion may be associated with the terminal stage of disease. Tumor-related effusion generally implies a poor prognosis.

11.25 Special Implications for the PTA: Pleural Effusion After transthoracic aspiration, encourage deep-breathing exercises to promote lung expansion and watch for respiratory distress or pneumothorax (sudden onset of dyspnea or cyanosis). In the presence of a chest tube, prevent kinking by carefully coiling the tubing on top of the bed and securing it to the bed linen, leaving room for the client to turn.

Position changes must be performed carefully to avoid disturbing the surgical site or the chest tube. The PTA may use or teach the client a splinting technique by applying firm support with both hands to the surgical site and chest tube area to help lessen muscle pull and pain as the client coughs. If the person has open drainage through a rib resection or intercostal tube, use hand and dressing precautions.

Pleural Empyema

Pleural empyema (infected pleural effusion) is an accumulation of pus that occurs occasionally as a complication of pleurisy or some other respiratory disease, usually pneumonia. It is a normal response to infection but may also occur after external contamination (penetrating trauma, chest tube placement, or other surgical procedure) or esophageal perforation. Symptoms include dyspnea, coughing, ipsilateral pleural chest or shoulder pain, malaise, tachycardia, cough, and fever. In addition to chest films, transthoracic aspiration biopsy may be done to confirm the diagnosis and determine the specific causative organism.

The condition is treated with intercostal chest tube drainage, rest, and sedative cough mixtures. Long-term antibiotics are generally needed, and attention must be paid to the person's nutritional status.[64] Intrapleural fibrinolytic agents may have some use reducing need for surgery in patients with empyema.[328] See in this chapter 11.25 Special Implications for the PTA: Pleural Effusion.

Pleural Fibrosis

Pleural fibrosis may follow inflammation (especially from asbestos), hemorrhagic effusion, and infection of the pleurae. It can manifest as localized plaques or diffusely. There appears to be a complex interaction of inflammatory cells, coagulation, profibrotic mediators, and growth factors in this process.[245] Early use of corticosteroids may decrease the incidence but is not effective in reducing established fibrosis. Surgical decortication can be effective in resolving symptoms.[157]

REFERENCES/SUGGESTED READINGS

To enhance this text and add value for the reader, references and suggested readings are included on the companion Evolve site that accompanies this textbook. The reader can view the source and access it online whenever possible.

The Hepatic, Pancreatic, and Biliary Systems

VOCAB BUILDERS

Albumin	Dehydrogenase	Oculocephalic reflex
Alkalinizing	Emulsification	Paracentesis
Ascites	Fulminant	Pruritus
Asterixis	Hemangiomas	Sjögren's syndrome
Charcot's triad	Hepatomegaly	Varices
Coagulopathy	Icterus	Xanthelasmas
Colic	Jaundice	
Decerebrate posturing	Neoadjuvant	

The *liver* has more than 500 separate functions such as the conversion and excretion of bilirubin (red bile pigment, which is an end-product of heme from hemoglobin in red blood cells). The liver is the sole source of *albumin* and other plasma proteins and also produces 500 to 1500 mL of bile each day. Other important functions of the liver include production of clotting factors and storage of vitamins. The liver and gut are the key organs in nutrient absorption and metabolism; nutrients bind to toxins in this pathway and aid in eliminating these toxins from the body.

The liver contributes to a functional immune system by reducing the amount of toxins that could impair the gut lining, which in turn helps prevent the entry of bacteria and viruses into the system. Bile acids, drugs, chemicals, and toxins undergo extensive enterohepatic circulation during the processes of metabolism. The liver also filters all of the blood from the gastrointestinal (GI) system and is therefore the primary organ for metastasis of intestinal cancer.

The *pancreas* is both an exocrine and an endocrine gland. Its primary function in digestion is exocrine secretion of digestive enzymes and pancreatic juices, transported through the pancreatic duct to the duodenum. Proteins, carbohydrates, and fats are broken down in the duodenum, aided by pancreatic and other secretions, which also help to neutralize the acidic substances passed from the stomach to the duodenum. The endocrine function involves the secretion of glucagon and insulin by islet of Langerhans cells for the regulation of carbohydrate metabolism. Pancreatic disease may result in a variety of clinical presentations, depending on whether the exocrine or endocrine function has been impaired.

The *gallbladder,* acting as a reservoir for bile, stores and concentrates the bile during fasting periods and then contracts to expel the bile into the duodenum in response to the arrival of food. Bile helps in *alkalinizing* the intestinal contents and plays a role in the *emulsification,* absorption, and digestion of fat. The signal for the gallbladder to contract comes from the release of cholecystokinin (CCK), a hormone released into the bloodstream from the wall of the duodenum and upper small intestine.

SIGNS AND SYMPTOMS OF HEPATIC DISEASE

Primary signs and symptoms of liver diseases vary and can include GI symptoms, edema or ascites, dark urine, light-colored or clay-colored feces, and right upper abdominal pain (Box 12.1). Impairment of the liver can result in *hepatic failure* when either the mass of liver cells is sufficiently diminished or their function is impaired as a result of cirrhosis, liver cancer, or infection and/or inflammation. Hepatic failure does not refer to one specific morphologic change but rather to a clinical

---

BOX 12.1   Most Common Signs and Symptoms of Hepatic Disease

- Gastrointestinal symptoms
- Edema, ascites
- Dark urine
- Light-colored or clay-colored stools
- Right upper quadrant abdominal pain
- Skin changes
  - Jaundice
  - Bruising
  - Spider angioma
  - Palmar erythema
- Neurologic involvement
  - Confusion
  - Sleep disturbances
  - Muscle tremors
  - Hyperreactive reflexes
  - Asterixis
- Musculoskeletal pain (see text for sites)
- Hepatic osteodystrophy
- Jaundice

---

syndrome that includes hepatic encephalopathy, renal failure (hepatorenal syndrome), endocrine changes, and jaundice.

Dark urine and light stools occur in association with *jaundice* (yellow pigmentation of skin, sclerae, and mucous membranes). Any damage to the liver impairs bilirubin metabolism from the blood. Normally, bile converted from bilirubin causes brown coloration of the stool. Light-colored (almost white) stools and urine the color of tea or cola indicate an inability of the liver or biliary system to excrete bilirubin properly.

Skin changes associated with the hepatic system include jaundice, pallor, and orange or green skin. The changes described here in urine, stool, or skin color may be caused by hepatitis, gallbladder disease, pancreatic cancer blocking the bile duct, hepatotoxic medications, or cirrhosis. Other skin changes may include bruising, spider angiomata, and palmar erythema. The person may complain of throbbing, tingling palms.

Neurologic symptoms, such as confusion, sleep disturbances, muscle tremors, hyperreactive reflexes, and asterixis may occur. When liver dysfunction results in increased serum ammonia and urea levels, peripheral nerve function can be impaired. *Asterixis* and numbness or tingling (misinterpreted as carpal tunnel syndrome) can occur as a result of this ammonia abnormality, causing intrinsic nerve pathology. Asterixis is the inability to maintain wrist extension with forward flexion of the upper extremities. A test for asterixis is asking the client to extend the wrist and hand with the rest of the arm supported on a firm surface or with the arms held out in front of the body. Observe for

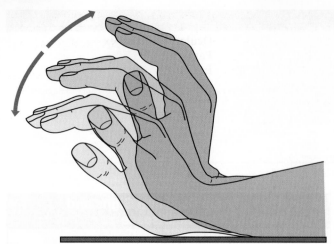

FIG. 12.1 Flapping tremor. The flapping tremor elicited by attempted wrist extension while the forearm is fixed is the most common neurologic abnormality associated with liver failure. It can also be observed in uremia, respiratory failure, and severe heart failure. The tremor is absent at rest, decreased by intentional movement, and maximal on sustained posture. It is usually bilateral, although one side may be affected more than the other. (Redrawn from Dooley J, Sherlock S: Sherlock's diseases of the liver and biliary system, ed 12, West Sussex, U.K., 2011, Wiley-Blackwell.)

quick, irregular extensions and flexions of the wrist and fingers (Fig. 12.1). Altered neurotransmission, in the form of impaired inflow of joint and other afferent information to the brainstem reticular formation, causes the movement dysfunction.

Musculoskeletal locations of pain associated with the hepatic and biliary systems include thoracic pain between scapulae, right shoulder, right upper trapezius, right interscapular area, or right subscapular area.

Hepatic osteodystrophy, abnormal development of bone, can occur in all forms of cholestasis (bile flow suppression) and hepatocellular disease, especially in the alcoholic. Hepatic osteoporosis is secondary to osteoblastic dysfunction rather than to excessive bone resorption.

Vertebral wedging, vertebral crush fractures, and kyphosis can be severe; decalcification of the rib cage and pseudofractures occur frequently. Painful osteoarthropathy may develop in the wrists and ankles as a nonspecific complication of chronic liver disease.

Portal hypertension, ascites, and *hepatic encephalopathy* are three other major complications of liver disease that are discussed in greater depth in this chapter as distinct clinical conditions.

12.1 Special Implications for the PTA: Signs and Symptoms of Hepatic Disease Active, intense exercise should be avoided when the liver is compromised (i.e., during jaundice or any other active liver disease) because the cornerstone of medical treatment and promotion of healing of the liver is rest.

An increased risk of *coagulopathy* (decreased clotting ability) also occurs with liver disease, necessitating precautions. Easy bruising and bleeding under the skin or into the joints in response to the slightest trauma can occur when coagulation is impaired. This condition necessitates extreme care in the therapy setting, especially with any intervention requiring manual therapy or the use of any

---

equipment, including modalities, resistive exercise or weight-training devices, and potentially gait belts.

The most common neurologic abnormality associated with liver failure (liver flap or asterixis) (see Fig. 12.1) also can be observed in uremia, respiratory failure, and severe heart failure. The rapid flexion extension movements at the metacarpophalangeal and wrist joints often are accompanied by lateral movements of the digits. Sometimes movement of arms, neck, and jaws; protruding tongue; retracted mouth; and tightly closed eyelids are involved, and the gait is ataxic. The tremor is absent at rest, decreased by intentional movement, and maximal on sustained posture. It is usually bilateral, although not bilaterally synchronous, and one side may be affected more than the other. It may be observed by gentle elevation of a limb or by the client's gripping the hand of the physical therapist assistant (PTA). In coma, the tremor disappears.

AGING AND THE HEPATIC SYSTEM

The liver decreases in size and weight with advancing age, requiring more time to process substances, medications, and alcohol. Liver function test results remain unchanged and within normal limits established for the adult. However, these tests often measure hepatic damage rather than overall function; abnormal values for these tests in older adults reflect disease rather than the effects of aging.

The decreased liver weight is accompanied by diminished blood flow. This combination of decreased liver mass and blood flow may account for some changes in drug elimination observed in the older adult. Dose adjustments to compensate for pharmacokinetic and pharmacodynamic changes that occur in the older adult are being studied and adjustments for specific drugs presented.[38]

The pancreas undergoes structural changes, such as fibrosis, fatty acid deposits, and atrophy, but the pancreas has a large reserve capacity, and 90% of its function would have to be lost before any observable dysfunction would occur. Much remains unknown about the gallbladder in the aging process, but aging apparently has little effect on gallbladder size, contractility, or function. The gallbladder releases less bile into the liver, allowing more time for gallstones to develop. There is some evidence that moderate and vigorous physical activity enhances the function of the gallbladder as measured by reduced risk of gallbladder removal in physically active women.[35]

HEALING IN THE HEPATIC SYSTEM

Generally, older organs may not adapt to injury as well as younger organs, so severe hepatic illnesses (e.g., severe hepatitis) may not be tolerated as well by the older person. Delayed or impaired tissue repair may require longer time for recovery of homeostasis.

Liver injury is followed by complete parenchymal regeneration, the formation of scars, or a combination of both. Chronic hepatic injury, such as chronic viral hepatitis or alcoholic liver injury, destroys the extracellular matrix framework. This type of destruction results in a combination of regenerated nodules separated by bands of fibrous connective tissue (fibrosis), which is termed *cirrhosis.*

Orthotopic liver transplantation has become an established therapy for end-stage liver disease. Biliary atresia is the most common indication for pediatric liver transplantation. Theoretically, anyone with advanced, irreversible liver disease with

---

BOX 12.2   Classification of Jaundice

Diseases Associated with Overproduction of Bilirubin
- Hemolysis
  - Thalassemia, sickle cell anemia,
  - Autoimmune hemolytic anemia
- Reabsorption of hematoma
- Blood transfusion

Decreased Uptake or Conjugation in Bilirubin Metabolism
- Gilbert's syndrome
- Jaundice of newborns
- Drugs

Hepatocyte Dysfunction
- Hepatitis
  - Viral
  - Alcohol-related
  - Autoimmune
  - Toxic, drug-induced
  - Ischemia
- Chronic hepatic disease
  - Wilson's disease
  - Hemochromatosis

Impaired Bile Flow
- Cholelithiasis
- Primary sclerosing cholangitis
- Pancreatic cancer
- Pancreatitis

---

certain mortality may be considered for a liver transplant, provided the disease could be corrected by liver transplantation.

Current animal research is centered on identifying and harvesting specific stem cells from the bone marrow that under special conditions will convert into functioning liver tissue. In human research, a new procedure called *hepatocyte transplantation* is being pioneered. An effective temporary liver support system could improve the chance of survival with or without a transplant as the final treatment.

LIVER

Liver Disease Complications

As a result of the extraordinary number of vital functions the liver performs, severe complications result when the liver has been damaged or is no longer functioning. Jaundice is a symptom that occurs with many types of diseases and disorders (both acute and chronic). End-stage complications occur most often because of cirrhosis and include portal hypertension, hepatic encephalopathy, ascites, and the hepatorenal syndrome. Any illness, toxin, or infection that leads to end-stage liver disease can display these complications.

Jaundice (Icterus)

Jaundice, or *icterus*, is not a disease but is rather a common symptom of many different diseases and disorders (Box 12.2). It is clinically characterized by yellow discoloration of the skin, sclerae, and mucous membranes. Jaundice occurs either as a result of an overproduction of bilirubin, defects in bilirubin metabolism (in uptake by the liver or conjugation), the presence of liver disease, or obstruction of bile flow.

Diseases, toxins, infections, and ischemia can cause generalized liver disease (acute and chronic), which reduces the capability of the liver to function normally and process bilirubin. Finally, bile ducts can be obstructed by diseases, tumors, and stones, leading to an elevation in bilirubin that has been conjugated.

Laboratory testing can aid in the specific diagnosis of jaundice. Elevations in liver transaminases (aspartate aminotransferase and alanine aminotransferase) suggest that liver disease is involved. Many other tests are available for the specific diagnosis of jaundice, depending on the suspected process, and are included in the specific disease sections in this chapter.

12.2 Special Implications for the PTA: Jaundice (Icterus) With successful treatment of the underlying cause, jaundice usually begins to resolve within 4 to 6 weeks. After this time, activity and exercise can be resumed or increased per individual tolerance, depending on the overall medical condition and presence of any complications. The return of normal stool and urine colors is an indication of resolution.

Cirrhosis

Cirrhosis is the final common pathway of chronic, progressive inflammation of the liver. There are many diseases, medications, and toxins that can damage the liver and ultimately lead to cirrhosis, but the most common in the United States include alcohol abuse and hepatitis C virus (HCV).

Overall, in the United States cirrhosis is the twelfth leading cause of death, accounting for about 28,000 deaths a year.[4] Cirrhosis of the liver occurs when inflammation (from disease or toxin) causes liver tissue damage and/or necrosis. With continued cycles of inflammation and healing, fibrous bands of connective tissue replace normal liver cells. Once 80% to 90% of the liver has been replaced with scar tissue, there is also significant loss of function, associated with decompensation of homeostasis.

The signs and symptoms of cirrhosis (Figs. 12.2 and 12.3) are multiple and varied, representing interference with major functions of the liver. Clients with cirrhosis exhibit fatigue, weight loss, jaundice, coagulopathies, loss of ability to metabolize drugs, and hypoalbuminemia (the remaining serious complications are discussed later). History, physical examination, laboratory tests, and imaging tests aid in diagnosing the specific cause. Once cirrhosis has developed, it is usually not reversible, although each disease may have a specific therapy to reduce the risk of development of cirrhosis. Typically, complications are treated on an individual basis and transplantation provides the best therapy for long-term survival.

12.3 Special Implications for the PTA: Cirrhosis One of the most common symptoms associated with cirrhosis is *ascites*, an accumulation of fluid in the peritoneal cavity surrounding the intestines. The distention often occurs very slowly over a number of weeks or months and may be associated with bilateral edema of the feet and ankles. The client may be unable to put on a pair of shoes, preferring to leave the shoes unlaced or to wear slippers. In a home health or inpatient hospital setting, this change in dress may not be as noticeable as it would be in a private practice or outpatient clinic. It is always important to remain alert to these potential signs

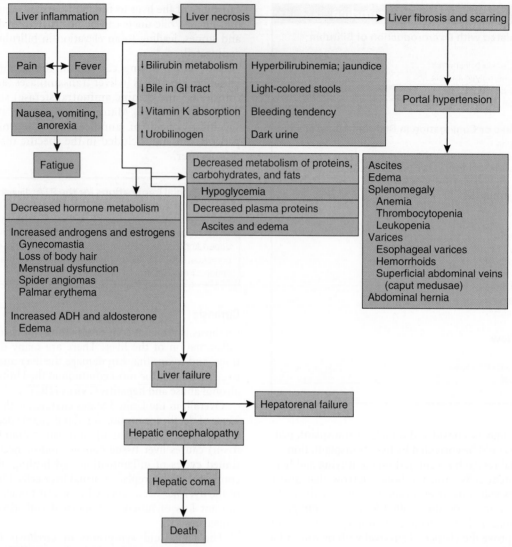

FIG. 12.2 Pathologic basis *(purple boxes)* and resultant clinical manifestations *(green boxes)* associated with cirrhosis of the liver.

of fluid retention and to ask about any changes in health status or weight gain.

Detection of blood loss in the form of hematemesis, tarry stools, bleeding gums, frequent and heavy nosebleeds, or excessive bruising must be reported to the physician. Preventing increased intraabdominal pressure (see Box 12.1) and preventing injury from falls require client education regarding safety precautions.

Alcohol causes whole-body and tissue-specific changes in protein metabolism. Chronic alcohol use reduces skeletal lean tissue mass. Loss of skeletal collagen contributes to alcohol-related osteoporosis. The loss of skeletal muscle protein (i.e., chronic alcoholic myopathy) occurs in up to two-thirds of all chronic alcohol users. Most clients with cirrhosis have significantly reduced aerobic capacity. Rest to reduce metabolic demands on the liver and to increase circulation often is recommended for clients with cirrhosis. Frequent rests during therapy and avoiding unnecessary fatigue are also important. Chronic alcoholic myopathy affecting the proximal muscles is usually mild and results in muscle atrophy and measurable decrease in muscle strength. The PTA must remain alert to any potential medical complications in any client, regardless of the physical therapy diagnosis.

Portal Hypertension

Portal refers to the area in which blood vessels enter into the liver. Venous blood returning from the stomach, large and small intestine, pancreas, and spleen is transported via the portal vein to the liver (the splanchnic circulation). Most cases of portal hypertension are related to cirrhosis. Other causes include thrombus, tumor, and infection, or the condition may be idiopathic.

Fibrosis, nodularity, and abnormal liver architecture combine to form mechanical barriers to blood flow and increase the resistance.

As a result of this increased portal pressure, blood that normally flows to the portal vein is reversed and blood begins to flow back to the stomach, esophagus, umbilicus, and rectum. These engorged vessels give rise to rectal varices, prominent vessels around the umbilicus, and gastroesophageal varices.

Gastroesophageal varices are one of the most serious complications of portal hypertension, occurring in 40% of people with cirrhosis. Endoscopy should be performed in all clients with cirrhosis to screen for varices. Clinical manifestations of gastroesophageal bleeding include hematemesis or melena (or both).

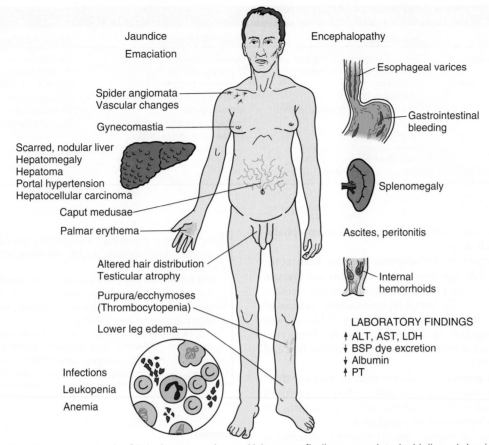

Jaundice
Emaciation

Encephalopathy

Esophageal varices

Gastrointestinal
bleeding

Spider angiomata
Vascular changes

Gynecomastia

Scarred, nodular liver
Hepatomegaly
Hepatoma
Portal hypertension
Hepatocellular carcinoma

Caput medusae

Palmar erythema

Splenomegaly

Ascites, peritonitis

Altered hair distribution
Testicular atrophy

Internal
hemorrhoids

Purpura/ecchymoses
(Thrombocytopenia)

Lower leg edema

LABORATORY FINDINGS
↑ ALT, AST, LDH
↓ BSP dye excretion
↓ Albumin
↑ PT

Infections
Leukopenia
Anemia

FIG. 12.3 Liver cirrhosis. Clinical presentation and laboratory findings associated with liver cirrhosis. *ALT,* alanine aminotransferase; *AST,* aspartate aminotransferase; *BSP,* sulfobromophthalein; *LDH,* lactate dehydrogenase; *PT,* prothrombin time. (From Black JM, Matassarin-Jacobs E, editors: Medical-surgical nursing: clinical management for continuity of care, ed 5, Philadelphia, 1997, Saunders.)

The blood is usually dark red in color. Over half of bleeds stop spontaneously, and over 90% of bleeds can be controlled with therapy. However, serious bleeding can quickly result in hypovolemia, shock, and death. Treatment is aimed at preventing bleeding by decreasing portal blood flow and intrahepatic pressure.

Prognosis is poor for clients with repeated esophageal varices, and liver transplantation should be pursued.

12.4 Special Implications for the PTA: Portal Hypertension Patterns will depend on complications associated with portal hypertension. For example, some people with varices develop anemia or toxic neuropathy, whereas others may develop ascites and encephalopathy. The PTA should refer to the practice patterns for each of those (or other) conditions on an individual basis.

Portal pressure in individuals is dynamic, with highest pressures during the night, after eating, and in response to coughing, sneezing, and exercise. Such variations may combine with local factors in vessel walls to contribute to a pressure surge that can lead to a variceal bleed. The PTA can teach the individual how to modify and reduce pressure, especially anything that increases intraabdominal pressure (see Box 12.1) such as coughing, straining at stool, or lifting improperly. Any therapy program for a client with known varices must take this factor into account when presenting active or active-assisted exercises, or unsupported gait training.[20]

Hepatic Encephalopathy

Hepatic encephalopathy refers to a potentially reversible, decreased level of consciousness in people with severe liver disease. This complication can occur with both acute and chronic liver disease. People with chronic end-stage liver disease often have an insidious onset; initially there are mild changes in the ability to concentrate and complete complex tasks. As the hepatic encephalopathy progresses, mental status changes become more obvious and are classified in stages I to IV, depending on the severity of neurologic involvement (Table 12.1).

Stage I is characterized by impaired attention, depression, and some personality changes; neurologic signs include tremor and incoordination. Stage II displays drowsiness, sleep disorders, changes in behavior, and poor short-term memory; accompanying signs are asterixis (flapping tremor; see Fig. 12.1), ataxia, and slurred speech. The motor apraxia in stage II can be best observed by keeping a record of the client's handwriting and drawings of simple shapes such as a circle, square, triangle, and rectangle. Progressive deterioration is apparent in these handwriting samples.

Confusion and somnolence are indicative of stage III encephalopathy associated with nystagmus, clonus, muscular rigidity, and hypoactive reflexes. Stage IV reflects severe encephalopathy; the person is in a comatose state and exhibits abnormal reflexes, such the *oculocephalic ("doll's eye") reflex; decerebrate posturing* may be present; pupils may be dilated; and there is no

TABLE 12.1	**Stages of Hepatic Encephalopathy**		
Stage I (Prodromal)	**Stage II (Impending)**	**Stage III (Arousal)**	**Stage IV (Comatose)**
Slight personality changes	Tremor progresses to asterixis	Hyperventilation	No asterixis
Slight tremor	Resistance to passive movement	Marked confusion	Positive Babinski's reflex
Bilateral numbness or tingling	Myoclonus	Incoherent speech	Oculocephalic (doll's eye) reflex
Muscular incoordination	Lethargy	Asterixis (liver flap)	Decerebrate posturing
Apraxia	Unusual behavior (abusive, violent, and noisy)	Muscle rigidity	Dilated pupils
	Apraxia	Hyporeactive deep tendon reflexes	Lack of response to stimuli
	Ataxia	Sleeps most of the time	
	Sleep disorders		
	Slow or slurred speech		

response to stimuli. There are characteristic electroencephalogram findings at each stage.

The cause of hepatic encephalopathy has not been completely elucidated, although several key elements are known. Ammonia is created by bacteria in the colon from the metabolism of protein and urea. The liver is typically able to metabolize ammonia, but with liver disease and shunting of blood away from the liver (particularly to the brain), ammonia levels rise. In the brain, ammonia appears to directly alter the function and signaling of nerve cells.

Although serum ammonia levels are used to monitor therapy, the level does not correspond well with the severity of encephalopathy, reinforcing the fact that other mechanisms are involved in the development of encephalopathy.

The development of hepatic encephalopathy warrants a careful evaluation and correction of the cause. Serious and common causes include bleeding, infection (particularly spontaneous bacterial peritonitis [SBP]), hypovolemia, or electrolyte abnormalities (hypokalemia). Other common factors that may precipitate or severely aggravate hepatic encephalopathy include constipation, diuretics, increased dietary protein, and central nervous system–depressant drugs, such as alcohol, benzodiazepines (e.g., Librium, Valium, Dalmane, and Tranxene), and opiates.

Because protein can precipitate or worsen encephalopathy, many of the symptoms can be improved by eliminating or reducing sources of protein (i.e., stopping any internal bleeding and restricting dietary protein to 60 g/day). Health care providers must also be aware of any subtle changes in mental status, because the ability to drive is often impaired. Driving must be assessed on a case-by-case basis.

Ammonia-lowering therapy in suspected encephalopathy cases can be beneficial even when the ammonia level is normal, because the production is tied to other toxins.

Reversal of hepatic encephalopathy is typically successful when a source is identified, corrected, and treated appropriately. However, without intervention, mortality is high, as the person's condition progresses into coma. As with most complications of end-stage liver disease, liver transplantation provides the best long-term treatment.

12.5 Special Implications for the PTA: **Hepatic Encephalopathy** The inpatient or homebound client with hepatic encephalopathy has difficulty ambulating and is extremely unsteady. Protective measures must be taken against falls. The home health PTA must be alert for any report of GI bleeding that will result in protein accumulation in the GI tract, exacerbating this condition (e.g., blood in stools or black or tarry stools). The client should be following a low-protein diet.

Skin breakdown in a client who is malnourished from liver disease and is immobile, jaundiced, and edematous can occur in less than 24 hours. Careful attention to skin care, passive exercise, and frequent changes in position are required.

Rest between activities is advocated, and strenuous exercise is to be avoided. The PTA should watch for (and immediately report) signs of anemia (e.g., reduced hemoglobin, weakness, dyspnea on exertion, easy fatigability, skin pallor, or tachycardia).

Ascites

Ascites is the abnormal accumulation of fluid within the peritoneal cavity. It is most often caused by cirrhosis (85% of cases), but other diseases associated with ascites include heart failure, abdominal malignancies, nephrotic syndrome, infection, and malnutrition.

The mechanism for the accumulation of fluid in the case of cirrhosis is principally a result of portal hypertension. High pressure in the vessels attempting to pass blood through the cirrhotic liver leads to vasodilatation of the splanchnic vessels (vessels to the gut or viscera), which in turn decreases the filling of the vessels going to the kidney.

Ascites becomes clinically detectable when more than 500 mL has accumulated, causing weight gain, abdominal distention, increased abdominal girth, and, eventually, peripheral edema (Fig. 12.4). Dyspnea with increased respiratory rate occurs when the fluid displaces the diaphragm.

Diagnosis of ascites is usually based on clinical manifestations in the presence of liver disease. *Paracentesis* is used as the initial test in people with new-onset ascites to determine the cause. Fluid is sent to the laboratory for chemical and microscopic evaluation. Abdominal ultrasonography can aid in locating pockets of ascitic fluid.

In people with established cirrhosis, paracentesis can be diagnostic and therapeutic. Large-volume paracentesis with administration of albumin is the treatment of choice for tense ascites (i.e., when a person is no longer able to breathe or eat comfortably), followed by the use of diuretics to reduce reaccumulation of fluid.

Treatment of mild to moderate ascites includes sodium restriction accompanied by diuretic use.[68]

Prophylactic antibiotics may be used in some clients with a history of SBP and are often administered to people with a GI

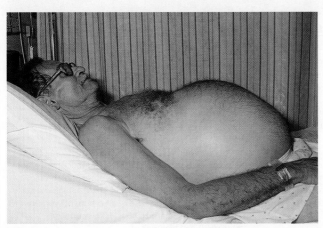

FIG. 12.4 Ascites in an individual with cirrhosis. Distended abdomen, dilated upper abdominal veins, and inverted umbilicus are classic manifestations. Peripheral edema associated with developing ascites may be observed first by the therapist. (From Swartz MH: Textbook of physical diagnosis, ed 7, Philadelphia, 2014, Saunders.)

bleed.[78] The development of refractory ascites is associated with a poor prognosis, with a 12-month survival of 25%. Liver transplantation provides the best treatment option but is not always readily available.

Complications include hepatorenal syndrome (discussed later) and SBP. The microbial source of SBP (infection of the ascitic fluid) is the gut in which organisms (typically *Escherichia coli*, streptococci [mostly pneumococci], and *Klebsiella*) are translocated into lymph nodes and then into the ascitic fluid. Bacterial peritonitis is symptomatic in 87% of cases (fever, chills, abdominal pain, mental status changes, and tenderness), but symptoms can often be subtle. Without diagnosis by paracentesis and antibiotic treatment, the infection can be fatal.

12.6 Special Implications for the PTA: Ascites Most people with ascites are more comfortable in a high Fowler's position (head of the bed raised 18 to 20 inches above level with the knees elevated). Breathing techniques are important to maintain adequate respiratory function and to prevent the development of atelectasis or pneumonia. The homebound person who has ascites should be monitored for the possible development of bacterial peritonitis. Onset of fever, chills, abdominal pain, and tenderness should be reported to the physician.

The edema associated with ascites may mask muscle wasting that occurs when the body does not have an adequate intake of protein to maintain structure and facilitate wound healing. The client must be encouraged to change position to maintain integrity of the skin and promote circulation. Small pillows or folded towels can be used to support the rib cage and the bulging flank while the client is lying on his or her side.

The abdominal distention associated with ascites may develop very slowly over a number of weeks or months and may be accompanied by bilateral edema of the feet and ankles. The client may be unable to put on a pair of shoes, preferring to leave the shoes unlaced or to wear slippers. In a home health, inpatient hospital, or nursing home setting, this change in dress may not be as

---

noticeable as it would be in a private practice or outpatient clinic. It is always important to remain alert to these potential signs of fluid retention and to ask about any changes in health status or weight gain.

Fluid intake and output are usually carefully measured and restricted, so in any setting the PTA is encouraged to know the individual's limits and to participate in reporting measurements as well. This is especially important because clients frequently ask the PTA for fluids in response to perceived exertion or increased exertion after exercise or ambulation. The person who is noncompliant or in denial requests fluids because of the false belief that fluids provided but not recorded do not count. For the homebound client who is receiving diuretics, the bedroom should be close to the bathroom.

Hepatorenal Syndrome

Hepatorenal syndrome is characterized by renal dysfunction in people with portal hypertension and advanced liver failure. About 7% to 15% of people with end-stage cirrhosis will develop this syndrome, which portends a poor prognosis. This leads to constriction of the vessels in the limbs and to the brain, as well as the kidneys. The total effect is that the vasoconstrictors have a greater effect than the vasodilators, and kidney dysfunction develops.[21]

Common illnesses found in people with cirrhosis that can cause renal insufficiency include infection (particularly SBP), shock, medications, bleeding, and fluid losses. Renal obstruction should be ruled out by ultrasonography.

Hepatorenal syndrome is classified into two types. Type 1 is rapid both in onset and in progression to renal failure and carries a poor short-term prognosis. Type 2 is more insidious in onset with progression over months; ascites is often the key feature of this type. Because of the intense vasoconstriction, treatment centers around the use of vasodilators and albumin, which aid in increasing blood flow to the kidneys. Transjugular intrahepatic portosystemic shunts may also be of benefit.[5]

Optimal treatment consists of liver transplantation, which has a 5-year posttransplant survival rate of 70%. Although many people will improve with medical treatment, liver transplantation should be pursued because of poor long-term prognosis. Hemodialysis may be required to bridge treatment until a transplant is available.

Hepatitis

Hepatitis is an acute or chronic inflammation of the liver caused by a virus, a chemical, a drug reaction, or alcohol abuse. Classifications of hepatitis are listed in Table 12.2.

Viral causes of hepatitis include Epstein-Barr virus (mononucleosis), herpes simplex virus types I and II, varicella-zoster virus, measles, or cytomegalovirus (CMV). Hepatitis from any cause produces very similar symptoms and usually requires a careful client history to establish the diagnosis.

People with mild to moderate acute hepatitis rarely require hospitalization. The emphasis is on preventing the spread of infectious agents and avoiding further liver damage when the underlying cause is drug-induced or toxic hepatitis. Persons with fulminant hepatitis (which has a severe, sudden intensity and is sometimes fatal) require special management because of the rapid progression of the disease and the potential need for urgent liver transplantation.

TABLE 12.2   Types of Viral Hepatitis

	Hepatitis A	Hepatitis B	Hepatitis C	Hepatitis D	Hepatitis E
Incidence	Less than 4500 cases reported to CDC in 2005 Reduced incidence with introduction of hepatitis vaccine A (approximately 42,000 new cases occurred)	Reduced incidence; 51,000 new acute cases in the United States (2005); 1.5 million carriers	Transfusion-related cases decreasing with blood screening but increased incidence expected related to risk behaviors in the 1960s and 1970s; 3.2 million chronically infected	Uncommon in United States; most common in drug addicts, sexually active young adults, individuals receiving multiple transfusions	Epidemic in developing countries; rare in United States; risk greatest to persons traveling to endemic regions
Morbidity	Results in acute infection only; does not progress to chronic hepatitis or cirrhosis; small risk of fulminant hepatitis; lifetime immunity	Most common cause of chronic hepatitis and liver cancer; second major cause of cirrhosis in the United States after alcohol abuse	Accounts for 60%-70% of all chronic hepatitis; 30% of chronic cases progress to cirrhosis; associated with liver cancer	Coinfection with HBV and HDV leads to more severe acute disease (fulminant hepatitis 2%-20%) but low risk of chronic disease Superinfection (acquire HDV after HBV) has high risk of severe chronic disease (70%-80%)	Causes acute self-limiting infection; does not progress to chronic hepatitis; high mortality in pregnant women, 10% mortality
Transmission	Fecal–oral route; spread by feces, saliva, and contaminated food and water	Parenteral Sexual contact Vertical Unidentified exposure	Parenteral Unidentified exposure	Parenteral Sexual contact (same as HBV) Perinatal rare, requires coinfection with HBV to reproduce	Same as HAV; fecal–oral (contamination of water)
Treatment	Immune globulin before or within 2 weeks of exposure; supportive; most people recover within 4-8 weeks	α-Interferon and antiviral agents for chronic HBV; HBIG for exposed, unvaccinated persons	Combination therapy (interferon, ribavirin) in select cases	Interferon alfa-2b can inhibit HDV replication but effect ends when therapy ends	None; preventive measures
Diagnosis	Blood test to identify antibody; IgM; anti-HAV	Blood tests to identify antigen and antibodies; HBsAg; HBeAg; HBcAg	Blood test to identify antibody; does not distinguish between current and past infection; anti-HCV Limited use of nucleic acid test (polymerase chain reaction)	Blood test to detect antigen and antibody; anti-HDV	Blood test to detect anti-HEV IgM antibodies
Vaccine	Vaccine available; combined HAV and HBV vaccine available (Twinrix)	Vaccines available	None available	Immunization against hepatitis B can prevent hepatitis D infection	Recombinant vaccine IgM; antibodies under investigation

CDC, Centers for Disease Control and Prevention; *HAV,* hepatitis A virus; *HBcAg,* hepatitis B core antigen; *HBeAg,* hepatitis B antigen; *HBIG,* hepatitis B immune globulin; *HBsAg,* hepatitis B surface antigen; *HBV,* hepatitis B virus; *HCV,* hepatitis C virus; *HDV,* hepatitis D virus; *HEV,* hepatitis E virus; *IgM,* immunoglobulin M.
Data from Centers for Disease Control and Prevention (CDC): National Center for Infectious Diseases (online). www.cdc.gov/hepatitis. Accessed August 25, 2016.

Chronic Hepatitis

Chronic hepatitis comprises several diseases that are grouped together because they have common clinical manifestations. The disease is defined as chronic with evidence of ongoing injury for 6 months or more.

Chronic hepatitis is described in diagnostic terms that include the cause, degree of active inflammation and injury (i.e., grade: mild, moderate, severe, or I, II, III), and the degree of scarring or how advanced the process is (i.e., stage: I, II, or III; IV represents cirrhosis). Stages of disease are usually irreversible.

Chronic hepatitis has multiple causes, including viruses, medications, metabolic abnormalities, and autoimmune disorders. Despite extensive testing, some cases cannot be attributed to any known cause and are probably the result of as yet unidentified viruses. Hepatitis B virus (HBV), with or without hepatitis D virus (HDV); HCV; and hepatitis G virus (HGV) can progress to chronic hepatitis.

Most people with chronic hepatitis are asymptomatic, and when symptoms occur, these are nonspecific and mild, with fatigue, malaise, loss of appetite, polyarthralgias, and intermittent right upper quadrant discomfort. Some people report sleep disturbances or difficulty in concentrating. Symptoms of advanced disease or an acute exacerbation include nausea, poor appetite, weight loss, muscle weakness, itching, dark urine, and jaundice. Once cirrhosis is present, weakness, weight loss, abdominal swelling, edema, easy bruising, muscle wasting and weakness, GI bleeding, and hepatic encephalopathy with mental confusion may arise.

The diagnosis of chronic viral hepatitis is based on serologic testing. The diagnosis can usually be made from clinical features and blood test results alone.

Liver biopsy is important to assess the severity of underlying liver disease (grade and stage) and to determine the need for antiviral treatment. The treatment for chronic viral hepatitis has improved substantially in the last decade and depends on the underlying cause and grade and stage of disease.

The prognosis in chronic hepatitis is variable depending on the development of cirrhosis and other complications such as hepatocellular carcinoma (HCC). Male gender, moderate to heavy alcohol consumption, and other coexistent liver disorders are the factors that increase the rate of progression to cirrhosis; HCV is the major risk factor of development of liver cancer. The 5-year survival rate for compensated cirrhosis is greater than 90%, but the prognosis and survival rate for decompensation (characterized by development of variceal bleeding, ascites, and hepatic encephalopathy) are extremely poor. Progression of chronic hepatitis to decompensated cirrhosis is an indication for liver transplantation.

Fulminant Hepatitis

Fulminant hepatitis is the generic term for any rapidly progressing form of liver inflammation that results in hepatic encephalopathy (confusion, stupor, and coma) within a few weeks of developing infection. This type of hepatitis is rare, occurring in less than 1% of persons with acute viral hepatitis, but it can be fatal. The most common causes are acetaminophen hepatotoxicity (20% to 25% of all cases of fulminant hepatitis),[37] idiosyncratic drug reaction, hepatitis A virus (HAV) and HBV, and hepatic ischemia. Encephalopathy may progress to cerebral edema, which is the most common cause of death.

Diagnosis is made in the presence of a combination of hepatic encephalopathy, acute liver disease (elevated serum bilirubin and transaminase levels), and liver failure. Treatment is supportive because the underlying etiologic factors of liver failure are rarely treatable short of liver transplantation.

Prognosis is determined in part by the cause of the condition. If the prognosis is deemed poor and no contraindications to transplantation are present, the person should be immediately considered for transplantation. Short-term prognosis without liver transplantation is very poor, and the mortality rate is high (80%). Despite the poor prognosis, complete recovery can occur as a result of liver cell regeneration with recovery of liver function. The development of artificial liver support devices has not been shown to improve outcome, and they are not widely available.

Viral Hepatitis

Overview. Each of the recognized hepatitis viruses belongs to a different virus family, and each has a unique epidemiology.[9] Characteristics of these strains of viruses are presented in Table 12.2. The identification of the specific virus is made difficult by the fact that a long incubation period often occurs between acquisition of the infection and development of the first symptoms. Not all causative agents have been identified, and because hepatitis can be easily spread before symptoms appear, morbidity is high in terms of loss of time from school or work. More than half and possibly as many as 90% of all cases go unreported because symptoms are mild or even subclinical.

The virus that causes hepatitis A, formerly known as *infectious hepatitis,* is transmitted by the oral–fecal route. This route of transmission is primarily from poor or improper handwashing and personal hygiene, particularly after using the bathroom and then handling food for public consumption. Transmission also may occur through the shared used of oral utensils such as straws, silverware, and toothbrushes.[16] The illness can last from 4 to 8 weeks; it generally lasts longer and is more severe in persons older than 50 or in people with chronic, underlying liver disease.[18]

HBV is transmitted percutaneously (i.e., via puncture of the skin) or through mucosal contact. It is highly infectious: 100 times more infectious than HIV and 10 times more infectious than HCV. Because HBV can be transmitted through heterosexual or homosexual intercourse, it is considered a sexually transmitted disease. The average incubation period is 90 days (with a range of 60 to 150 days), with symptoms occurring around 60 days.[46]

HCV is now most commonly associated with injection drug use. As with HAV, the period of infectivity begins before the onset of symptoms, and the person may become a lifetime carrier of this virus. Clinically, HCV is very similar to HBV and often is asymptomatic; the acute HCV infection is usually mild. Chronic HCV varies greatly in its course and outcome from asymptomatic with normal liver function to a mild degree of liver injury and overall good prognosis to severe symptomatic HCV with complications of cirrhosis and end-stage liver disease.

HDV, or delta virus, manifests as a coinfection or superinfection of HBV. Only individuals with HBV are at risk for hepatitis D. Risk factors and transmission mode are the same as for HBV; parenteral drug users have a high incidence of HDV. The symptoms of HDV are similar to those of HBV except that clients are more likely to have fulminant hepatitis and to develop chronic active hepatitis and cirrhosis.

Hepatitis E virus (HEV) is transmitted by contaminated water via the oral-fecal route and clinically resembles HAV. It is believed to be nonfatal, although it has been clearly associated with liver damage. A 20% to 25% mortality rate exists in pregnant women from fulminant hepatitis.[2] This virus tends to occur in poor socioeconomic conditions, primarily occurs in developing countries (contaminated waste water and sewage), and is rare in the United States. No specific treatment is available for HEV, but ensuring clean drinking water remains the best preventive strategy.

HGV is most prevalent in African countries. It is parenterally transmitted, although vertical and sexual transmissions are well documented. *Parenteral* refers to transmission in some other mode than via the alimentary canal (enteric system), such as by subcutaneous, intramuscular, intraorbital, intracapsular, intraspinal, intrasternal, or intravenous injection. It may cause acute or chronic infection, but little information about this viral cause of hepatitis is known.[72]

Incidence and risk factors. Each year, approximately 500,000 Americans are infected with some form of hepatitis virus; annually about 15,000 persons die of its complications. Hepatitis A is the predominant type of hepatitis, comprising 40% to 60% of acute viral hepatitis cases.

Because HAV is transmitted via the fecal–oral route, one risk factor for acquiring the virus is working at a daycare center; children who attend daycare centers are also at higher risk. Because of the HAV vaccine the infection rate in this population has improved; this may change the prevalence of the disease, with more cases being reported in adults (adults display a more severe clinical course than children).[15] Another risk factor for HAV is visiting or living in an underdeveloped country in which the rate is high.

Prevalence of HBV infection has significantly decreased in most ethnic populations except blacks, who continue to demonstrate an elevated prevalence of three times that of other racial or ethnic populations.[46] Common risk factors for HBV infection include sexual relations, injection drug use, sharing of needles, needlesticks, and perinatal (vertical) transmission from mother to child. Injection drug use and intimate contact with another person with HBV are the two most frequent sources of HBV in the United States. Transfusion-related hepatitis B is rare, because the initiation of donor screening for HBV and the HBV vaccine have improved the incidence in dialysis clients and workers.

Men traditionally were more likely to contract HCV than women, but the incidence was fairly equal among various ethnic groups and populations. In the past, HCV infection was commonly acquired through blood transfusion. Currently, because of donor screening, the incidence of HCV from transfusion is uncommon. The number of people with chronic HCV is significant: about 3.2 to 4 million people are chronically infected with HCV. Most of these cases were acquired during the 1970s and 1980s when the rates were the highest.

Risk factors for HCV are similar to those for HBV. Currently, 68% of the new cases of HCV occur among injection drug users sharing needles. See Table 12.3 for other risk factors.

The number of people who develop HBV and HCV infection from dialysis or work-related exposure is low. People undergoing chronic hemodialysis are at risk for HBV and HCV infection because the process of hemodialysis requires vascular access for prolonged periods. Furthermore, individuals receiving hemodialysis are immunosuppressed, which increases their susceptibility to infection, and they require frequent hospitalizations and surgery, which increases their opportunities for exposure to nosocomial infections.[52]

HBV is relatively stable in the environment and remains viable for at least 7 days on environmental surfaces at room temperature. Blood-contaminated surfaces that are not routinely cleaned and disinfected represent a reservoir for HBV transmission.

HEV is most common in developing countries. On the basis of serologic tests, an estimated one-third of the world's population has been infected with HEV. In India the lifetime prevalence is more than 60%.[73]

Pathogenesis. The viruses associated with hepatitis are not typically cytopathic (destroy cells), yet the body's reaction to the virus often creates significant inflammation; the intensity of the disease depends on the degree of immune response. Antibodies prevent spread of virus and provide immunity against further infection. In adults with intact immunity, this response is able to clear the virus. However, in infants, young children, and the immunosuppressed, the immune system is unable to mount an adequate defense and the virus continues to replicate and reside in the liver, leading to a chronic state.

Clinical manifestations. Most cases of acute viral hepatitis are asymptomatic and never reported. Classic symptoms of acute hepatitis are often the same, regardless of the responsible virus. Most individuals present with malaise, fatigue, mild fever, nausea, vomiting, anorexia, right upper quadrant discomfort, and occasionally diarrhea. Jaundice, dark urine, and clay-colored stools may also be observed. Most people who acquire HCV become chronic carriers of the disease (60% to 85%). Some people may develop extrahepatic manifestations. Rheumatologic and skin manifestations are the most common.

TABLE 12.3   Risk Factors for Hepatitis

Hepatitis A	Hepatitis B	Hepatitis C	Hepatitis D	Hepatitis E
Household contacts or sexual contacts of infected persons	Injection drug use	Current or previously used injected illegal drugs (even if only one or two times years ago); intranasal cocaine use with shared equipment	Same as B	Same as A
Unprotected homosexual or bisexual activity	Unprotected homosexual or bisexual activity; persons with multiple sex partners or diagnosis of sexually transmitted disease			
Injection or noninjection illegal drug use (regional outbreaks reported)	Incarceration in correctional facilities—adults and youth (drug use and unsafe sexual practices)	Received blood transfusion or organ transplant before July 1992 or blood clotting products made before 1987		
Living in areas with increased rates of HAV infection (children at greatest risk)	Certain ethnic groups and adoptive families with adoptees from these areas: Asia, South America, South Africa, Mexico, Eastern and Mediterranean Europe			
Travel in areas in which HAV is epidemic	Travel to high risk areas			
Tattoo inscription or removal; body or ear piercing with shared or unsterile needles	Occupational risk[a]: morticians, dental workers, emergency medical technicians, firefighters, health care workers in contact with body fluid or blood	Tattooing and body piercing as a risk factor for HCV infection has not been completely evaluated in the United States but does not appear likely		
	Liver transplant recipient	Evidence of liver disease, liver transplant recipient		
	Infants born to mothers with HBV infection	Infants born to HCV-infected mothers (low risk; 5%)		
	Immunocompromised individuals; receiving or administering chronic kidney dialysis (clients and staff)	Long-term kidney dialysis (clients and staff)		
Blood clotting factor disorder (no new cases from 1998–2002)	Multiple blood products or blood transfusions before July 1992			

[a]HBV can also survive in dried blood at least 1 week.
HAV, Hepatitis A virus; *HBV,* hepatitis B virus; *HCV,* hepatitis C virus.
Data from Centers for Disease Control and Prevention (CDC): National Center for Infectious Diseases. http://www.cdc.gov/hepatitis. Accessed August 25, 2016.

Medical Management

Prevention

Prevention takes place at three levels: primary, secondary, and tertiary.

Primary prevention involves primary immunization (HAV, HBV, and HEV), education regarding food preparation and proper handwashing, avoiding needle punctures by contaminated needles (or other similar infective material), and practicing protective sex or avoiding sexual contact during the period of hepatitis B surface antigen (HBsAg) positivity.

Secondary prevention involves passive immunization after exposure to HAV or HBV, travel precautions when visiting areas in which hepatitis is endemic (e.g., avoid drinking unbottled water or beverages served with ice; avoid eating foods rinsed in contaminated water, such as fruits and vegetables; and avoid eating shellfish).

Tertiary prevention involves education of infected persons about preventing possible infectivity to others and self-care during active infection (e.g., avoid strenuous activity and ingestion of hepatotoxins, such as alcohol and acetaminophen; some advocate alternative treatment such as herbs, acupuncture, and dietary measures).

Diagnosis

History, clinical examination, and serologic and molecular testing help provide an accurate diagnosis (see Table 12.2). A liver biopsy provides information about the severity of disease and establishes grading and degree of fibrosis but is necessary only in the case of chronic hepatitis.

Treatment

Treatment options have expanded, and prevention methods are available for two of the six viruses, although no cure is available for the viruses that are responsible for chronic liver disease (HBV, HDV, and HGV). The development of new antiviral agents that inhibit steps in the viral replication process is under investigation.[54] Any hepatic irritants, such as alcohol, medications, or chemicals (e.g., occupational exposure to carbon tetrachloride), must be avoided in all types of hepatitis. Surveillance by ultrasonography every 6 to 12 months is recommended to detect HCC. Administration of HAV and HBV vaccine is recommended for anyone with chronic HCV because of the potential for increased severity of acute hepatitis superimposed on existing liver disease.[74]

Prognosis

Prognosis varies with each type. A substantial proportion of HBV morbidity and mortality that occurs in the health care setting can be prevented by vaccinating health care workers against HBV. In addition, health care workers must practice infection control measures. Other prophylactic strategies are based on avoidance of high-risk behavior and use of immunoglobulin.

against HBV. All PTAs should follow standard precautions at all times to protect themselves and must wear personal protective equipment whenever appropriate. Such gear should never be worn in the car or laundered at home to avoid contamination of those sites.

The frequency of arthralgia as a symptom associated with hepatitis increases with age. Joint pains affected only 18% of children, compared with 45% of adults older than 30 years.

No known studies have been published regarding the benefit of physical therapy in providing symptomatic joint relief until these symptoms resolve as the person recovers from the underlying pathology. Overall, in the recovery process, adequate rest to conserve energy is important. The affected individual is encouraged to gradually return to levels of activity before illness. Fatigue associated with hepatitis may interfere with activities of daily living and may persist even after the jaundice resolves. A careful balance of activity is important to avoid weakness secondary to prolonged bed rest; a reasonable activity level is more conducive to recovery than is enforced bed rest. Whenever possible, rehabilitation intervention or increased activity should not be scheduled right after meals.

Watch for signs of fluid shift, such as weight gain and orthostasis; dehydration; pneumonia; vascular problems; and pressure ulcers and any signs of recurrence. After the diagnosis of viral hepatitis has been established, the affected individual should have regular medical checkups for at least 1 year and should avoid using any alcohol or over-the-counter (OTC) drugs during this period.

α-Interferon (antiviral used in the treatment of some hepatitis) has bone marrow suppressive effects necessitating careful monitoring of platelet or neutrophil count. Other side effects of combination therapy may include increased fatigue, increased muscle pain and potential inflammatory myopathy, headaches, local skin irritation (site of injection), irritability and depression, hair loss, itching, sinusitis, and cough. These symptoms usually subside in the first few weeks of treatment; prolonged or intolerable side effects must be reported to the physician.

Hepatitis B and the Athlete

For most of the infections considered, the athlete is more at risk during activities off the playing field than while competing. Inclusion of immunizations against measles and HBV as a prerequisite to participation would eliminate these two diseases from the list of dangers to athletes (and all individuals). Although the risk of blood-borne pathogen infection during sports is exceedingly small, good hygiene practices concerning blood are still important. The American Academy of Pediatrics has made recommendations to minimize the risk of blood-borne pathogen transmission in the context of athletic events and has issued safety precautions. The PTA in this type of setting is encouraged to review these guidelines.[3]

The presence of HBV infection does not contraindicate participation in sports or athletic activities; decisions regarding play are made according to clinical signs and symptoms such as fatigue, fever, or organomegaly. Chronic HBV infection with evidence of organ impairment necessitates reduction in intensity and duration of activity.

12.7 Special Implications for the PTA: Viral Hepatitis Any direct contact with blood or body fluids of clients with HBV or HCV infection requires the administration of immunoglobulin (Ig), a preparation of antibodies, in the early incubation period. PTAs at risk for contact with HBV because of their close contact with the blood or body fluids of carriers should receive active immunization

---

Drug-Related Hepatotoxicity
Overview and Incidence

Injury to the liver can be caused by many drugs or toxins. More than 600 medicinal agents, chemicals, and herbal remedies are recognized as producing hepatic injury.[37]

Although OTC and prescription medications are often thought to be the only agents to cause liver injury, complementary or alternative medications are also known to be hepatotoxic.[75]

Drugs are currently the most common cause of acute liver failure.[33,56] Hepatotoxicity has also been the principal reason for removing several new drugs from the market.[24]

Etiologic and Risk Factors

A host of factors may enhance susceptibility to drug-induced liver disease, including age (adults more so than children), gender (women have a higher risk than men), obesity, malnutrition, pregnancy, concurrent medication use, history of drug reactions, and genetic variability (probably the most important factor). Preexisting liver diseases and comorbidities appear to alter the rate of recovery rather than affect the risk of developing hepatotoxicity.[69] Alcohol use and fasting may increase the likelihood of acetaminophen-related hepatotoxicity.[77]

Pathogenesis

Drugs and toxins can result in liver injury via numerous mechanisms. The pattern of injury is often drug dependent. Patterns of liver injury include hepatocellular, cholestatic, mixed, hypersensitivity (or immunologic), and mitochondrial injury. Hepatocellular injury is defined by inflammation of the hepatocytes, breakup of the hepatic lobule (composed of the central vein, portal vein, hepatic artery, bile duct, and hepatic cords), and hepatocellular necrosis. Mitochondrial injury is demonstrated by small droplets of fat (or microvesicular steatosis) within the hepatocyte. Valproic acid has been known to cause this type of cellular change.

Clinical Manifestations

The manifestations of drug-related liver disease can range from mild symptoms to fulminant liver failure. Vague symptoms, including fatigue, nausea, and right upper quadrant pain or discomfort, may be the first indications of hepatotoxicity. Other symptoms associated with liver injury are jaundice, pruritus, and dark urine. Fever and rash are often present with a hypersensitivity reaction. As discussed, drugs often cause a specific pattern of injury. The most readily identifiable patterns are hepatocellular and cholestatic.

Hepatocellular liver disease frequently manifests with abdominal discomfort or pain, fatigue, and jaundice; the clinical course is acute and can be severe. Cholestatic liver disease manifests clinically by jaundice and pruritus. In contrast to the hepatocellular pattern, cholestatic disease is often less acutely serious, but healing may be prolonged and chronic, taking weeks to months.

> **12.8 Special Implications for the PTA: Drug-Related Hepatotoxicity** PTAs should be alert to the possibility of drug toxicity or drug reactions in clients taking multiple medications or reactions in people who are combining prescription medications or OTC medications with complementary or alternative medications. Many people do not consider OTC drugs as medications and may take the same drug with different names or combine OTC drugs with prescription medications. People with memory loss or short-term memory deficits may take multiple doses in a short amount of time because they cannot remember when or whether they took their medication. Other guiding principles for the recovery process are as mentioned for viral hepatitis.

Autoimmune Hepatitis
Overview and Incidence

Autoimmune hepatitis is a chronic progressive, inflammatory disorder of the liver of unknown cause. It occurs in adults and children and is characterized by the presence of abnormal liver histology, autoantibodies, elevated levels of serum immunoglobulins, and frequent association with other autoimmune diseases.

Etiologic Factors and Pathogenesis

The cause and pathogenesis of autoimmune hepatitis are not known. The disease appears to occur among genetically predisposed individuals.

Purported triggering agents include viruses (such as measles virus, hepatitis viruses, CMV, and Epstein-Barr virus) and drugs. It is uncertain if drugs actually trigger autoimmune hepatitis or merely cause a drug-mediated hepatitis with features similar to autoimmune hepatitis. Most people with autoimmune hepatitis, however, have no identifiable trigger.

Clinical Manifestations

Autoimmune hepatitis is represented by a wide spectrum of clinical manifestations. Autoimmune hepatitis is usually progressive and chronic, although a minority of cases are characterized by a fluctuating course.

The most common presenting symptoms are fatigue (85%), jaundice (46%), anorexia (30%), myalgias (30%), and diarrhea (28%). The presence of another autoimmune disorder, such as thyroiditis, ulcerative colitis, type 1 diabetes, rheumatoid arthritis, and celiac disease,[1] is seen in one-third of affected individuals. Physical examination findings may be normal, but 78% of clients have hepatomegaly. Individuals with fulminant hepatitis often have profound jaundice.

Complications of autoimmune hepatitis are similar to those of other chronic liver diseases, particularly the development of cirrhosis.

> **12.9 Special Implications for the PTA: Autoimmune Hepatitis** Management of a client who has an autoimmune disease with liver involvement is a challenge. Energy conservation and maintaining quiet body functions during active liver disease must be balanced by activities to prevent musculoskeletal deconditioning with accompanying loss of strength, flexibility, and/or mobility.

Alcohol-Related Liver Disease
Overview, Incidence, and Risk Factors

Although over two-thirds of Americans drink alcohol, only a minority develop problems leading to chronic alcohol abuse and severe liver disease. Yet alcohol problems result in significant morbidity and mortality; over 40% of deaths from cirrhosis are alcohol related and 30% of HCC cases are a result of alcohol-related liver disease.

More men than women acquire liver disease, but women develop the disease after a shorter exposure to alcohol and while consuming lower quantities of alcohol compared with men. In men, six to eight alcohol-containing beverages daily (60 to 80 g/day) over a 5-year period can lead to liver disease, whereas only three to four drinks per day are needed to cause the same effect in women.

Women are more vulnerable to the effects of alcohol than men. Women produce substantially less of the gastric enzyme alcohol *dehydrogenase,* which breaks down ethanol in the stomach. As a result, women absorb 75% more alcohol into the bloodstream. About 90% of heavy drinkers develop fat accumulation in the liver (the first sign of alcohol abuse). Research suggests that genetics may play an important role in preventing liver damage despite chronic alcohol exposure.

Alcohol-related liver disease encompasses alcoholic hepatitis and alcoholic cirrhosis. Alcoholic hepatitis occurs in only 10% to 35% of heavy drinkers and is the precursor for the development of alcoholic cirrhosis. People with alcoholic hepatitis are nine times more likely than people with fatty liver infiltration to develop cirrhosis.[39]

Some cofactors that may predispose to cirrhosis include coexisting HCV, smoking, and obesity. Although much progress has been made in understanding potential causes, many questions remain such as determining which factors lead to severe liver damage and the mechanisms that protect other heavy drinkers.

Pathogenesis

The initial physiologic change observed in the liver with alcohol exposure is the accumulation of fat, which is reversible with abstinence. In some people, with continued exposure to alcohol, there is a progression of damage to the liver consisting of inflammation, necrosis of individual cells, and early fibrosis, termed *alcoholic hepatitis*. With continued heavy drinking, micronodular fibrosis (small bands of fibers) can develop and eventually progress to large bands of fibrosis, creating large nodules of fibrotic liver tissue (macronodular cirrhosis). Once cirrhosis has developed, HCC may result. Alcohol can also alter the balance between prooxidants and antioxidants, causing oxidative stress and liver injury.

Clinical Manifestations

The initial histologic change noted in heavy drinkers is fatty liver infiltrate. This is often asymptomatic and detected only on laboratory evaluation. Even clients with alcoholic hepatitis and/or cirrhosis may be asymptomatic. Others may experience nausea, vomiting, abdominal pain, jaundice, anorexia, fever, and weight loss.

The most common sign in people with fatty liver or alcoholic hepatitis is hepatomegaly; 60% of all people with alcohol-related liver disease exhibit jaundice and ascites (typically in clients with severe disease). Splenomegaly is more common as the disease worsens, and hepatic encephalopathy can exist in varying degrees, ranging from mild cognitive impairment to coma. Clients with alcoholic hepatitis or cirrhosis often display spider angiomata, liver tenderness, and edema.[48]

Medical Management

Diagnosis

The diagnosis of alcoholic hepatitis is made using the appropriate history of heavy drinking, consistent laboratory values, and no evidence of other diseases that could cause liver injury. Because alcohol can worsen preexisting diseases, such as viral hepatitis, the diagnosis of alcohol-related liver disease should not be made without a thorough evaluation.

A history of heavy drinking may not be present because of client denial. Only 50% of clients who abuse alcohol are identified by their physician. Often, despite advanced disease, laboratory levels may be only mildly elevated. Because the diagnosis of alcohol-related liver disease can competently be made using history, physical examination findings, and laboratory information, liver biopsy is rarely needed.

Treatment and Prognosis

Treatment of alcoholic hepatitis centers on cessation of alcohol use, nutritional support and education, and prevention of the complications of end-stage disease. Corticosteroids can be used for severe cases of alcoholic hepatitis, whereas *S*-adenosylmethionine, an antioxidant, may reduce mortality and decrease the need for liver transplantation.[47]

Alcoholic hepatitis carries a poor prognosis if the person continues to drink alcohol. Frequently the disease will stabilize if the person stops drinking.

Clients who develop cirrhosis (but are asymptomatic) and are able to abstain from alcohol have a prognosis of 80% at 5 years. Liver transplantation is offered to clients who have end-stage liver disease and are able to stop drinking, typically for at least a period of 6 months. This often allows for sufficient improvement to the point of not requiring a liver transplant. Prognosis depends on the severity of disease, other coexisting illnesses (e.g., HCV), nutritional status, the client's ability to abstain from alcohol, and the presence of end-stage liver disease.

12.10 Special Implications for the PTA: Alcohol-Related Liver Disease Follow the same guidelines regarding liver protection as are discussed in 12.7 Special Implications for the PTA: Viral Hepatitis. Increased susceptibility to infections necessitates careful handwashing before treating clients with alcohol-related liver disease. (See also 12.3 Special Implications for the PTA: Cirrhosis.) The presence of coagulopathy necessitates additional precautions. (See 12.1 Special Implications for the PTA: Signs and Symptoms of Hepatic Disease.)

Primary Biliary Cirrhosis
Overview and Incidence

Primary biliary cirrhosis (PBC) occurs most frequently in women (80% to 90% of cases) from 40 to 60 years of age.

PBC is a slowly progressive (irreversible), chronic liver disease that causes inflammatory destruction of the small intrahepatic bile ducts, decreased bile secretion, cirrhosis, and ultimately liver failure. An autoimmune attack against the bile duct is probably an important pathogenetic element, but the precipitating event and contribution of genetic and environmental factors are uncertain. The disease is associated with other autoimmune disorders, including scleroderma, Sjögren's syndrome, thyroiditis, pernicious anemia, and renal tubular acidosis. Although it is most common in whites from North America and Europe, cases have occurred in all races.

Etiologic Factors and Pathogenesis

The underlying cause of PBC has a basis in aberrant autoimmunity. As the ducts are destroyed, toxic substances build up in the liver, intensifying the damage. Chronic inflammation leads to fibrosis, cirrhosis, and eventually, without treatment, liver failure.

Research has also been investigating factors that lead to the production of antimitochondrial antibodies.

Clinical Manifestations

Most people with PBC are asymptomatic (50% to 60%) at diagnosis. The most common presenting symptom is fatigue, which is noted in over 20% of affected clients at diagnosis. With progression of the disease, fatigue becomes more significant, occurring in about 80% of people,[19] and may be disabling.[62]

Other symptoms of the disease include hyperlipidemia, osteopenia, and the presence of other autoimmune diseases (e.g., *Sjögren's syndrome* and scleroderma).[36,80] In the later stages of the disease, clients may exhibit portal hypertension, malabsorption, fat-soluble vitamin deficiencies, and steatorrhea (the result of impairment of excretion of bile into the intestine). Complications from advanced liver disease include ascites, bleeding from esophageal varices, and hepatic encephalopathy.

The physical examination findings are typically normal in asymptomatic people, but skin manifestations often occur as the disease progresses. Pruritus frequently leads to excoriations of the skin, and spider nevi, thickening of the skin, and increased skin pigmentation are often detected with advancement. Xanthelasmas are seen in 5% to 10% of persons with the disease (Fig. 12.5). Hepatomegaly is noted in 70% of

clients, yet splenomegaly is uncommon at presentation, often developing only near the end stages of PBC. Jaundice is observed later in the illness, often months to years after diagnosis. Muscle wasting, edema, and ascites often herald liver failure.

Medical Management

Diagnosis

A probable diagnosis of PBC can be made with only the presence of antimitochondrial antibodies and elevated liver enzymes, but a definite diagnosis requires a liver biopsy. The hallmark of PBC is asymmetric inflammation and destruction of the bile duct within the portal triads.

The clinical course of the disease is variable, and early diagnosis is important to initiate therapeutic measures before the development of advanced disease.

Treatment

Most people with PBC are now treated with ursodeoxycholic acid (UDCA), or ursodiol, a bile acid taken in capsules.

UDCA has also been shown to reduce the risk of death or need for liver transplantation after 4 years of therapy and can be effective for up to 10 years.[60,63] It appears to be safe and has few adverse effects. If used in clients with early-stage disease, it may delay the development of hepatic fibrosis and esophageal varices, with survival rates slightly lower than seen in an age-sex–matched control population.[10,11,61]

Colchicine and methotrexate are two drugs that are often used when UDCA is no longer efficacious; other drugs are under investigation.[66]

Liver transplantation is considered for clients with end-stage liver disease (i.e., hepatorenal syndrome, diuretic-resistant edema, bleeding esophageal varices, and hepatic encephalopathy), unacceptable quality of life caused by intractable symptoms, or anticipated death in less than 1 year.[44]

Many laboratory values and factors are followed to aid in determining the appropriate time for liver transplantation. Clients who receive a liver transplant often have difficulty weaning from immunosuppressants, and evidence of recurrent disease appears in 15% of clients at 3 years and 30% at 10 years.[55]

Liver transplantation leads to an initial worsening of osteopenia, but bone mineral density typically returns to baseline after 1 year and can subsequently continue to improve. Because of a lack of bile acid secretion, fat-soluble vitamins (i.e., vitamins D, A, and K) are not absorbed in the intestine. This typically occurs in the later stages of the disease, and clients can be given supplements as needed.

Prognosis

Clients who are diagnosed with stage 1 or 2 disease typically have a better response to treatment.

Liver transplantation offers persons with liver failure improved survival. The survival rate at 1 year is 92%, and the 5-year rate is 85%. Death is usually a result of hepatic failure or complications of portal hypertension associated with cirrhosis.

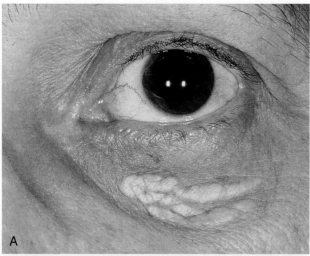

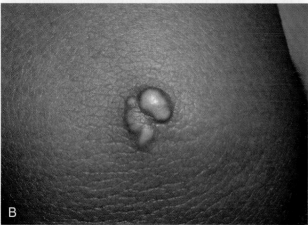

FIG. 12.5 Xanthelasma. Multiple, soft yellow plaques involving the eyelid (A, lower and upper). Lipid-laden foam cells seen in the dermis tend to cluster around blood vessels. Lipid deposits can also be seen along the extensor surfaces of the body such as the heels, elbows (B), and dorsum of the hands. (A, From Yanoff M, Duke JS: Ophthalmology, ed 4, Edinburgh, 2014, Saunders. B, From Bolognia JL, Jorizzo JL, Schaffer JV: Dermatology, ed 3, London, 2012.)

12.11 Special Implications for the PTA: Primary Biliary Cirrhosis The most significant clinical problem for clients with PBC is bone disease characterized by impaired osteoblastic activity and accelerated osteoclastic activity. Calcium and vitamin D should be carefully monitored and appropriate replacement instituted. Physical activity after an osteoporosis protocol should be encouraged but with proper pacing and energy conservation. Occasionally, sensory neuropathy (xanthomatous neuropathy) of the hands and/or feet may occur. Cholesterol-laden macrophages accumulate in the subcutaneous tissues and create local lesions, termed *xanthomas*, around the eyelids and over skin, tendons, nerves, joints, and other locations.

Intrahepatic Cholestasis of Pregnancy

Intrahepatic cholestasis (suppression of bile flow) of pregnancy is characterized by pruritus and cholestatic jaundice; it usually occurs in the last trimester of each pregnancy and promptly resolves after delivery.

Cholestasis of pregnancy is most likely related to the inhibitory effect estrogen has on bile formation in susceptible women. Maternal health is unaffected by this condition, but the effects on the unborn child can be serious, including fetal distress, stillbirth, prematurity, and an increased risk of intracranial hemorrhage during delivery. UDCA can be used to relieve symptoms and is well tolerated by both mother and fetus. No significant effects are apparent on the liver of the mother, although the risk of developing gallstones is increased.

Vascular Disease of the Liver

Congestive heart failure is the major cause of liver congestion, especially in the Western world, where ischemic heart disease is so prevalent. Backward congestion of the liver and the decreased perfusion of the liver secondary to decline in cardiac output result in abnormal liver function test results. Hepatic encephalopathy may contribute to the altered mentation seen with severe congestive heart failure. Decreased cerebral perfusion, hypoxemia, and electrolyte imbalance are usually the major contributors to the confused state that can be seen in people with severe congestive heart failure.

Portal vein obstruction can be the result of thrombosis, infection, constriction, or invasion. Thrombosis of the portal system is typically caused by a hypercoagulable state or secondary to inflammation, cirrhosis, trauma, or cancer. Inflammatory diseases that affect thrombosis of the portal vein include pancreatitis and inflammatory bowel disease. HCC and pancreatic cancer are the two most common malignancies to cause thrombosis; they also lead to constriction and invasion of the vein.

Ischemic hepatitis or hypoxic hepatitis results when tissue of the liver does not receive adequate oxygen. This may occur in any disease process that reduces blood flow (cardiac failure), reduces oxygen supply (respiratory failure), or increases oxygen requirements (sepsis).

Liver Neoplasms

Hepatic neoplasms can be divided into three groups: benign neoplasms, primary malignant neoplasms, and metastatic malignant neoplasms. Cancer arising from the liver itself is called *primary;* liver cancer that has spread from somewhere else is labeled *secondary* or *metastatic.*

Primary liver tumors may arise from hepatocytes, connective tissue, blood vessels, or bile ducts and are either benign or malignant (Table 12.4). Primary malignant cancer is almost always found in a cirrhotic liver and is considered a late complication of cirrhosis. Benign and malignant neoplasms can also occur in women taking oral contraceptives. A few rare tumors arise from the bile ducts within the liver and are associated with certain hormonal drugs and cancers. *Cholangiocarcinomas* are discussed later in this chapter.

Benign Liver Neoplasms

Cavernous hemangioma. About 7% of autopsied livers contain hemangiomas, making this lesion the most common benign liver tumor. It is of unknown cause and occurs in all age groups, more commonly among women. The pathology is similar to that of *hemangiomas* anywhere in the body; it is a blood-filled mass of variable size and can be located anywhere in the liver.

Most hepatic hemangiomas are asymptomatic until they become large enough to cause a sense of fullness or upper abdominal pain. Hepatomegaly or an abdominal mass is the most common physical finding. Hepatic hemangiomas are often discovered coincidentally on computed tomography (CT) scan, by magnetic resonance imaging (MRI), or during laparotomy. Treatment is not usually recommended because most hepatic hemangiomas have a benign course with negligible risk of malignancy and minimal chance of spontaneous hemorrhage. Surgical resection may be performed if the hemangioma is consistently symptomatic, producing pain or fever, or if the tumor is large enough for traumatic rupture to be considered a risk (e.g., a palpable lesion in an athlete).

12.12 Special Implications for the PTA: Cavernous Hemangioma Most liver hemangiomas are small, are found incidentally, and require no special precautions. In the case of a known large liver hemangioma, the client must be cautioned to avoid activities and positions that will increase intraabdominal pressure to avoid risk of rupture (see Box 12.1). For the same reason, throughout therapy and especially during exercise, the client must be instructed in proper breathing techniques.

Liver adenomas. Liver cell adenomas are most common in the third and fourth decades, almost exclusively in women. Although the incidence remains low in men, oral contraceptives have significantly increased the incidence in women. Most remain asymptomatic, although with growth, right upper quadrant abdominal pain may be present. Although classified as benign tumors, they are highly vascular and carry a risk for rupture and subsequent hemorrhage. The clinical presentation is often one of acute abdominal disease because of necrosis of the tumor with hemorrhage. Pain, fever, and circulatory collapse occur in the presence

TABLE 12.4	Classification of Primary Liver Neoplasms	
Origin	**Benign**	**Malignant**
Hepatocytes	Adenoma	Hepatocellular carcinoma
Connective tissue	Fibroma	Sarcoma
Blood vessels	Hemangioma	Hemangioendothelioma
Bile ducts	Cholangioma	Cholangiocarcinoma

of hemorrhage. Most adenomas are evaluated with hepatic angiography, MRI, or CT. Liver function test results are usually within normal limits. Because of the risk of rupture and, rarely, malignant transformation to HCC, resection is usually recommended. Affected women should refrain from taking oral contraceptives.

> **12.13 Special Implications for the PTA: Liver Adenomas** The PTA is most likely to see clients with liver adenomas postoperatively after the danger of rupture and hemorrhage has passed. Standard postoperative protocols are usually sufficient.

Malignant Liver Neoplasms

Primary hepatocellular carcinoma

Overview and incidence. HCC is the fifth most common cancer in the world; it is also the most common primary liver cancer, constituting about 90% to 95% of primary liver cancers in adults. In Western countries, HCC is linked to cirrhosis. It is seen more often in men, and the incidence increases with age. In many countries, including the United States, a definite increase in the incidence of HCC has been reported, largely attributable to the increasing incidence of HCV infection.[53]

Etiologic and risk factors. Epidemiologic and laboratory studies have firmly established a strong and specific association between HBV and HCV with HCC. Cirrhosis is typically a prerequisite for HCC development in association with HCV.

In all parts of the world, there is a strong correlation between HCC and cirrhosis (of any cause). Another risk factor is dietary exposure to aflatoxin B_1, which is derived from the fungi *Aspergillus flavus* and *A. parasiticus*. This is a major concern in Africa and Asia. Up to 45% of individuals with hemochromatosis (an iron overload disease) can develop HCC. Although the tumor is more likely to arise with the development of cirrhosis, it is not necessarily true (i.e., HCC can develop in the absence of cirrhosis).

Pathogenesis and clinical manifestations. The exact events leading to malignant transformation of the hepatic cell remain unknown, but it does appear that HBV is both directly and indirectly carcinogenic. Indirect carcinogenic effects are the result of the chronic necroinflammatory hepatic disease.

Most people who develop HCC are unaware of it until advanced stages. Abdominal pain (60% to 95%) and weight loss (35% to 70%) are the most common initial symptoms. Other symptoms include weakness, fatigue, poor appetite, early satiety, fullness of the abdomen, diarrhea, and constipation. Jaundice is observed in only 5% to 25% of cases. Metastases occur to the bone and lungs, resulting in back pain and cough. Physical examination may demonstrate an enlarged liver, ascites, or splenomegaly. Unfortunately, many of these signs and symptoms may already be present because of cirrhosis and not distinguished as HCC.

> **12.14 Special Implications for the PTA: Primary Hepatocellular Carcinoma** Liver tumors that cause elevation of the diaphragm can cause right shoulder pain or symptoms of respiratory involvement. Peripheral edema associated with developing ascites may be observed first by the PTA (see the section on ascites in this chapter). As the tumor grows, pain may radiate to the back (midthoracic region).

Metastatic Malignant Tumors

The liver is one of the most common sites of metastasis from other primary cancers (e.g., colorectal, stomach, pancreas, esophagus, lung, and breast cancers, melanoma, Hodgkin's disease, and non-Hodgkin's lymphoma). Metastatic tumors occur 20 times more often than primary liver tumors and constitute the bulk of hepatic malignancy.

As with other types of cancers, secondary liver cancer can occur as a result of local invasion from neighboring organs, lymphatic spread, spread across body cavities, and spread via the vascular system. The liver filters blood from everywhere in the body, but because all blood from the digestive organs passes through the liver before joining the general circulation, the liver is the first organ to filter cancer cells released from the stomach, intestine, or pancreas.

Metastatic tumors to the liver originating in some organs (e.g., stomach or lung) never give rise to hepatic symptoms, whereas others produce hepatic symptoms or jaundice with less than 60% replacement of the liver. Certain tumors (colon, breast, or melanoma) typically replace 90% of the liver before jaundice develops. Melanomas are associated with such minimal tissue reaction that almost complete hepatic replacement occurs before hepatic symptoms develop.

Clinical manifestations, diagnosis, and treatment are the same as for the primary (original) neoplasm. Treatment is the same as for unresectable liver cancer (see the section on HCC in this chapter).

Liver Abscess

Liver abscess most often occurs among individuals with other underlying disorders. Most common underlying causes include *bacterial cholangitis* secondary to obstruction of the bile ducts by stone or stricture; *portal vein bacteremia* secondary to bacterial seeding via the portal vein from viscera infected after bowel inflammation or organ perforation; *liver flukes*, a parasitic infestation; or *amebiasis,* an infestation with amebae from tropical or subtropical areas.

Other predisposing factors are diabetes mellitus, infected hepatic cysts, metastatic liver tumors with secondary infection, and diverticulitis. Pyogenic (pus-filled) abscesses may be single or multiple; liver cirrhosis is a strong risk factor for single pyogenic liver abscess, and multiple abscesses often arise from a biliary source of infection.

Clinical manifestations are commonly right-sided abdominal and shoulder pain, nausea, vomiting, rapid weight loss, high fever, and diaphoresis. The liver's close proximity to the base of the right lung may contribute to the development of right pleural effusion. Complications of hepatic abscess relate to rupture and direct spread of infection. Diagnosis is accomplished by a variety of possible tests including liver function tests, chest x-ray examination, contrast-enhanced CT scan of the abdomen, ultrasonography of the right upper quadrant, liver scan, and arteriography. Treatment may consist of antimicrobial therapy alone or percutaneous aspiration of the abscess with antimicrobial therapy. Surgery may be required to relieve biliary tract obstruction and to drain abscesses that do not respond to percutaneous drainage and antibiotics.

Unrecognized and untreated, pyogenic liver abscess is universally fatal. The mortality from hepatic abscess in treated cases remains high, ranging from 40% to 80%. Amebic abscesses are an exception; when treated, the mortality rate is less than 3%. Early diagnosis and aggressive treatment can significantly reduce the mortality in some cases. Specific antibiotics are required whenever abscess is caused by amebic infestation.

> **12.15 Special Implications for the PTA: Liver Abscess** Clients with liver abscess are very ill and usually are seen only by the PTA assigned to an intensive care unit team. In such situations vital signs are assessed regularly to detect high fever and rapid pulse, which are early signs of sepsis (a common complication). Movement, coughing, and deep breathing are important to prevent or limit pulmonary complications related to hepatic abscess, and skin care in the presence of high fever is essential. Careful disposal of feces and careful handwashing to avoid transmission are required when abscess is caused by amebic infestation.

Liver Injuries

Toxic liver injury can occur as a result of drugs or from occupational exposure to chemicals and toxins. Hepatotoxic chemicals produce liver cell necrosis. Agents responsible for toxic liver injury include yellow phosphorus, carbon tetrachloride, phalloidin (mushroom toxin), and acetaminophen (analgesic). Reye's syndrome in children may be related to aspirin toxicity. In addition to jaundice, other symptoms of liver toxicity may occur (e.g., cholestasis or chronic hepatitis).

Toxic liver injury produces toxic hepatitis (discussed earlier in this chapter). The prognosis is usually good if the toxin is withdrawn and never reintroduced. Whatever drug is responsible, it is well documented that liver toxicity becomes more severe with advancing age.

Liver injury by trauma may be either penetrating or blunt, leading to laceration and hemorrhage. Penetrating injuries are usually knife or missile wounds (gunshots). A knife wound leaves a sharp clear incision, whereas gunshot wounds enter and exit with greater damage. Blunt trauma from a fall or from hitting a steering wheel has varying effects, from small hematomas to large lacerations, as a result of severe impact forces.

> **12.16 Special Implications for the PTA: Liver Injuries** The PTA will likely be treating clients with liver injury secondary to trauma postoperatively in the trauma unit. Common postoperative problems include pulmonary infections and abscess formation. Clients are assessed postoperatively for manifestations of infection (e.g., fever, chills, or difficulty breathing). Physical therapy intervention is focused on prevention of respiratory complications, especially pneumonia, and provision of skin care and extremity movement until the client can begin progressive transfer and mobility skills.

PANCREAS

Diabetes Mellitus

The pancreas has dual functions, acting as both an endocrine gland in secreting hormones insulin and glucagon and as an exocrine gland in producing digestive enzymes. The cells of the pancreas that function in the endocrine capacity are the islets of Langerhans, constituting 1% to 2% of the pancreatic mass. Defective endocrine function of the pancreas resulting in ineffective insulin (whether deficient or defective in action within the body) characterizes diabetes mellitus.

Pancreatitis

Pancreatitis is a potentially serious inflammation of the pancreas that may result in autodigestion of the pancreas by its own enzymes. Pancreatitis may be acute or chronic; the acute form is brief, usually mild, and reversible, whereas the chronic form is recurrent or persisting. Because the hormones and enzymes provided by the pancreas perform many vital functions, acute pancreatitis causes systemic problems and complications that affect the entire body. Approximately 15% of all cases of acute pancreatitis develop into chronic pancreatitis.

Acute Pancreatitis

Incidence and etiologic factors. Acute pancreatitis is an inflammatory process of the pancreas that can involve surrounding organs, as well as cause a systemic reaction. Pancreatitis can arise from a variety of factors and conditions (Box 12.3) or as a result of an unknown cause (10% of cases). The most common cause is gallstones, followed by chronic alcohol consumption. Other causes include hypertriglyceridemia (levels over 1000 mg/dL), trauma, duct obstruction (neoplasms), and medications. The incidence has increased over the past few decades, but the mortality rate has remained fairly constant at 7%.

Pancreatitis can involve only the interstitium of the pancreas (termed *interstitial pancreatitis*), or it can involve necrosis of pancreatic tissue (called *necrotizing pancreatitis*). Interstitial pancreatitis accounts for 80% of cases and has a milder course and few complications, whereas necrotizing pancreatitis occurs in 20% of cases and can result in significant complications and higher mortality.

Pathogenesis. Acute pancreatitis is thought to result from the inappropriate activation of trypsinogen within acinar cells to the enzyme trypsin. Trypsin is the principal enzyme responsible for activating other pancreatic enzymes. The buildup of pancreatic enzymes can trigger pancreatic autodigestion. The release of enzymes leads to an out-of-proportion inflammatory response with associated edema and inflammation.[81]

> ## BOX 12.3   Conditions and Situations Associated with Acute Pancreatitis
>
> - Alcohol abuse[a]
> - Autoimmune diseases
> - Cystic fibrosis
> - Gallstones[a]
> - Hereditary (familial) pancreatitis
> - Hypercalcemia
> - Hyperlipidemia (hypertriglyceridemia)
> - Infection
> - Ischemia
> - Medications (oral estrogens, antibiotics, AZT, thiazide diuretics, corticosteroids)
> - Neoplasm
> - Peptic ulcers
> - Post-ERCP
> - Postoperative inflammation
> - Pregnancy (third trimester)
> - Blunt or penetrating trauma (including ischemia and perfusion that occur during some surgical procedures)
> - Vasculitis
> - Viral infections
> - Unknown
>
> *AZT*, Azidothymidine; *ERCP*, endoscopic retrograde cholangiopancreatography.
> [a]Most common causes.

Pancreatitis becomes severe when a systemic response[6,70] leads to multiorgan failure and occasionally death. Severe ischemia and inflammation can result in the leakage of pancreatic fluid and the formation of fluid collections and pseudocysts. A pseudocyst is a liquefied collection of necrotic debris and pancreatic enzymes. Complications of pseudocysts include infection, bleeding, and rupture into the peritoneum.

Infection can occur secondary to the breakdown of normal barriers in the gut because of hypoperfusion of the colon. Also, under investigation are multiple genes that, coupled with the appropriate environmental conditions, may be responsible for the development of pancreatitis.[76]

Clinical manifestations. Symptoms in clients with acute pancreatitis can vary from mild, nonspecific abdominal pain to profound pain accompanied by systemic symptoms. Most people with mild to moderate disease have pain, nausea, anorexia, and vomiting. Abdominal pain, the cardinal symptom of acute pancreatitis, may be dull at first but can increase in quality and intensity to sharp and severe.

Quality of pain can vary, depending on the cause and severity of disease, but the pain often involves the entire upper abdomen. Right upper quadrant pain with radiation to the back may be more prevalent with gallstones. The pain is typically steady and at maximal intensity within 10 to 20 minutes. Pain can be triggered or made worse by eating fatty meals or drinking alcohol. Position changes usually do not alleviate the discomfort. Nausea and vomiting occur in 90% of people with pancreatitis and can be severe.

In a minority of cases the condition develops into severe pancreatitis with serious complications. Symptoms that warn of worsening condition include tachycardia, hypoxia, tachypnea, and changes in mental status. Complications of pancreatitis include pancreatic fluid–filled collections (57% of cases), pseudocysts, and necrosis. These fluid collections can enlarge, leading to worsening pain. Bacteria can infect these collections and necrotic areas, resulting in pain, leukocytosis, fever, hypotension, and hypovolemia. Often the first sign of a complication is a failure to improve followed by unexpected deterioration. Ascites and pleural effusions are rare complications.

Medical Management

Diagnosis

Diagnosis is based on clinical presentation, laboratory tests, and imaging studies. Early in the disease process (within 24 to 72 hours), pancreatic enzymes released from injured acinar cells result in elevated serum amylase and lipase levels, which are diagnostic for acute pancreatitis.

Lipase levels are more specific to acute pancreatitis, rising in 4 to 8 hours, peaking around 24 hours, and staying elevated for at least 14 days.

Treatment

For most persons (about 80% of cases), acute pancreatitis is a mild disease that subsides spontaneously within several days. Treatment for mild pancreatitis is largely symptomatic and designed to preserve normal pancreatic function while preventing complications and includes intravenous fluids for hydration, analgesics for pain control, and eating nothing by mouth to allow the pancreas to rest. If after 2 to 3 days there is no improvement, a CT scan should be obtained to determine whether complications are present.

Clients are allowed to return home once the pain is under control and they are able to eat, drink, and take oral analgesics. Food intake progresses from clear liquids for 24 hours to small, low-fat meals with a slow increase in quantity over several days as tolerated.[81] If pancreatitis is secondary to gallstones, laparoscopic cholecystectomy can be performed. If fluid collections are present, surgery should be delayed until they have resolved. Endoscopic retrograde cholangiopancreatography (ERCP) with endoscopic sphincterotomy may be performed if common bile duct stones are present or for clients who are not surgical candidates.

Severe pancreatitis is defined by the presence of organ failure, local complications, or both. It is important to identify clients with severe pancreatitis at admission to provide aggressive care and close observation for complications. People admitted to the hospital with severe pancreatitis require admittance to an intensive care unit, aggressive intravenous hydration, and pain control. Enteral nutrition (within 2 to 3 days) is preferred to decrease infectious complications.[45] Severe pancreatitis can be accompanied by significant complications, including the formation of pancreatic fluid collections, pseudocysts, necrosis, bacterial cholangitis, and infected fluid collections and necrotic areas.

Prognosis

Prognosis of individuals with acute pancreatitis depends on the severity of the condition. Individuals with mild pancreatitis (80% of cases) have a better outcome than those with necrotizing or severe disease. The clinical course of mild disease follows a self-limiting pattern, resolving within 2 weeks of onset. The risk of dying from severe pancreatitis is 10% to 30%; death is the result of complications such as infection. Yet most people who experience severe pancreatitis are able to recover, and at 6 years about 65% of people are able to work full time. Recurrences and the development of diabetes mellitus are common in alcoholic pancreatitis, particularly with continued drinking of alcohol.

12.17 Special Implications for the PTA: Acute Pancreatitis

The PTA is most likely to see acute pancreatitis either when the early presentation is back pain (undiagnosed) or when acute respiratory distress syndrome develops as a complication, necessitating assisted respiration and pulmonary care. Pancreatic inflammation and scarring occurring as part of the acute pancreatic process can result in decreased spinal extension, especially of the thoracolumbar junction. This problem is difficult to treat and requires the therapy team to make reasonable goals (e.g., maintain function and current range of motion), especially when the pancreatitis is in an active, ongoing phase.

Even with client compliance with treatment intervention and subsiding of inflammation, the residual scarring is difficult to reach or affect with mobilization techniques and continues to reduce mechanical motion. Back pain associated with acute pancreatitis may be accompanied by GI symptoms such as diarrhea, pain after a meal, anorexia, and unexplained weight loss. The client may not see any connection between GI symptoms and back pain and may not report the additional symptoms.

The pain may be relieved by heat initially (decreases muscular tension); preferred positions include leaning forward, sitting up, or lying motionless on the left side in a fetal-flexed position. Promoting comfort and rest as part of the medical rehabilitation process may necessitate teaching the client positioning (side-lying, knee-chest position with a pillow pressed against the abdomen, or sitting with the trunk flexed may be helpful) and relaxation techniques.

For the client who is restricted from eating or drinking to rest the GI tract and decrease pancreatic stimulation, even ice chips can stimulate enzymes and increase pain. In such cases the PTA must be careful not to give in to the client's repeated requests for food, water, or ice chips unless approved by nursing or medical staff. Clients with acute pancreatitis are allowed to resume oral intake when all abdominal pain and tenderness have resolved.

Monitor the individual with acute pancreatitis for signs and symptoms of bleeding; alert the health care team about bruising or prolonged bleeding.

Chronic Pancreatitis

Overview, incidence, and etiology. Chronic pancreatitis is characterized by the development of irreversible changes in the pancreas secondary to chronic inflammation. The principal causes are chronic alcohol consumption, a history of severe acute pancreatitis, autoimmune, hereditary factors, and idiopathic origin. In Western industrialized nations, the most common cause of chronic pancreatitis is alcohol abuse, accounting for more than 50% of cases.

The typical person with alcohol-related chronic pancreatitis is male, is aged 35 to 45 years, and has consumed large quantities (150 g or more per day) for more than 6 years. Hereditary pancreatitis is found in clients who have two or more relatives with the disease, including those with cystic fibrosis.

Pathogenesis. Several hypotheses have been published to explain the development of chronic pancreatitis. Most are directed toward alcohol-related chronic pancreatitis but have some applicability to other types. The first one suggests that alcohol consumption leads to release of pancreatic fluid that is high in protein, creating plugs in the pancreatic ducts, which may calcify and produce pancreatic stones. Pancreatic stones are seen in several types of chronic pancreatitis, although damage is noted in areas without obstruction.

A second hypothesis proposes that alcohol or one of its metabolites acts as a direct toxin on pancreatic tissue. Alcohol may also stimulate the release of CCK, which, in the presence of alcohol, leads to the transcription of inflammatory enzymes.[57]

A third hypothesis explains that after repeated bouts of acute pancreatitis, areas of necrosis heal with the formation of scar tissue or fibrosis. In persons without a history of acute episodes, the pathogenesis of chronic pancreatitis may relate to persistent necrosis and insidious scarring, similar to the progression of cirrhosis of the liver. Theories continue to evolve, and the pathogenesis most likely depends on both genetic and environmental factors.

Clinical manifestations. Most clients with chronic pancreatitis have abdominal pain, which is also the most significant problem. Chronic pain often leads to an abuse of opioids, decreased appetite, weight loss, and poor quality of life; it is also the most common reason for surgery in people with this disease. Pain is typically epigastric in location, often with radiation to the back. It is made worse with meals but can be relieved by bringing the knees to the chest or bending forward. Nausea and vomiting are often associated with the pain. Pain during the course of the disease varies; many people will experience acute attacks followed by periods of feeling well. As the number of attacks increases and they occur more frequently, pain becomes more chronic in nature. Others have continual pain that gradually increases in intensity.

Chronic destruction of pancreatic tissue contributes to the loss of pancreatic function, resulting in diarrhea, steatorrhea, and diabetes mellitus. Diabetes is also seen later in the course of the disease, particularly after surgical removal of the pancreas. This can lead to severe and prolonged hypoglycemia with the use of insulin.

History is often significant for alcohol abuse; other clients may have a history of pancreatitis or family history of chronic pancreatitis. Physical examination is usually significant for abdominal tenderness, with few other findings.

Medical Management

Diagnosis

The diagnosis of chronic pancreatitis may be difficult to make, particularly in the early stages of the disease when the pancreas lacks significant functional or structural changes. Routine laboratory test values, such as lipase and amylase levels, are often not elevated except during an acute episode of pancreatitis.

Imaging tests can demonstrate structural changes. Some of the changes seen in chronic pancreatitis include dilated pancreatic ducts, strictures, pancreatic stones, lobularity, and atrophy. Various imaging modalities can be used to diagnose chronic pancreatitis. Often the least invasive test is used, such as transabdominal ultrasonography or CT.

Other tests are used as needed, such as endoscopic ultrasonography (EUS), ERCP, or magnetic resonance cholangiopancreatography (MRCP) and MRI.

Treatment

The treatment of chronic pancreatitis is directed toward prevention of further pancreatic injury, pain relief, and replacement of lost endocrine or exocrine function. Cessation of alcohol intake is essential in the management of chronic pancreatitis in clients with alcohol-related pancreatitis. Smoking has also been linked with increased risk of mortality in people with alcohol-related pancreatitis and should be avoided.[43]

Pain can be initially treated with nonnarcotics, advancing to narcotics as needed. Narcotics are useful for persons with established chronic pancreatitis, but the risk of addiction is about 10% to 30%. Nerve blocks can also aid in the reduction of pain.

Treatment of a dominant stricture in the pancreatic duct with stents and pancreatic duct sphincterotomy improves pain in over half of clients with large duct disease[67]; surgical drainage for persistent pseudocysts, as well as surgical intervention to eliminate obstruction of pancreatic ducts, may be indicated for severe pain, although the pain often returns.

A pancreatectomy may be performed as a last means of relieving refractory pain. Oral enzyme replacements are taken before, during, and after meals to correct enzyme deficiencies and to prevent malabsorption. Insulin may be required in the case of islet cell dysfunction but is used with care secondary to the loss of glucagon-producing cells.

Prognosis

Complications include the development of large pseudocysts, bleeding from pseudoaneurysms, splenic vein thrombosis, and fistula formation. Pancreatic cancer develops in about 3% to 4% of people with chronic pancreatitis and is often difficult to distinguish from chronic changes of pancreatitis. Chronic pancreatitis is a serious disease, often leading to chronic disability. Alcohol-related chronic pancreatitis carries a poor prognosis without alcohol cessation and increases the risk of mortality by 60%. Overall, the 10-year survival of persons with chronic pancreatitis is 70%, and the 20-year survival rate is 45%.[43]

12.18 Special Implications for the PTA: Chronic Pancreatitis

Back pain in the upper thoracic area or pain at the thoracolumbar junction may be the presenting symptom for some individuals with chronic pancreatitis, but past medical history including the presence of pancreatitis should raise a red flag and suggest that careful screening is required in these cases. People with alcohol-related chronic pancreatitis often have peripheral neuropathy.

The clinical presentation with aggravating and relieving factors (e.g., alcohol consumption, food intake, or positional changes noted) or failure to improve with therapy intervention adds additional red flag symptoms.[22] The person with known pancreatitis and/or pancreatectomy may need monitoring of vital signs and/or blood glucose levels depending on complications present. Education about the effects of malabsorption and associated osteoporosis should be included.

Pancreatic Cancer
Overview and Incidence

Pancreatic cancer is the fourth leading cause of cancer mortality in the United States, with more than 32,000 deaths each year.[29] It also has the lowest 5-year survival rate (3% to 5%) of any type of cancer.

Most pancreatic neoplasms (90%) arise from exocrine cells and are *adenocarcinoma* (70% in the proximal or head of the pancreas, 10% in the pancreas body, and 15% in the tail). Adenocarcinoma is the focus of this discussion.

Pancreatic cancer is more common in black men and women than in whites, occurs in the Western world most often, and has a peak incidence in the seventh and eighth decades.

Etiologic and Risk Factors

Clear evidence of increased risk of pancreatic cancer has been shown related to advancing age. Pancreatic adenocarcinoma is rare in people under the age of 45 years; however, the risk increases after the age of 50 years. Of people with pancreatic adenocarcinoma, 7% to 8% have a family history.

Tobacco use, exposure to certain chemicals, obesity, diets high in fats and meat, history of familial chronic pancreatitis, history of nonfamilial chronic pancreatitis, and a history of partial gastrectomy are also risk factors.[32] The presence of adult-onset diabetes mellitus and impaired glucose tolerance (especially in women), chronic pancreatitis, and prior gastrectomy may be contributing factors. Obesity and physical activity (both linked with abnormal glucose metabolism) are associated with increased risk of pancreatic cancer. Higher consumption of red and processed meat is also associated with elevated pancreatic cancer risk.[32]

No support exists for any direct effect from exposure to radiation, socioeconomic status, alcohol intake, or coffee consumption, although these risk factors remain under investigation.[40]

Pathogenesis

Although the specific cause of pancreatic cancer is unknown, many genes are under investigation as possibly being linked to its development. Many adenocarcinomas infiltrate into vascular spaces, lymphatic spaces, and perineural spaces. Pancreatic cancer appears to progress from flat ductal lesions to papillary ductal lesions without irregularities then with irregularities (atypia) and finally to infiltrating adenocarcinoma. The existence of such a progression suggests that it may be possible to detect a curable precursor lesion and early cancer with a molecular test in the future.[40]

Clinical Manifestations

The clinical features of pancreatic cancer are initially nonspecific and vague, which contribute to the delay in diagnosis. Most clients are seen for pain (80% to 85%), weight loss (60%), and jaundice (47%). These symptoms suggest advanced disease. Typically, people with significant pain have tumor in the body or tail of the pancreas, whereas jaundice and weight loss are more suggestive of tumor in the head of the pancreas.

Pain is a common symptom of pancreatic carcinoma because of invasion of tumor into nerves. In later stages of the disease, pain may be intractable. Pain is often epigastric in location, radiating to the back (thoracic or lumbar regions). Jaundice accompanied by pruritus, dark urine, and acholic stools occurs and is caused by compression of the biliary tree by tumor.

Pancreatitis may also develop from obstruction of the duct. In some people, pancreatitis may be the first sign of the disease. Deep venous thrombosis can occur as a result of tumor presence.

Metastasis. Pancreatic adenocarcinomas metastasize via the hematologic and lymphatic systems to the liver, peritoneum, lungs and pleura, and adrenal glands. These metastasized tumors may grow by direct extension, causing further involvement of the duodenum, stomach, spleen, and colon. Tumors of the body and tail of the pancreas are twice as likely to metastasize to the peritoneum compared with tumors in the head of the pancreas.

Medical Management

Prevention

At the present time, the best advice to reduce the risk of pancreatic cancer is to avoid tobacco use, maintain a healthful weight, remain physically active, and eat five or more ½-cup servings of vegetables and fruits each day.[32]

Diagnosis

Spiral CT with intravenous contrast of the abdomen is the most common test in the assessment of pancreatic adenocarcinoma. These CT scans also provide staging information that aids in determining resectability.

If a tumor is felt to be resectable by CT and is in the body or tail of the pancreas, laparoscopy may be performed. Laboratory test results can be abnormal, including elevated bilirubin level if biliary tree obstruction is present. The *tumor, node, metastases* (TNM) staging system classifies pancreatic carcinoma according to tumor size, extent of local invasion, presence or absence of regional lymph node metastases, and presence or absence of distant nonnodal metastatic disease. Preoperative staging provides information required for determining surgical resectability and prognosis.

Treatment

Treatment of pancreatic adenocarcinoma is based on the stage of the tumor. Surgical resection provides the only curative therapy, yet this is appropriate for only a minority of clients. For people with resectable disease, pancreaticoduodenectomy (Whipple procedure) is the procedure of choice.

Chemoradiation can be provided to people with locally advanced disease, and chemotherapy for those with metastatic disease. *Neoadjuvant therapy* (given before surgery) consists of chemoradiation and can be given for local tumors that have a high probability of not being entirely resectable. Much of the therapy offered to clients with pancreatic carcinoma is palliative to improve quality of life. Pain control is a significant part of therapy. Long-lasting opioids and celiac plexus neurolysis can substantially improve quality of life. Pancreatic enzyme replacement aids clients with malabsorption and steatorrhea problems. For clients who experience jaundice and will receive neoadjuvant therapy or may not be a candidate for surgery, ERCP-guided stent placement in the biliary ducts can help relieve obstruction, or biliary bypass surgery can be performed.

Prognosis

Surgical resection is currently the only treatment that provides long-term survival; yet only 20% of people with tumor deemed to be resectable are alive at 5 years; this is most likely related to microfoci of tumor still present outside the main mass. For clients with locally advanced or metastatic disease, long-term survival is rare and the mortality rate is nearly 100%. Chemoradiation therapy can prolong survival to a median of 1 year for people with locally advanced disease, whereas chemotherapy offers clients with metastatic disease approximately 6 months.

Factors associated with a more favorable outcome include tumor size less than 3 cm, lymph nodes without tumor, surgical margins free of tumor, and pathology consistent with a well-differentiated tumor.

12.19 Special Implications for the PTA: Pancreatic Cancer
Vague back pain may be the first symptomatic presentation, and cervical lymphadenopathy (called Virchow's node) may be the first sign of distant metastases. The PTA is most likely to palpate an enlarged supraclavicular lymph node (usually left sided), a finding that should always alert the PTA that a screening for medical disease should be conducted by the therapy team. Paraneoplastic syndrome associated with pancreatic carcinoma may manifest as neuromyopathy, dermatomyositis, or thrombophlebitis associated with abnormalities in blood coagulation (coagulopathy). The presence of coagulopathy is an indication for caution in the administration of certain therapeutic interventions (see 12.1 Special Implications for the PTA: Signs and Symptoms of Hepatic Disease).

The PTA is most likely to be involved with the client with diagnosed pancreatic cancer who experiences intractable back pain. Referral to chronic pain clinics or hospice centers likely includes physical therapy services. Repeated nerve blocks may be performed after a reasonable effort to manage pain through the use of transcutaneous electrical nerve stimulation, biofeedback, analgesics, or other pain control techniques. Indwelling infusion pumps implanted to deliver analgesics directly to the site of visceral afferent nerves in the epidural or intrathecal spaces may be used for short periods (i.e., 1 to 3 months).

BILIARY CONDITIONS (Table 12.5)

Cholelithiasis (Gallstone Disease)
Overview, Definition, and Incidence

Cholelithiasis, or gallstone disease, is one of the most common GI diseases in the United States, occurring in an estimated 20 million people (about 14 million women and 6 million men). Most gallstones are asymptomatic and are detected only on radiologic examinations performed for other reasons. Yet in about 25% of cases, significant symptoms and complications develop because of the presence of gallstones, requiring surgery or other treatment. Age appears to play a role in the development of cholelithiasis; gallstones are present in 20% to 35% of people by age 55 years.

Cholelithiasis occurs when stones form in the bile. These gallstones form in the gallbladder as a result of changes in the normal components of bile. Symptoms occur when these stones block bile flow in any of the ducts, the most common being the cystic duct.

Etiologic and Risk Factors

Many risk factors are associated with the development of gallstones (Box 12.4). Advancing age is a significant risk factor. Genetics plays a role in gallstone formation.

Obesity is a well-known risk factor, particularly in women. Women are also more than twice as likely to develop gallstones as men. This trend is seen until the fifth decade when the risk for women approaches that of men, suggesting estrogen may be the principal factor.

Because of the prevalence of gastric bypass surgery and other methods of extreme weight loss, rapid weight loss has emerged as a risk for cholelithiasis. People who receive total parenteral nutrition (TPN) often develop cholelithiasis; after 3 to 4 months of TPN about 45% of people form gallstones. Pregnancy is another common factor in cholelithiasis. As pregnancy progresses, the bile is more lithogenic (i.e., more prone to stone formation); up to 2% of pregnant women develop gallstones.

Many drugs contribute to the formation of gallstones. Estrogen is the most studied (i.e., oral contraceptives [excluding newer, low-dose products], estrogen replacement therapy),[78] but reports have shown ceftriaxone, clofibrate, and octreotide are also lithogenic.

TABLE 12.5	Biliary Tract Terminology
Term	**Definition**
Chole-	Pertaining to bile
Cholang-	Pertaining to bile ducts
Cholangiography	X-ray study of bile ducts
Cholangitis	Inflammation of bile duct
Cholecyst-	Pertaining to the gallbladder
Cholecystectomy	Removal of gallbladder
Cholecystitis	Inflammation of gallbladder
Cholecystography	X-ray study of gallbladder
Cholecystostomy	Incision and drainage of gallbladder
Choledocho-	Pertaining to common bile duct
Choledocholithiasis	Stones in common bile duct
Choledochostomy	Exploration of common bile duct
Cholelith-	Gallstones
Cholelithiasis	Presence of gallstones
Cholescintigraphy	Radionuclide imaging of biliary system
Cholestasis	Stoppage or suppression of bile flow

Pathogenesis

In the formation of cholesterol gallstones, the cholesterol is obtained principally from the diet.

The liver produces bile to aid in excreting excess cholesterol. If the bile contains more cholesterol than it is able to aggregate, the bile becomes oversaturated with cholesterol and forms cholesterol crystals. In the presence of gallbladder-secreted glycoproteins, there is a precipitation of the crystal aggregates, and gallstones are formed.[27]

Environmental and genetic factors most likely affect the amount of biliary cholesterol. Excess dietary cholesterol consumption may lead to an increase in the amount absorbed into the liver from the blood, but studies are conflicting.[30,50]

Clinical Manifestations

The majority of gallstones remain asymptomatic once formed in the gallbladder. Only a minority (approximately 25%) cause painful symptoms. This occurs when the stone attempts to pass down the ducts leading to the duodenum, becoming wedged. The most common location of obstruction is the cystic duct (Fig. 12.6). This causes abdominal pain (often referred to as *biliary colic*). Obstruction of the cystic duct distends the gallbladder while the muscles in the duct wall contract, trying to expel the stone. The pain of biliary colic may be intermittent or steady; it is usually severe and is located in the right upper

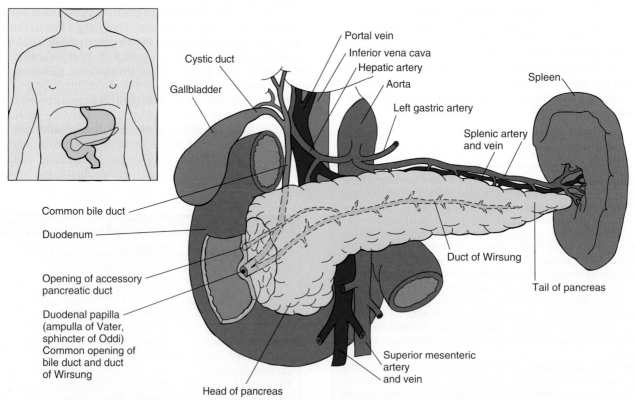

FIG. 12.6 The pancreas. The pancreas (located behind the stomach) and gallbladder are anterior to the L1-L3 vertebral bodies. Attaching to the duodenum to the right, the pancreas extends horizontally across to the spleen in the left abdomen, coming in contact with the duodenum, kidneys, liver, and spleen. Obstruction of either the hepatic or common bile duct by stone or spasm blocks the exit of bile from the liver, in which it is formed, and prevents bile from ejecting into the duodenum. (Redrawn from Black JM, Matassarin-Jacobs E, editors: Luckmann and Sorensen's medical-surgical nursing, ed 4, Philadelphia, 1993, Saunders.)

quadrant just below or slightly to the right of the sternum, with abdominal tenderness and muscle guarding. In more severe cases, rebound pain may be present. Painful symptoms are frequently related to meals, although not exclusively post-prandial. The pain often radiates to the right shoulder and upper back (60% of cases) and is associated with nausea and vomiting.

Episodes can last from 20 minutes to several hours and may develop daily or as infrequently as once every few years. Complicated cases often feature jaundice, fever, nausea and vomiting, and leukocytosis.

Other symptoms are vague, including heartburn, belching, flatulence, epigastric discomfort, and food intolerance (especially for fats). Gallstones in the older adult may not cause pain, fever, or jaundice; instead, mental confusion may be the only manifestation of gallstones.

Serious complications occur in 20% of cases when a stone becomes lodged in the lower end of the common bile duct, causing inflammation (cholangitis) leading to bacterial infection and jaundice (indicating the stone is in the common bile duct). Sometimes acute pancreatitis develops when the duct from the pancreas that joins the common bile duct also becomes blocked (see Fig. 12.6). About 15% of clients with gallstones also have stones in the common bile duct (choledocholithiasis).

Medical Management

Diagnosis

Diagnosis is based on history, physical examination, and radiographic evaluation. Physical examination often reveals tenderness to palpation in the right upper quadrant of the abdomen. The radiologic test of choice is transabdominal ultrasound. Ultrasonography reveals gallstones in more than 95% of cases (when 1.5 mm or greater in size). Ultrasound can also provide information concerning the gallbladder and ducts and can aid in predicting possible technical difficulties during surgery.[59]

Treatment and Prognosis

Asymptomatic gallstones typically do not require treatment, except in populations at high risk, such as people with sickle cell anemia. Prophylactic cholecystectomy may be recommended in these cases. Other groups requiring prophylactic treatment include those experiencing rapid weight loss or receiving TPN.

Once gallstones cause pain, there is a 1% to 2% annual risk of developing complications, and 50% of people with symptomatic cholelithiasis will have a recurrent episode. Cholecystectomy therefore is recommended for most symptomatic clients. Laparoscopic cholecystectomy is the preferred surgical approach because the complication rate is decreased compared with an open procedure. When the gallbladder is removed, bile drains directly from the liver into the intestine, eliminating the opportunity for stone formation.

Medical treatment is used only in select clients and consists of oral dissolution with UDCA, with or without extracorporeal shock-wave lithotripsy. Even with successful medical treatment, 30% to 50% of stones recur within 5 years.

> **12.20 Special Implications for the PTA: Cholelithiasis (Gallstone Disease)** Physical activity may play an important role in the prevention of symptomatic gallstone disease in up to a third of all cases. Based on a limited number of studies, increasing exercise to 30 minutes of endurance-type training five times per week is recommended.[34,35] The loss of the gallbladder itself does not appear to have an impact on physical activity and exercise.
>
> The closed procedure (laparoscopic cholecystectomy) can be performed as outpatient (day) surgery without complications.
>
> The usual postoperative exercises (e.g., breathing, turning, coughing, wound splinting, compressive stockings, and leg exercises) for any surgical procedure apply, especially in case of complications. Early activity helps to prevent pooling of blood in the lower extremities and subsequent development of thrombosis. It also assists the return of intestinal motility; thus the client is encouraged to begin progressive movement and ambulation as soon as possible.

Complications of Cholelithiasis
Choledocholithiasis

Defined as calculi in the common bile duct, choledocholithiasis occurs in 5% to 10% of persons with gallstones and has the same cause and pathogenesis. Common duct stones usually originate in the gallbladder, but they also may form spontaneously in the common duct and can therefore occur after a person has had a cholecystectomy. When symptomatic, duct stones produce right upper quadrant pain, often with radiating pain to the shoulder and/or back (see previous discussion of clinical manifestations in the section on cholelithiasis).

Diagnosis is based on clinical picture and radiologic or endoscopic evidence of dilated bile ducts, ductal stones, or impaired bile flow. ERCP is very sensitive and provides the means to extract the stone during the procedure.[17] It consists of the introduction of radiopaque medium into the biliary system by percutaneous puncture of a bile duct to permit x-ray examination of the bile ducts. Laparoscopic transcystic bile duct exploration can detect and remove common bile duct stones in more than 90% of clients, and laparoscopic choledochotomy can be performed if transcystic bile duct exploration is not successful.

Complications of choledocholithiasis can be severe, including pancreatitis and cholangitis. Choledocholithiasis is currently the most common cause of pancreatitis in the world. Clients with mild pancreatitis typically will pass the stone spontaneously but require cholecystectomy to prevent another episode of pancreatitis (see the discussion of acute pancreatitis in this chapter and acute cholangitis in the next section).

> **12.21 Special Implications for the PTA: Choledocholithiasis** Special considerations for the PTA are the same as with the client with cholelithiasis. When choledocholithiasis occurs in the absence of a gallbladder (primary common duct stones), the presenting symptom can be shoulder pain. The PTA must be alert to this possibility in anyone who has had a cholecystectomy (see also the section on Jaundice in this chapter).

Acute Cholangitis

In 6% to 9% of cholelithiasis cases, obstruction and stasis of bile leads to a suppurative infection of the biliary tree, which is termed *acute cholangitis*. Acute cholangitis symptoms include those of cholelithiasis plus fever and jaundice. These three symptoms of pain, fever, and jaundice are referred to as *Charcot's triad* and are noted in 50% to 100% of people with cholangitis.

Reynolds' pentad (seen in only 14% of cases) includes Charcot's triad plus hypotension and mental confusion. The presence of Reynolds' pentad is an ominous sign, with mortality approaching 100% unless there is emergent decompression of the biliary tree. Acute cholangitis can be categorized into three stages: mild grade I (responds to medical therapy), moderate grade II (no organ dysfunction but not responding to initial medical treatment), and severe grade III (at least one new organ dysfunction).[79]

CT scans and ultrasonography can aid in distinguishing cholecystitis from cholangitis, as well as in identifying possible abscesses in the liver. EUS can identify stones in the common bile duct.

Treatment is given according to the grade of illness. Grade I is mild and can typically be treated with appropriate antibiotics with subsequent laparoscopic cholecystectomy. Clients with grade II disease are treated with antibiotics and early biliary drainage. Once the client's condition is stable, this therapy is followed by open or laparoscopic cholecystectomy. Stage III disease requires appropriate intensive care support with urgent endoscopic or percutaneous transhepatic biliary drainage once the person's hemodynamics are stable. Endoscopic biliary drainage can be achieved with either endoscopic nasobiliary drainage or tube stent placement.

A complication of cholangitis and biliary drainage includes biliary peritonitis. This can occur because of perforation of the gallbladder with leakage of bile into the abdominal cavity. This requires immediate cholecystectomy and/or drainage.

Cholecystitis

Cholecystitis is the most common complication of gallstone disease, with 700,000 cholecystectomies performed in the United States each year.[41] Cholecystitis, or inflammation of the gallbladder, may be acute or chronic and occurs most often as a result of impaction of gallstones in the cystic duct (see Fig. 12.6), causing obstruction to bile flow and painful distension of the gallbladder.

Acute cholecystitis caused by gallstones accounts for the majority of cases, and acalculous cholecystitis (i.e., gallstones not present) makes up the remaining 10%. Acute cholecystitis from stones is most common during middle age (particularly in women), whereas the acute acalculous form is most common among older adult men and carries a worse prognosis.

Some of the causes of acalculous cholecystitis include ischemia; chemicals that enter biliary secretions; motility disorders associated with drugs; infections with microorganisms, protozoa, and parasites; collagen disease; and allergic reactions. Acute acalculous cholecystitis is associated with a recent operation, trauma, burns, multisystem organ failure, and TPN.[31]

Gallbladder attacks are usually caused by gallbladder and/or cystic duct distention because the stone causes obstruction to the flow of bile. The increased pressure and stasis of bile lead to damage of the mucosa with subsequent release of inflammatory enzymes. Gallbladder inflammation causes prolonged pain characterized as steady right upper quadrant abdominal pain with abdominal tenderness, muscle guarding, and rebound pain. Upper quadrant pain often radiates to the upper back (between the scapulae) and into the right scapula or right shoulder. Accompanying GI symptoms usually include nausea, anorexia, and vomiting, and there may be signs of visceral or peritoneal inflammation (e.g., pain worse with movement and locally tender to touch).

Diagnosis is made on the basis of clinical history, examination, laboratory findings, and imaging. The white blood cell count is usually elevated (12,000 to 15,000 cells/mL). Total serum bilirubin, serum aminotransferase, and alkaline phosphatase levels are often elevated in the acute disease, but they are normal or minimally elevated in the chronic form. X-ray films of the abdomen show radiopaque gallstones in only 15% of cases. Abdominal ultrasonography often shows stones, thickened gallbladder wall, and pericholecystic fluid.

Biliary scintigraphy (hepatoiminodiacetic acid [HIDA] scan) is useful in demonstrating an obstructed cystic duct. Any stone detected can be removed immediately. The same information can be obtained by passing a thin needle into the abdominal wall through which dye is injected into the ducts. This procedure is called *percutaneous transhepatic cholangiography*.

Laparoscopic cholecystectomy (gallbladder resection) is the treatment and procedure of choice, because it is less invasive than an open procedure and healing and hospital time are reduced.[8] Prognosis for both acute and chronic cholecystitis is good with medical intervention. Acute attacks may resolve spontaneously, but recurrences are common, necessitating cholecystectomy. Complications can be serious and usually are associated with cholangitis. The mortality of acute cholecystitis is 5% to 10% for clients older than 60 with serious associated diseases.

An infrequent complication of laparoscopic cholecystectomy is injury to the bile duct (0.4% to 0.6% of all cases), causing leakage of bile into the abdomen. Symptoms postoperatively include fever, abdominal pain, ascites, nausea, elevated bilirubin levels, and rarely, frank jaundice. Intraperitoneal bile fluid collections can be seen on ultrasonography, CT scanning, or HIDA scan. ERCP can be used to detect the site of injury and treat the obstruction. Prompt repair requires less treatment than delayed diagnosis, which often requires a more complex reconstruction.

12.22 Special Implications for the PTA: Cholecystitis Special considerations for the PTA are the same as for the client with cholelithiasis (see also the section on Jaundice in this chapter). It is possible for a person to develop acholelithiasis cholecystitis, or inflammation of the gallbladder without gallstones. The PTA may see a clinical picture typical of gallbladder disease, including mid upper back or scapular pain (below or between the scapulae) or right shoulder pain associated with right upper quadrant abdominal pain. Close questioning may reveal accompanying associated GI signs and symptoms.

The person may have been evaluated for gallbladder disease, but ultrasonography does not always show small stones. Unless further and more elaborate testing has been performed to examine gallbladder function, the individual may end up in therapy for treatment of the affected musculoskeletal areas. Lack of results from therapy and/or progression of symptoms corresponding to progression of disease necessitates further medical follow-up.

Primary Biliary Cirrhosis

See the discussion of PBC earlier in this chapter, in the section on the liver.

Primary Sclerosing Cholangitis

Sclerosing cholangitis is a chronic cholestatic disease of unknown origin characterized by progressive destruction of intrahepatic and extrahepatic bile ducts. It has been linked to altered immunity, toxins, ischemia, and infectious agents in people who are genetically susceptible. Approximately two-thirds of cases occur in clients 20 to 40 years of age, and the incidence is believed to be rising; it is seen more commonly in men than in women (3:1 ratio). Eighty percent of clients with primary sclerosing cholangitis (PSC) also have inflammatory bowel disease, most frequently ulcerative colitis; yet only 5% of people with ulcerative colitis develop PSC.[49]

The inflammatory process associated with this disease results in hepatitis, fibrosis, and thickening of the ductal walls. This fibrosing process narrows and eventually obstructs the intrahepatic and extrahepatic bile ducts; the basic mechanisms of disease pathogenesis in PSC remain unknown.

Over 40% of people are asymptomatic at the time of diagnosis. With the progression of disease, symptomatic presentation usually includes pruritus and jaundice accompanied by abdominal pain, fatigue, anorexia, and weight loss. Complications associated with the disease include bacterial cholangitis, pigmented bile stones, steatorrhea, malabsorption, and metabolic bone disease; severe complications involve the development of cirrhosis and portal hypertension, and the risk of developing cholangiocarcinoma (10% to 30% lifetime risk), HCC, and colon cancer.[64]

Diagnosis is made on the basis of clinical, laboratory, and radiologic findings. The diagnosis is confirmed by ERCP or MRCP, which demonstrate the characteristic "beads on a string" appearance of the bile ducts (strictures and dilatation of the ducts). Liver biopsy is performed for staging rather than diagnosis. Causes of secondary sclerosing cholangitis (such as chronic bacterial cholangitis, biliary neoplasms, and drug-induced bile duct injury) should also be excluded.

Medical therapy is based on managing symptoms, correcting dominant strictures, and treating bacterial cholangitis when it occurs. UDCA improves biliary secretion and laboratory parameters but has not been shown to significantly improve survival. Currently, liver transplantation is the only therapeutic option for people with end-stage liver disease resulting from this disorder.[28,71] The results of transplantation for PSC are excellent, with 1-year survival rates of 90% to 97% and 5-year survival rates of 80% to 86%.[25] Optimal timing for liver transplantation is still not well defined, but the goal of therapy is to treat people as early as possible to prevent progression to the advanced stages of this disease or the development of cancer. Recurrence of PSC after liver transplantation occurs in about 4% of clients per year but appears to have little effect on survival.[26] Clients who develop cholangiocarcinoma and undergo liver transplant have a poor prognosis.[23]

12.23 Special Implications for the PTA: Primary Sclerosing Cholangitis Special considerations for the PTA are the same as for the client with cholelithiasis (see also in this chapter the section on Jaundice).

Neoplasms of the Gallbladder and Biliary Tract
Benign Neoplasms

Biliary neoplasms, whether benign or malignant, are rare. Most nonmalignant tumors of the gallbladder and biliary tree are polyps. These polyps are found incidentally by ultrasonography or during cholecystectomy (for gallstone symptoms). Because polyps that are 1 cm or larger have a greater potential to be malignant, treatment consists of cholecystectomy.

Malignant Neoplasms

Cancers of the biliary tract are divided into gallbladder cancer, cholangiocarcinoma, and adenocarcinoma of the ampulla of Vater. *Gallbladder cancer* is the sixth most common GI cancer, causing about 2800 deaths per year, and it is the most common cancer of the biliary tree.[29]

Risk factors for gallbladder cancer include age (the elderly are most often affected), female gender (women are three times more likely to develop gallbladder cancer), and gallstones (80% to 90% of people with gallbladder cancer have gallstones). Other factors include obesity, gallbladder wall calcification (porcelain gallbladder), chronic typhoid carriers, and gallbladder polyps. However, despite these known risk factors, many cases of gallbladder cancer occur in people without obvious risk factors.[14]

Adenocarcinoma of the gallbladder is the most common type of gallbladder cancer (over 80% of cases), with squamous cell and small cell carcinoma accounting for the remaining cases. Clinical presentation of malignant gallbladder diseases depends on the stage of disease and the location and extent of the lesion, but it is often insidious. By the time the tumor becomes symptomatic, it is often incurable.

Symptoms most often mimic gallstone disease (acute and chronic cholecystitis). Right upper quadrant pain radiating to the upper back is the most common symptom (80% of cases), with weight loss, progressive (obstructive) jaundice (30% of cases), anorexia, fatty food intolerance, and right upper quadrant mass (in advanced disease).

Pruritus and skin excoriations are commonly associated with the presence of jaundice. Gallbladder cancer is usually found either as an incidental finding at surgery, as a suspected tumor (because of symptoms) with the prospect of resectability, or as advanced unresectable disease.

Ultrasonography is the most common initial test for diagnosis, although CT and MRI can be used to detect the extent of disease. CT scans and cholangiography are used preoperatively to determine resectability of the tumor. Disease can be metastatic to lungs and bones and usually involves the liver. Simple cholecystectomy is appropriate only for stages 0 and 1; the remainder require extended or radical cholecystectomy (with removal of lymph nodes, adjacent hepatic tissue, and/or portions of the extrahepatic biliary tree).[16]

For clients with unresectable disease and jaundice, a biliary bypass (hepaticojejunostomy) can be performed to relieve obstruction. Overall prognosis is poor, with a 5-year survival rate of 5% to 10%. Cures are obtained only when all detectable tumor is surgically removed in the early stages of the disease. Stage I tumors have an overall survival rate of 100% and nearly 50% for node-negative stage II and stage III disease. Chemotherapy and radiation provide little benefit.

Cholangiocarcinoma, or cancer of the bile ducts, is a rare tumor. Cholangiocarcinoma occurs more frequently in people aged 50 to 70 years. Affected persons most often have jaundice secondary to obstruction of the bile duct (90% of cases) with associated acholic stool (light colored) and pruritus. Other symptoms include weight loss, anorexia, and fatigue.

On physical examination, hepatomegaly or a palpable gallbladder (Courvoisier's sign) may be present with advanced disease. Laboratory values are consistent with biliary obstruction. CT scans or MRCP can be used to detect the disease, and ERCP with brushings or biopsy may be diagnostic and relieve obstruction (a presurgical histologic diagnosis is often difficult to obtain).

Resectability is determined by a lack of metastatic disease, local invasion of the vascular structures around the liver, or the ability to completely resect the tumor. Laparoscopic surgery may be done initially to determine whether metastatic disease is present (metastatic disease is found in 25% of cases that were felt to be resectable after imaging studies). A pancreaticoduodenectomy is performed for tumors in the distal portion of the biliary tree. However, because most cholangiocarcinomas are near the liver and large vessels, surgery must be tailored to the location of the tumor, with 35% actually resectable.

Radiation therapy may be of some survival benefit. Endoscopic or percutaneous stent placement for biliary decompression often relieves symptoms for clients with nonresectable disease. Cure is obtained by complete surgical resection of tumor. Survival rates are determined by extent of disease and involvement with large vessels and structures around the liver.

Adenocarcinoma of the ampulla of Vater is a rare, distal bile duct tumor. The ampulla of Vater is a small area (about 1 cm in diameter) located at the common opening of the pancreatic and bile ducts into the duodenum (see Fig. 12.6). This cancer has an incidence of 2.9 cases per million people in the United States.

Because of its location, this tumor causes obstructive jaundice early in the disease process (80% of cases). Abdominal pain (50%), weight loss (75%), and occult GI bleeding (30%) are other common symptoms.

Diagnosis is made by EUS, CT scan, and ERCP. Surgical resection, typically a pancreaticoduodenectomy, is the treatment of choice, with no clear benefit to chemoradiation. Resection is feasible in over 85% of cases with a 5-year survival of up to 45%.[13,65]

12.24 Special Implications for the PTA: Gallbladder and Biliary Tract Neoplasm Special considerations for the PTA are the same as for the client with cholelithiasis (see also in this chapter the section on Jaundice).

REFERENCES/SUGGESTED READINGS

To enhance this text and add value for the reader, references and suggested readings are included on the companion Evolve site that accompanies this textbook. The reader can view the source and access it online whenever possible.

Introduction to Pathology of the Musculoskeletal System

VOCAB BUILDERS

Chemotaxis	Pavementing	Resistance training
Endurance training	Phagocytosis	Sarcopenia
Margination	Psychoneuroimmunology	Strength training

The new century, characterized by increasing individual participation in high-speed travel, complex industry, and competitive and recreational sports, also is marked by significant increases in primary musculoskeletal system injury and conditions that have enormous impact on society.

The fact that the skeletal system, with its associated soft tissues, provides a protective covering for important structures such as the brain and heart and essentially makes up the limbs puts this system at risk for traumatic and repetitive insults and injuries (Box 13.1).

More than ever, the gap between science and clinical applications of therapeutic exercise has been narrowed. New diagnostic technology, the genome project, and a new branch of study called genomics are providing an increasing understanding of the molecular basis for disease and injury. This new knowledge is changing the approach for health care intervention in many areas, including the musculoskeletal system.

The ability to document the influence and effects of exercise at the molecular and cellular levels has resulted in early functional rehabilitation, preventive exercise programs, and the use of exercise as first-line intervention for many conditions. Maintaining good musculoskeletal health and recovering quickly from musculoskeletal injury or disease contribute to an individual's overall health, welfare, and quality of life.

More than 50% of injuries in the United States are to the musculoskeletal system; 28.6 million Americans incur musculoskeletal injuries each year. Fractures, sprains and strains, and dislocations account for nearly half of all musculoskeletal injuries.

Annually, an estimated 7 million Americans receive medical attention for sports-related injuries.[27] Children younger than 15 years old account for more than 3.8 million sports-related injuries in the United States each year. Violence-related sports and recreational injuries (e.g., being pushed, hit) are increasing among children and adolescents.[26]

BOX 13.1   Common Musculoskeletal Disorders

- Fracture
- Dislocation
- Subluxation
- Contusion
- Hematoma
- Repetitive overuse, microtrauma
- Strain, sprain
- Degenerative disease

Severe cerebral palsy and other developmental disorders are more common than ever before, because many infants with these complications at birth now survive and live into adulthood. The age span of humans has become progressively longer, with a variety of accompanying age-related conditions such as osteoporosis and degenerative joint or disk disease. Arthritis is the leading chronic condition reported by Americans age 65 years and older.[75]

In addition, the musculoskeletal system often is confronted with immobilization secondary to major illness or injury, bed rest, or casting or splinting of a specific body region. It reacts quickly to the lack of mechanical stress and normal loading (immobilization) in ways that may adversely affect recovery and rehabilitation.

The physical and physiologic responses of the musculoskeletal tissues and resultant deterioration occur within days but take many months to reverse. In fact, 3 weeks of bed rest has a more profound impact on physical work capacity than three decades of aging.[36,43]

Like all other body systems, the musculoskeletal system does not function in isolation. Therefore primary disease of the musculoskeletal system can significantly affect other body systems and vice versa. In addition, certain diseases are systemic, meaning that all body systems, including the musculoskeletal system, can be involved to some degree. The challenge to develop an effective rehabilitation program is heightened when one is faced with complex, multisystem disorders.

The purpose of this section is to provide an overview of the musculoskeletal system, including the biologic response to trauma and examples of how primary diseases in other organs affect the musculoskeletal system, and vice versa, and to begin to examine the local (musculoskeletal) and systemic (e.g., immune system, endocrine system, gastrointestinal system) effects of exercise. An approach that assesses all the systems and considers underlying pathology is essential when identifying the source of dysfunction.

ADVANCES IN MUSCULOSKELETAL BIOTECHNOLOGY

Over the past 10 years, advances in molecular biology techniques have extended the potential for understanding musculoskeletal disorders from the microscopic (histologic) level down to the molecular level of gene expression within individual cells. These advances are initiating new avenues of research and, ultimately, novel clinical interventions.[6]

Orthopedic surgery has been revolutionized by tissue engineering, including biologic manipulation for spinal fusion[35]; synthetic skeletal substitute materials[13]; preservation and restoration, transplantation, or fabrication of avascular tissue

(e.g., meniscus, articular cartilage)[69,77]; and joint restoration instead of joint replacement.[52]

Other technologic advances are under scientific investigation, such as bone implants to stimulate bone development and prevent limb loss associated with cancer[16,86]; injectable bone substitute that eliminates the need for bone grafts, strengthens osteoporotic vertebral bodies, or heals compression and nonunion fractures[32,35]; synthetic muscle regeneration; and new materials and plastics making it possible to replace spinal disks or extend joint replacements by an additional 10 years or more.

Recently the influence of biopsychosocial–spiritual stress on the physical body has come to the forefront of research in a field of study referred to as *psychoneuroimmunology*. Approximately 40% to 80% of adults in primary care report only their physical symptoms (including musculoskeletal manifestations), leaving a large portion of clients with significant psychologic distress undiagnosed.[54]

Gender discrepancies in rates of injuries and muscle mass response to *strength training* or deconditioning are also under investigation.[12,29] Differences in ligamentous laxity, muscle strength, endurance, muscle reaction time, and muscle recruitment time in males versus females and athletes versus nonathletes may provide additional important information for prevention and rehabilitation of musculoskeletal injuries.[59]

Women double their rate of injury during ovulation, when levels of estrogen are the highest. Training and conditioning differently during different times of the month may help protect women from injury.[23,30,50] The effectiveness of neuromuscular and proprioceptive training in preventing anterior cruciate ligament injuries in female athletes has been demonstrated.[61]

Men increase their muscle volume about twice as much in response to strength training compared with women; men also experience larger losses in response to detraining than women.[53,62]

BIOLOGIC RESPONSE TO TRAUMA

The immediate biologic response to trauma is a generalized inflammatory reaction regardless of what tissue is damaged or the nature of the injury.[8] The response is marked by vascular, chemical, and cellular events, with the ultimate purpose being to prepare the area for repair. The primary objective of the vascular response to injury is to mobilize and transport the body's defenses (white blood cells).

Vasoconstriction occurs initially along with reduced fluid flow through the injured area, resulting from development of fibrinogen clots in the tissue spaces and lymphatic channels (which prevents the spread of bacteria and toxins). Vasoconstriction allows for the white blood cells to migrate to the periphery of the vessel in a process called *margination*. These white blood cells eventually adhere to the walls of the damaged capillary, a process called *pavementing*.

Shortly after the injury and vasoconstriction, vasodilation of the local blood vessels occurs. The increased blood flow is accompanied by increased permeability of the small blood vessels. The permeability changes are secondary to direct trauma to the vessels and to the presence of chemical mediators such as histamines, serotonin, and bradykinins.

The increased permeability allows for the white blood cells to squeeze through the blood vessel wall. This process is called *diapedesis*. The increased blood volume and vessel permeability also result in a significant transfer of fluid into the injured area.

The fluid shift occurs because of the heightened intravascular hydrostatic pressure and the altered osmotic pressure gradient (as larger molecules escape into the tissues).

Once beyond the blood vessel walls the white blood cells are guided to the site of injury by a process called *chemotaxis.* Numerous elements of the damaged tissue (i.e., bacterial toxins and tissue polysaccharides) draw the white blood cells to the area of highest concentration of these elements.

Upon arriving at the site of damage, the white blood cells begin to clean up the area by the process of *phagocytosis.* The neutrophils, monocytes, and macrophages recognize, engulf, and digest debris, necrotic tissue, red blood cells, and proteins to prepare the area for repair and growth of new tissue.

Clinical findings of acute inflammation include increased muscle tone or spasm and loss of function. Movements of the involved area are generally slow and guarded. Cyriax described two components of passive movement testing that also suggest acute inflammation: a spasm end feel and pain reported before resistance is noted by the practitioner as the limb is moved passively.[28]

If surgery is not indicated, the most effective interventions for acute inflammation are pharmacotherapy and physical therapy. Salicylates (except aspirin) and nonsteroidal antiinflammatory drugs are the most commonly administered medications for pain and inflammation.

The antiinflammatory effect is attained chiefly by inhibition of the biosynthesis of prostaglandins. Other antiinflammatory mechanisms include decreasing the release of chemical mediators from granulocytes, basophils, and mast cells; decreasing the sensitivity of vessels to bradykinin and histamine; and reversing or controlling the degree of vasodilation.

13.1 Special Implications for the PTA: Biologic Response to Trauma See the section on Specific Tissue or Organ Repair in Chapter 3 and 3.6 Special Implications for the PTA: Specific Tissue or Organ Repair.

THE MUSCULOSKELETAL SYSTEM THROUGHOUT THE LIFE SPAN

There has recently been an increased emphasis on research for childhood and adolescent exercise in part because of the rising rate of childhood obesity.[67] There has been a false belief that children should not exercise intensely or strength train. This has been disproven and in fact it has been shown that children older than age 8 years can safely exercise and strength train with sufficient supervision.[9]

Much has been written about the effects of aging on the musculoskeletal system, especially in light of exercise as an effective intervention for so many diseases and conditions. Participation in a regular exercise program is an effective intervention to reduce or prevent a number of functional declines associated with aging.

Endurance training can help maintain and improve various aspects of cardiovascular function (as measured by maximal VO_2, cardiac output, and arteriovenous oxygen difference) and enhance submaximal performance. In the case of children, they are not smaller versions of adults.[9] They have different physiologic responses to exercise, different musculoskeletal structure, and thus are susceptible to different injuries.

There are many physiologic differences between the adult and the child during exercise. The child has a smaller heart size than the adult; thus there is a smaller stroke volume, or in simple terms a smaller heart pushes less blood. A child has a higher heart rate during submaximal and maximal exercise. This increased heart rate offsets some of the decreased stroke volume but not enough to compensate for the size difference.[95] Because of these factors, the child cannot exercise as efficiently as an adult can and must be watched very closely. However, exercise for children should be encouraged with the proper supervision.

Importantly, reductions in risk factors associated with disease states (e.g., heart disease, diabetes) improve health status and contribute to an increase in life expectancy.[10,11]

A common question among parents is when and if children can safely begin strength training. There is no exact chronological age when this should begin. Instead, strength training can begin when the child is able to understand and follow detailed instructions on proper technique and progression of the program.[40]

Strength training for adults helps offset the loss in muscle mass and strength typically associated with normal aging. Additional benefits from regular exercise include improved bone health and therefore reduction in risk for osteoporosis; improved postural stability, which reduces the risk of falling and associated injuries and fractures; and increased flexibility and range of motion.

Although not as abundant, evidence also suggests that involvement in regular exercise also can provide a number of psychologic benefits related to preserved cognitive function, alleviation of depressive symptoms and behavior, and an improved concept of personal control and self-determination.[11,12]

Sports-related injuries among people born between 1946 and 1964, now referred to as "boomeritis,"[7] are on the increase as older adults continue to participate actively in sports of all kinds. Physical therapist assistants (PTAs) can provide valuable preventive education regarding the aging process as it relates to the musculoskeletal system and exercise. This presentation is a brief summary of the findings to date; more in-depth discussion is available.[33,47,68,87]

Muscle
Sarcopenia

Overview and definition. Age-related loss in muscle mass, strength, and endurance accompanied by changes in the metabolic quality of skeletal muscle is termed *sarcopenia.* Sarcopenia involves both the reduction of muscle mass and/or function as well as the impairment of the muscle's capacity to regenerate.[34]

Muscle mass is lost at a rate of 4% to 6% per decade starting at age 40 years in women and age 60 years in men.[51] The greatest decline in both men and women occurs with inactivity, acute illness, and after age 70 years, at which time the mean loss of muscle mass has been measured as 1% per year.[90] At all ages, females appear to be more vulnerable to loss of lean tissue than males; however, in men and women, muscle strength can be maintained through exercise well into the eighth decade.[42,55]

Etiology. The etiology is multifactorial, involving changes in muscle metabolism, endocrine changes (e.g., low testosterone levels), nutritional factors, and mitochondrial and genetic factors.[66,71] It remains uncertain how much age-related loss of muscle function is an inevitable consequence of aging, nutritional status, or dysregulation of neurologic, hormonal, and/or immunologic homeostasis.

Likewise, it remains unknown how much sarcopenia reflects a decline in physical activity and exercise capacity, and as part of a broad cycle, whether this decline is a function of age, lack of motivation, decline in neuromuscular function from disuse or loss of motoneurons, age-associated decreases in metabolism, or other factors such as anemia or high levels of inflammatory markers.[22,91]

Pathogenesis. The identification of the molecular chain able to reverse sarcopenia is a major goal of studies on human aging. Animal studies suggest that myofiber regeneration in sarcopenic muscle is halted at the point in which reinnervation is critical for the final differentiation into mature myofibers.

Combined evidence points to a decreased capacity among motoneurons to innervate regenerating fibers. There are also changes observed in the expression of several cytokines known to play important roles in establishing and maintaining neuromuscular connectivity during development and adulthood.[37]

The decline in muscle mass previously thought to be the result of proteins breaking down faster than they were being created and restored may be linked instead to other potential reasons such as diet and nutrition, the body's ability to use protein from food, and hormonal changes.[89] For example, inadequate dietary intake of protein also results in loss of skeletal muscle mass; the current recommended daily allowance may not be adequate to completely meet the metabolic and physiologic needs of virtually all older people.[20]

Loss of muscle function appears to be caused by decreased total fibers, decreased muscle fiber size, impaired excitation–contraction coupling mechanism, or decreased high-threshold motor units. For example, at midthigh, muscle accounts for 90% of the cross-sectional area in young, active adults. However, this same measurement taken in older adults is only 30%.[43]

Effects of sarcopenia. From a clinical perspective, loss in muscle mass accounts for the age-associated decreases in basal metabolic rate contributing to metabolic disorders such as type 2 diabetes mellitus and osteoporosis and decreases in muscle strength and activity levels, which, in turn, are the cause of the decreased energy requirements of the aging adult.[39]

Loss of muscle mass (i.e., atrophy) and definition and loss of muscle function resulting in subsequent muscle weakness are implicated in difficulty accomplishing activities of daily living (e.g., rising from a chair, climbing stairs, carrying groceries), slow gait speed, impaired balance reactions, and increased risk of vertebral compression (and other) fractures. There does not appear to be a relationship between age-related sarcopenia and the bone mass loss also prevalent in the same age group.[24]

Aging workers notice increasing difficulty continuing a job they have previously performed without trouble. Slowing down of reflexes and coordination combined with loss of muscle mass and strength can make it difficult to remain in the same job or train for a new job.

By age 65 years, changes in the muscle mass, muscle weakness, and decreased levels of physical activity are evident in the increased numbers of falls and injuries. Injuries in an aging musculoskeletal system take longer to recover from, contributing to further physical deconditioning, potentially creating additional comorbidities.

Exercise and sarcopenia. Appropriate exercise can alter, slow, or even partially reverse some of the age-related physiologic changes that occur in skeletal muscle, including sarcopenia.

Skeletal muscle adaptations in response to strength training in older adults occur with progressive *resistance training* or high-intensity training (e.g., two to six sets of eight repetitions at approximately 80% of the person's one-repetition maximum).[92]

Understanding muscle fiber types and the impact of physical therapy interventions on muscle fiber type conversions is becoming increasingly important in today's evidence-based practice. An excellent review of these concepts is available.[76] We know, for example, that age-related changes can be counteracted and physical function improved by increased physical activity of a resistive nature.[84] Mechanical load on muscle can increase the cross-sectional area of the remaining fibers but does not restore fiber numbers characteristic of young muscle.[1]

Strength training has been shown to improve insulin-stimulated glucose uptake both in healthy older adults and in individuals with diabetes. Strength training also improves muscle strength in healthy adults and in those who have chronic diseases. Increased strength leads to improved function and a decreased risk for falls, injuries, and fractures.[31] These results also promote increased independence and improved quality of life.[97]

Aging muscle may be resistant to insulin-like growth factor I (IGF-I), which promotes myoblast proliferation, differentiation, and protein assimilation in muscle through multiple signaling mechanisms. Exercise may be able to help aging muscle that is resistant to IGF-I by reversing this effect.[1]

High-resistance training exercise has been of significant benefit to sarcopenia.[66] In fact, after 6 months of exercise training, resistance exercise has been shown to reverse mitochondrial dysfunction for genes that are affected by both age and exercise.[65] Combinations of resistance exercise, aerobic exercise, and stretching have shown beneficial effects on sarcopenia, but the optimum regimen for older adults remains unclear.[46,57]

Many older adults would like to be more physically active but do not have the experience or knowledge to develop and build up an exercise regimen without appropriate supervision such as the PTA can offer. Others have participated in athletics throughout adulthood and continue to train and remain in good health. The therapist can help educate older adults about the importance of maintaining strength training and endurance with the emphasis on strength, which decreases more rapidly than endurance.[44]

Joint and Connective Tissue

At the same time as changes in bone and muscle are taking place, a progressive loss of flexibility and changes in connective tissue starts contributing to an increased incidence of joint problems beginning in middle age and progressing through old age. Loss of flexibility also contributes to increased risk of falls and other injuries. Connective or periarticular tissue, including fascia, articular cartilage, ligaments, and tendons, becomes less extensible, with resultant decreased active and passive range of motion. Conversely, studies have shown that weight bearing and gentle shear forces stimulate and improve the health of all of the previously mentioned tissues throughout the life span.[5]

Increased Stiffness and Decreased Flexibility

It is not clear whether this decreased flexibility occurs as a consequence of biologic aging, inactivity, degenerative disease, adhesion molecules, or a combination of all these factors.[93] One possible cause is related to fibrinogen, produced in the liver and converted to fibrin, which constantly circulates throughout the body to serve as a clotting mechanism (with superglue-like effects) should an injury occur.

Fibrinogen normally leaks out of the vasculature in small amounts into the intracellular space and then adheres to cellular structures, causing microfibrinous adhesions among the cells. Activity and movement normally break down these adhesions along with macrophagic activity to dissolve unused fibrinogen and fibrin.

In the aging process, less fibrinogen and fewer (less efficient) macrophages are available. These factors, along with less physical activity and movement, allow these microadhesions to accumulate in muscle and fascia, resulting in an increased sense of overall stiffness.

Others have shown that aging collagen has increased cross-links between molecules, increasing the mechanical stability of collagen but also contributing to increased tissue stiffness.[73] Increased collagen content in the endomysium of animal intramuscular connective tissue has been shown to correlate with increased stiffness of the whole muscle.[4]

Regardless of the exact physiologic mechanism for the gradual increase in stiffness associated with aging, physical activity has an important influence in alleviating stiffness. Further research is needed to understand how and what kind of physical activity influences or possibly prevents stiffness.[68,94]

Changes in Articular Cartilage

Articular cartilage, which cushions the subchondral bone and provides a low-friction surface necessary for free movement, contains few cells, is aneural and avascular, and often starts to break down with increasing age.[15,33] The main proteoglycan in articular cartilage (aggrecan) binds with hyaluronan to form massive aggregates that expand the collagen matrix of the tissue to provide it with its compressive and tensile strength.

With age, proteoglycan aggregation is reduced and smaller proteoglycans are synthesized with an increase in keratin sulfate and reduced chondroitin sulfate content. The hydrophilic proteoglycans have been shown to become shorter in aged tissue and therefore lose their ability to hold water in the matrix.[19] Dehydrated articular cartilage may have a reduced ability to dissipate forces across the joint.[68]

Degeneration and thinning or damage of articular cartilage with loss of water content contributes to a significant increase in incidence of osteoarthritis with aging. By age 60 years, as much as 80% of the population shows evidence of such changes, although only about 15% present with symptoms.[93]

Knowledge of these changes has resulted in new interventions such as glucosamine-chondroitin supplementation and joint viscosupplementation for osteoarthritis. With or without a symptomatic presentation, educating adults about the importance of joint protection is an important role of the PTA.

Tendons

Tendons exhibit a lower metabolic activity associated with aging that has implications for injury and healing in the aging population.[2,3] Also, an age-related decrease occurs in the tensile strength of some tendons and ligament–bone interfaces, and loss of integrity of some joint capsules occurs. For example, rotator cuff impairment with loss of joint function is common in older people. A gradual loss of connective tissue resistance to calcium crystal formation occurs in the older adult, leading to an increase in the incidence of crystal-related arthropathies[33] (e.g., gout, pseudogout).

Proprioception.   Joint proprioception, described as sensations generated to increase awareness of joint orientation at rest and in motion, declines with age, especially in the knee and ankle.[70] Joint proprioception provides both a sense of joint position and sense of joint movement. Mechanoreceptors located in the joint capsules, ligaments, muscles, tendons, and skin provide the sensory information needed for a sense of joint position.

The presence of osteoarthritis seems to make joint proprioception even worse, although it is unclear whether impaired joint sense promotes arthritic change or whether arthritic change causes the sensory loss. There is some evidence that proprioception may be reduced before the development of joint degenerative change.[56]

Bone

The skeletal system serves numerous functions in the human body throughout the life span. Bone is the primary storage depot for calcium, phosphate, sodium, and magnesium. Bones are the hosts for the hemopoietic bone marrow (growth and development of elements of blood). They also serve important mechanical functions, such as protection of components of the nervous system and visceral organs; provision of rigid internal support for the trunk and extremities; and provision of attachment sites for numerous soft tissue structures.

Bone is remodeling constantly throughout life. Although osteoclasts resorb the existing bone, new bone is being formed by osteoblasts. Three primary influences affect this remodeling process: (1) mechanical stresses; (2) calcium and phosphate levels in the extracellular fluid; and (3) hormonal levels of parathyroid hormone, calcitonin, vitamin D, cortisol, growth hormone, thyroid hormone, and sex hormones.

The osteology of a child varies from the adult in many ways. The bone is more porous and is more susceptible to compression and greenstick fractures. Another injury unique to the child is a physeal or growth plate fracture. A growth plate is in a long bone most commonly found near a joint. These growth plates provide for axial and circumferential growth of bones. These areas are the weakest point around joints; thus injuries usually occur in the growth plate not the joint.[58]

Aging adversely affects the "quality" of human bone material, both the stiffness and strength of bone and its "toughness." These effects are caused by factors such as architectural changes, compositional changes, physiochemical changes, changes at the micromechanical level, and the degree of prior in vivo microdamage.[98]

The bone density of the skeleton reaches its peak during an adult's twenties and remains stable for about two decades. Around the time of menopause for women, resorption (the process by which bone is broken down and calcium is released from the bone for use by the body), increases, whereas formation (the bone-rebuilding process), fails to keep pace. This imbalance, which is triggered by declining estrogen levels, leads to rapid bone loss during the first decade after menopause, with moderate bone loss thereafter. In women with low peak bone mass, it can result in osteoporosis with increased potential for vertebral, hip, or other fracture.[48]

The same progressive decrease of calcium can occur in men, only at a reduced and slowed rate. In women, loss occurs at a rate of approximately 1% per year after age 35 years, with acceleration especially during the first 5 years after menopause. Men lose 10% to 15% by age 70 years and 20% by age 80 years.

In women the loss is greater, amounting to about 20% by age 65 years and 30% by age 80 years.[5,81] In both genders, by age 65 years, bone loss generally has progressed to a point in which the older adult is predisposed to fractures, especially when other comorbidities exist (e.g., diabetes, balance or vestibular impairment, renal impairment, immobilization).[93]

THE MUSCULOSKELETAL SYSTEM AND EXERCISE

There are two general classifications of musculoskeletal differences between children and adults: bone and muscle. The differences in these structures at varying maturation stages leads to a separate set of common injury patterns.[67]

By the year 2030, 70 million people in the United States will be age 65 years or older; people age 85 years and older will be the fastest growing segment of the population. As more individuals live longer, the importance of exercise and physical activity to improve health, functional capacity, quality of life, and independence will increase in this country.[10,11]

Strength training is considered a promising intervention for reversing the loss of muscle function and the deterioration of muscle structure that is associated with advanced age. The capacity of older men and women to adapt to increased levels of physical activity is preserved, even in the most aged adult.[18,88]

For example, the relationship of exercise to insulin action is important because increased body fat (especially abdominal obesity) and decreased exercise is linked to the increased incidence of diabetes in the aging population.

Regularly performed exercise can affect nutritional needs and functional capacity in the older adult, contributing a preventive effect.[37] Combining knowledge of exercise principles with nutrition is important for all people but especially in the older adult population; disabled individuals; athletes; adolescents; and anyone with a medical condition, disease, or illness.[96]

Muscle

Typical human muscles contain two different types of muscle fibers based on speeds of shortening and morphologic differences. Type I muscle fibers, known also as *slow oxidative* or *slow twitch* fibers, are the fatigue-resistant red fibers. The red color is the result of high amounts of myoglobin and a high capillary content. Greater myoglobin and capillary content contributes to the increased oxidative capacity of red muscles compared with white muscles (type II).[76]

Type II fibers, or fast twitch fibers, have two different characteristics. Type IIa, which are bigger and faster than type I, are also fatigue resistant and are referred to as *fast oxidative fibers*. Type IIb fibers are the classic white fibers, which lack aerobic enzymes and therefore fatigue rapidly. Each muscle contains type I and type II fibers in various proportions.

The basic distribution of fiber types is thought to be an inherited characteristic. Although distribution varies among individuals, the average ratio of fast to slow twitch fibers is 50:50. Individuals trained in endurance activities usually have a higher proportion of slow-twitch fibers, and those trained for high-intensity, high-speed activities have more high-twitch fibers. The oxidative capacity of both fibers can be increased greatly by endurance training, but the glycolic capacity and contractile properties are not modified.[78]

Muscle function can be described in terms of strength and endurance, which is also how we focus the training of muscle.

Strength can be defined in several ways depending on the specific method of measurement but is usually related to the diameter of the muscle fiber, which has been consistently shown to increase with strength training.

Endurance can be measured as the ability to work over time; local muscle endurance is distinguished from general body endurance as the ability of an isolated muscle group to continue a prescribed task rather than the ability to continue an activity such as running, swimming, or jogging for an extended period of time.[78]

As a result of specificity of training and the need for maintaining muscular strength and endurance, and flexibility of the major muscle groups, a well-rounded training program including aerobic and resistance (strength and endurance) training and flexibility exercises is recommended.

Strength Training

Strength training refers to exercise directed at improving the maximum force-generating capacity of muscle. A key difference in the response to exercise for the younger age group is the effect on muscle mass. It has been shown that a limited amount of weight lifting improves strength in the child muscle, but there is little gain in muscle mass. The strength increase is from improved coordination and neuromuscular recruitment. Strength training can assist the normal muscle development occurring throughout puberty. The recommended weight-lifting program for adolescents is low weight–high repetition activity because of the decreased muscle mass. This is especially true in the beginning stages of weight lifting. Proper lifting technique is the key to avoiding injuries in the adolescent population.[67]

There is evidence that strength training has a positive effect on aging skeletal muscle.[92] Collectively, studies indicate that strength training in the older adult (1) produces substantial increases in the strength, mass, power, and quality of skeletal muscle; (2) can increase endurance performance; (3) normalizes blood pressure in those with high-normal values; (4) reduces insulin resistance; (5) decreases both total and intraabdominal fat; (6) increases resting metabolic rate in older men; (7) prevents the loss of bone mineral density with age; (8) reduces risk factors for falls; and (9) may reduce pain and improve function in those with osteoarthritis in the knee.

Significant strength gains are possible in all populations, including older adults, when exposed to an adequate strength training program. Strength gains occur from enhanced neuromuscular activation over the initial 8 weeks and from increased fiber density and hypertrophy during subsequent weeks.[60]

Considerable evidence exists that sarcopenia can be prevented, reduced, and reversed with prescriptive strength training programs that emphasize gradual, progressive, high-intensity resistance exercises (e.g., high load–low repetition) for the upper and lower extremities.[14,74,76]

Resistance training significantly increases muscle size and increases energy requirements and insulin action in adults older than age 65 years. A program of once- or twice-weekly resistance exercise (performed at a level described as "reasonably difficult" or "difficult") achieves muscle strength gains similar to 3 days/week training in older adults and is associated with improved neuromuscular performance.[85] The goal is to design a program for each individual to provide the proper amount of physical activity and exercise to attain maximal benefit at the lowest risk.[10,11]

Strength training does not increase maximal oxygen uptake beyond normal (i.e., individuals attain the same maximal VO_2 before and after training).[63,64] In postmenopausal women, muscle performance, muscle mass, and muscle composition are improved by hormone replacement therapy (HRT). The beneficial effects of HRT combined with high-impact physical training appear to exceed those of HRT alone.[79,80,83] Long-term results remain under investigation.

Endurance Training

Endurance training refers to exercise directed at improving stamina (the duration that a person can maintain strenuous activity) and aerobic capacity (VO_{2max}). Endurance training places a high metabolic demand on the muscle and will increase the oxidative capacity of all muscle fiber types.[76]

Endurance exercise can reverse the decline in physical conditioning associated with aging. An endurance training program using relatively modest intensity of training can reverse 100% of the loss of cardiovascular capacity, returning some healthy older adults to levels of aerobic power present in young adulthood. Even an older person who has failed to maintain fitness over time can benefit from an exercise program.[63,64]

In middle-aged adults, the mechanism responsible for decline in cardiovascular capacity appears to be a reduced plasticity of heart muscle; improved aerobic power after training appears to be directly related to peripheral oxygen extraction (i.e., the muscles' ability to take up and use oxygen).

Aerobic exercise results in improvements in functional capacity and reduced risk of developing type 2 diabetes mellitus in the older adult. Aerobic endurance training for fewer than 2 days/week at less than 40% to 50% VO_2 and for less than 10 minutes is generally not a sufficient stimulus for developing and maintaining cardiovascular fitness in healthy adults.

Joint

As discussed earlier, tendons, ligaments, and muscles around the joints have less water content, resulting in increased stiffness, with increasing age. Articular cartilage has less tensile strength and biochemical composition changes, often leading to osteoarthritis.[72]

Joint changes with deterioration of subchondral bone and atrophy of the synovium also can occur. Well-regulated exercise does not produce or exacerbate joint symptoms and actually may improve them.[25] This concept is discussed in greater detail in the section on osteoarthritis.

Bone

The relationship between bone mass and activity is well established. Complete immobilization and weightlessness result in rapid onset of accelerated bone resorption; bone mass recovers when activity resumes, but whether bone loss is completely reversible is unknown. Immobilization also leads to changes in collagen, ligaments, and the musculotendinous junction at the joint, causing reduced range of motion. Evidence has shown that these same concepts apply to children as well. An increased activity level is associated with increased bone mineral density and positive changes in collagen and ligaments.[67]

Osteopenia, osteomalacia, and osteoporosis affect the mineralization of bone matrix and can impact the bone health of the aging adult. Older adults are at greater risk for osteoporosis-related fractures, both age related for all adults and postmenopause related for women.

Specific Exercise Guidelines

Resistance training is an integral component in the comprehensive health program promoted by major health organizations such as the American Heart Association, American College of Sports Medicine, Surgeon General's office, and others. Population-specific guidelines have been published. For children, as stated earlier, the most important concept is doing the exercise with proper technique and supervision. Once the technique has been perfected, 8 to 15 repetitions should be performed. The weight should then be increased in small increments. The weight should not be increased until 8 to 15 repetitions can be performed with good technique. This is why supervision is essential for adolescent strength training. Strength training should be done two to three times per week. There is evidence showing that there is no benefit to strength training more than four times per week.[95]

The American Academy of Pediatrics Committee on Sports Medicine and Fitness[1] has a list of recommendations that should be followed:

a. A thorough medical examination should be completed before a strength training program begins.
b. If general health benefits are the goal, aerobic exercise should be included.
c. Warm-up and cool-down periods are an essential part of the strength training regimen.
d. Specific strength training exercise should be learned with no weight to perfect the technique. Small increments of weight should be added in 8 to 15 repetition sets.
e. All muscle groups should be included, and the activities should include full range of motion.
f. If any sign of injury occurs, all activity should stop and a thorough medical examination should be completed.[67]

Current research indicates that for healthy people of all ages and many people with chronic diseases, single-set programs of up to 15 repetitions performed a minimum of twice per week are recommended.

Each workout session should consist of 8 to 10 different exercises that train the major muscle groups. Single-set programs are less time-consuming and generally result in greater compliance. The goal of this type of program is to develop and maintain a significant amount of muscle mass, endurance, and strength to contribute to overall fitness and health.

Although age in itself is not a limiting factor to exercise training, a more gradual approach in applying prescriptive exercise at older ages may be necessary because exercise programs also can cause injury, especially in the presence of comorbidities such as arthritis, obesity, neurologic disease, postural instability, cardiovascular impairment, previous joint injuries, joint deformity, or other musculoskeletal complications, such as tendonitis or shoulder impingement syndrome. High-intensity resistance training (at more than 60% of the one-repetition maximum) has been demonstrated to cause large increases in strength in the older adult (older than age 65 years).[17,38]

People with chronic diseases may have to limit range of motion for some exercises and use lighter weights with more repetitions.[41,49] Otherwise, older adults do not have to "take it easy" when performing exercise. The presence of heart disease, diabetes, cancer, or other comorbidities may require some initial progression in the prescribed program.[92]

Overall, PTAs should pay careful attention to finding exercise intensities that are optimally suited to induce the desired training effects. The skeletal muscle of older people is more easily damaged with the loading that occurs during training compared with the skeletal muscle of younger adults. Care should be taken to monitor soreness and prevent muscle injuries after exercise.[92]

Recommendations for the quantity and quality of exercise for developing and maintaining cardiorespiratory and muscular fitness and flexibility in healthy adults also have been published. A certain combination of *frequency* (3 to 5 days/week), *intensity* (55% or 65% to 90% of maximum heart rate or 40% or 50% to 85% of VO_{2max}), and *duration* (20 to 60 minutes continuously or 10-minute bouts intermittently throughout the day) of exercise performed consistently over time has been found effective for producing a training effect.[10,11]

Fatigue, the inability to continue to maintain a given activity, may develop as a result of depletion of muscle and liver glycogen, decreases in blood glucose, dehydration, and increases in body temperature. In a strength training program for adults older than age 65 years, repeated maximum voluntary contractions resulting in fatigue may differ from those for younger populations. This may be relevant for designing optimal strength training programs for older adults specifically requiring closer supervision to ensure that each repetition is completed without substitution or incomplete range of motion and to adjust rest times between contractions. Alternatively, electrical stimulation may provide more consistent muscle activation during strength training in this age group.[82]

Exercise guidelines for the very old (older than age 85 years) also have been published by the American College of Sports Medicine as follows: *frequency* of at least 2 days/week, preferably 3 days; *intensity* of 40% to 60% of heart rate reserve; and *duration* of at least 20 minutes. Walking, leg/arm ergometry, seated stepping machines, and water exercises are recommended.

Additional recommendations for resistance training include two to three sets of 8 to 12 repetitions performed with good form and through the entire range of motion for each exercise performed on each training day (one set may be sufficient); some standing postures with free weights and balance training should be included.[10,11] When 12 repetitions can be completed without difficulty (observe for increased respiration, extremity tremors, facial grimacing), the weight can be increased by 5% with a lower number of repetitions to begin a new training cycle.

MUSCULOSKELETAL SYSTEM DISEASE

Although not nearly as common as traumatic and repetitive or overuse injuries, musculoskeletal system diseases are significant from the standpoint of disability, mortality, and cost in terms of health care dollars.[21] The most serious of these diseases are cancer and infection. The pathogenesis of these two types of diseases illustrates the intricate interrelationships between the musculoskeletal system and other body systems.

The primary highways or communication networks connecting the musculoskeletal and other body systems are the circulatory and lymphatic systems. These pathways are the routes used by disease to travel from one system to another. In addition, these highways deliver the nutrients and other supplies needed by the musculoskeletal system.

Cancer

Although primary malignant bone and soft tissue tumors are rare, metastatic disease of the musculoskeletal system is relatively common. Bone is one of the three most favored sites of solid tumor metastasis, indicating that the bone microenvironment provides fertile ground for the growth of many tumors. Although lung, breast, and prostate are the three primary sites responsible for most metastatic bone disease, tumors of the thyroid and kidney, lymphoma, and melanoma also can metastasize to the skeletal system.

Cancer cells typically invade the thin-walled lymphatic channels, capillaries, and venules as opposed to the thicker walled arterioles and arteries. Once the cancer cells enter the bloodstream, they must lodge in the vascular network of the host tissue before the secondary cancer can develop.

Organs with extensive circulatory or lymphatic systems, like the lungs and liver, are the most common sites of metastasis. Of the other potential sites of metastasis, the axial skeleton is among the most common. The blood supply to the axial skeleton is extensive compared with that to the distal components of the extremities, and the spinal blood flow through the thin-walled, valveless veins is slow and sluggish. This gives the circulating cancer cells ample opportunity to attach to the vessels' endothelia. The bony thorax, lumbar spine, and pelvis are the most common components of the axial skeleton for seeding of cancer to occur, and the vertebral bodies, because of the extensive venous plexus, appear to be the initial site for development of disease.

As with primary bone tumors, the major manifestation of metastatic bone cancer is pain, especially on weight bearing and at night. The pain can be caused by stretching of the periosteum or irritation of a nerve root or spinal cord, or can be secondary to bone collapse (pathologic fracture).

Once the cancer begins to spread, clients report fatigue, malaise, fever, nausea, and other symptoms. Therapists working with clients diagnosed with cancer must be vigilant for symptoms or signs suggestive of systemic compromise and be aware of common sites of metastasis for the particular primary tumor.

An awareness of signs and symptoms associated with the potential target organs is important, and any suspicious findings should be reported to the physician. Unfortunately, often the initial presenting symptom associated with the disease is pain from the bone metastasis (back pain), which can result in a delay in the diagnosis.

Infection

As with cancer, infection can originate in the musculoskeletal system or it can spread to the musculoskeletal system from elsewhere in the body. The most common cause of osteomyelitis is direct extension of bacterial organisms by penetrating wounds, fractures, or surgical intervention. Staphylococci and streptococci are the most common infecting agents.

The other common mechanism by which bacterial organisms reach the musculoskeletal system is via the hematogenous route. The original infection could be of the urinary tract (adults) or skin or teeth (children). In adults, the most common site of osteomyelitis is the vertebral body or intervertebral disk. The sluggish blood flow through the valveless veins facilitates bacterial seeding. Cases have been described illustrating the lengthy delay in diagnosis of vertebral osteomyelitis when back pain is the primary presentation.

Back pain can occur as a symptom of many diseases. Anyone with back pain of nontraumatic or unknown origin must be screened for medical disease, especially possible gastrointestinal or abdominal involvement related to infections (e.g., diverticulitis, appendicitis, pelvic inflammatory disease, Crohn's disease).

If infection occurs and penetrates the pelvic floor or retroperitoneal tissues (i.e., those organs outside the peritoneum such as the kidneys, colon, and bladder), abscesses may result in isolated referred hip or thigh pain and antalgic gait.

A variety of objective test procedures may be used by the therapist to assess for iliopsoas abscess formation, including the pinch-an-inch test, the iliopsoas muscle test, the obturator test, and palpation of the iliopsoas muscle.

Approximately 25% of all clients with inflammatory bowel disease (IBD; e.g., Crohn's disease, ulcerative colitis, diverticulitis) may present with migratory arthralgias, monarthritis, polyarthritis, or sacroiliitis. The joint problems and gastrointestinal disorders may appear simultaneously, the joint problems may manifest first (sometimes even years before bowel symptoms), or intestinal symptoms may present along with articular symptoms but be disregarded as part of the whole picture by the client.

Any time a client presents with low back, hip, or sacroiliac pain of unknown origin, the therapist must screen for medical disease by asking a few simple questions about the presence of accompanying intestinal symptoms, known personal or family history for IBD, and possible relief of symptoms after passing stool or gas.[45]

Joint problems usually respond to treatment of the underlying bowel disease but in some cases require separate management. Interventions for the musculoskeletal involvement follows the usual protocols for each area affected.

REFERENCES/SUGGESTED READINGS

To enhance this text and add value for the reader, references and suggested readings are included on the companion Evolve site that accompanies this textbook. The reader can view the source and access it online whenever possible.

14

Genetic and Developmental Disorders

CHAPTER OBJECTIVES

1. Review major pathologies associated with genetic and developmental conditions.
2. Consider anatomic and physiologic aspects that affect treatment choices for persons with genetic and developmental conditions.
3. Theorize treatment interventions according to goals for each genetic and developmental condition discussed.

OUTLINE

VOCAB BUILDERS

Arthrogryposis multiplex congenita
Atlantoaxial instability
Down syndrome
Erb's palsy
Hydrocephalus
Hypotonia

Kyphoscoliosis
Meningocele
Muscular dystrophies
Myelomeningocele
Myopathies
Osteogenesis imperfecta

Scoliosis
Spina bifida occulta
Spinal muscular atrophy
Subluxation
Torticollis
Ventriculoperitoneal shunt

Pediatric diseases and disorders comprise a large number of conditions. Entire volumes have been devoted just to pediatric pathologies. Given the format of this book and space limitations, in this chapter we have included as many of the more commonly encountered genetic and developmental disorders as possible.

A brief discussion of several other rare but important diagnoses is included. Because physical and occupational therapy intervention is not the focus here, the reader is referred to other, more appropriate resources for specific and thorough intervention guidelines for these conditions.[19,76,114,136]

DOWN SYNDROME

Definition and Incidence

Down syndrome was the first genetic disorder attributed to a chromosomal aberration and is referred to as *trisomy 21* (also *Down's syndrome*). It is characterized by muscle *hypotonia*, cognitive delay, abnormal facial features, and other distinctive physical abnormalities.

Down syndrome is the most common inherited chromosomal disorder, occurring once in every 800 live births. The incidence of Down syndrome rises with maternal age. Before maternal age 30 the incidence is 1 in 1000 births; it is 1 in 50 for mothers aged 35 to 39, and 1 in 20 for mothers over 40 years old. There is a 1% risk of recurrence for a couple who have had a child with Down syndrome.[105]

Etiologic Factors and Pathogenesis

Trisomy 21 produces three copies of chromosome 21 instead of the normal two because of faulty meiosis (cell division by which reproductive cells are formed) of the ovum or sometimes the sperm. This results in a karyotype (chromosomal constitution of the cell nucleus) of 47 chromosomes instead of the normal 46.

The faulty cell division can also occur after fertilization, leading to only a portion of cells being affected, with a milder clinical picture. This situation is referred to as *mosaicism*. Because of the positive correlation between increasing age and Down syndrome, it is hypothesized that deterioration of the oocyte (immature ovum) or environmental factors such as radiation and viruses may cause a predisposition to mistakes in meiosis and the resulting chromosomal abnormality.

In a small number of cases Down syndrome occurs as a result of a translocation of chromosome 15, 21, or 22 (i.e., the long arm of the chromosome breaks off and attaches to another chromosome). Chromosomal translocation can be hereditary or associated with advanced parental age. The third copy of chromosome 21 is the cause of the phenotypic characteristics that are observed in people with Down syndrome. There are presumably many genes that are present in triplicate in individuals with Down syndrome. Only a few of these have been identified as causative of specific pathology in Down syndrome; most likely there are many more that will be identified in the future.

Alzheimer's disease is also more common in people with Down syndrome, occurring at an earlier age than that of the Alzheimer population in general. By the age of 40 symptoms of Alzheimer can be seen in almost everyone with Down syndrome.

The resulting gross pathology in people with Down syndrome is an overall reduction in brain weight. This especially affects the size of the cerebral and cerebellar hemispheres, the

TABLE 14.1 Down Syndrome: Clinical Characteristics	
Most Frequently Observed Manifestations	**Associated Manifestations**
Flattened nasal bridge (90%)	Other congenital anomalies
Almond eye shape	Absence of kidney
Flat occiput	Duodenal atresia
Muscle hypotonia and joint hyperextensibility	Tracheoesophageal fistula
Congenital heart disease	Feeding difficulties
Language and cognitive delay	Atlantoaxial instability
Short limbs, short broad hands and feet	Sensory impairment
Epicanthal folds	Hearing loss (conductive)
High arched palate; protruding, fissured tongue	Visual impairment
Delayed acquisition of gross motor skills	• Strabismus
Simian line (transverse palmar crease)	• Myopia
	• Nystagmus
	• Cataracts
	• Conjunctivitis
	Delayed growth and sexual development
	Obesity
	Diabetes mellitus
	Otitis media
	Hepatitis B carriers
	Thyroid dysfunction
	Constipation associated with gastrointestinal tract anomalies
	Atrioventricular and ventricular septal defects

hippocampus, the pons, and the mammillary bodies. Additional abnormal findings may include smaller convolutions within the brain, structural abnormalities in the dendritic spines of the pyramidal neurons of the motor cortex, and abnormalities of the pyramidal system as a whole, including decreased pyramidal neurons in the hippocampus.

This last finding and the decreased size of the amygdala in people with Down syndrome who develop dementia have particular significance, as they relate to the increased incidence of Alzheimer's symptoms in older adults with Down syndrome.[3]

Clinical Manifestations

Children with Down syndrome are readily identified by their flattened nasal bridges, eye shape, short limbs, and mild to moderate hypotonia. The most frequently observed clinical characteristics are listed in Table 14.1.

Children with Down syndrome frequently have a variety of musculoskeletal or orthopedic problems believed to be acquired secondary to soft tissue laxity and muscle hypotonia. Some of the more common findings include recurrent patellar dislocation, excessive foot pronation, scoliosis, slipped capital femoral epiphyses (secondary to persistent hip abduction associated with hypotonia), and late hip dislocation (after 2 years).

Atlantoaxial instability (AAI) of the cervical spine (*subluxation* between C1 and C2) is a characteristic in some children with Down syndrome.

Children with Down syndrome predictably experience feeding difficulties and delayed acquisition of motor skills. These skills, however, improve with age. Because of the hypotonia and decreased strength, midline upper extremity movement is difficult, and gait usually is characterized by smaller step lengths, increased knee flexion at contact and hyperextension in stance, decreased single limb support, and an increased hip flexion posture. These children have slower reaction times and slower postural reactions.

Secondary disorders often develop after age 30 or 35, including obesity, diabetes mellitus, and cardiovascular disease. Other significant problems can include osteoarthritic degeneration of the spine and osteoporosis with vertebral or long bone fractures. Recent research indicates a high prevalence of Alzheimer's disease in older adults with Down syndrome.

Medical Management

Diagnosis

Measurement of α-fetoprotein (AFP), human chorionic gonadotropin, and unconjugated estrogen in maternal serum (triple screen) allows detection of an estimated 60% to 70% of fetuses with Down syndrome. Using this screening test, prenatal diagnosis may be made during the second trimester (15½ to 20 weeks' gestation).

Ultrasound identification based on nuchal translucency provides a good way to identify the fetus with Down syndrome at 10 to 14 weeks' gestation. Ultrasound carries a 6% false-positive rate and will identify only 77% of affected fetuses.[85]

Postnatal diagnosis usually begins with suspected physical findings at birth. Genetic studies showing the chromosomal abnormality can confirm the diagnosis. Specific diagnostic testing for the secondary problems discussed earlier varies depending on the involved organ systems suspected of dysfunction.

Treatment

Because no known cure exists for Down syndrome, treatment is directed toward specific medical problems (e.g., antibiotics for infection, cardiac surgery, monitoring of thyroid function, monitoring for development of Alzheimer's disease). The overall goal of treatment intervention is to help affected children develop to their full potential. This involves a team of experts, including physical therapist assistants (PTAs).

Prognosis

The improved life expectancy of people with Down syndrome as a result of the greater availability of surgery and advances in medical care has been documented, but life expectancy still remains lower than for the general population.[80]

The presence of congenital malformations, especially of the heart and gastrointestinal tract, can result in high mortality rates in the affected population[47]; lack of mobility and poor eating skills are also predictors of early death.[39] Respiratory tract infections are very common secondary to hypotonicity of chest and abdominal muscles and contribute significantly to morbidity and mortality. Immune system dysfunction also may be present and is associated with a higher incidence of acute myeloid leukemia than in the general pediatric population.[59]

Significant health problems contributing to mortality have been reported in the adult population with Down syndrome, including untreated congenital heart anomalies, acquired cardiac disease, pulmonary hypertension, recurrent respiratory infections, and aspiration leading to chronic pulmonary inter-

stitial changes, and complications from presenile dementia and Alzheimer's disease.

Over the last 40 years the life span of those with Down syndrome has increased significantly. In 1968 the average age of death was 2 years of age and by 1997[104] it had increased to 55 years of age. Unfortunately this degree of improvement has not occurred for everyone with Down syndrome. There is a significant disparity that exists based on race, with Caucasians with Down syndrome having a significantly longer life span than nonwhites.[21]

14.1 Special Implications for the PTA: Down Syndrome

Precautions

Because AAI is a potential problem, radiographs should be considered before any type of event that could result in a direct downward force on the cervical area (e.g., surgery, especially head and neck surgery; manual therapy; tumbling; diving; horseback riding). Transportation in a car or bus or on a bicycle alone or with an adult may be considered a potentially risky activity in which specific support is required. Likewise, riding carnival-type rides such as fast-moving carousels, roller coasters, and so on must be discussed with the family.

Subluxation of the cervical vertebrae more than 4.5 mm (occurs in 1% to 2% of cases) with or without neurologic symptoms is considered to be an indicator for intervention (e.g., cervical fusion). The therapist professional is an important source of information for increasing family and community awareness regarding the potential precautions and contraindications associated with AAI.

Decreased muscle tone compromises respiratory expansion. In addition, the underdeveloped nasal bone causes a chronic problem of inadequate drainage of mucus. The constant stuffy nose forces the child to breathe by mouth, which dries the oropharyngeal membranes, increasing susceptibility to upper respiratory tract infections.

Low oral motor tone and a protruding tongue can interfere with feeding, especially solid foods. Because the child breathes by mouth, sucking for any length of time is difficult. When eating solids, the child may gag on food because of mucus in the oropharynx.

The parents should be instructed in taking measures to lessen these problems, such as clearing the nose with a bulb-type syringe, especially before each feeding; providing frequent feedings with opportunities for rest; rinsing the mouth with water after feedings; changing the child's position frequently; practicing good handwashing; and performing postural drainage and percussion if necessary.

Gross and Fine Motor Development

The PTA concerned with motor development as well as other clinical, educational, psychosocial, or vocational issues relevant to people with Down syndrome is referred to other, more intervention-oriented resources.[15,60,153]

Physical Activity and Exercise[81]

Developing an active lifestyle early in childhood is important given the risk factors for the development of obesity, diabetes mellitus, and cardiovascular disease in this group. The presence of cardiac defects may affect the client's overall level of activity, fitness, and endurance training, especially in the school setting.

Some evidence suggests that individuals with Down syndrome physiologically work harder when engaged in physical activity or exercise (e.g., higher heart rate, greater oxygen consumption and minute ventilation) compared with peers who are without impairment or who are developmentally delayed but do not have Down syndrome.[40]

Anyone with Down syndrome interested in participating in the Special Olympics must work closely with the therapy staff, support staff, and physician to establish guidelines for safety. These individuals can benefit from aerobic conditioning, but the frequency, intensity, and duration must be modified from the general recommendations of the American College of Sports Medicine.

Lower peak heart rate and lower VO_2 in this population necessitate a lower level of aerobic conditioning. Vital signs should be monitored throughout the exercise program as a means of determining workload levels and progressing the activity or exercise.

SCOLIOSIS

Definition

Scoliosis is an abnormal lateral curvature of the spine. The curvature may be toward the right (more common in thoracic curves) or the left (more common in lumbar curves). Rotation of the vertebral column around its axis occurs and causes the associated rib cage deformity. Scoliosis is often associated with kyphosis and lordosis.

Overview and Incidence

Scoliosis is classified as idiopathic (unknown cause; 80% of all cases), osteopathic (a result of spinal disease or bony abnormality), myopathic (a result of muscle weakness), or neuropathic (a result of a central nervous system [CNS] disorder).

Age of onset can vary from birth onward, and the condition is referred to as *infantile* (0 to 3 years), *juvenile* (ages 3 to 10), *adolescent* (age 10 until bone maturity at 18 to 20 years of age), or *adult* (after skeletal maturation).[45] From 0.4% to 5.5% of children may have some type of scoliosis,[132] with 3% to 5% of children requiring some type of treatment intervention. The incidence is increased with associated neuromuscular impairments such as cerebral palsy, spina bifida, neurofibromatosis, and muscular dystrophy (MD).[23]

Infantile idiopathic scoliosis (rare in the United States) is characterized by curvatures that are most often thoracic and toward the left and most commonly affects boys. Juvenile idiopathic scoliosis is characterized most often by a right thoracic curvature and can be rapidly progressive. Adolescent idiopathic scoliosis of greater than 30 degrees is seen most often in girls without any neurologic impairments in a 10:1 ratio.[151] In its milder forms (10-degree curve or less), scoliosis affects boys and girls equally, but girls are more likely to develop more severe curvatures requiring intervention.

Etiologic Factors

Scoliosis may be functional or structural. Functional (postural) scoliosis may be caused by factors other than vertebral involvement, such as pain, poor posture, leg length discrepancy, or muscle spasm induced by a herniated disk or spondylolisthesis. These curves disappear when the cause is remedied. Functional scoliosis can become structural if untreated.

Structural scoliosis is a fixed curvature of the spine associated with vertebral rotation and asymmetry of the ligamentous supporting structures. It can be caused by deformity of the vertebral bodies and may be congenital (e.g., wedge vertebrae, fused ribs or vertebrae, hemivertebrae), musculoskeletal (e.g.,

osteoporosis, spinal tuberculosis, rheumatoid arthritis), neuromuscular (e.g., cerebral palsy, polio, myelomeningocele, MD), or, most commonly, idiopathic.

At the present time, despite extensive study, the cause of idiopathic scoliosis remains unknown. Researchers hypothesize that this type of scoliosis relates to the maturation disturbances of the CNS, including neurohormonal transmitters or neuromodulators secondary to genetic defect.[84]

Pathogenesis

The pathogenesis of scoliosis remains unclear but may be better understood in relation to the underlying cause. Abnormal embryonic formation and segmentation of the spinal column are possible pathologic pathways in congenital scoliosis. Neuromuscular scoliosis is often the result of an imbalance or asymmetry of muscle activity through the trunk and spine.

The earliest pathologic changes associated with idiopathic scoliosis occur in the soft tissues as the muscles, ligaments, and other tissues become shortened on the concave side of the curve. Some hypothesize[132] that scoliosis sets up abnormal forces across the spine because of the differences in length–tension relationships, with the muscles on the convexity being in a lengthened position and those on the concavity positioned in a relatively shortened state, and as a result a muscle imbalance is present.

Evidence establishes the existence of hypertrophy of the muscles on the side of the convexity[78]; however, the muscles on the concavity still are at a mechanical advantage and facilitate the progression of a curve once it is established. In time, bone deformities occur as compression forces on one side of the vertebral bodies apply asymmetric forces to the epiphyseal ossification center, resulting in increased bone density on that side. The compressive force is greatest on the vertebrae in the apex of the concavity, so the apical vertebrae become most deformed. A scoliometer can also be used to measure the degree of curvature (Figs. 14.1 and 14.2).

Clinical Manifestations

Curvatures of less than 20 degrees (mild scoliosis) rarely cause significant problems. Severe untreated scoliosis (curvatures greater than 60 degrees) may produce pulmonary insufficiency and reduced lung capacity, back pain, degenerative spinal arthritis, disk disease, vertebral subluxation, or sciatica.

Back pain is not typical in children or adolescents with mild scoliosis and should be evaluated by a physician who can rule out spondylolisthesis, tumor, infection, or occult trauma. Back pain may be associated with curve progression after institution of brace treatment for idiopathic scoliosis.[116]

The adult with scoliosis often has back pain that is considered multifactorial, arising from muscle fatigue, trunk imbalance, facet arthropathy, spinal stenosis, degenerative disk disease, and radiculopathy. Although the incidence of back pain in adults with scoliosis is similar to that in the general population, the pain in the group with scoliosis is greater and more persistent.[11]

Common characteristics of scoliosis are asymmetric shoulder and pelvic position, often identified when clothes do not hang evenly. Curves are designated as right or left depending on the convexity (e.g., right thoracic scoliosis describes a curve in the thoracic spine with convexity to the right). Usually one primary curvature exists with a secondary or compensatory curvature that develops to balance the body. Two primary curvatures may exist (usually right

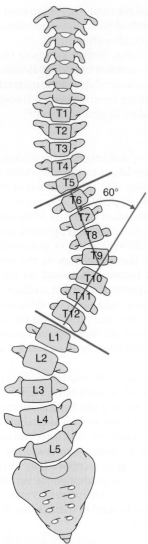

FIG. 14.1 Cobb's method of measuring scoliosis. This is the method most commonly used because it is readily reproduced. The top vertebra used in the measurement is identified as the uppermost vertebra whose upper surface tilts toward the curvature's concave side. (The superior surface of the vertebra above it usually tilts in the opposite direction or may be parallel to it.) The bottom vertebra is the lowest vertebra whose inferior surface tilts toward the curvature's concave side. (Likewise, the inferior surface of the vertebra below it usually tilts in the opposite direction or may be parallel to it.) A line is drawn parallel to each of these vertebrae. The angle formed by the intersection of lines drawn perpendicular to each of the parallel lines is the angle of the curvature.

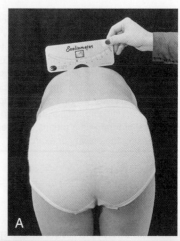

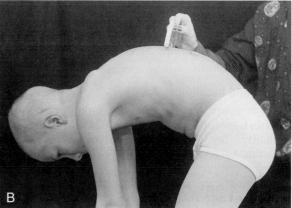

FIG. 14.2 (A and B) The scoliometer. This device can be used by any health care worker trained to screen for scoliosis. Some medical personnel also use this device to monitor curvatures over time, avoiding unnecessary radiographs. Ask the client to bend forward slowly (Adam's position), stopping when the shoulders are level with the hips. View the client from both the front and back, keeping your eyes at the same level as the back. Before measuring with the scoliometer, adjust the height of the person's bending position to the level at which the deformity of the spine is most pronounced. This position varies from one person to another depending on the location of the curvature (e.g., a low lumber curvature requires further bending than an upper thoracic curvature). Lay the scoliometer across the deformity with the 0 mark over the top of the spinous process. A measurement of 5 degrees or more in the screening test is considered positive and requires medical follow-up. Visually observe for asymmetry of the ribs or paravertebral muscles. In this child, hamstring tightness (greater on the left) accounts for the positional shift to the left. The scoliometer reading was zero. (Courtesy Todd Goodrich, University of Montana, Missoula.)

thoracic and left lumbar). If the curvatures of the spine are balanced (compensated), the head is centered over the center of the pelvis; if the spinal alignment is uncompensated, the head is displaced to one side.

Paraspinal muscles become asymmetric as the muscles on the convex side of the curve become rounded, appearing prominent or bulging, while the muscles on the concave side flatten. Rotational deformity on the convex side is observed as a rib hump (gibbus) sometimes seen in the upright position but always apparent in the forward bend position.

Medical Management

Treatment

Prevention of postural or idiopathic structural scoliosis is the key to management of the majority of scoliosis cases. Early detection allows for early treatment without surgical intervention and with good long-term results. Overall goals of management are to prevent severe and progressive deformities that might lead to decreased cardiorespiratory function.

Conservative care in the past has included exercise and electrical stimulation; however, this has not been proven effi-

TABLE 14.2	Scoliosis: Bracing Options
Brace	**Use**
Milwaukee (CTLSO)	Best with curvature at T8 or above
Boston (TLSO)	Best with curvature apex lower than T9 or T10
Lyon	For idiopathic scoliosis with thoracic hypokyphosis
Charleston	For idiopathic curves fabricated in maximum side-bend correction

CTLSO, Cervicothoracolumbosacral orthosis; *TLSO,* thoracolumbosacral orthosis.

cacious.[103] Observation and monitoring every 4 to 6 months for curvatures less than 25 degrees, spinal orthoses for curvatures 25 to 45 degrees (Table 14.2), and surgery for curvatures greater than 45 degrees have been recommended.[96,119] The goal of the use of spinal orthoses is to serve as a passive restraint system to maintain curvatures within 5 degrees of the curvature measurement at the time of initial application. This is accomplished successfully in 85% to 88% of cases.[152] Curvatures with an apex between T8 and L2 and compensated thoracolumbar curves respond the most favorably to bracing,[108] whereas curvatures with an apex at T6 or above have the poorest outcome.

Researchers continue to explore improved dynamic orthotics and holistic treatment approaches. Exercise has not traditionally been viewed as efficacious for scoliosis; however, there is some renewed interest in its potential effect on the flexibility of an existing scoliotic curve.[61] Progressive resistive exercises specifically aimed at decreasing muscle imbalances of the trunk rotators and extensors are effective for curves less than 45 degrees.[98]

Orthotic regimens have varied for late-onset idiopathic scoliosis, and the existing research on bracing demonstrated about a 33% success rate using the Charleston brace.[79]

Interventions in the adult with scoliosis should include a conservative nonoperative course of physical therapy to improve aerobic capacity, strengthen muscles, and improve flexibility and joint motion; nonnarcotic analgesics; nutritional counseling; smoking (or tobacco-use) cessation; and nerve root blocks, facet injections, and epidural steroid injections before surgery. Bracing has never been shown to have an effect on the natural history of adult scoliosis but may be used for certain people who are not operative candidates to stop health-threatening progression.[11] Customized seating systems can be used to maintain skeletal alignment and correct flexible contractures.

Surgical intervention (e.g., fusion with posterior segmental spinal instrumentation) may be necessary for curvatures greater than 45 degrees, in the presence of chronic pain, or when the curvature appears to be causing neurologic changes. Surgical goals are to halt progression of the curvature, improve alignment, decrease deformity, prevent pulmonary problems, and eliminate pain. The surgical options include a variety of segmental instrumentation systems including Luque, Cotrel–Dubousset, and unit rod instrumentation and Harrington rods. These are combined with posterior fusion and, in more severe cases, anterior fusion. Minimally invasive surgery can be used in the population to decrease the morbidity associated with open thoracotomy in those people who need an anterior release along with spinal fusion. This procedure is designed to maximize the stability of thoracic curves with a minimal incision. This technique uses an endoscope to enter the chest anteriorly and remove the disk material to destabilize the spine and obtain correction of the curve to the greatest degree possible.[34,111] This endoscopic approach may result in better spinal alignment with faster recovery, fewer complications, and less pain.[5]

Prognosis

Postural curvatures resolve as the primary problem is treated. Structural curvatures are not eliminated but rather increase during periods of rapid skeletal growth. If the curvature is less than 40 degrees at skeletal maturity, the risk of progression is small. In curvatures greater than 50 degrees, the spine is biomechanically unstable, and the curvature will likely continue to progress at a rate of 1 degree per year throughout life.[11]

Ill-fitting or inappropriate seating systems can contribute to this progression.[75] In severe kyphoscoliosis, pain and uncomfortable positioning can complicate care, and resultant pulmonary compromise can lead to death.

14.2 Special Implications for the PTA: Scoliosis

Therapeutic Interventions

Key roles of the PTA include the education of the public about scoliosis. Consumer education must include recommendations for adequate calcium intake and participation in weight-bearing activities. This is especially important for girls; studies show girls have a higher risk of developing osteoporosis in this population.[24]

Traditional exercise programs of stretching and general strengthening continue to be used but have not been found to halt or improve scoliosis even when used in conjunction with orthoses. When strengthening programs are used, their focus is on trunk extensors, abdominals, and gluteal muscles (especially hip extensors) focused on reducing muscle imbalances. Progressive resistive exercises for the trunk should be done to both sides using exercise equipment for this purpose. The program should start out with weight equal to one-fourth the child's body weight. When the client can do 20 repetitions of each exercise, then the resistance can be increased by 5%. The exercises should be done twice weekly for 15 minutes. Adults with scoliosis also can be helped by this program.[99] It may not change the degree of the curvature, but it can help control back pain.[98]

Stretching activities focus on the iliopsoas and low back extensors and lateral trunk flexors on the concave side of the curvature.

Postoperative

During the hospital stay after spinal surgery the therapy and nursing staff must check sensation, color, and blood supply in all extremities to detect neurovascular deficit, which is a serious complication after spinal surgery that is monitored intraoperatively. The person should be logrolled often and deep-breathing exercises encouraged to avoid pulmonary complications.

For ambulatory patients, upright mobility can begin within 24 hours depending on the surgeon's protocol. Adults are treated with antiembolic stockings and sequential compression devices until they are ambulatory, and most operative clients (depending on the instrumentation used) are fitted soon after surgery with a custom-molded lightweight plastic orthosis. The brace is to be worn full time when the patient is out of bed, but in some cases a progressive tolerance schedule may be required. A vigilant preventive skin care program is instituted.

Activities of daily living (ADLs; even brushing the hair or teeth can be beneficial) and active range-of-motion (ROM) exercises of the extremities help maintain circulation and muscle strength. Patients should be instructed in quadriceps arcs, calf pumping, and other ROM exercises and should perform the exercises frequently on their own throughout the day.

Cast syndrome is a rare but serious complication that can follow spinal surgery and application of a body cast. It is characterized by nausea, abdominal pressure, vomiting, and vague abdominal pain; cast syndrome probably results from hyperextension of the spine. This hyperextension accentuates lumbar lordosis with compression of a portion of the duodenum between the superior mesenteric artery and the aorta and vertebral column posteriorly. The PTA encountering anyone in a body jacket, localizer cast, or high hip spica cast must be aware of this condition, because it can develop as late as several weeks to months after application of the cast. Medical treatment is necessary for this condition.

The incidence of other postsurgical complications is low but may include infection at the surgical site, dislodgment of instrumentation, failure of fusion, and urinary tract infection, among other common postoperative complications. Osteophytes and foraminal narrowing in the concavity of the lumbar curvature may develop in older clients, causing nerve root impingement and radicular pain. Recovery in the adult may take 6 to 12 months, with improvement continuing for up to 2 years.[11]

Precautions

Precautions after spinal fusion depend on the type of fusion, segmental stabilization versus Harrington rod, and physician preference. Segmental stabilization provides some advantages over the traditional Harrington rod, including the ability to get out of bed on the first day after surgery and to go home from the hospital as soon as the fourth or fifth day after surgery. The more rigid segmental stabilization may make osteoporosis more likely to occur; however, the rate of pseudarthrosis is lower.[71]

Segmental instrumentation provides a better correction of the scoliosis, and postoperative casting or bracing often is not required. Precautions generally include avoiding excessive bending, trunk rotation, or hyperextension. Lifting limitations are often imposed depending on type of fusion, and the PTA can provide necessary instructions for safe lifting. These precautions are to help prevent breaking or dislodging of the hardware while promoting bony union in the corrected position.

Functional mobility is severely limited for the first 4 weeks after surgery. Typically, after 3 months any type of noncontact sport is acceptable, including aerobic exercise such as walking or stationary bicycling. Swimming especially is encouraged and can be started early after some types of fusions; however, diving is contraindicated.

By 1 year after surgery, the individual typically may participate in other noncontact activities such as horseback riding, skating, or skiing. Vigorous activities and contact sports usually are avoided unless the client is directed otherwise by the physician, and restrictions can vary from one physician to another and with various types of fixation devices. The same guidelines usually are followed for the child or adolescent who is wearing a brace but has not had surgery. The physical therapy team should work closely with the physicians when determining the postsurgical plan of care.

Skin care and prevention of breakdown are essential for anyone wearing a cast or spinal orthosis or brace. The patient should be taught good skin care and how to recognize signs of irritation that can lead to lesions. In addition, the PTA and patient should seek medical care if concerns regarding skin integrity develop.

KYPHOSCOLIOSIS

Overview and Etiologic Factors

Scheuermann's disease (juvenile kyphosis, vertebral epiphysitis) is a structural deformity classically characterized by anterior wedging of 5 degrees or more of three adjacent thoracic bodies and affecting adolescents aged 12 to 16 years. Scheuermann's disease is the most common cause of structural kyphosis in

adolescence. The mode of inheritance is likely autosomal dominant, but the etiologic factors and pathogenesis of this excessive kyphosis remain unknown.

In the aging population, *kyphoscoliosis* (adult round back) is more likely to develop as a result of poor posture, aging, degeneration of the intervertebral disks, vertebral compression fractures or osteoporotic collapse of the vertebrae, endocrine disorders (e.g., hyperparathyroidism, Cushing's disease), arthritis, Paget disease, metastatic tumor, or tuberculosis.

Clinical Manifestations

Adolescent kyphosis is usually asymptomatic, although some adolescents experience mild pain at the apex of the curvature, fatigue, prominent vertebral spinous processes, and tenderness or stiffness in the involved area or along the entire spine. The pectoral, hamstring, and hip flexor muscles are often tight, producing a crouched posture with anterior pelvic tilt and lumbar lordosis. Signs and symptoms associated with adult kyphosis are similar to those of the adolescent form but rarely produce local tenderness unless caused by vertebral compression fractures.

Medical Management

Diagnosis

Similar to individuals with scoliosis, adolescents may be referred for medical evaluation as a result of school screening, or they may seek treatment because of concerns over posture and appearance. Adults more commonly seek treatment because of increased pain. Diagnosis is based on clinical examination and confirmed by radiographic findings.

Treatment

Indications for treatment remain controversial, because the true natural history of this disease has not been clearly defined. Presently, the choice of treatment in kyphosis is based on the severity and progression of the curve, the age of the individual, and the symptomatology present.

Bracing appears to be very effective if the diagnosis is made early and in adolescents who have not reached skeletal maturity and have curves of less than 50 degrees.[83] Surgical management is warranted in those with more severe curves and in adults who continue to show progression of the curve or who have progressive neurologic symptoms or unmanageable pain.

14.3 Special Implications for the PTA: Kyphoscoliosis Kyphosis usually responds to physical therapy intervention combined with antiinflammatory medications and behavioral modifications.[140] Exercises (e.g., postural exercises, soft tissue mobilization, stretching, thoracic hyperextension, exercises to strengthen abdominal and gluteal muscles) are helpful to maintain flexibility and improve strength in the thoracic musculature.

Precautions and implications for postoperative care are similar to those for scoliosis.

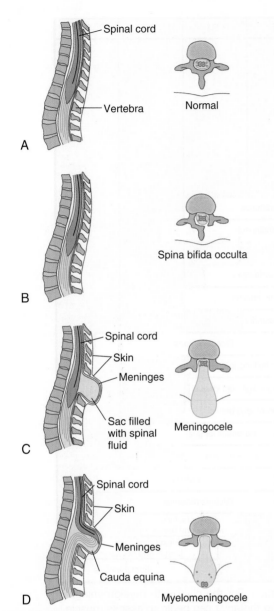

FIG. 14.3 Various degrees of spina bifida. (A) Normal anatomic structure. (B) Spina bifida occulta results in only a bony defect, with the spinal cord, meninges, and spinal fluid intact. (C) Meningocele involves the bifid vertebra, with only a cerebrospinal fluid (CSF)–filled sac protruding; the spinal cord or cauda equina (depending on the level of the lesion) remains intact. (D) Myelomeningocele is the most severe form because the spine is open and the protruding sac contains CSF, the meninges, and the spinal cord or cauda equina.

SPINA BIFIDA OCCULTA, MENINGOCELE, AND MYELOMENINGOCELE

Definition

Congenital neural tube defects (NTDs) encompass a variety of abnormalities. The term *spina bifida* is the one most often used to describe the more common congenital defects of neural tube closure. Normally the spinal cord and cauda equina are encased in a protective sheath of bone and meninges (Fig. 14.3). Failure of neural tube closure produces defects that may involve the entire length of the neural tube or may be restricted to a small area.

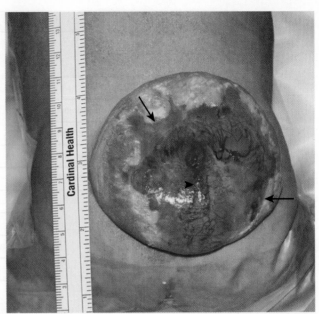

FIG. 14.4 Myelomeningocele in a newborn. The neural placode is visible at the surface *(arrowhead)* in this lumbosacral myelomeningocele. A placode is an area of thickening in the embryonic epithelial layer in which the spinal cord develops later. Abnormal epithelium lines the edges of the cerebrospinal fluid–filled cyst *(arrows)*. (From Swaiman KF, Ashwal S, Ferriero DM: Swaiman's pediatric neurology: principles and practice, ed 5, Edinburgh, 2012, Saunders.)

The three most common NTDs presented here are *spina bifida occulta* (incomplete fusion of the posterior vertebral arch), *meningocele* (external protrusion of the meninges), and *myelomeningocele* (protrusion of the meninges and spinal cord). Generally these defects occur in the lumbosacral area but also may be found in the sacral, thoracic, and cervical areas (Fig. 14.4).

Incidence and Etiologic Factors

After it was recommended that childbearing-aged women consume daily folic acid supplements, the birth prevalence of spina bifida in the United States decreased 6.9%. Notably, the prevalence of NTD-affected pregnancies remained higher among Hispanic women than among women in other racial or ethnic populations.

The incidence of NTDs varies by ethnic background, geographic area, and socioeconomic status. Data collected by the Centers for Disease Control and Prevention place the incidence in Atlanta at 1.9 per 10,000 live births of Caucasian or Hispanic children. The incidence is 1.7 per 10,000 African American children.[10] Spina bifida occurs more frequently on the East Coast of the United States than on the West Coast. Regional variations are significant, however, and in Scandinavia the rate can be as low as 2 per 10,000, whereas in China it can be as high as 100 per 10,000.[127] A study showed that because of the focus on weight loss in Japanese women, the incidence of spina bifida increased as a result of reduced intake of dietary folic acid.[134]

Evidence supports the hypothesis that the cause of NTDs is multifactorial and related to the interaction of a genetic predisposition, teratogenic exposure, and an essential folic acid deficiency or folic acid metabolic disorder. Folic acid is a B vitamin found chiefly in yeast, orange juice, and green leafy vegetables and bread products, which are now fortified with folic acid.

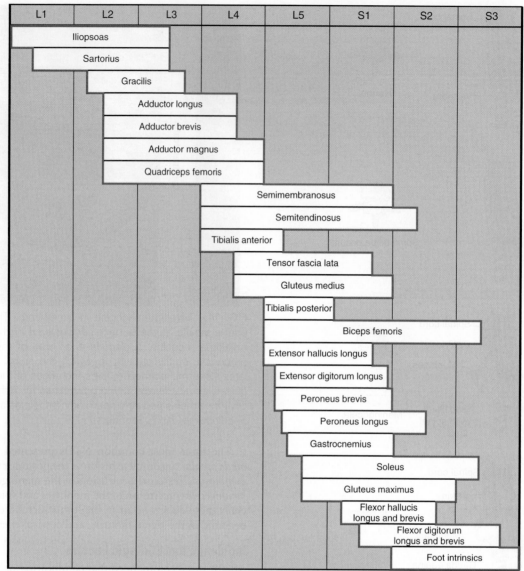

| L1 | L2 | L3 | L4 | L5 | S1 | S2 | S3 |

Iliopsoas
Sartorius
Gracilis
Adductor longus
Adductor brevis
Adductor magnus
Quadriceps femoris
Semimembranosus
Semitendinosus
Tibialis anterior
Tensor fascia lata
Gluteus medius
Tibialis posterior
Biceps femoris
Extensor hallucis longus
Extensor digitorum longus
Peroneus brevis
Peroneus longus
Gastrocnemius
Soleus
Gluteus maximus
Flexor hallucis longus and brevis
Flexor digitorum longus and brevis
Foot intrinsics

FIG. 14.5 Normal lumbar and sacral segmental innervation. For the child with myelomeningocele, once the level of the lesion has been identified, the therapist can begin to assess muscle involvement above and below that level. (Redrawn from Sharrard WJ: The segmental innervation of the lower limb muscles in man, Ann R Coll Surg Engl 35:106–122, 1964.)

Multivitamins containing folic acid taken when planning a pregnancy and during the first 6 weeks of pregnancy prevent 50% to 70% of NTDs.[95,97] Women must be cautioned that half of all pregnancies are not planned and that folic acid must be taken before conception to be effective. Taking supplements containing folic acid is the safest and most effective way of preventing NTDs.[93]

Many genetic disorders are associated with NTDs, either with recessive, dominant, or X-linked inheritance patterns. Couples who have had one child with spina bifida have a recurrence rate of 3% to 8%.[94] Increased rates of spina bifida are found in individuals with trisomy 13 and 18[30] and in chromosome 13q deletion syndrome.[82]

Teratogenic exposure also has been associated with an increased incidence of NTDs. Exposure to vitamin A, valproic acid, solvents, lead, herbicides, glycol ether, clomiphene, carbamazepine, aminopterin, and alcohol has been linked to increased rates of NTDs. A number of occupations have also

been linked to NTDs, presumably because of teratogenic exposure. Finally, insulin-dependent diabetes has been associated with increased risk of NTDs as well.[58]

Clinical Manifestations

NTDs are typically divided into two groups, occulta (hidden) and aperta (visible). Approximately 75% of vertebral defects are located in the lumbosacral region, most commonly at the L5 to S1 level. Motor dysfunction depends on the level of involvement and sparing of sensory and motor innervation (Fig. 14.5 and Table 14.3).

The loss of motor function is not evenly distributed over the limbs and spine, resulting in muscle imbalance contributing to the development of scoliosis and various musculoskeletal deformities that are related to the specific muscles not innervated. Clinical features and other associated characteristics are listed in Table 14.4.

TABLE 14.3 Myelomeningocele: Functional Mobility

Motor Level Spinal Cord Segment	Critical Motor Function Present	Bracing or External Support for Ambulation	Typical Functional Activity
≤T10	No LE movement	Standing brace or equipment	Supported sitting[a]
T12	Strong trunk No LE movement	HKAFOs Sometimes with thoracic corset	Sliding board transfers Good sitting balance[a] Therapeutic ambulation Independent wheelchair mobility
L1-L2	Unopposed hip flexion, some adduction	Standing brace or equipment HKAPOs, KAFOs, or RGOs Crutches once ambulating with walker	Household ambulation[a] May community ambulate if motivated
L3-L4	Quadriceps[b] Medial hamstrings Anterior tibialis	KAFOs Crutches Floor reaction AFOs, twister cables	Household and short community ambulation[a] Wheelchair for long distances
L5	Weak toe activity	KAFOs Crutches (yes and no) Floor reaction AFOs (yes and no)	Household and short community ambulation[a] Community ambulation[c]
S1	Lateral hamstring Peroneals	Usually no AFOs or upper limb support	Community ambulation
S2-S3	Mild intrinsic foot weakness	Possible crutch or cane with increased age	Community ambulation

[a]Do not usually walk as adults.
[b]Approximately 50% probability of long-distance ambulation with muscle grade 4/5.
[c]Able to use ambulation as the primary means of locomotion outside the home.
AFO, Ankle-foot orthosis; *HKAFO,* hip-knee-ankle-foot orthosis; *KAFO,* knee-ankle-foot orthosis; *LE,* lower extremity; *RGO,* reciprocating gait orthosis.

TABLE 14.4 Myelomeningocele: Clinical Features and Associated Characteristics

Clinical Features	Associated Characteristics
Hydrocephalus	90% have intelligence within the normal range (intelligence quotient >80) Increased incidence of learning disabilities 10%-30% risk of seizures Increased cerebrospinal fluid pressure
Arnold–Chiari malformation	Weakness, pain, sensory changes, vertigo, ataxia, diplopia
Bowel and bladder incontinence	Small spastic bladder: reflux Large flaccid bladder: residual urine, infection
Sensory impairment below the lesion	Lack of response to pain and touch Trophic ulcers of the sacrum and/or lower limbs
Flaccid paralysis below the lesion	0-2 years: truncal hypotonia Delayed automatic reactions Vasomotor insufficiency Obesity
Absence of deep tendon reflexes	
Clubfoot (talipes equinovarus)	Altered biomechanics
Hip subluxation, dislocation	30% demonstrate decreased ambulation status by age 12 years
Scoliosis	Late childhood and early adolescence: kyphoscoliosis

BOX 14.1 Signs and Symptoms of Hydrocephalus

- Full, bulging, tense soft spot (fontanel) on top of the child's head
- Large, prominent veins in the scalp
- Setting sun sign (child appears to look only downward; the whites of the eyes are obvious above the colored portion of the eyes)
- Behavioral changes (e.g., irritability, lethargy)
- High-pitched cry
- Seizures
- Vomiting or change in appetite

but occasionally bowel and bladder disturbances or foot weakness occurs.

In spina bifida aperta (meningocele and myelomeningocele), a saclike cyst protrudes outside the spine. Like spina bifida occulta, meningocele rarely causes neurologic deficits, whereas myelomeningocele causes permanent neurologic impairment depending on the level of involvement.

Myelomeningocele may be accompanied by flaccid or spastic paralysis, various combinations of bowel and bladder incontinence, musculoskeletal deformities (e.g., scoliosis, hip dysplasia, hip dislocation, clubfoot [talipes equinovarus], hip and knee contractures), hydrocephalus, and cognitive limitations. During the first 2 years of life, children with myelomeningocele often manifest various degrees of truncal hypotonia and delayed automatic postural reactions, even those children with sacrum-level lesions.

Approximately 90% of children born with this condition have an associated *hydrocephalus* (Box 14.1). Hydrocephalus accompanying spina bifida usually occurs in the presence of a type I or type II Arnold–Chiari malformation; that is, the cerebellar tonsils are displaced through the foramen magnum (Fig. 14.6), resulting in obstruction of

Spina bifida occulta does not protrude visibly but is often accompanied by a depression or dimple in the skin, a tuft of dark hair, soft fatty deposits (subcutaneous lipomas or dermoid cyst), port-wine nevi, or a combination of these abnormalities on the skin at the level of the underlying lesion. Spina bifida occulta usually does not cause neurologic dysfunction,

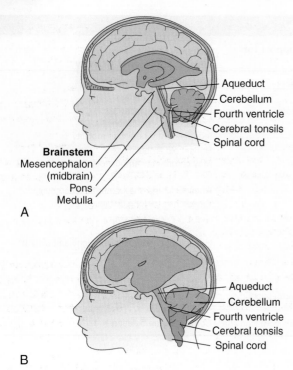

Brainstem
Mesencephalon
(midbrain)
Pons
Medulla

A

B

FIG. 14.6 Arnold–Chiari malformation. (A) Normal brain with patent cerebrospinal fluid (CSF) circulation. (B) Arnold–Chiari type II malformation with enlarged ventricles, which predisposes a child with myelomeningocele to hydrocephalus. The brainstem, the fourth ventricle, part of the cerebellum, and the cerebral tonsils are displaced downward through the foramen magnum, leading to blockage of CSF flow. In addition, pressure on the brainstem housing the cranial nerves may result in nerve palsies.

cerebrospinal fluid (CSF) flow and increased CSF pressure and hydrocephalus.

Cranial nerve involvement with feeding difficulties, choking, pooling of secretions, aspiration, and stridor is also a common finding. Vertigo, ataxia, or spasticity as well as pain, progressive weakness, and diplopia can also be presenting findings in the older child. Tethered cord syndrome is also a common comorbidity after surgical closure of the primary lesion and can occur at any time during growth. As the child grows, the spinal cord can become tethered or bound down, resulting in progressive neurologic compromise. The presenting features are consistent with neurologic compromise and include incontinence, progressive weakness, and back pain. Tethered cord syndrome occurs in 3% to 5% of children with spina bifida.[70]

Sensory disturbances usually parallel motor dysfunction. Pressure ulcers at the sacrum, ischial tuberosities, knees, and the dorsum of the feet can be a significant comorbidity. Factors contributing to pressure ulcers in this population are listed in Box 14.2. Many of the same risk factors are present in other conditions associated with pressure ulcers (e.g., diabetic neuropathy).

Bowel and bladder problems are present in virtually all children with myelomeningocele because these functions are controlled at the S2 to S4 levels. Even children with sacral lesions and normal leg movement often have bowel and bladder problems.

BOX 14.2   Factors Contributing to Pressure Ulcers in Myelomeningocele

- Ammonia from urine burns
- Friction burns (feet and knees of young active children)
- Pressure from casts or splints
- Bony prominences
- Vascular problems
- Poor transfer skills
- Obesity
- Asymmetric weight bearing or posture (scoliosis, orthopedic deformities)

Problems with urinary incontinence and infection can occur if the bladder is small and spastic (bladder holds little urine) or large and hypotonic (incomplete emptying of the bladder and ureteral reflux). Bladder dyssynergy occurs with either a flaccid or a spastic sphincter. Normally when the bladder contracts, the sphincter relaxes, allowing urine to flow. In a dyssynergistic state, the bladder and sphincter contract together, predisposing the child to urethral reflux.

Medical Management

Diagnosis

Frequently NTDs are detected prenatally with ultrasonic scanning and serum AFP testing. Elevated AFP usually occurs by 14 weeks' gestation in the presence of NTDs. This type of screening will not detect skin-covered (closed) neural defects such as spina bifida occulta. The potential for false-positive results with this test may result in unnecessary intervention.

Amniocentesis can detect only open NTDs and is recommended for pregnant women who have previously had children with NTDs or in the case of a large lesion noted with ultrasonic scanning. The need for more accurate, noninvasive imaging of the CNS has been recognized, and fetal magnetic resonance imaging (MRI) has become an effective, noninvasive means of assessing fetal CNS anatomy with superior ability to resolve posterior fossa anatomy over ultrasonography. However, to date fetal MRI has not surpassed ultrasonography in evaluation of hydrocephalus and the level and nature of the spinal lesion.[86] Fetal surgery techniques are being developed to correct the spinal deformity via cesarean section or fetoscope before the due date. After the corrective spinal surgery, the fetus is returned to the mother's uterus and allowed to continue to develop in utero. This surgery has shown dramatic improvements in the amount of limitation experienced by the child.

Postnatally, meningocele and myelomeningocele are obvious on examination. Transillumination of the protruding sac usually can distinguish between these two conditions. In meningocele, the sac with its CSF contents is transilluminated (light shines through the sac); in myelomeningocele, the light does not shine through the neural bundle. Spinal films can be used to detect defects, and computed tomography scans demonstrate the presence of hydrocephalus. Other laboratory tests may include urinalysis, urine cultures, and tests for renal function.

Treatment

Timing of the closure is important. Prenatal diagnosis has made planned cesarean sections, fetal repair, and therapeutic abortion possible. A cesarean section is the preferred method of birth to avoid trauma to the neural sac that occurs during vaginal delivery.

Prenatal closure is now available by fetal surgery or abdominal scope and has been found to decrease the incidence of shunt-dependent hydrocephalus and reverse Chiari malformation from above 90% in each case to 59% and 38%, respectively.[14,144] By interrupting the flow of CSF during gestation, intrauterine repair enables the cerebellum and brainstem to resume a normal (or nearly normal) configuration.

Prospective parents should be cautioned not to expect improvement in leg function as a result of this surgery. The potential benefits of surgery must be weighed carefully against the potential risks of preterm labor and delivery, potential infection, and blood loss.[143]

If postnatal closure is chosen, infection and drying of the nerve roots can lead to further loss of function and necessitate surgical closure within 48 hours of birth. *Ventriculoperitoneal shunting* (Figs. 14.7 and 14.8) is recommended in the presence of hydrocephalus; shunt revision is often required as the child grows or if the shunt becomes obstructed, infected, or separated.

The timing of the operative repair of the lesion remains under heavy debate. Some centers are repairing the defect before birth and are having good results. In most centers early closure (within the first 24 to 48 hours) after birth is the standard, with the goal of preventing local infection, avoiding trauma to the exposed tissues, and avoiding stretching of other nerve roots, thus preventing further motor impairment.

Other experts contend that surgical repair is best delayed until after further assessment of neurologic function, intellectual potential, and extent of complications. This delay increases the infant's ability to tolerate the surgical procedure, allows for better epithelialization of the sac (reducing the risk of infection), and permits easier mobilization of skin for closure.

A variety of plastic surgical procedures can be used for skin closure. The goal is to place the sac and its contents back in the body with good skin coverage of the lesion and careful closure. Excision of the membranous covering or removal of any portion of the sac may damage functioning neural tissue and is avoided completely. Although this corrective procedure may prevent an infection of the spinal cord or brain, the surgery has little or no effect on the neurologic function of the infant.

A variety of orthopedic surgical interventions may be required throughout the child's growing years. Surgical correction for hip dislocation rarely is indicated, except in the case of ambulatory clients with unilateral dislocation.[46] Investigation has shown that a level pelvis and good ROM of the hips are more important for ambulation than reduction of bilateral hip dislocation.[62]

Spinal fusion for kyphotic deformity of the spine offers mixed results and frequent complications. Hip flexion and knee flexion contractures often are addressed with muscle releases, and foot deformity correction often is achieved with soft tissue surgical procedures and, in more severe cases, with bony surgical procedures (Figs. 14.9 through 14.11).

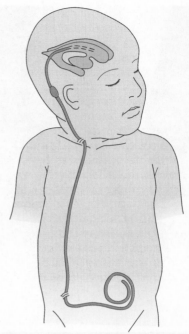

FIG. 14.7 Ventriculoperitoneal shunt. This provides primary drainage of cerebrospinal fluid from the ventricles to an extracranial compartment (usually either the heart [ventriculoatrial] or the abdominal or peritoneal [ventriculoperitoneal] cavity, as shown here). Extra tubing is left in the extracranial site to uncoil as the child grows. A unidirectional valve designed to open at a predetermined intraventricular pressure and close when the pressure falls below that level prevents backflow of fluid.

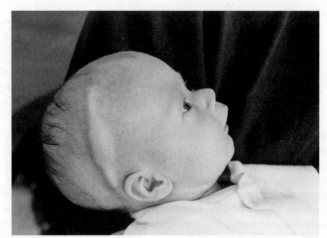

FIG. 14.8 Placement of the shunt. The shunt is placed very superficially, necessitating caution when handling the infant. The physical therapist assistant must be careful to avoid placing pressure over the shunt, stretching the neck, or placing the child in the head-down position. Parents may be distressed initially by the cosmetic appearance of the shunt, but as the child grows, and with hair growth, the shunt is no longer visible. Fig. 14.10 shows this same child with no obvious signs of a shunt. (Courtesy Todd Goodrich, University of Montana, Missoula.)

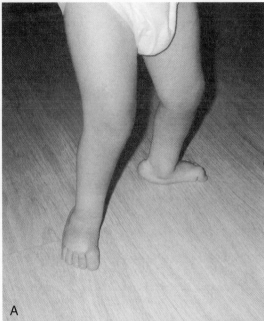

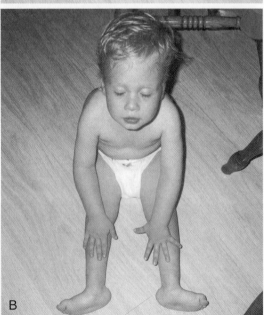

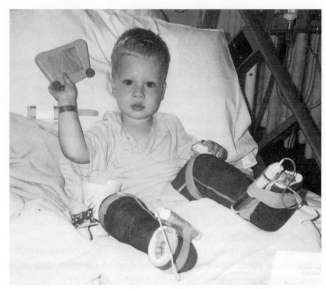

FIG. 14.10 Postoperative inpatient after orthopedic reconstructive surgery for congenital vertical talus deformity. Drainage tubes directly from the incision sites were used for 12 hours. (Courtesy Zane and Dianna Kuhnhenn, Missoula, Montana.)

FIG. 14.9 Orthopedic involvement. (A) Three-year-old boy with bilateral congenital vertical talus resulting in rocker-bottom foot deformities caused by an L4 to L5 myelomeningocele. Note the compensatory knee flexion and genu valgus along with developing toe flexion contractures (the latter from loss of motor control). (B) Rocker-bottom foot deformity seen more clearly in the non–weight-bearing position. (Courtesy Zane and Dianna Kuhnhenn, Missoula, Montana.)

Medical management of the bowel and bladder dysfunction is of critical importance from both a medical and a social standpoint. The muscles of the bladder can show either spasticity or flaccidity, leading to either a condition in which the bladder is small and under high pressure from urine or large and stretched out and under low pressure.

In children with spastic bladders under high pressure, vesicoureteral reflux and decreased bladder volume and compliance are critical factors that contribute to damage to the upper urinary tract

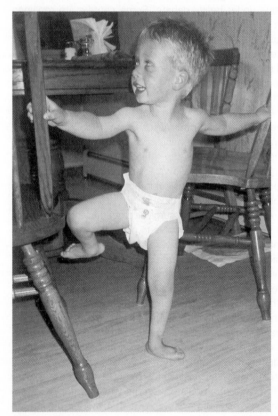

FIG. 14.11 Postoperative result. Risk for skin breakdown is reduced around the great toe (no longer contracted into flexion), and base of support is improved for ambulation and allows the child to stand on one leg with support (note the more neutral alignment of lower extremity, especially the knee). The child wears ankle-foot orthoses to maintain proper alignment; there may be some regression of alignment in time because of the continued lack of motor control. (Courtesy Zane and Dianna Kuhnhenn, Missoula, Montana.)

and kidneys. Children with hypotonic bladders often have more residual urine and are more prone to infection.

Infection is treated prophylactically in most children with spina bifida, with antibiotics and high fluid intake as a critical part of an overall management program. Kidney damage is unusual in children with hypotonic bladders because bladder urine is under low pressure and reflux is less of a problem.

Complete bladder emptying using clean intermittent catheterization provides a means to manage urine flow. Manual pressure on the bladder (Credé's method) is used less often because of its tendency to cause reflux. Implantation of an artificial urinary sphincter has been used in the older child or adolescent,[110] and bladder augmentation or urinary diversion are options for the child with high pressures and insufficient volume.

In most of these devices, the opening and closing of the bladder outlet are accomplished by a cuff placed around the outlet. The cuff can be constricted to close the outlet or relaxed to open the outlet and allow urine to flow. Intravesical electrical stimulation remains controversial; however, it has been used at some centers, with increased bladder compliance and increased bladder volume being the most common positive outcomes.[72]

Stool incontinence is managed most commonly by a program to regulate bowel movements using diet, timed enemas, or suppositories. In some centers the Malone antegrade continence enema procedure is being used to aid in bowel control. This procedure places a cecostomy, bringing the cecum to the abdominal wall in a procedure similar to the placement of a percutaneous endoscopic gastrostomy tube. Antegrade enemas are then used to control bowel function.[29]

Prognosis

Early, aggressive care of NTDs has now improved the overall prognosis associated with this condition. Prognosis varies with the degree of accompanying neurologic deficit, but researchers are evaluating quality-of-life issues as a possible predictor of prognosis.[74]

At present, prognosis is poorest for those children who have total paralysis below the lesion, kyphoscoliosis, hydrocephalus, and progressive loss of renal function secondary to chronic infection and reflux. At present, survival to adulthood is approximately 85%; most deaths occur before age 4.

Approximately two-thirds of children with myelomeningocele and shunted hydrocephalus have intelligence that falls in the normal range. The remaining one-third fall into the range for mental retardation, usually mild. Irrespective of intelligence quotient (IQ), children with spina bifida still have difficulties in perceptual organizational abilities, attention, speed of motor response, memory, and hand function in addition to mental flexibility, efficiency of processing, conceptualization, and problem solving. Overall cognitive delays occur less often as a result of improved medical treatment for these children.

Adult outcome data are incomplete at this time. Most adults over 40 years of age survived the preshunt era of the 1950s and are without hydrocephalus, whereas adults now in their thirties include people with more severe disabilities who benefited from the advances in medical and surgical management.

Adults with myelomeningocele continue to need therapy and medical management secondary to joint and spinal deformities, joint pain, pressure ulcers, neurologic

deterioration, depression, and poor social interaction and adjustment skills.

Prognosis for Motor Function

The child's motor abilities vary according to the level of the lesion, but delay in achieving ambulation can be expected in all children with spina bifida, including those with low neuro-segment-level lesions.

A child's ability to walk outdoors and use a wheelchair by age 7 usually suggests a good ambulation prognosis.[31] If functional ambulation is not present by 7 to 9 years of age, it is unlikely to occur subsequently.[2,42] A third of all people with myelomeningocele demonstrate a decline in ambulatory status with increasing age, usually beginning around age 12. These losses in ambulatory status often correlate with a variety of adolescent changes, including increasing body size and composition, loss of upper and lower extremity strength, or immobilization for varied periods of time secondary to musculoskeletal surgery or fracture healing. In addition, as children enter the junior high and high school grade levels they may desire a faster means of mobility, and even those who were previously ambulatory may seek wheeled mobility options, including power mobility.

The ambulatory status of adults with spina bifida is highly determined by two variables: motor level and sitting balance. Overall ambulation status declines over time.

14.4 Special Implications for the PTA: Spina Bifida Occulta, Meningocele, Myelomeningocele Throughout the life span of an individual with spina bifida occulta, meningocele, or myelomeningocele, the PTA participates actively in providing direct intervention, preventive care that can reduce complications and morbidity (and the associated costs of these), adaptive equipment, and client and family education. The PTA participates in both preoperative and postoperative care throughout the life of the individual. Functional rehabilitation provided by the PTA facilitates functional outcomes.

Neonatal Intensive Care Unit
Before surgery to repair the meningocele, pressure of any kind against the sac must be avoided. Whenever the (unrepaired) infant is held, the spine must be maintained in good alignment without tension in the area of the defect. The infant must be kept in the prone position to minimize tension on the sac and to reduce the risk of trauma.

The prone position allows for optimal positioning of the legs, especially in cases of associated hip dysplasia. The infant is placed flat with the hips slightly flexed to reduce tension on the defect. The legs are maintained in abduction with a pad (a folded diaper or towel) between the knees, and a small diaper roll is placed under the ankles to maintain a neutral foot position.

The prone position is maintained after operative closure, although many neurosurgeons allow a side-lying or partial side-lying position unless it aggravates a coexisting hip dysplasia or permits undesirable hip flexion. The side-lying position offers an opportunity for position changes, which reduces the risk of pressure sores and facilitates feeding.

In all handling procedures, care must be taken to avoid pressure on the sac preoperatively or on the operative site postoperatively. If permitted, the infant can be held upright against the body. For the infant with hydrocephalus, until the shunt is in place and draining well, activities that position the head above the body tend to decrease intracranial pressure. Activities that position the head below the body increase intracranial pressure; as a result, care should be taken with handling. In the older child positional headaches may be indicative of shunt malfunction.

Therapeutic Interventions
Skin Care
Areas of sensory and motor impairment are subject to skin breakdown and require meticulous care. The loss of skin sensation, especially decreased pain awareness, can lead to injury and pressure ulcers. Inadequate circulation results in wounds not healing properly.

Placing the infant on a soft foam or fleece pad reduces pressure on the knees and ankles. Periodic cleansing, application of lotion, and gentle massage aid circulation, which often is compromised. Bath water must be tested carefully because the child cannot feel the water temperature. The family should be advised to use sunscreen to prevent sunburn and to observe for tight-fitting shoes or braces. The skin should be checked daily for reddened or blotched areas that do not disappear within 10 minutes of relieving pressure.

Exercise
Passive ROM exercises must be performed slowly and cautiously, given the tendency toward fracture in this population. When the hip joints are unstable, stretching into hip flexion or adduction may aggravate a tendency toward hip subluxation.

Philosophic differences exist regarding the extent and direction of management programs for children with myelomeningocele. Children whose programs emphasize upright activities and ambulation show better outcomes (compared with children whose programs focus primarily on wheelchair mobility) in transfer skills (even after they have stopped ambulating), greater bone density, fewer lower extremity fractures, and a smaller incidence of pressure ulcers.[88] High-level lesions do not preclude ambulation; however, this may be a relatively energy-intensive activity compared with wheeled mobility and may have a negative impact on some aspects of school performance.[44]

Shunt Care
Ongoing intervention includes an awareness of signs and symptoms associated with changes resulting from increased CSF pressure in the presence of hydrocephalus with or without a shunt (Box 14.3). A shunting mechanism is used for hydrocephalus associated with a variety of conditions other than myelomeningocele.

Depending on the underlying condition, shunts can become obstructed or stop functioning for many reasons (e.g., occlusion resulting from blood clots or brain fragments, tumor cell aggregates, bacterial colonization, or other debris; the tube itself can become kinked or blocked at the tip; or growth of the infant or child or physical activities can result in disconnection of the shunt components or withdrawal of a distal catheter from its intended drainage site).

Shunt systems also may fail because of mechanical malfunction, including fracture of the catheters, leading to underdrainage or overdrainage.

Infants do not show typical signs of increased intracranial pressure, because skull suture lines are not fully closed. In this age group, a bulging fontanelle is the most obvious sign of pathology. Once the skull bones have fused and the anterior fontanelle is no longer palpable (9 to 16 months of age), pressure can build inside the closed space, resulting in a variety of symptoms, including headache, vomiting, eyes drifting downward, and irritability.

Tethered Cord
Tethering of the spinal cord may develop with myelodysplasia. The cord becomes caught or tethered from scar tissue and is stretched as the vertebral canal continues to elongate (Box 14.4). Other causes of a tethered cord may include meningomyelocele repair, obstructed CSF shunt, syringomyelia (a disease of the spinal cord in which the nerve tissue is replaced by a cavity filled with fluid), benign tumor, and spinal cord hypoplasia (i.e., the cord is progressively shorter than the canal and pulled as a result).

Latex Sensitivities
Children with spina bifida have been identified as having the greatest risk of becoming allergic to latex.[56] Typical symptoms include watery eyes, wheezing, hives, rash, swelling, and, in severe cases, anaphylaxis, a life-threatening reaction. These responses occur when items containing latex touch the skin, mucous membranes (mouth, genitals, bladder, or rectum), or open areas. Latex precautions must be paramount when treating a child with spina bifida. The PTA must avoid using toys, feeding utensils, or other items made of latex that the infant or child might put in the mouth. Parents must be advised to read all labels and avoid products, especially toys and utensils, containing latex. If latex content is not indicated, the manufacturer should be contacted for verification before purchase or use of the item.

Adaptive Equipment
Controversy also exists regarding the best choice of lower extremity bracing and ambulation method. One area of contention involves the hip-knee-ankle-foot orthosis (HKAFO) for swing-through gait only versus the reciprocating gait orthosis (RGO), which allows the individual options of a swing-to, swing-through, or reciprocating gait.

Precautions when considering HKAFO or RGO include severe spinal deformity, spasticity, decreased upper extremity strength, moderate obesity, knee flexion or plantar flexion contractures greater than 15 to 20 degrees, and hip flexion contracture greater than 35 degrees.

Another area of bracing consideration is whether to brace high, providing a more normal-appearing pattern and protecting against progressive orthopedic deformity, or to brace low, allowing more freedom of movement. Given the many improvements and number of bracing options available, the key to maintaining ambulatory status is good lower extremity ROM and a level pelvis. The choice of bracing depends on a careful evaluation of the individual's ROM, strength, and gait pattern.

Children should be positioned in weight-bearing positions to deter hip malformation and to increase bone density. This can be accomplished by the use of standing frames. As is age appropriate, the child should be introduced to standing mobility either via a parapodium or mobile standing frame.

NEUROMUSCULAR DISORDERS

Neuromuscular disorders including the MDs, congenital *myopathies*, and spinal muscular atrophy (SMA) are presented in this chapter. Other neuromuscular disorders such as Charcot-Marie-Tooth disease, amyotrophic lateral sclerosis, Guillain-Barré polyneuritis, and chronic inflammatory demyelinating polyneuropathy are discussed in other chapters in this text.

Muscular Dystrophies
Definition and Overview
The MDs make up the largest and most common group of inherited progressive neuromuscular disorders of childhood. They affect all population types, even animals. Signs of MD can occur at any point in the life span.

MDs, in general, have a genetic origin and are characterized by ongoing, typically symmetric, muscle wasting with increasing

BOX 14.3 Signs and Symptoms of Shunt Malfunction

- Congestion of scalp veins
- Firm or tense soft spot on cranium (fontanel)
- Listlessness, drowsiness, irritability
- Vomiting, change in appetite
- Marked depression of the anterior fontanel (overdrainage)
- Disturbance in urinary and bowel patterns
- Increasing head circumference
- Swelling along the shunt
- Seizures
- Nuchal (nape of the neck) rigidity
- Additional symptoms for older children and adults
  - Gradual personality change
  - Headaches
  - Blurring vision
  - Memory loss
  - Progressive coordination problems
  - Declining school or work performance
  - Decrease in sensory or motor functions

BOX 14.4 Signs and Symptoms of Tethered Cord Syndrome

- Changes in bowel and bladder function
- Scoliosis
- Increased spasticity
- Increased asymmetric postures or movement
- Altered gait pattern
- Decreased upper extremity coordination
- Changes in muscle strength (at or below the lesion)
- Back pain

deformity and disability. Paradoxically, in some forms (e.g., Duchenne's, Becker's) wasted muscles tend to hypertrophy because of connective tissue and fat deposits, giving the visual appearance of muscle strength.

Six major types of MD are included in this text discussion: (1) Duchenne's muscular dystrophy (DMD), (2) Becker's muscular dystrophy (BMD), (3) facioscapulohumeral (Landouzy–Dejerine) dystrophy (FSHD), (4) limb-girdle dystrophy (LGMD), (5) myotonic dystrophy, and (6) muscular dystrophy congenita (MDC), also known as congenital muscular dystrophy (CMD). These forms of MD involve a primary degeneration of muscle with a gradual loss of strength, but each type differs as to which muscle groups are affected (Fig. 14.12).

Incidence and Etiologic Factors

The incidence of DMD is approximately 1 in 3500 live births. Rates of occurrence for each type are listed in Table 14.5. All dystrophies are genetically based disorders.

DMD and BMD are X-linked recessive disorders caused by mutations in the dystrophin gene. In these two forms of MD, males are affected clinically and females are usually only carriers.

FSHD is an autosomal dominant disorder with onset in early adolescence. The son or daughter of a person affected with FSHD is at 50% risk for inheriting the defective gene. FSHD occurs with an incidence of 1 in 20,000.

LGMD may be inherited in several ways depending on the type. LGMD type 2 (A through L) disorders are autosomal recessive disorders of late childhood or adolescence, and type 1 (A through G) disorders are autosomal dominant disorders. Dominant disorders carry a 50% risk of inheritance if one parent is affected; recessive disorders carry a 25% risk of disease when both parents are carriers and a 50% chance of carrier status.

Myotonic dystrophy demonstrates an autosomal dominant inheritance pattern, with each generation being somewhat more severely affected than the last. MDC is a group of recessively inherited disorders that can be divided into two groups based on the presence of brain involvement. Only the most common forms are included here. The overall incidence has been placed at 4.65 per 100,000 in the Italian population.[101] In Japan, however, Fukuyama MD, one form of MDC, is as common as DMD.

Pathogenesis

Knowledge of the MDs and understanding of their increasing complexities escalated dramatically in the late 1980s when the protein dystrophin was identified as the causative factor in DMD and BMD. Subsequently, other members of the dystrophin glycoprotein transmembrane complex were identified as causative proteins in many other forms of MD.

These discoveries, along with advances in research and technology, have brought new information on the molecular pathogenesis of these disorders, including the genetic and molecular characterization of many forms of MD.

Duchenne's and Becker's muscular dystrophy. The affected gene in DMD and BMD encodes mRNA for the adhesive protein dystrophin, which is located in the muscle membrane, the sarcolemma. Muscle membrane lesions play an early role in the pathogenesis of MD, involving skeletal, cardiac, and smooth muscle membranes.

Dystrophin is the protein that links the muscle surface membrane (sarcolemma) with the contractile muscle protein (actin). Lack of normal dystrophin makes the sarcolemma susceptible to damage during contraction–relaxation cycles. Disruption of the muscle membrane and muscle fiber necrosis is initiated by muscle contraction, especially eccentric contraction.[109]

Males with undetectable levels of dystrophin have Duchenne-type MD, whereas those with nearly normal levels but dystrophin of an abnormal size or low levels have the Becker-type MD. The absence or altered state of dystrophin destabilizes the membrane and allows the influx of calcium, which triggers the destruction of the cell.[8] Muscle cells are replaced by fatty and connective tissues, and contractures develop.

Limb-girdle muscular dystrophy. LGMD is a collection of genetically heterogeneous disorders that can be broadly divided on a genetic basis into two groups. LGMD type 1 (LGMD1A through LGMD1G) are all inherited dominantly, and LGMD type 2 (LGMD2A through LGMD2L) are inherited recessively.

LGMD type 1A is the result of the absence of myotilin and is very rare. Myotilin is a thin filament protein associated with the Z disk and is involved in assembly of the contractile mechanism of the cell.[123] LGMD1B results from the absence of lamins A C, which are part of a large class of proteins. They are nuclear membrane proteins that are involved in stability of the nuclear membrane and cell differentiation.[55]

LGMD1C results from the absence of caveolin-3. Caveolin-3 is found as part of the muscle membrane and acts in cell signaling. The remaining dominant forms of LGMD (2D through 2F) have genetic characteristics but as yet have no protein identified.[55]

The second group of LGMDs (2A through 2K) are more common than the dominant forms and are inherited recessively.

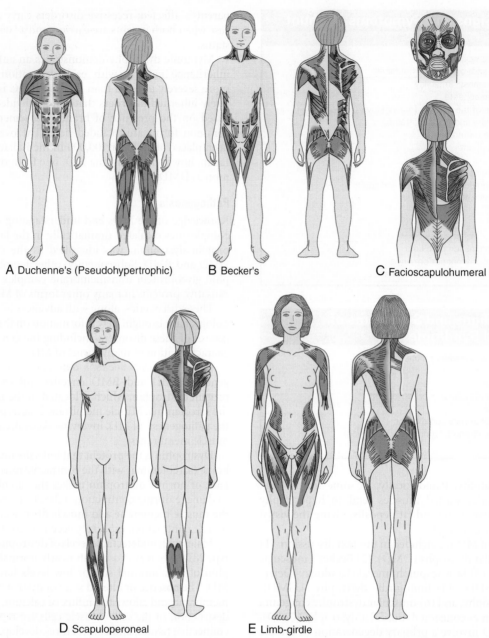

A Duchenne's (Pseudohypertrophic)   B Becker's   C Facioscapulohumeral

D Scapuloperoneal   E Limb-girdle

FIG. 14.12 Muscle groups involved in muscular dystrophies. These are presented in relative terms; that is, unlike spinal cord injury with definitive muscle involvement, in muscular dystrophy, proximal or distal muscle groups are affected in varying ways with individual differences noted. For example, in the facioscapulohumeral form the lower erector spinae is featured here but may be spared, and in limb-girdle dystrophy the lower abdominal muscles may be involved but are not shown in this illustration. (A) Duchenne's: shoulder girdle (trapezius, levator scapulae, rhomboids, serratus anterior), pectoral muscles, deltoid, rectus abdominis, gluteals, hamstrings, calf muscles. (B) Becker's: neck, trunk, pelvic and shoulder girdles. (C) Facioscapulohumeral: muscles of the face and shoulder girdle. (D) Scapuloperoneal: muscles of the legs below the knees (first), shoulder girdle (later). (E) Limb-girdle: upper arm (biceps and deltoid) and pelvic girdle.

TABLE 14.5 Disorders of Muscle

Type	Incidence	Onset	Inheritance	Course
Duchenne's (pseudohypertrophic) muscular dystrophy	20-30 in 100,000 live male births; female carrier	Becomes apparent at 2-4 years	X-linked; recessive; mutation in the dystrophin gene; 30% arise from mutation	Rapidly progressive; loss of walking by 9-10 years; death in 20s
Becker's muscular dystrophy	5 in 100,000 live births; female carrier	Variable, initial diagnosis 5-10 years	X-linked; recessive; mutation in the dystrophin gene	Slowly progressive; walking maintained past early teens; life span until adulthood
Facioscapulohumeral dystrophy	5 in 100,000 live births (males more often affected than females); female carrier	Any age: usually early adolescence	Autosomal dominant; 10%-30% arise from mutation	Slowly progressive; loss of walking in later life; variable life expectancy
Limb-girdle	1 in more than 100,000 live births	Early childhood to late adolescence	Autosomal recessive or dominant	Slowly progressive; mild impairment
Myotonic dystrophy	13 in 100,000 live births	Variable onset; classically adolescence	Autosomal dominant	Rate of progression dependent on age of onset; mild involvement, greater functional independence, greater longevity
Congenital muscular dystrophy	4.65 in 100,000	Birth or shortly after	Autosomal recessive or de novo autosomal dominant	Progressive; death for some in first years, in others more slowly progressive and individual achieves ambulation
Congenital myopathies	2 in 100,000 (nemaline myopathy)	Onset at birth	Autosomal recessive or dominant	Initial improvement static to slowly progressive

LGMD2A is one of the most common, with an estimated carrier frequency of 1 in 103.[112] The underlying defect in LGMD2A is that of a cellular regulatory enzyme P94, calpain 3, in the calpain family of molecules (calcium-activated protein enzymes). The function of calpain 3 is not well understood, but it appears to play a role in the organization of the muscle cell as it forms.[106]

LGMD2B is caused by an absence of dysferlin (chromosome 2p13). This is also the protein defect in Miyoshi myopathy, which has a different dystrophic distal phenotype.[150] Dysferlin acts as a membrane repair molecule and interacts with other molecules at the muscle membrane.[18]

The absent gene in LGMD2C, LGMD2D, LGMD2E, and LGMD2F codes for a specific protein in the sarcoglycan–glycoprotein complex. This glycoprotein complex is found in close association with dystrophin in the muscle membrane. These proteins act to stabilize the membrane. As a group these are known as sarcoglycanopathies, because each is named for the missing sarcoglycan protein (γ, α, β, and δ).

The pathogenesis of fiber demise in some types of LGMD is presumably similar to that of DMD and BMD. The absence of some of the sarcoglycans affects the integration of other sarcoglycans and the dystroglycan complex in the muscle membrane.[57,141]

LGMD2G is the result of a genetic defect on the seventeenth chromosome (17q11-12), which codes for the protein telethonin. Telethonin is a protein that acts closely together with titin (discussed later) in the formation of the muscle cell. In the adult muscle it is found at the Z disk in the sarcomere.[100]

LGMD2H results from the absence of TRIM 32, which belongs to a family of similar proteins. TRIM 32 is not well understood but acts in conjunction with other enzymes in the muscle and is found to be upregulated in situations in which muscle remodeling is occurring, as is the case when changes in weight bearing occur. LGMD2I is also a common form of LGMD caused by a mutation in the fukutin-related protein (FKRP) gene (19q13.3). FKRP encodes for an enzyme that is involved in glycosylation of α-dystroglycan.[139] α-Dystroglycan is a component of the dystrophin–glycoprotein complex.

The clinical picture of individuals with abnormalities of this protein is widely distributed, ranging from mild, late-onset disease in the fourth or fifth decade of life to a severe form of MDC with brain abnormalities in addition to severe weakness at birth.[9]

LGMD2J results from a mutation at 2q24.3 in the titin gene. Titin is a large intracellular protein that is responsible for elasticity and stability of the sarcomere. In addition, it plays a role in the assembly of the sarcomere in the developing muscle cell. LGMD2K has been designated to identify the milder phenotypic variants of the POMT1 mutation. This is the same mutation that is found in some of the more severe MDC cases with Walker–Warburg syndrome (WWS). LGMD2L is a mutation in the fukutin gene.

Congenital muscular dystrophy. The pathogenesis of the MDCs with brain involvement is related to the glycosylation of α-dystroglycan. Glycosylation is the addition of sugars or chains of sugars (glycans) to proteins and lipids. This process takes place in the endoplasmic reticulum and Golgi complex and is regulated by a series of enzymes that control the addition of glycans.

Five of the MDCs have been linked to mutations in the process of glycosylation. Different mutations in the same gene can produce widely varied phenotypes, which in some cases result from the varied amounts of residual enzyme activity. Glycosylation has been identified as necessary for the binding of laminin 2 to dystroglycan in the extracellular matrix.

WWS is the most severe MDC and is the result of defects in the first step in the glycosylation process. The gene that is responsible is the *POMT1* gene. In addition, defects in fukutin and FKRPs can also be seen in WWS and presumably occur in the glycosylation pathway, although FKRP defects can produce a wide range of clinical phenotypes. Muscle-eye-brain disease can be caused by mutations in the *POMgNT1* gene, which encodes for the transferase in the next step in the pathway.

Facioscapulohumeral dystrophy. FSHD is less well understood. The genetic defect has been found at 4q35 in 90% to 95% of individuals with FSHD.[17,148] However, the abnormal protein

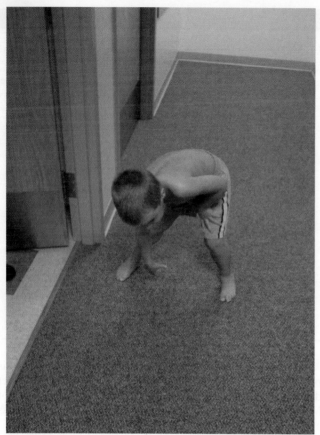

FIG. 14.13 Gowers' sign. This boy adopts the typical movement seen with proximal weakness, such as myopathies, when arising from the floor or a chair or even when climbing stairs. During Gowers' maneuver the client places the hands on the thighs and walks up the legs with the hands until the weight of the trunk can be placed posterior to the hip joint. This sign is characteristic of weakness of the lumbar and gluteal muscles. (Courtesy Allan Glanzman, Children's Seashore House of the Children's Hospital of Philadelphia, Pennsylvania.)

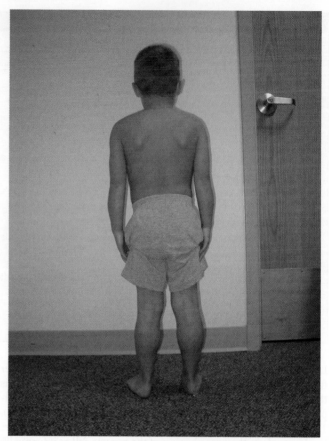

FIG. 14.14 Duchenne's muscular dystrophy with pseudohypertrophy of calves and lordotic posture that places the weight of the trunk behind the hip joint. Even though weakness occurs symmetrically, habitual standing postures may create asymmetries in flexibility in some cases. (Courtesy Allan Glanzman, Children's Seashore House of the Children's Hospital of Philadelphia, Pennsylvania.)

has not been identified, because it is coded for at some distance from the genetic defect and has yet to be cloned.

Myotonic dystrophy. There are three forms of myotonic dystrophy. The major form of myotonic dystrophy, also known as Steinert type or MD1, has been linked to chromosome band 19q13.3 and represents 98% of the cases. Two other types of myotonic dystrophy have been identified. Myotonic dystrophy type 2 (MD2) has been linked to chromosome band 3q21.3 (MD2),[92] and a third type has been linked to chromosome band 15q21-24. People with myotonic dystrophy have muscular weakness, wasting, and hypotonia. The degree of severity and age of onset vary with the type of myotonic dystrophy present (see Table 14.5).

Clinical Manifestations

Duchenne's muscular dystrophy. DMD is usually identified when the child has difficulty getting up off the floor (Gowers' sign; Fig. 14.13), falls frequently, has difficulty climbing stairs, and starts to walk with a waddling gait (proximal muscle weakness) and an increased lumbar lordosis (compensation for abdominal and hip extensor weakness). At the same time, the child begins to walk on the toes because of contracture of the

posterior calf musculature and weakness of the anterior tibial, peroneal, and proximal muscles.

Hip abductor weakness produces a positive Trendelenburg's sign, which eventually changes to a compensated gluteus medius gait as hip abductor weakness progresses. Classically ambulation continues to deteriorate up to the age of 10 to 12 years, at which time the majority of people with DMD are no longer able to walk.[12,130] However, with more recent medical treatment with prednisone or deflazacort children may walk beyond their twelfth birthday.

The shoulder girdle becomes involved, with excessive scapular winging and muscle hypertrophy (especially the upper arms but also the calves and thighs; Fig. 14.14). One of the major problems in gait occurs when the affected person requires upper extremity support. Shoulder girdle weakness and the need to maintain the weight line posterior to the hips and anterior to the knees often prevents the use of crutches to support the body weight.

Weakness of the shoulder girdle also causes difficulty in performing overhead activities related to hygiene and work. Bicipital tendinitis or other impingement disorders at the shoulder occur as the children get older as the result of weakness and the repeated manual lifts that become necessary for transfers. Muscle imbalances create biomechanical dysfunction, and weakness impairs the ability to stabilize the shoulder girdle, contributing to shoulder problems.

With the progression of weakness, scoliosis occurs at a rate of 80% to 90% and usually progresses more rapidly after the person is wheelchair bound. Spinal fusion is usually considered when the spinal curve approaches 40 degrees. Early fusion, when a good correction and level pelvis can be obtained, and when the individual's respiratory status is relatively more intact, produces the best result.

Common comorbidities associated with DMD include cognitive, respiratory, cardiac, and gastrointestinal dysfunction. The average IQ of individuals with DMD is 1 standard deviation below the mean, with specific reading disorders noted irrespective of IQ. Even so, many children with DMD have normal or above-normal intelligence.

Children with DMD develop a progressive restrictive respiratory impairment secondary to weakness and contracture of the respiratory muscles. Respiratory problems become more of a problem after the children become wheelchair bound. Nocturnal hypoventilation is one of the earlier manifestations of respiratory involvement and is usually accompanied by headaches, sleep disturbance, or nightmares. Chest muscle deterioration combined with joint contractures and involvement of the spine results in diminished ventilation and ability to produce pressure to cough up secretions, leading to pneumonia, other respiratory infections, and even death.

Disruption of sarcoglycan complexes in vascular smooth muscle also can result in vascular irregularities of the heart, diaphragm, kidneys, and gastrointestinal tract. Gastrointestinal problems are common, and constipation and pseudoobstruction can result from the smooth muscle deterioration and gastric dilatation that can occur.

Becker's muscular dystrophy. Signs and symptoms of BMD resemble those of DMD but with a slower progression and longer life expectancy. Ambulation is preserved into midadolescence or later but often is marked by toe walking with bilateral calf muscle hypertrophy.

Proximal muscles tend to be affected to a greater degree and before the involvement of the distal musculature, with primary effects observed in the neck (relatively preserved in BMD versus DMD), trunk, pelvis, and shoulder girdle. Muscle cramps are a common complaint in late childhood and early adolescence.

Scoliosis and contractures (elbow flexors, forearm pronators, and wrist flexors in the upper extremity; and plantar flexors, knee flexors, and hip abductors in the lower extremity) and other comorbidities also found in DMD are common; however, these occur less frequently and with less severity in BMD.

Limb-girdle muscular dystrophy. LGMD affects both proximal and distal muscles and follows a slow course, often with only mild impairment, although the course can vary widely even in a given family. Early symptoms develop as a result of muscle weakness in the upper arm (biceps and deltoid muscles) and pelvic muscles, usually noticed in late adolescence or early adulthood but as late as the person's forties.

Winging of the scapulae, lumbar lordosis, abdominal protrusion, waddling gait, poor balance, and inability to raise the arms may also develop. The lack of consistent clinical features makes this type of MD more difficult to diagnose.

Congenital muscular dystrophy. MDC is a spectrum of disease states that most commonly manifest at the more severe end of the spectrum in infancy with rapidly progressive muscle strength loss and progressive respiratory symptoms.

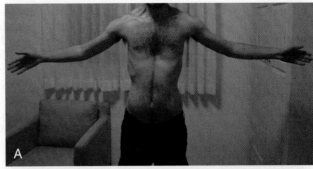
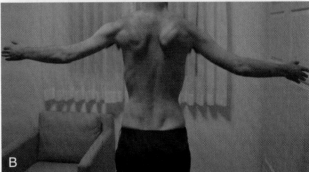

FIG. 14.15 Facioscapulohumeral dystrophy. Weakness of subscapular musculature makes it difficult to perform overhead activities; wasting also causes the clavicles to jut forward and the shoulders to have a drooping appearance (A). During humeral movement the scapulae wing and ride up over the thorax (B). (From Dori Z, Sarig Bahat H: Unusual scapular winging—A case report, Man Ther 24:75–80.)

Clients demonstrate a mixed central and peripheral picture with involvement of both the brain and muscle in addition to involvement of the visual system. WWS is the most severe of the MDCs and manifests at birth with a rapidly progressive course, with death most commonly occurring before a year of age. Ocular impairments include retinal abnormalities, microphthalmia, glaucoma, cataracts, and anterior chamber abnormalities.

The CNS complications include a cobblestone lissencephaly with agyria as well as areas of macrogyria and polymicrogyria. Cerebellar abnormalities are also present and include hypoplasia in addition to fourth ventricular dilatation. Common phenotypic presentation includes onset at or shortly after birth with weakness and delayed gross motor skills with progressive contractures and additional weakness, with very few individuals achieving ambulation and those typically requiring a wheelchair by the age of 10.

Cognitive impairment is common and often severe, with MRI findings somewhat similar to those found in WWS. The most prominent feature of the phenotype is the prominent distal laxity mixed with proximal contractures, particularly of the knee.

Facioscapulohumeral dystrophy. FSHD is a mild form of MD beginning with weakness and atrophy of the facial muscles and shoulder girdle, usually manifesting in the second decade of life. Phenotypic expression is more common in males than in females (95% versus 69%), with more females being carriers. Inability to close the eyes may be the earliest sign; the face is expressionless even when laughing or crying, forward shoulders and scapular winging develop, and the person has difficulty raising the arms overhead (Fig. 14.15).

Other changes in the face include diffuse facial flattening, a pouting lower lip, and inability to pucker the mouth to whistle or, for the infant, an inability to suckle. Progression is descending, with subsequent involvement of either the distal anterior leg or hip girdle muscles.[135] Weakness of the lower extremities may be delayed for many years. Contractures, skeletal deformities, and hypertrophy of the muscles are uncommon.

There is wide variability in age at onset, disease severity, and side-to-side symmetry, even within affected members of the same family. Associated non–skeletal muscle manifestations include high-frequency hearing loss and retinal telangiectasias (a group of retinal vascular anomalies characterized by retinal vessel dilation and tortuosity), both of which are usually asymptomatic.[135,148]

A variation of FSHD is scapuloperoneal MD, involving the proximal muscles of the shoulder girdle with sparing of the face. The process slowly spreads to the distal part of the lower extremities in several years or decades. Early symptoms may include shoulder weakness characterized by scapular winging; foot drop develops later.

Myotonic dystrophy. The clinical presentation of myotonic dystrophy occurs along a spectrum of disease severity that is based on the size of the genetic triple repeat. Three phenotypes have been identified. The most severe is congenital myotonic dystrophy with weakness and myotonia at birth. The classic form is characterized by weakness and some degree of disability, with mild myotonia and cataracts.

The clinical symptomatology of myotonic dystrophy includes muscle weakness and wasting with a delayed relaxation of the muscle and increased excitability. Ocular cataracts are also a defining factor; cardiac conduction defects are a serious comorbidity. A wide variety of other symptoms, including sensorineural hearing loss, hypersomnia, testicular atrophy (and sterility), and endocrine dysfunction, are also found in myotonic dystrophy.[6]

Medical Management

Treatment

At present no known treatment halts the progression of MD. Despite recent advances in our understanding of the MDs, current therapy for these disorders remains primarily supportive. Research in the area of molecular biology that has brought specific information about the molecular pathogenesis involved may one day lead to effective treatment.

Presently, treatment intervention is directed toward maintaining function in unaffected muscle groups for as long as possible, using supportive measures such as physical and occupational therapy, orthopedic appliances, orthopedic surgery, nutritional supplements, and pharmaceuticals. Children who remain active as long as possible avoid the complications (e.g., contractures, pressure ulcers, infections) and deconditioning that are common once they are wheelchair bound.

It is important to remember that there is an active muscle degeneration underlying the MDs. Strengthening, especially eccentric exercise, is not helpful and may cause increased weakness, particularly in DMD. Contracture management is the focus of treatment for the PTA and is important in maintaining function in clients with MD. Splinting, stretching, and serial casting are mainstays of treatment in

this group and should be considered when approaching these clients.

The effective use of glucocorticoid therapy (e.g., prednisone and deflazacort) to slow the progression of DMD and BMD has been reported. The use of glucocorticoids has become the mainstay of treatment for many individuals with these forms of dystrophy. It has been shown to improve muscle force and function in children with DMD. The functional advantage of this medical treatment is the child's ability to maintain independent ambulation, respiratory function, and spinal alignment for longer periods of time.

Stem cell and gene therapy for MD is currently under investigation, with researchers exploring a variety of ways to exogenously deliver healthy copies of the dystrophin gene to dystrophic muscles[77,91] or pharmacologically treat the effects of this disease.[22] Experiments in the mdx mouse have investigated the use of viruses to implant a miniature version of the dystrophin gene into dystrophin-deficient muscles to delay or stop muscle degeneration.

In other research models, attempts have been made to inject skeletal muscles with donor cells, a gene transfer method referred to as *myoblast transfer therapy*. These myoblasts fuse with diseased muscle fibers and provide the missing gene to replace dystrophin. There have been no reports of improved strength in people with DMD with this procedure.[102,131,149]

Prognosis

Prognosis varies with the type of MD present. As a general rule, the earlier the clinical signs appear, the more rapid, progressive, and disabling the dystrophy. DMD generally occurs during early childhood with rapid progression of symptoms and results in death in the third or later decade of life.

Pulmonary complications, resulting from respiratory muscle dysfunction, and cardiac dysfunction in the form of conduction defects or myopathy, are the common sources of morbidity and mortality. People with BMD usually live into the fifth decade (their forties) or beyond; death occurs secondary to respiratory dysfunction or heart failure. Those with FSHD involvement may appear almost stable over a period of years; variable progression occurs among those with LGMD. People with both FSHD and LGMD have a relatively normal life span.

14.5 Special Implications for the PTA: Muscular Dystrophy

Precautions When people with MD become ill or injured and are on bed rest (at home or in the hospital) even for a few days, they may lose many of their functional abilities. For example, a child who falls and breaks a leg and is on bed rest or otherwise immobilized may never regain the ability to ambulate. These children should be encouraged to be as mobile as possible, and if possible to ambulate for even a few minutes per day during the course of any illness.

Although activity helps the client maintain functional abilities, strenuous exercise may facilitate the breakdown of muscle fibers, so exercise must be approached cautiously. Low-repetition maximum weightlifting, especially eccentric strengthening, is not recommended. Exercise is best done in the pool, where exercise is concentric. Any exercise program should produce only minimal fatigue with no postexercise soreness, because the amount of damage to the muscle membrane with exercise is related directly to the magnitude of the stress placed on it during contraction.[109]

Respiratory involvement necessitates careful monitoring of breathing techniques, respiratory movements, and oxygen saturation levels. Monitoring oxygen during exercise and activity is recommended. The client should be instructed in diaphragmatic, deep-breathing exercises. Airway clearance techniques, including the use of percussion and postural drainage and mechanical insufflator–exsufflator for assisted cough, are especially useful during illness.[4]

Investigators have shown that the inspiratory muscles can be trained for both force and endurance in this population. These training-related improvements in inspiratory muscle performance are more likely to occur in those who are less severely affected by the disease. In those clients who have disease to the extent that they are already retaining carbon dioxide, little change occurs in respiratory muscle force or endurance with training.[90]

In the later stages of respiratory compromise nighttime mechanical ventilation (e.g., continuous positive airway pressure [CPAP] or bilevel positive airway pressure [BiPAP] delivered by face mask) is an intervention used to rest the respiratory muscles. A major priority for these children is to avoid or delay the need for intubation and full-time mechanical ventilation; these noninvasive methods can aid in this goal.[28]

Therapy Interventions

For individuals with the more disabling forms of MD such as DMD, the PTA can provide anticipatory guidance about the course of the disease and valuable information regarding the use of various types of adaptive equipment. Initially, grab bars provide for safety, but eventually a rolling commode or combination commode and bath chair is needed. As DMD progresses, a power wheelchair provides functional mobility once ambulation is no longer possible.

Eventually, adapted controls (minijoystick, touch pad, or fiberoptic switches) may be required for the power chair to accommodate the severe weakness and contracture that develop in the later stages of DMD. Power rotational wheelchair systems allow for pressure relief where pressure-relieving cushions are no longer sufficient.

In the individual who no longer has access to a computer for school or work secondary to severe weakness, environmental control systems allow computer access for control of the mouse from the wheelchair control or completely hands-free control through the use of voice recognition software.

Overhead slings and mobile arm supports are helpful with feeding and other upper extremity activities, especially after spinal surgery, when axial flexibility is removed and greater active ROM is required for these functional tasks.

Splinting and night positioning in addition to active and passive ROM exercises will aid in delaying the onset of contractures and reducing the associated morbidity. Home environmental assessment and careful family and client interviews are important in planning out the appropriate adaptive equipment and home modifications.

Both children and adults can benefit from ambulation and pool therapy programs aimed at improving endurance.

Spinal Muscular Atrophy

Overview and Incidence

SMA is a neuromuscular disease characterized by progressive weakness and wasting of skeletal muscles resulting from anterior horn cell degeneration. SMA is the second most common fatal autosomal recessive disorder after cystic fibrosis. The overall prevalence is 1 in 15,000 live births, and 1 in 50 individuals carry the genetic defect (Table 14.6).

Childhood SMA is divided into severe (type I), intermediate (type II), and mild (type III). Type I, the more severe or acute form, is referred to as Werdnig–Hoffmann disease and causes respiratory failure and early death in the first few years of life if respiratory support is not provided.

Kugelberg–Welander disease, or type III SMA, is the mildest form. These individuals learn to walk without assistance; a relatively slow progression is noted in type III. Type II is an intermediate form; affected individuals demonstrate the ability to sit independently at some point, but significant functional impairment and reliance on power mobility are typical (see Table 14.6). Despite the classification system into three types, SMA really involves a continuous spectrum of severity.

Etiologic Factors and Pathogenesis

The basis of this inherited pathologic condition (autosomal recessive trait) is gene deletions in the SMA critical region of the long arm of chromosome 5 (5q13.1).[49] The *SMN1* gene is defective in 99% of all cases of SMA and is the cause of SMA.

Progressive degeneration of anterior horn cells of the spinal cord is noted in SMA, with selected motor nuclei of the brainstem being variably affected. In the remaining axons, sprouting occurs, resulting in enlarged motor units. The underlying pathogenesis of anterior horn cell loss appears to be the persistence of programmed cell death in the anterior horn cells.[128]

Clinical Manifestations

Progressive atrophy of skeletal muscles is noted, with a variable degree of hypotonia, weakness, and fatigue reported. Often fatal restrictive lung disease is present. There is a slowly progressive loss of motor function. Explanations for this loss of function remain undetermined, but decrease in motor function could be caused by factors such as increased body size.[67]

Other factors that may contribute to weakness and fatigue include chronic respiratory insufficiency with hypoventilation and carbon dioxide retention and chronic malnutrition.[68]

Children with SMA type I manifest features of this disorder within the first 3 to 4 months of life. The child has marked hypotonia and severe generalized weakness and is unable to sit unsupported. Children with type II manifest chronic weakness before 18 months of age and attain sitting but never walk without assistance.

By definition, individuals with type III SMA are able to ambulate at some point in their lives, although they often require the use of assistive devices and orthotics to maintain proper skeletal alignment. Clinical problems associated with the muscle weakness seen in SMA include feeding and nutrition, respiratory, cardiac, and orthopedic problems.

Medical Management

Diagnosis

The diagnosis should be suspected on the basis of clinical manifestations but is established from muscle biopsy and an electromyogram in which a neuropathic pattern is found. Nerve conduction velocities can be normal (slowing may be

TABLE 14.6 **Spinal Muscular Atrophy**

Type	Incidence	Onset	Inheritance	Features	Course
SMA type I (Werdnig–Hoffmann), acute or severe form	1 in 15,000-20,000 live births	0-3 months old	Autosomal recessive	LEs flexed, abducted, and externally rotated (frog position) (UEs abducted, externally rotated, unable to move to midline against gravity Poor head control Significantly decreased muscle tone, weakness Decreased newborn movements, decreased diaphragmatic movements High risk of scoliosis Proximal muscle weakness greater than distal weakness Weak cry and cough Normal sensation and intellect	Rapidly progressive Severe hypotonia Death within first 3 years 32% survive second year 8% survive 10 years[97]
SMA type II, intermediate form	Same as type I	6-12 months old	Autosomal recessive	LEs flexed, abducted, and externally rotated Limited trunk control Weakness Increased risk of scoliosis Normal sensation and intellect	Progress that stabilizes Moderate to severe hypotonia Shortened life span[97] Patient attains the ability to sit at some point Reliance on power mobility
SMA type III, Kugelberg–Welander, mild form	6 in 100,000 live births	2-15 years old	Autosomal recessive	Proximal weakness (greatest with trunk, hip, knee extension) Trendelenburg's gait, especially with running Slow continued development progression Sits independently Walks independently (lumbar lordosis, waddling gait, genu recurvatum, protuberant abdomen) Wheelchair bound in early adulthood (dependent on age of onset) Good UE strength	Slowly progressive Mild impairment Patient attains the ability to ambulate at some point Wheelchair dependent in adulthood

LE, Lower extremity; *SMA,* spinal muscular atrophy; *UE,* upper extremity.

noted later in the course); motor action potentials are decreased in magnitude.

Genetic testing for SMA also confirms the diagnosis.

Treatment

Treatment is symptomatic and preventive, primarily preventing pulmonary infection and treating or preventing orthopedic problems, the most serious of which is scoliosis. Feeding problems are common, especially in individuals with bulbar muscle weakness; gastrostomy tube feedings are often necessary to optimally manage nutrition.

Respiratory problems (involvement of the intercostals) are common, and percussion and postural drainage and treatments with an insufflator–exsufflator (also known as "coughalator," a machine that helps in the removal of bronchial secretions from the respiratory tract) can aid in airway clearance, especially during intercurrent illness. Positive pressure ventilatory support, typically by BiPAP (initially at night), can extend the life span in these clients. Cardiac involvement is often secondary to the chronic respiratory insufficiency typical of this disease.

The majority of people with SMA type I or II develop some type of scoliosis; individuals with type III who become nonambulatory are also likely to develop scoliosis. Bracing has not been found to delay the progression of scoliosis but might help with sitting balance (Fig. 14.16). Care should be taken to allow good diaphragmatic movement and not create

increased respiratory effort if a soft spinal orthosis is chosen to manage sitting posture.

Spinal fusion is the primary means of management for scoliosis. Although fusion is often necessary, there is some consequence to function. Many individuals will not return completely to their prior functional level.[48] Individuals with type II SMA can develop hip subluxation or dislocation, but this is not typically painful and the literature on surgical correction is not supportive.

Individuals with type II SMA should participate in a standing program (Fig. 14.17). Knee-ankle-foot-orthoses (KAFOs) with ischial weight bearing are ideal for this in the younger age group. However, as contractures develop, standing will become more difficult despite the most aggressive splinting, ROM, and serial casting program.

SMA type III clients are most likely to ambulate, although about half of individuals in this group lose ambulatory skills in childhood or adolescence. Fractures are common and a significant source of morbidity and loss of functional skills.

Prognosis

Prognosis varies according to age of onset or type of SMA (see Table 14.6). The earlier the disease occurs, the faster the progression of muscle weakness and the poorer the prognosis. The presence of respiratory distress also contributes to a poorer prognosis.

SMA type I is the most severe and carries a very poor prognosis, with death likely in the first 2 years of life as a result of respiratory failure or respiratory infection. Most children with this form of SMA do not survive past 3 years without the aid of mechanical ventilation. Clients with type III (with onset after 2 years of age) remain independently ambulatory throughout adult life; onset before 2 years results in loss of ambulatory ability at an average age of 12 years.[121]

14.6 Special Implications for the PTA: Spinal Muscular Atrophy A variety of opinions exist regarding the usefulness or effectiveness of an active developmental program for children with SMA. However, often children with SMA type I or II outlive predictions, and therapy intervention is helpful in improving function and preventing musculoskeletal problems.

Precautions

The infant or child with SMA who is immobile requires frequent changes of position to prevent skin problems and other complications, especially pneumonia. The pharynx may require suctioning to remove secretions in the more severe cases, and feeding must be performed slowly and carefully with good positioning to prevent aspiration in those individuals with oral motor involvement.

The involvement of a therapist with specialization in feeding (usually an occupational therapist or speech-language pathologist) is essential for these children. These children are intellectually normal and require verbal, tactile, and auditory stimulation and various types of assistive technology.

Respiratory weakness or diminished head control may prevent the child from benefiting from prone positioning. This is especially problematic when the child cannot lift the head to clear the airway. The use of prone positioning must be evaluated and monitored carefully by the PTA; vertical positions (sitting and standing) tend to be the most functional.

Monitoring oxygen saturation levels may be necessary in evaluating programming effectiveness. Observe how much work is required to breathe, and whenever possible use a pulse oximeter to measure oxygen saturation noninvasively. Pulse oximetry can provide an outcome measure for documentation.

Therapy Interventions

Specific treatment protocols for this condition are beyond the scope of this book. An overall management program should include positioning to encourage head and trunk control and to promote functional strengthening, in addition to splinting and orthotics to maintain ROM and skeletal alignment. Appropriate assistive technologies and adapted devices can provide the maximum possible independence for children with SMA.

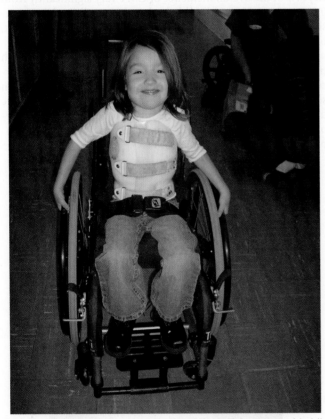

FIG. 14.16 Spinal muscular atrophy (SMA). This 4-year-old child with SMA type II is fitted with a one-piece body jacket or thoracolumbosacral orthosis (TLSO). The TLSO offers support and control of the trunk and lower spine for improved sitting posture, balance, and greater stability. Full body jackets of this type may increase the work of breathing; an abdominal cutout to allow diaphragmatic excursion is typically provided for individuals with SMA who rely on diaphragmatic respiration because of the pattern of muscular weakness. The chair is a titanium ultralight wheelchair, which this child can propel for independent mobility. (Courtesy Tamara Kittelson-Aldred, Specialty Occupational Therapy PLLC, Missoula, Montana.)

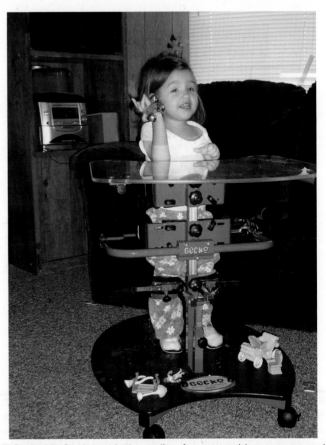

FIG. 14.17 Static vertical standing frame provides support and stability in the upright position for the child with spinal muscular atrophy. Ankle-foot orthoses provide support for weight bearing through the lower extremities. (Courtesy Tamara Kittelson-Aldred, Specialty Occupational Therapy PLLC, Missoula, Montana.)

Power mobility for the child with SMA who has no independent mobility is essential and should be considered in the child as young as 2 years of age (Fig. 14.18).[137] Low-technology solutions such as "slings and springs" also may be very liberating for the child who has limited antigravity upper extremity movement by providing a wide variety of exploratory opportunities.

Facilitation and active assistive work toward standing and ambulation have been found to be effective in increasing forced vital capacity and in reducing the incidence of hip dislocation and contracture. More severely involved clients may benefit from positioning in a standing frame or instruction in standing to assist with or perform transfers independently.[133] Children may also benefit from using a heavy model gait trainer or wheeled walker for assisted ambulation.

Elastic abdominal binders similar to those used with spinal cord injury patients can be used to provide increased trunk, abdominal, and diaphragmatic stability, especially if there is evidence of decreased oxygen saturation in sitting.[133] Inspiratory muscle training also has been found to be effective in neuromuscular disorders in improving maximal voluntary ventilation, maximal inspiratory mouth pressure, and respiratory load perception[52,154] and should be considered in this population.

Aquatic therapy can be a valuable adjunct to traditional intervention strategies for people at all levels of the SMA continuum. By using the physical properties of water such as buoyancy, hydrostatic pressure, viscosity, and turbulence, the PTA provides additional tools for intervention, especially in the case of extreme weakness characteristic of this disorder.[41]

TORTICOLLIS

Definition and Overview

Torticollis (congenital muscular torticollis [CMT]; wry neck) means *twisted neck* and is a contracted state of the sternocleidomastoid muscle (SCM), producing head tilt to the affected side with rotation of the chin to the opposite side (Fig. 14.19). Four types of muscle abnormalities have been identified on ultrasonography: 15% had a fibrotic mass in the SCM (type I), 77% had diffuse fibrosis mixed with normal muscle (type II), 5% had fibrotic tissue without normal muscle (type III), and the last group (type IV) had a fibrotic cord and included only 3% of the population.

Torticollis often is confused with a separate disorder known as *cervical dystonia* (also referred to as *acquired torticollis* or *spasmodic torticollis*). These are two separate entities. CMT as it is presented in this section is a musculoskeletal phenomenon, whereas cervical dystonia is a movement disorder with an underlying CNS pathology.

Incidence and Etiologic Factors

Reports of the overall incidence of CMT vary significantly from 0.6 to 400 per 100,000 live births, but this condition is not considered uncommon.[64] A variety of possible causes of CMT exist, but the precise cause remains unknown.

Initially it was thought that the fibrosis was related to birth trauma, because incidence is increased in breech (19%) and forceps (6%) delivery, vacuum extraction (30.5%), and cesarean section (17.9%).[25] Predisposing factors can include restrictive intrauterine environment, poor muscle tone, or cervical-vertebral abnormalities. A genetic contribution also has been proposed in a portion of cases of CMT.[38]

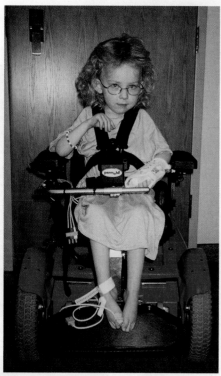

FIG. 14.18 Spinal muscular atrophy (SMA). Three-year-old with SMA in her power wheelchair, which allows her to adjust the seat height so that she can be on the floor to aid with transfers or at eye level with her peers. The adjustable seat allows the child to participate in activities at elevated surfaces (e.g., counter or table heights), retrieve objects from a shelf, or help decorate the tree at Christmas. (Courtesy Allan Glanzman, Children's Seashore House of the Children's Hospital of Philadelphia, Pennsylvania.)

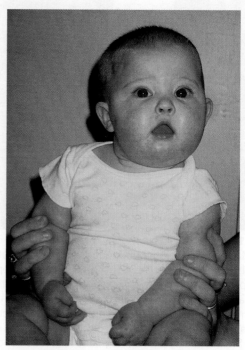

FIG. 14.19 Torticollis. Five-month-old with torticollis (head tilt toward the involved side and rotation away from the involved side). (Courtesy Allan Glanzman, Children's Seashore House of the Children's Hospital of Philadelphia, Pennsylvania.)

Pathogenesis

The possible pathogenesis of the muscular fibrosis seen in CMT has been explored experimentally in animal models and has been produced through venous occlusion, and this, in addition to arterial occlusion, has been proposed as the possible pathogenesis.[64]

One theory postulates that the malposition of the head potentially leads to a compartment syndrome. In this scenario, the SCM is not stretched or torn but rather kinked or compressed. With the head and neck in a position of forward flexion, lateral bend, and rotation, the ipsilateral SCM kinks, causing an ischemic injury and subsequent edema at the site of the kink.[27]

Clinical Manifestations

The first sign of CMT identified in a portion of affected children is a firm, nontender, palpable enlargement of the SCM often referred to as a *sternocleidomastoid tumor of infancy*. A portion of cases demonstrate bulbous fibrotic tissue at the base or midportion of the involved SCM. This local lesion usually reaches its maximal size by 1 month and then slowly regresses within 4 to 8 months and does not always result in torticollis.[142]

The typical position observed of lateral head tilt and rotation to the opposite side predominates regardless of whether a fibrotic mass is present (estimated in 15% to 66% of cases[64,66]) or no mass is palpated and the muscle is uniformly fibrotic and shortened.

If the deformity is severe, the infant's face, ear, and head flatten from resting on the affected side, a condition referred to as *plagiocephaly* ("oblique head"); this cranial asymmetry gradually worsens. The infant's chin turns away from the side of the shortened muscle, the head tilts to the shortened side, and the shoulder is elevated on the affected side, further limiting cervical movement.

The side of the plagiocephaly (best observed by looking down on the head from above) is usually defined by the side of the flattened forehead. When torticollis and plagiocephaly occur together, this condition is referred to as *plagiocephaly torticollis deformation sequence* (Fig. 14.20).

The incidence of other deformities such as hip dislocation and positional clubfoot is elevated in cases of CMT.[25,53] Subluxation of the cervical spine can also be associated with CMT and should be ruled out by cervical spine radiographs.[64,129]

Medical Management

Diagnosis

Clinical observation combined with the history forms the basis of the initial diagnostic process. Medical evaluation including radiographic studies of the spine is always indicated to rule out congenital deformities of the cervical spine, ocular anomalies, and less frequently tumors or other CNS pathology in children with presumed torticollis.

Treatment

Initial management involves a period of active observation for spontaneous resolution. During this time physical therapy to correct the positional and deformational effects is the mainstay of treatment for CMT. Interventions include twice daily passive ROM exercises to stretch the shortened muscle, preceded by warm compresses, massage, and slight

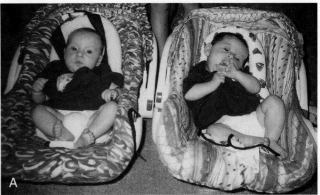

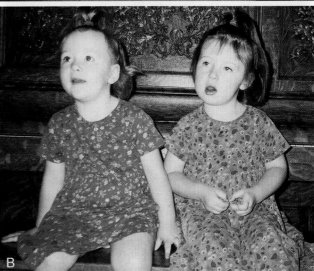

FIG. 14.20 Plagiocephaly torticollis deformation. (A) Four-month-old fraternal twins: the child on the right has marked untreated congenital muscular torticollis with plagiocephaly. Note the positional pelvic asymmetry from placement in a car seat. (B) The same twins (2 years old) after physical therapy (PT) intervention at age 6 months for the child on the right. PT intervention over a 3-month period of time included passive range of motion, facilitated active range of motion, positioning, and a cervical collar. A home exercise program was prescribed with periodic rechecks. Eventually the use of a helmet was instituted to remodel craniofacial asymmetry (see Fig. 14.22). Some craniofacial asymmetry persists, although full active and passive range of motion are present. (Courtesy Laurie Matteson, Great Falls, Montana. Used with permission.)

traction to relax the muscle before stretching; stabilization of the proximal attachment of the SCM and trapezius is important during ROM exercises.

Positioning is also important to encourage erect and midline head posture. Strengthening activities should include both active and active assistive exercises in addition to the incorporation of postural reactions in treatment when these reactions begin to develop.[73] When working with infants and toddlers it is best to embed their therapy program into a daily routine, thus allowing the caregiver to accomplish the stretching at diaper change, and to encourage the parent to position everything toward the unshortened side. For instance, if a child has a torticollis of the right SCM, the head rotates to the left and sidebends to the right. In such a case the child would tend to look toward the left. Along with manually stretching the tight muscles, people and objects should be presented to the child's right, thus encouraging the child to turn the head to the right. Similarly, the child should be positioned in the bed or when sleeping such that the wall is to the left and the door and activity are to the right. That way the child will wake up and gain immediate motivation to try to look toward the activity and not be encouraged to look left at the boring wall.

Splinting has been advocated by some for older children (older than 4 months) who continue to demonstrate head tilt.[69] A cervical collar or tubular orthosis for torticollis can be helpful in providing tactile cueing for movement in the direction opposite the lateral tilt. Usually these collars are the most effective at a time that is compatible with active head control (Fig. 14.21). Kinesio taping is also very effective if the child tolerates the tape and the adhesive. The tape is applied in an inverted Y shape over the contralateral SCM to help activate it and hold the head in a neutral position.

In cases of delayed treatment or when craniofacial asymmetry persists, nonsurgical remodeling of the skull using externally applied pressure can be used (Fig. 14.22). With advances in computer software and technology (e.g., pressure scanners), trained clinicians can determine the pressure in pounds per square inch that applies the appropriate force needed to achieve the remodeling process for each individual head diameter, volume, and topography.[145,147] The helmets are usually worn 23 hours per day for several months.

Surgical intervention is rare (e.g., SCM tenotomy, plastic surgery for craniofacial asymmetry) and is considered only if the individual continues to demonstrate significant motion restrictions of 30 degrees after 6 months of age or if the deformity persists past 12 months of age. Increased thickening of the SCM and increased deformity are also indications that warrant consideration of surgical intervention.[73]

Prognosis

CMT usually resolves with conservative treatment. Complete recovery, including full passive ROM, can be expected to take approximately 3 to 12 months, with fewer than 16% of children presented in the first year requiring surgery.[35] Left untreated or poorly managed, chronic, unresolved torticollis can result in persistent deformity and asymmetry of the shape and position of the head as well as the temporomandibular joint and cervical spine.

14.7 Special Implications for the PTA: Torticollis The prognostic information provided makes it possible for therapists to better predict treatment duration at the time of initial assessment. When parents are provided with more precise information about the length of treatment, parents may be more willing to adhere to the exercise program.[36]

The PTA must remain alert to recognize cervical subluxation in cases of CMT. This may be observed as residual head-neck posturing problems, even after successful neck muscle therapy; usually no neurologic deficits are present.

Likewise, torticollis that does not respond to physical therapy may have a nonorthopedic cause such as ocular torticollis, requiring further medical evaluation. Do not hesitate to ask for reevaluation if and when a child does not respond to therapy.

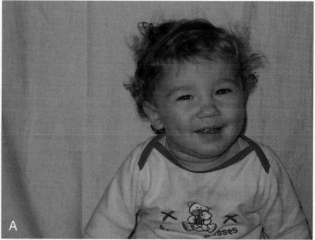
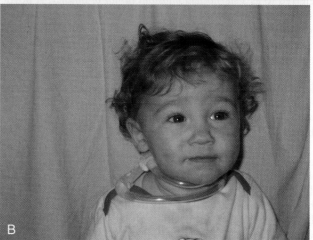

FIG. 14.21 Congenital torticollis. (A) Note the head tilt in this toddler with right-sided congenital torticollis. Despite his full range of motion, he has an occasional residual head tilt to the right and turn to the left. (B) The same child wearing a tubular orthosis for torticollis collar to encourage a more vertical head position. (Courtesy Allan Glanzman, Children's Seashore House of the Children's Hospital of Philadelphia, Pennsylvania.)

ERB'S PALSY

Definition and Overview

Erb's palsy is a paralysis of the upper limb typically resulting from a traction injury to the brachial plexus. It actually comprises three distinct types of brachial plexus palsies: (1) Erb–Duchenne palsy, affecting the C5 to C6 nerve roots (95% to 99% of all cases); (2) whole-arm palsy, affecting C5 to T1; and (3) Klumpke's palsy, affecting the C8 and T1 (lower plexus) nerve roots.

Incidence

The incidence of brachial plexus injuries has decreased secondary to improved obstetric management of difficult labors. Traction injuries are most common in newborns, occurring in 0.1% of spontaneous, 1.2% of breech, and 1.3% of forceps deliveries. Overall, the incidence of birth-related traction injuries is 0.3 to 2 per 1000 births.[146]

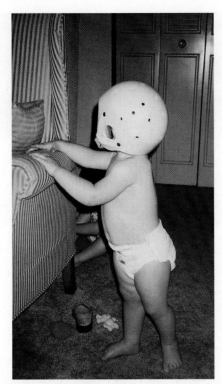

FIG. 14.22 Fourteen-month-old girl wearing a polypropylene helmet lined with durometer foam. This helmet applied remodeling pressure on the cranium to reshape unresolved craniofacial asymmetry that persisted as a result of delayed medical intervention and inconsistent use of a cervical collar. The helmet was accepted readily by the child and worn at all times (except for bathing) for approximately 4 months. Pressure was applied to the right posterior occiput to bring the head and neck into midline alignment while space was created in which the skull was flattened in the left posterior occipital area to allow for bony growth in that area. See Fig. 14.20, B for intervention outcome. (Courtesy Laurie Matteson, Great Falls, Montana. Used with permission.)

Etiologic and Risk Factors

The major contributing factor to these injuries has been found to be forced stretching of the brachial plexus, that is, a pulling away of the shoulder from the head secondary to a traction maneuver during the birth process.

The lower plexus injury resulting in Klumpke's palsy usually is caused by manipulation during delivery resulting from hyperabduction of the arm at the shoulder; that is, the head and trunk remain relatively immobile in the pelvis while the upper extremity is stretched severely. However, some question remains about the role of the obstetrician compared with the position of the infant and the forces encountered in the canal before birth.

Evidence suggests that the propulsive nature of the birth process when stretching of the involved nerves occurs is something over which the birth attendant has no control.[125]

Obstetric history associated with Erb's palsy is characterized by high birth weight or vertex delivery with shoulder dystocia (i.e., during delivery the baby's shoulder impinges on the mother's symphysis pubis). Klumpke's palsy more commonly is associated with heavy sedation, difficult breech delivery, and brow or face presentation. Brow or face presentation makes

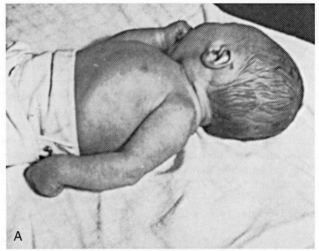

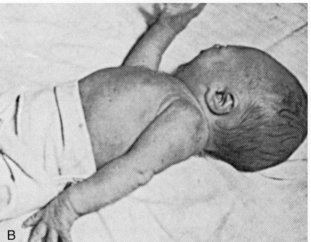

FIG. 14.23 Erb's palsy. (A) In this infant with Erb's palsy, the arm is maintained in a position of adduction and internal rotation at the shoulder with the lower arm pronated and fingers flexed. (B) Same infant demonstrating an asymmetric Moro reflex with opening of the left hand but still in the "waiter's tip" position. (From Kliegman RM, Stanton BMD, St. Geme J, et al. (eds): Nelson textbook of pediatrics, ed 20, Philadelphia, 2016, Elsevier.)

vaginal delivery impossible. Brow presentation rarely persists; in face presentation, the head is hyperextended and the chin is the presenting part.

Rarely, neoplasm present at birth results in brachial plexus palsy. The absence of signs of a traumatic injury accompanied by the onset of weakness and progressive course in the first few days of life must be investigated by MRI.[1]

Adults may acquire an Erb's palsy injury as a result of a severe trauma such as after a motorcycle accident or secondary to a work injury. The sequelae are similar to those in infants, and surgery is recommended to repair the damage, if possible.

Clinical Manifestations

Children with brachial plexus injuries are unlikely to demonstrate postural or placing responses with the involved upper extremity when tested. In Erb's palsy the arm is maintained in adduction and internal rotation at the shoulder with the lower arm pronated and fingers flexed, assuming the waiter's tip position (Fig. 14.23). Children with this type have difficulty with activities such as hand-to-mouth, hand-to-head, and hand-to-back of neck movements but usually have control of the wrist and fingers.

In Klumpke's palsy, paralysis of the small muscles of the hand and wrist flexors causes a claw hand appearance. Proximal shoulder control is good, but voluntary wrist and hand control is difficult. In severe forms of brachial palsy (whole-arm palsy), the whole plexus can be affected but to a varying degree (Fig. 14.24). In this case careful examination is necessary to identify affected muscles. In all three cases (Erb's, Klumpke's, and whole-arm palsy) normal sensation is diminished; however, gross pain sensation may not be decreased to the same degree as movement.

The clinical characteristics of brachial plexus injury are summarized in Table 14.7.

Medical Management

Diagnosis

Some injuries are recognizable readily at or soon after birth. Radiographs may be taken to rule out associated fractures of the clavicle. Imaging of the brachial plexus using MRI is not invasive and can demonstrate proximal and distal lesions.

MRI can be used to detect nerve root avulsions, nerve ruptures, brachial plexus scarring, posttraumatic neuroma, brachial plexus edema, spinal cord damage, abnormalities of the shoulder joint, trauma, neoplasms, and infection. This type of imaging allows diagnosis and careful preoperative evaluation of children with brachial plexus injuries.[7,20]

Electromyography can be used to delineate the extent of injury, aid in the prognosis, and assist the surgeon in identifying appropriate surgical procedures. Electromyography usually is delayed until 4 to 6 weeks after birth and may be followed serially over time to track recovery. Conduction studies can aid in separating actual axonal loss from conduction block. Needle electromyography can help determine the portion of the plexus damaged as well as the severity of the damage.[32]

Treatment

Although medical intervention may include the use of botulinum toxin (Botox) to address contractures that may develop over time[120] or surgery, treatment is primarily with a PTA following the strategies outlined in Table 14.7. Surgery has found renewed favor because evidence is increasing that microneurosurgical intervention at an early stage can improve the outcome. For example, some children have no chance of recovery unless they undergo early aggressive surgical reconstruction of the injured brachial plexus. In children with global or total paralysis, surgery is performed by 3 to 4 months to maximize ultimate extremity function and minimize disability.[54,138]

Surgery should be performed by an experienced pediatric neurosurgical team. Options for surgical care include tendon transfers, considered after a plateau in recovery has occurred, and microneurosurgery (e.g., nerve decompression, neurolysis, nerve repair, nerve reconstruction with grafts or tubes). The latter procedure is best considered for individuals aged 6 to 12 months for optimal functional results.[122]

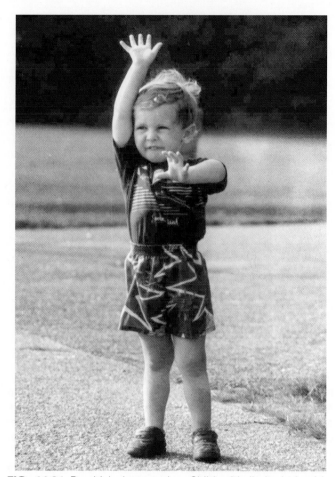

FIG. 14.24 Brachial plexus palsy. Child with limited shoulder external rotation and abduction of the left arm associated with whole-arm palsy. Full motion of the upper extremity is demonstrated on the right side. (From Green DP, Hotchkiss RN, Pederson WC: Green's operative hand surgery, ed 5, London, 2005, Churchill Livingstone.)

Prognosis

In most instances full recovery can be expected; however, some children do have long-term disability as an outcome and require careful follow-up to prevent the development of contractures and facilitate active motor control.

The first muscles to return are the elbow, wrist, and finger extensors, followed by the deltoid and biceps and later the external rotators. The timely recovery of these muscles (beginning at 6 weeks and continuing through 3 months) is prognostic of good functional recovery.[32]

The long-term prognosis for recovery of motor control is poor beyond 18 months (Table 14.8), and probably 15% of infants experience significant disability, with reports showing a wide range of long-term impairments.[122] Recovery of shoulder external rotation is highly indicative of a good long-term outcome; this is a key movement for performing a variety of functional tasks. Almost half of those with the Erb-Duchenne type of injuries do not recover shoulder external rotation, and contractures of the shoulder and elbow joint with atrophy of the affected muscles can occur.

TABLE 14.7 Brachial Plexus Injury: Clinical Characteristics

Type	Typical Posture	Strength Losses	Sensory Losses	Skeletal Changes	Treatment Strategies
Erb's (C5-C6)	Shoulder IR, adduction, finger flexion (difficulty with hand to mouth, hand to head, and back of neck)	Deltoid, supraspinatus, infraspinatus, teres minor, biceps, brachialis, brachioradialis, supinator	C5-C6 deficits	Flattening of glenoid fossa and humeral head Elongating deformity of coracoid process hooking down and lateral Scapular winging potential Posterior shoulder dislocation	Active or active assistive exercise: shoulder abduction; elbow flexion; forearm supination and shoulder ER
Klumpke's (C8-T1)	Pronation, elbow flexion contractures; no grasp reflex	Wrist flexors, long finger flexors; hand intrinsics	Diminished sensation	Hypertrophy of olecranon and coronoid process: elbow flexion contracture; posterior dislocation of radial head (25%)	Active or active assistive exercise: forearm supination, elbow extension, finger flexion Positional splint to assist with elbow extension; combined with upper extremity weight bearing
Total plexus injury (whole arm)	Combinations of previously mentioned postures	Combination of Erb's and Klumpke's types	Moderate losses	Posterior glenohumeral dislocation	Combination of previously mentioned treatment strategies

ER, External rotation; *IR,* internal rotation.

TABLE 14.8 Key Indicators of Recovery of Motor Control[a]

Muscle	Time Since Birth (Mo)
Elbow, wrist, and finger extensors	1½
Deltoid, biceps	2
Shoulder external rotators	3

[a]Good functional recovery is expected if the child achieves a strength grade of 3 or better within the listed time frames.

14.8 Special Implications for the PTA: Erb's Palsy An integrated team approach to congenital brachial plexus injuries is imperative. Each child must be carefully evaluated, therapy interventions maximized, and the surgical approach (when required) individualized to obtain the best outcome.

An aggressive and integrated physical and occupational therapy program is essential in the treatment of these injuries. The PTA uses a problem-solving approach and continually adjusts the interventions based on each child's unique needs. The maintenance of full passive mobility during the period of neurologic recovery is essential for normal joint development.

Early surgical correction of shoulder contractures and subluxations reduces permanent disability. Postoperative rehabilitative therapy can preserve and build on gains made possible by medical or surgical interventions.[115,117]

Treatment should focus on activities that encourage active and active assistive movement and that maintain the normal joint kinematics. The shoulder requires particular attention to maintain the normal scapulohumeral and scapulothoracic relationships in addition to maintaining the normal "roll and glide" of the glenohumeral joint and preventing subluxation.

Some strategies used to maintain functional upper extremity ROM, prevent subluxation, and improve active movement include neuromuscular electrical stimulation, biofeedback, myofascial release techniques (sometimes referred to as *soft tissue mobilization*), joint mobilization, and positioning using splints. Carefully applied neurodynamic techniques to physically challenge the nervous system in Erb's palsy may contribute to the physical health of the nervous system,

OSTEOGENESIS IMPERFECTA

Overview and Incidence

Osteogenesis imperfecta (OI), sometimes referred to as *brittle bones,* is a rare congenital disorder of collagen synthesis affecting bones and connective tissue. Four primary types of OI exist, with varying degrees of severity and clinical presentations (Table 14.9). Clinical features vary widely among types, within types, and even within the same family. Although the exact figure is unknown, experts estimate that 20,000 to 50,000 people have OI in the United States (prevalence).

Etiologic Factors and Pathogenesis

Most children with OI inherit the disorder from a parent (autosomal dominant inheritance). Genetic counseling requires recognition that the parent can be a carrier of the dominant gene by parental mosaicism (i.e., the parent carries the mutation in a portion of his or her germ cells).

Approximately 25% of children with OI, however, are born into a family with no history of the disorder. In these cases, the genetic defect occurred as a spontaneous mutation. Because the genetic defect is usually dominant (whether inherited from a parent or resulting from a spontaneous mutation), affected people have a 50% chance of passing on the disorder to each of their children.[107]

leading to optimum physiology. Scapulothoracic stabilization for winging of the scapula using taping may be helpful, but no reported outcomes have been published for these last two interventions.

Passive ROM exercises should be performed three times a day in the direction of limited movement to help prevent the development of contractures, and a well thought out home program that embeds stretching opportunities into the daily routine is an integral part of the therapy program. When splints are used, careful follow-up and family education are necessary, especially if sensory impairment is present.

TABLE 14.9	**Sillence Classification of Osteogenesis Imperfecta**	
Type	**Severity**	**Description**
I (most common form)	Mildest form of osteogenesis imperfecta	Mild to moderate fragility without deformity Most fractures occur before puberty Associated with blue sclerae, triangular face, hearing loss (beginning in 20s or 30s), easy bruising
II	Most severe form (perinatal lethal)	Stillbirth or death during infancy or early childhood Extreme fragility of connective tissue Multiple in utero fractures Usually intrauterine growth retardation Severe bone deformity Soft, large cranium Micromelia: long bones crumpled and bowed; ribs beaded
III	Moderately severe	Progressive deformities Scoliosis Triangular face, large skull Severe osteoporosis Severe fragility of bones; usually in utero fractures Fractures heal with deformity and bowing Associated with tinted sclerae (blue, purple, or gray) Extreme short stature Usually wheelchair bound by teenage years
IV	Variable but usually milder course; normal or near-normal life span	Mild to moderate skeletal fragility and osteoporosis (more severe than type I) Associated with bowing of long bones Barrel-shaped rib cage Bones fracture easily before puberty; some children improve at puberty Light or normal sclerae; may or may not have moderate short stature and joint hyperextensibility

More than 150 mutations have been identified as causative in OI, all affecting the genes (*COL1A1* and *COL1A2*) that code for type I collagen. Type I collagen is found in the extracellular matrix of bone, skin, and tendon and is the major structural protein (scaffolding) of these tissues.

When the defective gene instructs the body to make too little type I collagen or abnormal polypeptide chains that cannot form the triple helix of type I collagen, the symptomatology of OI becomes apparent. In type I, the least severe form of OI and more often the result of acquired rather than hereditary mutation, collagen production is reduced by 50%. The remaining collagen is produced normally, creating a relatively mild clinical picture. In the most severe form (type II) only 20% of collagen is produced and the phenotypic result is devastating.

In endochondral and intramembranous bone formation the final structure of bone is similar, despite different mechanics of formation. Collagen is produced by osteoblasts that in normal bone become surrounded by a collagen matrix. Once the matrix is formed, calcium is laid down, trabeculae develop, and cancellous bone is formed. As the trabeculae become thicker and the density increases, a cortex of compact bone is formed.

Bone modeling in OI appears to be defective, with a smaller cross-sectional area observed and thinner cortex noted in the long bones, leading to diminished strength. The overall mass of cancellous bone also is decreased in OI.

In individuals with OI cancellous bone volume does not increase with age as it does in children who do not have OI. This is related primarily to decreased rates of trabecular thickening in people with OI. In type I OI the annual rate of trabecular thickening is decreased, and in type III and type IV no trabecular thickening is noted over time.

The rate at which matrix is laid down in these three types of OI is slowed compared with the normal rate. Because this slowing is uniform across types I, III, and IV of OI, severity probably is not related to the decreased rate of matrix production.[118]

The underlying causes of the bony abnormalities seen in people with OI are not entirely understood but probably result from one or a combination of factors. These factors have a potential role in the ultimate phenotypic expression in OI and include the unique structural characteristics of the abnormal collagen created by the mutation, the absence of other connective tissue proteins that affect the assembly of the extracellular matrix, and the degree to which the collagen is incorporated into that matrix.[33,87]

Clinical Manifestations

This disease has a wide range of clinical presentations ranging from a normal appearance with occasional fractures to severe involvement with growth retardation and long bone and spinal deformities (Fig. 14.25; see Table 14.9). In its severe forms, OI is evident at birth because of the fractures and deformity that have occurred in utero.

The less severe forms may not become evident until the child begins to walk and fractures develop. The tendency to fracture declines after puberty when cortical bone density increases despite trabecular density remaining low. The fracture rate in women increases after menopause. Some children with OI can be mistaken for abused children until the diagnosis is made.

Shortened stature is common in children with OI. This is a result, at least in part, of the abnormal development of epiphyseal growth plates, deformity after fractures, osteoporosis, and vertebral collapse, which contribute to loss of height with increasing age. Lower extremities tend to be more involved than upper extremities. These children often bruise easily, and ligaments tend to show increased laxity.

Additional clinical features may include thin skin, joint hypermobility, deformity of bony auditory structures with subsequent hearing impairment, scoliosis, pectus deformity, deformed teeth, a tendency toward recurrent epistaxis, excess diaphoresis, cardiovascular complications (e.g., aortic and

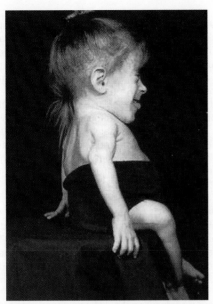

FIG. 14.25 Child with osteogenesis imperfecta type III. This shows defect of all four limbs and increased anteroposterior diameter of the chest. Note the spinal deformity. (From Bullough PG: Bullough and Vigorita's orthopaedic pathology, ed 3, St Louis, 1997, Mosby.)

mitral valve insufficiency, aortic dissection), and metabolic defects (e.g., elevated serum pyrophosphate, decreased platelet aggregation). Children with type III or IV OI are born with a triangular face, a feature that makes them easily identifiable.

Blue or tinted (purple, gray) sclerae are present. The sclerae are blue or tinted because they are abnormally translucent like thin skin, and consequently they filter the red color of the underlying choroid plexus of blood vessels, just as a bruise or a subcutaneous hematoma appears blue through thin translucent skin.[124]

Developmental motor skills often are delayed because of poorly developed muscles (atrophy), hypermobility of joints, and multiple fractures requiring immobilization. The majority of children with type I OI ambulate either as functional or household ambulators, and approximately 50% walk without any type of assistive device as community ambulators.

Almost half of children with type III OI are dependent on power mobility, with only 27% becoming household ambulators. Of children with type IV disease, 26% are community ambulators and 57% household ambulators. The best predictors of ambulatory status are disease type and the ability to sit by 9 or 10 months of age.[26,37]

Medical Management

Diagnosis

Diagnosis of OI is based on clinical manifestations and skin biopsy that looks at collagen. The collagen defect is used to determine what type of OI the person has according to the Sillence classification. Bone scans and x-ray films show evidence of multiple old fractures and skeletal deformities. Skull radiographs show wide sutures with small, irregularly shaped islands of bone called *wormian bones.*

Treatment

Orthopedic management is central to the overall care of symptomatic OI. Fracture prevention and control are the primary focus; careful positioning and handling are required to prevent fractures in the neonate. Lightweight HKAFOs and splints also may be used to help support the limbs, prevent fractures, and aid in ambulation. HKAFOs are used more often than KAFOs because KAFOs have a longer lever arm for rotational force, resulting in greater risk for proximal femur fractures.[50]

Fracture immobilization is as minimal as possible to prevent disuse atrophy. A repeated cycle of fracture and immobilization of the same bone can inhibit progress in mobility and the development of strength (Fig. 14.26). The use of intramedullary rods is one way of managing recurring fractures (Fig. 14.27). Indications for this procedure include more than two fractures in the same long bone within a 6-month period, lower extremity bone angles greater than 40 degrees, or very unstable lower extremities in a child who appears ready to walk. Telescoping intramedullary rods are used to stabilize the bones, elongating as the bone grows, although this procedure is not without risk.

The reoperation rate is significant, with complications related to osteopenia that occur around the rods (greater around thicker rods), rod migration, and bony growth even beyond the available expansion. Osteotomies also are performed to help control rotational deformities, with appropriate bracing to prolong the time period between potential surgeries.

Medical management has included the use of bisphosphonates, a class of medications (including pamidronate) that inhibit osteoclast function, improve bone mineral density, and decrease the incidence of fractures. Some data exist on the use of growth hormone in OI, but reports of an increased rate of fractures have prevented the use of growth hormone as a first-line drug in the treatment of OI.[155]

Initial reports of allogeneic bone marrow transplantation of mesenchymal cells (progenitors of osteoblasts) have been promising, with increased bone mineral content and histologic evidence of new bone formation 3 months after engraftment.[65] Studies in cell cultures and in mice have raised the possibility that several additional strategies may be developed to treat OI through the use of gene therapy; a review of current gene therapy strategies under investigation is available.[43]

Prognosis

People with OI types I and IV have a milder course and live a relatively normal life span. In type III OI, mortality can be related to cardiorespiratory failure stemming from kyphoscoliotic deformity. A significant risk also exists of basilar invagination of the skull and intracranial bleeding.[89]

Incomplete and relatively painless fractures after birth that receive no treatment can produce deformities from bones healing in poor alignment. Short stature and deformities give some individuals with OI the appearance of having achondroplasia. Milder forms of this condition cause fewer clinical problems, and these children survive into adulthood. All caregivers should be provided with medical documentation confirming the diagnosis of OI. This is especially helpful if the child is being treated by a medical professional unfamiliar to them. Often, previous healed fractures are mistaken for abuse and neglect.

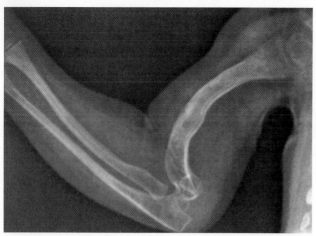

FIG. 14.26 Radiograph of upper extremity in a person with osteogenesis imperfecta. This radiograph shows severe osteoporosis, slender bones, and multiple healed fractures. (From Bullough PG: Bullough and Vigorita's orthopaedic pathology, ed 3, St Louis, 1997, Mosby.)

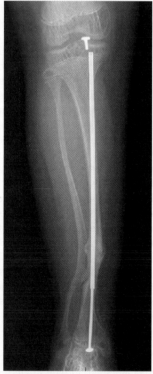

FIG. 14.27 AP x-ray of a 9-year-old girl with osteogenesis imperfecta (OI) after treatment of a tibia fracture with a Bailey-Dubow rod. (From Laron D, Pandya NK: Advances in the orthopedic management of osteogenesis imperfecta, Orthop Clin North Am 44(4):565–573, 2013.)

14.9 Special Implications for the PTA: Osteogenesis Imperfecta

Precautions

Infants and children with OI require careful handling to prevent fractures. They must be supported when they are being turned, positioned, moved, burped, and cuddled or held. Diaper changing must be performed gently, never lifting the legs by the ankles but rather by gently lifting the buttocks.

With the older child, passive ROM exercises (especially to obtain hip extension) can be used with caution and are considered safe if used in moderation. Rotational forces are contraindicated, but gentle stretching in straight planes and myofascial stretching are acceptable if done carefully and with the client's participation.

The child must be encouraged to use full active ROM without force. Strengthening activities should avoid placing weight near joint lines, and if manual resistance is applied, long lever arms should be avoided. The children do well with strengthening and stretching activities built into everyday routines, such as reaching for things on a higher shelf or carrying objects of varying weights.

Family Education

Educational material and information can be obtained from the Osteogenesis Imperfecta Foundation (www.oif.org). The family must be instructed in handling and positioning techniques. Precautions should be taken to avoid lifting the child under the arms or by the hands. The young child should not be tossed into the air or be involved in roughhouse play.

At the same time, families should be encouraged to hold and play with their child appropriately and to help the child develop interests that do not require strenuous physical activity. Fine motor skills are encouraged, and modifications in ADLs for personal hygiene may be necessary.

Swimming frequently is recommended, but the child must be monitored carefully to avoid falls in the shower and pool area. Nonskid aquatic shoes can be worn (by the child or by the caregiver carrying a nonambulatory child in the aquatic area) to assist with this precaution.

Family members must also be instructed to assess for fractures daily. The child may bruise easily, but it is common for a child to have no bruises around the fracture site. Symptoms to look for include limited use of an extremity, malposition of an extremity, focal swelling or tenderness, or crying when a body part is moved or when the child attempts to move.

In the case of diagnosed OI involving child abuse allegations, the parents are encouraged to carry a letter from the primary care physician documenting the diagnosis. Even so, any suspicion of actual abuse in the case of a child with OI requires careful documentation and appropriate referral.

Therapy Interventions

Therapy helps to prevent disuse weakness or loss of bone stock and strengthens muscles and builds bone density. Light resistance to exercise or movement can be used; aquatic programs are especially helpful in allowing exercise with light resistance.

Strengthening programs emphasize hip extension, hip abduction, trunk extension, and abdominal muscles. A hip extension, hip abduction, and spinal muscular strengthening program complemented by a swimming program two times per week has been found to correlate with an increased ability to assume and maintain an upright position and subsequent ambulation.[8]

Positioning is a significant part of the overall management program for these children. Positioning emphasizes a neutral position of the head, trunk, and lower extremities; neutral hip rotation; and hip extension. In fragile individuals, the prone position should be avoided except when fully supported or while being supported in the swimming pool.

The ability to stand is important and should be implemented at approximately 10 to 14 months' chronologic age. Standing can be initiated in a standing frame for 30 minutes twice daily. Special care must be taken to avoid fractures when placing and securing the child in the stander. Aquatic therapy also can be used as a medium for initiating standing activities in more severe cases. Throughout any standing activity the PTA must continue to monitor for lower extremity bowing secondary to bone instability.

Mobility

The PTA may have to use a significant amount of creativity to adapt ambulating devices and to accommodate for various musculoskeletal deficiencies while fostering the skills necessary for independent mobility. If ambulation is unlikely, the PTA should not hesitate to move quickly toward a wheelchair as the child's primary means of mobility.

When upper extremities are not involved (or are minimally affected) manual propulsion chairs offer a functional means of strengthening. Wheelchair fit is extremely important, because bones can bow around supporting surfaces such as armrests. Although children as young as 2 years old cognitively can use and benefit from powered mobility,[137] whenever possible, powered mobility is delayed in this population until the child is older (e.g., 5 or 6 years).

ARTHROGRYPOSIS MULTIPLEX CONGENITA

Definition and Overview

Arthrogryposis multiplex congenita (AMC; sometimes known as *multiple congenital contracture* [MCC]) is the MCC that is present at birth, resulting from decreased fetal movement in an intact skeleton. Contracture can result from any number of underlying pathologies. They may occur either in flexion or extension, and the muscles may be nothing more than fibrous bands.

Three different types of AMC exist: (1) contracture syndromes; (2) amyoplasia (lack of muscle formation or development); and (3) distal arthrogryposis, primarily affecting the hands and feet. Occasionally the child has associated abnormalities such as cleft palate, cardiac lesions, urinary tract malformations, and cryptorchidism (failure of testes to descend into the scrotum); however, their presence or absence depends on the underlying cause of the arthrogryposis.

Incidence and Etiologic Factors

AMC affects 1 in 5000 to 10,000 births. It can result from any condition that limits fetal movement. Various investigations have attributed the basic defect to an abnormality of muscle, CNS, lower motor neuron, or fetal environment. Hereditary factors have been identified in a number of isolated cases of AMC, with autosomal dominant, recessive, X-linked recessive, and mitochondrial inheritance patterns being identified.[51]

Other possible causes are prenatal viral infection, drugs, maternal hyperthermia, vascular compromise between mother and fetus, and decreased amniotic fluid in utero (oligohydramnios) limiting fetal movement. The joint deformities present in AMC appear to be secondary to the lack of active motion during intrauterine development and the presence of joint contractures and abnormal weight bearing across the joint.

In rare cases, maternal myasthenia gravis (MG) is a possible cause. MG is an autoimmune disorder caused by antibodies to the nicotinic acetylcholine receptor (AChR) and has been linked to the development of AMC. Maternal antibodies cross the placenta and block the function of the fetal isoform of the AChR, leading to fetal paralysis. This condition is potentially treatable and can be diagnosed by a routine antibody test in any pregnant woman who has MG.[113] However, asymptomatic cases of MG causing AMC have been reported.[13]

BOX 14.5   Arthrogryposis: Clinical Picture

- Speech, cognition usually within average limits
- Facial asymmetry
- Oral–motor: hypotonia, congenitally absent muscles, jaw stiffness contribute to oral–motor difficulties
- Trunk: thoracolumbar scoliosis (20%), rigid movement, slow responses, minimal rotation, all affecting equilibrium and balance
- Lower extremity jackknife posture (55%)
  - Flexed dislocated hips with extended knees
  - Clubfeet (talipes equinovarus)
- Lower extremity frog posture (45%)
  - Abducted, externally rotated hips
  - Knee flexion
  - Clubfeet (talipes equinovarus)
- Upper extremity posture
  - Shoulder adduction and internal rotation
  - Extended elbow, wrist ulnar deviation
  - Flexed wrists with stiff straight fingers; poor thumb control
- Functional reach impaired, requiring multiple muscle substitution, cocontraction of flexors and extensors, use of opposite arm or hand to assist
- Delayed motor development
  - Sitting independently: approximately 15 months
  - Ambulation: approximately 2 to 3 years if musculoskeletal limitations allow

---

Pathogenesis

The underlying cause of AMC is unknown; however, an underlying condition in all cases causes decreased fetal movement. Specifically, a disturbance may occur in the development of the anterior horn cells of motor neurons leading to an association with SMA.[16]

AMC also has been associated with a variety of CNS disorders, including migrational brain disorders and neurodegenerative disorders. MDC also is associated with a smaller percentage of cases of AMC.

Clinical Manifestations

The dominant features of AMC include joint contracture, articular rigidity, muscle weakness, and in some cases replacement of the muscle with fibrous and fatty tissue. Arthrogryposis can affect all joints of the body but tends to have a preference for the feet, hips, wrists, knees, elbows, and shoulders (in order of decreasing frequency). A typical clinical picture of a child with arthrogryposis is outlined in Box 14.5.

Because many of these children demonstrate average or above average intelligence, they are able to accommodate for loss of motion with a variety of alternative mobility patterns such as seat-scooting or rolling. They usually do not choose (or are unable to assume or maintain) the quadruped position.

The jackknife or frog posture also affects the child's ability to accommodate for movement. Children with knee flexion (frog-leg posture) are typically slower to roll but quicker to sit and scoot. Many of the children are unable to make the transition from sitting to standing but can maintain a standing position once placed upright.

As adults, these people commonly develop arthritis in a variety of different joints as a result of overuse. Many benefit from some type of wheeled or powered mobility for long distances, either because of the wear and tear on malaligned joints and the amount of energy required to move in a malaligned position or to improve functional mobility (often considered as an option at an early age).

Medical Management

Diagnosis

Prenatal diagnosis may be made by ultrasonic examination based on diminished fetal movement and detection of joint contractures. These findings usually do not become evident until 16 to 18 weeks' gestation.[126] A definitive diagnosis is made by neonatal examination and, if needed, radiographs. However, congenital joint contractures may be secondary to many conditions, necessitating differential diagnosis.

Treatment and Prognosis

Physical therapy and occupational therapy are the mainstays of early treatment, with passive mobilization of the joints, positioning, strengthening, and enhancement of functional adaptation skills (e.g., prevention of falls, mobility training, movement up and down stairs or on uneven terrain).

Orthopedic surgery often is used to address the many musculoskeletal limitations associated with AMC and often is combined with serial casting. Some of the more common surgical procedures include posterior spinal fusion for thoracolumbar scoliosis; quadriceps lengthening to increase knee flexion for functional movement; and posterior capsulotomies, hamstring lengthening, and wedge osteotomies to allow for increased functional knee extension.

Clubfoot deformity (Fig. 14.28) often is treated with heel cord lengthening and capsulotomy in addition to a talar procedure if needed to achieve a good correction. Hip procedures are associated with a fairly high risk of avascular necrosis and failed reduction.

The long-term prognosis depends on the underlying cause of joint contractures. The contractures found in this condition are nonprogressive and not life-threatening; however, the underlying cause can be both.

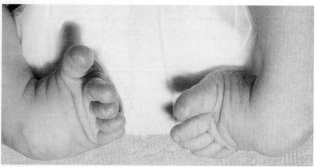

FIG. 14.28 Clubfoot deformity, talipes equinovarus (bilateral deviation). This 4-month-old child was diagnosed with spina bifida, hemivertebrae, and clubfoot. Early intervention can include serial casting to provide stretch to the contracted structures and to provide a more normal plantigrade foot position. Clubfoot is a common morbidity found in children with spina bifida. The casts are typically changed every 1 to 2 weeks and followed by the use of a molded ankle-foot orthosis to maintain the corrected position. Often as the child grows, surgical releases and osteotomies also are required to achieve an optimal correction. (From Zitelli BJ, McIntire SC, Nowalk AJ: Zitelli and Davis' atlas of pediatric physical diagnosis, ed 6, Philadelphia, 2012, Saunders.)

REFERENCES/SUGGESTED READINGS

To enhance this text and add value for the reader, references and suggested readings are included on the companion Evolve site that accompanies this textbook. The reader can view the source and access it online whenever possible.

14.10 Special Implications for the PTA: Arthrogryposis Multiplex Congenita

Therapeutic Interventions

The child benefits maximally from therapy from 0 to 2 years of age and during periodic growth spurts, with functional goals related to optimal functional mobility and ADLs. Strengthening programs focus on weak muscles or movement in opposition to typical resting postures.

Removable splints such as ankle-foot orthoses are recommended for positioning and stretching. These must be worn a minimum of 6 to 8 h/day and preferably up to 22 h/day. In children who are nonambulatory, power mobility should be considered as early as 2 years of age. A variety of adaptive equipment (including powered feeding devices)[63] is available to aid in the completion of ADLs.

15

Infectious Diseases of the Musculoskeletal System

CHAPTER OBJECTIVES

1. Review primary infections of the musculoskeletal system.
2. Discuss infection control following surgery of the musculoskeletal system.
3. Discuss infectious diseases that can affect the musculoskeletal system.

OUTLINE

VOCAB BUILDERS

Diskitis
Myositis
Myositis ossificans
Osteomyelitis
Polymyositis
Rhabdomyolysis
Septic arthritis
Skeletal tuberculosis
Tenosynovitis

Although chronic disease accounts for the majority of morbidity and mortality in the United States, infectious diseases of the musculoskeletal system are still common in the general population.[18] Fortunately, most of the microorganisms that humans encounter do not produce disease. In fact, *Staphylococcus* is part of the natural flora found in healthy individuals. The interaction between host and organism is complex but is responsible for determining whether an infectious disease ensues.

The body has a number of defense systems in place to prevent an infection from becoming established. These are important in understanding musculoskeletal infections. The skin serves as an effective barrier to invasion by microorganisms but can be easily breached by trauma, invasive procedures, or the bites from insects[80] and animals.[61] Even the best defense systems can fail or be overwhelmed by the sheer numbers of invading microorganisms. When bacteria become established in the host, the multiplication of the organism is what triggers the inflammatory response.

Understanding the epidemiology, pathogenesis, and treatment of musculoskeletal infections will allow the clinician to play an active role in all phases of diagnosis and intervention. From early detection of signs and symptoms that identify those clients who are at risk and need of further medical evaluation to the rehabilitation of those clients who undergo surgical intervention for musculoskeletal infections, the role of physical therapist assistants (PTAs) and their impact on the outcome of treatment cannot be underestimated.

 ## OSTEOMYELITIS

Definition

Osteomyelitis is an inflammation of bone caused by an infectious organism such as bacteria, but fungi, parasites, and viruses can also cause skeletal infections. *Acute osteomyelitis* is the clinical term for a new infection in bone that can develop into a chronic reaction when intervention is delayed or inadequate. It is a rapidly destructive pyogenic infection often seen in children, older adults, and intravenous (IV) drug abusers. The infection has the capability to spread quickly through the bloodstream, resulting in septicemia or a septic infectious joint.

Chronic osteomyelitis is often the result of a relapse, persistent bone infection, or acute disease remaining undiagnosed.

Incidence

Acute osteomyelitis is relatively uncommon, occurring more often in children than adults and affecting boys more often than girls. Chronic osteomyelitis is more common in adults and immunocompromised people. With the use of antibiotics the incidence of osteomyelitis was expected to decline. However, with the presence of drug-resistant organisms, the number of IV drug abusers, and the increased use of implantable prosthetic devices, osteomyelitis is actually becoming more common.[73]

See Box 15.1 for a list of risk factors. Infection is the second most common cause of prosthetic joint failure, after mechanical loosening. The incidences of prosthetic joint infection are higher after a revision.[75]

Etiologic Factors

Staphylococcus aureus is the usual causative agent of acute osteomyelitis.[68] Other organisms such as group B *Streptococcus, Pneumococcus, Pseudomonas aeruginosa, Haemophilus influenzae,* and *Escherichia coli,* and *Salmonella* infection are associated with osteomyelitis.

Osteomyelitis is either exogenous or hematogenous. *Exogenous osteomyelitis* is acquired by invasion of the bone by direct extension from the outside as a result of inoculation into the bone by a penetrating or puncture wound, extension from an overlying abscess or burn, or other trauma such as an open fracture.[6,14] *Hematogenous osteomyelitis* is acquired from spread of organisms from preexisting infections.

Osteomyelitis of the arm and hand bones may occur in drug abusers, and vertebral osteomyelitis is seen in adults from hematogenous spread from pelvic or urinary tract infections.

Pathogenesis

The pathophysiology of osteomyelitis is complex and poorly understood. Key factors include the virulence of the infecting organism; the person's immune status; any underlying disease; and the type, location, and vascularity of the involved bone. Regardless of the source of the pathogen, the pathogenesis of bone infection initially involves an inflammatory response. Acute osteomyelitis may develop in the metaphysis of long bones because of the decreased amount of phagocytosis and/or slower rate of blood flow in the terminal arterioles. The

---

> **BOX 15.1   States Associated with Musculoskeletal Infection**
>
> **Congenital**
> - Chronic granulomatous disease
> - Hemophilia
> - Hypogammaglobulinemia
> - Sickle cell hemoglobinopathy
>
> **Acquired**
> - Diabetes mellitus
> - Hematologic malignancy
> - Human immunodeficiency virus infection
> - Pharmacologic immunosuppression
>   - Organ transplantation
>   - Collagen-vascular diseases
> - Uremia
> - Myelopathy (spinal cord injury)
> - Alcoholism
> - Malnutrition; poor nutritional status

Modified from Brennan PJ, DeGirolamo MP: Musculoskeletal infections in immunocompromised hosts, Orthop Clin North Am 22:390, 1991.

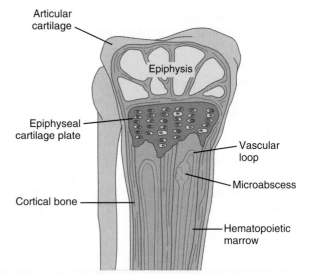

FIG. 15.1 The vascular loop in growing bone is a common initial site of bacterial seeding.

vascular loop in growing bone is a common site of bacterial seeding because the arterioles form a loop and then drain into the medullary cavity without establishing a capillary bed (Fig. 15.1). Trauma, including microtrauma, may also increase susceptibility to infection by slowing the blood flow.

Once bacteria gain access to these channels, they are able to proliferate unimpeded, forming a subperiosteal abscess that deprives the bone of its blood supply and eventually may cause necrosis. Necrotic cells then become a fertile bed for the organisms to multiply. Because sensory nerve endings are absent in cancellous bone, this process can progress without pain. Necrosis then stimulates the periosteum (osteoblasts) to create new bone.

The sheath of new bone, called an *involucrum*, forms around the *sequestrum,* necrotic tissue that has become separated, which works its way out through an abscess or the sinuses (Fig. 15.2). By the time the sequestrum forms, the osteomyelitis is chronic.

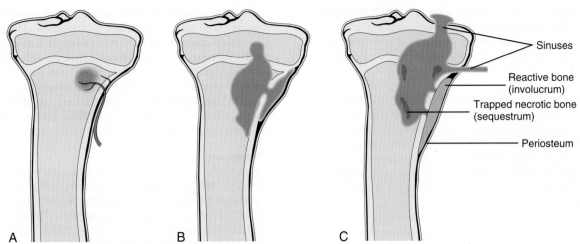

FIG. 15.2 Osteomyelitis. (A) Initial infection. The bacteria reach the metaphysis through the nutrient artery. (B) First stage: bacterial growth results in bone destruction and formation of an abscess. (C) Second stage: from the abscess cavity, the pus spreads between the trabeculae into the medulla, through the cartilage into the joint, or through the Haversian canals of the compact bones to the outside. These sinuses traversing the bone persist for a long time and heal slowly. The pus destroys the bone and sequesters part of it in the abscess cavity. Reactive new bone is formed around the focus of inflammation. (From Damjanov I: Pathology for the health-related professions, ed 4, St Louis, 2012, Saunders.)

In adults, this complication is rare because the periosteum is firmly attached to the cortex and resists displacement. Instead, infection disrupts and weakens the cortex, which predisposes the bone to pathologic fracture.

Clinical Manifestations

The primary manifestations of osteomyelitis vary between adults and children. Back pain is typically the chief complaint in adults, but once the infection becomes systemic (as opposed to an abscess) a low-grade fever may be present. Children are more likely to present with acute, severe complaints, such as high fever and intense pain, but in some cases, local manifestations will predominate, such as edema, erythema, and tenderness. These signs are easier to detect in the extremities, unlike vertebral osteomyelitis in which the infected structures lie much deeper.

In the initial phases of the infection, pain may not be a factor because of the lack of pain fibers in cancellous bone. This makes diagnosis and intervention difficult because of the potential rapid spread of the infectious agent, which is facilitated by the delay in the administration of appropriate antibiotics. When the infection extends into the periosteum, increased joint pain; diminished function; and systemic signs, such as fever, swelling, and malaise, may rapidly develop.

The pain will likely be described as deep and constant, increasing with weight bearing when the infection is anywhere in the lower extremity. Clients presenting with chronic osteomyelitis complain of local pain and swelling but otherwise are often asymptomatic. The clinical sign of "sausage toe" has been used to detect underlying pedal osteomyelitis. This clinical sign has been demonstrated to have good sensitivity and specificity in clients with diabetes.[64]

Once present, spinal osteomyelitis can produce intermittent or constant back pain. The pain can be aggravated by motion but is also present regardless of activity level in some individuals and throbbing at rest. It may radiate in a radicular distribution and is commonly accompanied by spinal tenderness and rigidity; accessory motions of the spine are often difficult to perform. Pyogenic vertebral osteomyelitis may result in a psoas abscess causing painful hip extension and/or an antalgic limp. Cervical abscess formation may lead to torticollis or dysphagia.[74]

Radiculopathy, myelopathy, or even complete paralysis can occur with neural compression as a result of abscess, instability, or spinal deformity associated with vertebral osteomyelitis. Direct spread of the infection into the epidural space can cause meningitis.[74]

Any unexplained cellulitis should be considered a sign of osteomyelitis in children, even if no other contributing signs or symptoms are evident.[73]

Medical Management

Prevention

Because chronic osteomyelitis is also recognized as a complication of treatment of open fractures, prevention of infection is important. The risks can be minimized if the wound is thoroughly debrided, irrigated, and left open for delayed primary closure. Delayed primary closure allows the wound bed to be inspected, and further debridement can be performed if necessary. Clients with any of the conditions listed in Box 15.1 or with any additional risk factors should be taught proper preventive measures and be aware of early warning signs. Anyone with biomaterial implants will have an increased risk of infection, especially in the immediate postoperative period. Although rare, late infections occurring 1 year postoperatively have been reported.[38]

Diagnosis

The diagnosis of infection in total joint revisions is challenging. An aspirate with a white blood cell (WBC) count higher than 50,000 is considered infected without an implant. A total knee replacement is considered infected with 2500 WBC/mL.[52] Medical diagnosis is often delayed because of the lack of specific signs and symptoms, especially in chronic osteomyelitis. Signs and symptoms that are generally associated with infection may be masked by (or mistaken for) normal postoperative changes.

Diagnosis and antimicrobial and surgical treatment of prosthetic joint infection are complex, and the recovery can be arduous and prolonged.[75] A careful history and a thorough physical examination are important. Laboratory values and radiographs are often negative in the early stages. Positive cultures are obtained in only 50% to 80% of cases; however, this is improving because of advancements in molecular techniques.[16,68,75]

Radiographs may not detect bony abnormality in infections of less than 10 days' duration. Lytic lesions may be demonstrable on radiographs within 2 weeks of onset of the disease. A periosteal reaction develops later (Fig. 15.3). Magnetic resonance imaging (MRI) and isotope bone scans are the procedures of choice in delineating the disease's anatomic extent.[73] Imaging tests are often used to localize or confirm the presence of infection. MRI is sensitive and provides valuable detail of *septic arthritis*, spinal osteomyelitis, and diabetic foot infections.[58] Radionuclide bone scan can detect early-stage disease and is helpful in detection and identifying multiple sites of involvement.[13] This procedure may be used as an alternative when MRI cannot be performed or as an adjunct diagnostic tool in people with an uncertain diagnosis.

Identification of the infectious pathogen is of utmost importance because the type of medication used often depends on the infecting microorganism. Specimens are obtained for culture or stains by aspiration, needle biopsy, or swab. Accurate identification is often difficult because of the technical problems of obtaining an acceptable sample. Image-enhanced needle biopsy can improve the specimen quality.

Treatment

Immediate treatment is called for, especially in acute osteomyelitis. The successful use of sequential IV and high-dose antibiotic therapy is now an accepted modality and has lessened the role of surgery in these infections. The choice of antibiotics is based on the culture results. Other factors to consider in choosing an antibiotic are the client's age and health status, site of infection, and previous antimicrobial therapy.

Antibiotics are delivered intravenously to hasten their effect when faced with serious infection that can progress rapidly. Evaluation of response to treatment by monitoring C-reactive protein levels has decreased the average duration of therapy to 3 to 4 weeks with few relapses.[45,68]

Surgery is indicated if the infection has spread to the joints. This is considered an orthopedic emergency. Articular cartilage can be damaged in a matter of hours. The goal of surgery is to drain exudate or pus from the bone or joint. Often, extensive debridement of both bone and surrounding soft tissue is required. These include soft tissue procedures to provide well-vascularized soft tissue coverage of defects and revascularized bone for stabilization of the affected area. In adults, both surgery and antibiotics are often required.

The goals for treatment of chronic osteomyelitis are to eliminate the infection by use of antibiotics if possible or by surgically removing infected tissue. If surgery is indicated, then the current trend is toward more radical surgery rather than serial debridements. Generally, chronic osteomyelitis is more difficult to treat than the acute type because it is difficult to eradicate completely. Exacerbations may respond well to treatment with rest and antibiotics, only to flare up again months later.

In the spine, surgery may be necessary to treat the infection and to address spinal deformity. Deformity of the spine from the infection or subsequent surgery may lead to pain or neurologic compromise. If surgery is not indicated, the person may be treated with short-term bed rest or the use of a brace for immobilization.

The use of appropriate antibiotics prophylactically is standard for some procedures, such as total joint replacements, and in open wounds that are contaminated. Antibiotic bead chains can be implanted in the infected area to achieve concentrated levels of antibiotics in the local tissue without raising serum levels to toxic ranges. These bead chains can be an effective method of prophylaxis and treatment of established infections.[46,69]

Prognosis

The risk of death in the majority of the population is negligible, but treatment remains a challenge to the orthopedic surgeon, radiologist, infectious disease specialist, and therapy team.[73] With early medical interventions, an infection arrest rate of 90% can be expected, even in chronic cases.[60]

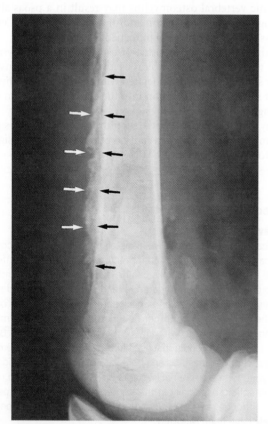

FIG. 15.3 Chronic osteomyelitis. A lateral view of the knee shows the periosteal reaction *(arrows)* suggestive of chronic osteomyelitis. The bone of the distal femur has a mottled appearance as a result of the infection. (From Mettler FA: *Essentials of radiology,* ed 3, Philadelphia, 2014, Saunders.)

If the process is unattended for a week to 10 days, some permanent loss of bone structure almost always occurs, as does the possibility of growth abnormality in the pediatric population. When osteomyelitis is diagnosed in the early clinical stages and treated with antibiotics, the prognosis is excellent. However, it is more often the case that the infection remains undetected for months, during which time it establishes itself in the affected bone and surrounding soft tissues.

When osteomyelitis persists for a long period of time, infected necrotic bone serves as an isolated reservoir for infection that will not respond well to systemic antibiotics. Reduced blood flow will facilitate the likelihood that an infection will be established and the pharmacologic agent will be prevented from reaching the locus of infection. The emergence of antibiotic resistance, particularly resistance to methicillin and vancomycin by *S. aureus* organisms, contributes to long-term sequelae and morbidity.[68]

Chronic osteomyelitis has a poor prognosis, even when treated surgically. People with chronic osteomyelitis are often in great pain, require prolonged medical care, and may, although rarely, require amputation of an extremity.

15.1 Special Implications for the PTA: Osteomyelitis

Anyone reporting recent onset of hip pain in the presence of risk factors associated with osteomyelitis or who has a recent history of surgery now presenting with hip pain may be experiencing a referred pain pattern from an abscess or infectious process affecting the psoas muscle. The therapist can perform several tests to help identify this condition.

PTAs working with clients with a recent history of infection, trauma, or surgery (within the previous 12 months) need to be vigilant for manifestations of infection (see Special Implications for the PTA 15.2: Infections of Prostheses and Implants), especially in cases of prostheses or in the presence of hardware for open reduction and internal fixation. Regular inspection will reveal drainage from the wound, pain with rehabilitation exercises or movement, low-grade fever, and swelling or redness. The increased chance of infection is thought to be a result of the enhanced ability of the infectious organism to attach to the implant.[73]

Preventing Complications

Preventing complications is best done by beginning rehabilitation early. PTAs should first recognize the possible side effects of medical intervention that may lead to complications such as contractures, atrophy, impaired joint mechanics, and loss of function. Treatment of osteomyelitis is complex, and rehabilitation is sometimes perplexing under the best of circumstances.

Sequelae of hip joint sepsis can include joint destruction, avascular necrosis, and fracture. When complications such as these arise, a full recovery is jeopardized. In addition to the musculoskeletal problems, the therapy team should consider other involved organ systems, such as the cardiovascular system, and what impact the comorbidities may have on healing, rehabilitation, and return to a high level of function.

Strict aseptic technique must be used when changing dressings and performing wound care. Reconstructive surgery to cover bone or soft tissue defects requires careful monitoring, dressing changes, and protection. If the client is in skeletal traction for fractures, the insertion points of pin tracks should be covered with small, dry dressings.

Pins used in external fixators also deserve close inspection. The PTA and client must avoid touching the skin around the pins and wires. Assess vital signs, wound appearance, and any new pain daily for signs of secondary infection. During the acute phase of this illness, any movement of the affected limb will cause discomfort or pain. The affected limb should be firmly supported and kept level with the body.

Active, active assisted, and passive range of motion (ROM) exercises of adjacent joints are essential. Good skin care is essential with proper positioning, frequent (but careful and gentle) position changes (at least every 2 hours), and skin assessment for any signs of developing pressure ulcers. Massage or any technique that can possibly spread the infection through mechanical means is to be avoided.

INFECTIONS OF PROSTHESES AND IMPLANTS

Overview

Over the last decades, joint replacement surgery has become commonplace, which is largely attributed to the success of these procedures in restoring function to people with disabling arthritis. People receiving total joint replacements number in the hundreds of thousands each year worldwide, and millions of people have indwelling prosthetic joints. Likewise, during the past 30 years, many new instrumentation systems for internal fixation of the spine have been developed.[10]

Implant infection remains the primary cause of prosthetic failure, occurring either acutely within the first month postoperatively or months to years after the joint replacement.[4] Nearly 80% of these infections are caused by *Staphylococcus* organisms, which enter by perioperative, hematogenous, or contiguous means. Perioperative infections occur around the time of surgery and are probably caused by contaminated hands at the surgical site. Hematogenous infections occur as a result of a primary infection somewhere else in the body. Contiguous infections occur secondary to a nearby infection.[78]

Other types of prostheses or implants susceptible to infection include breast implants, penile implants, dental implants, cardiac implants, other orthopedic devices and hardware, shunts, and even contact lenses (external to epithelial surfaces that can give rise to serious life-threatening infections).

Incidence

With improvements in surgical procedures and prophylactic antibiotics, the incidence of infection has been reduced to less than 1.5%. The incidence of infection does increase with longer procedures and revisions.[59] However, as the number of people undergoing replacements has grown, reoperations have become increasingly common. Bioprostheses, implanted in large numbers in the 1970s and early 1980s, have now gone into the second decade of life since implantation, a time when biodegradation becomes more common. Multiple reoperations carry a higher risk of infection. Likewise, as the population ages, an increasing number of total hip, knee, shoulder, elbow, wrist, and finger arthroplasties are coming up for revision.

Infection of a prosthetic joint causes loosening of the prosthesis and sepsis with significant mortality and morbidity. Two-thirds of prosthetic joint infections occur within 1 year of surgery and are the result of intraoperative inoculations of bacteria into the new joint or postoperative bacteremias. Early infections have been substantially reduced by preoperative use of antibiotics, the use of laminar flow in operating rooms, and improved surgical technique.[59]

Risk Factors

Certain groups have been identified as predisposed toward infection of their prosthetic joints, including those with prior surgery at the site of the prosthesis, rheumatoid arthritis, corticosteroid therapy, diabetes mellitus, poor nutritional status, low albumin, obesity, and extremely advanced age.[10]

Any factor that delays or impairs wound healing increases the risk of infection. Psoriasis, steroids, diabetes mellitus, and immunodeficiency increase the risk of prosthetic infection. Immunodeficiency can be either local (e.g., wear debris from the implant) or systemic (e.g., *Candida albicans*, rheumatoid arthritis, or immunosuppressive medications). Risk factors for infection of spinal instrumentation may include IV drug use, paraplegia with neurogenic bladder, and pyelonephritis (inflammation of the kidney and its pelvis) secondary to renal calculi.

Certain factors or events can enhance the ability of bacteria to multiply rapidly and increase the risk of infection (e.g., wound hematomas, seromas, hemarthroses, fresh operative wounds, ischemic wounds, and tissues in diabetic and steroid-treated people). In the early postimplantation period the fascial layers have not yet healed, and the deep, periprosthetic tissue is not protected by the usual physical barriers. Any superficial infection that develops, such as an infected wound hematoma, wound infection, or suture abscess, can become a preceding event for joint prosthesis infection.

Etiologic Factors and Pathogenesis

Prosthetic joints and other implants become infected by two different pathogenic routes: the hematogenous route and the locally introduced route. Any bacterium can induce infection of a total joint replacement by the hematogenous route, which accounts for 30% of prosthetic joint infections. Hematogenous spread may occur from dental, skin, respiratory tract, and urinary tract infections or procedures.

Locally introduced forms of infection account for about 70% of all prosthetic joint infections and occur as a result of wound infection next to the prosthesis, or to operative contamination. Operative contamination may be a result of direct implantation at the time of the operation by the operating team, from environmental sources, or from contaminated implant materials. Holes in the implants (e.g., press fit acetabular cups) are potential pathways through which debris can gain access to the implant–bone interface, resulting in infection, creating periprosthetic bone loss, and potentially initiating loosening.[56] Generally, these infections are caused by a single pathogen, but polymicrobial sepsis can occur.

Clinical Manifestations

Persistent joint pain may be the only symptom with no clinical signs of infection at all. *Staphylococcus* infections are usually characterized by symptoms similar to wound infection such as edema, hematoma, fever, and local pain. Late-onset or delayed infections usually present as increasing joint pain followed by rapid onset of systemic symptoms.[77]

Prosthetic joint infections can be divided into the following three categories: early (infection that develops less than 3 months after surgery), delayed (3 to 24 months after surgery), and late (more than 24 months).[66]

Early infections typically present with acute symptoms such as fever, joint pain, warmth, and redness. These individuals may form a sinus tract from the prosthesis to the skin with purulent drainage.

People who present with delayed infections often lack systemic symptoms, making diagnosis difficult. They display joint pain and/or joint loosening. Early and delayed infections are typically acquired at the time of surgery, whereas late infections develop from hematogenous seeding. In one study of 63 infected hip prosthesis, 29% were early infections, 41% delayed, and 30% were late infections.[34]

When a blood-borne infection arises in a prosthetic joint several months or years after implantation surgery, the fully healed connective tissue often is capable of restricting the septic process to a relatively small focus at the bone–cement interface. Joint pain is the principal symptom of deep tissue infection, irrespective of mode of presentation, and suggests either acute inflammation of the periarticular tissue or loosening of the prosthesis caused by subacute erosion of bone at the bone–cement interface.

Medical Management

Prevention

Sterilization and attention to infection control guidelines reduces the risk of infection.[4] Proper handwashing remains the key to reducing the transmission of pathogens to others and the spread of antimicrobial resistance. Despite this well-known fact, adherence by surgeons and other important health care workers remains low.[76] Researchers are working to design self-sterilizing materials and more effective infection-resistant materials. New coatings with an antiadhesive or biocide capabilities are the next step.

Diagnosis

Clinical manifestations of joint pain, swelling, erythema, and warmth all reflect an underlying inflammatory process in the surrounding tissues but are not specific for infection. When a painful prosthesis is accompanied by fever or purulent drainage from overlying cutaneous sinuses, infection is likely. The physician must differentiate infection from aseptic and mechanical problems (e.g., hemarthrosis, mechanical loosening, dislocation). Constant joint pain is suggestive of infection, whereas mechanical loosening commonly causes pain only with motion or weight bearing.

The diagnosis of joint prosthesis infection is dependent on isolation of the pathogen by aspiration of joint fluid or by obtaining tissue at arthrotomy. Gram stain and culture will typically identify the responsible organism in 65% to 94% of cases.[82] Special media may be required if fungus or atypical organisms are suspected. Culture of sinus tract drainage or overlying skin should be avoided. Elevated serum leukocyte count, erythrocyte sedimentation rate, and C-reactive protein level are suggestive but not diagnostic of joint infection. Ultrasound-guided (ultrasonography) aspiration in suspected sepsis of arthroplasty has been developed to facilitate this process.

Radiologic abnormalities may be helpful when changes are noted over serial radiographs, but some changes can lag behind symptoms 3 to 6 months. When both the distal and proximal components of a prosthetic joint demonstrate pathology on radiography, infection is more likely than simple mechanical loosening. However, such radiographic changes are not specific for infection and may also be seen with aseptic processes.

Typical radioisotope scans demonstrate increased uptake in areas of bone with enhanced blood supply or increased metabolic activity (a normal finding during the first 6 months postimplantation). Positive scans at 6 months after implantation are abnormal but do not differentiate among inflammation, possible loosening, and infection. However, newer technetium scans using labeled monoclonal antibodies appear to be more accurate for detecting prosthetic joint infection.[43]

A series of tests before, during, and after surgery are needed for early detection of implant infection. Periimplant infection does not respond well to oral antibiotic therapy because of antibiotic resistance from widespread clinical use of broad-spectrum antibiotics. The biofilm-forming strains of *Staphylococcus* seem to have an even higher degree of resistance to antibiotics. The person is at risk for implant failure and possible death.[4]

Treatment

Prosthesis removal accompanied by extensive and meticulous surgical debridement of surrounding tissue and effective antimicrobial therapy are usually necessary to treat deep infections, especially infections involving the interface between prosthesis and bone. Surgical debridement with retention of the prosthesis, followed by a course of antibiotics, may be appropriate for a limited and select group or people.[51]

For more predictably effective treatment of prosthetic joint replacement sepsis, complete removal of all foreign materials (metallic prosthesis, cement, and any accompanying biofilm) is essential. This can be done in a one-stage or two-stage exchange. The most successful protocol incorporates standardized antimicrobial therapy with a two-stage surgical procedure: (1) removal of prosthesis and cement and placement of an antibiotic-impregnated cement spacer, followed by a 6-week course of bactericidal antibiotic therapy, and (2) reimplantation of a new prosthesis using cement impregnated with an antibiotic at the conclusion of the 6-week antibiotic course.[22,57] Cementless two-stage hip procedures may result in infection rates similar to total hip arthroplasties done with cemented components, but studies are pending.[47,79]

Sometimes, surgical intervention is not possible because of a medical or surgical condition or refusal on the part of the affected individual. In such cases, lifelong oral antibiotic treatment may be required to suppress the infection and retain function of the joint. Serial radiographs are needed to monitor progressive bone resorption at the bone–cement interface. In such cases, the localized septic process may still extend into adjacent tissue compartments or become a systemic infection, or the person may develop side effects of chronic antibiotic administration.

Prognosis

Infection associated with prostheses and implants can produce significant morbidity and occasionally death. Early recognition and prompt therapy for infection in any location is critical to reducing the risk of seeding the joint implant hematogenously. Situations likely to cause bacteremia should be avoided.[10]

The American Dental Association and the American Academy of Orthopedic Surgeons have jointly advised that a single dose of prophylactic antibiotic be given to selected individuals undergoing dental procedures associated with significant bleeding and potential hematologic bacterial contamination. The selected populations include people with inflammatory arthropathies, immunosuppression, diabetes mellitus, malnutrition, hemophilia, or previous prosthetic joint infection and anyone undergoing these dental procedures within 2 years after joint replacement.

Perioperative antibiotic prophylaxis has been shown to reduce deep wound infection effectively in total joint replacement surgery. Cephalosporins continue to be the antibiotic of choice for orthopedic surgeons because of the broad spectrum of activity against the most common pathogens. The antibiotic is given within 60 minutes before the incision is made (120 minutes if vancomycin or a fluoroquinolone is added), and if the procedure is long, another dose is administered during surgery. The medication is then continued for less than 24 hours after surgery.[9]

Although only 2% to 3% of prostheses become infected within 10 years after implantation, there is considerable risk of morbidity (e.g., hospitalization, amputation, disability) and even death.[2]

15.2 Special Implications for the PTA: Infections of Prostheses and Implants Many cases of infection after instrumentation occur within months to years after surgery. The PTA may not be aware of existing hardware and should inquire about previous implants. A recent history of infection from dental caries, pulmonary or upper respiratory tract, gastrointestinal tract, or genitourinary tract in such a person requires medical evaluation. Any spontaneous drainage from previous scars or sites of surgery may be a sign of infection and must also be evaluated by a physician.

Anyone with implants of any kind with onset of increasing musculoskeletal symptoms (especially in the area of the surgery) must be screened for the possibility of infection. Normal radiographs and negative needle aspirates can delay medical diagnosis of infection. Knowing the risk factors for developing an antibiotic-resistant infection and recognizing red flag symptoms of infection can help the PTA in recognizing the need for persistence in obtaining follow-up medical care.

Breast Implantation

Silicone breast implants are medical devices implanted subcutaneously or subpectorally for cosmetic breast augmentation or reconstruction after mastectomy. Infection is the most common complication of breast implantation surgery, occurring in about 2% of cases. Factors that increase the risk for infection have not been well studied but surgical technique and underlying disease appear to be the principal reasons.

Women who undergo reconstruction with placement of implant after mastectomy for cancer are up to 10 times more likely to develop an infection than women receiving cosmetic augmentation. This is often the result of the side effects of chemotherapy and radiation therapy required with surgery.[32,62,67]

DISKITIS

Overview and Incidence

Although spinal infections are rare, for both children and adults, the disk is the most common site. *Diskitis* can range from a self-limiting inflammatory process to a pyogenic infection. It may involve the intervertebral disk or vertebral endplates, or both. The infection rate in adults 2 to 8 weeks postdiskectomy is less than 3%.

Etiologic and Risk Factors

A bacterial origin is usually the cause of the infection. *S. aureus* is commonly found, but in some cases, no organism can be isolated. *Mycobacterium tuberculosis* is also detected in disk infections. Children as young as age 2 years can develop diskitis, which may be confused with vertebral osteomyelitis. The origin of the infection in children may be traumatic, but the source of infection is more likely to be the hematogenous spread of a bacterial infection preceding the diskitis, such as in the upper respiratory or urinary tract. Fungal/yeast infections can also lead to diskitis.[21]

In adults the disk is relatively avascular, contributing to diskitis as the most common postoperative complication after diskectomy. The infection may involve the adjacent vertebrae and spread to the disk through the cartilaginous endplates. Other procedures capable of directly inoculating the disk, such as diskography, also carry the risk of infection. Direct inoculation is the only method by which an infection can arise from within the disk. As with children, urinary tract infections as the result of catheterization or cystoscopy may also be the underlying source of disk space infections.

Pathogenesis

If the infection arises within the disk itself, formation of a peridural abscess is not common. However, an infection extending to the disk from the cartilaginous plate can spread to cause an epidural abscess posteriorly or a paravertebral abscess anteriorly.[36]

Clinical Manifestations

Diskitis presents in different ways at different ages, but fever and spinal pain are classic symptoms in children. In the very young child, back pain or a refusal to walk and pain with hip extension may be the first symptoms and must be taken seriously. Abdominal pain and weight loss may occur, and the child may not be able to flex the lower back.[12] In children presenting with diskitis the concern is whether the diagnosis is actually vertebral osteomyelitis. Those with vertebral osteomyelitis often appear more ill and febrile.[11,31]

In adults, disk infection after spinal procedures usually is noted within a few days, whereas those developing from an infection at a distant site may not be evident for months. Spinal pain will be common and sometimes severe with radiation of the pain into the lower extremities. The lower extremity pain is not usually radicular; instead, it may involve multiple nerve levels. People may present with unusual posture and movement patterns that could be erroneously labeled pain of psychogenic origin. In both children and adults the back pain may range from mild to severe. The client will often report that the pain is made worse with activity and that rest does not relieve the pain.

Medical Management

Diagnosis

In children, routine radiographs are positive and often diagnostic but may not become so until 2 weeks have passed. Disk space narrowing, endplate irregularity, and a loss of lumbar lordosis are noted. Bone scans are also used for initial evaluation. Inflammatory markers may be elevated, but often laboratory tests are unhelpful, and cultures of blood and disk tissue are negative. In an 18-year retrospective study, plain x-rays were found to provide adequate

diagnostic information in 75% of the cases reviewed. However, MRI is essential in providing the differential diagnosis when vertebral osteomyelitis is a possibility; MRI reduces diagnostic delay and may help avoid the requirement for a biopsy.[12,21,31]

In adults the use of MRI in conjunction with bone scans using gadolinium enhancement has been found to be useful in differentiating normal postoperative disk space changes from those caused by infection. MRI is most useful in determining the extent of the infection and the required duration of oral antibiotic therapy after initial IV antibiotics but less valuable in demonstrating the type of infection (e.g., pyogenic versus tuberculous). The sclerosis present later in the disease course may be confused with a benign degenerative process or even with metastatic disease. MRI and biopsy may be used to differentiate chronic cases.

Treatment

Treatment for the younger person may consist of bed rest, hip spica casting, and bracing. Antibiotics are used but do not appear to radically alter the natural course of the infection in children.[12] In adults a removable body jacket can be used along with specific or empiric antibiotic therapy. The use of antibiotics prophylactically is common after spinal surgery in adults to prevent this condition from developing. Antifungal agents may first be tried for *Candida* diskitis. Surgery may be necessary.[21]

Prognosis

In both adults and children the prognosis is good, although pain may persist for several months up to several years. In children, long-term follow-up care has shown a resolution of the pain in spite of persistent radiographic changes.[24]

Late radiographic changes in adults include vertebral collapse, kyphosis, and eventually, bony ankylosis, which can take up to 2 years to run its course. Adults can expect similar spontaneous healing to occur, especially in those individuals with a strong immune response.

Complications can arise when the infection spreads or when an abscess forms. An epidural abscess can result in paralysis and is noted in older people, in those who have involvement of the cervical region, and in those with associated medical problems, such as diabetes.

15.3 Special Implications for the PTA: Diskitis Because very young children can be affected, diskitis must be considered a possible cause of spinal pain or refusal to bear weight or walk. Because the pain is usually related to activity and increases with weight bearing, it is easy to mistakenly attribute the symptoms to musculoskeletal origins. The presence of hip or back pain of unknown cause, especially after spinal surgery or recent infection, must be evaluated by a physician.

INFECTIOUS (SEPTIC) ARTHRITIS

Overview and Incidence

Infectious causes of fever and arthritis can be divided into four groups by causative agent (Box 15.2). This section is confined to the discussion of bacterial arthritis (also called *septic* or *infectious arthritis*), which differs from reactive arthritis in several ways. *Bacterial arthritis* may be a local response with joint destruction and sepsis, whereas *reactive arthritis* is defined as the occurrence of an acute, *aseptic,* and inflammatory arthropathy arising after an infectious process but at a site remote from the primary infection. Some of the other infectious causes of arthritis are discussed in other chapters.

Etiologic and Risk Factors

Bacteria, viruses, and fungi are all capable of infecting a joint by invading and inflaming the synovial membrane.[42] Predisposing factors for development of septic arthritis are listed in Box 15.3. Microorganisms can be introduced into the joint by direct inoculation, direct extension, or by hematogenous (through the bloodstream) spread, which is the most common route (Box 15.4). In addition, direct penetrating trauma, joint arthroplasty, and chronic joint damage as seen in diseases such as rheumatoid arthritis are also considered to put a joint at risk.[30]

Pathogenesis

After being directly inoculated into the joint cavity, bacteria rapidly multiply in the liquid culture medium of the synovial fluid and are phagocytosed by synovial lining cells. Bacteria are either killed by the synovial cells or form microabscesses within the synovial membrane. Organisms that reach the synovium through the bloodstream multiply in enlarging microabscesses of the synovium until they break into the articular cavity.

The infection process causes synovial, ligament, and cartilage damage. Bacterial toxins also activate the coagulation system, causing microvascular obstruction that leads to ischemia and necrosis, further permitting abscess formation, which destroys the cartilage matrix.

Finally, after the acute necrotic inflammatory synovitis, the synovial membrane proliferates, forming an inflammatory exudate called *pannus* that erodes articular cartilage of the joint capsule and subchondral bone. All of this can take place in 17 days, quickly destroying a joint in the process. This underscores the need for urgency in detection and intervention in septic arthritis.

A chronic inflammatory synovitis may persist even after antibiotics have eradicated the infection. The threshold for starting empiric therapy with antibiotics for those individuals with acute joint pain and swelling should therefore be low.[26]

Clinical Manifestations

People with infectious arthritis can be any age and can present with an acute onset of joint pain, swelling, tenderness, and loss of motion. Fever, chills, and other systemic symptoms depend on the stage of the illness. Physical examination may reveal the classic signs of infection such as increased temperature of the joint, swelling, redness, and loss of function. Pus may drain outside through a sinus formed from the joint to the outside. Only the severity and the nature of these signs will differentiate the septic joint from more mundane causes such as tendinitis and other noninfectious inflammatory diseases.

A child with a septic joint will often refuse to bear weight and be extremely tender to palpation at the joint and along the metaphysis. Destruction of the joints can proceed rapidly and have long-lasting effects.[15] In addition to the infection, the WBCs that enter the joint to combat the infection release enzymes that have a deleterious effect on articular cartilage. In a series of children studied younger than age 2 years with septic knees, 24% had a varus or valgus deformity at long-term follow-up care.[71]

In adults, *S. aureus* produces a monarticular sepsis, usually at the hip or knee. In children, the ankle and elbow are also common sites. Although not as common, polyarticular septic infectious arthritis has been reported. *Gonococcus* affects mostly women and may produce skin lesions, *tenosynovitis,* and polyarthralgias, in addition to systemic symptoms. Prosthetic joints are also sites of infection, which is probably introduced at the time of surgery. *S. epidermidis* is often the cause.

Generally, the coexistence of fever and the signs and symptoms of an acute exacerbation of arthritis must arouse suspicions of a septic joint and be managed as a medical emergency until proved otherwise.[30,41]

Medical Management

Diagnosis

Along with a detailed history and physical examination, the confirmation of the diagnosis is made by analysis of the joint fluid obtained by aspiration. The decision to aspirate the joint, however, is made on the basis of history and physical examination. The method to obtain a sample of the aspirate depends on the joint that is involved. Needle aspiration when possible is often considered the method of choice.[50] Aspiration of the sacroiliac and hip joints is difficult, and fluoroscopy is sometimes used. Decisions on treatment and appropriate antibiotics are aided by the results of cultures, stains, and laboratory studies such as the WBC count and erythrocyte sedimentation rate.

With the development of advanced DNA analysis techniques, identification of traces of bacterial genomes may eventually make it possible to develop specific vaccines or pharmacologic agents to prevent or treat septic arthritis.

Treatment

As already mentioned, any joint infection is considered a medical emergency. Admission to the hospital for treatment with specific IV antibiotics is required. Continued treatment with oral medication for an additional 2 to 3 weeks is standard.

Aspiration of the joint is critical. Along with needle aspiration, more aggressive techniques of tidal irrigation, arthroscopy, or arthrotomy may be used depending on the situation.[50] Open drainage is indicated for hip joint infections. In prosthetic joints the infection may require removal of the hardware and cement, along with a more prolonged course of antibiotics.

Early in the course of intervention, the joint should be rested. This may be accomplished by splinting, traction, or casting. Care in application of the splint will preserve function, and the splint should be removed periodically for ROM exercise. The importance of these simple ROM exercises cannot be overlooked because the risk for joint contracture as a complication of immobilization is a concern, especially in the older adult. More vigorous types of exercise and aggressive mobilization activities are performed when signs of infection have resolved.[42,50]

The aggressiveness of intervention is dictated by the specific organism, the joint involved, duration of symptoms, and the health of the individual. Surgical drainage is often required to preserve function and prevent complications. In some cases, joint instability (e.g., chronic or repeated hip subluxation) may require more extensive surgical intervention.

Prognosis

As for other infectious diseases, prompt treatment is the key to a successful outcome. If treatment is initiated within 5 to 7 days of onset, a good or excellent long-term result can be expected.[50,72] Currently, the mortality rate has dropped considerably for infections caused by nongonococcal agents; however, sequelae in the form of destructive changes in the bone or joint can result in significant functional limitations.

Mortality is higher in the older adult (increases after age 65 years) even with quick and correct interventions.[50] Overall mortality from septic arthritis ranges from 10% to 25%, and permanent joint disability occurs in 25% to 50% of survivors. Septic arthritis of the knee is associated with better outcomes than that of the hip.[26] The more common complications include osteomyelitis, abscess formation, and permanent loss of joint motion and joint instability. If the infection is not controlled, toxemia and septicemia can cause death.

15.4 Special Implications for the PTA: Infectious (Septic) Arthritis Immediate referral of a client with a suspected septic joint to a specialist may save the joint from unnecessary destruction. Being aware of client history, potential risk factors, and assessing for signs and symptoms of infection are essential. Including joint infection in the differential diagnosis of some clients with joint pain may expedite early intervention. This is important because the prognosis is related to the time between onset of symptoms and definitive treatment.

INFECTIOUS (INFLAMMATORY) MUSCLE DISEASE

Myositis

Overview

Myositis is a general term used to describe inflammation of the muscles that can be an autoimmune condition or directly caused by viral, bacterial, and parasitic agents. Infection-induced myositis is most often caused by *S. aureus* and parasites such as *Trichinella* and the tapeworm larva, *Taenia solium*.

When affecting skeletal muscle, these infectious agents result in inflammatory changes with sequela, ranging from significant functional losses to a minor self-limiting condition. Autoimmune conditions can be activated or aggravated by infections, which may explain the link between myositis, infections, and autoimmune processes.

The most common forms are dermatomyositis (DM), *polymyositis* (PM), and inclusion body myositis (IBM) (Box 15.5). DM appears to occur more often in children and older adults.

IBM is the most common acquired muscle disease in adults older than age 50 years and often misdiagnosed. This form is often progressive and debilitating and often does not respond to available treatments.[8,28]

Incidence

Myositis is diagnosed in 1 in 100,000 people a year, although some experts suspect that many cases may go unidentified because it is so often mistaken for the symptoms of aging or in women, depression.[55]

BOX 15.5 Types of Myositis

- Dermatomyositis
- Polymyositis
- Inclusion body myositis
- *Myositis ossificans*
- Idiopathic inflammatory myopathies
- Rhabdomyolysis
- Pyomyositis

Etiology and Pathogenesis

Myositis can be the first sign of a malignancy. Recent studies have quantified the risk, finding that people with DM face a threefold risk of cancer, whereas those individuals with PM face a 40% increase in risk.[48]

The antigens that produce the immune response are present in normal muscle tissue but at low levels. They are much more prevalent in myositis cells of individuals with autoimmune myositis and in muscle cells that are regenerating such as occurs after an injury. It is hypothesized that a feedforward loop occurs when damaged muscle cells start to repair themselves. These cells express higher amounts of the antigens, causing the immune system to respond; the immune response causes further damage to the muscle, which in turn repairs itself, its regenerating cells expressing even more antigens, and continuing the feedforward cycle.[17]

Inflammation is a major cause of muscle damage. Numerous drugs may induce myopathies, including cholesterol-lowering statins. Lipid-lowering drugs associated with myotoxicity can cause symptoms ranging in severity from myalgias to *rhabdomyolysis*, resulting in renal failure and death.[5,23,53]

Myositis caused by parasites is considered a relatively uncommon condition; however, the parasitic infection trichinosis is reported to affect up to 4% of the population.

Clinical Manifestations

The common symptoms of this family of conditions are as would be expected for any inflammatory process. The nonspecific symptoms include malaise, fever, muscle swelling, pain, tenderness, and lethargy. Specifically, the inflammatory response found in PM and DM is in connective tissue and muscle fibers.

Other than the symptoms associated with these infections, there is a risk of tissue necrosis and extensive muscle tissue damage with atrophy and weakness, especially if left untreated. Other clinical features of myositis are dysphagia, decreased esophageal motility, vasculitis, Raynaud's phenomenon, cardiomyopathy, and interstitial pulmonary fibrosis. A purple skin rash and eyelid edema are often associated with DM. The distribution of the rash includes the eyelids, face, chest, and extensor surfaces of the extremities. In adults, subcutaneous calcium deposits are a sign of severe long-term DM.

In most cases, IBM progresses slowly over months or years and is characterized by frequent falling episodes and trouble climbing stairs or standing from a seated position. Drop foot and subsequent tripping may be reported. Weak grip, difficulty swallowing, and muscle atrophy and weakness are often accompanied by functional decline and pain or discomfort secondary to weakness.[55]

Medical Management

Diagnosis

In addition to a careful and thorough history, a muscle biopsy is the primary diagnostic tool. A differential diagnosis requires muscle biopsy, electromyography, and laboratory values.

The muscle biopsy will make the differentiation between PM, DM, and IBM and exclude other myotonic diseases. Electromyography will demonstrate muscle irritability and myopathic changes. Because of the associated release of creatine kinase (CK) into the blood with skeletal muscle damage, this enzyme can be a useful measure of the extent of the infection. CK levels are 5 to 10 times higher than normal in PM, but only mildly increased in IBM.[8]

Treatment and Prognosis

Aggressive early treatment of any of these conditions will lead to an improved prognosis. Trichinosis can be very successfully treated with pharmacologic agents. The treatment of PM and DM often includes immunosuppressive therapy and corticosteroids. There is no established treatment that improves, arrests, or slows the progression of IBM; it is resistant to treatment with antiinflammatory, immunosuppressant, or immunomodulating agents.[37] Because of the resulting muscle weakness and possible extensive skeletal muscle damage associated with myositis, the client must be prepared for an aggressive and prolonged rehabilitative process.

The role of the physical and occupational therapy teams should not be underestimated in the attainment of a successful outcome. Submaximal exercise has been shown to be effective, although eccentric or intense exercise is not recommended.[8,39]

Other clinical trials are testing new drugs to add to the arsenal of corticosteroids, immunosuppressants, and IV immunoglobulin, which is a plasma product. For people with PM and DM, existing medications work well, although many of the drugs have serious side effects and may cease being effective over time.

> **15.5 Special Implications for the PTA: Myositis** Muscle pain and weakness in anyone at risk for myositis and especially for individuals taking lipid-lowering statins should be a red flag for the PTA. Underlying neuromuscular diseases may become clinically apparent during statin therapy and may predispose the individual to myotoxicity.[5] Exercise may be an additional risk factor for the symptomatic presentation of myotoxicity.[3] The alert PTA will recognize this potential condition and make an appropriate medical referral sooner rather than later.

Infections of Bursae and Tendons
Overview and Incidence

Acute infections affecting the bursae and tendons are uncommon and must be treated appropriately to avoid complications. The hand is very susceptible to scratches, bites, and subsequent infections. Hand infection can range from cellulitis to tenosynovitis. Because of the superficial nature of these tissues and the potential for dysfunction, hand infections are given special attention in this section.

Etiologic and Risk Factors

The bursae and tendons that lie close to the skin surface are most susceptible to infection from direct contact with microorganisms. Trauma to the elbow and knee is common, especially in sports such as wrestling. Anaerobic bacteria are more common in wounds from bites and in people with diabetes. The bacteria enter the body by direct inoculation through a local skin abrasion or with common procedures such as a cortisone injection into the inflamed bursae. *S. aureus* is the most common organism isolated and may cause up to 80% of infections.

Hand infections often develop from untreated injuries. Up to 60% of hand infections are related to trauma, 25% are caused by human bites, and 10% are a result of animal bites.[11] As with all infections, people with diabetes or who are immunocompromised have a greater risk of developing an infection in the hand. In addition, the risk of osteomyelitis is also of concern because of the close proximity of bone.

Pathogenesis

Infection in the hand can spread along synovial sheaths, fascial planes, and via lymphatic channels. Bursae are lined with a membrane similar to synovium and are therefore subject to the same pathologic processes, namely, inflammatory conditions caused by acute or chronic infections.

Clinical Manifestations

The olecranon and prepatellar bursae can be sites of localized infection. An olecranon bursal infection will cause pain, loss of function, and swelling, which may be accompanied by cellulitis. Infections of other bursae, such as the prepatellar and subdeltoid bursae, have similar presentations.

Tendon sheaths of the extremities can also become infected. As mentioned earlier, the hand is a common site because of its susceptibility to minor trauma. The anatomy of the hand determines the nature and presentation of the infection. For example, the tendon sheaths of the thumb and small finger extend proximally to the wrist, whereas the sheaths of the index, long, and ring fingers stop at the proximal pulley.

An infection of the flexor tendon of the thumb could rapidly spread to the small finger. Common signs associated with an infectious tenosynovitis include a finger maintained in slight flexion, fusiform (spindle-shaped) swelling, pain on extension (passive or active), and tenderness along the tendon sheath into the palm.

Medical Management

Diagnosis, Treatment, and Prognosis

In most joints, examination will identify a localized swelling not a joint effusion. Aspiration of fluid for laboratory analysis is performed before treatment. The use of antibiotics is often adequate, but surgical incision and drainage are sometimes required; occasionally, bursectomy is required. Prompt treatment with drainage, irrigation, and antibiotics is crucial.

Early and aggressive rehabilitation is essential, especially for a structure as complicated and integrated as the hand. Both physical and occupational therapists may play a role in this process. Given the potential complications of surgery and immobilization and the potential for tissue loss, a comprehensive rehabilitation program is necessary to maximize function.

> **15.6 Special Implications for the PTA: Infections of Bursae and Tendons** Early immobilization must be done with eventual recovery and function in mind. Active ROM exercise is initiated early, as soon as the infection begins to subside and treatment appears to be successful, which is often within 48 hours.

EXTRAPULMONARY TUBERCULOSIS

Tuberculosis (TB) is an acute or chronic infection caused by *M. tuberculosis* that can affect multiple organ systems via lymphatic and hematogenous spread during the initial pulmonary infection. Disseminated or miliary TB involves not only the lungs but also most other organ systems. Systems involved may

include the pulmonary, genitourinary, musculoskeletal, and lymphatic systems. Of these, the lymphatic system is most commonly involved in immunocompromised hosts such as those with HIV.

Extrapulmonary TB is more difficult to diagnose and treat than pulmonary TB. Extrapulmonary TB is often in inaccessible areas, which makes aspiration or biopsy and therefore diagnosis, more difficult. Also, smaller numbers of bacilli can cause extensive damage to joints but are harder to detect. TB involving the bone is usually transferred hematogenously from some other organ, usually the lung. Only one-fourth of people with skeletal TB have a known history of TB.

Skeletal Tuberculosis
Overview and Incidence

After a 40-year decline, the incidence of TB has increased over the past several decades. The World Health Organization estimates that more than 8 million new cases of TB occur annually, and approximately 3 million individuals die of TB and associated complications every year.[1] More than 15 million people in the United States are estimated to be infected with TB. Although TB is found in all 50 states, New York, California, and Hawaii have had the highest incidence. Skeletal TB is uncommon, but infection rates have held constant over the years. About 10% to 15% of TB is extrapulmonary, and only 10% of extrapulmonary TB is skeletal.

Pathogenesis and Clinical Manifestations

Extrapulmonary TB is spread hematogenously from other organs. In adults, the onset of *skeletal TB* is insidious, developing 2 to 3 years after the primary infection. Early signs and symptoms include pain and stiffness; the pain may be localized or referred. The lower thoracic and lumbar spine is commonly involved (Pott's disease), but other sites (e.g., weight-bearing joints, elbows) have been reported.[25] Systemic signs, such as fever, chills, weight loss, and fatigue, are not common in the early phase. Joint effusion often occurs with TB arthritis and has been shown to affect muscles and nerves around the joint.[20,81]

In the case of spine involvement (occurring 5% in the cervical spine, 25% in the thoracic spine, and 20% in the lumbar and lumbosacral spine), infection begins in the cancellous bone of the vertebral body and eventually spreads to the intervertebral disk and adjacent vertebrae. As the disease progresses, nerve root irritation, pressure from abscess, and collapse of the vertebral body will cause a progressive increase in pain and protective spasm with cord compression and possible paraplegia.[29,54] The abscess may extend from the lumbar region to the psoas muscle, producing hip pain.

Medical Management

Diagnosis

Early diagnosis is very helpful in preserving articular cartilage and the joint space but is often delayed for several months to years after the initial presentation because there are no symptoms pathognomonic of extrapulmonary TB. Treatment may be delayed because symptoms are consistent with chronic sciatica, when the true cause of the radiating pain is tuberculous sacroiliitis with an anterior synovial cyst.[19]

Conventional radiographs are important in the initial detection, and computed tomography and MRI can assist in further evaluation. Confirmation of skeletal TB requires microbiologic assessment with smear and culture. In the spine, this confirmation can be accomplished with fine-needle aspiration. Tissue biopsy is more often required for extrapulmonary disease.

Treatment and Prognosis

Treatment does not differ for pulmonary and extrapulmonary TB. Although surgical debridement is sometimes necessary, usually pharmacologic treatment is sufficient. Chemotherapy is the mainstay in the management of TB spondylitis.[54]

Extraarticular infections can sometimes be treated with curettage and bone grafting. For more advanced infections, resection of bones and joints, arthrodesis, and limb salvage or amputation may be indicated. Factors to be considered include the affected bone, extent of surgical excision, and involvement of soft tissue, articular cartilage, or bone.

In the spine, surgery is more often needed to address nerve compression or deformity secondary to collapse of the vertebral body rather than the infection. The resultant deformity often includes a marked kyphotic curve with a gibbus formation (Fig. 15.4). Paralysis can be a serious complication of vertebral TB and can be a result of the disease process or a secondary spinal deformity. Paralysis persisting longer than 6 months is unlikely to improve, and late paralysis with inactive disease and significant kyphosis is much less responsive to treatment.[54]

In the joint, if TB is diagnosed early when the infection is confined to the synovium, rest, medication, and joint protection may be adequate. In advanced disease with caseation, fibrosis, and scarring, the vascularity is reduced (Fig. 15.5), which makes medications less effective. Surgical excision or curettage of the affected areas may be necessary. In joints, the granulomatous tissue acts to separate the articular cartilage from the underlying bone.

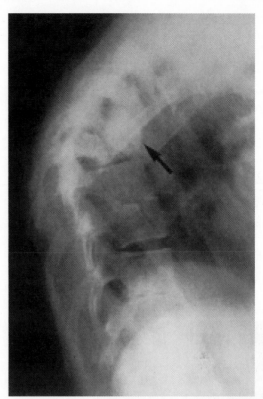

FIG. 15.4 Tuberculous spondylitis. Involvement at multiple levels. Gibbus deformity is seen in the upper thoracic region *(arrow)*. (From Yao D, Sartoris D: Musculoskeletal tuberculosis, Radiol Clin North Am 33:681, 1995.)

> **15.7 Special Implications for the PTA: Extrapulmonary (Skeletal) Tuberculosis** Extrapulmonary (skeletal) TB is not often seen in a physical therapy practice but can present as arthritis or other musculoskeletal manifestations of unknown cause. Anyone with this type of clinical presentation with a compromised immune system, especially AIDS/HIV, past or recent release from incarceration, a history of immigration to the United States from an area in which TB is endemic, or any other risk factor for TB listed in Chapter 11, should be screened for medical disease.

SUMMARY OF SPECIAL IMPLICATIONS FOR THE PTA

Rehabilitation after medical intervention for infectious diseases must proceed in a comprehensive and coordinated fashion. The pathology of each type of infectious disease process and every medical decision made in treatment will have some bearing on rehabilitation and outcome. Many questions such as these must be addressed when planning the rehabilitation program.

The hip joint is commonly affected and has been alluded to in several chapters as a site of infectious processes of many origins and will be used here again to illustrate some factors that should be considered in planning rehabilitation. Early in the course of intervention, rest may be a predominant feature but even this calls for therapy intervention. All health care providers must be made aware of the potentially adverse effects of apparently simple movements. For example, using a bedpan and performing isometric exercises produce acetabular contact pressure close to that of walking.[40] Therefore clinicians should not assume that a client who is on bed rest is not producing elevated joint compressive forces. Clients must be instructed in proper methods of moving, transferring, and positioning themselves.

Active ROM exercise is often the first type of supervised exercise permitted. Even simple movements must be done while noting limits set by pain, spasm, or apprehension. Active hip flexion has been found to increase acetabular contact pressure similar to that of full weight bearing.[70] However, passive ROM exercise has been found to have a beneficial effect on healing joints.[33,65]

Continuous passive ROM as a means of early mobilization in a postoperative rehabilitation regimen has been investigated and found to have no long-term benefit compared with daily standardized exercises.[7,48,49] However, the data on the effect of continuous passive motion on overall analgesic use and prevalence of deep vein thrombosis remain under investigation.

It may be worth remembering the motion requirements of certain positions so that functional goals can be set; for example, ascending stairs requires just over 65 degrees of hip flexion, whereas sitting in a chair requires about 105 degrees.[44] Restoring full ROM may not be as realistic or as necessary as obtaining the ROM required to restore function.

Exercise after prolonged immobilization should take these factors into consideration. Often, a non–weight-bearing status is used with the intention of minimally loading the joint. In fact,

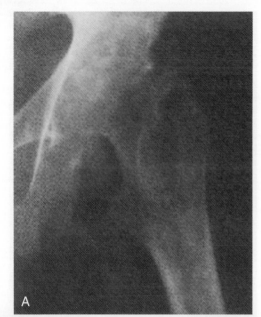

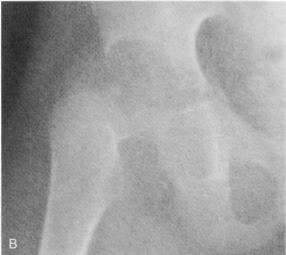

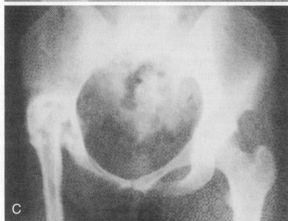

FIG. 15.5 Tuberculous arthritis. (A) Bony erosion of acetabulum and femoral head with joint space loss. There also is evidence of periarticular osteopenia. (B) Similar findings to (A) but with further destruction of the femoral head and acetabulum. (C) Advanced TB of the hip with superior displacement and ankylosis of the right hip joint. (From Yao D, Sartoris D: Musculoskeletal tuberculosis, Radiol Clin North Am 33:687, 1995.)

the compressive forces may actually increase compared with those of a touch-down, weight-bearing gait pattern.[63] Other factors, such as the weight of the limb and muscular contraction, must be considered. Long-term use of an ambulatory aid may be indicated even for as much as a 2- to 3-year period.[35] The use of a cane in the contralateral hand can reduce weight-bearing forces by up to 15%.[27]

REFERENCES/SUGGESTED READINGS

To enhance this text and add value for the reader, references and suggested readings are included on the companion Evolve site that accompanies this textbook. The reader can view the source and access it online whenever possible.

16

Musculoskeletal Neoplasms

CHAPTER OBJECTIVES

1. Review the pathophysiology of neoplasms.
2. Review the properties of benign and malignant growths.
3. Differentiate bone and soft tissue tumors with regards to both benign and malignant properties.
4. Consider physical therapy approaches and rehabilitation frameworks for specific musculoskeletal neoplasms.

OUTLINE

VOCAB BUILDERS

Angiography
Baker cyst
Chondrosarcoma
Ewing's sarcoma
Ganglia
Hematogenous

Lipoma
Multiple myeloma
Neurofibroma
Osteoblastoma
Osteochondroma
Osteoid osteoma

Osteosarcoma
Primary tumors
Radiograph
Schwannomas
Ultrasonography

Neoplasm is defined as a new or abnormal growth of cells and is often used interchangeably with *tumor,* which means any swelling or mass. Neoplasms are divided into two broad categories: benign and malignant. Benign neoplasms show no tendency to metastasize, are noninvasive, and are usually slow growing. A malignant neoplasm is one that can be invasive or can metastasize.

Although neoplasms represent a small portion of the spectrum of pathology seen in clinics, their severity and potential for serious consequences necessitate an understanding of their detection and treatment.

The purpose of this chapter is to review the characteristics of primary and secondary musculoskeletal neoplasms. Those that may be encountered by physical therapist assistants (PTAs) are highlighted. It is hoped that increasing awareness of the clinical manifestations will make earlier detection possible.

 PRIMARY TUMORS

Overview

Description

Primary musculoskeletal tumors are those that have developed from or within tissue in a localized area. Primary musculoskeletal neoplasms can be benign or malignant, soft tissue or bone. A soft tissue tumor may originate from muscle, cartilage, nerve, collagen, adipose, lymph or blood vessel, or skin. Common sites

in the body and location within the bone vary depending on the type of tumor (Table 16.1 and Fig. 16.1).

Modern classification of soft tissue tumors recognizes more than 200 benign and approximately 70 malignant (sarcomatous) lesions with a ratio of benign tumors to malignant sarcomas of 100:1. The focus of this chapter will remain on the most common bone and soft tissue tumors encountered in the PTA's practice.

Benign Neoplasm

Benign tumors are well differentiated, resemble normal tissue, rarely invade locally, and have low potential for autonomous growth. However, benign does not necessarily mean innocuous. For example, osteoblastomas in the spine may produce serious neurologic problems requiring resection, with additional complications possible from the surgical procedure.

Some benign bone tumors pose difficult evaluation and management problems and can result in a significant level of impairment. For example, large fibrous defects in weight-bearing bones can cause pathologic fractures. A *pathologic fracture* refers to bone that has been weakened by local destruction (osteoclastic resorption) from any cause; bone with this type of impairment is more readily fractured than normal bone.

Although the occurrence is rare, some benign lesions can develop into a malignancy. Benign lesions usually do not cause the constant, severe pain that is commonly associated with

TABLE 16.1	Classification of Soft Tissue and Bone Tumors	
Tissue of Origin	**Benign Tumor**	**Malignant Tumor**
Connective Tissue		
Fibrous	Fibroma	Fibrosarcoma
		Malignant fibrous histiocytoma
Cartilage	Chondroma	Chondrosarcoma
	Enchondroma	
	Chondroblastoma	
	Osteochondroma	
Bone (osteogenic)	Osteoma; osteoblastoma (giant osteoid osteoma)	Osteosarcoma (osteogenic sarcoma)
Bone marrow (myelogenic)		Leukemia
		Multiple myeloma
		Ewing's sarcoma
		Hodgkin's lymphoma of bone
Adipose (fat)	Lipoma	Liposarcoma
Synovium	Ganglion, giant cell of tendon sheath	Synovial sarcoma
Muscle		
Smooth muscle	Leiomyoma	Leiomyosarcoma (uterus, gastrointestinal system)
Striated muscle	Rhabdomyoma	Rhabdomyosarcoma (can occur anywhere)
Endothelium (Vascular, Lymphatic)		
Lymph vessels	Lymphangioma	Lymphangiosarcoma
		Kaposi's sarcoma
		Lymphosarcoma (lymphoma)
Blood vessels (angiogenic)	Angioma	Angiosarcoma
	Hemangioma	Hemangiosarcoma
Neural Tissue		
Nerve fibers and sheaths	Neurofibroma	Neurofibrosarcoma
	Neuroma	Neurogenic sarcoma (also known as *neurosarcoma* or *schwannoma*)
	Neurinoma (neurilemmoma)	
Glial tissue	Gliosis	Glioma
Epithelium		
Skin and mucous membrane	Papilloma	Squamous cell carcinoma
	Polyp	Basal cell carcinoma
Glandular epithelium	Adenoma	Adenocarcinoma

progressive malignant disease, but benign tumors can impair blood supply or compress nerve tissue.

Malignant Neoplasm

Malignant *primary tumors* of bone by definition have the capacity to spread to other sites and often do so aggressively by invading locally and destroying adjacent tissues and by metastasizing to distant sites. Skeletal neoplasms often metastasize to the lungs through the bloodstream.

Fortunately, malignant tumors are not as common as benign lesions; however, this rarity has made it difficult to standardize treatment interventions and management. For this reason, most individuals with malignant primary tumors are referred to regional centers, where valuable experience concerning evaluation and treatment can be gained and then applied to future cases.

Incidence

Primary tumors of the musculoskeletal system are uncommon, although the incidence is difficult to determine because these lesions often escape diagnosis (Table 16.2). Excluding myeloma and skin cancer, as few as 2400 new cases of primary bone tumors and 9200 cases of soft tissue sarcomas are detected annually in the United States with a 3:1 ratio of men to women affected.[39]

Risk Factors

Little progress has been made in our knowledge of the risk factors involved in the etiopathogenesis of malignant bone tumors. The main factors implicated are Paget's disease, Li-Fraumeni syndrome, antineoplastic drugs, ionizing radiation, and hereditary retinoblastoma.[27]

Several genetic conditions are related to the development of soft tissue sarcoma (e.g., neurofibromatosis, tuberous sclerosis, basal cell nevus syndrome), but this applies only to a small number of cases.[74] Soft tissue tumors also may be associated with high doses of radiation or exposure to toxic chemicals in the workplace (herbicides, dioxin, preservatives, and so on).

Etiologic Factors and Pathogenesis

The histogenesis of tumors is generally poorly understood, although significant progress has been made toward understanding tumor development as a biologic phenomenon.

Bone tumors. To grasp the concepts of tumor formation, one must understand that bone metabolism is a balancing

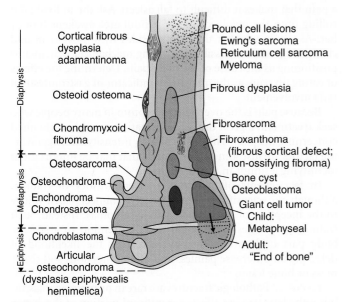

FIG. 16.1 Composite diagram illustrating frequent sites of bone tumors. The diagram depicts the end of a long bone that has been divided into the epiphysis, metaphysis, and diaphysis. The *epiphysis* refers to the articular end of the long bones, which is primarily cartilaginous in the growing child. The *metaphysis* is the wider part of the shaft of the long bone. The *diaphysis* refers to the shaft itself. The typical sites of common primary bone tumors are labeled. (Redrawn from Madewell JE, Ragsdale BD, Sweet DE: Radiologic and pathologic analysis of solitary bone lesions: I. Internal margins, Radiol Clin North Am 19:715, 1981.)

TABLE 16.2	Relative Frequency of Primary Bone Tumors[a]
Benign	
Osteochondroma	35% of benign tumors; 10% of all bone tumors
Osteoid osteoma	10%–12% of benign bone tumors
Enchondroma	10% of benign bone tumors; some report as high as 24%
Osteoblastoma	1%–2% of benign bone tumors
Chondroblastoma	<1% of all bone tumors
Hemangioma	<1% of all bone tumors
Malignant	
Metastatic neoplasm	Most common form of bone malignancy; *secondary* neoplasm of bone
Multiple myeloma	Most common *primary* neoplasm of bone; plasma cell malignancy (bone marrow)
Osteosarcoma	35% of all malignant bone tumors; 15%–20% of primary sarcomas (excluding multiple myeloma)
Chondrosarcoma	25% of malignant bone tumors (excluding multiple myeloma)
Ewing's sarcoma	16% of malignant bone tumors; second most common in children; fourth overall *primary* bone tumor for adults and children (after myeloma)
Malignant fibrous histiocytoma	2%–5% of malignant bone tumors (excluding multiple myeloma)
Fibrosarcoma	1.4% of malignant bone tumors (excluding multiple myeloma)

[a]Listed by decreasing order of frequency; with the exception of metastatic neoplasm listed, these statistics refer to primary bone tumors.
Data from Dorfman HD, Czerniak B: Bone cancers, Cancer 75(1 Suppl):203–210, 1995; Dorfman HD, Czerniak B: Bone tumors, St Louis, 1998, Mosby.

act of bone formation and resorption. The coupling of these two processes usually results in a balance of bone resorption and formation. When metabolic bone disease and neoplastic formations occur, this balance is upset.

Under normal circumstances, bone remodeling involves a fine balance between osteoblast activity, which promotes new bone synthesis, and osteoclasts, which stimulate bone resorption. This balance is disrupted by the presence of malignant cells, resulting in uncoupling of the process of remodeling.

Cortical bone is most abundant in the outer walls of the shafts of long bones and is quite dense. The haversian canal system, which refers to the concentric rings of lamellae, is found in cortical bone. Cortical bone surrounds the trabecular or cancellous bone, which is the honeycomb-like bone found in the ends of long bones. Trabeculae are aligned with applied stresses in the bone. The metabolic activity is higher in cancellous bone than cortical bone, which accounts for why many disorders that create disturbances in metabolic activity are first noted in cancellous bone.

Bone tumors are considered to be either osteoblastic or osteolytic, although most have characteristics of both processes. The osteoblastic process can be preceded by tumor cells or by normal cells in the host bone reacting to the tumor. Because the host bone continues with the normal process of resorption and bone formation, there will likely be a variety of cell types within the lesion. This makes histologic interpretation difficult.

Neoplastic cells do not themselves destroy bone, but their presence incites local osteoclastic resorption of bone. The cells of certain neoplasms also incite local osteoblastic deposition of normal bone, referred to as *reactive bone*. The neoplastic cells of the osteogenic group of neoplasms are capable of producing osteoid (young bone that has not undergone calcification) and bone, which are then referred to as *tumor bone* or *neoplastic bone*. The radiographic appearance of lesions affecting bone reflects varying proportions of bone resorption (osteolysis) and bone deposition (osteosclerosis)—some of the latter being reactive bone, and some being neoplastic bone.[59]

Soft tissue tumors. Four types of genetic disorders underlying soft tissue sarcomas have been identified: translocations, gene amplifications, mutations, and complex genetic imbalances. Detection of these molecular changes can guide treatment and may predict response to treatment. Techniques used to detect translocations are very sensitive and in some cases may be used to detect microscopic metastasis.[10]

Soft tissue sarcomas have a predictable growth pattern, beginning as small masses and often growing in a centripetal pattern. The leading edge of the tumor (reactive zone) contains edema, fibrous tissue, inflammatory cells, and tumor cells. Uncontrolled growth often causes loss of blood supply at the center of the tumor.

Benign soft tissue tumors also have a centripetal growth pattern, but the expansion is more controlled and much slower. Benign lesions tend to be more superficially located compared with malignant lesions, which often grow within tissues under the deep fascia.[67]

Clinical Manifestations

The clinical features must be well understood to ensure that the diagnostic evaluation proceeds expeditiously. Unfortunately, many tumors are not diagnosed on their initial presentation. This is because of the ambiguous presentation of most tumors in their early stages; rarely does one actually find the case that is described as typical for a given lesion.

Pain. Pain is a hallmark of tumor development, especially with malignant lesions. Constant pain that is not dependent on position or activity and is increased with weight-bearing activities is a red flag symptom. The presence of night pain is considered an additional important finding. When the client reports night pain, further questioning is required.

The PTA should ensure that the client is reporting true night pain, which awakens the person from sleep, rather than a pain that makes it difficult to fall asleep. Ask the individual if rolling onto the involved side or painful area awakens him or her. Ascertain whether the pain subsides with movement and change in position, possibly indicating mechanical ischemia or positioning as the cause of the night pain. Determine the effects of eating on pain, as this may be an indicator of gastrointestinal (GI) involvement.

Because pain is the overriding symptom in many people who seek treatment, a great deal of information should be obtained concerning the pain. The onset, nature, intensity, and aggravating factors are just some of the aspects that may be important in identifying a tumor in the early stages.

In fact, clients often report a recent history of trauma, although no scientific evidence directly connects such injury to the inception of soft tissue or bone sarcomas. Instead, such traumatic episodes are thought to call attention to a specific body part or location, thereby increasing the likelihood of detecting an otherwise painless and often innocuous soft tissue mass or bone lesion.[74]

Fractures. Pathologic fractures are rare in primary neoplasms, but if the lytic process affects a significant portion of the cortex (over 50%) or occupies 60% of the bone diameter, the risk of fracture increases. A relatively small lytic lesion in the femoral neck that destroys the inferior cortex of the femoral neck also places the client at increased risk. In benign lesions, no other symptoms may warn of the impending fracture.

A history of sudden onset of severe pain may be an indication of a pathologic fracture. In addition to the tumor itself, other factors such as disuse, treatment (biopsy, radiation), and other health problems (osteoporosis) may increase the risk of pathologic fracture.

Miscellaneous. Other signs and symptoms often encountered include swelling, fever, and the presence of a mass. Other factors that are useful in screening for serious pathology include unexplained weight loss, failure of rest to provide relief of pain, age, and history of cancer. The history will often give more meaningful information regarding the possibility of skeletal neoplasms than the physical examination.

Swelling. Swelling surrounding a tumor may not be detectable in a bone tumor, but with soft tissue tumors close to the skin surface, swelling may be one of the first presenting signs. The nature of swelling, including the location, amount, temperature, and tenderness, is somewhat dependent on the vascularity of the lesion.

Mass. A careful physical examination may reveal a mass or other signs of an inflammatory process. The presence of a mass should raise questions concerning the location, mobility, tenderness, dimensions, and recent changes in any of these factors. As with pain, the size of the mass is not indicative of the severity of the lesion but is one factor to consider. Any change in size, appearance, or other characteristics of a lump, local swelling, or lesion of any kind within the previous 6 weeks to 6 months should be reported to the physician.

Metastases. Sarcomas spread by *hematogenous* routes rather than through the lymphatics. The most common site of metastases for individuals with extremity sarcomas is the lung, followed by liver and other bone sites. Anyone diagnosed with soft tissue sarcoma has an approximately 50% chance of local recurrence, because these tumors spread along tissue planes and involve adjacent tissue. Lymph node involvement is uncommon and is often associated with poor prognosis.[41]

Medical Management

Diagnosis

Physical examination, imaging studies (e.g., x-ray examination, computed tomography [CT], magnetic resonance imaging [MRI]), and biopsy are the primary diagnostic tools.

Physical Examination

Many tumors cannot be observed or palpated during the physical examination, but if a mass is present its characteristics must be noted. The presence of café-au-lait spots (associated with neurofibromatosis), skin ulceration, or neurologic findings (e.g., footdrop, calf pain) may be significant.

Because synovial sarcoma, rhabdomyosarcoma, and epithelioid sarcoma can metastasize via the lymphatics, examination of the lymph nodes is essential.[67] A tumor overlying bone and muscle can be evaluated by contracting the muscle and checking for movement or change in consistency of the tumor.

Radiographic Examination

Radiographs also help differentiate between bone and soft tissue involvement. Plain radiographs are a mainstay in the detection and evaluation of many skeletal tumors. In many cases, skeletal tumors are found incidentally on routine radiographs for associated injuries. The radiograph provides unique information concerning skeletal tumors.

The location of the tumor will give many clues to the type of lesion (see Fig. 16.1). Some tumors develop exclusively in the epiphysis, whereas others develop in the diaphysis of long bones. Bone tumors tend to predominate in those ends of long bones that undergo the greatest growth and remodeling and hence have the greatest number of cells and amount of cell activity (shoulder and knee regions).

A tumor with a permeated or moth-eaten appearance (i.e., an area with multiple holes with irregular edges randomly distributed) with an expansive cortical shell indicates an aggressive malignant lesion (Fig. 16.2). Codman's triangle, a triangular-shaped area of reactive bone, is formed when the neoplasm has eroded the cortex, elevating the periosteum and producing reactive bone in the angle where it is still attached (Fig. 16.3).

The tumor's location, its effect on bone, and the local bone response to the lesion are just some of the radiographic features to be noted and will help in planning the rest of the evaluation.

Imaging

Radionuclide bone scan (scintigraphy), CT, MRI, angiography, and ultrasonography all have a place in the evaluation of bone lesions. *Bone scans* help locate skip metastases and the presence of bone metastases as well as metastatic bone lesions, and they assess tumor activity by the amount of ra-

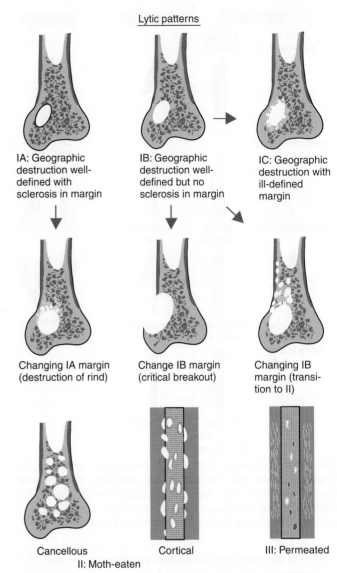

Lytic patterns

IA: Geographic destruction well-defined with sclerosis in margin

IB: Geographic destruction well-defined but no sclerosis in margin

IC: Geographic destruction with ill-defined margin

Changing IA margin (destruction of rind)

Change IB margin (critical breakout)

Changing IB margin (transition to II)

Cancellous   Cortical   III: Permeated
II: Moth-eaten

FIG. 16.2 Schematic diagram of patterns of bone destruction (types IA, IB, IC, II, and III) and their margins. Arrows indicate the most common transitions or combinations of these margins. Transitions imply increased activity and a greater probability of malignancy. (Redrawn from Madewell JE, Ragsdale BD, Sweet DE: Radiologic and pathologic analysis of solitary bone lesions: I. Internal margins, Radiol Clin North Am 19:715, 1981.)

dioisotope uptake in and around the tumor. Greater uptake indicates a more aggressive and malignant tumor.

CT scans are the most sensitive technique in detecting pulmonary metastases and also provide detailed information about the interaction between the tumor and various components of the bone (e.g., bone cortex, cancellous bone, reactive bone).

MRI has emerged as the most useful imaging tool for evaluating soft tissue tumors and is valuable in determining the extent of the marrow involvement and soft tissue masses outside the bone. The surgical team uses the information provided by MRI to help visualize the involvement of the tumor and to plan limb salvage techniques.

Angiography plays an important role when limb-sparing surgery is being considered by providing information regard-

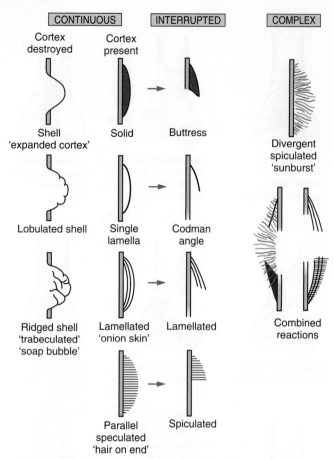

FIG. 16.3 Schematic diagram of periosteal reactions. The arrows indicate that the continuous reactions may be interrupted. (Redrawn from Ragsdale BD, Madewell JE, Sweet DE: Radiologic and pathologic analysis of solitary bone lesions: II. Periosteal reactions, Radiol Clin North Am 19:749, 1981.)

ing the neovascularity of the tumor and mapping the vascular anatomy.

Ultrasonography is a noninvasive imaging method that can be used to determine the size and consistency of a soft tissue mass. It may be used to establish intraarterial access for subsequent chemotherapy.[40]

Biopsy

A biopsy is the definitive diagnostic procedure in both bone and soft tissue tumors and is usually performed after physical examination and imaging. This procedure can take many forms. The decision to do an open or incisional core needle or fine-needle biopsy or an excisional biopsy is based on the location and type of tumor.

Laboratory Tests

Various laboratory studies are used to detect, diagnose, and differentiate musculoskeletal neoplasms. Laboratory tests that may be of value include the complete blood count (CBC), urinalysis, erythrocyte sedimentation rate (ESR) (elevated in Ewing's sarcoma), serum calcium (elevated in metastatic bone disease), phosphorus (decreased with "brown tumors" associated with hyperthyroidism), alkaline phosphatase (elevated in osteosarcoma and Paget's disease), and serum protein electrophoresis (abnormal in metastatic bone disease).

Serum levels of alkaline phosphatase and calcium are often elevated with metastatic disease. Elevated alkaline phosphatase and lactic dehydrogenase (LDH) also occur with osteosarcoma.

Staging and Grading

The purpose of much of the extensive workup once a tumor has been identified is to determine the grade and stage of the tumor. Grading determines the histologic characteristics, such as the extent of anaplasia or differentiation of the cells from grade I, indicating cells that are very differentiated, to grade IV, those that are undifferentiated.

Staging of a tumor is concerned with the extent of its growth, both local and distant. The tumor-node-metastasis (TNM) staging system reflects the degree of local extension at the primary tumor site, involvement of local nodes, and presence of metastasis. This classification group is strongly correlated with survival.

No universally accepted staging system for musculoskeletal neoplasms exists because of the low incidence of such tumors, their heterogeneous nature and unpredictable behavior, and disagreement as to the relative importance of prognostic factors.[53] The surgical staging system of Enneking is used for soft tissue and bone tumors and includes prognostic variables such as the histologic grade of the tumor, location of the tumor, and presence or absence of metastases (Table 16.3).[23] The American Joint Committee on Cancer (AJCC) also provides staging for soft tissue sarcomas.[3] Staging helps in planning and standardizing the intervention strategy for these rare lesions.

Grading sarcomas has been one of the most important contributions pathologists have made to the treatment of sarcomas. There is not one single grading scheme that works well for all sarcomas.

Treatment

Treatment ranges from *observation* in the case of some benign bone tumors to *surgical intervention*. Chemotherapy or surgery alone cures few people. Multimodal measures are needed for a long-term successful response.[4]

Complete tumor resection is the best surgical strategy and is attempted whenever possible. A marginal excision removes the tumor at its border, resulting in some of the tumor remaining. A wide excision (sometimes referred to as an *en bloc incision*) removes some of the normal surrounding tissue, leaving none of the tumor. Radical resection may be required, in which the entire involved bone and all the tissue compartments adjacent to the tumor are removed.

The spine, sacrum, pelvis, ankle, hand, mediastinum, and chest wall are just a few examples of bone cancer locations that make surgery difficult. When local excision has positive margins (not all the cancer was removed), local control may be increased with radiation and chemotherapy regimens. Immunotherapy and biotherapy are additional treatment methods used to prevent cancer recurrence.[4]

Limb salvage or limb-sparing procedures have largely replaced amputation as the principal method to eradicate primary sarcomas. The three phases to any limb-sparing procedure are (1) resection of the tumor, (2) reconstruction of the skeletal area involved, and (3) soft tissue and muscle transfer to complete the reconstruction.

TABLE 16.3   Enneking Staging System for Bone and Soft Tissue Tumors

Stage	Grade	Site
Stage 0	G_0 (benign neoplasm)	
Stage IA[a]	G_1 (low grade; locally inactive or latent tumor with low probability of metastases)	T_1 (tumor is contained within the bone and involves only one compartment; e.g., single compartment = individual bone with its medullary cavity)
Stage IB	G_1 (low grade; active, slow growth)	T_1 (tumor extends into soft tissue)
Stage IIA	G_2 (high grade; aggressive tumor with high metastatic potential	T_1 (tumor is contained within the bone)
Stage IIB	G_2 (high grade; aggressive)	T_2 (tumor extends beyond cortex into adjacent soft tissue, joint, epidural space, or other bone)
Stage III	Any grade	Metastases present

[a]The suffixes A and B in this system indicate A, intracompartmental or B, extracompartmental lesions.
From Dorfman HD, Czerniak B: Bone tumors, St Louis, 1998, Mosby.
For staging according to the American Joint Committee on Cancer (AJCC), see National Comprehensive Cancer Network (NCCN): Practice guidelines in oncology: soft tissue sarcoma, vol 2, 2007. http://www.globalgist.org/docs/NCCN_guidelines.pdf. Accessed September 27, 2016.

Obtaining a wide surgical margin while preserving limb viability and function remains the challenge to the medical team, requiring close coordination of surgical, medical, and oncologic staff. Often, soft tissue reconstruction is necessary to provide wound coverage after tumor removal.

The use of *radiation* is recommended for some tumors such as Ewing's sarcoma and myeloma, but many malignant tumors are not affected by radiation. For some soft tissue tumors, adjunctive radiation is used in an attempt to limit the degree of surgical excision needed. In general, radiation is not recommended for benign conditions. Irradiation creates a suboptimal tissue bed susceptible to wound breakdown, seroma, and hematoma formation and infection, which may complicate the success of soft tissue reconstruction.[74]

Because hematogenous spread occurs early in musculoskeletal tumors, *chemotherapy* is also used to help eradicate malignant tumors. For example, combination chemotherapy has resulted in increased survival rates in clients with Ewing's sarcoma and rhabdomyosarcoma as well. When chemotherapy is combined with other modalities such as surgery and radiation, less toxic doses can be used.

Prognosis

The prognosis is based in part on the type of tumor and whether it is benign or malignant. Survival is influenced by the grade of malignancy, tumor stage, and achieved surgical margins. A high grade and evidence of metastasis are associated with a poor prognosis for all neoplasms of bone or soft tissue regardless of the staging system that is used.[53] Tumor extension into both anterior and posterior columns of a vertebra is correlated with a poor outcome. Incomplete resections are more likely to result in tumor recurrence with subsequent surgeries and increased risk for complications and poor outcome.[76]

Slow-growing tumors should be followed for prolonged periods to determine the natural history and to identify the ultimate prognosis. Prognosis can vary from 3- to 5-year survival rates for clients with sarcomas and myeloma, to a better prognosis for tumors that are asymptomatic. Successfully treated individuals may develop severe late effects, including second cancers (e.g., radiation-induced sarcomas or treatment-related leukemia), particularly after high-dose therapy with an alkylating agent, and chemotherapy-induced cardiomyopathy.[6]

Recurrence

People with recurrent disease generally have a poor prognosis but need to undergo a complete reevaluation of the extent of the disease to determine this more specifically. The prognosis depends on the type of therapy given previously, duration of remission, and extent of metastases. Recurrence or progression of tumor during initial therapy is generally incurable.[6] The lung is the most common initial site of distant metastases for the majority of soft tissue and bone sarcomas. Other sites may include distant osseous sites, bone marrow, and lymph nodes.

16.1 Special Implications for the PTA: Primary Tumors Screening Assessment

A PTA's involvement with clients with musculoskeletal neoplasms should begin with increased efforts directed toward early detection and education. Although many musculoskeletal tumors produce symptoms that are also present with more mundane conditions, careful observation and monitoring of a client's response to intervention may lead to earlier detection and treatment.

Assessing for history of cancer, family history, and risk factors may alert the therapy team to the need to screen further for medical disease. This is especially true in the case of musculoskeletal symptoms of unknown cause or when the individual does not respond to physical therapy intervention as expected for a musculoskeletal problem.

The presence of suspicious lymph nodes or aberrant soft tissue masses maybe observed by the PT and PTA, but the client must be further evaluated by a physician. Through inclusion of the possibility of a primary musculoskeletal tumor in the differential diagnosis of clients who have continued pain despite appropriate rest and treatment, further medical evaluation may be recommended, which may help reveal other pathology.

Rehabilitation

Currently, an achievable goal for the majority of people with soft tissue and bone sarcomas is freedom from disease with long-term resumption of nearly normal function. PTAs are key to the successful attainment of this goal for individuals who are undergoing treatment for primary musculoskeletal neoplasms. A comprehensive approach should be used to ensure that both psychosocial–spiritual aspects and physical problems are addressed. Occupational status, family structure, and age are all important factors.[34]

Communication among the team members such as social workers, rehabilitation counselors, physicians, nurses, and therapists cannot be overemphasized. Communication is essential to coordination and follow-through in the treatment and rehabilitation program. A detailed approach to evaluation and treatment of clients with cancer should be formulated.[54]

Early postoperative mobilization is essential to prevent complications such as pressure ulcers, deep venous thrombosis, lymphedema, pneumonia, muscle wasting, and generalized weakness associated with prolonged bed rest. Surgical procedures will have an effect on multiple organ systems, as will chemotherapy and radiation therapy. A detailed assessment and description of pain is always indicated, because pain control is a critical component in successful acute rehabilitation.

Many other factors to consider before implementing a treatment plan after orthopedic procedures include controlling compressive forces and weight bearing. Wolf's law demonstrates that bone strength increases in response to imposed mechanical stress, such as the pulling force of muscles and the pressures of weight bearing. When bone resorption exceeds bone formation, osteopenia develops.

After excision of cancerous bone (sometimes accompanied by muscle resection), mechanical weakening and resultant bone instability may limit or contraindicate weight bearing and use of the involved extremity.[24] Remaining muscles should be strengthened and substitution patterns of muscle control implemented and encouraged where necessary.[34]

Other considerations in the rehabilitative process may include rehabilitation for the amputee, evaluation of adaptive equipment needs, ambulation devices, use of orthoses to support involved extremities, wound care management, environmental adaptations (e.g., access ramps, accessible doorways, bathroom grab bars), work site modifications, and quality-of-life issues. Client education is essential regarding proper body mechanics, energy conservation, side effects of treatment, and prevention and recognition of complications such as infection, deep vein thrombosis, skin breakdown, lymphedema, scar formation, and the loss of flexibility, strength, balance, or endurance.

Prescriptive Exercise

As discussed, treatment of tumors can result in amputation (sometimes as extensive as a hemipelvectomy[8]), prolonged immobilization, bone or muscle resection, or extensive surgical reconstruction, all of which require consideration of postoperative complications (e.g., ischemia, infection) and the involvement of many different types of rehabilitation.

An individualized program of exercise that takes into account the diagnosis, underlying pathology, physical condition of the individual, effects of various interventions, strength deficits, and structural instability is essential.

Limb-sparing techniques such as the endoprosthetic replacement (distal femoral replacement with rotating hinge device; expandable for pediatric population) continue to undergo modification and refinement. Surgeons are attempting to minimize muscle resection, maintain mechanical function, and successfully reattach the muscles to the endoprostheses or to surrounding soft tissue structures, thereby reducing functional impairment.

Rehabilitation techniques for these clients remain conjectural. Despite loss of range of motion (ROM) and muscle power, most clients report relatively good limb function. Early gait training and weight bearing with active assisted range are indicated, and isometric exercises about the joint are recommended.[4] General principles regarding energy conservation and exercise for the person with cancer, especially after chemotherapy or radiotherapy, should be followed.

PRIMARY BENIGN BONE TUMORS

Bone Island

Overview and Incidence

Bone islands are oval, usually small, sclerotic lesions of bone. They are one of the most common benign bone lesions. Bone islands have been observed in all bones and may manifest as solitary or multiple lesions. The lesion is well defined and made up of cortical bone with a well-developed haversian canal system. The borders blend in with the surrounding bone. The presence of spicules of cortical bone extending from the margins to the surrounding trabeculae is characteristic. A prevalence of 14% has been reported for spinal bone islands.[57]

Clinical Manifestations

Bone islands are always asymptomatic. They are seen on radiographs as incidental findings.

Medical Management

When the bone islands are small (less than 1 cm), diagnosis with plain radiographs is adequate. They are usually oblong and align themselves with the axis of the bone. A bone scan is usually normal, confirming the absence of malignancy. The emphasis is not on intervention but on the judicious use of diagnostic tools. Biopsies should be avoided, as they are usually unnecessary. Although some bone islands can enlarge, they do not transform into malignant lesions.

16.2 Special Implications for the PTA: Bone Islands Bone islands are seen in radiographs of clients with a variety of musculoskeletal traumas. If clients are aware of these lesions, they should be reassured that they pose no significant health concern. Many physicians do not inform clients that bone islands are present. Care must be taken not to alarm the client. The word *tumor* is foreboding and should be used sparingly.

Osteoid Osteoma

Overview, Incidence, and Etiologic Factors

Osteoid osteoma is a rare benign vascular osteoblastic lesion. It is often found in the cortex of long bones such as the femur and tibia but may occur in almost any bone except the skull. The tumors occur near the end of the diaphysis (Fig. 16.4). Osteoid osteoma accounts for about 10% to 12% of benign bone tumors. Most of these lesions are found in men under the age of 25. The cause of osteoid osteoma remains unknown.

Pathogenesis

Pathologic study shows areas of immature bone surrounded by prominent osteoblasts and osteoclasts. The lesion is vascular, but no cartilage is present. Osteoid osteoma is probably a "reactive" bone-forming lesion rather than a true neoplasm, consisting of a small, round nidus (nest) of osteoid tissue surrounded by reactive bone sclerosis.

The zone of sclerosis is not an integral part of the tumor and represents a secondary reversible change that gradually disappears after the removal of the nidus. Osteoid osteomas are not progressive and rarely grow larger than 1 cm in diameter. They are uncalcified and therefore radiolucent.

Spine involvement may result in an unexplained backache or painful type of scoliosis with unilateral spasticity of spinal muscles. Some people with vertebral lesions may have clinical symptoms suggestive of a neurologic disorder, lumbar disc disease, or both.[21] In the case of spine involvement, neurologic deficits can be caused by extradural compression.[75]

Medical Management

Diagnosis

Radiographs can be diagnostic for osteoid osteoma, although these are often normal early in the course. Later, a small (less than 1 cm) translucency or nidus forms, surrounded by sclerotic bone. When the tumor is not easily identified on radiographs (e.g., vertebral nidus), further testing is required, such as a bone scan, which will show a focal uptake of the radiotracer. Plain films may not be adequate when the tumor is intraarticular; in such cases CT or MRI can be used to accurately locate the nidus.

Treatment and Prognosis

In tumors that are symptomatic, surgical excision of the nidus may be indicated. Because the tumor is small, excision is usually sufficient, although bone grafting may be needed depending on the size and location of the tumor. Recurrence is rare, and a full recovery is common. Osteoid osteomas have no potential for malignant transformation.[75] Differences in the expected rate of recovery may occur depending on the location of the tumor and the extent of excision required. The size and extent of the resection may mandate some activity restrictions or weight-bearing limitations if the risk of fracture exists. Intraarticular lesions certainly require more extensive rehabilitation for restoration of normal function.

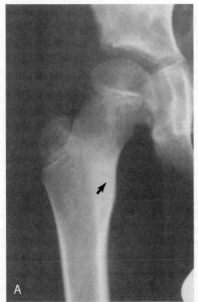
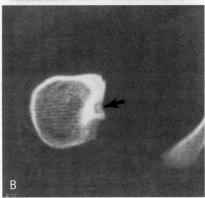

FIG. 16.4 Osteoid osteoma. (A) Bony sclerosis with cortical thickening is seen in this person with pain in the proximal femur. A faint lucency *(arrow)* can be seen in the area of sclerosis, which is the nidus of an osteoid osteoma. (B) A computed tomography (CT) scan through the nidus shows it to lie just dorsal to the lesser trochanter *(arrow)*. This is a characteristic appearance of an osteoid osteoma on CT scans. (From Helms C: Fundamentals of skeletal radiology, ed 4, Philadelphia, 2014, Saunders.)

Clinical Manifestations

Gradually increasing and persistent local pain in the area of the tumor, described as a dull ache, is the primary complaint. The pain is often worse at night and is characteristically relieved by aspirin and other nonsteroidal antiinflammatory drugs (NSAIDs). Pain relief may be a result of the inhibitory effect on prostaglandins produced by osteoid osteomas. Systemic symptoms are uncommon.

When the lesion is located near a joint, synovial effusion may develop and interfere with joint function, with local muscle atrophy developing.[59] A significant leg length discrepancy can occur, caused by the increased growth rate of affected bone in young individuals with open growth plates.

Though they occur rarely in the spine, if present they are found in the lower thoracic or lumbar spine located in the posterior vertebral arch. The tumor can lead to joint pain and dysfunction, often delaying the diagnosis by masquerading as a more common problem.[75]

Osteoblastoma
Overview

Osteoblastoma is another reactive but benign bone lesion similar to osteoid osteoma, only larger, with a tendency to expand. Some aggressive forms of osteoblastoma have been recognized. Unlike osteoid osteoma, osteoblastomas are often found in the spine, sacrum, and flat bones. Osteoblastomas involve the spine in approximately 35% of affected individuals, with the cervical spine affected in up to 39% of those people.[20]

Those found in the long bones are usually in the diaphysis, although as with most tumors they can be seen elsewhere (Fig. 16.5). The histologic makeup of osteoblastoma is very similar to that of an osteoid osteoma. In fact, sometimes it is size alone that differentiates the two, with osteoblastoma being the larger. The lesions are osteolytic and have a sclerotic border.

An aggressive osteoblastoma is a borderline lesion between benign osteoblastoma and osteosarcoma. It is very rare and not discussed further in this text.

Incidence

Osteoblastoma occurs most often in men younger than 30, but cases have been reported in children as young as 2 years old and adults in their seventies.[75] Osteoblastoma is a rare osteoblastic tumor that makes up only 1% to 2% of all benign bone tumors.

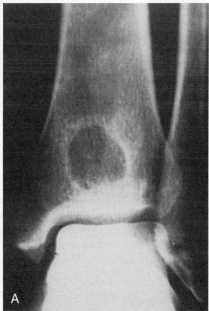

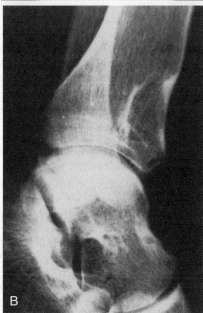

FIG. 16.5 Genuine (conventional) osteoblastoma of the tibia in a 24-year-old woman. Anteroposterior (A) and lateral (B) radiographs show a round radiolucent lesion with slightly sclerotic borders at the lower and anterior aspect of the tibia. (From Gitelis S, Schajowicz F: Osteoid osteoma and osteoblastoma, Orthop Clin 20:320, 1989.)

Clinical Manifestations

When the tumor is located in the spine, the pedicles are often affected. Pain is the common presentation; it is not relieved with aspirin as occurs with osteoid osteoma. In general, the pain of osteoblastoma is not as severe as with osteoid osteoma, especially at night. Tenderness over the lesion is expected. With a spinal location, a functional scoliosis may be observed. In some cases a neurologic deficit may be present, which can mimic other, more common causes of nerve compression. Metastases and even death have been reported with the aggressive variant, which can behave in a fashion similar to that of osteosarcoma.

Medical Management

Diagnosis

Osteoblastoma is seen on plain radiographs, but when it is located in the spine, other imaging techniques are also useful. The lesion can have variations in its appearance. Often it looks like a large osteoid osteoma with a well-defined radiolucency in the central portion and a thin, sclerotic border. It also can be similar to an aneurysmal bone cyst that is expansile and lytic and has a soap bubble appearance (see Fig. 16.3). CT and MRI are valuable in localizing the tumor and determining the extent of tissue involved.

Treatment

In the long bones, curettage (scraping to remove the contents of the bone cavity) is often adequate. A wider excision is sometimes recommended because of the unpredictable nature of osteoblastoma and high recurrence rate (up to 15%).

Extramarginal excisions can result in the need to perform reconstructive procedures using autografts or allografts and internal fixation when the tumor is located in the diaphysis of long bones. If the joint is affected, implants may be needed. In the spine, removal of the tumor may lead to instability, which may require fusion and internal fixation.

Prognosis

Ninety percent to 95% of osteoblastomas are cured by the initial treatment,[25] but even with careful removal of the tumors, they recur in about 10% of affected individuals.[61] There is a risk of malignant transformation into an osteosarcoma, which can sometimes be determined early. Appropriate intervention with adjunctive chemotherapy or radiation is the current standard of care.

PRIMARY MALIGNANT BONE TUMORS

Primary malignant bone tumors are relatively rare, representing about 6% to 7% of all pediatric neoplasms. Osteosarcomas are the most frequent type, followed by Ewing's sarcoma. Osteosarcomas make up over half of all malignant bone tumors; Ewing's sarcomas account for one-third of all primary malignant bone tumors (Table 16.4).[26]

Osteosarcoma

Overview

Osteosarcoma, also known as *osteogenic sarcoma*, is an extremely malignant tumor with destructive lesions and abundant sclerosis, both from the tumor itself and from reactive bone formation. A characteristic of osteosarcoma is the production of osteoid by malignant, neoplastic cells. This is seen on photomicrographs and is one of the features used to help differentiate this tumor. Resected specimens usually show that the cortex has been broken by the destructive tumor. Although various types of osteosarcoma exist, including parosteal, periosteal, telangiectatic, and small cell, only the most common, conventional intramedullary osteosarcoma, is discussed here.

Incidence

Osteosarcoma is the second most frequent malignant condition of bone, accounting for 15% to 20% of all primary bone tumors;

TABLE 16.4 Malignant Bone Tumors[a]

Tumor	Age (years)	Sex Ratio (M:F)	Common Sites	Location
Osteosarcoma	10–25	2:1	Long bones of extremities (knee joint), jaw	Metaphysis
Ewing's sarcoma	10–20	2:1	Long bones; multiple sites	No predilection for specific part of the bone; diaphysis most common
Chondrosarcoma	40–60	2:1	Pelvis, ribs, vertebrae, long bones (proximal)	Diaphysis or metaphysis

[a]In order of descending frequency.
Adapted from Damjanov I: Pathology for the health professions, ed 4, St. Louis, 2012, Saunders.

only myeloma is seen more often. Osteosarcoma occurs most often in male children, adolescents, and young adults under the age of 30, with a peak frequency during the adolescent growth spurt and another smaller peak in people older than 50.[21]

Osteosarcoma can develop in many bones but is more common in long bones, the site of the most active epiphyseal growth. The distal femur is the most common site, followed by the proximal tibia and proximal fibula (50% are located in the knee region), proximal humerus, pelvis, and occasionally the mandible, vertebrae, or scapula.

Etiologic and Risk Factors

Osteosarcomas can be primary or secondary. Certain genetic or acquired conditions increase the risk of osteosarcoma (e.g., retinoblastoma, Paget's disease of bone, enchondromatosis, ionizing radiation). Alterations of multiple chromosomes and their extra copies have been demonstrated but only in distinct clinical subsets of osteosarcoma. Secondary osteosarcomas are those that develop from other lesions such as Paget's disease, chronic osteomyelitis, osteoblastoma, or giant cell tumor.

Pathogenesis

Osteosarcoma grows rapidly and is locally destructive. It may be osteosclerotic (producing considerable neoplastic or tumor bone), or it may arise from more primitive cells and remain predominantly osteolytic, eroding the cortex of the metaphyseal region and resulting in pathologic fracture. As it continues to grow beyond the confines of the bone, the tumor lifts the periosteum, resulting in the formation of reactive bone in the angle between elevated periosteum and bone called *Codman's triangle* (see Fig. 16.3).

Clinical Manifestations

Osteosarcoma seems to appear in bones undergoing an active growth phase and appears at the epiphyseal plate of rapidly growing bone in adolescents. The long bones such as the distal femur, proximal humerus, and proximal tibia have a relatively more active growth period than other bones, which makes them more vulnerable (Fig. 16.6).

Pain that has continued for several weeks to months is the presenting complaint. The tumor is often located in the metaphysis but does not cross the physis. Even so, joint pain and tenderness can be present as the lesion penetrates the cortex and invades the joint capsule, also spreading to other nearby structures (e.g., tendons, fat, muscles).

Because osteosarcoma can be a rapidly destructive tumor, the pain increases, and swelling may develop in just a few weeks, accompanied by some limitation of motion. Systemic symptoms are rare, although occasional fever may occur. This aggressive neoplasm is very vascular, and the overlying skin is usually warm. Metastases appear in the lungs early in 90% of cases and occur in 20% to 25% of cases at the time of presentation.[6]

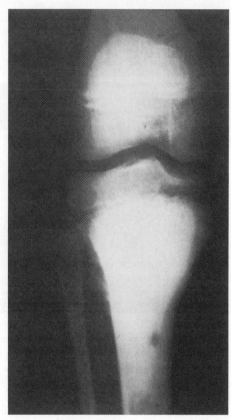

FIG. 16.6 Osteosarcoma. An extremely sclerotic lesion in the proximal tibia of a child is noted, which is characteristic of an osteogenic sarcoma. (From Helms C: Fundamentals of skeletal radiology, ed 4, Philadelphia, 2014, Saunders.)

Medical Management

Diagnosis

Diagnosis is often delayed, especially when swelling is minimal, as is often the case in early stages.[34] X-ray studies should be done with any complaint of bone pain, especially around the knee. Plain radiographs often reflect dramatic changes and obvious tumor formation, but important findings can also be subtle.

CT scans and especially MRI images are used to evaluate the extent of disease. In Fig. 16.7 plain films of a pelvis demonstrate minimal changes that could easily be dismissed as insignificant. The CT scan, however, reveals a large osteosarcoma involving the ilium. More commonly, radiographs show a rapidly growing lesion with poorly defined margins and a permeated or moth-eaten appearance in the lytic area.

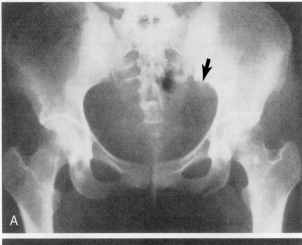

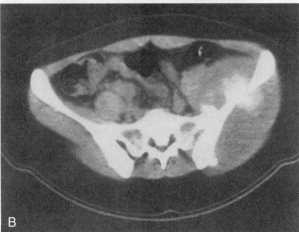

FIG. 16.7 Osteosarcoma. (A) A subtle sclerotic lesion is seen in the left ilium adjacent to the sacroiliac joint that was initially diagnosed as osteitis condensans ilii, a benign entity. Because of persistent pain, the person returned for a follow-up visit, and a small amount of cortical destruction on the pelvic brim was noted *(arrow)*. (B) A computed tomographic scan was performed, which showed a large tissue mass and new bone tumor around the ilium, which is characteristic of an osteogenic sarcoma. (From Helms C: Fundamentals of skeletal radiology, ed 4, Philadelphia, 2014, Saunders.)

A biopsy is performed to determine the histologic makeup of the lesion. Serum alkaline phosphatase level is often elevated, but this is not diagnostic.

Treatment

Because osteosarcoma is relatively resistant to radiation therapy, complete surgical removal of the primary tumor and any metastases is essential to cure.[6] The current surgical thinking is to use limb-sparing techniques whenever possible (Fig. 16.8).

The use of a noninvasive expandable prosthesis for skeletally immature children and adolescents after limb salvage for malignant tumors in the leg has been reported. The Repiphysis prosthesis for pediatric osteosarcoma is an expandable metal rod that replaces the bone and does not require repeated procedures to lengthen as the child's other leg grows. Painless electromagnetic rays are used to expand the rod slowly without compromise to the surrounding skin and muscle.[31]

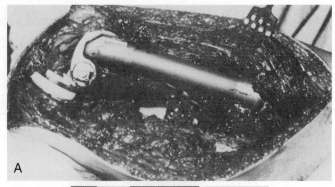

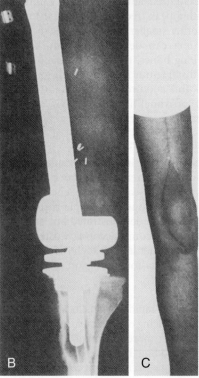

FIG. 16.8 Osteosarcoma of the distal femur in a 17-year-old boy. (A) Intraoperative photograph after resection of the distal femur. (B) Postoperative radiograph of custom-made, rotating-hinge prosthesis. (C) Follow-up clinical photograph (3 years after surgery). Soft tissue coverage of the prosthesis by latissimus dorsi myocutaneous free flap with acceptable cosmesis. (From Klein M, Kenan S, Lenis M: Osteosarcoma: clinical and pathologic considerations, Orthop Clin 20:343, 1989.)

Another creative procedure called *rotationplasty* removes the cancerous portion of the bone below the knee then uses the remaining bottom segment of the leg and ankle joint as a new knee. The surgeon removes the affected bone, rotates the lower portion of the leg 180 degrees so the foot faces the opposite direction, and reattaches it to the upper femoral area. Nerves, muscles, and blood supply are preserved. The posterior-facing ankle now functions as a weight-bearing knee joint in a specially fitted prosthesis (Fig. 16.9). Although the outcome is visually unusual, such a procedure improves gait and knee function and prevents amputation.[71]

Owing to the cosmesis of seeing a foot turned backward not being acceptable in some cases, children and families may still prefer endoprosthetic reconstruction or even amputation.

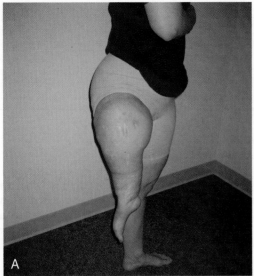

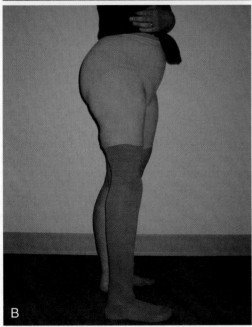

FIG. 16.9 Rotationplasty for osteosarcoma. The primary reason for rotationplasty is to enhance the person's mobility as a prosthesis user. Placing the ankle joint in the position of the knee creates a functional, natural knee, and the toes provide important sensory feedback to the brain. (A) Rotationplasty removes the cancerous portion of the femur (proximal to the midshaft of the femur), then rotates the lower portion of the leg 180 degrees so the foot faces the opposite direction. The proximal tibia is fused to the distal femur; the remaining bottom segment of the leg and ankle joint function as a new knee. (B) Standing on the prosthesis with the cover on it. (Courtesy Kevin Carroll, Hanger Prosthetics and Orthotics, Orlando, FL.)

Younger children (less than 10 years old) seem better able to adapt psychologically and physically to the rotationplasty.[46]

The tibia turn-up is another important procedure that is an option in cases of osteosarcoma (Fig. 16.10). The leg is amputated above the knee, and the tibia bone from the lower leg is inverted, or turned up, making it possible for the ankle end of the tibia to be fused to the bottom of the femur. The muscles are then sutured back onto the tibia.[16]

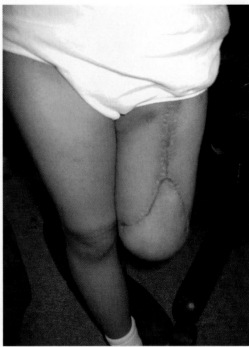

FIG. 16.10 Tibia turn-up procedure. Sarcoma just below lesser trochanter in a 7-year-old girl. There were three surgical options for this client: (1) transtrochanteric amputation (major loss of limb), (2) tibia turn-up procedure (shown here), or (3) rotationplasty (see Fig. 16.9). The tibia turn-up procedure was chosen for cosmetic reasons with excellent functional outcomes with the use of a prosthesis. The tibia turn-up procedure avoids high-level transfemoral amputation and provides an outcome similar to that of a knee disarticulation amputation. (Courtesy Kevin Carroll, Hanger Prosthetics and Orthotics, Orlando, FL.)

Tibia turn-up is an alternative that people may consider when the appearance of a rotationplasty seems too extreme. Tibia turn-up is also an option when cancer occurs in the thigh that might otherwise require a high-level above-knee amputation (Fig. 16.11). By having the tibia fused to the femur, these individuals now have a long residual limb that will be easier to fit with a prosthesis, providing them with increased function. Although these individuals will wear an above-knee prosthesis with a mechanical knee, their comfort and mobility will usually exceed that of above-knee prosthesis users with a short residual limb.[16]

When done in skeletally immature individuals, the rotationplasty and tibia turn-up techniques both make allowances for the natural process of growth that extends into young adulthood.

Chemotherapy often precedes surgery. Chemotherapy is evaluated by its effect on the client and tumor. Chemotherapy may also help lessen the chance of skip lesions, or multiple foci of tumor that can cause recurrence of the tumor after surgery.

Prognosis

Adjunctive (preoperative) chemotherapy and surgery results in 5-year cure rates of 70% to 80% for osteosarcoma. The majority of affected individuals (more than 90%) have limb-sparing surgery.[72] Surgery alone will probably allow pul-

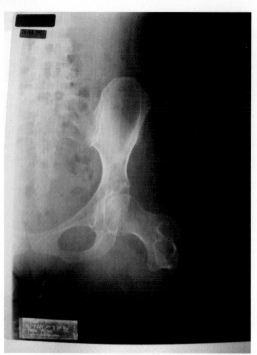

FIG. 16.11 Rotationplasty or tibia turn-up can be a good alternative to high-level above-knee amputations such as this. (Courtesy Kevin Carroll, Hanger Prosthetics and Orthotics, Orlando, FL.)

monary metastasis to occur. Individuals who develop lung metastases have a 20% to 30% 5-year survival rate.

Even with chemotherapy, the outcome is dependent on the stage at diagnosis and the ability of the surgeon to achieve a tumor-free margin. Local recurrence is a poor prognostic sign. Local recurrence of craniofacial lesions after treatment is 50% for mandibular tumors and even higher for maxillary and skull lesions (80% and 75%, respectively); metastases occur in about one-third of craniofacial osteosarcomas.[21]

In older people, osteosarcoma may develop as a complication of Paget's disease, in which case the prognosis is extremely grave.[59]

16.3 Special Implications for the PTA: Osteosarcoma Malignant neoplasms usually necessitate aggressive intervention, and therefore rehabilitation is more intensive, prolonged, and individualized. Extensive surgery, such as limb-sparing techniques, has provided PTAs with an opportunity to assist these clients in maximizing their function (Fig. 16.12). When musculoskeletal structures are involved, it is important to be aware of reduced tensile strength of malignant tissue compared with uninvolved bone tissue.

Postoperative Rehabilitation

Because these tumors are treated at regional medical centers, the initial phases of rehabilitation may involve physical therapists and PTAs with a great deal of experience working with clients with malignant neoplasms and those who have undergone various reconstructive surgical procedures.

When the client returns home a local PTA may be called on to continue the rehabilitation program. Communication with the therapy team at the regional medical center to confirm initial management plan, progression, and prognosis is recommended.

The use of a new tool, functional mobility assessment (FMA), has been examined in clients with lower extremity sarcoma. FMA

requires the individual to physically perform functional mobility tasks, provides a reliable and valid measure of objective functional outcome, and may help PTAs guide children and adolescents in returning to daily activities.[46]

As might be expected, rehabilitation after limb-sparing surgery or rotationplasty focuses on retraining muscles and increasing weight bearing and balance, ROM, and strength.

Chondrosarcoma
Overview and Incidence

Chondrosarcoma is usually a relatively slow-growing malignant neoplasm that arises either spontaneously in previously normal bone or as the result of malignant change in a preexisting non-malignant lesion, such as an osteochondroma or an enchondroma. The pelvic and shoulder girdles are common sites of tumor and related pain, as are the proximal and distal femur, proximal humerus, and ribs.

Chondrosarcoma is the second most common solid malignant tumor of bone in adults. These tumors can be primary or secondary. Primary chondrosarcomas are more common, but their origin is idiopathic. Secondary tumors are those that arise from previously benign cartilaginous tumors or from a preexisting condition such as Paget's disease.

Pathogenesis

In general, chondrosarcomas develop from cells committed to cartilaginous differentiation. The neoplastic cartilaginous cells produce cartilage rather than the osteoid seen with osteosarcoma. Alterations of programmed cell death (apoptosis) may play a significant role in the pathogenesis of low- to intermediate-grade chondrosarcomas, whereas high-grade lesions most likely develop by means of a multistep mechanism involving multiple transforming genes and tumor suppressor genes.[21]

Chondrosarcoma is classified by location of the lesion: central, peripheral, or juxtacortical. With *central chondrosarcoma*, the neoplastic tissue is compressed inside the bone, and areas of necrosis, cystic change, and hemorrhage are common. *Peripheral chondrosarcoma* arises outside the bone and then invades the bone. The *juxtacortical chondrosarcoma* is thought to be periosteal (affecting the periosteum) or parosteal (affecting the outer surface of the periosteum) in origin. Chondrosarcomas can be graded based on their microscopic appearance. The presence of a chondroid matrix, extent of necrosis, and type of cells are some of the grading standards used.

Clinical Manifestations

Pain is the most common presenting complaint, although this is a slow-growing tumor, so in some cases the tumor can exist for years without symptoms. The lesion can range from a slow-growing lesion to an aggressive malignancy capable of metastasizing to other organs. The metastatic potential of chondrosarcoma is less than for osteosarcoma. When metastasis occurs, it is via the hematogenous route to the lungs, other bones, or organs.

Medical Management

Diagnosis

On radiographs the tumor often shows an expansile lesion in the diaphysis of long bones with cortical thickening and destruction of the medullary bone (Fig. 16.13). The appear-

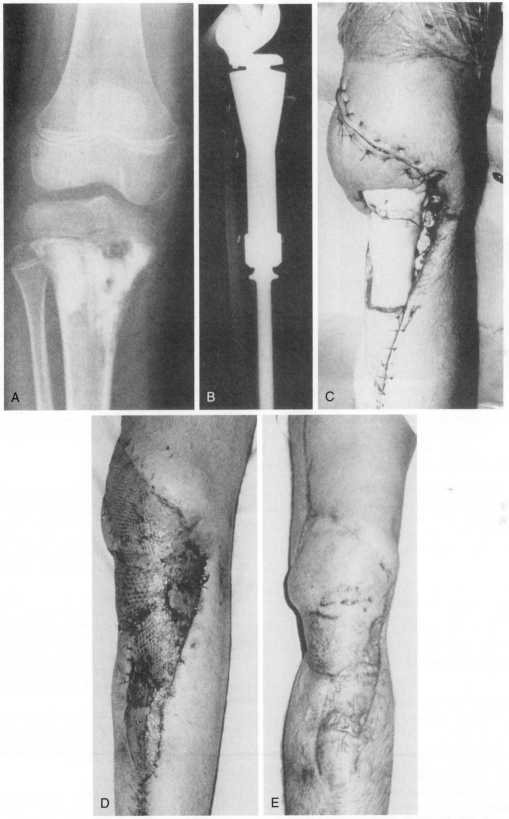

FIG. 16.12 Use of a free muscle transfer to salvage an infected massive prosthesis. (A) Preoperative radiograph of a 9-year-old boy with an osteosarcoma. (B) After radical resection, an expandable prosthesis was inserted. (C) When infection occurred, with subsequent breakdown of the wound, the prosthesis was removed, and the area was widely debrided. A spacer of antibiotic-impregnated methacrylate was inserted. (D) Infection was controlled, and the knee was reconstructed with another prosthesis and a free latissimus transfer. (E) A satisfactory result was obtained, sparing the leg. (From Hausman M: Microvascular applications in limb-sparing tumor surgery, Orthop Clin 20:434, 1989.)

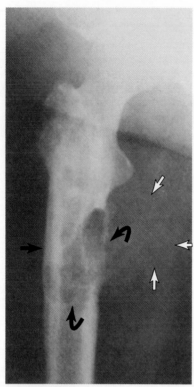

FIG. 16.13 Characteristic radiographic features of chondrosarcoma include thickening of the cortex *(closed arrow)*; destruction of the medullary and cortical bone *(curved arrows)*; and soft tissue mass *(open arrows)*. Note the characteristic punctate calcifications in the proximal part of the tumor. (From Greenspan A: Tumors of cartilage origin, Orthop Clin 20:359, 1989.)

ance is somewhat variable depending on the rate of growth and the host bone response. Biopsy is important not only for accurate diagnosis but also for guiding treatment. Chondrosarcoma can develop on the surface of bone or may be multicentric, involving several bones.

Treatment
Treatment of chondrosarcoma is surgical, with complete tumor removal. Wide resections or limb-sparing procedures are often required, and internal fixation after tumor removal to prevent fracture may be recommended. As with osteosarcoma, radiation therapy is ineffective. Owing to the slow-growing nature of this malignancy, chemotherapy is limited in its effectiveness.

Prognosis
The prognosis is dependent on the aggressiveness and stage of the lesion. For example, a grade I lesion is unlikely to metastasize, and if it is completely resected, a good prognosis follows with 80% chance of cure. A grade III lesion is much more likely to metastasize; however, the majority are grade I or II. Undifferentiated lesions found in the pelvis or any bone where complete resection is difficult carry a poorer prognosis. Secondary chondrosarcomas are usually of a low-grade malignancy and carry a good prognosis with adequate intervention.

Ewing's Sarcoma
Overview and Incidence
Ewing's sarcoma is a malignant nonosteogenic primary tumor that can arise in bone or soft tissue.[32] It is the second most

common primary malignant bone tumor of children, adolescents, and young adults and the fourth most common overall, although it accounts for only approximately 3% of all pediatric malignancies.[37] Most tumors of this type (80%) occur in young people under the age of 20; approximately 225 new cases are diagnosed each year in the United States.[7]

Although this type of bone tumor was noted as early as 1866, it was not until 1921 that James Ewing described his experience with the lesion. The pelvis and lower extremity are the most common sites. Unlike with many tumors, no predilection for a certain part of the bone is evident.

Risk Factors, Etiologic Factors, and Pathogenesis
Based on different levels of scientific evidence, the main risk factors related to Ewing's sarcoma include white race, parental occupation (exposure to pesticides, herbicides, fertilizers), and parental smoking.[26]

Cytogenetic studies show that 95% of these tumors are derived from a specific genetic translocation between chromosomes 11 and 22, although the molecular oncogenesis remains unknown.

The tumor is soft, sometimes viscous, with hemorrhagic necrosis caused by the rapid tumor growth outpacing its blood supply. The cortical bone is affected through the haversian canals. The medullary cavity is affected, and infiltration of the bone marrow can progress extensively without radiographic evidence of bone destruction. When the tumor perforates the cortex of the bone shaft and elevates the periosteum, the consequent reactive bone formation causes layered calcification referred to as an "onion-skin" appearance seen radiographically (Fig. 16.14).

Clinical Manifestations
As with other malignant bone tumors, local bone pain is the most common presenting symptom after an injury (e.g., sports-related injury), a factor that sometimes delays diagnosis. Ewing's sarcoma occurs most often in the long (tubular) bones (e.g., femur, tibia, fibula, humerus) and the pelvis. Less often, the ribs, scapula, vertebrae, feet, and craniofacial bones are involved.

Swelling occurs in approximately 70% of all cases, and both pain and swelling are usually progressive. The pain may be intermittent, which also delays diagnosis. There may be a palpable or observable mass. Pathologic fractures occur at the site of the tumor in long bones but only in 5% to 10% of cases. In young children, flulike symptoms, including a low-grade fever, may be present, which may lead to the mistaken diagnosis of osteomyelitis.[33]

Ewing's sarcoma frequently metastasizes to other bones, especially late in the course of the disease. When the cervical or lumbar spine is involved, neurologic deficit may lead to a mistaken diagnosis of disc disease.[33]

Medical Management
Diagnosis
Anyone suspected of having Ewing's sarcoma is staged for both local and metastatic disease. Radiographs show an obvious lytic process with a moth-eaten appearance involving a diffuse area of bone (Fig. 16.15). As mentioned, an onion-skin formation may be seen, which results from layers of reactive

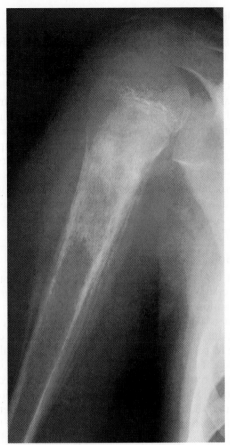

FIG. 16.14 Ewing's sarcoma of the humerus. Bone destruction is seen in the proximal metadiaphysis. The cortex is infiltrated and a multilaminar periosteal reaction with an onion-skin appearance is present medially; Codman's triangles are present on the lateral aspect. (From Grainger RG, Allison D: Grainger and Allison's diagnostic radiology: a textbook of medical imaging, ed 4, Philadelphia, 2001, Churchill Livingstone.)

bone (see Fig. 16.14). On radiographs the appearance of this lesion may not be sufficient to differentiate it from osteomyelitis or osteosarcoma.

An elevated ESR may be noted but is not diagnostic. CT, MRI, and bone scans can help diagnose and define the extent of the tumor. MRI is more sensitive than CT scan in assessing soft tissue involvement and bone marrow spread. The MRI or CT scan is repeated after several cycles of chemotherapy to better assess the response to chemotherapy and help plan further treatment of the local site with radiation or surgery.

Metastatic disease is evaluated at the time of presentation with chest radiographs or chest CT scan looking for pulmonary metastases. Bone scan to detect bone metastases, bone marrow aspirate at a site far from the local tumor site, and tumor biopsy are used to assess the spread of the disease and help with staging and treatment planning.

Treatment

Significant progress has been made in the management of Ewing's sarcoma in the past 25 years. Cure requires intensive therapy to control both local and distant disease. Multimodal treatment can include chemotherapy, radiotherapy,

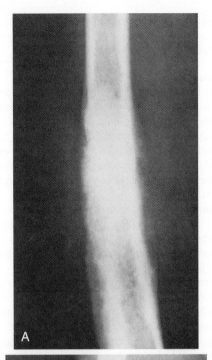

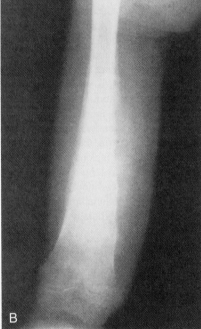

FIG. 16.15 Ewing's sarcoma. (A) A mixed lytic-sclerotic lesion in the femur of a child with the amorphous sunburst periostitis that is characteristic of Ewing's sarcoma. (B) This is a predominantly sclerotic process with large amounts of sunburst periostitis in the diaphysis of a femur that, on biopsy, was found to be Ewing's sarcoma. (From Helms C: Fundamentals of skeletal radiology, ed 4, Philadelphia, 2014, Saunders.)

immunotherapy or biotherapy, embolization, and surgery.[5,7] Local tumors are very responsive to high-dose radiation. In some cases radiation is associated with the additional morbidities of second malignancy and a significant adverse impact on both cardiac and pulmonary function.[63]

Effective combination chemotherapy has been developed to eradicate distant metastases. Selective surgery in the treatment of primary Ewing's sarcoma can result in amputation, but the development of limb-sparing techniques has reduced amputations considerably.

Prognosis

Although Ewing's sarcoma is extremely malignant with a high frequency of both metastatic spread and local recurrence, the prognosis for clients with this tumor is improving steadily. Just a few decades ago only about 5% to 10% of clients with Ewing's sarcoma lived longer than 5 years after detection. The 5-year survival rate is now in excess of 70% if metastasis has not occurred at the time of diagnosis and treatment.[37]

People with Ewing's sarcoma of distal sites such as the bones of the hands and feet have a much better prognosis than people with lesions in central sites such as the pelvis and sacrum. Tumors larger than 8 to 10 cm have a significantly poorer outcome than smaller tumors.[69]

Long-term survival is determined by the presence or absence of metastasis and the site and extent of the local tumor[42]; only about 25% of individuals with metastatic disease at the time of diagnosis survive 5 years.[7]

Many individuals without metastasis are remaining continuously disease free at 5 and 10 years. As many as 35% of clients will have metastatic disease at the time of diagnosis, usually to the lung. More than four metastatic nodules is a poor prognostic indicator, whereas good response to chemotherapy (e.g., decrease in the size of the tumor mass, greater than 95% tumor kill) is a favorable prognostic sign.[55,73]

There is much debate about the role of age at diagnosis. Some studies show older age to be associated with poorer outcome; others show no association between age and survival. It may be that younger children with small, well-defined, distal lesions have the best prognosis.[62] With the increase in long-term survival rates after improved treatment intervention, the problems of late local recurrence, late functional impairment secondary to complications of radiation therapy, and radiation-induced sarcomas are on the rise.[69]

16.4 Special Implications for the PTA: Ewing's Sarcoma As with osteosarcoma, initial intervention is aggressive, involving extensive surgical resection, limb salvage, and sometimes amputation. Saving the person's life is the first priority. After that, rehabilitation becomes the focus, including recovery of function, social reintegration, and return to work or school.

Analysis of rehabilitation suggests that clients with cemented modular oncologic endoprostheses recover faster than individuals treated using other techniques. The level of functional performance may be different depending on the treatment plan chosen. For example, sparing the extremity may lead to greater functional impairment compared with some people undergoing amputation who are provided with a modern prosthesis.

Some of the newer amputation surgeries and reconstructive techniques provide greater function but possibly less cosmetically acceptable results for some people. Some clients complete the entire course of rehabilitation but eventually decide that an amputation will provide greater functionality.

MULTIPLE MYELOMA

Multiple myeloma is a hematopoietic neoplasm involving bone marrow. It is a primary bone cancer with plasma cell proliferation and is one of a group of disorders called *plasma cell dyscrasias.*

Skeletal involvement is most common in the spine, pelvis, and skull, because bone marrow is found in high concentrations in these structures. Deep bone pain is often present clinically, and radiographs may demonstrate osteopenia and punched-out areas of bone with sclerotic borders (in flat bones) (Fig. 16.16).

The prognosis is generally poor, with most people dying from the disease within 1 to 3 years after the diagnosis is made.

PRIMARY SOFT TISSUE TUMORS

Benign Soft Tissue Tumors

Common benign soft tissue tumors include lipoma, ganglia, popliteal cyst (Baker cyst), nerve sheath tumor (neurofibroma and schwannoma), and desmoid tumors.

Lipoma is the most common soft tissue tumor, generally occurring during middle age and late adulthood and composed of mature fat cells. These tumors are usually superficially located in the subcutaneous tissue and remain asymptomatic. Occasionally a lipoma of the breast will grow large enough to cause tenderness and block lymphatic drainage, requiring removal. Even without surgical excision, lipomas are unlikely to ever undergo malignant transformation, but recurrence is possible if the lesion, including microscopic cells, is not completely removed.

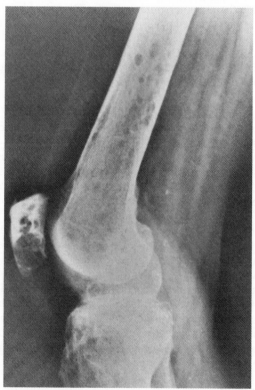

FIG. 16.16 Multiple myeloma. Small lucencies in the distal femur, proximal tibia, and patella. (From Ghelman B: Radiology of bone tumors, Orthop Clin 20:307, 1989.)

Ganglia arise from a joint capsule or tendon sheath, usually on the dorsal aspect of the wrist but sometimes on the volar aspect of the wrist or on the lower extremity. Pain or tenderness may or may not be present; pressure on a nerve can cause focal neurologic symptoms.

Popliteal cyst, more commonly referred to as a *Baker cyst*, is a subtype of ganglion that often communicates with a joint space. A Baker cyst is most often palpated behind the knee in older adults with osteoarthritis. Rupture of the cyst or hemorrhage from the joint into the cyst causes episodes of severe pain. Swelling distal to the lesion (calf and foot) may also occur.

Nerve sheath tumor is a tumor of the nerve sheath arising in a peripheral nerve and growing concentrically from the center of the nerve. Neurofibromas infiltrate the nerve and splay apart the individual nerve fibers. They are usually superficially located, painless, and benign but can sometimes degenerate into cancer.

Neurofibromas can occur as a single lesion or in greater numbers as part of a collection of symptoms in association with von Recklinghausen's disease (neurofibromatosis) and schwannomas. Neurofibromas contain cells and features of Schwann cells but also contain fibroblasts and perineural cells. Both neurofibromas and schwannomas are benign, grow slowly, and can be cured surgically.[1,43]

Schwannomas and neurofibromas arise from the coverings of peripheral and cranial nerves. Schwannoma is a rare tumor of the sheath or lining around the peripheral nerves. It starts in the Schwann cells, which is how it gets its name. Schwann cells help form the cover around the nerves called the *myelin sheath*. Schwannomas can be benign or malignant. The malignant type is called *neurosarcoma* or *neurogenic sarcoma*.

In the benign form, growth is slow and painless. The tumor stays on the outside of the nerve. The benign form does not spread to other areas and is not likely to cause death. But if it grows large enough to put pressure on the nerve, then pain, numbness, and even paralysis can occur.

Malignant Soft Tissue Tumors
Overview and Incidence

Soft tissue sarcomas are a heterogeneous group of rare tumors that arise predominantly from the embryonic mesoderm and manifest most often as an asymptomatic mass. They can occur anywhere in the body, but most originate in the extremities (59%), trunk (19%), retroperitoneum (15%), or head and neck (9%).[19]

Sarcomas account for 1% of all newly diagnosed adult cancers. In 2007 there were 9220 cases of soft tissue tumors, including heart tumors.[39] The incidence is much higher in children, constituting 15% of annual pediatric malignancies.

Types of soft tissue sarcomas. Currently there are more than 50 histologic types of soft tissue sarcoma that have been identified. The most common are malignant fibrous histiocytoma, leiomyosarcoma, liposarcoma, synovial sarcoma, and malignant peripheral nerve sheath tumors. Rhabdomyosarcoma is the most common soft tissue sarcoma of childhood (Table 16.5).[19]

Malignant schwannoma, also known as *neurosarcoma* or *neurogenic sarcoma*, is a rare nerve sheath tumor of the peripheral nerves arising from Schwann cells or within existing neurofibromas. Malignant schwannomas can occur anywhere in the body but are often located on the flexor surface of the extremities. They are usually slow growing and painless, often present for years.[67] When pressure is placed on the involved nerve, then pain, paresthesia, and paralysis may occur.

Rhabdomyosarcomas constitute more than half of all soft tissue sarcomas in children younger than 15. Occurrence in adults is possible but relatively rare.[52] Approximately 250 children in the United States are diagnosed each year with rhabdomyosarcoma.[6,51]

Rhabdomyosarcoma is a malignancy of striated muscle but can occur sporadically at any site in the body and is of unknown cause. Symptoms are site dependent, but the tumor manifests as a painless mass in the soft tissues. About one-third of all people with rhabdomyosarcoma have readily resectable tumors, half

TABLE 16.5 Soft Tissue Sarcoma[a]

Tumor	Age	Sex Ratio	Common Sites
Malignant fibrous histiocytoma	50–70	3:1 (male:female)	Leg, thigh, retroperitoneum; extremities (lower affected more frequently than upper)
Liposarcoma	40–60	1:1 (male:female)	Any site of adipose tissue; extremity, trunk, retroperitoneum, breast
Rhabdomyosarcoma	Children <15 years; Two peaks: 2–6 years and 15–19 years	1.4:1 (male:female)	Any site; four main areas: head and neck, genitourinary (bladder, prostate, testes), extremities, trunk
Leiomyosarcoma	50–70	Women affected more frequently than men	Skin, deep soft tissues of the extremities, retroperitoneum, uterus
Malignant schwannoma	20–50; can occur at any age	Men affected more frequently than women	Peripheral nerves, any site; flexor surface extremities
Synovial sarcoma	Young adult, 15–40	Men affected more frequently than women	Extremity, knee (popliteal area), feet, hands, forearm
Epithelioid sarcoma (rare)	Young adult	Men affected more frequently than women	Extensor surface of the extremities, tendon sheath, joint capsule (shoulder), hands, feet
Clear cell sarcoma (rare)	Young adult	Women affected more frequently than men	Deep to dermis; tendon, aponeuroses; spinal nerve root (rare)
Fibrosarcoma (rare)	35–55	Men affected more frequently than women	Fibrous connective tissue (thigh, posterior knee); scars, subcutaneous fibrous tissue, deep connective tissue, around tendons or nerve sheaths, ligaments, muscle fascia; can occur as bone tumors (periosteum)

[a]Listed in approximate descending order of prevalence. Most soft tissue sarcomas are rare; some (as labeled) are extremely rare.

do not, and in about half of all cases regional lymphatic spread at diagnosis is evident, with a much less favorable prognosis.[52] Over the last 30 years, the prognosis for children with rhabdomyosarcoma has improved dramatically with the use of multiagent chemotherapy, aggressive surgery for local disease, and more precise delivery of radiation therapy. Prognosis depends on the type of gross residual tumor (histology), location of the tumor, and the presence and number of metastases at the time of diagnosis.

Liposarcomas are slow-growing lesions that can achieve a large size (10 to 15 cm), usually located in the thigh but occasionally retroperitoneally, causing pain and weight loss. *Synovial sarcoma* occurs as a slow-growing mass of the extremities, often located near the knee. These lesions are painful and tender to palpation and often manifest similarly to a Baker cyst or ganglion. Reclassification of this sarcoma will eventually reflect the fact that the synovium is not involved in this type of sarcoma.

Epithelioid sarcoma, a small, firm, slow-growing mass, typically arises on the extensor surface of an extremity but can also occur on the shoulder. These masses can develop deep enough to be undetectable on physical examination. Epithelioid sarcoma can look like a rheumatoid nodule, ganglion, or draining abscess and is often mistaken for a benign lesion.

Clear cell sarcoma arises deep to the dermis, has a uniform growth pattern, and is often located on tendons or aponeuroses. In rare cases this type of tumor can also originate in the spinal nerve roots with dissemination to the vertebral bodies, resulting in cauda equina syndrome. In approximately 20% of individuals the tumor has a dark appearance resulting from production of melanin, and it is often confused with benign soft tissue tumors.[67]

Etiology and Risk Factors

Soft tissue sarcomas do not seem to develop from malignant changes of benign soft tissue tumors. Specific inherited genetic alterations are associated with an increased risk of soft tissue sarcomas. Distinct chromosomal translocations that code for oncoproteins are associated with certain histologic subtypes of soft tissue sarcomas.

Risk factors for soft tissue sarcomas include radiation therapy for cancer of the breast, cervix, testes, or lymphatic system with a mean latency period of approximately 10 years. Other risk factors include occupational exposure to chemicals, including herbicides and wood preservatives.

Pathogenesis

All sarcomas share a mesodermal cellular origin, but research has not been able to completely identify the pathogenesis involved. Sarcomas probably do not originate from normal tissue but arise from aberrant differentiated and proliferative malignant mesenchymal cell formations. There are some genetic origins that have been specifically identified for individual sarcoma types. Many sarcoma-linked oncogenes appear to be triggered by viruses; sequencing of these viruses may eventually allow for the development of specific antibodies against oncogenic activation.[68]

Clinical Manifestations

Soft tissue sarcomas manifest most often as painless, asymptomatic masses. They can grow quite large before being observed but do not usually produce pain when compressing surrounding structures. Metastasis occurs primarily hematogenously, with lymph node dissemination in rare cases.

Medical Management

Diagnosis

Diagnostic imaging, fine-needle aspiration, biopsy, and clinical studies are the mainstay of diagnosis. X-ray studies are used to look for lung metastases; CT scans and contrast-enhanced techniques provide details of high-grade lesions and large tumors and assess the extent of tumor burden and proximity to vital structures. MRI is the preferred imaging modality for sarcomas of the extremities.[35]

Staging of soft tissue sarcomas follows the AJCC method of staging based on anatomic location (depth), grade, size of the tumor, and presence of distant or nodal metastases (nodal status). Metastases occur to the lungs first, but also to the bone, brain, and liver. Intracompartmental or extracompartmental extension of extremity sarcomas is important for surgical decision making and planning.[49]

Treatment

Treatment depends on the type of tumor, stage, and location. Surgical excision with clear margins combined with radiation yields good local control, but metastasis and death remain significant problems, especially for individuals who have sarcomas at sites other than the extremities.

Systemic therapy (i.e., cytotoxic chemotherapy) is effective only for certain histologic subtypes; the adverse toxic side effects in individuals who do not respond to chemotherapy negate the routine use of this form of treatment. Many studies with randomized controlled trials have now shown that chemotherapy does not improve disease-free and overall survival in people with soft tissue sarcomas.[29,56,65]

Likewise, there are few supportive data to show that the use of preoperative chemotherapy can improve survival rates. Studies are underway to combine systemic chemotherapy with radiosensitizers and concurrent external beam radiation in hopes of treating microscopic disease, thus producing favorable local as well as systemic results.

There has been a gradual change in the local treatment of soft tissue sarcomas from amputation to a more conservative, limb-sparing, function-preserving approach combined with radiation.[56] Amputation may be required for high-grade extremity sarcomas in about 5% of people whose tumor cannot be removed while still preserving function using limb-sparing techniques.[9,19] See previous discussion under Primary Tumors in this chapter.

Prognosis

The overall 5-year survival rate for soft tissue sarcomas of all stages remains about 50% to 60%.[58] Death from recurrence and metastatic complications occurs within 2 to 3 years of the initial diagnosis in 80% of cases. Despite improvements in local control rates, individuals with high-risk soft tissue sarcomas have poor long-term results.

Advanced metastatic sarcomas are always incurable; management is palliative. Factors associated with a poorer prognosis include age older than 60, tumors larger than 5 cm, and high-grade histology.[49] Individuals with leiomyosarcomas, clear cell sarcomas, and malignant fibrous histiocytomas may have a poorer survival rate than individuals who have fibrosarcomas, liposarcomas, and neurofibrosarcomas.[45]

Cartilaginous Tumors

Many tumors of cartilaginous origin can occur. Three of the more common tumors of a cartilaginous origin are the enchondroma, osteochondroma, and chondrosarcoma. Cartilage tumors involving some parts of the skeleton (e.g., small bones of the hands and feet) are almost always benign, whereas cartilaginous lesions of the ribs, sternum, and flat bones such as the pelvis and scapula are more likely to be aggressive.[21]

Determining the aggressiveness of cartilaginous tumors is especially difficult, and even the histologic differentiation is troublesome. Sometimes the presence of pain or the development of pain in a previously diagnosed benign cartilaginous tumor such as an enchondroma is all that raises suspicion of a malignant process or transformation.

Osteochondroma

Overview and incidence. Osteochondroma is the most common primary benign neoplasm of bone, accounting for 90% of all benign bone tumors.[30] A continuous osseous outgrowth of bone with a cartilaginous cap is characteristic (Fig. 16.17). The outgrowth arises from the metaphysis of long bones and extends away from the nearest epiphysis. The metaphyses of long bones, especially the distal femur, proximal humerus, and proximal tibia, are common sites. The flat bones of the ilium and scapula can also be involved.[30]

The incidence of osteochondroma is unknown. Some reports indicate that men are affected more often, but this may be because it is often an incidental finding, and men may be more likely to have a radiograph taken during the second decade of life when the lesion is usually seen.

Pathogenesis. Osteochondromas appear to result from aberrant epiphyseal development. They are an extension of normal bone capped by cartilage that forms a prominent "tumor" (lump, swelling), sometimes referred to as *osteocartilaginous exostosis.* The younger the individual, the larger is the cartilage cap, because during the growing years, an osteochondroma has its own epiphyseal plate from which it grows.[59]

The lesion will usually cease growing when the individual reaches skeletal maturity. The central portion of the lesion is normal medullary bone. The lesion may begin as a displaced fragment of epiphyseal cartilage that penetrates a cortical defect and continues to grow.

Clinical manifestations. In some people a hard mass will be detected, sometimes present for many years. When the tumor is palpable it may, owing to the cartilaginous cap, feel much larger than is apparent on radiographs.

Osteochondromas are not painful lesions in themselves, but they may interfere with the function of surrounding soft tissues such as tendons, nerves, or bursae. Blood vessels can also be compromised by the tumors (Fig. 16.18), and if tumors are sufficiently large, they may even limit joint motion.

Synovial osteochondromatosis can occur secondary to benign proliferation of the synovium and manifests as multiple loose bodies within a joint.

Medical Management

Diagnosis

Plain radiographs may show a slender stalk of bone directed away from the nearest growth plate. This is referred to as

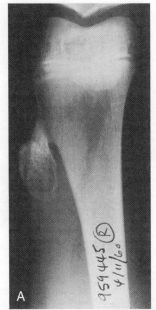
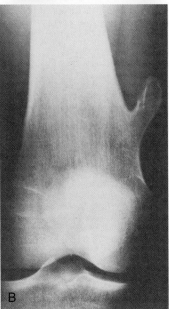

FIG. 16.17 Osteochondroma. Two radiographs (A and B) showing mature osteochondroma: stalked lesion pointing toward the diaphysis and away from the growth plate. (From Bogumill G, Schwamm H: Orthopedic pathology, Philadelphia, 1984, Saunders.)

a *pedunculated osteochondroma.* A sessile osteochondroma has a broad base of attachment (Fig. 16.19). In both types the most important feature to note is the continuity of the cortex between the host bone and the tumor.

CT and MRI are not commonly used in the diagnostic workup of benign lesions, but if atypical clinical manifestations or recent changes in the appearance of the lesion on plain radiographs are evident, MRI may be indicated. For example, MRI can demonstrate the continuity of the marrow between the tumor and the host bone, thereby ruling out a periosteal osteosarcoma.

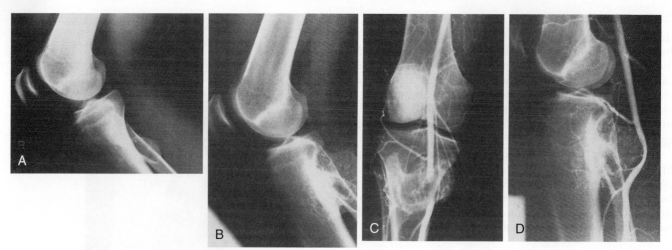

FIG. 16.18 Osteochondroma of the proximal fibula in a young man. (A) Lateral radiograph of the right knee obtained when the patient was 17 years old demonstrates an exophytic lesion arising from the proximal fibula. (B) Lateral radiograph obtained 8 years later shows considerable interim growth of the osteochondroma, although a smooth outline is maintained. (C) Anteroposterior and (D) lateral angiograms demonstrate displacement and marked narrowing of the distal popliteal artery by the tumor. (From Giudici M, Moser R, Kransdorf M: Cartilaginous bone tumors, Radiol Clin North Am 31:247, 1993.)

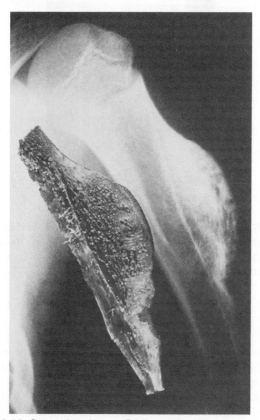

FIG. 16.19 Osteochondroma. Radiograph and gross specimen of the sessile osteochondroma. Note the cartilaginous component causing the radiographic defect in the distal portion. Note also incorporation of hematopoietic tissue into the base of the osteochondroma. (From Bogumill G, Schwamm H: Orthopedic pathology, Philadelphia, 1984, Saunders.)

Treatment and Prognosis

Because osteochondromas usually cease their growth at skeletal maturity, no intervention is needed unless they are symptomatic or interfering with normal limb function. Removal of the lesion is sometimes required when symptoms such as vascular compromise, chronic bursitis, or pain develop secondarily. Rarely, an osteochondroma can transform into a chondrosarcoma. Symptomatic lesions that are removed have a very low recurrence rate.

METASTATIC TUMORS

Overview

Cancer commonly metastasizes to bone; skeletal involvement represents the third most common site of metastatic spread (after lung and liver).[64] *Secondary* or *metastatic neoplasms* refer to those lesions that originate in other organs of the body. All malignant tumors have the capability to spread to bone; the skeleton is the third most common site of metastatic carcinoma, exceeded only by lung and liver. Malignant tumors that have metastasized to the bone are the most common neoplasm of the bone.

Although all of the factors that affect the timing and location of metastasis are not known, some patterns do exist. Cancer metastases (both carcinomas and sarcomas) to bone are a common clinical problem, because the cancers that cause them are prevalent and often metastasize.[12] Primary cancers responsible for 75% of all bone metastases include prostate, breast, lung, kidney, and thyroid.

Common sites for *breast* cancer to metastasize include the pelvis, ribs, vertebrae, and proximal femur. *Lung* cancer can metastasize to the bone early in the disease, remaining asymptomatic until widespread dissemination has taken place; therefore, treatment is often not successful. Neoplasms in the *kidney* metastasize to the vertebrae, pelvis, and proximal femur in about 40% of the cases. The *prostate* is the most common source of skeletal metastases in men.

Incidence and Etiology

Metastatic bone neoplasms are much more common than primary bone lesions; about half of all individuals with cancer (except skin cancer) will develop bone metastases at some point. Incidence increases to 80% of individuals with advanced cancer. The incidence of bone metastasis is expected to increase with the prolonged survival associated with improved antineoplastic therapies now available. The spine is the site most commonly affected, with more than 50% of the metastases involving the spine[66]—usually the thoracic or lumbar spine, much less often the cervical spine, and rarely the atlantoaxial region.[2]

In the spine, the size of the vertebral body may influence the distribution of metastases. The larger lumbar vertebral bodies are more commonly affected than the smaller thoracic or cervical vertebrae. Neurologic compromise is more likely to occur when metastatic lesions affect the thoracic spine because of the smaller ratio between the diameter of the spinal canal and the spinal cord within the thoracic spine.[70]

Risk Factors

Risk factors are those related to the primary cancer. For some cancers the risk factors are well documented, and efforts to educate individuals on health risks should be stressed. Adequate exercise, proper diet and nutrition, and avoidance of tobacco use are the primary preventive measures. It is likely that the increase in incidence of spinal (and other) metastases can be attributed to the improving survival of clients with cancer.[70]

Pathogenesis

The pathophysiology of metastasis is not completely understood, but new information on the biology of tumor metastases derived from advanced techniques in molecular pathology is contributing new insight daily. The development of metastatic disease, regardless of the eventual target organ, usually follows a common pathway.

Cancer can spread through the bloodstream, through the lymphatic system, or by direct extension into adjacent tissue. Hematogenous spread of the cancer is most common, and therefore skeletal metastases are found in areas of bones with a good blood supply. These include the vertebrae, ribs, skull, and proximal femur and humerus.

The development of skeletal metastasis involves a series of events that begins when a tumor cell separates from the primary site, enters the blood system, and then extravasates from the blood vessel to the secondary site.[70] Adhesion molecules control separation and clustering of cancerous cells. The presence or absence of certain molecules controls the ability of cells to metastasize.

Metastasis to bone often results in osteolysis, because cancer cells secrete a number of paracrine factors that stimulate osteoclast function. The cancer tries to destroy the bone (lytic process), and in response, the bone attempts to grow new bone (blastic process) to surround the cancer. If the cancer overwhelms the bone, it becomes weak and fractures easily. Bone metastases may be lytic (most common), blastic, or mixed. Lesions originating from the breast, lung, kidney, and thyroid are usually lytic. Blastic metastases are commonly associated with advanced carcinomas of the prostate and sometimes the breast.[48]

Clinical Manifestations

Although as many as 50% of people with breast or prostate metastasis have no bone pain, pain remains the most common presenting symptom, often characterized as sharp, severe, mechanical, worse at night, and transient or intermittent in the early course but eventually constant in more advanced cancer.

Bone pain of a mechanical nature associated with skeletal metastases occurs as a result of significant bone destruction, joint instability, mechanical insufficiency, and fracture. It is often incapacitating and persistent despite local and systemic therapies. Long bone or vertebral fractures with or without spinal cord compression may be the first indication of advanced disease. Spinal cord compression, the most serious complication of bone metastasis, occurs secondary to increased pressure on the spinal cord or as a result of vertebral collapse. Classic signs and symptoms of cord compression include pain, numbness, and/or paralysis.[24]

Pain may also arise from a biologic origin for a number of reasons. It may occur as a result of rapid growth of the tumor stretching the periosteum. Increased blood flow or angiogenesis (sometimes giving a throbbing or pulsatile sensation) and the release of cytokines at the site of the metastases gives rise to bone pain. Because the skeleton provides both form and support, growing tumors that deform the cortical bone contribute to activity-associated pain. This type of pain is often intermittent and related to weight bearing and movement.[47]

These pain syndromes contribute to increasing loss of mobility and bed rest, the effects of which are increasing generalized weakness, risk of thromboembolism, hypercalcemia, atelectasis, and pneumonia. Atelectasis and pneumonia occur particularly in anyone with painful rib metastases. Mechanical failure or pathologic bone fracture may occur as a result of prolonged immobilization (osteoporosis).

Medical Management

Diagnosis

A history of malignancy raises the suspicion of recurrent disease or a metastatic lesion. The evaluation of an individual with a previous history of cancer or a current malignancy and bone pain begins with a physical examination and basic radiographic studies. Spinal metastasis may be evident by the loss of the pedicle as seen in the anteroposterior view of a standard spinal radiograph.

Whole-body bone scans are much more sensitive for early detection of skeletal metastasis but are not useful in predicting fractures. Approximately one-third of those with skeletal metastatic disease have positive bone scan findings yet negative radiographic results. Scans are also used to determine the extent of dissemination.

CT and MRI also have roles in delineating various types of metastasis and assessing the size and extent of the lesion. More advanced technology using single-photon emission computed tomography (SPECT) allows for better determination of anatomic location of the areas of radioisotope uptake.[60,70] Biopsy is sometimes necessary to confirm a diagnosis when the primary source is not known. CT-guided biopsy is used to assess spinal lesions; diagnostic accuracy is greater for lytic lesions (93%) compared with sclerotic lesions (76%).[44]

Other diagnostic tests may include serum chemistries, urinalysis, serum protein electrophoresis, and prostate-specific antigen determination (for men). Biochemical markers of bone turnover such as N-telopeptide and pyridinium crosslinks (pyridinoline and deoxypyridinoline) may provide information on bone dynamics that reflect disease activity in bone.

Treatment

Therapeutic interventions may depend, in part, on the extent of involvement. The person with localized disease may be offered potentially curative therapy, whereas the individual with extensive skeletal and visceral involvement may benefit only from palliative treatment.[38]

Treatment of bone metastasis is problematic, costly, and primarily palliative. Prolonging survival is not always possible, so improving function with pain relief, local control of disease, and bone stability is often the primary goal. This is becoming more important as treatment for primary cancers improves. Individuals may die of the primary tumor or from the metastasis (e.g., breast cancer). When survival rates and longevity increase, the likelihood of skeletal metastasis increases.

Intervention for skeletal neoplasms requires a multidisciplinary approach to optimize therapy options and coordinate their sequencing. Intervention modalities may include endocrine therapy (for breast and prostate cancer), chemotherapy, biotherapy (immunotherapy), use of bone-seeking radioisotopes (a therapy that has analgesic and antitumor effects), and bisphosphonates to suppress bone resorption. These are often combined with other localized interventions such as surgery and site-directed radiation therapy.

Surgery is rarely curative but can be an effective therapy to decompress neural tissue for resolution of symptoms and/or restoration of function, reduce anxiety, improve mobility and function, facilitate nursing care, preempt fracture (i.e., repair bony lesions before they fracture), and control local tumor when nonsurgical therapies fail.[48,74]

Pathologic fractures that occur in the femur and humerus often require surgical stabilization. Intramedullary fixation with interlocking devices to limit motion at the fracture site is indicated in many instances. The desire to restore normal anatomy must be weighed against the reality that the individual may have a terminal disease. An estimated life expectancy of at least 6 months is desirable before extensive joint reconstructive procedures are carried out.[36]

Where the risk of fracture is great, as when more than 50% of the cortex is destroyed, prophylactic nailing of the femur may be indicated (Fig. 16.20).

Spinal metastases can cause severe pain, instability, and spinal cord compression with neurologic compromise. Pathologic fractures of the spine can be immobilized in an appropriate spinal brace, but a progressive neurologic deficit is an indication for surgical intervention. Surgery can take the form of decompression, posterior stabilization, excision, and reconstruction or prosthetic replacement. Vertebroplasty or kyphoplasty may be considered for the person with a vertebral compression fracture and minimal bone deformity.[27]

Prognosis

Although management of the skeletal metastasis may be successful in terms of restoring stability to a pathologic fracture, the prognosis for the primary cancer is still guarded. Only rarely is the skeletal metastasis actually the

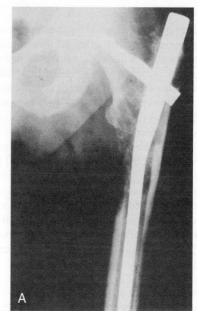

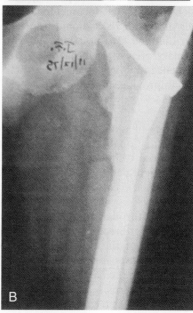

FIG. 16.20 (A) Prophylactic fixation in a 63-year-old woman with an impending fracture secondary to breast metastasis treated by Zickel nailing. (B) Complete healing of this subtrochanteric lesion 5 months after radiation and chemotherapy. (From Habermann E, Lopez R: Metastatic disease of bone and treatment of pathologic fracture, Orthop Clin 20:475, 1989.)

cause of death. Skeletal morbidity includes bone pain, hypercalcemia, pathologic fracture, spinal cord or nerve root compression, and immobility, all of which can affect mortality rates.[18]

The median survival for people with tumors that have metastasized to the bone is determined by the type of tumor (e.g., prostate, 29 months; breast, 23 months; kidney, 12 months; lung, less than 4 months). The overall median survival after detection of bone metastases is approximately 19 months; this significant amount of time allows for interventions that can dramatically improve a person's quality of life and functional independence.[22]

Favorable prognostic factors include indolent nature of the primary lesion (e.g., prostate cancer); well-differentiated tumor on histologic examination; a long recurrence-free survival (greater than 3 years); sclerotic lesion on radiograph as opposed to a lytic lesion, especially after treatment; a single bone lesion; a single system involved with metastatic disease; low tumor markers; no vital organ involvement; and general good condition of the individual.

Unfavorable prognostic factors include the following[22]:

- Aggressive nature of the primary lesion (e.g., lung cancer)
- Poorly differentiated tumor on histology
- Short recurrence-free survival (less than 1 year)
- Lytic lesion
- No sclerosis on radiograph following treatment
- Multiple bone lesions
- Multiple system metastases
- High tumor markers
- Vital organ involvement
- General poor condition of the individual

The risk of pathologic fracture is greater in osteolytic lesions of the long bones. A direct relationship exists between the degree of cortical destruction and the risk of pathologic fracture. When cortical destruction is less than 25% to 35%, the risk for fracture is low. Destruction greater than 50% correlates with a much higher risk for pathologic fracture. The presence of pain with weight-bearing activities indicates compromised structural integrity and therefore also places the individual at greater risk of fracture.[24,28]

16.5 Special Implications for the PTA: Metastatic Tumors
Early Detection

Metastases to the skeleton are important to the PTA because the presence of musculoskeletal pain may be the initial symptom of an undetected primary carcinoma elsewhere. Early detection is essential for effective intervention. A thorough history and a high index of suspicion can lead to the timely communication with a physician. In people with a history of cancer, the clinician should be vigilant regarding the likelihood and common sites of metastasis. Autopsy-based analyses of the distributions of bone metastases demonstrate that the most favored sites are the vertebrae, pelvis, femur, and bones of the upper extremity. Metastases distal to the elbow or knee are rare; when they do occur, the kidney is most likely the site of the primary tumor.[48]

Preoperative Intervention

Exercise is recommended for individuals with bone metastases before and after surgery, focusing on increasing muscle strength and endurance while maintaining bone protection. Exercise programs directed at strengthening and stretching are often needed; high-impact and high-torsion activities should be avoided.[22]

Chemotherapy for some cancers includes the use of steroids that can lead to muscle atrophy, especially of the type II fibers. Isometric exercises may prevent marked atrophy. Radiation therapy can lead to contracture of soft tissues, and clients should be taught to stretch and self-mobilize the soft tissues of susceptible areas before treatment.

Instruction in fall prevention strategies, including optimal body mechanics and exercises to maintain strength and balance, is essential before and after surgery.[22] This is especially true for anyone taking pain medication that causes drowsiness and decreased coordination.[24]

Rehabilitation

People who have had a pathologic fracture stabilized are often referred for rehabilitation. Hypercalcemia is common in the acute or subacute phase[13] and occurs when bone resorption is greater than new bone formation. The osteolysis that occurs with bone metastasis is one cause of hypercalcemia.

Treatment of the primary cancer with chemotherapy and/or radiation therapy often provides additional challenges, such as fatigue and increased risk of infection. For a client with lung cancer, baseline pulmonary status should be established and proper breathing techniques taught. Management of clients with metastatic disease is challenging because, in addition to these complications, clients often need extensive rehabilitation after the medical treatment.

Management of skeletal metastasis, including fracture, is aimed at improving or restoring function, especially maintaining ambulatory function to preserve quality of life and prevent the negative sequelae of immobility. If the bone has been compromised or fractures have occurred, surgical intervention will attempt to stabilize the defect.

After the surgery, early mobilization—including gait training, bed mobility, and transfers—is essential. Maximizing functional independence is the driving force behind all rehabilitation efforts. Safety and bone protection are important during mobility and strengthening activities. Evaluation of upper extremity function and coexisting upper extremity metastases before allowing weight bearing through the arms is important.[22]

There is a reluctance to ambulate clients who are at risk for pathologic fracture because a measure of risk has not been developed, but in fact an active rehabilitation program may not place a client at increased risk for fracture.[14] The risk of producing pathologic fractures in clients with cancer by increasing mobility and function is low.[15] Many individuals with skeletal metastases and pathologic fracture have been shown to be good candidates for intensive rehabilitation programs if they do not have hypercalcemia caused by lytic metastases or pain severe enough to require parenteral narcotics.[11]

Because many of the people with metastatic disease are at risk for pathologic fractures, the risk of falling must be considered when planning for ambulation training, especially in older adults. Assessments of mental status, balance, strength, ROM, endurance, vision, ambulation history, and symptoms of dizziness are all important and will help plan ambulation training. Even with the most critical analysis of the risks and benefits, PTAs who work with individuals who have serious medical conditions such as metastatic lesions and pathologic fractures must be prepared for setbacks and unexpected events to occur when attempting to preserve or maximize function.

Rehabilitative decision making in this area requires collaboration between the therapy team and the medical staff (e.g., oncologist, surgeon) and takes into primary consideration the degree of cortical involvement. It is very helpful if the therapy team has access to imaging studies with accurate information about the extent of involvement, specific levels affected, and knowledge of stability (or instability) of spinal segments to assist in treatment planning. The following guidelines are just that: a guide to be used as a template to begin with but modified by individual differences and interests, postoperative protocols, physician input, and so on.

For clients with less than 25% of the cortex invaded, submaximal isometrics and gentle aerobics (e.g., bicycling at low resistance, aquatics if approved by the physician for those with wounds or fractures that are healing) are generally permitted, and the involved limb most typically is cleared for weight bearing as tolerated.

When cortical involvement increases to 25% to 50%, restrictions tighten and allow for gentle ROM exercises without pressure into the end ROM and limb offloading to partial weight bearing. Finally, with greater than 50% cortical involvement, exercise may need to be deferred and the limb maintained non–weight bearing.[17,24]

REFERENCES/SUGGESTED READINGS

To enhance this text and add value for the reader, references and suggested readings are included on the companion Evolve site that accompanies this textbook. The reader can view the source and access it online whenever possible.

17

Bone, Joint, and Soft Tissue Diseases and Disorders

1. Review and outline the process of bone formation, maturation, resorption, and remodeling.
2. Review and outline the role of mechanical stress in stimulating bone growth, repair, and strength.
3. Discuss diseases affecting bone, articular cartilage, and joint spaces that affect movement and function.
4. Discuss diseases affecting soft tissue that affect movement and function.

OUTLINE

People presenting with muscle, joint, and bone disorders make up a significant percentage of a physical therapy practice. These conditions are primarily manifested by pain, deformity, and loss of mobility and function. Many of the people seen by therapists and physical therapist assistants (PTAs) have these conditions secondary to trauma or repetitive overuse; these conditions are generally self-contained or local in terms of involved tissues.

Although this book is primarily a compilation of diseases and conditions of all systems, this chapter contains both orthopedic and systemic conditions that affect the bones, joint, and muscles that may not fall into any other category. Because the focus of this text is not orthopedics, many orthopedic conditions have not been included. For the most part, those conditions with a more generalized effect or accompanied by a systemic component are included here.

Metabolic disorders can affect numerous body tissues, including bony structures. Primary metabolic diseases and their implications for the therapy professionals are discussed elsewhere. Metabolic disorders primarily affecting the skeletal system are the focus of the first section in this chapter. The remainder of the chapter is divided into three distinct anatomic areas: bone, joint, and soft tissue, with conditions and diseases placed in the area most notably affected. Frequently there is overlap, and one condition affecting more than one area is found in a single section. As always, the reader is encouraged to keep a broad perspective whenever studying an isolated condition or anatomic area.

BONE

Bone is composed of a meshwork of collagen fibers inlaid with calcium and phosphate. The human skeleton is composed of two main bone types: trabecular and cortical. The skeleton is a metabolically active organ that undergoes continuous remodeling throughout life with an annual turnover of cortical and trabecular bone of about 10% of the adult skeleton.[313] This remodeling is necessary both to maintain the structural integrity of the skeleton and to serve a metabolic function as a storehouse of calcium and phosphorus. These dual functions can come into conflict under conditions of changing mechanical forces or metabolic and nutritional stress.[295]

Bone Composition

The outer substance of bone mass is the *cortical* (compact) bone, found primarily in the shafts of the long bones and comprising roughly 80% of skeletal mass. The concentric orientation of lamellae deposited around a central nutrient canal in cortical bone forms very dense tissue. Of the total volume of cortical bone, 80% to 90% is calcified. *Trabecular*—also referred to as

spongy or cancellous—bone is the central meshwork of bones. Trabecular mass constitutes approximately 20% of the adult skeleton and is sensitive to influences relating to metabolic and hormonal implications. Fifteen percent to 25% of trabecular bone volume is calcified. The remaining volume is occupied by bone marrow, fat, and blood vessels.[337]

Because bone turnover is a surface event and trabecular bone has a high surface area, bones rich in trabeculae (e.g., vertebrae, metaphyseal segments of long bones, and the calcaneus) are more active, metabolically exhibiting a greater rate of turnover and resorption with loss of structural integrity during the aging process (Fig. 17.1). The ultimate strength of a specific bone appears to be related to the percentage of trabecular versus cortical bone, the structural integrity, and the trabecular interconnections of the bone.[407]

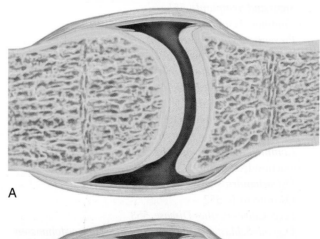

A

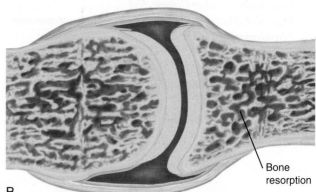

B

FIG. 17.1 Osteoporosis. (A) Normal bone and joint. (B) Osteoporotic changes shown with bone resorption greater than bone formation resulting in weakened trabeculae and increasing risk for fracture. (From Jarvis C: Physical examination and health assessment, ed 7, Philadelphia, 2016, Saunders.)

Bone Remodeling

Bone renews itself in a constant process called *remodeling*, a repeating cycle of *osteoclasts* breaking down the existing bone bit by bit (resorption) and *osteoblasts* laying down new cells (formation) for mineralization. The purpose of remodeling is to maintain the strength and integrity of the skeleton by replacing fatigue-damaged older bone with new bone and to act as a source of vital minerals (e.g., calcium) necessary for the maintenance of mineral homeostasis. Calcium's importance extends far beyond the bone. It circulates throughout the body to regulate heart rate, muscle contractions, blood pressure, and other systemic functions. When blood levels of calcium drop below the level necessary to carry out these functions, it is replenished from bone.

Bone mass is known to reach its maximum size and density (peak bone mass) by the time an adult reaches age 30 years. Women have a tendency to lose bone mass sooner than men, often beginning in their late 30s. Bone loss is accelerated for women during and after menopause; men are more likely to experience bone loss in their mid- to late 60s.

This section will review the presentation and interventions used for common conditions occurring to bone beginning with metabolic bone disease, then moving on to fractures and osteochondroses. The metabolic bone disease section will cover osteoporosis, osteomalacia, and Paget's disease. Later in the chapter, information will be provided about fractures, osteochondritis dissecans, osteonecrosis, Legg–Calvé–Perthes disease, Osgood–Schlatter syndrome, and Sinding–Larsen–Johansson syndrome.

Metabolic Bone Disease

Clinical disorders in which bone resorption is increased are common and include Paget's disease of bone, osteoporosis, and the bone changes secondary to cancer such as occur in myeloma and metastases from breast or prostate cancer. Clinical disorders of reduced bone resorption are less common and have a genetic basis (e.g., osteopetrosis).

Metabolic bone disease is typically manifested by diffuse loss of bone density and bone strength, but increased bone density and decreased bone strength can occur such as with Paget's disease. Significant disability—marked by bone pain, postural deformity, and fracture—can occur secondary to these bony changes. The commonly observed accentuated thoracic spine kyphosis in clients with vertebral collapse secondary to osteoporosis can compromise cardiopulmonary function, affecting the person's ability to participate in a rehabilitation program.

The most serious, potentially life-threatening, and costly complication of metabolic bone disease is fracture. Osteoporosis alone is estimated to be responsible for more than 1.5 million fractures annually (700,000 vertebral fractures, 300,000 hip fractures, 250,000 wrist fractures, and 250,000 other fractures); one in three women older than age 50 years experience a fracture in their lifetime.[115,261] The monetary cost of these fractures is estimated at $10 billion to $15 billion annually in the United States. This estimate does not include the indirect costs of lost wages or productivity of either the individual or the caregiver.[257]

Physical therapists (PTs) and PTAs have an important role in the primary prevention of disability secondary to the complications associated with metabolic bone disease. Client education regarding posture, body mechanics, and proper exercise is an important component of any prevention program. Physical therapy intervention is also a vital part of the rehabilitation of clients disabled by the resultant pain or postural deformities that can accompany these diseases. PTAs also treat many clients who have experienced traumatic injury precipitated by the presence of metabolic bone disease or conversely, people who are experiencing the metabolic consequences of trauma.

Osteoporosis

Osteoporosis develops when new bone formation falls behind resorption, possibly related to impaired new bone formation due to declining osteoblast function (Fig. 17.2). The onset of bone loss is likely to be genetically predetermined, and the subsequent rate of bone loss may also be influenced by genetic factors.

Bone loss increases at the time of menopause as a result of the marked reduction in the circulating concentrations of estradiol and progesterone (Fig. 17.3).[90] Small defects in formation remaining at the completion of a normal remodeling cycle accumulate and also contribute to age-related losses in bone mass. Thus the bone that experiences the greatest number of remodeling cycles is at the highest risk for age-related losses in mass.[337]

Bone demineralization. Bone *demineralization*, which can lead to osteopenia, takes place when a deficit in hormonal levels, inadequate physical activity (mechanical load), or poor nutrition occurs. Bone strength is a function of skeletal load—that is, bone responds to alterations in mechanical forces. Although the exact physiologic mechanism causing bone to sense and respond to alterations in mechanical loads is unclear, adaptations appear to be site specific.

Mechanical stimuli may be the only type of stimuli capable of inducing modeling in mature bone; young bone responds more favorably to mechanical loading than old bone, again emphasizing the importance of physical activity and exercise in the adolescent and young adult.[400] Physical activity transmits mechanical loads to the skeleton through gravitational forces and muscular pull at sites of attachment. In the absence of mechanical forces (space flight or prolonged bed rest), urinary calcium excretion increases and bone density decreases.[337] Bone mineral density (BMD) changes induced by loading are not maintained long term, which is why regular site-specific

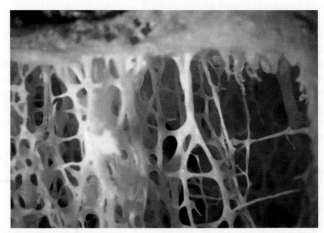

FIG. 17.2 Osteoporosis of the lumbar vertebra with generalized loss of bone. The vertical plates have become perforated and the number of horizontal cross-braces are decreased markedly in proportion to the vertical plates. (From McPherson RA: Henry's clinical diagnosis and management by laboratory methods, ed 22, Philadelphia, 2011, Saunders.)

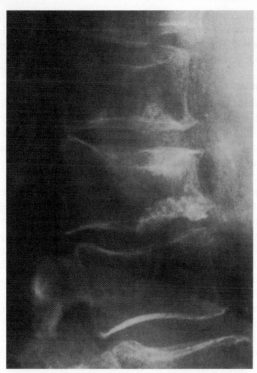

FIG. 17.3 Postmenopausal osteoporosis in a 59-year-old woman. Lateral view of the thoracolumbar spine shows protrusion of disk material through a weakened end plate (Schmorl's node). Note also the biconcave appearance of several vertebral bodies. (From Grainger, RG: Grainger & Allison's diagnostic radiology: a textbook of medical imaging, ed 4, Philadelphia, 2001, Churchill Livingstone.)

and weight-bearing exercises must be done routinely to prevent osteoporosis and reduce bone fracture risk.[400]

Hormonal levels, physical activity, and nutrition are the key factors that facilitate bone growth because they regulate the osteoblastic and osteoclastic remodeling cycles, initiate a natural cycle of microscopic bone damage and subsequent repair, and foster solid bone architecture.[54]

Definition and incidence. Osteoporosis is a combination of decreased bone mass and microdamage to the bone structure that results in a susceptibility to fracture. Osteoporosis can be classified as primary or secondary, depending on the underlying etiology. *Primary osteoporosis,* the most common, can occur in both genders at all ages but often follows menopause in women and occurs later in life in men.[338] Osteoporosis associated with medications, other conditions, or diseases is referred to as *secondary osteoporosis* (Box 17.1).

Osteoporosis is by far the most common metabolic bone disease, affecting approximately 10 million people living in the United States. An additional 34 million Americans already have low bone mass (osteopenia) that places them at increased risk of osteoporosis. With the aging of America, osteoporosis is expected to increase in prevalence.[258]

The disease is much more common in women, especially postmenopausal women who are estrogen deficient. However, osteoporosis in men represents a major public health problem, which until recently has received little recognition. Approximately 2 million men are affected by osteoporosis and another 12 million are at risk as a result of low bone mass.

According to the National Osteoporosis Foundation (NOF), this condition in men is underdiagnosed, undertreated, and underreported.[260]

One in every two women older than age 50 years will experience fragility fractures secondary to osteoporosis. One in four men will experience an osteoporosis-related fragility fracture during his lifetime, usually later (because of greater bone mass than women) at approximately age 70 years. Men who are affected have a higher morbidity and mortality rate of 30% compared with 9% for women.[24,365] This is because men are older at the time they sustain a fracture and are more likely to have comorbid disease, malnutrition, and complicated hospitalizations.[366]

The cause of *primary osteoporosis* is unknown, but many contributory factors exist, such as mild but prolonged negative calcium balance, declining gonadal and adrenal function, relative or progressive estrogen deficiency, or a sedentary lifestyle. *Secondary osteoporosis* may be caused by prolonged drug therapy with corticosteroids, heparin, anticonvulsants, and other medications; alcoholism, malnutrition, malabsorption, or lactose intolerance; endocrine disorders; or other conditions or diseases (see Box 17.1).

Risk factors. Bone mass peaks between the ages of 25 and 35 years, and the rate of bone resorption begins to exceed the rate of bone formation. This physiologic mismatch can progress to a point at which osteopenia (Box 17.2) may be noted radiographically and a diagnosis of osteoporosis made. Box 17.1 lists the many risk factors and conditions or diseases associated with osteoporosis. Chronic diseases, or medications used to treat these diseases, may have side effects that can damage bone or interfere with bone formation, leading to osteoporosis.

Hormonal status. Postmenopausal women are at higher risk for developing the disease. Diagnosis of primary postmenopausal osteoporosis occurs with increasing frequency from age 51 to 75 years. The increased risk of osteoporosis related to menopause is due primarily to the decreased production of estrogen. Women lose bone at the usual rate of 1% per year after peak bone density has been achieved; however, bone loss accelerates to a varying degree (depending on such factors as calcium intake and absorption, hormonal balance, and activity level) for about 5 to 8 years after menopause, increasing the risk of fracture. Researchers report a wide range from 2% to 11% loss for the 10 years after menopause, slowing after that to about 0.5% to 1% of bone mass per year.[55,267,304]

Men experience a gradual slowing of testosterone production with age, and below-normal testosterone levels have been associated with loss of bone mineral mass.

Heredity/genetics. Peak bone mass is partly genetically determined as evidenced by the varying prevalence of osteoporosis among different ethnic groups, but other variables also exist, such as differences in bone geometry and rate of bone loss. Individual differences among people of the same ethnic background can occur, possibly in part because of inheriting specific genes that affect bone mass and turnover.[321]

Body build is related to bone fragility. Thin women have less cortical bone and are therefore at greater risk of fractures. Obesity, by increasing the mechanical strain on bone, may result in increased peak bone mass, reducing bone fragility. In addition, obesity increases the amount of biologically available estrogen, protecting against fracture.[55] Women with a family history of osteoporosis are at high risk of developing osteoporotic fractures.

BOX 17.1   Risk Factors and Conditions Associated with Osteoporosis

Risk Factors

Nonmodifiable

- Age 50 years and older
- Caucasian/Asian
- Northern European ancestry
- Menopausal (occurs early in those younger than age 45 years and can be surgically induced through bilateral oophorectomy)
- Family history of osteoporosis; personal history of fragility, fracture; fragility fracture in first-degree relative
- Long periods of inactivity, immobilization
- Depression
- Femoral neck BMD

Risk Factors for Which Intervention Might Reduce Incidence of Osteoporosis and Fractures

- Immobility, long-term care
- Excess intake of:
  - Alcohol (>2 drinks/day)
  - Tobacco
  - Caffeine[a] (equivalent to >3 cups caffeinated coffee/day)
- Amenorrhea (abnormal absence of menses)
- Estrogen deficiency (women)/testosterone deficiency (men)
- Medications (>6 months)
  - Corticosteroids/steroids
  - Immunosuppressants
  - Anticoagulants (heparin, Coumadin)
  - Nonthiazide diuretics (furosemide)[b]
  - Methotrexate (MTX)
  - Cisplatin (chemotherapy)
  - Aromatase inhibiters (breast cancer treatment)
  - Antacids (containing aluminum)
  - Laxatives
  - Anticonvulsants
  - Benzodiazepines (Valium, Librium, Xanax)
  - Some antibiotics (e.g., tetracycline derivatives)
  - Buffered aspirin
  - Excessive thyroid hormones
  - Lithium
  - Androgen deprivation (prostate cancer)

- Depo-Provera (contraceptive)
- Low body weight and body mass index, thin, small body frame
- Diet and nutrition
  - Calcium and magnesium deficiency
  - Vitamin D deficiency
  - Vitamin C deficiency (helps with calcium absorption)
  - High ratio of animal to vegetable protein intake
  - High fat diet (reduces calcium absorption in the gut)
  - Excessive sugar (depletes phosphorus)
  - High intake of low-calcium beverages such as coffee and carbonated soft drinks
  - Eating disorders (bulimia, anorexia nervosa, binge eating)
  - Repeated crash dieting or "yo-yo" dieting

Associated Diseases and Disorders

- Endocrine disorders
  - Hyperthyroidism
  - Type 2 diabetes mellitus
  - Cushing's disease
  - Male hypogonadism (testosterone deficiency)
- Malabsorption
  - Celiac disease
  - GI disease; gastric surgery
  - Hepatic disease
- Medication related
  - Organ transplantation
  - Chronic pulmonary disease
  - Rheumatic diseases, including juvenile idiopathic arthritis
- Chronic renal failure
- Osteogenesis imperfecta
- Cancer and cancer treatment (children and adults), skeletal metastasis
- Eating disorders
- Spinal cord injury
- Cerebrovascular accident or stroke
- Acid–base imbalance (metabolic acidosis)
- Depression
- Erectile dysfunction (hypogonadism)
- HIV/AIDS

[a]Caffeine from any source in excess of 300 mg/day should be avoided.
[b]Some diuretics such as the nonthiazide diuretics have calcium-retaining properties with reduced incidence of hip fracture with long-term use.
BMD, Bone mineral density; *GI,* gastrointestinal; *HIV/AIDS,* human immunodeficiency virus/acquired immunodeficiency syndrome.

BOX 17.2   Terminology of Metabolic Bone Disease

Osteomalacia: Softening of the bones
Osteopenia: Too little bone; low bone mass
Osteopetrosis: Increased bone density
Osteoporosis: Decreased bone density

Ethnicity. Ethnicity is also considered a risk factor because bone mass correlates positively with skin pigmentation. Whites have the least amount of bone mass, whereas blacks have the greatest amount. Men have wider long bones than women, and blacks have wider long bones than whites. Therefore black men are at lowest risk of developing osteoporosis.[331]

Limited information available suggests that Native American women have lower bone densities than white non-Hispanic women, and Mexican American women have bone densities intermediate between those of white non-Hispanic women and black women.[257]

Physical inactivity. Inactivity and immobilization have been associated with decreased bone formation. The prolonged inactivity results in reduced gravitational and muscular forces acting on the skeletal system. The decreased mechanical stress on bony structures alters bone physiology, resulting in decreased bone mass.

Disuse osteopenia, which can be caused by immobilization (e.g., cast, bed rest, long-term care, or neurologic impairment), results from a change in cellular function. Residents in nursing homes or long-term care facilities have a fivefold to tenfold greater fracture risk than community dwellers.[74]

Tobacco and alcohol. Cigarette smoking is associated with a reduction of bone mass and is a well-known risk factor for spinal and hip fractures.[200,355] More than two "units" of alcohol per day is a risk factor for osteoporosis.[165] A unit is defined as one 12-oz beer, one 5-oz glass of wine, or 1.5 oz of hard liquor.

Medications. Long-term use of medications, including corticosteroids, has been associated with the presence of osteoporosis. Most bone loss occurs during the first 6 months of systemic corticosteroid therapy. Other medications have also been implicated (see Box 17.1).

Depression. Depression is now recognized as a risk factor for osteoporosis.[328,412] Individuals with a history of a major depressive disorder are more likely to have lower bone densities and higher levels of cortisol than people without depression, regardless of physical activity levels.[231] Poor nutrition as a result of loss of appetite may be another depression-related risk factor for osteoporosis.

Diet and nutrition. Different sources of dietary protein may have different effects on bone metabolism. Women age 65 and older with a high dietary ratio of animal-to-vegetable protein intake have more rapid femoral neck bone loss and a greater risk of hip fracture than do those with a low ratio.

Bone density is decreased in anorexic and bulimic women and is possibly the result of estrogen deficiency, low intake of nutrients, low body weight, early onset and long duration of amenorrhea, low calcium intake, reduced physical activity, and hypercortisolism. This type of reduced bone density is associated with a significantly increased risk of fracture even at a young age.[109] A new term, *female athlete triad,* has been coined to describe the combination of disordered eating, amenorrhea, and osteoporosis, which is a situation that often goes unrecognized and untreated.[322]

A significant number of people with osteoporosis also have celiac disease, a gastrointestinal (GI) disorder that impairs the absorption of calcium, various nutrients, and vitamin D needed for maintaining healthy bones. Identification and effective dietary therapy for celiac disease can lead to improved absorption of vital nutrients and potentially reverse the decline in BMD. Celiac disease increases the long-term risk of fracture, especially hip fracture.[134,207]

Structures involved. The vertebral bodies, hip, ribs, radius, and femur are the most common fracture sites (in that order), although any bone in the body can be affected. Fractures are often "silent" compression fractures of vertebral bodies, sacral insufficiency fractures, or complete fractures of the spine or femoral neck. Recently, metatarsal insufficiency fracture in

both men and women has been brought to the forefront as a previously unrecognized early sign of osteoporosis.[381]

Vertebral compression fractures (VCFs) are the most common osteoporosis-related spinal fractures presenting with clinical symptoms of back pain, posture change, loss of height, functional impairment, disability, and diminished quality of life (Fig. 17.4). These can occur without injury or fall when the bone becomes so porous or weak that it begins to compress. By age 90 years, the force required to produce failure of the L3 vertebrae is approximately one-fourth the compressive failure force at age 30 years.[167]

Signs and symptoms. Loss of height, postural changes, back pain, and fracture are the most common presenting features of osteoporosis. Postural changes may include lax abdominal musculature, protuberant abdomen, forward head, increased thoracic kyphosis, dowager's hump, loss of lumbar lordosis, posterior pelvic tilt, knee hyperextension, shoulder internal rotation, scapular forward rotation, palms facing backward, and other deviations in alignment observed when assessed by a PT. Marked thoracic spine kyphosis and loss of overall body height are common findings, especially after a VCF. Similarly, bone loss in the mandible can contribute to changes in facial appearance.

Muscular pain and spasm can occur in the lower back paravertebral muscles, as can burning pain in the midthoracic region lateral to the spine because of excess stretch placed on the rhomboid muscles from the compensatory forward rotation of the scapulae. Trigger points secondary to kyphoscoliosis, rhomboid imbalance, and paravertebral muscle spasm are common. Similar muscle imbalance and muscular symptoms are observed or reported in the lower quadrant with involvement of the lumbosacral and sacroiliac joints and surrounding musculature.

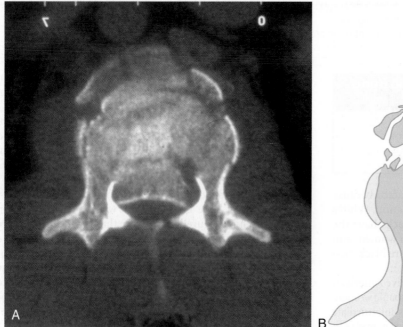
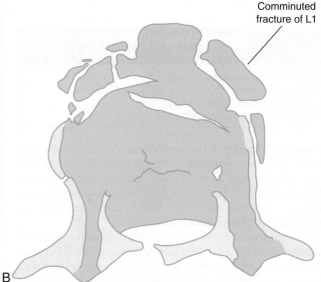

Comminuted fracture of L1

FIG. 17.4 Computed tomography of unstable comminuted vertebral compression (burst) fracture of the lumbar vertebra (L1). (From Marx JA: *Rosen's emergency medicine: concepts and clinical practice,* ed 8, St Louis, 2014, Mosby.)

The prevalence of vertebral fractures increases steadily with age, ranging between 20% for 50-year-old postmenopausal women and 64% for older women. The majority of vertebral fractures are not connected with severe trauma, and only one in three is diagnosed clinically. Almost 20% of women will experience another fracture within 1 year after a vertebral fracture.[115]

Pain associated with VCFs is usually severe and localized to the site of fracture, typically midthoracic, lower thoracic, and lumbar spine. Tenderness to palpation over the fracture is common in both symptomatic and otherwise asymptomatic cases. Pain may radiate to the abdomen or flanks and is aggravated by prolonged sitting or standing, bending, or performing a Valsalva maneuver. Side lying with hips and knees flexed may alleviate the pain. Generalized bone pain is more suggestive of metastatic carcinoma or osteomalacia. Neurologic symptoms may not occur immediately but rather develop insidiously over days to months.[26]

Common tests and measures. Careful assessment of the osteoporotic person is essential in developing a comprehensive plan that reduces fracture risk and improves quality of life. Assessment of the individual with osteoporosis includes history and physical examination, laboratory testing, and imaging studies. Information gathered during this assessment assists clinicians in targeting strategies to prevent fractures. Diagnosis and intervention are based on bone density and risk assessment[347]; in the case of secondary osteoporosis, the specific underlying cause must be determined through the diagnostic process before intervention can be initiated.

History. The medical history should contain the personal and family history of fractures, lifestyle, intake of substances such as vitamin D, calcium, corticosteroids, and other medications. Clinicians should be aware of problems with vitamin D measurement, including seasonal variation, variability among laboratories, and the desirable therapeutic range. The physical examination can reveal relevant information such as height loss and risk of falls.[186]

Bone mineral density testing. BMD is often used as a proxy measure and accounts for approximately 70% of bone strength.[257] A BMD test is the simplest way to assess for osteoporosis. Without this test, most people are unaware they have osteoporosis until a fracture occurs, although some fractures can be painless or the pain may be mistaken for arthritis, delaying diagnosis.

BMD is a measurement of the mineral content of bone in grams per square centimeter (g/cm^2) for the area of the body that has been scanned. Osteoporosis is now defined in terms of standard deviations from the average peak bone mass, also called a *T-score*. Sometimes a *Z-score* is also reported, which is the number of standard deviations by which the BMD differs from the mean value for the woman's age and ethnicity. Baseline BMD tests performed at the time of menopause (cessation of menstrual flow) or even earlier (during the perimenopausal phase) can provide a baseline assessment for future reference.

Multiple imaging modalities can be used to evaluate BMD and diagnose osteoporosis, including dual energy x-ray absorptiometry (DXA), which measures spine, hip, or total body density; peripheral DXA (pDXA), which measures wrist, heel, or finger density only; quantitative ultrasound (QUS), in which sound waves are used to measure calcaneal, tibial, or patellar density; computed tomography (CT); or radiographic absorptiometry, which is a radiograph of the hand. These methods are not interchangeable and do not provide equivalent information.

DXA is the preferred procedure because it measures bone density at the hip and spine where bone loss occurs more rapidly (Table 17.1).[186]

Radiography. Fractures are usually diagnosed by radiograph examination (x-ray) that demonstrates the fracture (Fig. 17.5) and also reveals the osteopenia leading to the diagnosis of osteoporosis. Once osteopenia is noted, other causes of metabolic bone disease must be ruled out, including hyperthyroidism, hyperparathyroidism, osteomalacia, testicular failure, malignancies, and so on. Diagnostic criteria for men with this condition are at present based on those for women, although the validity of this approach is under discussion; 30% or greater bone density loss must occur before such abnormalities can be noted on an x-ray film.

Laboratory testing. Laboratory testing can detect other risk factors and can provide clues to etiology. Selection of laboratory tests should be individualized because there is no consensus regarding which tests are optimal.

TABLE 17.1   World Health Organization (WHO) Classification for Bone Mineral Density

T-Score	Significance
−1.0 or higher	Normal, low risk for fracture
−1.0–2.5[a]	Osteopenia (low bone mass)
−2.5 or lower[b]	Osteoporosis

[a]Half of fragility fractures occur in this group.
[b]The National Osteoporosis Foundation (NOF) suggests that anyone with a T-score of −2.0 or less or −1.5 or less with at least one risk factor should be treated to reduce fracture risk.
From World Health Organization Study Group: Assessment of fracture risk and its application to screening for postmenopausal osteoporosis, Tech Rep Series 843, Geneva, 1994, WHO.

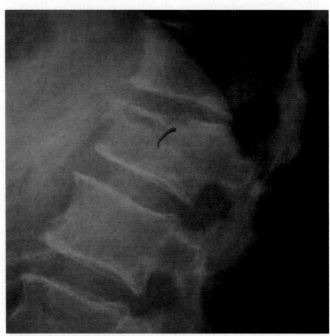

FIG. 17.5 Decreased bone density of vertebrae with compression fracture. (From Lavelle W, Carl A, Lavelle ED, et al: Vertebroplasty and kyphoplasty. Anesthesiology Clinics 25(4):913-928, 2007.)

BOX 17.3 **Management of Osteoporosis**

Prevention

Client education
Optimize calcium and magnesium intake (see Table 17.2)
Exposure to sunlight; vitamin D therapy
Regular physical activity (weight bearing) and prescriptive exercise
Other lifestyle changes (e.g., reduce or eliminate alcohol and tobacco)
Maintenance of menstrual cycles from youth through adulthood
Minimize intake of carbonated soft drinks and caffeine
Minimize use of medication(s) known to cause bone loss
Recognize and treat any medical conditions that can affect bone health
Adequate nutrition and calories; avoid chronic dieting or "yo-yo" dieting
Reduce animal sources of protein; increase vegetable sources of protein
Phytoestrogens (under investigation)
Psychosocial support

Management

Same as for prevention
Pharmacotherapy (single or combination)
Bisphosphonates
  • IV: pamidronate (Aredia), zoledronate (Zometa)
  • Oral: risedronate (Actonel), ibandronate (Boniva), etidronate (Didronel), alendronate (Fosamax sodium), tiludronate (Skelid)
  • Oral/IV: clodronic acid
Hormonal therapy (ERT/HRT for women, testosterone for men)
SERMs: raloxifene (Evista)
Calcitonin (nasal or injection):
  • Miacalcin
  • Calcimar
PTH, rhPTH: teriparatide (Forteo)
OPG
Osteoporosis education, balance assessment, and falls prevention
Psychosocial support
Falls and fracture prevention

ERT, Estrogen replacement therapy; *HRT,* hormone replacement therapy; *IV,* intravenous; *OPG,* osteoprotegerin; *PTH,* parathyroid hormone; *rhPTH,* recombinant human PTH; *SERMs,* selective estrogen receptor modulators.

Screening. Although osteoporosis was once called a "silent disease" because it was not recognized until a fracture signaled its presence, the widespread availability of technology to measure bone density has made it possible to identify people at risk for osteoporosis before fractures are imminent. Currently, no accurate measure of overall bone strength and standards of routine screening assessment have been established.

The NOF's guide for physicians suggests a bone density test for every woman age 65 years and older.[262] Additionally, the NOF has recommended testing for postmenopausal women younger than age 65 years who have sustained a bone fracture in adulthood, have a family history of osteoporosis, are thin, or smoke. Optimal intervals between tests have not been established. The measurements given here apply to white, adult women; it is not clear how to apply this diagnostic criterion to men and children and across ethnic groups. Because of the difficulty in accurate measurement and standardization between instruments and sites, controversy exists among experts regarding the continued use of this diagnostic criterion.[257]

Common management. Because no cure is available for osteoporosis, prevention and, more effectively, early intervention is essential for everyone (men, women, young, and old) but especially for those at risk (Box 17.3). By minimizing modifiable risk factors, people at high risk for developing osteoporosis may be able to achieve higher peak bone mass in the hope of delaying or preventing the onset of osteoporosis.[338] Because peak adult bone density depends on factors during growth and development, preventing osteoporosis in the aging adult begins by providing necessary dietary calcium intake during bone development and calcification in childhood and adolescence (Table 17.2).

Regular exercise and physical activity, combined with adequate calcium, is considered both a prophylactic and treatment measure for osteoporosis from childhood through the adult years. The risk of fractures can be reduced by 50% if vitamin and nutrient requirements are met in the first two to three decades of life.[132]

Diet. Dietary considerations, such as reducing animal sources of protein, increasing vegetable sources,[329,332] and increasing whole soy foods,[327] may result in reduced risk for both cardiovascular disease and osteoporosis. Low-fat dairy and other calcium- and magnesium-rich foods (e.g., broccoli or kale, sardines or salmon with the bones, fresh or dried apricots, figs, turnip greens, oranges or calcium-enriched orange juice, or tofu) and calcium supplements are the primary means of achieving an adequate calcium intake. Vitamin D helps the body absorb, synthesize, and transport calcium within the body, therefore necessitating adequate sunshine each day. Vitamin D requirements vary by geographic location and age. Additional vitamin D (food or supplementation) is recommended; many calcium supplements contain vitamin D.

Medications. Pharmacotherapy to reduce fracture risk in women with reduced BMD is initiated when the T-score is lower than 2 in the absence of risk factors or lower than 1.5 if other risk factors are present.[54,262]

Postmenopausal women need estrogen replacement with *selective estrogen receptor modulators* (SERMs), which maximize the beneficial effect of estrogen on bone. Raloxifene (Evista) is the only SERM approved by the Food and Drug Administration (FDA) at the time of this writing for the treatment and prevention of osteoporosis.

Bisphosphonates are a family of drugs that inhibit bone resorption and actually reverse bone loss. These drugs are currently being used in various bone conditions involving increased levels of bone resorption, such as osteoporosis and Paget's disease of bone.

All resorptive agents currently approved for treatment of osteoporosis (e.g., bisphosphonates, SERMs, or nasal calcitonin) decrease bone resorption but cannot induce new bone formation. Consequently, their effects are limited. The use of agents that stimulate new bone formation, such as recombinant human parathyroid hormone (rhPTH [teriparatide]), is under investigation as a single agent and in combination with antiresorptive agents.[106,311]

Combined administration of hormone replacement therapy (HRT) and bisphosphonates appears to have a more pronounced effect in the appendicular skeleton than the axial skeleton, with greater increases of bone mass at the lumbar spine and hip than for either of the therapies alone.[128]

Rehabilitation. Management goals are centered on stabilizing or increasing bone mass, preventing fractures, maximizing

TABLE 17.2   Daily Calcium Requirements

Age Group	Minimum Daily Requirements (Elemental Calcium)	Calcium Administration
Birth to 6 months	400 mg	Calcium supplements come in several preparations (e.g., carbonate, citrate, gluconate, lactate, phosphate). Calcium carbonate should be taken with meals that do not contain calcium-rich foods. Recommended daily requirements refer to elemental or actual calcium. Check the label for the *%Daily Value*, and note how many tablets or capsules are required to obtain this amount.
6 months to 1 year	600 mg	The body can absorb 500 mg of calcium at a time. Spread calcium intake (food or supplements) over the course of a day. Separate calcium supplements away from foods high in calcium or vitamins with calcium added.
Children ages 2–8 years	800 mg	Beware of foods containing wheat bran or oxalic acid (e.g., chocolate, cauliflower, rhubarb, beet greens, Brussels sprouts) that interfere with calcium absorption. Take calcium supplements away from these foods.
Children and adolescents ages 9–17 years[a]	1300 mg	Calcium can interfere with the effectiveness of a variety of tetracycline antibiotics and quinolones such as Cipro, Floxin, Maxaquin, Noroxin, and Penetrex. Avoid consuming calcium (food or supplements) within 2–4 hours of taking these drugs.
Adolescents and young adults (11–24 years)	1200–1500 mg; the NOF recommends 1000 mg for this age group	Calcium, especially in antacids, may interfere with certain calcium channel blockers and β-blockers and thyroid medication (thyroxine). Check with prescribing physician about how to take calcium.
Women, ages 25–50 years	1000–1200 mg	Calcium can interfere with bisphosphonate absorption. If taking bisphosphonates, delay consuming calcium (food or supplements) at least 30 minutes.
Pregnant or lactating females; women older than age 50 years	1200–1500 mg	Calcium just before bedtime can aid with reducing muscle cramps and improving sleep.
Postmenopausal women on estrogen therapy	1000 mg (some report 1200 mg)	Spend at least 10 minutes daily in the sun (longer if using sunscreen) to obtain vitamin D necessary for calcium absorption and bone formation.
Postmenopausal women not on estrogen therapy	1500 mg	For every ounce over 4 oz of animal protein, an additional 100 mg of calcium is required to stay even.
Men up to age 65 years[a]	1200 mg	Take calcium supplements with a meal rather than on an empty stomach, unless the foods contain significant amounts of calcium.
Men older than age 65 years[b]	1500 mg	Extrastrength antacid made with calcium carbonate in tablet form (e.g., Tums) is used by some people to obtain calcium. Beware of this antacid; decreased stomach acid alters food digestion and absorption. For the individual with reduced stomach acid and especially the older adult, this may not be a good choice.
All women and men older than age 65 years	1500 mg	

[a]This category is included by the Institute of Medicine.[44]
[b]Some sources recommend older than age 55 years.
NOF, National Osteoporosis Foundation.
From National Women's Health Information Center, US Department of Health and Human Services, 2000; Swan KG, Lobo M, Lane JM, et al.: Osteoporosis in men: a serious but underrecognized problem, J Musculoskelet Med 18:310–316, 2001.
Anyone receiving medications for osteoporosis prevention should also be taking at least 1200 mg calcium and 400 IU/day vitamin D (800 IU/day for men older than age 65 years) each day in addition to a weight-bearing exercise program that is site specific; calcium is best absorbed when taken several times a day in amounts of 500 mg or less.

physical performance and function, improving quality of life, and managing symptoms, especially in the presence of pain from fractures and deformity.[409]

Intervention begins with the identification of people at risk or who have been identified as osteoporotic but who have not received any education, training, or rehabilitation. An excellent document is available summarizing the various aspects of osteoporosis and outlining directions for future research that may be of interest to the PTA.[257]

PTAs should be aware of the symptoms and signs associated with osteoporosis, because they may be in a position to request a reassessment by the PT to refer a client to a physician for examination based on a change in the person's status, especially in the presence of significant risk factors. For example, a 65-year-old woman being treated for a rotator cuff disorder may report the onset of sharp midthoracic pain associated with sneezing since her last visit, but she now notes a constant, dull ache in the area. In addition, the client and therapist note an increase in the thoracic kyphosis. Communication with a PT

and a physician regarding these clinical changes is warranted because of the concern about a possible fracture.

The therapist should also be aware of the potential side effects common to osteoporosis medications. For example, calcium can cause constipation, calcitonin may be accompanied by nausea and flushing, raloxifene may cause leg cramps, and the bisphosphonates are associated with GI intolerance and/or esophagitis. Side effects of estrogen replacement therapy are listed in Box 17.4.

The results of numerous studies of exercise and bone health as they are presented here represent four different exercise-related issues: (1) building bone mass, (2) slowing the decline of BMD, (3) preventing fracture, and (4) maintaining muscle mass and strength. An excellent summary of many studies of specific types of exercise in differing populations is available.[393]

Intervention modalities may include therapeutic exercise, resistance bands, foam rolls or balance balls, electrotherapy modalities, spinal orthoses or corsets, soft tissue mobilization, and so on. During an acute symptomatic episode, local

BOX 17.4	**Side Effects of Estrogens**[a]

- Sudden onset of or change in headache, coordination, vision, breathing, speech, or extremity strength or sensation[a]
- Chest pain[a]
- Groin or calf pain[a]
- Change in vaginal bleeding
- Urinary incontinence
- Increased blood pressure
- Breast discharge or lumps
- Skin rash
- Extremity edema
- Jaundice
- Abdominal pain
- Tremors

These side effects warrant communication with a physician. Those marked with a superscript "a" call for *immediate* communication with a physician.

modalities are often used to control pain and improve movement and function. Using the osteoporosis disability index can help document improvements and positive outcomes.[272] Exercises combined with bracing or other rehabilitative measures aimed at reducing the anterior translation of the cervicothoracic spine and thoracic hyperkyphosis may be beneficial in reducing the risk or occurrence of osteoporotic fractures.[167]

Exercise. Although the effect of exercise on slowing the decline of BMD later in life is modest, epidemiologic evidence suggests that being active can reduce hip fracture incidence by 50% in the older adult population (age 65 years and older).[315] The level of exercise must be maintained because the benefits are lost if exercise is discontinued. A physical therapy professional understands the musculoskeletal system and the underlying pathologies and comorbidities and can implement an effective intervention plan that takes these variables into consideration.

Weighted exercise combined with calcium citrate supplementation has been shown in the Bone Estrogen Strength Training (BEST) study to increase bone density even in women who did not take HRT. Exercises, such as leg presses, seated rows, wall squats, and back extensions and latissimus pull downs, improve bone in the wrist, hip, and spine by 1% to 2% even in women who did not take a hormone replacement.[57]

Exercises to build bone density must be directed at the muscles supporting or attached to the affected bone. Both aerobic and resistance training exercise can provide weight-bearing stimulus to bone, but research indicates that resistance training has a more profound site-specific effect (directed at the areas that demonstrate bone loss) than aerobic exercise.[312,367,368]

In the past decade of research, many cross-sectional and longitudinal studies have shown a direct, positive relationship between the effects of resistance training and bone density.[188] On the other hand, aerobics, yoga, Pilates, and tai chi chuan are more likely to increase muscle strength and help maintain coordination and balance, which help prevent loss of balance and provide protection during loss of balance or falls.[185,209,293,366]

More studies are available now regarding the effects of tai chi on BMD, especially in postmenopausal women. Limited evidence suggests that tai chi may be an effective, safe, and practical intervention for maintaining BMD in postmenopausal women.[403]

Activity assessment is also important for the more active adult with osteoporosis. For those with vertebral osteoporosis or previous history of vertebral fractures, activities such as golfing, bowling, biking, rowing, sit-ups, or other exercise with a major component of spinal flexion, side bending, or spinal rotation should be excluded. Swimming is an excellent physical activity, especially for those individuals with arthritis or other joint involvement, but without a weight-bearing component, it is not beneficial to offset the complications of osteoporosis nor does it build bone density.

The minimal or most effective frequency, intensity, and duration of exercise have not been determined. Optimal overload at specific skeletal sites during various activities remains to be determined by future studies. The NOF recommends a preventive program of 45 to 60 minutes of weight-bearing exercise four times a week.[261]

Vibration. *Whole body vibration,* also known as *oscillating plate therapy,* is a new method of treatment being tested as a tool for the prevention of osteoporosis and bone fractures. Vibrating plates that are the size and shape of a bathroom scale have shown effectiveness in increasing BMD (and balance). Vibratory exercise may be more effective than walking to improve both these measures. Researchers continue to investigate the physiologic mechanisms involved and to identify the most appropriate parameters to use that are both safe and effective.[37,113,159]

The female athlete. The PTA working with elite female athletes must be aware of the documented decrease in bone density despite normal calcium intakes and regular exercise. A unique challenge exists with this population: the need to reduce bone stress while maintaining adequate muscular and aerobic conditioning in female athletes who are amenorrheic. The PTA can offer important client education, because many athletes do not realize the long-term orthopedic consequences of menstruation cessation. In the presence of bone density decline, the therapy staff should identify and initiate alternative training regimes. Non–weight-bearing and minimal weight-bearing activities such as aquatic therapy and cycling will significantly decrease the forces acting on the bone while still maintaining the training effect. Pool running is a viable activity for maintenance of cardiovascular and muscular training that closely simulates the sport itself.[234]

Aquatic exercise. Although swimmers have been shown to have higher mineral densities than those of control groups,[22,269] the protective effect of swimming as an effective exercise against osteoporosis and subsequent fractures has not been demonstrated. Activities with substantial muscular involvement but without gravitational forces are associated with lower BMD than those with a weight-bearing component.[370]

Although swimming and aquatic therapy are not weight-bearing activities and therefore are not preventive, they still help maintain range of motion (ROM), build strength, and increase cardiovascular fitness with minimal stress on bones and joints. Walking in the water against the resistive force of the water is a better alternative for those individuals participating in an aquatic exercise program.

Surgery. Because of the challenges of reconstruction of osteoporotic bone, open surgical management is reserved only for those rare cases that involve neurologic deficits or an unstable spine. As with other metabolic bone diseases, delayed healing and poor retention of internal fixation devices after fracture can occur in clients with osteoporosis. Postoperatively, the response to rehabilitation may be slowed, and adjustments may have to be made in the program to protect the injured area as recovery takes place. Close communication with the physician is called for to ensure safety.

Prognosis. Osteoporosis, once thought to be a natural part of aging among women, is no longer considered age- or gender-dependent. Although osteoporosis is one of the greatest detriments to women's health and accounts for significant morbidity and mortality, it is largely preventable because of the remarkable progress in the scientific understanding of its causes, diagnosis, and treatment. Even so, at the present time, 24% of women older than age 50 years die of complications (e.g., pneumonia, infections, and fracture emboli) in the first year after an osteoporotic-associated hip fracture.[261]

Medical treatment for osteoporosis has been shown to decrease the incidence of vertebral fractures by 40% to 60% after just 1 year of treatment. The occurrence of a single vertebral fracture substantially increases the likelihood of future fractures and progressive kyphotic deformity.[257] Even so, only 50% of women with VCFs diagnosed incidentally with chest radiographs are started on any pharmacologic treatment.[179]

Low bone density at the hip is a strong and independent predictor of all-cause and cardiovascular mortality in men age 65 years and older.[386]

Adherence to osteoporosis medications is relatively poor, with up to 30% of individuals suspending their treatment within 6 to 12 months of initiating therapy. Poor adherence is usually attributed to drug-induced adverse effects and results in increased risk of fracture and hospitalization.[277] Some women may discontinue pharmacologic treatment early because their BMD test results do not show osteoporosis (or they think that is the interpretation of the test results).[382]

Precautions and complications. Caution should be taken with using certain treatment techniques in people with known osteoporosis or those at high risk of having the disease. Although it is important that provocation and mobility information be collected and joint dysfunction be treated to improve functional abilities, precautions must be taken, including using other techniques or altering the person's position (e.g., side lying or sitting) so that the anterior thorax is not stabilized, which could result in a vertebral fracture.

Flexion exercises are clearly contraindicated for anyone with osteoporosis. Anterior compressive forces associated with forward flexion of the spine can contribute to VCFs. Posterior pelvic tilt and partial sit-ups (minimal abdominal crunches, lifting the head and upper torso only to the level of T6) do not appear to cause any anterior compressive force.[349,350]

Osteomalacia

Definition and incidence. In contrast to osteoporosis, which results in a loss of bone mass and brittle bones, *osteomalacia* is a progressive disease in which lack of mineralization of new bone matrix results in a softening of bone without loss of the present bone matrix. Osteomalacia is a generalized bone condition in which insufficient mineralization of the bone matrix results from calcium, vitamin D, and/or phosphate deficiency. The disease is sometimes referred to as the adult form of *rickets*, but the absence of epiphyseal plates in adults precludes the epiphyseal plate changes seen in rickets.

The two primary causes of osteomalacia are insufficient intestinal calcium absorption and increased renal phosphorus losses. The insufficient calcium absorption could occur because of either a lack of calcium or a resistance to the action of vitamin D. The increased renal phosphorus losses can occur associated

---

BOX 17.5 Risk Factors Associated with Osteomalacia

- Old age
- Residence in cold geographic area
- Vitamin D deficiency
- Gastrectomy
- Intestinal malabsorption associated with:
  - Diseases of the small intestine
  - Cholangiolitic disorders of the liver
  - Biliary obstruction
  - Chronic pancreatic insufficiency
- Long-term use of:
  - Anticonvulsants
  - Tranquilizers
  - Sedatives
  - Muscle relaxants
  - Diuretics
  - Antacids containing aluminum hydroxide
- History of:
  - Hyperparathyroidism
  - Chronic renal failure
  - Renal tubular defects (decreased reabsorption of phosphate)

---

with renal and renal tubular insufficiency. In addition, the long-term use of antacids and the presence of long-standing hyperparathyroidism can lead to phosphate deficiencies contributing to the development of osteomalacia.

The dietary deficiency type of osteomalacia has been eradicated in the United States for the most part by the widespread supplementation of dairy products with vitamin D. However, osteomalacia does occur in the malnourished aging adult who may not receive adequate nutrition or enough exposure to sunlight.[317]

Housebound and institutionalized individuals are especially at risk; thus the prevalence of osteomalacia is expected to increase with the aging of the American population.[69] Diseases of the small intestine, cholestatic disorders of the liver, biliary obstruction, and chronic pancreatic insufficiency increase the risk of developing osteomalacia because these conditions adversely affect the absorption of calcium and the action of vitamin D.

Osteomalacia is seen with greater frequency in cultures where the population has increased skin pigmentation and the diet is deficient in vitamin D (e.g., northern China, Japan, and northern India).[69] Osteomalacia is common in the aged adult because of calcium- and vitamin D–deficient diets and decreased sunlight exposure. This situation is worsened by the intestinal malabsorption problems associated with aging or the presence of systemic lupus erythematosus (SLE) that usually requires avoidance of sunlight to prevent ultraviolet-induced flare-ups.[321]

Long-term use of commonly prescribed medications also increases the risk of developing osteomalacia. Anticonvulsant medications, such as phenobarbital and phenytoin, accelerate breakdown of the active forms of vitamin D by inducing hepatic hydroxylases. As mentioned, antacids can cause phosphate deficiency. Box 17.5 summarizes the risk factors associated with osteomalacia.

Structures involved. Although the bone matrix remains intact (i.e., the bone structure remains unchanged) in osteomalacia, a generalized decrease in calcification of the matrix (calcification results in bone) and an increase in uncalcified matrix occur, leaving instead osteoid (bone that has not matured or calcified).

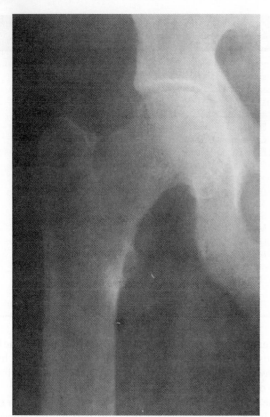

FIG. 17.6 Osteomalacia of the femur. Note the loss of the sharp interface between cortical bone and cancellous bone caused by demineralization of the cortex. (From Richardson JK, Iglarsh ZA: *Clinical orthopedic physical therapy*, Philadelphia, 1994, Saunders.)

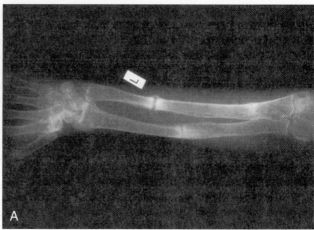

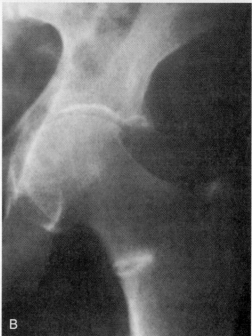

FIG. 17.7 Osteomalacia. (A) Forearm and (B) femoral neck. Looser's zones are seen as translucent zones with sclerotic margins. Usual sites include the medial femoral neck, pubic rami, lateral borders of the scapulae, and ribs. Complete fractures can extend through Looser's zones; these will heal with appropriate treatment. (From Bullough P: *Orthopedic pathology*, ed 5, St Louis, 2010, Mosby.)

Thus too little calcified bone occurs; failure of calcium salts to be deposited promptly in newly formed organic bone matrix (osteoid) results in osteomalacia.[317]

Demineralization results in an exaggeration of the osteoid seams seen radiographically adjacent to the relatively sparse areas of calcified bone (Fig. 17.6). As the osteoid accumulates, bone strength declines. These exaggerated seams occur because of the excessive time lag between collagen deposition and the appearance of the calcium salt. Areas of abundant osteoid appear radiographically as radiolucent stripes. These so-called pseudofractures, known as *Looser's zones*, occur most commonly on the concave side of long bones, the ischial and pubic rami, and the ribs and scapula (Fig. 17.7). These pseudofractures develop from the healing of multiple microstress fractures in the moderately severe form of osteomalacia sometimes referred to as *Milkman's syndrome*.[317]

Signs and symptoms. The diagnosis of osteomalacia is difficult and often delayed because many people present initially with diffuse, generalized aching and fatigue in the presence of anorexia and weight loss. Proximal myopathy and sensory polyneuropathy may also be present, resulting in a confusing clinical presentation. Bone pain and periarticular tenderness can occur in the spine, ribs, pelvis, and proximal extremities.

The combination of muscle weakness and softening of bone contributes to postural deformities, including increased thoracic kyphosis, a heart-shaped pelvis, and marked bowing of the femurs and tibias. The muscular weakness (proximal myopathy) may lead to a waddling gait and difficulties with transitional movements such as rising from sitting to standing, climbing stairs, or moving in and out of bed.[69]

Although not occurring nearly as often as in osteoporosis, acute fracture may be what leads to the diagnosis of osteomalacia. The radius, femur, vertebral bodies, ribs, and pubic ramus are common sites of fracture.

Common tests and measures. Osteomalacia may present with a variety of clinical and radiographic manifestations mimicking other musculoskeletal disorders (e.g., fibromyalgia or polymyalgia rheumatica).[299] For this reason, numerous methods are used to diagnose osteomalacia, including radiographs, bone scan, bone biopsy, and a laboratory workup (blood tests and urinalysis). Serum for levels of calcium, albumin, phosphate, alkaline phosphatase, and parathyroid hormone (PTH) are also obtained. Urine is collected to assess calcium and phosphate excretion rates.

Radiographically, osteomalacia, like osteoporosis, may present as osteopenia. A bone biopsy may be done at the site of osteopenia to evaluate the bone matrix. Besides osteopenia, radiolucent bands in the bone cortex (Looser's zones) may be revealed radiographically (see Fig. 17.7).

Common management. The treatment of osteomalacia depends on the cause. If inadequate nutrition is the problem, strengthening the dietary regimen with calcium and vitamin D is necessary. This step may be sufficient to improve the calcification of the organic matrix and thereby result in healing of the pseudofractures and strengthening the bones in general.

If osteomalacia is a result of intestinal malabsorption, treatment is directed to correct the primary disease. Phosphate supplementation can be prescribed in the presence of renal phosphate wasting. If used, vitamin D must be given to enhance calcium absorption impaired by the phosphate.

Considerable overlap occurs between osteomalacia and osteoporosis regarding implications for the PTA. The reader is directed to the section associated with osteoporosis for the discussion of client injury during examination and intervention, recognition of possible fracture, postoperative care, and side effects of calcium agents.

Paget's Disease

Sir James Paget, who described the disease more than a century ago, thought it was likely a bone infection. We know now that *Paget's disease* is a metabolic bone disease that is often inherited in an autosomal dominant pattern which results in overproduction of bone weakened tissue.[59,206]

Environmental factors, specifically slow viruses that take years to progress to a point where symptoms become evident, may play a role in the development of Paget's disease[181]; the hereditary factor may be the reason family members are susceptible to the suspected virus.[336] Exactly how the viruses affect osteoclasts remains unknown.[67]

Paget's disease has become less prevalent and people are presenting even later and with less severe disease than before, thus environmental factors may be an important etiologic factor in this disease. People born recently and presenting with Paget's disease have substantially less severe bone disease.[56]

Definition and incidence. Paget's disease (also known as *osteitis deformans*) is the second most common metabolic bone disease after osteoporosis. A progressive disorder of the adult skeletal system, this disease is characterized by abnormal bone remodeling with increased bone resorption and excessive, unorganized new bone formation caused by activated osteoclasts. Eventually, the normal bone marrow is replaced by vascular and fibrous tissue. Although Paget's disease is a state of high bone turnover, the excess bone that is formed lacks the structural stability of normal bone (enlarged bone but weakened), leading to complications such as deformity, fracture, arthritis, and pain. The disease may involve one or more sites.

Paget's disease is a common disease of the aging adult population, rarely presenting before age 35 years, with increasing prevalence among adults older than age 50 years. Approximately 3% to 4% of the population older than age 50 years and 10% of those older than age 70 years may be affected (up to 3 million people in the United States).[8]

Although still unclear, both prevalence and severity of Paget's disease seem to be declining. Current prevalence is only approximately 50% of that in 1983.[56] Men and women are both affected, although a slight increased prevalence is evident among men. The disease is often familial and has an unusual geographic distribution. Populations of the British Isles and countries where migration from Britain occurred (the United States, Australia, New Zealand, and Canada) have a greater incidence. The disease is almost nonexistent in Asia and in the native African and South American populations.

An initial osteoclastic, resorptive stage where abnormal osteoclasts proliferate unrestrained is evident. The bone resorption is so rapid that osteoblastic activity cannot keep up and fibrous tissue replaces bone. Radiographically, the resultant lytic areas are sharply defined and flame- or wedge-shaped. The initial resorption is followed by abnormal regeneration called the *osteoblastic sclerotic phase.*

In the sclerotic phase, the normal cancellous architecture is replaced by coarse, thickened struts of trabecular bone, and the cortical bone is irregularly thickened, rough, and pitted. The abnormal arrangement of the lamellar bone, separated by so-called cement lines, gives the bone the look of a mosaic. Although heavily calcified, the bone is now enlarged but weakened with a chaotic woven pattern rather than the well-organized lamellar structure seen in normal bone.

Involvement of the vertebral bodies presents with a picture-frame appearance radiographically as the cortical shell and endplates become greatly exaggerated in comparison to the coarse, cancellous bone portion of the vertebral body (Fig. 17.8). The final stage of the disease is characterized by little cellular activity.

Structures involved. The progressive deossification that weakens the bony structure primarily affects the axial skeleton. The lesions occur at multiple sites, particularly the skull, spine, pelvis, femurs, and tibias. Pathologic fractures can occur in any bone (Fig. 17.9), especially in the proximal femurs, pelvis, and lumbar spine.

Signs and symptoms. Paget's disease begins insidiously and progresses slowly; in mild cases, a person may have a few symptoms or may be symptom free over a very long period, eventually presenting with bone pain and skeletal deformities. When Paget's disease is active in several bones, overactive osteoclasts can release enough calcium in the blood to cause hypercalcemia, with fatigue, weakness, loss of appetite, abdominal pain, and/or constipation.[8]

If working with an aging adult population, PTAs need to be aware of the symptoms and signs of Paget's disease. Because pain is often the initial symptom and is usually a vague diffuse ache, difficulty in distinguishing this disease from degenerative joint disease of the lumbar spine, hips, or knees can be evident.

Affected bones change in shape, size, and direction, causing bone pain, arthritis, deformities, and fractures (Box 17.6). The most common presenting symptom is pain, which may be of headache, radicular, osteoarthritic, muscular, or other skeletal origin. Direct pain from periosteal irritation of involved bones is deep and boring, worse at night, and reduced but not eliminated with activity. In some people, this direct pain may be referred to nearby muscles and joints.[398]

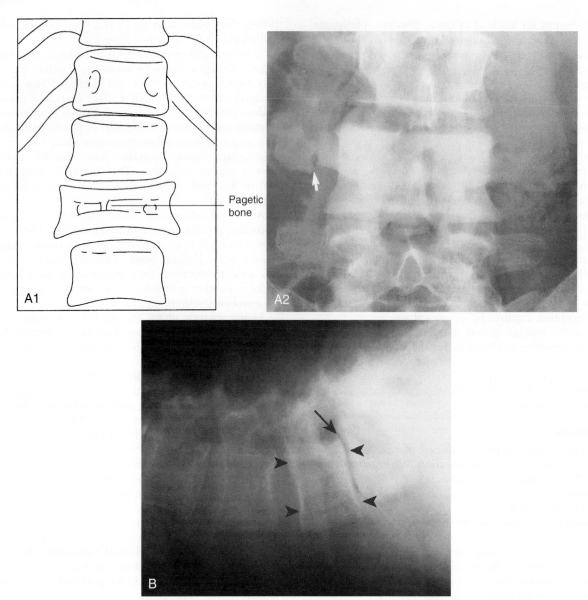

FIG. 17.8 (A) Clinical radiograph of the spine shows a solitary focus of pagetic bone. A loss of height of the vertebra (compression), some increases in the width of the vertebra, and a typical "picture-frame" appearance are evident. (B) Pathologic (type V) spondylolisthesis of L4 on L5 in a patient with Paget's disease *(arrow)*; observe the picture frame vertebra *(arrowheads)* and degenerative disk disease with vacuum phenomena of the L4 disk. (A2, From Taylor JAM, Hughes TH, Resnick D: Skeletal imaging: Atlas of the spine and extremities, ed 2, St. Louis, 2010, Saunders. B, From Marchiori D: Clinical imaging: With skeletal, chest, and abdominal pattern differentials, ed 3, St. Louis, 2014, Mosby.)

Clients may also experience fatigue, lightheadedness, and general stiffness. New onset of pain may be related to pathologic fracture of the vertebral bodies, pelvis, or long bones. Damage to the cartilage of joints adjacent to the affected bone and distortion of the normal joint alignment from bony changes may lead to osteoarthritis. This is often more disabling than the Paget's disease itself and will not respond to treatment of the underlying bone disease.[90]

Clinical findings also include postural deformities such as increased thoracic kyphosis and bowing of the femurs and tibias (Fig. 17.10). Bony softening of the femoral neck can cause coxa vara (reduced angle of the femoral neck) and may result

in a waddling gait. These changes may produce increased local mechanical stresses resulting in pain.

Paget's disease of the skull and spinal column can produce neurologic complications as a result of either direct impingement (myelopathy) or ischemia related to a *pagetic steal syndrome* (hypervascular pagetic bone "steals" blood from the neural tissue).[398]

Typical neurologic deficits may include eighth cranial nerve involvement (most common) with hearing loss related to involvement of the ossicles or bony foraminal encroachment. Headaches may occur if the skull is involved, and the forehead may enlarge as the amount of bone in the skull expands and the

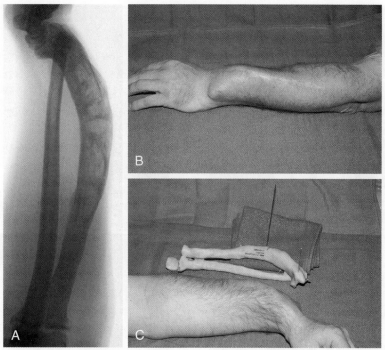

FIG. 17.9 Paget's disease. A complex malunion of the radius in a 62-year-old man after several fractures. (A) The presenting lateral radiograph of the severe deformity. (B) The clinical appearance. (C) A bone model made from computed tomographic scans and used for preoperative planning for correction of the deformity. (From Browner BD: Skeletal trauma: basic science, management, and reconstruction, ed 3, Philadelphia, 2003, Saunders.)

BOX 17.6   Clinical Manifestations of Paget's Disease

Pain
- Headache
- Muscular
- Osteoarthritis
- Radicular
- Skeletal

Skeletal
- Pain (bone pain that may be referred to nearby joints and muscles)
- Deformities
  - Kyphoscoliosis
  - Bone thickening or enlargement (including skull)
  - Bowing (outward bowed femur, forward bowed tibia)
  - Coxa varus (waddling gait); acetabular protrusion
  - Vertebral compression or collapse
- Fractures
- Osteoarthritis

Muscular
- Pain (myalgia)
- Stiffness

Neurologic
- Nerve compression syndromes (including cranial, spinal, and peripheral nerves)
- Mental confusion, deterioration in cognitive function
- Sensorineural hearing loss

Cardiovascular
- Increased cardiac output
- Increased vascularity (increased skin temperature over involved bone)
- Heart failure

Miscellaneous
- Fatigue
- Tinnitus
- Lightheadedness, dizziness, vertigo

---

foramen for the cranial nerves gets smaller (Fig. 17.11). Affected individuals also report tinnitus, vertigo, and hearing loss.

Other nerve or spinal cord compression syndromes may occur as enlarged pagetic bones put pressure on various nerve structures. Findings may include myelopathy, spinal stenosis, radiculoneuropathy, cauda equina syndrome, peripheral nerve entrapment, carpal and tarsal tunnel syndromes, and any of the effects of cranial nerve compression.[398] Thickening of the skull causes compression of the auditory nerves most often; other cranial nerves are only rarely involved in Paget's disease.

Other findings may include mental deterioration (Paget's disease causes reduced blood flow to the brain) and cardiovascular disease (rare). When one-third to one-half of the skeleton is involved, an increase in cardiac output may be severe enough to cause heart failure. This is the most common cause of death in people with advanced Paget's disease.[398]

Clients with diffuse headaches may present with undiagnosed Paget's disease. These clients may report hearing loss, tinnitus, incontinence, diplopia, or swallowing difficulties. Slurring of speech or the onset of signs or symptoms associated

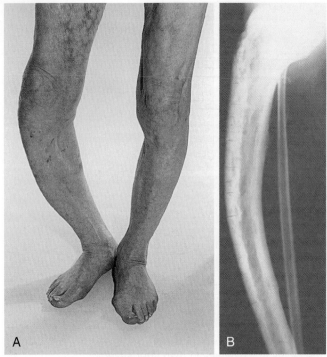

FIG. 17.10 (A) Bowing of the leg is often seen in Paget's disease. (B) X-ray of a person with Paget's disease affecting the tibia (but not the fibula). Diffuse osteosclerosis, cortical thickening, pseudofractures, and anterior bowing are the predominant findings. (A, From Kumar PJ, Clark ML: Kumar & Clark's clinical medicine, ed 8, Edinburgh, 2012, Saunders. B, From Taylor JAM, Hughes TH, Resnick D: Skeletal imaging: Atlas of the spine and extremities, ed 2, St. Louis, 2010, Saunders.)

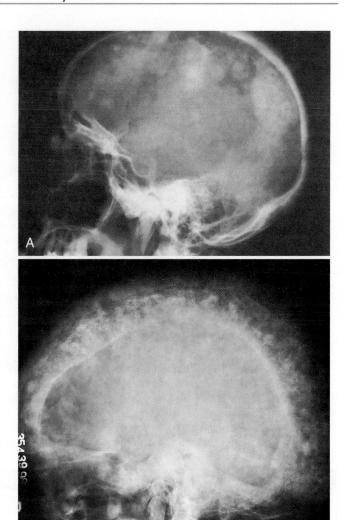

FIG. 17.11 Clinical radiographs of the skull in later stages of Paget's disease. (A) Marked patchy sclerosis appears in the bone, the organized architecture is lost, and the bone becomes extremely thick, on occasion several times thicker than normal. (B) Advanced involvement of the skull with marked thickening of the entire vault, areas of osteolysis, and patchy new bone formation resulting in a "cotton-wool" appearance called *osteoporosis circumscripta cranii*. This person experienced progressive hearing loss. (A, From Bullough P: Orthopedic pathology, ed 5, St Louis, 2010, Mosby. B, From Goldman L: Cecil textbook of medicine, ed 22, Philadelphia, 2004, Saunders.)

with heart disease is evident. The presentation of any of the above warrants communication with a physician and the PT on the case. Awareness of the side effects of antiinflammatory medications is also important. These side effects include indigestion, nausea, vomiting, melena, tinnitus, hearing loss, vertigo, and hyperpnea. Again, if any of these signs or symptoms are reported, communication with a physician is warranted.

Common tests and measures. Because Paget's disease progresses slowly and the severity of the disease varies considerably among individuals, it may be many years before a diagnosis is made or the person may be misdiagnosed with arthritis or other disorders. In fact, the diagnosis is often made incidentally on the basis of radiographs or laboratory tests done for other reasons.

If the disease is advanced, the diagnosis is made based on the characteristic bone deformities and radiologic bony changes. Bone scans are positive only if the disease is active and marked by rapid bone turnover but provide information that helps determine the extent and activity of the condition. Bone scans must be confirmed by radiographic examination as other conditions are also accompanied by a metabolically active lesion. A bone biopsy may occasionally be done to make a differential diagnosis ruling out hyperparathyroidism, bone metastasis, multiple myeloma, and fibrous dysplasia.

Common management. The goal of treatment is to normalize Paget's disease activity for a prolonged period. Because of the osteoclast involvement, inhibitors of bone resorption are the first line of treatment. These pharmacologic

agents (see Box 17.3) decrease bone turnover through the inhibition of osteoclastic activity, improve bone density, and reduce fracture incidence. Individuals under long-term oral bisphosphonate use are treated with caution because of the potential side effects, especially recently reported osteonecrosis of the jaw.[251]

Management of Paget's disease depends on the degree of pain and extent of the pathologic changes. Nonsteroidal and other antiinflammatory agents are used to control the pain. Surgical intervention may be indicated for reasons other than fracture repair. Interventions include occipital craniectomy to relieve basilar and nerve compression, tibial osteotomy if the deformity is severe, and joint replacement(s) if severe degenerative joint disease is present (Fig. 17.12).

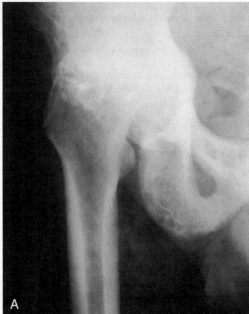

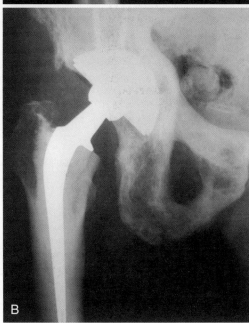

FIG. 17.12 Extensive Paget's disease of the acetabulum and femur in an 82-year-old man. (A) Protrusion deformity and varus femoral neck are seen. (B) After total hip replacement. Acetabulum required autogenous bone graft from femoral head. Cementless acetabular component appears bone ingrown 5 years after surgery. (From Canale ST: Campbell's operative orthopedics, ed 10, St Louis, 2003, Mosby.)

Although Paget's disease and osteoporosis can occur in the same person, these are completely different disorders with different causes. However, despite their marked differences, considerable overlap is evident between Paget's disease and osteoporosis regarding interventions and implications for the PTA. The overlap includes the discussion of client injury during examination and treatment, recognition of possible fracture, and postoperative care.

Exercise programs. Exercise is very important in maintaining skeletal health and is recommended for people with Paget's disease.

Joints adjacent to involved bone may function at a mechanical disadvantage, causing muscular pain that can be reduced with exercise. Strengthening muscles can also help minimize skeletal complications of Paget's disease with its mechanical stresses and resultant structural abnormalities of bone.[398]

The pain associated with Paget's disease often leads to less physical activity in daily life. Loss of muscle strength, joint motion, and cardiovascular endurance occur, leading to functional limitations such as slower walking and shorter distances. Exercise helps with weight control, improving cardiovascular function and cardiac output, and maintains muscular strength and joint motion.[342]

Severity of Paget's disease will determine the exercise program. Stretching, strengthening, endurance, aerobics, balance, and coordination exercises are all important. Some types of exercise should be avoided such as jogging, running, jumping, and if the spine is affected, forward bending and twisting exercises.[342]

Complications of orthopedic surgery on pagetic bone include hemorrhage, infection, pathologic fracture, delayed union or nonunion, and aseptic loosening of the hardware.[166] The PTA may be involved in management of extremity deformities requiring management with orthotics.

Prognosis. The course of Paget's disease varies widely from individual to individual. It may be completely stable and asymptomatic, or at the other end of the continuum, rapid progression can occur. The outlook is generally good, particularly if treatment is given before major changes have occurred. Biochemical remission with bisphosphonates is achievable in a majority of individuals.[351]

Although rarely fatal by itself, Paget's disease is accompanied by osteogenic sarcoma in less than 1% of all Paget's disease cases; this figure represents an increase in risk that is several-thousand-fold higher than the general population.[121,122] Prognosis for individuals with Paget's sarcoma is poor and is unrelated to the site or stage of presentation.[66] Little progress has occurred in the treatment of Paget's sarcoma over the years despite improvement in the treatment of standard osteosarcoma.[214]

Fracture

Definition and Incidence

A fracture is any defect in the continuity of a bone, ranging from a small crack to a complex fracture with multiple segments. Fractures can be classified into three general categories: (1) fracture by sudden impact (traumatic), (2) stress or fatigue fracture, or (3) pathologic fracture.

A *traumatic* fracture is the most common type of fracture and is usually associated with sudden impact, such as occurs with assault, abuse, traumatic falls, or motor vehicle accidents. Motor vehicle accidents involve fractures of the skull, nasal bone, and mandible most often; high-velocity injuries including automobile or motorcycle accidents often result in open fractures of the lower extremity. In the general population, radius and/or ulna fractures comprise the largest proportion of upper extremity fractures. The most affected age group is children ages 5 to 14 years as a result of accidental falls at home.[47]

Age is an important risk factor for fractures. The rate of hip fracture increases at age 50 years, doubling every 5 to 6 years. Increasing age and low BMD are the two most important independent risk factors for an initial vertebral or nonvertebral fracture.[24]

BOX 17.7   Risk Factors for Fractures

- Trauma
  - Motor vehicle accidents
  - Industrial or work-related accidents
  - Assault
  - History of falls; risk factors for falls (see also Box 17.8)
  - Overuse (marathon runners, military); sudden changes in training (duration, intensity)
  - Participation in sports, including dance (recreational or competitive)
- Advanced age
- Women: postmenopausal osteoporosis; military: stress fractures
- Men: hypogonadism (erectile dysfunction, prostate cancer)
- Any insufficiency[a] or fragility fractures, especially vertebral fractures
- Residence in a long-term care facility
- Poor self-rated health
- Low physical function
  - Slow gait speed; gait disorders or movement dysfunction; low levels of physical activity
  - Difficulty in turning while walking; inability to pivot
  - Use of a walking aid (cane, walker)
  - Decreased quadriceps strength (e.g., inability to rise from chair without using arms)
  - Increased postural (body) sway[b,306,340]
  - Impaired cognition, dementia
- Physical attributes
  - Low physical fitness
  - Decreased bone mineral density
  - Bone geometry (see text description)
  - Leg length discrepancy
  - Height
  - Low body mass index; low muscle mass
  - Poor nutrition; eating disorder; vitamin D deficiency
- Alcohol and/or substance use
- Other diseases or conditions
  - Osteoporosis; failure to treat or undertreatment of osteoporosis
  - Osteogenesis imperfecta
  - Osteonecrosis
  - Neoplasm; skeletal metastases; surgical resection for tumor
- Radiation treatment
- High-dose, long-term use of proton pump inhibitors

[a]Fracture in bones with nontumorous disease (e.g., rheumatoid arthritis, osteoporosis, following radiation) at normal load.[175]
[b]Postural sway is a corrective mechanism associated with staying upright and can be used as a measure of balance. Postural sway increases with age (reflecting decreased balance) and with the use of benzodiazepines.[306]

BOX 17.8   Risk Factors for Falls

Age Changes
- Muscle weakness or imbalance
- Decreased balance
- Age-related changes in peripheral vestibular mechanisms
- Impaired proprioception or sensation
- Delayed muscle response, increased reaction time

Pathologic Conditions
- Pathologic fractures
- Vestibular disorders
- Orthostatic hypotension (especially before breakfast)
- Dehydration
- Neuropathies
- Osteoporosis
- Arthritis
- Amputation
- Visual or hearing impairment
- Cardiovascular disease
- Urinary incontinence
- Central nervous system disorder (e.g., stroke, Parkinson's disease, multiple sclerosis, traumatic brain injury, spinal cord injury, amyotrophic lateral sclerosis)
- Altered neuromuscular reflexes
- Depression; dementia or other cognitive impairments
- Anemia

Medications
- Antihypertensives
- Sedatives–hypnotics
- Tricyclic antidepressants
- Diuretics
- Narcotics
- Benzodiazepines (antianxiety)
- Phenothiazines
- Polypharmacology (use of more than four medications)

Environmental
- Poor lighting
- Throw rugs, loose carpet, complex carpet designs
- Cluster of electrical wires or cords
- Stairs without handrails
- Bathrooms without grab bars
- Slippery floors (water, urine, floor surface)
- Restraints
- Footwear, especially slippers

Other
- History of falls (past month)
- Abuse or assault of older persons
- Sedentary lifestyle
- Nonambulatory status requiring transfers
- Gait changes or limitations
  - Decreased stride length or speed
  - Increased stride width
  - Muscular weakness
- Postural instability
- Fear of falling[380]
- Use of assistive devices (e.g., walkers, cane)
- Use of alcohol or other drugs
- Sleep disturbance, sleep disorder, or insomnia

A woman's risk of developing a hip fracture is equal to her combined risk of developing breast, uterine, and ovarian cancer.[259] Data collected from the U.S. Medicare population older than age 65 years revealed a pattern of rapidly rising rates with age for fractures of the pelvis, hip, and other parts of the femur among women. Fractures at the hip were most common, accounting for 38% of the fractures identified. The proximal humerus, distal radius/ulna, and ankle also were common fracture sites. Fractures distal to the elbow or knee had only small increases in incidence with age more than 65 years. Women have higher fracture rates than men of the same race, and whites generally have higher rates than blacks of the same gender.[18]

Fracture risk for adults has been consistently associated with a history of falls, including falls to the side, and attributes of bone geometry, such as tallness, hip axis, and femur length.[257] The way a person falls, laterally landing directly on the trochanter versus falling backward, is an independent risk factor for hip fractures.[108,278] Other risk factors for fracture are listed in

Boxes 17.7 and 17.8. Some risk factors for fracture, such as age, low body mass index, and low levels of physical activity, probably affect fracture incidence through their effects on bone density and propensity to fall and inability to absorb impact.[257] Vitamin D deficiency and its link with generalized muscle weakness leading to falls and fractures is likely more prevalent among older adults than previously thought.[101,395]

A *stress* (or fatigue) fracture, sometimes referred to as a stress reaction or bone stress injury, is caused by the bone's inability to withstand stress applied in a rhythmic, repeated, microtraumatic fashion. More simply stated, a fatigue fracture occurs if normal bone is exposed to repeated abnormal stress, or if normal stress is applied to abnormal bone. These types of overuse stress or fatigue fractures are most common in track and field athletes, distance runners, and soldiers in training. Most occur in the lower extremity and affect the tibial shaft and metatarsal bones, but they can also occur at the pubic ramus, femoral neck, or fibula; an increasing number of stress fractures have been reported in the knee (tibial plateau, proximal tibial shaft, femoral condyles).[266,310] The mechanism for injury in a stress fracture can be either compressive or distractive. Compressive stress fractures occur as a result of forceful heel strike during prolonged marching or running. Distractive stress reactions occur as a result of muscle pull on a bony insertion point and can become more serious if displacement occurs.

In the case of stress fractures, an abrupt increase in the intensity or duration of training (i.e., military trainees, athletes preparing for marathons) is often an additional risk factor.[266] Female recruits are at increased risk for pelvic and sacral stress fractures. The generally increased risk of bone stress injuries among females has been explained by anatomic (wide pelvis, coxa vara, genu valgum), hormonal, and nutritional factors.[221] Leg length discrepancy may also increase the risk of stress fracture, especially in female athletes. Decreased muscle mass and strength may play a role in the developing stress fractures by absorbing less of the force and distributing or exerting more load to the bone. Good muscle strength may decrease the strain on bone and delay muscle fatigue. Muscle fatigue may cause alterations in running mechanics that could increase ground reaction forces exerted on the bone.[169,221]

Pathologic fracture is a term used to describe a fracture that occurs in bone that is abnormally fragile because of another disease condition, most commonly cancer or reduced bone density. A subset of pathologic fractures would be *insufficiency fractures*, which occur in bones with structural alterations due to osteopenia, osteoporosis, or disorders of calcium metabolism. Insufficiency fractures (sometimes referred to as insufficiency stress fractures) result from a normal stress or force acting on bone that has deficient elastic resistance or has been weakened by decreased mineralization. Reduced bone integrity can result from many factors but occurs most commonly from the effects of radiation, postmenopausal or corticosteroid-induced osteoporosis, or other underlying metabolic bone disease. Insufficiency fractures arise insidiously or as a result of minor trauma. It has been proposed that weight bearing alone can be enough "trauma" to transmit a traumatic force to the compromised spine.[191]

Vertebral compression fracture (VCF) is one of the most common osteoporosis-related pathologic fractures, accounting for approximately 700,000 injuries. VCFs often occur with only minor trauma. Only 20% to 25% of people who sustain a VCF develop symptoms severe enough to seek medical attention.[198] VCFs are classified as wedge, crush, or biconcave according to their appearance.[157] The greater prevalence of wedge fractures may be related to degenerative disk disease, a condition that causes normal intradiskal pressure to shift and concentrate load to the peripheral aspects of the vertebral body.[182]

The incidence increases with age and with decreasing bone density. Factors that increase the risk of a first vertebral fracture include previous nonspine fracture, low BMD at all sites, low body mass index, current smoking, low milk consumption during pregnancy, low levels of daily physical activity, previous fall(s), and regular use of aluminum-containing antacids.[264] Men are less likely to develop osteoporosis and subsequent fracture, but they are not immune to this condition and are frequently undertreated for osteoporosis even after a fracture. Epidemiologic studies have confirmed that osteoporosis in men is an increasing health problem, possibly attributable to increased longevity and increased awareness of the problem.[97]

Decreased BMD associated with osteoporosis accounts for the largest number of fractures among the older adult population. In fact, a fracture may be the first sign of an underlying diagnosis of osteoporosis, and a serious fracture is a risk factor itself for future fractures in high-risk groups. There are an estimated 1.5 million osteoporosis-related fragility fractures in the United States each year.

Signs and Symptoms

Point tenderness over the site of the fracture is usually present, but not all fractures are equally painful. Pathologic and insufficiency fractures of the spine, pelvis, or sacrum often present with nonspecific low back, groin, or pelvic pain, mimicking other clinical conditions such as local tumor or metastatic disease or disk disease. With many fractures, attempts to move the injured limb will provoke severe pain, but in the presence of a fatigue fracture (stress reaction) active movement is typically painless. Resistive motions or repetitive weight bearing will cause pain, and the area will be exquisitely tender to local palpation. There may be edema observed in the area of the fracture. Clinical manifestations are most severe when the fracture is unstable.

Stress fractures typically present as vague achy pain that is worse after an activity. Specific point tenderness is rare and the source of the pain may be difficult to distinguish during the examination.

The deformity associated with an extremity fracture is often obvious, but the deformity of a spinal fracture is not always so. For example, a compression fracture of a thoracic vertebral body may result in an anterior wedging of the body but only a mildly accentuated thoracic kyphosis. When thoracic kyphosis does occur, decreased trunk strength and decreased pulmonary function are possible.[190] In the presence of a compression fracture of a thoracic vertebra, the initial pain may be sharp and severe, but after a few days it may become dull and achy. The pain may be reproducible on examination with pressure over the spinous process of the involved level. Pain associated with VCFs tends to be postural (i.e., worse with spinal extension or even standing up straight); it can be debilitating enough to confine some older adults to a wheelchair or bed.

Older adults with VCF are two to three times more likely to die secondary to pulmonary causes (e.g., congestive heart failure, pneumonia) and have an increased risk for hospitalization and mortality.[75] Urinary retention and GI symptoms are also common manifestations in people with VCFs. Neurologic deficits can also occur, but these symptoms usually resolve; less than 5% of affected individuals need surgical decompression.[338]

Occasionally, in an adolescent or young adult who has not achieved mature bone growth, a persistent but painless prominence may occur 1 to 3 months after a *minimally displaced fracture.* It is located on the compression side of the fracture within the newly formed subperiosteal bone as a result of encapsulation or calcification of a hematoma. This transient postfracture cyst is benign but must be medically diagnosed as such, because it cannot be distinguished clinically from infection or tumors.[374]

Common Tests and Measures

Traumatic fractures are often diagnosed by visual inspection and confirmed by plain radiographs. They can further be classified as stable (nondisplaced) if the fragments are in alignment or classified as unstable if the fragments are displaced. Bone fragments that pierce the skin are part of an open fracture, whereas the term *closed* refers to fragments that remain within the skin. Displaced, open fractures are most likely to be unstable, requiring immediate surgical intervention. Fractures can often involve surrounding soft tissue, vascular, and neurologic structures, requiring careful assessment at the time of injury and follow-up as healing progresses.

In the case of stress fractures conventional radiographic studies (x-rays) are usually inadequate; often the lag time between manifestation of symptoms and detection of positive radiographic findings ranges from 1 week to several months; therefore additional studies such as a bone scan or magnetic resonance imaging (MRI) may be necessary to determine the diagnosis. Up to 35% of sacral fractures are undetected on plain radiographs; cross-sectional imaging such as CT or MRI may be needed to identify and confirm sacral fractures. Radionuclide bone scanning (scintigraphy) has become a useful imaging study because it can demonstrate subtle changes in bone metabolism long before conventional radiography. MRI is also sensitive for detecting pathophysiologic changes associated with stress injuries but is more expensive and is reserved for cases in which other imaging findings are indeterminate.[107] CT is the imaging technique of choice to identify pathologic fractures.[221,405] Many VCFs are detected incidentally on chest radiographs.

Prevention Management

PTAs play a key role in the prevention of falls. Education and fall risk assessments are two important variables in preventing fractures from occurring. Fall prevention is important in adults older than 60 years of age (Box 17.9).

Common Management

The medical approach to management of all fractures is based on the location of the fracture, assessment of fracture type, need for reduction, presence of instability after reduction, and functional requirements of the affected individual. Individual factors such as age, activity level, the person's general health and overall condition, and the presence of any other injuries must also be taken into consideration. The goal of treatment is to provide stable positioning, promote bone healing, comfort, and early mobilization to prevent potential complications from immobility (e.g., constipation, deep vein thrombosis, pulmonary embolism, pneumonia).

In the case of stress fractures, the initial period of rest is followed by a gradual return to activity. Attention should be paid to modifying the activities that precipitated the stress fracture. The progression of return to sports is based on symptomatic response to increasing activity.[216]

The presence of osteoporosis complicates the need for immobilization or spinal fusion. Nonoperative treatment for VCFs

---

BOX 17.9 **Prevention of Falls**

- Wear low-heeled, closed footwear with rubber soles or good gripping ability; avoid smooth-bottomed shoes or boots. This applies to slippers; wear slippers or shoes when getting out of bed at night.
- Provide adequate lighting for hallways, stairways, bathrooms; use a flashlight outdoors. Wear glasses at night when getting out of bed for any reason.
- Conduct a home safety evaluation. Remove loose cords, slippery throw rugs; repair uneven stairs, steps, and sidewalks.
- Avoid oversedation; carefully monitor medications (especially sleep medications and antidepressants) and drink alcohol in moderation (never drink alcohol if taking medications without your physician's approval).
- Provide sturdy handrails on both sides of stairways.
- Provide grab bars on bathroom walls and nonskid strips on mats in tub or shower and beside tub or shower.
- Avoid going outdoors when it is wet, icy, or slippery; wear footwear with good traction or clip-on ice grippers; avoid walking on wet leaves or garden or yard clippings or debris.
- Carry items close to the body and leave one hand free to grasp railings or for balance.
- Know the location of pets before walking through a room or area of the house or apartment; maintain floors free of clutter and small objects.
- Put aside pride and use an appropriate assistive device as recommended by the therapist (e.g., cane, walking stick, walker); walkers equipped with a seat work well for people with limited endurance.
- Encourage a program of physical activity and exercise that is attainable.
- Avoid changing position quickly, such as when getting out of a chair or bed. Stand for a moment to see if you are dizzy so that you can sit down again if necessary.
- Keep items on shelves in the kitchen and elsewhere within reach. Do not stand on a chair or stepladder to reach items. Consider the consequences of a fall and broken hip if you are tempted and if you are thinking, "Nothing will happen, I will be fine."

---

includes activity modification, bracing, assistive devices, pharmacology (e.g., narcotic analgesics, calcitonin), and physical therapy. Hospital admission and bed rest is required for up to 20% of the population for whom conservative care is not possible or adequate. The debilitating effects of immobilization and keeping older adults bed bound is well recognized, with increased risks for developing pulmonary complications, pressure ulcers, deep vein thrombosis, and urinary tract infections. BMD is further reduced by immobility and bed rest, thereby increasing the risk of additional VCFs and other fragility fractures.[338]

Surgery. Surgical intervention may be required for traumatic displaced fractures, open fractures, or VCFs. Surgical techniques may include internal fixation (e.g., metal plating, wiring, screws), traction, bone grafts, or bone graft substitutes. After surgical reduction, a cast or other immobilization device may be applied. Some surgical techniques allow for a shortened period of immobilization and earlier movement. All members of the rehabilitation team should review the surgical reports to understand the technique that was used and which structures were involved.

VCFs also may be treated by surgical decompression and fusion, vertebroplasty, and kyphoplasty. Analgesic therapy is effective for most people with VCFs from bone metastases.[287] Newer minimally invasive procedures for the management of acute vertebral fracture have been developed. Injection of FDA-approved polymethylmethacrylate bone cement into the fractured vertebra is being used around the United States in procedures known as *vertebroplasty* or *kyphoplasty.*

General rehabilitation principles. Following bone fracture, there is usually a period of immobilization using casting, splinting, or bracing to remove longitudinal stress. This period allows for the phagocytic removal of necrotic bone tissue and the initial deposition of the fibrocartilaginous callus.

For any type of fracture, management during this postfracture period is directed toward blood clot prevention (mechanical and/or pharmacologic), promoting fracture repair by avoiding substances that can inhibit fracture repair (e.g., nicotine, corticosteroids), and possibly increasing caloric intake for soft tissue healing. Additional soft tissue injuries may manifest as the fracture heals; the PT and PTA should monitor clients for complaints of numbness and tingling or temperature changes in extremities that may indicate neurologic or vascular injury.

Gradually progressive stress will be applied to stimulate fracture callus formation and healing. In the case of pelvic or lower extremity fractures, the timing and extent of mobilization depend on the type of fixation used. For example, if an external fixation is applied for fracture stabilization, mobilization can occur within tolerance of the person's symptoms almost immediately. If casting or rigid bracing was used, mobilization may not occur until the cast is removed.

Partial weight bearing following a lower extremity fracture is usually considered 30% to 50% of body weight. Touch or touch-down weight bearing is 10% of body weight, but this is a subjective decision that is not easily determined. Allowing for unrestricted weight bearing according to the client's tolerance (WBAT) is less restrictive, but the PT and PTA must assess for intact cognition and decision-making abilities, intact sensation, upper body strength, vestibular function and balance, and proprioception before allowing unsupervised WBAT.

The literature supports recommending follow-up for strength and functional assessment 7 to 9 months after fracture.[324,339] Muscle strength around the hip remains weak after hip fracture, with joint arthroplasty requiring an exercise program for strengthening for 1 year or longer.[115,341] Short-term intervention with physical therapy can be very cost effective in reducing refracture rates.[339,340]

There are some widely accepted guidelines and rehabilitation protocols for various types of fractures (e.g., Neer rehabilitation program for shoulder fractures, Vanderbilt program, Tinetti protocol of balance exercises for rehabilitation from hip fractures).[194,379] The American Academy of Orthopaedic Surgeons offers guidelines for the rehabilitation of many different types of fractures. Several publications with fracture rehabilitation protocols are available specifically for the physical therapy professional.[30,193,195,222,271]

Rehabilitation in the acute care setting. Early repair and physical therapy have been shown to reduce hospital stays, increase chances of returning home (rather than being discharged to a nursing facility or rehabilitation facility), reduce complications, and improve functional mobility and independence at discharge,[111,172] and are associated with higher rates of 6-month survival.[52,143] PTAs are encouraged to share the results of studies such as these with hospital administrators when developing fall and fracture prevention programs.

Early mobilization accompanied by transfer training and maintaining strength and ROM after fracture surgery are essential to reduce the risk of deep vein thromboembolism, pulmonary or infectious complications, skin breakdown, and decline in mental status.

Following a fracture anywhere in the lower extremity (including the hip), some orthopedic surgeons advocate unrestricted weight bearing, advising the client to decide himself or herself how much weight to put on the leg. Stable fractures can usually tolerate weight bearing. Rotationally stable but potentially long unstable femur fracture may be allowed toe-touch weight bearing. Clients with vertically and rotationally unstable femoral fractures may be restricted to non–weight-bearing status using a wheelchair or electric scooter (if not in a spica hip cast).[297]

Although immediate weight bearing may cause initial bone loss, the long-term success of achieving bone growth remains unchanged,[339] and the short-term benefits of functional recovery and quicker return to independent living that accompany unrestricted weight bearing are important.[176,279]

Depending on the type of fracture, some movements may be restricted to allow for proper fracture consolidation. Most importantly, a non–weight-bearing status can actually place greater forces on the hip as a result of the biomechanics involved in maintaining correct positioning of the lower extremity.[148,250] In the case of femoral neck or intertrochanteric fractures, there is little biomechanical justification for restricted weight bearing; indeed, there is far greater pressure generated from performing a hip bridge while using a bedpan that is almost equivalent to the effect of unsupported ambulation.[176]

Older adults who receive physical therapy while still in the hospital following hip replacement for hip fracture are more likely to be discharged directly home rather than to a rehabilitation or assisted living facility.[124] People with hip fractures who receive additional home health visits are less likely to be hospitalized and more likely to need fewer medical visits, which usually translates into lower Medicare costs.[156] Mortality rates following hip fractures in older adults may be improved by a more intensive rehabilitation program immediately after the operation. The best predictor of mortality immediately after hip fracture up to 1 year after fracture is the inability to stand up, an indicator of frailty.[133] Older adults admitted for care of a fall-related hip fracture should be evaluated early in their hospital stay to determine risk for falls following discharge. Indicators may include a previous history of falls and prefracture use of an assistive device for ambulation. The plan of care should include balance and mobility training to prevent future falls. A previous history of falls is a risk factor for future falls; poor balance, slow gait speed, and decline in activities of daily living (ADLs) have been identified in older adults who fall within 6 months following a hip fracture.[343]

Rehabilitation for vertebral compression fractures. Individuals with acute VCFs can be difficult to treat, because pain and fear can be severe. Even when extra care is taken with logrolling techniques, transitional movements can be exquisitely painful, with the client crying and begging the PTA to stop. Arranging for premedication 45 to 60 minutes before treatment is advised, followed by modalities to modulate the pain and promote relaxation before attempting movement or exercise. Adaptive equipment, from wheelchair modifications to spinal orthotics to assistive devices (e.g., reachers/grabbers, stocking aids, raised toilet seats, bed grab bars), helps to improve posture, function, mobility, confidence, and independence. For clients with VCFs, the plan of care should include trunk extension strengthening and a cognitive–behavioral component to improve coping, especially for older adults. Improvements have been retained for at least 6 months in one randomized, controlled trial.[103]

Modalities and fractures. Many studies carried out on the effect of ultrasound waves on fracture healing show that bone heals faster when it responds to applied pressure. Low-intensity

(0.1 W/cm^2) pulsed ultrasound (2-millisecond bursts of sine waves of 1.0 MHz [frequency]; duration of 20 minutes daily) is an established therapy for fracture repair.[402]

In both animal and human trials, such ultrasounds have been shown to facilitate fresh fracture repair and initiate healing in fractures with repair defects. However, the mechanism by which ultrasound achieves these outcomes is not clear. One possible mechanism is the direct stimulation of bone formation. Ultrasound has a direct effect on blood flow distribution around a fracture site, resulting in greater callus formation. This increased circulation serves as a principal factor facilitating the acceleration of fracture healing by ultrasound.[15,371,402]

Ultrasound and electromagnetic stimulation are used most often for fracture healing where physicians anticipate healing problems or where nonunion has already occurred. A relatively new fracture management tool that incorporates the application of a specifically modified diagnostic ultrasound unit to heal fractures with the intention of accelerating repair is available.[401] Therapists in some parts of the United States are involved in the use and study of this modality.

Bone grafting. Bone grafting to enhance bone repair can be applied during the repair stage of bone formation. *Autogenous* bone grafting takes bone from another part of the body and implants it in the bony defect that requires healing. The graft is most often taken from the iliac crest or fibula and contains all the components needed for bone healing. Donor site pain is a common complaint and the primary reason why some people prefer to use *allogenic* bone graft material from a donor such as a bone bank. The use of biodegradable plastics has been developed to provide scaffolding for the regrowth of tissue with the potential for healing fractures and repairing bone lost to tumors, osteoporosis, trauma, and other disorders.

Commercially available demineralized bone matrix can be used to enhance bone healing, especially in people with nonunions or after the removal of bone cysts or fibrous lesions. Demineralized bone matrix still retains some of the original trabecular structure, which can function as a scaffold for osteoconduction.[119]

Complications. The healing of a fracture can be abnormal in one of several ways. The fracture may heal in the expected amount of time but in an unsatisfactory position with residual bony deformity, called *malunion.* The fracture may heal, but this may take considerably longer than the expected time *(delayed union);* or the fracture may fail to heal *(nonunion),* with resultant formation of either a fibrous union or a false joint *(pseudoarthrosis).* Loss of blood supply to the fracture fragments may impede healing by preventing adequate revascularization. Motion at the fracture site or an excessively wide gap can also contribute to nonunion. Individuals with nonunion often have pain, heat, and tenderness at the fracture site.

Other complications may include associated soft tissue injury, complications secondary to treatment, infection, skin ulceration, growth disturbances, posttraumatic degenerative arthritis, soft tissue or connective tissue adhesions, arthrodesis, myositis ossificans, osteomyelitis, refracture, nerve injury and neurologic complications, and vascular compromise.[317]

Complications of fractures require vigilance on the PTA's part and possibly quick action. Significant swelling can occur around the fracture site, and if the swelling is contained within a closed soft tissue compartment, *compartmental syndrome* may occur. Because of the progressively increased intracompartmental pressure, nerve and circulatory compromise can occur.

This condition may be acute or chronic. The compartment becomes exquisitely painful. Immediate action is required to relieve the stress and pressure during an acute episode of compartment syndrome.

Thorough sensory and motor examination may be warranted. If the PTA notes skin changes, decreased motor function, burning, paresthesia, or diminished reflexes, contact with the PT and the physician is necessary. Permanent damage and loss of function may result if this condition is not treated.[63]

Another complication associated with fractures is *fat embolism,* a potentially fatal event. The risk of developing this condition is related to fracture of long bones and the bony pelvis, which contain the most marrow. The fat globules from the bone marrow or from the subcutaneous tissue at the fracture site migrate to the lung parenchyma and can block pulmonary vessels, decreasing alveolar diffusion of oxygen. The initial symptoms typically appear 1 to 3 days after injury, but this complication can occur up to a week later. Subtle changes in behavior and orientation occur if there are emboli in the cerebral circulation. There may also be complaints of dyspnea and chest pain, diaphoresis, pallor, or cyanosis. A rash may develop on the anterior chest wall, neck, axillae, and shoulders. The onset of any of these symptoms warrants immediate physician contact.

The PTA must be alert to other complications that can occur following fracture, such as *loss of fixation* because of breakage of wires or displacement of screws. Other concerns include the possibility of *refracture, delayed union, malunion,* and *infection.*[335] Monitoring of delayed or nonunion fracture is usually done via regular radiographs; however, symptoms such as continued high pain levels or point tenderness may indicate that additional follow-up with the physician is necessary. Infection at the fracture site can delay healing; therefore fever or increased redness, tenderness, or irritation of the fracture site should be examined by the physician for possible infection. Anyone on bed rest is at risk for complications from immobility, including constipation, deep vein thrombosis, pulmonary embolism, and pneumonia.

Heterotopic Ossification
Definition and Incidence
Heterotopic ossification (HO) is defined as bone formation in nonosseous tissues (usually muscles and other soft tissue areas). It is considered a benign condition of abnormal bone formation in soft tissue that occurs most commonly after trauma such as fractures, surgical procedures (especially total hip replacements), spinal cord and traumatic brain injuries, burns, and amputations. HO is the most common complication of total hip arthroplasty.[43] Classification of HO is based on the anatomic location and effect on functional motion (Box 17.10).

There is an increased incidence of HO among military personnel with blast injuries. The extreme force destroys bone,

---

BOX 17.10   Classification of Heterotopic Ossification

Class I: Presence of heterotopic ossification but without functional range-of-motion limitations
Class II: Heterotopic ossification with limitations in all planes of motion
Class III: Heterotopic ossification with ankylosis preventing motion

Data from Hastings H: Classification and treatment of heterotopic ossification about the elbow and forearm, Hand Clin 10:417–437, 1994.

muscles, and tendons, resulting in amputation. Bone growth associated with HO in the residual limb does not follow a predictable pattern, and bone may grow into long spikes or develop more like cobwebs.

In addition to acquired forms of HO, there are forms due to hereditary causes such as fibrodysplasia ossificans progressiva, progressive osseous heteroplasia, and Albright's hereditary osteodystrophy. These conditions are extremely rare but do provide helpful information on the pathophysiology of the condition.[390]

Heterotopic ossification and *myositis ossificans* (MO) are terms often used interchangeably. Both conditions represent the deposition of mature lamellar bone and share radiographic and histologic characteristics, but the locations in which they occur are different. HO develops in nonosseous tissues, whereas MO is isolated to formation in bruised, damaged, or inflamed muscle.[39]

HO in people with spinal cord injuries is often referred to as *neurogenic heterotopic ossification* (NHO). NHO appears to be related more to the degree of completeness of spinal cord injury than the level involved; individuals with complete transverse spinal cord injuries are more likely to develop HO compared with those with incomplete spinal cord injuries.[39]

Risk factors for HO include a serious traumatic injury, previous history of HO, hypertrophic osteoarthritis, ankylosing spondylitis (AS), and diffuse idiopathic skeletal hyperostosis (DISH). Men seem to be at higher risk for HO than women. Other risk factors may include Paget's disease, rheumatoid arthritis (RA), posttraumatic arthritis, neural axis and thermal injuries, and osteonecrosis.[39,43]

Surgery-related factors may contribute to the formation of HO. Individuals who have undergone multiple surgical interventions over a short period are at increased risk of HO. This may be attributed to the extensive damage to soft tissues, presence of disseminated bone dust, or formation of hematoma. Length of time in surgery has also been implicated.[39]

HO occurs in 1% to 3% of the burn population. It appears to be related more to the degree of thermal injury than to the location of the burn. Individuals with third-degree burns affecting more than 20% of the total body surface are at greatest risk for the development of HO. Systemic physiologic factors in conjunction with local factors are the likely underlying etiology.[77,151]

Structures Involved

Sites affected most often include the hip, elbow, knee, shoulder, and temporomandibular joints. The elbow is the most common site of HO in burn clients; of the 1% to 3% of burn clients affected, the elbow is involved more than 90% of the time.[151] Typically, a bridge of ectopic bone forms across the posterolateral aspect of the elbow, possibly filling in the olecranon fossa.

Direct trauma is the most common cause of heterotopic bone formation in the elbow. It appears that there is a link between the severity of injury and the amount of ectopic bone formation that develops. Someone who sustains a massive traumatic injury is very likely to develop HO; HO is five times more likely if there is both fracture and dislocation of the elbow.[39]

Individuals with traumatic brain injury are predisposed to HO, most likely due to osteoinductive factors released at the site of the brain injury, although little is known about this process.[95] In the case of bone fracture or reaming of the bone during joint replacements, bone marrow (which is capable of forming bone) may spread into well-vascularized muscle tissue. Bone marrow combined with growth factors from traumatized tissues may set off a series of steps leading to bone development and HO.[17,43]

In the acute phase, the inflammatory process results in edema and degeneration of muscle tissue. After a few weeks, the inflamed tissue is replaced with cartilage and bone, with the bone undergoing intensive turnover as if forming bone callus in fractures.[362]

In HO, the ectopic bone is not enveloped by periosteum. Instead there are three zones. The center is made up of dense cells and is surrounded by a layer of osteoid. The outermost layer consists of highly organized bone, although ectopic bone has twice the number of osteoclasts compared with normal bone and a higher number of osteoblasts as well.[408]

Signs and Symptoms

HO may be asymptomatic and without pain, but pain and loss of motion are the most common presenting symptoms, often within 2 weeks of the precipitating trauma, surgery, burn, or neurologic insult. Swelling, warmth, erythema, and tenderness mimic a low-grade infection or, in the case of surgery, the normal postoperative inflammation that is often present. The hallmark sign of HO is a progressive loss of joint motion at a time when posttraumatic inflammation should be resolving.

As the ectopic ossification advances, the acute symptoms described may subside, but motion continues to decrease, even with intervention such as dynamic and/or static progressive splinting. Over the next 3 to 6 months, the HO matures and the individual develops a rigid or abrupt end feel, with pain at the end ROM. Delayed nerve palsy is common when the elbow is affected.[39]

Common Tests and Measures

Different classification schemes are used depending on the site affected. Most grade the condition based on a scale from 0 to 3 or 0 to 4. Grade 0 is no islands of bone visible on x-ray. The final grade is bony ankylosis, with progressive involvement between the lowest and highest grade (e.g., bone spurs, periarticular bone formation).

Radiographic evidence with mineralization may be observed 4 to 6 weeks after the trauma (sometimes as early as 2 weeks after the incident event). X-rays show both the location, extent, and maturity of pathologic bone. HO must be differentiated from metastatic calcification, most often associated with hypercalcemia, and from dystrophic calcifications in tumors. History and radiographic examination usually provide the tools needed to diagnose this condition. Ultrasound may prove useful in diagnosing HO around the hip or elbow.

A CT scan may be best to show the exact location and involvement of the articular surfaces. Laboratory tests to measure the level of serum alkaline phosphatase are used by some, but they are not consistently accurate.

Common Management

Radiation applied to the damaged limb site within a few days after the injury may respond but there is always the risk of impaired healing for those with bone fractures. Surgical resection is delayed until the bone matures and develops a distinct fibrous capsule in order to minimize trauma to the tissues and reduce the risk of recurrence and may only be done in cases where ADLs are compromised by loss of motion.[151]

Indication for surgery may not be just the presence of HO but rather the severity of functional restriction when loss of motion prevents the individual from using the affected extremity. A comprehensive rehabilitation program is needed to maximize motion, restore function, and reduce the risk of developing ankylosis. Once surgical removal is done, radiation and non-steroidal antiinflammatory drugs (NSAIDs) are continued to prevent recurrence.

Prevention. Prevention is recommended for individuals at high risk of ectopic ossification, including those with neurologic injury, burns, history of HO, and/or a history of other conditions previously mentioned. The best prevention for HO is to avoid soft tissue trauma, especially among high-risk individuals undergoing surgery of any kind. Complete wound lavage and the removal of all bone debris and reamings may help prevent HO.[43]

Measures can be taken to prevent HO, such as radiation treatment and pharmaceuticals such as NSAIDs or diphosphonates, which inhibit osteoid cells from calcifying. The effect lasts only as long as the drug is taken. GI disturbance and osteomalacia are adverse side effects of this treatment, making it less than optimal.

NSAIDs (e.g., indomethacin) are effective in reducing the frequency and magnitude of ectopic bone formation in some areas (e.g., hip). Used during the first 3 weeks postoperatively, indomethacin inhibits precursor (undifferentiated) cells from developing into osteoblasts.

Low-dose external beam radiation is another effective preventive measure. Fractionated radiation has been shown to be effective in preventing HO from developing when delivered within 72 hours after surgery.[201] It can be used alone or in combination with NSAIDs.

17.1 Special Implications for the PTA: Heterotopic Ossification The PTA's management of HO has evolved in the recent past based on knowledge of the condition. Traditional thinking that passive ROM is contraindicated with HO has been abandoned. There was concern that passive ROM could lead to further bone growth, but this has not proven accurate.[39]

A specific program of physical therapy intervention can be planned based on the timing of the referral. During the acute and edematous phase (first 1 to 2 weeks postoperatively), proper measures are taken to reduce swelling, minimize scar formation, and provide pain management to allow for maximum participation in the program. ROM exercises (passive and active) can begin but must take into account the type and extent of injury present (e.g., fracture, joint instability). Forcible joint manipulation can lead to muscle tears and ossification within the muscle and is contraindicated.

Phase 2 occurs during the inflammatory stage approximately 2 to 6 weeks after the injury or incident event. Unorganized scar tissue forms during this phase but remains soft and deformable so that ROM gains can be made. The soft tissues still respond to various modalities, and self-passive stretching with weighted stretches and/or dynamic or static progressive splinting is most likely to recapture lost motion. Specific recommendations for HO affecting the elbow are available.[39]

The PTA should continue to encourage functional use of affected areas, including strengthening when appropriate, and emphasize motion throughout all motions, even if x-rays show HO developing around week 4 to 6 in this phase. By week 6, bone fractures are typically healed, allowing for more aggressive splinting. Scar tissue is fully formed but still malleable during this third (fibrotic) phase from 6 to 12 weeks. Splinting and resistive exercises can continue to maximize gains in motion.

Finally, during the last phase, 3 to 6 months after injury or surgery, scar tissue is organized and fibrotic. The individual may continue to make small gains, but often motion has reached a plateau and splints are discontinued gradually. Clients should be encouraged to continue a home strengthening program for at least another 6 months.[39]

Complications

Areas of calcification and bone spurs may progress to ankylosis. Pressure from the bone formation can result in pressure ulcers and interfere with skin grafts. Loss of motion can have serious consequences for daily function, especially for those individuals who are already neurologically compromised.

Osteochondroses

A number of clinical disorders of ossification centers (epiphyses) in growing children share the common denominator of avascular necrosis and its sequelae. These disorders are grouped together and referred to as the *osteochondroses*[317] with multiple synonyms (epiphysitis, osteochondritis, aseptic necrosis, ischemic epiphyseal necrosis). There are additional eponyms based on the name of the person or persons who described the disorder as well, such as Kohler's disease (tarsal-navicular bone disease), Osgood-Schlatter disease, and Legg–Calvé–Perthes disease. The underlying etiologic factors and pathogenesis are similar in all these entities, and the clinical manifestations are determined by the stresses and strains present. Most susceptible areas are the epiphyses, which are entirely covered by articular cartilage and therefore poorly vascularized.

Osteochondritis Dissecans

Definition and incidence. Osteochondritis dissecans (OCD) is a disorder of one or more ossification sites with localized subchondral necrosis followed by recalcification. This condition affects the subchondral bone and the layer of articular cartilage just above. A piece of articular cartilage and fragment of bone separate and pull away from the underlying bone. These fragments can become loose bodies in the joint; the most common site of involvement is the medial femoral condyle.

Structures involved. OCD is caused by repetitive microtrauma resulting in ischemia and disruption of the subchondral growth. The articular cartilage softens, and fragment separation leads to cartilage injury that can progress to form a crater. Although this process can occur in any joint, it is most commonly found at the knee, elbow, or ankle. Approximately 70% to 80% of cases occur on the posterior aspect of the medial femoral condyle.[173]

Signs and symptoms. Activity-related pain, swelling, and giving way are common symptoms. Pain is increased with passive knee extension and tibial internal rotation and relieved with tibial external rotation. This test is called Wilson's sign.

Common tests and measures. Radiologic studies are usually the first step toward a diagnosis of OCD and are useful in predicting prognosis. MRI is more accurate for estimating the size of the lesion and the extent of the damage to cartilage and subchondral bone.[173]

Antalgic gait and tenderness to palpation may be the primary complaints. PTs should focus on measuring ROM loss, tenderness to palpation, changes in posture or gait pattern, and functional involvement. The Lysholm scale may be used as an outcome measure for these clients.

Common management. Management varies with the person's age and the severity of the lesion. Nonoperative management is favored for juvenile OCD, which will usually heal in 10 to 18 months. There is debate about the best method and length of immobilization for these clients, and research continues to develop a comprehensive protocol that includes activity modification, protected weight bearing, or immobilization for 4 to 6 weeks.[173]

Operative management is recommended for adults with detached or unstable lesions or juveniles who do not respond to conservative care. Surgical interventions involve removal of loose bodies from the joint, fixation of unstable fragments, and restoration of the integrity of the articular cartilage. Surgeons may use arthroscopic drilling, debridement, internal fixation (using screws, pins or plugs), or transplantation of periosteum depending on the size and extent of the lesion.[173]

Physical therapy interventions may include modalities to control effusion and pain while providing instruction in the use of braces and assistive devices. Later, physical therapy will include quadriceps strengthening and gradual return to activities.

Osteonecrosis

Definition and incidence. The term *osteonecrosis* refers to the death of bone and bone marrow cellular components as a result of loss of blood supply in the absence of infection. *Avascular necrosis* and *aseptic necrosis* are synonyms for this condition.

The femoral head is the most common site of this disorder (sometimes called Chandler's disease), but other sites can include the scaphoid, talus, proximal humerus, tibial plateau, and small bones of the wrist and foot. Avascular necrosis is the underlying cause for 10% of total hip replacement surgeries[256] and overall affects approximately 20,000 people annually, often between the second and fifth decades of life.[187]

Structures involved. Osteocytic necrosis results from tissue ischemia brought on by the impairment of blood-conducting vessels. A minimum of 2 hours of complete ischemia and anoxia is necessary for permanent loss of bone tissue.[160] The bony ischemia may be secondary to trauma disrupting the arterial supply or to thrombosis disrupting the microcirculation. Bones or portions of bones that have limited collateral circulation and few vascular foramina are susceptible to avascular necrosis. Box 17.11 lists conditions associated with osteonecrosis. A number of these conditions are linked to osteonecrosis by the development of fat emboli (caused by altered fat metabolism) in the vascular tree of the involved bone. The conditions associated with the development of fat emboli include alcoholism, obesity, pregnancy, pancreatitis, medications (e.g., oral contraceptives, corticosteroids), and unrelated fractures. Many cases of femoral head osteonecrosis are idiopathic (i.e., no known cause or risk factor can be identified).

Osteonecrosis has also been recognized as a complication in human immunodeficiency virus (HIV)–positive individuals; in fact, individuals who are HIV positive have a 100-fold greater risk of developing osteonecrosis than the general population.[249] The exact mechanism for this remains unknown. More recently, the use of bisphosphonates has been linked with osteonecrosis of the jaw (sometimes referred to as "dead jaw syndrome"), especially after trauma to the teeth or bones of the jaw such as occurs with dental surgery (e.g., tooth extraction). The reason this happens is not entirely clear. This phenomenon is most likely to occur in individuals treated for bone cancer with intravenous bisphosphonates. The dosage of intravenous bisphosphonates can be as much as 12 times more than the oral bisphosphonate dosage prescribed for osteoporosis. Individuals with cancer treated this way also undergo other bone-weakening treatments (e.g., chemotherapy, radiation therapy).

Certain bones are more vulnerable to osteonecrosis than others. These bones are covered extensively by cartilage, have few vascular foramina, and have limited collateral circulation. The femoral head is a prime example of a bone at risk. The superolateral two-thirds of the femoral head receives its blood supply almost entirely from the lateral epiphyseal branches of the medial femoral circumflex artery (Fig. 17.13). The only other source of blood for the femoral head is the medial epiphyseal artery (contained within the ligamentum teres), which has limited anastomoses with the lateral epiphyseal vessels. Hip dislocation or fracture of the neck of the femur can compromise the precarious vascular supply to the head of the femur.

The talus, scaphoid, and proximal humerus are also susceptible to osteonecrosis.

As the ischemia progresses, repair processes occur but are not capable of preventing necrosis and deformation of the

---

BOX 17.11 Conditions Associated with Osteonecrosis

- Idiopathic
- Trauma (e.g., fall)
- Systemic lupus erythematosus
- Pancreatitis
- Diabetes mellitus
- Hyperlipidemia
- Cushing's disease
- Gout
- Sickle cell disease
- Alcoholism
- Obesity
- Pregnancy
- Medications
  - Oral contraceptives
  - Corticosteroids
  - Bisphosphonates (under investigation)
- Organ transplantation (medication related)
- Human immunodeficiency virus (HIV) infection
- Radiation therapy (less common)
- Dysbaric disease (deep sea diving; rare)

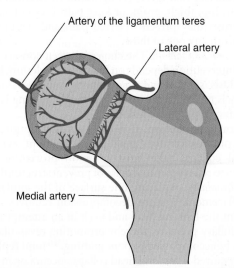

FIG. 17.13 Blood supply to the femoral head in a child. (From Bullough PG: Orthopedic pathology, ed 5, London, 2010, Mosby.)

Artery of the ligamentum teres

Lateral artery

Medial artery

bone, such as flattening and collapse of the femoral head. The articular cartilage and acetabulum are usually spared until late in the disease process, but the articular cartilage may be lifted off the underlying bone, resulting in irreparable damage to the joint.[146] The entire process extends over many years, and unlike in osteochondrosis of immature bone (e.g., Legg–Calvé–Perthes disease), spontaneous healing never occurs.

Signs and symptoms. Often no symptoms are observed during the initial development of osteonecrosis even though an ischemic condition of the bone exists.[146] Hip pain is the usual initial presenting complaint, with a gradual onset—sometimes of many weeks' duration—before diagnosis. The pain may be mild and intermittent initially but will progress to become severe, especially during weight-bearing activities.

If the femur is involved, the pain may be noted in the groin, thigh, or medial knee area. An antalgic gait is noted, and pain provocation occurs with weight-bearing activities and hip ROM exercises, especially internal rotation and flexion and adduction. The affected individual will report a slowly progressive stiffening of the joint. When fracture occurs, it is usually at the junction between necrotic bone and reparative bone, possibly extending down through the reparative interface to the healthy inferior cortex of the femoral neck.[237]

Eventually degenerative joint changes and osteoarthrosis occur at the involved hip joint; the pathologic process is often relentless, with collapse of the femoral head imminent in spite of medical intervention.[146]

Osteonecrosis of the jaw is characterized by exposed bone in the mouth, numbness or heaviness in the jaw, pain, swelling, infection, and loose teeth. Delayed or poor wound healing after dental surgery may be the first indication of a problem. Crepitus as the jaw opens and closes may be present and is often described as like the sound of someone walking on ice.

Common tests and measures. Plain films may be normal initially. Bone scan, MRI, and CT scans are much more sensitive procedures and detect subtle bony changes.

PTs are always advised to obtain a thorough and complete history from clients, especially in the presence of musculoskeletal manifestations of apparently unknown cause. Because osteonecrosis is difficult to identify early, knowledge of causative factors (see Box 17.11) is important. Differential diagnosis of lumbar, hip, thigh, groin, or knee pain is essential, because osteonecrosis may present referred pain and symptoms as if coming from any one of these.

Common management. The choice between conservative and surgical intervention depends on the size of the lesion, how early the diagnosis is made, and whether bony collapse has occurred. If surgery is not indicated, protected weight bearing is essential to prevent collapse of the lesion.

Surgical intervention. If needed, surgical options include core decompression for small lesions without evidence of structural collapse (the most common procedure in early diagnosis) to relieve pain and delay or prevent structural collapse, *hemi-arthroplasty* (replacing one surface of the joint), or total joint replacement.[202] Core decompression removes a core of bone from the femoral head and neck in an attempt to relieve intermedullary pressure, thereby promoting revascularization. This may be accompanied by bone grafting.[360] Joint replacement may be required if femoral head collapse occurs or in order to prevent this complication. However, this procedure is limited by young age and high activity level as well as the limited life expectancy of the prosthesis.

New techniques for bone stimulation may be used, such as replacing the dead bone with living bone from the individual's fibula to give added strength to the damaged area and possibly prevent or postpone joint arthroplasty in young individuals; see also the section Fracture: Common Management in this chapter.

An osteotomy may be performed to shift the site to where maximal weight bearing occurs on a particular joint surface. Analgesics and NSAIDs are used for symptomatic relief of pain.

Prognosis. The prognosis depends on the extent of damage that has occurred before diagnosis in the case of nontraumatic disease. Unfortunately, many cases are diagnosed in an advanced stage of disease, when minimally invasive surgical procedures are no longer helpful.[187] Early intervention (both surgical and nonsurgical) has definitely improved the outcome, but many people with femoral head osteonecrosis experience irreversible damage to the joint and will need total arthroplasty.

17.2 Special Implications for the PTA: Osteonecrosis When treating people at risk for osteonecrosis, PTAs must consider the possibility of fracture if there is a sudden worsening of pain complaints followed by a sudden, dramatic loss in ROM. Once the diagnosis is made, close communication with the physician is important for safe progression of weight bearing and exercise.

Following surgical intervention, the usual postoperative precautions and indications apply for minimization of complications (e.g., deep vein thrombosis), early mobilization, assessment for gait-assistive devices, gait training, demonstration of motion restrictions, and pain management.

In the case of microvascular bone transplantation, some physicians caution clients to avoid high-impact activities such as jumping, skiing, competitive tennis, and carrying more than 100 lb, although long-term studies of these stresses on repaired or reconstructed bones have not been carried out.

Legg–Calvé–Perthes Disease

Definition and incidence. Legg–Calvé–Perthes disease, also known as *coxa plana* (flat hip) and *osteochondritis deformans juvenilis*, is epiphyseal aseptic necrosis (or avascular necrosis) of the proximal end of the femur. It is a self-limiting disorder characterized by avascular necrosis of the capital femoral epiphysis (the center of ossification of the femoral head). Complete revascularization of the avascular epiphysis occurs over time without any treatment.

This condition occurs in approximately 1 in 1200 children, primarily boys (5:1 ratio of boys to girls) between the ages of 3 and 12 years, making it the most common of the osteochondroses. Legg–Calvé–Perthes disease occurs 10 times more often in whites than in blacks.

Deformation of the epiphysis with changes in the shape of the femoral head and the acetabulum occur during the process of revascularization in a significant portion of affected individuals. This may lead to degenerative arthritis in young adult life.[164]

Structures involved. The direct cause is a reduction in blood flow to the joint, though what causes this is unknown. It may be that the artery of the ligamentum teres femoris closes too early, not allowing time for the circumflex femoral artery to take over. Genetic coagulopathy has been suggested,[361] possibly triggered by exposure to cigarette smoke in utero and during childhood.[102]

Delay in bone age relative to the child's chronologic age suggests a possible general disorder of skeletal growth with focal

TABLE 17.3 Stages of Legg–Calvé–Perthes Disease

Stage	Time Period	Pathogenesis
Avascular (stage I)	1–2 weeks	Quiet phase: Spontaneous vascular interruption to the epiphysis causes necrosis of the femoral head with degenerative changes; hip synovium and joint capsule are swollen, edematous, and hyperemic; joint space widens; cells of the epiphysis die, but bone remains unchanged.
Revascularization (stage II; fragmentation stage)	6–12 months	Vascular reaction: New blood supply causes bone resorption and deposition of new bone cells; deformity from pressure on weakened area occurs; the entire or anterior one-half of the epiphysis of the femoral head is necrotic; increased blood supply and decalcification of bone cause softening at the junction of the femoral neck and the capital epiphyseal plate; granulation tissue and blood vessels invade the dead bone, now detectable on radiographic examination.
Reparative (stage III; residual stage)	2–3 years	New bone replaces necrotic bone; the necrotic: femoral head is replaced or surrounded by new bone (sometimes giving it an appearance of a head inside a head; see Fig. 17.14); collapse and flattening of the femoral head causes the femoral neck to become short and wide, with subluxation, progressive deformity, and even fracture possible.
Regenerative (intravascular)	Final months	Completion of healing or regeneration gradually reforms the head of the femur into live spongy bone; restoration of the femoral head to a normal shape is more likely in younger children and only if the anterior epiphysis was involved; residual deformity may exist in some cases that can lead to the gradual development of joint disease (osteoarthritis).

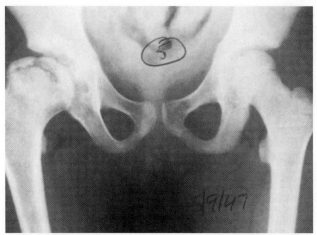

FIG. 17.14 Radiograph of lower pelvis in Legg–Calvé–Perthes disease after revascularization of the necrotic femoral head shows enlargement of the head, with the original necrotic ossification center seen as a "head within a head." (From Bullough PG: Orthopedic pathology, ed 3, London, 1997, Mosby-Wolfe.)

expression in the hip. Mechanisms proposed to explain the delay in bone maturation include genetic, endocrine, nutritional, and socioeconomic factors.[189]

The disease process consists of four stages lasting from 2 to 5 years (Table 17.3 and Fig. 17.14). Because the growth plate of the femoral head lies above the insertion of the capsule of the hip joint in children and because the epiphyseal plate acts as a firm barrier to blood flow between the metaphysis and epiphysis, the femoral head depends on vessels that track along the surface of the neck of the femur to enter the epiphysis above the growth plate.

Delays in bone maturation observed with this disease are correlated with the stage of the disease. The decrease in bone age delay in the later stages of the disease indicates that as the disease progresses, bone maturation accelerates and tries to catch up with the chronologic age. This phenomenon is referred to as *bone maturation acceleration*. This process occurs earlier in the epiphyses of the lower ends of the radius and ulna and short bones of the hands compared with the carpal bones.[189]

Signs and symptoms. The Legg–Calvé–Perthes condition is characterized by insidious onset, initially presenting as the intermittent appearance of a limp on the involved side with hip pain described as soreness or aching with accompanying stiffness. The pain may be present in the groin and along the entire length of the thigh following the path of the obturator nerve or referred pain just in the area of the knee. There is usually pinpoint tenderness over the hip capsule.

Painful symptoms are aggravated by activity and fatigue and relieved somewhat by rest. Mild Legg–Calvé–Perthes disease is characterized by partial femoral head collapse, retention of a full range of hip abduction and rotation, and lack of subluxation on radiographic examination.

Delay in bone maturation is a common feature of this condition. Skeletal development is unevenly timed in the growing bones, with the maximum delay occurring in the distal limb segments. As the condition progresses, there are decreases in active and passive ROM, as well as limited physiologic (accessory) motion affecting walking and running.

Severe Legg–Calvé–Perthes disease begins later and involves collapse of the whole femoral head, stiffness, and subluxation. Atrophy of the thigh musculature and restriction of hip abduction and rotation may develop. Short stature may develop as a result of epiphyseal dysplasia, and in those individuals who are left untreated, a flat femoral head will develop that is prone to degenerative joint disease.[296]

Late complications in adults with a childhood history of Legg–Calvé–Perthes include early osteoarthritis of the hip and acetabular labral tears. Hip, groin, or back pain may be the first symptom in affected adults. Postural asymmetry, leg length discrepancy, decreased ROM, and decreased strength may be accompanied by an abnormal gait pattern.[20]

Common tests and measures. Physical examination, clinical history, and radiographic examination (Fig. 17.15) confirm the diagnosis. MRI is widely accepted as the imaging method of choice, allowing early diagnosis and providing staging information necessary for adequate management.

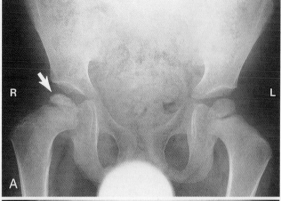

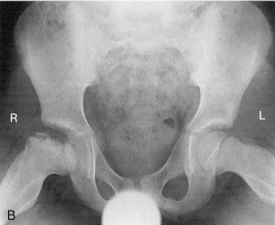

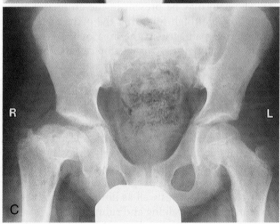

FIG. 17.15 Legg–Calvé–Perthes disease. (A) Anterior view of the pelvis demonstrates fragmentation and sclerosis of the right femoral epiphysis *(arrow)* in a 6-year-old male. (B) Follow-up film obtained 8 years later shows continuing deformity resulting from osteonecrosis. (C) The child developed significant degenerative arthritis by age 12. (From Mettler FA: *Essentials of radiology,* ed 3, Philadelphia, 2014, Saunders.)

There are several different classifications used to determine severity of disease and prognosis. The Catterall classification specifies four different groups defined by radiographic appearance during the period of greatest bone loss. The Salter–Thomson classification simplifies the Catterall classification by reducing it down to two groups: group A (Catterall I, II), in which less than 50% of the ball is involved, and group B (Catterall III, IV), in which more than 50% of the ball is involved. Both classifications share the view that if less than 50% of the

ball is involved, the prognosis is good, whereas more than 50% involvement indicates a potentially poor prognosis.

Many doctors use these classifications because they provide an accurate method of determining prognosis and help in determining the appropriate form of treatment.

Common management.

General principles. The goal of treatment is to limit deformity and preserve the integrity of the femoral head. Mild disease may not require intervention, but careful follow-up with radiographic examination every 3 months is needed to observe for deterioration and progression of the disease.[226]

Current methods of treatment attempt to prevent deformation of the femoral head and restore the spherical and congruent femoral head contour of the acetabulum. This is done by ensuring that the vulnerable anterolateral part of the avascular capital femoral epiphysis is contained within the acetabulum, a process called *containment.* The femoral head can be molded to a normal shape as it heals. The idea is to accomplish this while the bone is biologically plastic and before it is irreparably deformed.[164]

The closer to normal the femoral head is when growth stops, the better the hip will function in later life. The way that surgeons achieve this goal is through containment. In the past, weight bearing was minimized, but more recently, therapy allows the child to continue weight bearing with the femur in an abducted and internally rotated position. Keeping the head of the femur well seated in the acetabulum decreases focal areas of increased load and minimizes distortion, thereby maintaining ROM and preventing deformity.

The femoral head must be held in the joint socket (acetabulum) as much as possible. It is better if the hip is allowed to move and is not held completely still in the joint socket. Joint motion is necessary for nutrition of the cartilage and for healthy growth of the joint. All treatment options for Legg–Calvé–Perthes disease try to position and hold the hip in the acetabulum as much as possible. This healing process can take several years.

Conservative care is usually continued for 2 to 4 years. A variety of splints, braces, and positional devices may be used to maintain the proper position. When lack of motion has become a problem, the child may be admitted to the hospital and placed in traction. Traction is used to quiet the inflammation. Anti-inflammatory medications may be prescribed. Physical therapy is used to restore the hip motion as the inflammation comes under control. This process usually takes about a week. Home traction may also be an option.

In some cases, surgery will be required to obtain adequate containment. Sometimes adequate motion cannot be regained with traction and physical therapy alone. If the condition is longstanding, the muscles may have contracted or shrunk and cannot be stretched back out.

Surgical interventions. To help restore motion, the surgeon may recommend a *tenotomy* of the contracted muscles. When a tenotomy is performed, the tendon of the muscle that is overly tight is cut and lengthened. This is a simple procedure that requires only a small incision. The tendon eventually scars down in the lengthened position, and no functional loss is noticeable.

Surgical treatment for containment may be best in older children who are not compliant with brace treatment or where the psychologic effects of wearing braces may outweigh the benefits. Surgical containment does not require long-term use of braces or casts. Once the procedure has been performed and the bones have healed, the child can pursue normal activities as tolerated.

Surgical treatment for containment usually consists of procedures that realign either the femur (thighbone), the acetabulum (hip socket), or both. Realignment of the femur is called a *femoral osteotomy*. This procedure changes the angle of the femoral neck so that the femoral head points more toward the socket. To perform this procedure, an incision is made in the side of the thigh. The bone of the femur is cut and realigned in a new position. A large metal plate and screws are then inserted to hold the bones in the new position until the bone has healed. The plate and screws may need to be removed once the bone has healed.

Realignment of the acetabulum is called a *pelvic osteotomy*. This procedure changes the angle of the acetabulum (socket) so that it covers or contains more of the femoral head. For this procedure, an incision is made in the side of the buttock. The bone of the pelvis is cut and realigned in a new position. Large metal pins or screws are then inserted to hold the bones in the new position until the bone has healed. The pins usually must be removed once the bone has healed.

If there is a serious structural change in the anatomy of the hip, there may need to be further surgery to restore the alignment closer to normal. This is usually not considered until growth stops. As a child grows, there will be some remodeling that occurs in the hip joint. This may improve the situation such that further surgery is unnecessary.

In severe cases, both femoral osteotomy and pelvic osteotomy may be combined to obtain even more containment.

Prognosis. Legg–Calvé–Perthes disease may vary in severity from a mild self-healing problem with no sequelae to a condition that will destroy the hip unless serious action is taken. Early on, it may be difficult to determine which course the disease will follow. Even though the disease is self-limiting, the prognosis varies according to the age of onset (better prognosis in children whose onset is before age 5 years). Children older than age 8 years at the time of onset have a better outcome with surgical treatment than with nonoperative care.[136] There is some evidence to suggest that early delay in bone age (stage I of the disease) is linked with more severe disease.[189]

Older age, complete involvement of the femoral head, and noncompliance with treatment contribute to a poorer prognosis. Although girls are less likely to develop Legg–Calvé–Perthes disease compared with boys, they often have a poorer prognosis. The reason for this difference is unknown.

A delay in bone age maturation of more than 2 years in stage I of the disease has been linked with greater severity of the disease. However, children with Legg–Calvé–Perthes disease have a normal onset of puberty, and by the time they are 12 to 15 years old, their stature and bone age are the same as those of their peers.[178]

17.3 Special Implications for the PTA: Legg–Calvé–Perthes Disease PTAs may be involved in gait training, aquatic therapy, and ROM exercises during this period. It should be emphasized to the child and family that Legg–Calvé–Perthes disease is a long-term problem, with treatment aimed at minimizing damage while the disease runs its course. Performing exercises daily is essential during the healing process to ensure that the femur and hip socket have a perfectly smooth interface. This will minimize the long-term effects of the disease. As sufferers age, problems in the knee and back can arise as a result of the abnormal posture and stride adopted to protect the affected joint.

Surgery may be performed to contain the femoral head in the acetabulum, especially in children older than age 6 years with serious involvement of the femoral head. Hip replacements are relatively common during the sixth decade as the already damaged hip suffers routine wear; this varies from individual to individual.

Osgood–Schlatter Syndrome/Sinding–Larsen–Johansson Syndrome

Definition and incidence. Osgood–Schlatter syndrome (osteochondrosis) results from fibers of the patellar tendon pulling small bits of immature bone from the tibial tuberosity. In the past, Osgood–Schlatter was considered a form of osteochondritis (inflammation of bone and cartilage), but more recent thinking suggests that the process is one part of the spectrum of mechanical problems related to the extensor mechanism. Rather than being an actual degenerative "disease," Osgood–Schlatter is considered a form of tendinitis of the patellar tendon and therefore referred to as a "syndrome." It is most commonly seen in active adolescent boys ages 10 to 15 years but can also affect girls ages 8 to 13 years. The ratio of boys to girls affected by Osgood–Schlatter disease is 3:1.

Sinding–Larsen–Johansson syndrome involves the same mechanism acting at the proximal patellar attachment and resulting in fragmentation of the patella rather than the tibial tuberosity. It usually occurs in younger children than Osgood–Schlatter syndrome, but the general principles of examination and treatment are essentially the same.[227]

Structures involved. Both Osgood–Schlatter syndrome and Sinding–Larsen–Johansson syndrome are probably the result of indirect trauma, such as a force produced by the sudden, powerful contraction of the quadriceps muscle during an activity or repetitive stress before complete fusion of the epiphysis to the main bone has occurred. It is further aggravated by traction associated with bone growth in adolescents and the presence of external tibial torsion. Other causes include local deficient blood supply and genetic factors.

Another possible cause is abnormal alignment in the legs. Children who are knock-kneed or flat-footed seem to be most prone to the condition. These postures put a sharper angle between the quadriceps muscle and the patellar tendon. This angle is called the *Q angle*. A large Q angle puts more tension on the bone growth plate of the tibial tuberosity, increasing the chances for an Osgood–Schlatter lesion to develop. A high-riding patella, called *patella alta*, is also thought to contribute to development of Osgood–Schlatter lesions.[225]

In young athletes, the tendon is attached to immature bone that is weaker than normal adult bone. With excessive stresses on the tendon from running and jumping, the structure becomes irritated and a tendinitis begins. Often fragments representing cartilage or bone formations are found on the surface of the patellar tendon and are a potential cause of pain. These patellar tendon fibers can actually pull fragments away from the tibial epiphysis (Fig. 17.16).

Signs and symptoms. Clinically, clients with Osgood–Schlatter syndrome report constant aching and pain at the site of the tibial tubercle (just below the kneecap), which is often enlarged on visual examination. Besides the obvious soft tissue swelling, there may be localized heat and tenderness, the latter elicited with direct pressure over the tibial tubercle.

In contrast, clients with Sinding–Larsen–Johansson syndrome are usually 9 to 12 years old and report pain and tenderness at the distal pole of the patella.[227]

For both groups, symptoms are aggravated by any activity that causes forceful contraction of the patellar tendon against the tubercle, such as active knee extension or resisted knee flexion (e.g., going up or down stairs, running, jumping, biking, hiking, kneeling, squatting). Many children with this condition also have significant tightness in the hamstrings, iliotibial

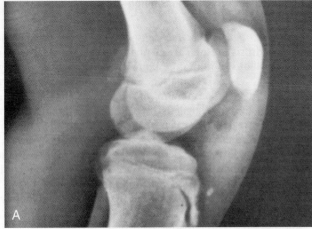

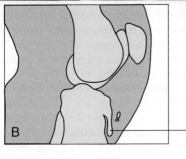

— Avulsed and
fragmented
tibial tubercle

FIG. 17.16 Clinical radiograph of the knee in a 12-year-old child shows fragmentation and avulsion of the tibial tubercle. Swelling below the knee and an enlarged tibial tuberosity may be observed clinically. This condition, known as Osgood–Schlatter disease, is probably posttraumatic. (From Bullough PG: Orthopedic pathology, ed 5, London, 2010, Mosby.)

band, triceps surae (bellies of the gastrocnemius and soleus), and quadriceps muscles. Tightness in these areas can potentially increase the flexion moment and subsequent stresses at the tibial tubercle.

Common tests and measures. Clinical diagnosis may be confirmed by radiograph or ultrasonography. Although the films may be normal, epiphyseal separation, soft tissue swelling, and bone fragmentation can be visualized in many cases. It is important to differentiate it from similar conditions such as patellar tendinitis, chondromalacia patella, or synovial plica.

17.4 Special Implications for the PTA: Osgood–Schlatter Syndrome/Sinding–Larsen–Johansson Syndrome The PTA should record loss of joint ROM, location of tenderness to palpation, and joint effusion. Current activity levels and response to exercise should also be recorded.

The management of Osgood–Schlatter and Sinding–Larsen–Johansson syndromes are essentially the same. Activity modification is recommended until symptoms have subsided. Immobilization is no longer advocated with this condition, although rest from aggravating activities is necessary. The time frame for decreased activity ranges from 2 to 3 weeks in some individuals to 2 to 3 months or more in others. Enough time must be allowed for revascularization, healing, and ossification of the tibial tubercle before resumption of unrestricted athletic participation. NSAIDs and ice are used regularly.

Treatment should include exercises to address the mechanical inefficiencies of the extensor mechanism, stretching for any areas of inflexibility (usually the hamstrings), and strengthening areas of weakness such as ankle dorsiflexion, and pain-free quadriceps strengthening.

Balance and coordination should be assessed and rehabilitation provided as appropriate. Support may be provided through the use of a knee sleeve or brace.

About 90% of children with this condition respond well to nonoperative treatment. Complete recovery is expected with closure of the tibial growth plate.[100] Conservative measures are usually sufficient to provide pain relief and resolution of local swelling. Some individuals experience mild discomfort in kneeling; activity restriction is imposed until the individual is symptom free.

When conservative care fails to resolve painful symptoms, full-extension immobilization of the leg through reinforced elastic knee support, cast, or splint may be prescribed for 6 to 8 weeks. In chronic, unresolved cases, surgery may be necessary to remove the epiphyseal ossicle that forms in the tendon. In extreme cases, the epiphysis may actually be removed or holes drilled into the tibial tubercle to facilitate revascularization of the area.

JOINT

This section presents information on common disorders that effect joint functioning. Many of these processes compromise the joint space and cause pain. Included in this section are chondrolysis, osteoarthritis, and rheumatic diseases. PTAs are likely to manage clients with these disorders as their primary or secondary diagnosis.

Chondrolysis
Definition and Incidence
Chondrolysis is a process of progressive cartilage degeneration resulting in narrowing of the joint space and loss of motion. It is seen most often as a complication of slipped capital femoral epiphysis (SCFE) but can occur in association with infection, trauma, and prolonged immobilization for any reason. Trauma can also include orthopedic procedures such as arthroscopic meniscectomy, shoulder arthroscopy, anterior cruciate ligament reconstruction, and thermal capsulorrhaphy.[44,120,192,284]

Structures Involved
The hip is the most likely location for chondrolysis to occur, but cases have been reported affecting the knee, shoulder, and ankle. Spontaneous chondrolysis without known risk factors occurs occasionally, most commonly in adolescent girls. In fact chondrolysis occurs five times more often in females than in males; adolescence is the most common period of onset.[411]

The etiology is unknown; many theories have been proposed, including nutritional abnormalities, mechanical injury, ischemia, abnormal chondrocyte metabolism, ischemia, and abnormal intracapsular pressure. There may be some evidence to support an autoimmune mechanism responsible for the cartilage destruction. Clearly, some disruption of the cartilage extracellular matrix occurs, leading to chondrolysis, but the key to the process has not been discovered.

Signs and Symptoms
Regardless of the underlying cause of this condition, the affected individual presents with progressive joint stiffness with progressive loss of motion and pain. Chondrolysis of the hip

causes anterior hip and/or groin pain accompanied by an antalgic gait. Soft tissue contracture can result in an apparent leg length discrepancy and pelvic obliquity with muscle atrophy. Painful ankylosis may develop in some individuals, whereas others experience an improvement in pain and ROM.[411]

Common Tests and Measures

Imaging studies are used to make the diagnosis. Plain radiographs are the first choice, but in difficult cases, the definitive diagnosis may be made on the basis of scintigraphy and/or MRI.

Common Management

Treatment begins with NSAIDs to control synovial inflammation. Protected weight bearing and maintaining joint motion are important components of the treatment plan. Surgery may be indicated, usually a capsulectomy tendon release of the adductor and iliopsoas, but the best course of operative treatment is unknown.[411]

Osteoarthritis

Definition and Incidence

Osteoarthritis (OA), or degenerative joint disease, is a slowly evolving articular disease that appears to originate in the cartilage and affects the underlying bone, soft tissues, and synovial fluid. OA is divided into two classifications: primary and secondary. *Primary OA* is a disorder of unknown cause, and the cascade of joint degeneration events associated with it is thought to be related to a defect in the articular cartilage. *Secondary OA* has a known cause, which may be trauma, infection, hemarthrosis, osteonecrosis, or some other condition.

OA is present worldwide as a heterogeneous group of conditions that lead to slow, progressive degeneration of joint structures with defective integrity of articular cartilage and related changes in the underlying bone. OA can lead to loss of mobility, chronic pain, deformity, and loss of function.

OA is the single most common joint disease, with an estimated prevalence of 60% in men and 70% in women later in life after the age of 65 years, affecting an estimated 40 million people in the United States. In fact, it is the most common musculoskeletal disorder worldwide affecting the hands and large weight-bearing joints such as the hip and knee and causing disability.[216] And the overall prevalence is expected to increase dramatically over the next 20 years as the population ages.[112]

Before age 50 years, the prevalence of OA in most joints is higher in men than in women, but this changes after age 65 years. In the United States OA is second only to ischemic heart disease as a cause of work disability in men older than 50 years.[70]

In the United States about 6% of adults older than age 30 years have OA of the knee and 3% have OA of the hip; incidence rises with increasing age. Both incidence and prevalence are expected to rise in the coming decades as a result of the aging of America combined with more extreme sports and activities. OA is the most common indication for total joint replacements.

Structures Involved

The most commonly involved joints associated with this disorder are the weight-bearing joints, especially the hip and knee but also the shoulder, lumbar and cervical spine and the first carpometacarpal and metatarsophalangeal joints.

The etiology of OA is multifactorial, including many components of biomechanics and biochemistry. Evidence is growing for the role of systemic factors such as genetics, nutrition and weight control, estrogen use, bone density, and local biomechanical factors, such as muscle weakness, obesity, and joint laxity, as causative.[83] Serious injury and an inherited predisposition account for 50% of all cases of OA in the hands, hips, and knees.[82,96,308] Smokers with knee OA sustain greater cartilage loss and have more severe knee pain than those who do not smoke, suggesting a role for tobacco in cartilage degeneration.[11]

There is low or no additional risk of OA from regular, moderate running, but sports that involve high-intensity, acute, direct joint impact from contact with other players do carry an increased risk of OA, especially when repetitive joint impact and twisting are combined. Football players, soccer players, hockey players, and baseball pitchers are especially at increased risk. Anterior cruciate ligament injury may predispose athletes to knee OA, especially when accompanied by meniscectomy.[51,235] Much of the OA in men is attributable to occupational activities, particularly kneeling or squatting, along with heavy lifting and repetitive use of heavy machinery.[82,83]

Generalized ligamentous laxity appears to be a predisposing factor; this may be related to the presence of estrogen receptors on the ligaments. Postmenopausal women appear to be at increased risk.[375] Some women have a condition called *hypermobility joint syndrome* or *hypermobility syndrome* with loose, unstable joints resulting from a dominant inherited connective tissue disorder. Hypermobility syndrome is characterized by excessive laxity of multiple joints, a condition that is separate from the generalized hypermobility associated with disorders such as Ehlers–Danlos syndrome, RA, SLE, or Marfan's syndrome.[314]

Muscle weakness can also cause joint changes leading to OA, such as occurs with prolonged immobilization, polymyositis, multiple sclerosis, or any of the myopathies listed in Box 17.12.

Recent research into the pathophysiologic events associated with OA indicates that OA is a disorder of the whole synovial joint organ, not just "wear and tear" on the cartilage. In fact, it may be that damage to the articular cartilage is the byproduct of a disease process that is centered in subchondral bone in particular. Emphasis is now on the joint as a whole rather than just the cartilage. The view of OA has shifted to that of both a local and systemic condition in which inflammation plays an important part in determining the symptoms and disease progression.[81,213] The former wear-and-tear concept already mentioned has been replaced by the idea that OA is an active disease process with joint tissue destruction and aberrant repair as a result of alterations in cellular function.

Articular cartilage has an important role in joint physiology by providing a smooth, relatively friction-free surface between the bony ends making up the joint. In addition, the cartilage disperses the mechanical load transmitted through the joint. With progressive loss of cartilage, inflammation develops, with resultant bony overgrowth, ligament laxity, and progressive muscle weakness and atrophy accompanied by joint pain.

Once the cartilage begins to break down, excessive mechanical stress begins to fall on other joint structures. That stress causes fissuring, thinning, and eventually loss of the articular cartilage, which exposes the subchondral bone. The bone then becomes denser, with the surface becoming worn and polished. The joint space narrows as the cartilage thins, and sclerosis of the subchondral bone occurs as new bone is formed in response to the now excessive mechanical load. New bone also forms at the joint margins (osteophytes) (Fig. 17.17), with the result

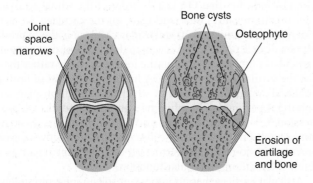

FIG. 17.17 (A) Early degenerative changes associated with osteoarthritis include joint space narrowing and articular cartilage erosion. (B) Late degenerative changes associated with osteoarthritis include osteophyte formation and articular cartilage fissuring and eburnation.

being mechanical joint failure and varying degrees of loss of joint function.

Immobilization is another factor that can result in articular cartilage degeneration. Secondary to the lack of vascular supply, articular cartilage depends on repetitive mechanical loading and unloading for the nutritional elements to reach the chondrocytes and the cellular waste products to return to the synovial fluid and eventually to the bloodstream. This nutritional mechanism of articular cartilage is interrupted by immobilization. If the nutritional cycle is interrupted long enough, structural changes will occur.

Although joint cartilage is the final target of the pathologic processes, the underlying subchondral bone may be the primary etiologic agent. New research focused on modifying changes in the bone may alter the pathologic processes observed in the adjacent cartilage.[325] Tissue changes in OA are the result of active joint remodeling processes involving an imbalance in repair activity; people with OA may have a general tendency toward increased bone metabolic activity, especially in response to biomechanical or other stimuli such as occurs with obesity and injury. As OA develops, loss of cartilage, hypertrophic changes in neighboring bone and joint capsule, mild synovial inflammation, and degenerative changes in the menisci, ligaments, and tendons all contribute to pain and loss of joint function, resulting in joint failure.[334]

Signs and Symptoms

The most common symptoms of OA include bony enlargement, limited joint ROM, crepitus on motion, tenderness on pressure, joint effusion, malalignment, and joint deformity. Inflammation is a prominent sign that plays a role in symptom generation. Soft tissue inflammation and edema are observed during acute exacerbations.[81]

The onset of symptoms related to OA can occur slowly or suddenly. Only a portion of people who have radiographic evidence of OA have associated pain. For most people the pain complaints progress slowly and gradually. Because the cartilage is not innervated, pain is not perceived until the bone or other structures surrounding the joint are involved. The primary cause of joint pain is attributed to a breakdown in the mechanics of movement rather than inflammation. The pain is often described as a deep ache that is worse with activity and better after rest; pain can occur at rest and at night with advanced disease.[88,163]

Pain with activity is most likely due to pulling on the attachment of tendons and ligaments to bone and other mechanical factors, whereas pain at rest may be caused by synovial inflammation. Night pain is a poor prognostic indicator and may occur as a result of intraosseous hypertension, which stretches periosteal pain neurons.[105]

Stiffness of relatively short duration, generally less than 30 minutes, can occur after periods of inactivity, including sitting and sleeping. Morning stiffness, referred to as the *gel phenomenon* or "joint gelling," usually only lasts 5 to 10 minutes after awakening. Movement and activity dissipate this stiffness until the individual sits or rests for a long period. This differs from RA, in which the morning stiffness or gelling can last until noon or even midafternoon.

Swelling, if present, is mild and localized to the joint. *Loss of flexibility* is usually associated with significant disease and can occur secondary to soft tissue contractures, intraarticular loose bodies, large osteophytes, and loss of joint surface congruity.

Crepitus, which is an audible crackling or grating sensation produced when roughened articular or extraarticular surfaces rub together during movement, may be noted on physical examination. Enlarged joint surfaces, including osteophytes, may be palpable. Although many people have physical and radiographic findings of OA, they may not have symptoms, whereas others with minimal changes observed develop significant symptoms. The reasons for this remain unknown.

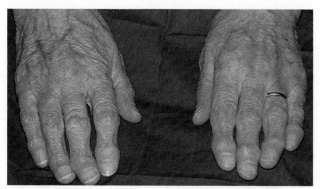

FIG. 17.18 Typical hand deformities in osteoarthritis. Heberden's nodes are seen on the distal interphalangeal joints, and Bouchard's nodes are at the proximal interphalangeal joints. (From Forbes CD, Jackson WF: Color atlas and text of clinical medicine, ed 3, London, 2003, Mosby.)

For many women, OA typically develops within a few years of menopause and is often associated with mild inflammation for the first year or two that a particular joint is involved. The joints may intermittently be warm and tender. The disease is strikingly symmetric, although the degree of involvement may vary somewhat. OA of the hands affecting the distal interphalangeal and proximal interphalangeal joints occurs most often in this group of women. The gradual loss of joint motion can assume major significance, with the person finding it difficult to grasp small objects.

After 1 or 2 years of inflammation, the joints enlarge with osteophyte (spur) formation, referred to as Heberden's nodes (affecting the distal interphalangeal joints) and Bouchard's nodes (affecting the proximal interphalangeal joints) (Fig. 17.18) and become unsightly. Pain may also be noted with loss of joint articular cartilage. Lateral deformities of the joints are common, with stretching of the collateral ligaments and bone resorption. This leads to overlapping of the fingers and considerable loss of functional ability.

Common Tests and Measures

OA is diagnosed by correlation of history, physical examination, radiologic findings (Figs. 17.19 and 17.20), and laboratory tests, which rule out rheumatic disease. Box 17.13 lists radiographic changes associated with OA. The history of location of symptoms, symptom duration, functional limitations, trauma, medical comorbidities, and family history helps guide the physician in making the diagnosis.

The American College of Rheumatology guidelines for the diagnosis of knee OA include knee pain with radiographic changes of osteophyte formation and at least one of the following: age more than 50 years, morning stiffness lasting less than 30 minutes, or crepitus on motion.[7]

Other symptoms diagnostic of OA include a locking or a "giving way" sensation in the knees, swelling, and exacerbation of symptoms with inactivity or overactivity. Walking on uneven ground and climbing stairs also aggravate knee and/or hip OA.[388]

The physician also relies on findings from the physical examination, such as joint line or bony tenderness, joint effusion (not always present), quadriceps muscle atrophy, varus or valgus deformity (knee), and any abnormalities such as Heberden's nodes, a classic osteoarthritic change

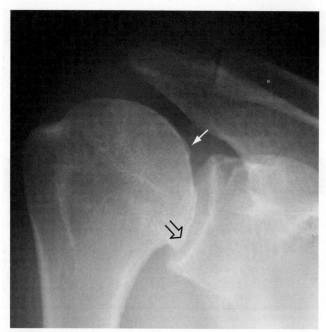

FIG. 17.19 Osteoarthritis of the shoulder. There is osteophytic lipping (open arrow) from the humeral head, including new bone formation deep to the cartilage (closed arrow). (From Harris ED: Kelley's textbook of rheumatology, ed 7, Philadelphia, 2005, Saunders.)

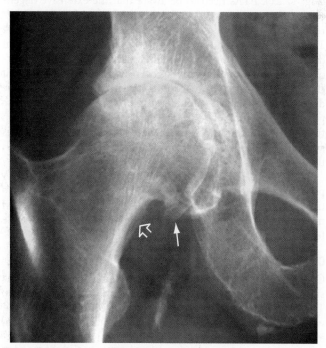

FIG. 17.20 Osteoarthritis of the hip. The anteroposterior view of the hip shows complete cartilage space loss superiorly. There is osteophytic lipping from the femoral head, especially medially (arrow), and buttressing bone (open arrow) is present along the femoral neck. (From Harris ED: Kelley's textbook of rheumatology, ed 7, Philadelphia, 2005, Saunders.)

observed in the distal interphalangeal joints of the hands (see Fig. 17.18).

OA is classified based on clinical information and radiologic evidence. The radiographic classification used most often is the 0 to 4 grading system proposed by Kellgren and Lawrence

BOX 17.13   Osteoarthritis: Radiographic Findings[a]

- Joint space widening (early evidence)
- Subchondral bone sclerosis
- Subchondral bone cysts
- Osteophytes
- Joint space narrowing

[a]Listed in order of progression.

TABLE 17.4   Kellgren and Lawrence Grading System for the Knee

Grade	Radiographic Findings
1	Possible osteophytes; no joint space narrowing
2	Definite osteophytes; possible narrowing of joint space
3	Moderate multiple osteophytes; definite joint space narrowing; some sclerosis and possible deformity of bone ends
4	Large osteophytes; marked joint space narrowing; severe sclerosis and definite deformity of bone ends

Data from Kellgren J, Lawrence J: Radiologic assessment of osteoarthritis, Ann Rheum Dis 16:494–501, 1957.

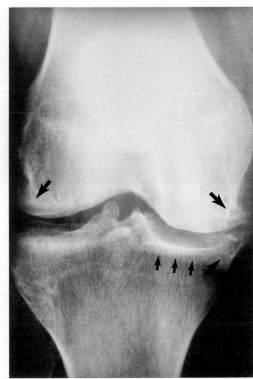

FIG. 17.21 Osteoarthritis of the knee. Proliferative marginal osteophytes *(larger arrows),* narrowing of the medial weight-bearing joint space, and eburnation (exposure of the subchondral bone, surface becomes smooth and polished as it wears down) *(smaller arrows).* (From Noble J: Textbook of primary care medicine, ed 3, St Louis, 2001, Mosby.)

(Table 17.4).[168] Grade 4 changes include large osteophytes, severe joint space narrowing, bony sclerosis, and bone exposure (Fig. 17.21). PTAs need to be aware that the extensive degenerative changes demonstrated on radiographs MAY NOT correlate to complaints of pain and the presence of symptoms. The assumption that a person with significant, extensive joint degeneration will not improve should not be made until a thorough rehabilitation program has been attempted. Conversely, it should not be assumed that someone with minor radiographic degenerative changes cannot be experiencing severe, intense pain. PTs should rely primarily on the clinical examination findings for direction regarding the development of prognosis and intervention and relay concerns to the PTA involved with the case.

MRI is becoming increasingly helpful in determining OA pathology because of its ability to show the condition of cartilage and the surrounding soft tissues. Laboratory evaluation may include ESR and rheumatoid factor, but generally these tests are not needed.[388]

Common Management

OA is managed on an individual basis, and treatment consists of a combination of conservative and surgical options. Treatment is modified based on response and should begin with conservative care, including education, weight loss, exercise, orthotics and/or braces, medications, and complementary approaches.

The combination of modest weight loss and moderate exercise provides better overall improvements in function, pain, and mobility in older adults who are overweight or obese with knee OA.[229] Greater improvements in function have been observed in older obese adults with the most weight loss.[236] Surgery is avoided and considered only when debilitating pain and major limitation of functions interfere with walking and daily activities or impair the ability to sleep or work.[153]

Physical therapy has been shown effective in OA of the knee to reduce pain; improve physical function; increase isometric muscle strength, gait speed, and stride length; and improve quality of life. A combination of manual physical therapy and supervised exercise provides beneficial effects that are still present 1 year later and delays or prevents the need for surgical intervention, with fewer joint replacements reported.[65,91] Such supervised exercise/manual therapy programs have been shown to increase improvement and provide greater symptomatic relief compared with a similar unsupervised home exercise program.[64,208]

Optimizing existing and potential joint function by improving flexibility and strength is important. In fact, exercise combined with self-management appears to have a similar effect to drug treatments and is generally safer.[78,292] Low-intensity, controlled movements that do not increase pain can help individuals regain or maintain motion and flexibility.[82,83]

The PT and PTA can use the same guidelines for all individuals when establishing frequency, intensity, and duration by following well-known general concepts (e.g., establish *intensity* by calculating heart rate at 60% of the heart rate maximum, begin at the individual's level of *duration* anywhere from 1 to 2 minutes and build up to 30 minutes, work toward a *frequency* of five to seven times per week). Clients should be taught how to monitor and progress frequency, intensity, and duration. Use good biomechanics and avoid exacerbating musculoskeletal symptoms.

In the presence of mild joint swelling, the client should be taught to use ice before exercise and to incorporate a program of submaximal exercise to warm up before beginning the prescribed exercise program.[224] If there is joint effusion, the surrounding muscles cannot contract maximally because of reflex inhibition caused by joint distention. Submaximal exercise for 3 or 4 minutes on a swollen joint decreases this inhibition mechanism, allowing for continued strength training. Moderate to severe joint effusion may require additional physical therapy intervention, such as electrical stimulation.

Resistance and low-intensity aerobic exercise may reduce the incidence of disability related to ADLs and prolong autonomy in adults older than age 60 years, specifically those with knee OA. The lowest ADL disability risks were found for participants with the highest compliance to the exercise program.[282] Long-term weight training and aerobic walking programs significantly improve postural sway in older adults with OA, thereby improving static postural stability.[230]

In the case of the frail older adult, progressive resistive exercises have been shown to be safe and effective following an acute illness when monitored carefully (e.g., measuring vital signs, observing for signs of physiologic distress).[363] Other specific exercise recommendations and safety considerations are available,[9,65,239,242] but the optimal type of exercise and duration for the prevention and treatment of OA remain under investigation.

Successful management of degenerative joint disease may require evaluating and treating dysfunction of other body regions. For example, someone with OA of the knee and pain on ambulation may have significant foot or ankle dysfunction. Treating joint and soft tissue hypomobility and muscle imbalances and fabricating orthoses may considerably alter the mechanical stresses on the arthritic knee.

For those individuals who do not seem to respond, progress, or improve with physical therapy intervention, a number of factors should be considered. Mode of treatment delivery is not the only parameter. Treatment compliance, mechanical characteristics (e.g., joint laxity, malalignment), and radiographic severity should be carefully considered. Research is needed to focus on predictive factors and outcomes for individual characteristics and type of exercise protocols prescribed.[87]

Pharmacotherapy. For many years, analgesics and NSAIDs have been the first-line medical treatment approach for OA. Newly discovered information about the pathophysiology of OA is paving the way for researchers to design medical therapy that targets specific sites of pathophysiologic pathways involved in the pathogenesis of OA. Medical attention has shifted from easing the pain of OA to slowing the disorder's progression and actually preventing it.

Antiresorptive drugs aimed at altering the increased metabolic states of the subchondral bone may have an effect in altering damage done to the overlying cartilage. This approach is based on the hypothesis that the underlying subchondral bone, either indirectly through biomechanical effects or directly via release of cytokines, is responsible for driving the release of degradative enzymes and, ultimately, the destruction of overlying cartilage.

A fairly recent nondrug, nonsurgical treatment known as *viscosupplementation* has been developed. This intervention involves direct injections into the knee of substances derived from sodium hyaluronate (hylan G-F 20 [Synvisc], Hyalgan), a principal component of natural synovial fluid. These injections help restore some of the viscosity and elasticity of the diseased joint fluid and offer pain relief for 6 to 12 months. Viscosupplementation is used when standard conservative treatments for knee OA (e.g., medications, physical therapy, behavioral therapy) have been inadequate or ineffective.

Education. The United States Centers for Disease Control and Prevention has launched a major public health initiative, called the National Arthritis Action Plan, to identify and change behaviors that may cause OA, calling for a significant change in the way this disease is treated. Medical interventions involving expensive medications, joint injections, and surgery are now suggested for use in the 10% to 30% of cases where OA will progress to severe joint damage.

Multimodal treatment should include client education and self-management. Two excellent resources for consumer education and self-management of OA are available: *The Arthritis Cure*[376] and *Maximizing the Arthritis Cure.*[377] More attention is recommended to exercise and to psychosocial problems (e.g., isolation, depression) that may influence the person's perception of pain. The value of a well-designed exercise program including training for strength and endurance also has been recognized.[68,82,83,389] Aquatic therapy is especially helpful as a gravity-eliminated resistive exercise. Behavioral interventions directed toward enhancing self-management are important, including prevention, diet and weight control, and low-impact exercise.

Complementary or alternative therapy. Glucosamine and *chondroitin* sulfate are components of cartilage taken with the hope of decreasing pain and improving function while halting the progression of disease by stopping an enzyme that is believed to break down cartilage. Glucosamine is derived from the shells of lobster, shrimp, and crabs; chondroitin sulfate is derived from cow cartilage. These are available as a nutritional supplement, sometimes referred to as a *nutraceutical.* Long-term use of these agents may provide combined structure-modifying and symptom-modifying effects, making these potentially disease-modifying agents for OA.[135,301,302,376] Investigators in various trials report a range of results with this treatment, making conclusions difficult. Differences in studies are too great to make comparisons or meta-analysis conclusive. Different glucosamine preparations add to the complexity of comparative studies.[300,396] The safety of this product used over a long period of time has also been questioned.[205]

Best available evidence suggests that acupuncture, several herbal preparations (e.g., devil's claw root, white willow bark), and capsaicin cream are beneficial. Evidence is weak or contradictory for homeopathy, magnet therapy, tai chi, leech therapy, music therapy, yoga, imagery, and therapeutic touch. Many other treatments have not been scientifically tested.[76]

The Arthritis Foundation has published an excellent resource on alternative therapies[12]; some experts advise people not to think of these therapies as "alternative" but rather as synergistic measures that can be integrated into a total care plan. An area of medicine called complementary and integrative medicine has developed as more medical doctors have started incorporating these treatment methods into their overall management plans.

Surgery. Surgical intervention is considered when pain and loss of function are severe. Arthroscopic management, including lavage and debridement, abrasion arthroplasty, subchondral penetration procedures such as drilling and microfracture, and laser/thermal chondroplasty, may benefit some individuals, potentially delaying reconstructive procedures (e.g., osteotomy, joint arthrodesis or fusion, total joint replacement). Each of these procedures is under investigation for efficacy and long-term results.[152] To help joint replacements last longer, intense research is focusing on more wear- and corrosion-resistant materials as well as investigating how the tissue around the replacement responds. Replacement of damaged cartilage is also under investigation using one of three types of cartilage: one's own cartilage, donor cartilage, and cartilage produced by tissue engineering of progenitor cells.

Prevention. Arthritis (including OA and rheumatic conditions) is the leading cause of disability in the United States, affecting a total of more than 43 million people in the United States, with an estimated prevalence of nearly 60 million by the year 2020.[40,42] The Arthritis Foundation, Centers for Disease Control and Prevention, and *Healthy People 2020* are working together to implement the National Arthritis Action Plan to promote progress toward reaching arthritis-related national objectives for 2020.[131]

Arthritis research is providing a growing body of knowledge about prevention as well as slowing the disease's progression and new, more effective combinations of drug and behavioral interventions. Education is a cornerstone of prevention and management for this condition. A healthy lifestyle helps prevent OA, and exercise can lessen disability if OA has developed. Moderate exercise has been shown to improve the knee cartilage in individuals at high risk of developing OA.[309] Strengthening the quadriceps muscle and maintaining an appropriate body weight for height reduce risk of OA at the knee by 30%.[82,83]

Sports officials and athletes need to work with athletic trainers, exercise physiologists, and physical therapy professionals to evaluate and modify rules, equipment, and playing surfaces while providing adequate training to help reduce injuries. Early diagnosis and intervention with complete rehabilitation of joint injuries can decrease the risk of subsequent OA.[82,83] High intakes of vitamin C are associated with lower rates of OA on radiograph examination and less knee pain from OA. High levels of vitamin D protect against new and progressive OA.[82,83]

Joint protection. People with symptoms associated with OA must understand their role in minimizing the mechanical stresses on the involved joint or joints. The diseased joints need to be protected from excessive mechanical forces. Educating the client on how to reduce the daily wear and tear on the joint is essential. This may include the use of postural supports, braces, an assistive device, or an exercise program to vary the stresses with which the involved joints are dealing. Proper posture and avoidance of prolonged stressful postures, use of supports, varying of physical activities to vary the stresses (i.e., alternating biking with swimming or walking), and following through with a flexibility and strengthening exercise program are all components under the affected individual's control.

Wearing shoes that fit properly and are appropriate for the activity may help avoid injury. Good alignment of the joints is important, especially in the knee. Evaluating the need for an assistive ambulatory device, a shock-absorbent shoe insert, brace, or other orthotic devices is important to unload the pressure on affected joints. A simple lateral wedge insole of 5 or 10 degrees directly reduces the knee varus torque in individuals with medial knee OA and can interrupt the OA cycle, slowing the progression of the disease and disability.[170]

Aquatic physical therapy is used often in the management of individuals with hip and knee OA. Compared with no intervention, a 6-week program of aquatic therapy resulted in significantly less pain with improved physical function, strength,

and quality of life. In studies with only short-term follow-up, aquatic exercise did not make the joint condition worse or result in injury.[141,399] Compared with a gym-based resistance exercise program, aquatic therapy yields equal results.[89]

Prognosis. OA is a major contributor to functional impairment and reduced independence in adults older than age 65 years. It is a chronic condition with unpredictable symptoms that often cause fluctuations in pain and function.[1] Mobility disability (defined as needing help walking or climbing stairs) is common for those with hip and/or knee OA. The social burden in terms of personal suffering and use of health resources is expected to increase with the increasing prevalence of obesity and the aging of the American population.[153]

Although there is no known cure for OA, by following the guidelines for lifestyle changes, pain management, and self-management incorporating exercise and weight loss, affected individuals can substantially decrease the pain and dysfunction associated with OA.

Complications. The medications commonly prescribed for OA have significant potential side effects. The NSAIDs have the potential to cause ulcers, especially when taken with over-the-counter drugs. Peptic ulcer disease can be manifested by a multitude of complaints, including indigestion, nausea, vomiting, thoracic pain, and melena (black tarry stools). The onset of any of these complaints calls for communication with a physician.

Nutraceuticals, such as chondroitin, can also cause problems in some individuals. Chondroitin is chemically similar to blood-thinning drugs, such as heparin, warfarin (Coumadin), and even aspirin, and could cause excessive bleeding. Anyone taking these supplements with unexplained back or shoulder pain or excessive bruising or bleeding from any part of the body (nose, gums, vagina, urine, rectum) must be evaluated by a physician.

Anyone taking these supplements who also has diabetes should be aware that some studies in animals have shown that glucosamine increases blood glucose levels. Preliminary studies in humans remain inconclusive.[245]

Rheumatic Diseases

Rheumatic disorders are systemic diseases encompassing more than 100 different diseases divided into 10 classification categories. These disorders can affect any and all body systems. The onset of joint pain and loss of function may be accompanied by fever, rash, diarrhea, scleritis, or neuritis symptoms that are not typically associated with joint or muscle conditions normally brought on by repetitive overuse or trauma.

Rheumatic disorders are also often marked by periods of exacerbation and remission. During a period of exacerbation, the PT and PTA will often need to modify the treatment approach considerably. In addition, aggressive medical intervention (i.e., medications) may need to be initiated to prevent or minimize the tissue destruction that can occur with these disorders. Many of the rheumatic conditions are chronic and progressive, requiring long-term rehabilitation and ongoing adjustment of functional goals.

PTAs must be able to differentiate between degenerative joint disease (OA) and rheumatic joint conditions (Table 17.5). If there is any suspicion of the presence of a rheumatic disorder, immediate referral to a physician is warranted. When someone with RA presents with systemic symptoms or if existing complaints worsen, communication with a physician is advised.

TABLE 17.5   Osteoarthritis and Rheumatoid Arthritis

	Osteoarthritis	Rheumatoid Arthritis
Onset	Usually begins at age 40 years Gradual onset over many years; affects majority of adults older than age 65 years	Initially develops between ages 25 and 50 years Onset may be sudden over several weeks to months; intermittent exacerbation and remission
Incidence[41]	12% of U.S. adults; 21 million people	1%–2% of U.S. adults; 600,000 men, and 1.5 million women; estimated prevalence rate of juvenile RA in children under 16 is between 30,000 and 50,000
Gender	Most common in men before age 45 years; after 45 years more common among women	Affects women 3:1 compared with men but more disabling and severe when present in men
Etiology	Etiology remains unknown; immunologic reaction with massive inflammatory response; possible genetic and environmental triggers	Multifactorial; local biomechanical factors, biochemistry, previous injury, inherited predisposition
Manifestations	Usually begins in joints on one side of the body Primarily affects hips, knees, spine, hands, feet Inflammation with redness, warmth, and swelling in 10% of cases Brief morning stiffness that is decreased by physical activity movement	Symmetric simultaneous joint distribution Can affect any joint (large or small); predilection for upper extremities Inflammation almost always present Prolonged morning stiffness lasting 1 hour or more
Associated signs and symptoms	No systemic symptoms; possible associated trigger points	Systemic presentation with constitutional symptoms (e.g., fatigue, malaise, weight loss, fever)
Laboratory values	Effusions infrequently, synovial fluid has low WBC and high viscosity ESR may be mildly to moderately increased Rheumatoid factor absent New biomarkers under investigation (e.g., C-telopeptide, CTX, C-reactive protein, cartilage glycoprotein 39 [YKL-40])	Synovial fluid has high WBC and low viscosity ESR markedly increased in the presence of an inflammatory process but not specifically diagnostic for RA Rheumatoid factor usually present but is not specific or diagnostic for RA (can be elevated in other diseases) C-reactive protein, a true indicator of systemic inflammation, strong predictor of disease outcome (RA progresses more rapidly in the presence of elevated C-reactive protein) Other biomarkers are under investigation (e.g., vascular endothelial growth factor [VEGF],[a] matrix metalloproteinase 3 [MMP-3])

[a]VEGF is an angiogenetic cytokine; its presence supports the theory that expansion of the synovial vasculature is important for the development of joint destruction in RA.

ESR, Erythrocyte sedimentation rate; *RA,* rheumatoid arthritis; *WBC,* white blood cell count.

Rheumatoid Arthritis

Definition and incidence. Rheumatoid arthritis is a chronic systemic inflammatory disease presenting with a wide range of articular and extraarticular findings. Chronic arthritis in multiple joint is responsible for gradual destruction of joint tissues, resulting in severe deformity and disability. RA affects more than the musculoskeletal system; the cardiovascular, pulmonary, and GI systems also may be involved. Eye lesions, infection, and osteoporosis are other potential manifestations.

RA is a major subclassification within the category of diffuse connective tissue diseases that also includes juvenile arthritis, SLE, progressive systemic sclerosis (scleroderma), polymyositis, and dermatomyositis.[110]

RA has a worldwide distribution and affects all races. Approximately 1% to 2% of the U.S. adult population (2.1 million people) has RA, which is the second most prevalent form of arthritis after OA.

Risk factors. Age and *female gender* are the two primary risk factors associated with RA. Although the onset of the disorder can occur at any age, the peak onset is usually between 20 and 50 years; with the aging of America, the prevalence of RA is expected to rise. Women are affected two to three times more frequently than men; although it is less common, children can also develop the disorder (see the section Juvenile Idiopathic Arthritis in this chapter).

Pregnancy and oral contraceptives appear to influence the incidence and severity of the disease. The incidence of RA in women who have borne a child is lower, and oral contraceptives diminish the incidence of severe arthritis. A woman who has never been pregnant and does not use oral contraceptives has a fourfold increased risk of developing RA.[40,129,356]

Prophylactic administration of recombinant hepatitis B vaccine may trigger the development of RA in previously healthy people. Vaccine-related arthritis may be linked to genetic factors.[289] An association between autoimmune thyroid diseases and rheumatic diseases has been established, although its precise mechanism is unclear. For example, RA often occurs in association with Graves' disease and Hashimoto's thyroiditis.[220]

Drinking decaffeinated coffee (four or more cups per day) may be an independent risk factor among older women, especially in the presence of seropositive disease, but the mechanism for this remains unknown.[233]

Little is known about the exact causes of RA, except that joint inflammation is a consequence of massive infiltration of immune cells (especially T lymphocytes) into the synovial fluid. Genetic predisposition and environmental triggers, such as a bacteria, are both considered possible etiologic factors in the stimulation of T cells.[79,147]

Structures involved. RA is considered an autoimmune disease, with inflammation and destruction targeted at the joint capsule (articular) and elsewhere throughout the body (extraarticular). Approximately 80% of people with RA are rheumatoid factor positive.[126]

Rheumatoid factors are autoantibodies that react with immunoglobulin antibodies found in the blood. Rheumatoid factor has also been found in the synovial fluid and synovial membranes of those with the disease.

RA begins attacking the joint in the synovium. In RA, the cells of the synovial lining multiply, there is an influx of leukocytes from the peripheral circulation, and the synovium becomes edematous. The synovial lining thickens, resulting in the clinical synovitis seen so often.

These changes can result in the development of thickened synovium, a destructive vascular granulation tissue called *pannus*. The inflammatory cells found within the pannus are destructive, preventing the synovium from performing its two primary functions: lubricating the joint and providing nutrients to the articular cartilage. As this pannus tissue proliferates, encroaching on the joint space at the margins where the hyaline cartilage and synovial lining do not adequately cover the bone, it dissolves collagen, cartilage, subchondral bone, and other periarticular tissues in its path (Fig. 17.22).

Multiple joints are usually involved, with symmetric, bilateral presentation. The most frequently involved joints are the wrist, knee, and joints of the fingers, hands, and feet, although RA can affect any joint, including the temporomandibular joints. The metacarpophalangeal and proximal interphalangeal joints of the hand are involved early. There is a potential for atlantoaxial subluxation (usually anterior) and brainstem or spinal cord compression. The upper cervical spine is affected most commonly because the occiput-C1 and the C1–C2 articulations are purely synovial and are thus primary targets for rheumatoid involvement. In addition, because the C1 and C2 facets are oriented in the axial plane, there is no bony interlocking to prevent subluxation in the face of ligamentous destruction.[303]

Signs and symptoms. RA is a systemic disease typically manifested by articular and extraarticular complaints (Box 17.14). The symptoms usually begin insidiously and progress slowly as the disease process moves from cartilage damage to ligamentous laxity and, finally, synovial expansion with erosion. Complaints of fatigue, weight loss, weakness, and general, diffuse musculoskeletal pain are often the initial presentation. Deconditioning and depression are common complications of this disease.

The course of RA can vary considerably from mild to severely disabling and is difficult to predict, but it appears that adults with RA today have less severe symptoms and less functional disability than even a decade ago. This positive trend and more favorable course of disease may be attributed to earlier diagnosis with a shorter duration of symptoms at the time of diagnosis and more aggressive use of drug therapy.[404]

Joint. The musculoskeletal symptoms gradually localize to specific joints. The involved joints can be swollen, warm, painful, and stiff. After periods of rest (e.g., prolonged sitting, sleeping), intense joint pain and stiffness may last 30 minutes to several hours as activity is initiated.

As the disease progresses, joint deformity can progress to subluxation. Deformities in the fingers are common, including ulnar deviation, swan-neck deformity, and boutonnière deformity. The ulnar deviation occurs as the extensor tendons slip to the ulnar aspect of the metacarpal head. Hyperextension of the proximal interphalangeal joint and partial flexion of the distal interphalangeal joint make up the swan-neck deformity (Fig. 17.23). The boutonnière deformity is marked by flexion of the proximal interphalangeal joint and hyperextension of the distal interphalangeal joint (Fig. 17.24).

Soft tissue. Soft tissue manifestations of RA can include synovitis, bursitis, tendinitis, fasciitis, neuritis, and vasculitis. These problems are often overlooked but can be very debilitating. Soft tissue imbalance combined with joint involvement can result in significant deformity, especially in the hands and feet.

Spine. Early involvement of the spinal column is common and typically limited to the cervical spine, with deep, aching neck pain radiating into the occipital or temporal areas, or behind the eyes reported in 40% to 88% of persons.[23,171,303] Neck movement precipitates or aggravates neck pain; facial and ear pain and occipital headaches occur frequently with active disease.[171]

The natural history of cervical instability in people with RA is variable, and only some develop neurologic deficits.[72] Symptoms of C1–C2 subluxation include a sensation of the head falling forward with neck flexion, loss of consciousness or syncope, dysphagia, vertigo, seizures, hemiplegia, dysarthria, nystagmus, and peripheral paresthesias and loss of dexterity of the hands.[28] Urinary retention and later incontinence are symptoms of more severe involvement. Sleep apnea may be caused by brainstem compression associated with atlantoaxial impaction.[283]

There may be a positive *Lhermitte's* sign with shocklike sensations of the torso or extremities with neck flexion. Atlantoaxial instability may result in vertebrobasilar insufficiency with visual disturbances, loss of equilibrium, vertigo, tinnitus, and dysphagia.[303] Asymmetric destruction of the lateral atlantoaxial joints may result in a clinical presentation of head tilt down and to one side. When the neck is flexed, the spinous process of the axis may be prominent.

Pain associated with RA in the subaxial segments of the cervical spine is located in the lateral aspects of the neck and clavicles (C3–C4) and over the shoulders (C5–C6). Neurologic symptoms include burning paresthesias and numbness, which may be attributed to carpal tunnel syndrome, delaying the diagnosis of cervical myelopathy.

Cutaneous. The visible rheumatoid nodule is a characteristic skin finding in RA, occurring in approximately 25% of all cases. These granulomatous lesions usually occur in areas of repeated mechanical pressure, such as over the extensor surface of the elbow, Achilles tendon, and extensor surface of the fingers (Fig. 17.25). Nodules are usually asymptomatic, but they can become tender or cause skin breakdown and become infected. Nodules that cannot be seen visibly can also occur in the heart, lungs, and GI tract, causing serious problems such as heart arrhythmias and respiratory failure.

Neurologic. One-third of adults with RA have cervical spine involvement leading to compressive cervical myelopathy

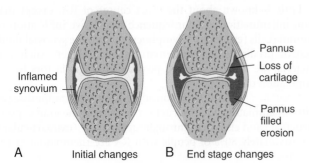

FIG. 17.22 (A) Early synovial changes associated with rheumatoid arthritis. (B) Late joint changes associated with rheumatoid arthritis, including pannus formation and articular cartilage eburnation.

BOX 17.14   Articular and Extraarticular Manifestations of Rheumatoid Arthritis

Cardiac

- Conduction defects (usually asymptomatic)
- Pericarditis
- Interstitial myocarditis
- Coronary arteritis
- Vasculitis
- Aortitis

Hematologic

- Anemia of chronic disease
- Felty's syndrome (splenomegaly, neutropenia)
- Lymphoma, leukemia

Musculoskeletal

- Osteopenia, osteoporosis (associated fractures)
- Joint pain (reflects severity of synovitis; may not be present at rest)
- Joint stiffness (present in most cases, especially after inactivity; duration reflects degree of synovial inflammation; improves with physical activity)
- Joint contracture (extension of involved joints most commonly affected)
- Swelling (synovial tissue)
- Muscle atrophy (hands, feet; occurs rapidly in severe disease)
- Muscle weakness; often out of proportion to the degree of muscular atrophy
- Tenosynovitis, tendonitis, tendon triggering, tendon rupture
- Joint deformity

Neurologic

- Compression neuropathies; nerve entrapment syndromes (e.g., carpal tunnel syndrome, tarsal tunnel syndrome)
- Polyneuropathy
- Peripheral neuropathy (mononeuritis multiplex, stocking-glove peripheral neuropathy)
- Myelopathy; subluxation or instability of C1-C2
- Lhermitte's sign (upper extremity paresthesias that increase with neck flexion)

Integumentary

- Nodulosis (see Fig. 17.25; subcutaneous nodules, especially over olecranon and proximal ulna, extensor surfaces of fingers, Achilles tendon ["pump bumps"])

- Nodules can occur in tendon, bone, sclerae, over pinna or ear, and in visceral organs, especially lung
- Palmar erythema (identical to changes found in liver disease and pregnancy; persists even in remission)
- Sweet's syndrome
- Vasculitis

Ocular

- Episcleritis (inflammation of the superficial sclera and conjunctiva)
- Scleritis (inflammation of the sclera)
- Sicca syndrome (dry eyes)

Psychologic

- Depression (common); other mood disorders

Pulmonary

- Effusions
- Interstitial pneumonia
- Interstitial fibrosis
- Nodules (rheumatoid nodulosis)
- Pleurisy, pleuritis
- Empyema
- Pulmonary hypertension

Renal

- Interstitial nephritis, nephritic syndrome
- Vasculitis

Vascular

- Skin changes (rash, ulcers, purpura, bullae)
- Infarctions (brain, viscera, nail folds; see Fig. 17.26)
- Digital gangrene
- Medium-vessel arteritis
- Small-vessel vasculitis

Other

- Unexplained weight loss, anorexia
- Malaise, fatigue
- Lymphadenopathy (lymph node enlargement; more common in men)
- Colon cancer

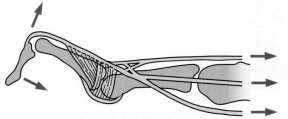

FIG. 17.23 Swan-neck deformity. (Redrawn from Richardson JK, Iglarsh ZA, editors: Clinical orthopedic physical therapy, Philadelphia, 1994, Saunders.)

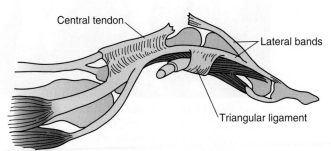

FIG. 17.24 Boutonnière deformity. (Redrawn from Richardson JK, Iglarsh ZA, editors: Clinical orthopedic physical therapy, Philadelphia, 1994, Saunders.)

presented as neck pain and stiffness, Lhermitte's sign, weakness of the upper or lower extremities, hyperactive distal tendon reflexes, and presence of Babinski's sign. In severe cases, urinary and fecal incontinence and paralysis can occur.[92]

Peripheral neuropathies are common as the nerves become compressed by inflamed synovia in tight compartments. Pain, dysesthesias, motor loss, and muscle atrophy can occur, leading to dysfunction and disability. Rheumatoid vasculitis involving medium-sized arteries to the muscles can lead to mononeuritis multiplex, whereas small-vessel vasculitis causes stocking-glove peripheral neuropathy.[92]

Extraarticular. The extraarticular manifestations are numerous and affect men and women equally (Fig. 17.26; see also Box 17.14). Many of these manifestations impair cardiopulmonary function, restrict activity, decrease endurance, and are disabling; some are life threatening. They could easily hamper rehabilitation efforts, delaying or preventing progress.

Individuals with RA are also at increased risk for severe infection, including tuberculosis, requiring hospitalization.[38,71,94] There is also a greater risk of cardiovascular and cerebrovascular

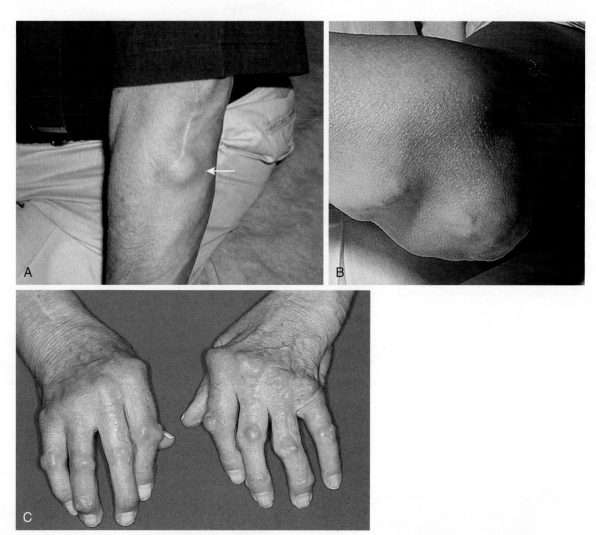

FIG. 17.25 (A) Rheumatoid nodule(s) *(arrow)* may be firm, raised, nontender bumps over which the skin slides easily. Common sites are in the olecranon bursa (elbow), along the extensor surface of the forearm, and behind the heel (calcaneus). (B) These nodules are also associated with rheumatoid arthritis and are firm, nontender, and freely movable. These are most common in people with severe arthritis, high-titer rheumatoid factor, or rheumatoid vasculitis. (C) Multiple rheumatoid nodules of the digits with typical ulnar deviation deformity from long-standing rheumatoid arthritis. Histologically identical lesions have been found in the sclera (eye), larynx, heart, lungs, and abdominal wall. The lesions develop insidiously and may regress spontaneously but usually persist. (A, From Hochberg MC, Silman AJ, Smolen JS, et al., editors: Rheumatology, ed 4, Philadelphia, 2008, Mosby. B, From Walker BR, Colledge NR, Ralston SH, et al., editors: Davidson's principles and practice of medicine, ed 22, Edinburgh, 2014, Churchill Livingstone. C, From Hochberg MC, Silman AJ, Smolen JS, et al., editors: Rheumatology, ed 6, Philadelphia, 2015, Mosby.)

morbidity and mortality among adults with RA compared with adults with OA.

Common tests and measures. In the early stages of RA the diagnosis can be difficult because of the gradual, subtle onset of the complaints. The symptoms may wax and wane, delaying the visit to a physician's office. Early diagnosis can help prevent or reduce erosive and irreversible joint damage as well as reduce morbidity and mortality associated with this chronic disease. The diagnosis is ultimately based on a combination of history, physical examination, imaging studies, and laboratory tests, with careful exclusion of other disorders.

Table 17.6 lists the diagnostic criteria for RA proposed by the American College of Rheumatology. Although the criteria require that signs and symptoms be present for at least 6 weeks before a definitive diagnosis can be made and that this period represents a delay in diagnosis, the truth is that many individuals suffer symptoms much longer than this before seeing a physician. At least half of all adults with RA are not referred for rheumatologic consultation until they have had their disease for at least 6 months (sometimes more than 1 year).[248]

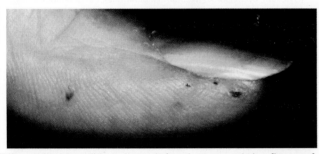

FIG. 17.26 Vasculitis splinter infarction around the finger of a person with systemic vasculitis associated with rheumatoid arthritis (extraarticular manifestation). Clinical features are diverse, because virtually any blood vessel anywhere in the body can be affected. (From Moots RJ, Bacon PA: Extraarticular manifestations of rheumatoid arthritis, J Musculoskelet Med 11:10–23, 1994.)

Conventional radiography, ultrasonography, and MRI studies are allowing more accurate diagnosis of RA. The earliest joint changes (periarticular swelling and cortical thinning with erosion at the margins of the articular cartilage and joint space narrowing) are seen on plain radiographs (Fig. 17.27). Screening cervical spine radiographs should be considered for all individuals with RA but especially for those with advanced peripheral joint disease.[171]

MRI is more sensitive than conventional radiography for detecting early RA and can show lesions of the synovium and cartilage and joint effusions.[73] MRI has the ability to visualize synovitis and detect bone edema, which is emerging as a predictor of future erosive bone changes.[29] Ultrasonography now allows the visualization of small superficial structures and can reveal synovial inflammation and tenosynovitis as well as effusions and bone erosions.

PTAs must be aware of the symptoms and signs associated with RA to differentiate it from other musculoskeletal conditions, particularly osteoarthritis. Being aware of the clinical signs and symptoms of RA will help the PTA make an early referral. The distribution of joint involvement is an important clue. RA usually affects the small joints of the feet and hands symmetrically; generalized pain ("I hurt all over") is not characteristic of RA.

Quick, aggressive medical treatment is necessary to minimize joint destruction. Unexplained joint pain for 1 month or more, especially accompanied by systemic complaints, skin rash, or extensor nodules, no matter how mild, should raise concern on the PTA's part. Cervical pain with reports of urinary retention or incontinence warrants immediate medical evaluation. Also, insidious onset of polyarthritis or joint pain within 6 weeks of taking a medication should raise suspicion regarding the nature of the pain complaints. Any of these red flags suggests the need for a medical referral if a physician has not recently evaluated the affected individual.

When distinguishing articular pain from periarticular involvement, remember that true arthritis produces pain and limitation during both active and passive ROM, whereas limitation from tendinitis is much worse during active than during passive motion. Inflammatory joint involvement

TABLE 17.6 Criteria for the Classification of Acute Rheumatoid Arthritis[a]

Criterion	Definition
1. Morning stiffness	Morning stiffness in and around the joints, lasting at least 1 hour before maximal improvement
2. Arthritis of three or more joint areas	At least three joint areas simultaneously have had soft tissue swelling or fluid (not bony overgrowth alone) observed by a physician; the 14 possible areas are right or left PIP, MCP, wrist, elbow, knee, ankle, and MTP joints
3. Arthritis of hand joints	At least one area swollen (as defined above) in a wrist, MCP, or PIP joint
4. Symmetric arthritis	Simultaneous involvement of the same joint areas (as defined in criterion 2) on both sides of the body (bilateral involvement of PIPs, MCPs, or MTPs is acceptable without absolute symmetry)
5. Rheumatoid nodules	Subcutaneous nodules over bony prominences or extensor surfaces or in juxtaarticular regions, observed by a physician
6. Serum rheumatoid factor	Demonstration of abnormal amounts of serum rheumatoid factor by any method for which the result has been positive in <5% of normal control subjects
7. Radiographic changes	Radiographic changes typical of rheumatoid arthritis on posteroanterior hand and wrist radiographs, which must include erosions or unequivocal bony decalcification localized in or most marked adjacent to the involved joints (osteoarthritis changes alone do not qualify)

MCP, Metacarpophalangeal; *MTP*, metatarsophalangeal; *PIP*, proximal interphalangeal.

[a]For classification purposes, a person shall be said to have rheumatoid arthritis if he or she has satisfied at least four or these seven criteria. Criteria 1 through 4 must have been present for at least 6 weeks.

Data from Arnett FC: The American Rheumatism Association 1987 revised criteria for the classification of rheumatoid arthritis, Arthritis Rheum 31:315–324, 1988.

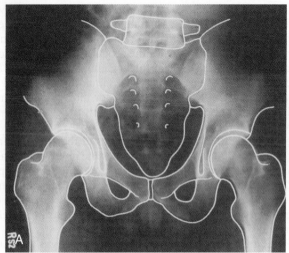

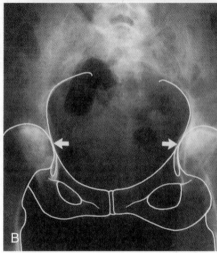

FIG. 17.27 (A) Radiograph of normal hips and pelvis. (B) Radiograph of rheumatoid arthritis of the hips. Note the narrowed joint space (loss of articular cartilage) and periarticular bone density changes. (From Richardson JK, Iglarsh ZA, editors: *Clinical orthopedic physical therapy*, Philadelphia, 1994, Saunders.)

typically produces warmth, erythema, and tenderness. Frequently, there is bogginess related to underlying synovitis or effusion. These indicators are not present with joint pain of a mechanical cause.

Before initiating any rehabilitation program for this group of individuals, a thorough limb and joint examination must be done to provide an objective way to assess and document disease activity and progression or, conversely, remission and improved function. Numerous resources are available to assist the clinician in carrying out a thorough clinical assessment of the individual with RA, including a helpful joint-by-joint guide (describing where and how to palpate).[243,318,334,345] Physical therapy examination should also include observation of functional performance, limitations, impairments, and a systems review as outlined in the *Guide to Physical Therapist Practice*.[10]

The feet are often overlooked in people with RA, but foot involvement occurs frequently, can impair gait, and can prevent safe participation in an exercise program. Careful assessment of the feet may reveal uneven or pathologic weight-bearing patterns. Gait analysis and assessment of shoe wear can provide

BOX 17.15   Pharmacotherapy for Rheumatoid Arthritis

Analgesics
- Various over-the-counter and prescription drugs, including acetaminophen (Tylenol), tramadol (Ultram), and codeine

Nonsteroidal Antiinflammatory Drugs
- Over-the-counter and prescription formulas, including aspirin, ibuprofen (Advil, Motrin), naproxen (Aleve, Anaprox, Naprelan, Naprosyn), ketoprofen (Orudis, Oruvail), diclofenac (Voltaren), diflunisal (Dolobid), indomethacin (Indocin)

Corticosteroids
- Oral or injection formulas, including prednisone (Cortan, Deltasone, Meticorten), methylprednisolone (Medrol)

Disease-Modifying Antirheumatic Drugs
- Antimalarials (hydroxychloroquine [Plaquenil])
- Antibiotics (sulfasalazine [Azulfidine], minocycline [Minocin, Dynacin])
- Injectable and oral gold (Ridaura)
- D-Penicillamine (Depen, Cuprimine)
- Methotrexate (Amethopterin, Rheumatrex)
- Immunosuppressants (azathioprine [Imuran], cyclophosphamide [Cytoxan], cyclosporine [Neoral, Sandimmune], Leflunomide [Arava])

Biologic Response Modifiers
Cytokine Inhibitors[a]
- Tumor necrosis factor (TNF) inhibitors[b] (etanercept [Enbrel], infliximab [Remicade], adalimumab [Humira])
- Interleukin-1 inhibitor (anakinra [Kineret])

Lymphocyte Inhibitors
- Rituximab (Rituxan) (antibody originally developed for the treatment of B-cell lymphoma)
- Abatacept (Orencia) (interrupts the activation of T cells, leading to T-cell anergy and apoptosis)

Investigational Drugs (in Clinical Trials)
- HuMax-CD20 (antibody that targets B cells)
- Belimumab (LymphoStat-B; inhibits B-cell growth and survival)
- Atacicept (inhibits B-cell growth and survival)
- Tocilizumab (anti–interleukin-6 receptor monoclonal antibody)
- Certolizumab (human monoclonal antibody to TNF-α)
- Golimumab (human monoclonal antibody to TNF-α)

[a]PEGylation is a new way to deliver anti–TNF-α agents that is site specific. Polyethylene glycol is added to enhance the pharmacokinetic properties of a molecule, decreasing its volume of distribution and clearance and increasing its half-life.
[b]May also be referred to as TNF-α antagonists.
Data from Yazici Y: Bright future for RA therapies, J Musculoskelet Med Suppl:32–35, 2006.

additional significant information regarding altered biomechanics. Providing assistive devices or orthotics before initiating an exercise program may be essential.[318,344,345]

Common management. Early treatment of RA is critical to improving long-term outcomes, because clinical evidence has clearly shown that joint destruction in RA begins early in the disease.[290] The treatment goals for someone with RA are to reduce pain, maintain mobility, and minimize stiffness, edema, and joint destruction. Aggressive combination drug therapy (Box 17.15) in conjunction with other management techniques, including physical therapy, is the mainstay of treatment.

The management approach is individualized, especially in the presence of extraarticular manifestation. The chronic nature of the disease makes client education and continual adherence to the treatment program vital. Because the inflammatory process results in progressive joint destruction, controlling inflammation is a primary goal. Medications, rest, ambulatory assistive devices, orthoses, and ice can be used during the acute phase.

Pharmacotherapy. Many medications are available now to help in the management of RA (see Box 17.15). Analgesics are used to help relieve pain. NSAIDs reduce pain, swelling, and inflammation. Corticosteroids help reduce inflammation and pain and can slow joint damage. Biotechnology has made new pharmacologic agents possible with genetically engineered products that can relieve symptoms and slow the progression of this disease. These new agents can "reset the inflammatory thermostat" and avoid joint damage.[276]

Disease-modifying antirheumatic drugs (DMARDs) and biologic response modifiers (BRMs) are two examples of newer types of drugs used in combination with analgesics, antiinflammatories, and steroids to alter the course and clinical presentation of RA. Some DMARDs block the activity of a protein that triggers and prolongs the inflammatory process, leading to joint destruction. Others block a protein present in excess in people with RA, thus inhibiting inflammation and cartilage damage.

Immunosuppressants, such as methotrexate (MTX; Rheumatrex), azathioprine (Imuran), and cyclophosphamide (Cytoxan), may be used. MTX is currently the most widely used immunosuppressant for RA management because of its long-term efficacy. Although its exact mechanism remains unknown, it has been shown to alleviate pain and morning stiffness. Effects tend to plateau after 6 months, and side effects can be numerous; regular serum monitoring of liver and renal function is required.

NSAIDs are effective for pain and swelling associated with inflamed joints caused by RA, but these pharmacologic agents do not affect disease progression. Corticosteroids may be prescribed in addition to DMARDs and NSAIDs to relieve pain and in clients with unremitting disease with extraarticular manifestations. Intraarticular injections can provide relief of acute inflammation. Administration of these drugs for periods of 3 to 6 months is often necessary for benefit to be noted.

Surgery. Surgery may be indicated if conservative care is insufficient in achieving acceptable pain control and level of function. Synovectomy (removal of damaged synovial tissue or pannus) to reduce pain and joint damage is the primary operation for the wrist. Total joint replacement procedures are performed at the shoulder, hip, knee, wrist, and fingers. The most common soft tissue procedure is tenosynovectomy of the hand. Studies support prophylactic stabilization of the rheumatoid cervical spine to prevent paralysis in high-risk individuals.[49,254]

17.5 Special Implications for the PTA: Rheumatoid Arthritis RA is a chronic, progressive disease requiring an interdisciplinary team approach that is individual to the client and comprehensive, with long-range planning that extends beyond the initial acute phase. The role of the physical therapy professional as an integral part of the management of RA has been well established,[33,199,265] with a renewed focus on outcome-based intervention.

The American College of Rheumatology has developed criteria for classification of functional status for individuals with RA that may help guide the PT and PTA in designing and monitoring the results of an appropriate plan of care (Box 17.16).

The Ottawa Panel has identified nine goals in the rehabilitation of individuals with RA, including decreasing pain, effusion (swelling), and stiffness; correcting or preventing joint deformity; increasing motion and muscle force (decreasing weakness); improving mobility and walking; increasing physical fitness; reducing fatigue; and increasing functional status.[273]

Complete bed rest is rarely indicated and is saved for those with severe, uncontrolled inflammation. For many people, a rest period of up to 2 hours during the day is important for dealing with general body fatigue and protection of involved joints. Splints can be applied to rest involved joints, prevent excessive movement, and reduce mechanical stresses. Crutches, canes, or walkers can be used to reduce weight-bearing stresses and enhance balance.

A home program of self-management will include instruction in proper body mechanics, positioning, joint protection, and energy conservation. Adaptive equipment designed to make tasks easier may include large key handle attachments allowing the person to use the whole palm to turn a key, spring-open scissors with big loops for anyone with hand involvement, jar openers and electric can openers, clip-on bottle openers, and ergonomic kitchen utensils with large handles and ergonomically angled handles.[223]

Instability at any joint, particularly at the atlantoaxial segment, requires caution on the PTA's part. Such a joint may present with a marked reduction in ROM, such as the shoulder or neck feeling stuck or caught with a certain movement. A history of periods of significant loss of ROM alternating with full ROM suggests joint hypermobility. Restoration of mobility is an important goal, but choosing techniques that are gentle or applying traction while stretching is necessary.

The extraarticular problems may affect the rehabilitation program. For example, if fatigue is present, the PTA may have to allow periods of rest during the treatment session. During periods of symptom exacerbation, there is a fine line between overextending the client and maximizing activity. There are times when active exercise may have to be curtailed, but passive stretching remains important to prevent contractures.

Splenomegaly may account for tenderness on palpation and fullness or increased resistance of the left upper abdominal quadrant. Deep soft tissue techniques are contraindicated in this area. Percussion techniques may help delineate the caudal boundaries of the spleen.

Exercise Programs

Exercises to prevent contractures, improve strength and flexibility, and enhance cardiorespiratory or aerobic conditioning are important components of the rehabilitation program.[125,174,265] Joint pain leads to a reflex inhibition of muscle surrounding the joints, causing disuse atrophy of these muscles. Use of corticosteroids may lead to an additional decrease in strength and function.[265]

Avoid overloading and overtraining. For the individual with active (acute) disease, adequate sleep is essential. Encourage 8 to 10 hours of rest each night. ROM exercises should begin with low repetitions several times throughout the day. Isometric exercises with short holds (4 to 6 seconds) have been suggested, once again using low repetitions (start with one or two and build up gradually to four to six).[158]

ROM exercises can be increased up to 8 to 10 repetitions in subacute cases, with the addition of dynamic strengthening exercises. Stable, quiescent, or inactive disease makes it possible to add an aerobic component such as walking, aquatics, or biking for at least 15 minutes each day three times a week. ROM and strengthening can be continued and monitored.[158]

A group of experts from the University of Ottawa reviewed comparative controlled trials and compiled evidence to suggest and support the conclusion that therapeutic exercises, including specific functional strengthening and whole-body functional strengthening, are a beneficial intervention for individuals with RA. The benefit may vary depending on the stage of disease (acute, subacute, inactive) but includes reduced pain, improved overall function, and decreased number of sick leaves.[274]

A helpful guide in establishing the level of acceptable exercise intensity is as follows: Acute pain during exercise indicates a need to modify the program; if joint pain persists for more than 1 hour after exercise is completed, the exercise was probably excessive.[98] Other recommendations and guidelines for including conditioning exercise in a comprehensive management program for RA are available.[9,14,241]

Regular, dynamic strength training combined with endurance-type physical activities improves muscle strength and physical function but not BMD in adults with early and long-standing RA without causing detrimental effects on disease activity.[117,118]

Low-load resistive muscle training has been shown to increase functional capacity and is a clinically safe form of exercise in mild to moderate RA.[174] Other studies report that moderate- or high-intensity strength training programs have better training effects on muscle strength in RA. It is essential to maintain the training routine to obtain long-term benefits.[116]

Aerobic exercises are safe to perform during the subacute and inactive stages of RA. Aerobic capacity can be estimated using a single-stage submaximal treadmill test.[240] Training programs begin at 50% (and work toward 80%) of maximal oxygen uptake based on the baseline test results. Without baseline testing, the PTA can rely upon (and teach the client to use) the Borg scale for rating of perceived exertion. Heart rate monitors are also helpful in enabling clients to track their cardiovascular responses.[158]

Aquatic therapy may be beneficial for conditioning, strengthening, and flexibility while reducing mechanical stress on the joints. Water exercise provides the means by which people with RA can reach needed training levels in a comfortable environment.

Client Education

Helping individuals affected by RA understand the disease, disease process, treatment, possible outcomes, and role of exercise and self-care is a major part of the PTA's task. Self-management includes learning pacing, joint protection, and energy conservation; monitoring symptoms; and maintaining or progressing an exercise program. The systemic nature of this disease produces global fatigue; the demand for energy to move joints may increase if biomechanics are altered.[158]

The need for frequent rest breaks, change in level of activity, and change in positions throughout the day should be taught and their use encouraged, but they should be balanced by the need to avoid muscle wasting and weakness from immobilization. ROM, stretching, and isometric exercises must be taught, monitored, and reinforced for as long as the PTA follows the individual, always teaching the client how to modify the program during periods of active inflammation.

Physical Modalities

Various modalities provide temporary pain relief and may be used in effectively and safely controlling symptoms of the acute inflammatory phase of RA. Information on the rationale for use and effectiveness of the various physical modalities is available.[35,232,242]

Although cold may be more suitable in acute inflammation, people with RA usually prefer heat. Superficial heat (e.g., paraffin baths, moist hot packs, hydrotherapy, or aquatic therapy) is recommended, whereas prolonged or deep heat is contraindicated, because it may increase intraarticular temperature, possibly contributing to joint destruction.[139] Electrotherapeutic modalities and thermotherapy physical agents are often used as part of a rehabilitation program mainly for pain relief, to control inflammation, and to reduce joint stiffness.

The Ottawa Panel recommends the use of low-level laser therapy, therapeutic ultrasound, thermotherapy, electrical stimulation, and transcutaneous electrical nerve stimulation for the management of RA. This recommendation is based on the analysis of systematic and literature reviews. Specifics of studies reviewed and a summary of the findings have been published in *Physical Therapy*.[273]

BOX 17.16 **ACR Criteria for Classification of Functional Status in Rheumatoid Arthritis**

Class 1: Completely able to perform usual activities of daily living (self-care, vocational, avocational)
Class 2: Able to perform usual self-care and vocational activities, but limited in avocational activities
Class 3: Able to perform usual self-care activities, but limited in vocational and avocational activities
Class 4: Limited in ability to perform usual self-care, vocational, and avocational activities

ACR, American College of Rheumatology.

Postoperative care. Surgical treatment of RA is often complicated by the client's generalized debilitated condition. People with RA tend to have poor skin condition, poorly healing wounds, and osteopenic bone. Generalized bone loss occurs early in the course of RA and correlates with disease activity. This condition is further affected by the use of corticosteroids.

Anyone with RA should be taught early on that if surgery is ever indicated, a program of isometric exercises and ROM before surgery is advised. Review dislocation precautions and restrictions before the surgical procedure. After arthroplasty, correction of deformity and relief of pain are typical, but recurrence of deformity can occur even with appropriate rehabilitation. Many clients are still very satisfied with the improved cosmesis, reduced pain, and improved function. Maximum benefit from arthroplasty may not occur for up to 1 year after surgery.[45]

Prognosis. There is no known cure for RA at this time, and joint changes are usually irreversible. Restrictions in the ability to perform specific actions and difficulty in performing ADLs can result in functional limitations and disability. It is now established that the longer a person has RA, the greater the likelihood of having cervical spine disease.[268]

Knowledge of the natural history of RA affecting the cervical spine is limited. Up to 80% of individuals with rheumatoid subluxations of the cervical spine demonstrate radiologic progression but may not experience corresponding clinical symptoms.[171] The presence of myelopathy increases the risk of mortality dramatically; without surgery, most people die within 1 year. Even with surgery to stabilize the spine, death from cord compression does occur.[263]

Quality-of-life issues are central to this disease when people who expected to be active and productive are severely incapacitated in early adulthood. The natural history of RA varies considerably, but people who present at an early stage and receive early intervention continue to do well years later, with reduced joint pain and inflammation and preservation of function.[369]

Mortality in adults with extraarticular manifestations of RA is significantly greater than in those whose disease is limited to the joints; in many people, the extraarticular manifestations are more debilitating than the arthritis itself.[92] Death from complications associated with RA and its treatment can occur. These

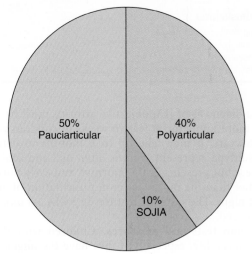

FIG. 17.28 Breakdown in types of juvenile idiopathic arthritis (JIA).

complications include subluxation of the upper cervical spine; infections; GI hemorrhage and perforation; and renal, heart, and lung disease. The same factors that contribute to joint inflammation also accelerate atherosclerosis and heart disease; early death resulting from coronary artery disease will be the focus of future treatment efforts.[62]

Juvenile idiopathic arthritis. Although the term *juvenile idiopathic arthritis* (JIA; formerly *juvenile rheumatoid arthritis* [JRA]) brings to mind a single disease similar to adult RA, it is actually an umbrella term for a heterogeneous group of arthritides (Box 17.17) of unknown cause that begin before age 16 years and occur in all races. Each subtype has a different presentation, genetic background, and prognosis.[27,298]

Definition and Incidence. Approximately 30,000 to 50,000 children in the United States are affected by one of the subtypes discussed here (Fig. 17.28). The general classification of JIA is based on the number of involved joints and the presence of systemic signs and symptoms. Many other forms of arthritis (e.g., SLE, dermatomyositis, scleroderma) that affect adults also occur in children, although less frequently.

Pauciarticular JIA (PaJIA; also known as oligoarthritis), meaning "few joints," generally affects four or fewer joints, usually in an asymmetric pattern, and most commonly involves the knees, elbows, wrists, and ankles. Girls are affected more often than boys, usually between the ages of 1 and 5 years. This type of JIA is relatively mild with few extraarticular features. Parents may notice a swollen joint and limp or abnormal gait, usually early after the child wakes up in

the morning. Leg length discrepancy is common. Pain is not a central feature at first, and the disease rarely manifests any constitutional symptoms.[247]

PaJIA is the most common type of JIA, comprising one-half of all JIA cases. Usually PaJIA runs a benign course; it recurs in up to 20% of children, most often during the first year but possibly delayed by as much as 5 years after the initial diagnosis. There are some children who develop persistent joint disease, referred to as extended oligoarthritis.[247]

Polyarticular JIA (PoJIA) affects five or more joints, most commonly including the large and small joints (wrists, cervical spine, temporomandibular joint, small joints of the hands and feet, as well as the knees, ankles, and hips). Joint involvement is usually symmetric and is most like that of adult RA, with the potential for severe, destructive arthropathy. PoJIA comprises 40% of all cases of JIA and affects girls more than boys. There are two subtypes, depending on whether children are rheumatoid factor positive or negative.[247]

Systemic-onset JIA (SoJIA; also called Still's disease; sometimes also affecting adults, although rare) affects boys and girls equally with involvement of any number of joints. This subtype has the most severe extraarticular manifestations, affecting many body systems, and comprises 10% of all cases of JIA. It often begins with a high-spiking fever and chills that appear intermittently for weeks and may be accompanied by a rash on the thighs and chest that often goes away within a few hours (Fig. 17.29). The fever pattern is marked by spikes exceeding 102° F (39° C) and periods between the spikes during which the child feels much better. Inflammatory arthritis typically develops at some point, and 95% of the children have joint complaints within 1 year of the initial presenting symptoms. Approximately half of the children who have SoJIA recover almost entirely; unfortunately, one-third of the children remain ill, with persistent inflammation manifesting as fever, rash, and chronic destructive arthritis.[247] In addition to inflamed joints, the child may experience enlargement of the spleen and lymph nodes; inflammation of the liver, heart, and surrounding tissues; and anemia.[23] Box 17.18 lists clinical manifestations associated with Still's disease.

Psoriatic JIA presents with psoriasis, arthritis, and at least two of the following: dactylitis, nail abnormalities, and a family history of psoriasis. Treatment with aggressive immunosuppressives may be required; uveitis (a potentially dangerous inflammation of the eye that can result in permanent damage or blindness) is a feature in some cases.

Enthesitis-related arthritis presents as inflammation of the tendon attachments to the bone, especially along the spine and Achilles tendon, along with arthritis and any two of the following: sacroiliac joint tenderness, inflammatory spinal pain, the presence of HLA-B27, positive family history, acute uveitis, and pauciarticular or polyarticular arthritis in boys older than 8 years.

Structures involved. The cause is still poorly understood, but JIA may be triggered by environmental factors and infection (viral or bacterial) in children with a genetic predisposition. Genomic studies hope to identify genetic traits that will predict disease risk and other characteristics such as disease course, age of onset, and disease severity. Eventually researchers may be able to identify molecular biomarkers to help diagnose and treat this group of arthritides.[285]

JIA can occur in boys or girls of any age (girls more often than boys) and most commonly begins during the toddler or

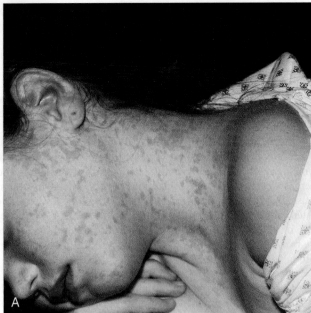

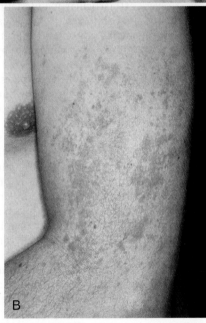

FIG. 17.29 (A) and (B) Skin rash associated with juvenile idiopathic arthritis. (A, From Paller AS, Mancini AJ: Hurwitz clinical pediatric dermatology: a textbook of skin disorders of childhood adolescence, ed 3, Philadelphia, 2006, Saunders. B, From James WD, Berger T, Elston D: Andrews' diseases of the skin: clinical dermatology, ed 10, Philadelphia, 2006, Saunders.)

early adolescent period. The pathogenesis is similar to that of adult RA, with immune cells mistakenly attacking the joints and organs, causing inflammation, destruction, fatigue, and other local and systemic effects.

Signs and symptoms. Early disease recognition is needed to help improve the clinical outcome, but symptoms of rheumatic disease are often mistaken for "growing pains," delaying diagnosis by many months. Diagnosis involves a medical history, physical examination, and laboratory tests, including serum evaluation to measure inflammation and to detect ANAs, rheumatoid factor, or sometimes HLA-B27.

BOX 17.18 Clinical Manifestations Associated with Still's Disease

Systemic
- Fever
- Rash
- Lymphadenopathy
- Polyarthritis
- Pericarditis
- Pleuritis
- Peptic ulcer disease
- Hepatitis
- Anemia
- Anorexia
- Weight loss

Musculoskeletal
- Polyarthritis, polyarthralgias
- Myalgia, myositis
- Tenosynovitis
- Skeletal growth disturbances (short stature, failure to thrive)

For a diagnosis of JIA, objective arthritis must be seen in one or more joints for at least 6 weeks in children younger than 16 years; it may take up to 6 months to determine which subtype is present. Pain is often dull and aching and less severe but presents in the morning and early during the day rather than the more common presentation of growing pains at night. The systemic features in SoJIA are more readily diagnosed.

Common tests and measures. Children with JIA may have no disability, especially if they have the oligoarticular form of the disease. Severe disability is seen most often in cases of rheumatoid factor–positive polyarticular and systemic disease, followed by rheumatoid factor–negative polyarthritis, enthesitis-related arthritis, and psoriatic arthritis. Physical therapy is an important adjunctive therapy for JIA.[27]

Efforts have been made to identify early predictive clinical, laboratory, demographic, genetic, or treatment-related factors for functional disability. It appears that there are complex interactions between disease subtypes but with specific predictors of outcome for each disease subtype.

The 6-minute walk test has been shown to be a good test for measuring functional exercise capacity in a small study of children (boys and girls) with JIA ages 7 to 17 years.[275] This might be a good place to begin baseline studies and evaluate response to the aerobic component of the plan of care for individuals with JIA.

Common management. Some of the immunomodulatory medications used in adult RA can be used in cases of JIA, but none of the current medications used has a curative potential. The goal of treatment is to control pain, preserve joint motion and function, minimize systemic complications, and assist in normal growth and development.

Medications. Early aggressive combination medications are replacing the previous gradual add-on approach to treatment (i.e., start with one drug and slowly add another and another to gain the desired effects without too many side effects).[397] Medications are administered to control the systemic and articular complaints and, in some cases, halt the progression of the disease. These agents may include immunosuppressives, DMARDs (e.g., MTX), and biologic agents such as TNF inhibitors (etanercept [Enbrel], infliximab [Remicade]).[114]

Corticosteroids are indicated if severe anemia, unrelenting fever, or vasculitis is present.

Invasive procedures. Bone marrow transplantation may be used in cases of JIA that are resistant to standard medical management.[364] Autologous stem cell transplantation (ASCT) is used for some individuals whose disease does not respond to MTX and other DMARDs. Complete remission is possible for up to half of the individuals receiving ASCT, with improvement reported in those individuals who are not resistant. Infection is a common morbidity associated with this treatment, observed in up to 71% of cases, in addition to an associated death rate of 15%.[61]

Conservative care. Physical therapy and occupational therapy are utilized for pain control, facilitation of mobility, and function. Equally important is the role of exercise in improving strength, endurance, and aerobic capacity. In children with JIA, resistive exercise produces a change in the immune response, with significantly lower levels of cytokines and higher levels of antiinflammatory compounds compared with those who did not exercise.[394]

With respect to joint impairment, loss of joint motion is the strongest indicator of functional disability in children with systemic JIA, and loss of joint motion has a greater effect on lower limb function than on upper limb function.[21] By the time children become adults, only 20% of them have moderate to severe limitations.

The role of the PTA in preventing joint loss should not be underestimated. Cervical spine involvement can occur in PoJIA and systemic JIA, with cervical stiffness as the most common finding. Neck pain is uncommon, and neurologic complications are less likely to develop in JIA than in adult RA.

If the PTA is seeing a young child with joint pain who has not been diagnosed, sensitivity to soft tissue manipulation despite improved or restored joint ROM warrants further medical investigation. For children with a known diagnosis, the use of physical modalities may be appropriate but must be used with caution as children are not always able to perceive and/or report discomfort.

Aquatic physical therapy is an excellent way to complete exercises while providing joint protection and engaging the child in a fun activity. One study engaged 54 children with JIA ages 5 to 13 years in a supervised aquatic training program 1 hour/week for 20 weeks. Measures of functional ability, health-related quality of life, joint status, and physical fitness showed no improvement, but there were also no signs of worse health status, suggesting that swimming is a safe exercise program.[372]

Strengthening programs for children with rheumatic disease can be part of the exercise program, even for children younger than age 6 years. Twice-daily sessions of 15 to 20 minutes are advised.[305] Research at the University of Buffalo showed significant improvement in function and better strength, endurance, and aerobic capacity. Equally important, pain, disability, and use of medications decreased significantly.[86]

Active exercise is not advised during flare-ups when joints are inflamed, but most children usually self-limit their physical activity according to symptoms. Passive stretching and modified aquatic physical therapy are better choices during exacerbations.

Children with dormant JIA can participate in some sports activities. With improved medical therapies, children with JIA are able to lead a more active lifestyle compared with similar children even 10 years ago. The PTA can be helpful in observing each child for abnormal biomechanics that can place him or her at increased risk for injury or future articular damage. Neuromuscular training may be needed to improve neuromuscular function and biomechanics. Proper technical performance during athletics may allow children with JIA to use joint-loading techniques (e.g., during jumping and landing) in a safe and controlled manner.[253]

Low BMD is a common secondary condition associated with JIA. Weight-bearing exercise programs to reduce the risk of low BMD are safe and effective for children with JIA who are healthy and should be included in the plan of care.[93]

The role of physical activity and an active lifestyle in cardiorespiratory fitness has been documented, but long-term follow-up is still needed to show if such a program protects from loss of aerobic fitness in this population group.[373]

Client education. The PTA should keep in mind the significant impact JIA has on the children and their families. The cost of this disease can be staggering, with pharmacotherapy, hospitalizations, medical visits, and other professional services, including physical and occupational therapy. Parents and children should be educated on the importance of avoiding forced or deep flexion of inflamed joints. Some activities may need to be modified or avoided.

Psychosocial–spiritual and quality-of-life issues should also be addressed. Appearance and body image are affected directly by JIA (e.g., generalized growth failure, local growth anomalies such as micrognathia), side effects of drug therapy, surgical scars, and severity of pain and fatigue. The PTA may be the first one to recognize overall problems with adjustment reflected by anxiety, depression, and/or social withdrawal.[27]

For those children with JIA who reach adulthood, significant problems can result from arthritis and uveitis, medication morbidity, and lifelong disability.[238] Young women may face the issue of pregnancy and childbirth with fears of transmitting JIA to the offspring, and possible reduced ability to conceive along with increased rates of miscarriages have been reported by some.[270]

Prognosis. The prognosis has greatly improved as a result of substantial progress in disease management, especially the use of particular medications. Early onset, progressive forms of JIA have a guarded prognosis. Between 25% and 70% of children with JIA will still have active arthritis 10 years after disease onset; more than 40% enter adulthood with active arthritis.[203]

The mortality risk for children with JIA has been estimated to be three to five times higher than in the general population.[378] Morbidity and mortality may be improved (including increased rates of disease remission) with the changes in treatment approaches, but this has not been documented as yet.[203]

Spondyloarthropathies

Spondyloarthropathies (SpAs), a group of disorders formerly considered variants of RA, are in fact distinct entities with similar features affecting the spine (Box 17.19). SpAs are characterized by inflammation of the joints of the spine and include several distinct entities: AS, psoriatic arthritis, and reactive arthritis, including arthritides that accompany inflammatory bowel disease (IBD), and Reiter's syndrome. Inflammatory eye disease (e.g., uveitis, conjunctivitis, iritis) occurs in approximately 25% of clients. Arthritic symptoms flare with IBD and usually affect the lower extremities in an asymmetric pattern. Vasculitis, clubbing of the fingers, and skin changes may be present.

Ankylosing Spondylitis

Whenever someone presents with new onset of back, sacroiliac, or hip pain in the absence of trauma or overuse that is accompanied by associated signs and symptoms of systemic disease (e.g., fever, fatigue, respiratory compromise), the PTA must recognize that these are not symptoms typically associated with mechanical causes of back pain. If present, these features are considered red flags that should raise concern regarding the underlying cause of the complaints.

Definition and incidence. AS, sometimes referred to as *Marie–Strümpell disease,* is an inflammatory arthropathy of the axial skeleton, including the sacroiliac joints, apophyseal (facet) joints, costovertebral joints, and intervertebral disk articulations.

Prevalence of AS is 0.1% to 0.2% in the U.S. general population. Nearly 2 million people in the United States have this condition, making it almost as common as RA. It is higher in Caucasians and some Native Americans than in African Americans, Asians, or other nonwhite groups.[2] AS typically affects young people, beginning between the ages of 15 and 30 years (rarely after age 40 years). This differs from back pain of mechanical origin, which is much more likely to develop between ages 30 and 65 years. Men are affected two to three times more often than women, although this disorder may be just as prevalent in women but diagnosed less often because of a milder disease course with fewer spinal problems and more involvement of joints such as the knees and ankles.[392,410] Overall, sibling risk is about 5.9%.[196]

Gender, age, race, and family history are all important factors related to the risk of developing AS. Although it is more prevalent in males, there is significantly less disparity in incidence between the genders than was once thought. The belief is that the disorder has been grossly underdiagnosed in women because the disease tends to be milder and peripheral joint involvement is more common, confusing the clinical picture.

Structures involved. Approximately one-third of those with AS have asymmetric involvement of the large peripheral joints, including the hip, knee, and shoulder. Fig. 17.30 shows the most commonly involved joints. The disorder can ultimately lead to fibrosis, calcification, and ossification with fusion of the involved joints. The pain, resultant postural deformities, and complications associated with this disease can be disabling.

The pathogenesis of AS is poorly understood, but the fundamental lesion appears to be chronic inflammation at sites of attachment of cartilage, tendons, ligaments, and synovium to

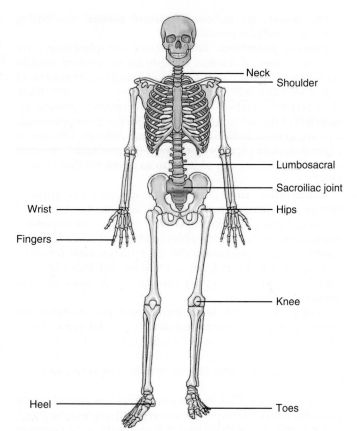

FIG. 17.30 Joints most commonly involved in ankylosing spondylitis and incidence of involvement. Neck, 75%; shoulder, 30%, lumbosacral, 50%; hips, 30%; knee, 30%; heel, 30%; toes, fingers, and wrist, less than 5% each; sacroiliac joint, 100%. Not shown: jaw, 15%; eye, 20%; ribs, 20%; costovertebral junction, 70%. (Data from Ramanujan T, Schumacher HR: Ankylosing spondylitis: early recognition and management, J Musculoskelet Med 1:75–91, 1992. Illustration modified from Lampignano J, Bontrager KL: Textbook of radiographic positioning and related anatomy, ed 8, St Louis, 2014, Mosby.)

the bone.[291] AS is marked by a chronic inflammation at the area where the ligaments attach to the vertebrae, initially in the lumbar spine and then in the sacroiliac joint.

Disruption of this ligamentous–osseous junction results, and reactive bone formation occurs as part of the repair process. Cartilage of the sacroiliac joints may also be involved (Fig. 17.31). The replacement of inflamed cartilaginous structures by bone contributes to progressive ossification with bony growth between the vertebrae, leading to a fused, rigid, or bamboo spine, characteristic of end-stage disease (Fig. 17.32).

Signs and symptoms. Insidious onset of low back, buttock, or hip pain and stiffness lasting for at least 3 months are often the initial presenting complaints. Early onset of back pain, stiffness, and fatigue during childhood often goes unrecognized for what it is. Onset of symptoms leading to a diagnosis occurs most often during early adulthood.[291]

At first the pain is described as a dull ache that is poorly localized, but it can be intermittently sharp. Over time, pain can become severe and constant, increased by prolonged rest or immobility and decreased by active movement. Coughing, sneezing, and twisting may worsen the pain.[196] Pain may radiate to the thighs but does not usually go below the knee.[3]

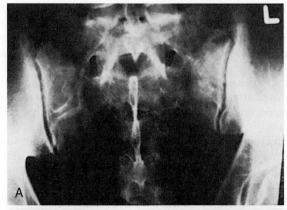

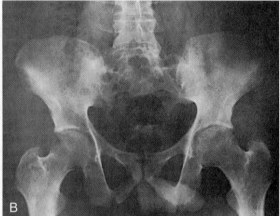

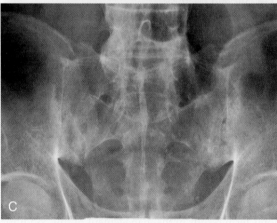

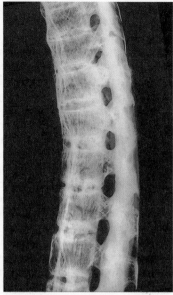

FIG. 17.32 Radiograph of a sagittal vertebral column in a person with ankylosing spondylitis. There is complete fusion of the spine, accentuated kyphosis, and loss of lumbar and cervical lordosis. There is also complete fusion of the intervertebral disk spaces. (From Bullough PG: Orthopedic pathology, ed 5, St Louis, Mosby, 2010.)

FIG. 17.31 Progression of ankylosing spondylitis of the sacroiliac joints. (A) Normal sacroiliac joints. (B) Fusion of sacroiliac joint spaces; the sclerosis has resorbed, and there is slight narrowing of the left hip joint. (C) Advanced ankylosing spondylitis with generalized osteoporosis and fusion of the spinous process, intervertebral disks, sacroiliac joints, and symphysis pubis. The entire skeletal unit has been transformed into one continuous osseous mass. (A, From Magee D: Orthopedic physical assessment, ed 6, St Louis, 2014, Saunders. B, From Rothman RH, Simeone FA: The spine, Philadelphia, 1982, Saunders. C, From Hamblen DL, Simpson H: Adam's outline of orthopaedics, ed 14, Edinburgh, 2010, Churchill Livingstone.)

Buttock pain is often unilateral but may alternate from side to side. Significant morning stiffness lasting more than 1 hour is often present. There may be tenderness over the spinous processes and sacroiliac areas with associated paraspinal spasms.

Enthesitis, which is inflammation of the tendons, ligaments, and capsular attachments to bone, may produce tenderness, pain and/or stiffness, and restricted mobility in the costosternal, costovertebral, and manubriosternal joints, iliac crest, ischial tuberosities, greater trochanters, spinous processes, or ligamentous attachments at the calcaneus.

Other clinical features include early loss of normal lumbar lordosis with accompanying increased kyphosis of the thoracic spine, painful limitation of cervical joint motion, and loss of spine mobility (flexibility) in all planes of motion.

In some cases, the initial complaints may occur in the extremities (e.g., hips or knees) with back symptoms appearing on average 3 years after onset of the peripheral involvement. Shoulder symptoms and loss of shoulder mobility are common but are rarely disabling. Involvement of the shoulder joint in AS correlates with involvement of other peripheral joints as well as the extent of radiographic change on shoulder films.[406]

Common tests and measures. AS is not easily detected in the early stages without a specialized MRI; early, accurate diagnosis allows treatment to start before the onset of permanent rigidity and deformity.

Diagnosis is usually based on identification of the clinical manifestations and radiographic findings.[2] History, physical examination, radiography, and laboratory tests are all used in the diagnosis.

Radiographs may be negative in the early stages of the disease; MRI enables the examiner to identify sacroiliitis earlier than plain radiography. However, radiographic findings of symmetric, bilateral sacroiliitis include blurring of joint margins, juxtaarticular sclerosis, erosions, and joint space narrowing are evident later in the disease process. The replacement of ligamentous tissue by bone at the site where the annulus fibrosus of the intervertebral disk inserts into the vertebral body results in a characteristic square-shaped vertebral body. In addition, as bony tissue bridges the vertebral bodies and posterior arches, the thoracic and lumbar spine takes on the appearance of a bamboo spine on radiographs (see Fig. 17.32).

Earlier in the disease process, intraarticular inflammation, early cartilage changes, and underlying bone marrow edema and osteitis can be seen with a specific MRI technique called short tau inversion recovery sequences.[291] No laboratory test is diagnostic of AS; laboratory tests assist primarily by ruling out other diseases.[291,346]

In the physical examination, ROM tests provide important information. The Schober test, chest expansion, and military stand against the wall are clinical tests used most often. The *Schober test* begins in the standing position by placing a mark at the lumbosacral junction, which is represented by the intersection of a line joining the dimples at the posterosuperior iliac spines. Place a second mark 5 cm below and 10 cm above the lumbosacral junction. The client is then asked to bend forward and attempt to touch the toes so the therapist can measure the distance between the upper and lower marks. The distance between these two marks has been found to correlate very closely with anterior flexion measured radiologically. The distance increases more than 5 cm in the absence of AS and less than 5 cm when AS is present.

Chest expansion involves circumferential measurements taken at the fourth intercostal space (or just below the breasts in women) before and after full inspiration and should reveal an excursion of 4 to 5 cm. Excursion less than 4 cm, and especially anything less than 2.5 cm, is a suspicious finding.

Hip flexion contractures are often present bilaterally and can be assessed using the Thomas test (in the supine position, ask the individual to maximally flex the contralateral hip joint; observe for loss of lumbar lordosis and flexion of the opposite leg, signaling a positive Thomas test result for the presence of a hip flexion contracture; repeat on the other side). Loss of hip mobility can result in reduced functional ability.

The Bath Ankylosing Spondylitis Functional Index along with the Dougados Functional Index score, Bath Ankylosing Spondylitis Metrology Index, and Bath Ankylosing Spondylitis Disease Activity Index are self-assessment tools that can be used both by the PTA and by the client to establish a baseline and document improvement or decline.[19,34,255]

Common management. The primary focus of intervention is to reduce inflammation and stiffness in the joints, maintaining mobility and proper postural alignment of the spine to prevent structural damage, while providing pain relief. Effective education is essential, because much of the management requires lifestyle adjustments and cooperation, especially compliance with the exercise program.[196]

Medical management. Joint involvement can be managed with NSAIDs, but in some cases DMARDs such as MTX or sulfasalazine may be used for peripheral disease. Spondylodiskitis or spinal fracture may require surgical intervention.[28] Spinal fusion may be needed but is not routinely recommended. The most valuable surgical intervention is total joint arthroplasty, especially a total hip replacement.[196] It is expected that with the new biologic therapies, the need for surgical intervention will become a rare event.[28]

Physical therapy. Exercising has been shown to benefit people with AS, but consistency, not quantity, seems to be the key factor in influencing posture, strength, motion, mobility, fitness, and overall health.[323] Home programs and group programs have both been shown to be beneficial for individuals with AS.[58,85]

A multimodal physical therapy program including aerobic, stretching, and pulmonary exercises along with routine medical management has been shown to yield greater improvements in spinal mobility, work capacity, and chest expansion compared with medical care alone. Individuals in a 50-minute, three-times-a-week multimodal exercise program were significantly improved after 3 months in chest expansion, chin-to-chest distance, occiput to wall distance, and the modified Schober flexion test.[155]

Functional and breathing capacity as well as balance should be assessed and developed. Stretching of the shortened muscles and chest expansion exercises should be encouraged. Improving and/or maintaining cardiovascular fitness is important.

Strengthening of the trunk extensors is equally important, so that if and when spinal fusion occurs, the spine is aligned in the most functional position possible. This requires a coordinated effort among all team members, including the affected individual and family.

High-impact and flexion exercises should be avoided, whereas low-impact aerobic exercise with extension and rotational components can be emphasized. Each individual will need to identify personal limitations and safe levels of participation.

In general, contact sports and high-risk activities such as downhill skiing, horseback riding, boxing, football, soccer, and water skiing should be avoided; aquatic therapy is an excellent option for most people provided extension principles are emphasized. In the presence of spinal fusion and osteoporosis, other activities requiring high levels of balance, agility, and coordination (e.g., bicycling, ice skating, rollerblading) can result in falls and fractures.

Overexercising can be potentially harmful and can exacerbate the inflammatory process; principles of relaxation, proper body mechanics, and energy conservation should be a part of the education program offered, including assessment of ADLs and providing necessary aids or devices such as long-handled reaching tools, adaptations for the car, special garden tools, or elastic shoelaces. Learning and using proper breathing techniques throughout all activities will help maintain chest expansion, improve oxygenation, and minimize muscle fatigue.

At present, aggressive but careful stretching to address the areas of hypomobility and the muscle imbalances is purported to help maintain as optimal a posture as possible. An exercise program focusing on specific strengthening and flexibility exercises of the shortened muscle chains offers promising short- and long-term results in the management of this condition.[84]

Client education. With the fragility of the spine in AS and the risk of fractures from even a minor injury or fall, falls prevention is important. This is an area for careful attention, because a number of people with AS suffer neurologic deficit after injury, especially spinal fracture.[142]

Trunk ROM and strengthening exercises to minimize thoracic kyphosis are essential. The more severe the kyphosis, the more hindered pulmonary function will be and the more pronounced the compensatory forward head posture. Postural deformities contribute to cervical pain and headaches and may also affect balance; these can be addressed with a comprehensive home exercise program. Avoiding obesity is recommended to reduce stress on weight-bearing joints and the cardiopulmonary system.

Body mechanics. The affected individual may need help modifying home or work situations. Resting in the prone position is advised to help avoid hip and spine flexion contractures. The

Spondylitis Association of America[357] recommends a firm, supportive sleeping surface to maintain good spinal alignment. Soft mattresses or waterbeds can contribute to excessive flexion and stooped postures.

The PTA can provide additional recommendations for the use of pillows or towel rolls for proper alignment in the various positions. The person may not stay positioned all night, but with time and training, changing positions and realigning props can be incorporated into the sleep cycle at least part of the time.

Proper lifting techniques can be demonstrated, with return demonstration provided by the client. The PTA should observe the work area or instruct the individual in appropriate ergonomics given the diagnosis of AS. Appropriate footwear advice should be provided; some people benefit from functional foot orthoses.

Prognosis. The extent of disability in persons with AS varies considerably, but fewer than 1% experience complete remission and more than 80% who are ill for longer than 20 years still have daily pain.[13,410] Periods of exacerbation and remission are common during the course of the disease.

The severity of symptoms during the first decade indicates the long-term severity and disabling nature of the disorder. Severe disease is usually marked by peripheral joint and extraarticular manifestations. The onset of hip disease in anyone with AS at any stage of the disease is a major prognostic marker for long-term severe disease and is more common in people with onset at a young age.[31]

Individuals with AS have an increased mortality rate. The impact of this disease can be seen in various aspects of workforce participation, such as needing more assistance, withdrawal from the workforce, and reduced quality of life. Early diagnosis and management will likely help prevent functional disability and improve outcomes.[25]

Complications. Long-standing AS disease is associated with multiple complications. Skeletal complications include osteoporosis, fracture, atlantoaxial subluxation, and spinal stenosis. In the most severe cases, the spine becomes so completely fused that the person may become locked in a rigid upright or stooped position, unable to move the neck or back in any direction. Flexion contractures, rigid gait, and flexing at the knees in order to maintain an upright position are not uncommon findings.

The stiff and osteoporotic spinal column is prone to fracture from even a minor insult; a significant proportion of individuals with AS experience vertebral fracture during the course of the disease. Fracture sites range from T7 to S1.[80,142] In fact, the incidence of thoracolumbar fractures in AS is four times higher than in the general population.[53,142]

AS is a systemic disease with widespread effects. In addition to arthritis in the spine, arthritis in other joints may be accompanied by inflammatory bowel syndrome with fever, fatigue, loss of appetite, weight loss, and other extraarticular complications. These clinical features distinguish AS from mechanical pain. The most common extraarticular manifestation is uveitis, occurring in 20% to 30% of affected individuals. Cardiomegaly, pericarditis, aortic regurgitation or insufficiency, amyloidosis (rare), and pulmonary complications may also occur. Pulmonary problems include upper lobe fibrosis and decreased total lung capacity and vital capacity (late stages of AS).[218]

Reactive arthritis. This section is confined to the discussion of reactive arthritis, which is defined as the occurrence of an acute, *aseptic,* inflammatory arthropathy arising after an infectious process but at a site remote from the primary infection. It is different from bacterial arthritis, which may be a local response with joint destruction and sepsis. The most common form of reactive arthritis is Reiter's syndrome, which will be discussed separately.

The borderline between reactive arthritis and true septic arthritis may be obscure, because several organisms can cause both, with overlapping symptoms and laboratory features. Other infectious causes of arthritis are discussed in other chapters (e.g., HIV, Lyme disease and Epstein–Barr virus, and rheumatic fever).

Definition and incidence. Reactive arthritis is a recognized result of infection with a number of intestinal pathogens, such as *Campylobacter jejuni* (GI tract), *Salmonella typhimurium,* *Shigella* (dysentery), *Chlamydia trachomatis* (genitourinary tract), *Chlamydia pneumoniae* (respiratory tract), *Yersinia,* *Mycoplasma fermentans,*[147] and *Clostridium difficile* (colitis associated with antibiotic therapy).

The overall prevalence of reactive arthritis has declined, although an increase has been seen in a small population group composed of intravenous drug users with acquired immunodeficiency syndrome. Reactive arthritis is most common in young, sexually active adults, especially men who have been infected with *C. trachomatis.* Reactive arthritis following urogenital infection is underdiagnosed in women.[252]

Structures involved. Bacteria in the joint may stimulate the immune system to produce antibodies and protein factors (cytokines), several of which produce local inflammation and tissue damage, leading to an arthritic joint. Reactive arthritis is usually asymmetric, affecting more than one joint, typically the large and medium joints of the lower extremities. Sacroiliac joint involvement occurs in about 10% of acute cases and 30% of chronic cases.

Signs and symptoms. The arthritis first manifests 1 to 4 weeks after the infectious insult. The client may report mild arthralgia and arthritis to incapacitating illness that may result in bed rest for several weeks. Joint pain may be minimal with no signs of inflammation, but stiffness, pain, tenderness, and loss of motion are often present.[252]

Associated findings may include uveitis, enthesitis (inflammation involving the sites of bony insertion of tendons and ligaments), sacroiliitis, urethritis, and conjunctivitis. Reactive arthritis encompasses a subgroup that demonstrates the classic clinical triad of arthritis, urethritis, and conjunctivitis, which is called Reiter's syndrome (see further discussion in the next section).

Extraarticular manifestations of reactive arthritis may include onycholysis of the fingernails or toenails, dactylitis (sausage-like swelling of the toes and fingers because of joint and tenosynovium inflammation), painless mucosal ulcers in the mouth, discharge from the vagina or penis, urologic symptoms (urgency, frequency, difficulty starting or continuing a flow of urine), or various types of skin lesions.

Common tests and measures. Laboratory evaluation, synovial fluid aspiration, cultures for bacteria, antibody testing, measurement of serum immunoglobulin, and imaging studies contribute to the differential medical diagnosis. Physical therapy examination should include a through history and muscle and joint testing.

The relationship of infections of the GI or genitourinary system to the joint is well documented, so that anyone with new onset of joint involvement must be medically evaluated for an underlying bacterial or infectious cause.

Medical history may reveal a recent infectious process, use of antibiotics, presence of a sexually transmitted disease, or bowel disease to alert the physician. The presence of joint involvement accompanied by (or alternating with) GI signs and symptoms such as diarrhea, abdominal pain, or bloating; constitutional symptoms (e.g., fever, night sweats); or positive iliopsoas or obturator sign must be reported to the physician.

Common management. NSAIDs and disease-modifying drugs are the basis of medical management. A short course of corticosteroids may be necessary in some cases, and antirheumatic agents may be beneficial in chronic reactive arthritis. Antibiotics are recommended if the infection is identified.

The overall prognosis for reactive arthritis is good even in severe cases, but full recovery does not always occur. Many people will experience some form of persisting symptoms that can lead to chronic disability.

Recurrence is possible, and a chronic form of this condition can develop, characterized by recurring arthritis that is accompanied by tendinitis or tenosynovitis. Sacroiliitis and spondylitis may not resolve but may persist, with ongoing pain and stiffness of the neck and back.[252]

Physical therapy intervention is very valuable during convalescence to regain full motion, strength, and function. Temporary splinting may be advised in the most painful cases, but muscle atrophy can be rapid, and therefore immobilization should be minimized.[252]

Reiter's syndrome.

Definition and incidence. Reiter's syndrome is one of the most common examples of reactive arthritis. Reiter's syndrome usually follows venereal disease or an episode of bacillary dysentery and is associated with typical extraarticular manifestations.

The prevalence and incidence of Reiter's syndrome are difficult to establish because of (1) the lack of consensus regarding diagnostic criteria, (2) the nomadic nature of the young target population, (3) the underreporting of venereal disease, and (4) the asymptomatic or milder course in affected women.

Age, gender, and medical history are important risk factors associated with Reiter's syndrome. The peak onset of this disorder occurs during the third decade of life, although children and older adults can also develop this disease.

A history of infection, especially venereal or dysenteric, is associated with increased risk of developing this condition. Men and women are equally affected by enteric infections. Reiter's syndrome is the most common form of reactive arthritis observed in HIV-infected adults and appears to be more strongly associated with male homosexuality than with injection drug use or other risky behaviors.[333]

Structures involved. Reiter's syndrome is primarily marked by inflammatory synovitis and inflammatory erosion at the insertion sites of ligaments and tendons (enthesitis). Heterotopic bone formation can occur at these sites. Synovial findings include edema, cellular invasion (lymphocytes, neutrophils, plasma cells), and vascular changes.

Signs and symptoms. The triad of symptoms classically associated with Reiter's syndrome includes urethritis, conjunctivitis, and arthritis. The urethritis and conjunctivitis often occur early in the disease. Other ocular manifestations include uveitis and keratitis (fungal infection of the cornea).

Three musculoskeletal manifestations are acute inflammatory arthritis, inflammatory back pain, and enthesitis. Only about one-third of individuals affected by Reiter's syndrome have all three. As discussed in the previous section, the arthritis is usually asymmetric, is often acute, and typically involves joints of the lower extremity, including the knees, ankles, and first metatarsophalangeal joint. Isolated hand joints can be involved. Although most of the symptoms and signs disappear within days or weeks, the arthritis may last for months or years.

Skin lesions may be indistinguishable from those of psoriasis. Low back pain is also a common complaint. The arthritis can progress and spread to the spine and even to the upper extremities.

Common tests and measures. The diagnosis of Reiter's syndrome may require months to establish, because the various manifestations can occur at different times. The combination of peripheral arthritis with urethritis lasting longer than 1 month is necessary before the diagnosis can be confirmed.

Laboratory tests typically reveal an aggressive inflammatory process. Elevated ESR and C-reactive protein are detected, and thrombocytosis and leukocytosis are common findings. Urine samples, genital swabs, and stool cultures are useful laboratory tests for identifying the triggering infection.

Up to 70% of those with established Reiter's syndrome may have radiographic abnormalities, including (1) asymmetric involvement of the lower extremity, (2) ill-defined bony erosions with adjacent bony proliferation, and (3) paravertebral ossification.

New-onset inflammatory joint disease with a history of recent enteric or venereal infection or new sexual contact strongly suggests a systemic origin of symptoms. Reiter's syndrome is one condition in which medical history and general health status may provide the most important information.

Common management. Although Reiter's syndrome is precipitated by an infection, there is no evidence that antibiotic therapy changes the course of the disorder. Treatment in general is largely symptomatic, with NSAIDs being the primary intervention.

If the arthritis persists, joint protection and maintenance of function become important. Immobilization and inactivity are usually discouraged, whereas ROM and stretching exercises are emphasized. Typically the arthritis resolves in 3 to 12 months but can recur. Chronic articular or spinal disease occurs in 30% of the population affected; severe disability occurs in less than 15% of those afflicted.[2]

Gout.

Although *gout* is a metabolic disorder and could be presented in earlier chapters, it is predominantly viewed as a form of arthritis because of its clinical presentation. Gout can be manifested as a joint disorder characterized by acute or chronic arthritis. Crystals other than uric acid crystals can also form inside joints, such as occurs in a condition called *pseudogout* when calcium pyrophosphate dihydrate crystals are present.

Definition and incidence. Gout represents a heterogeneous group of metabolic disorders marked by an elevated level of serum uric acid and the deposition of urate crystals in the joints, soft tissues, and kidneys. Gout is the most common crystalopathy in the United States.

The presence of calcium pyrophosphate dihydrate crystals in the synovial fluid can cause symptoms identical to those of acute gout. Unlike gout, however, calcium pyrophosphate dihydrate most often affects the knees of older women and may have polyarticular involvement. Pseudogout, also known as chondrocalcinosis, is associated with a number of metabolic disorders, such as hypothyroidism, hemochromatosis, hyperparathyroidism, and diabetes mellitus.

Primary gout is predominantly associated with middle-aged men, with a peak incidence during the fifth decade of life. It is the most common inflammatory disease in men older than age 30 years, affecting 2.1 million people in the United States, generally becoming symptomatic after a period of hyperuricemia lasting 10 to 20 years.[244]

Gout is rare in children, and less than 10% of the cases occur in women. Most women with gout are 15 years or more post-menopausal (later for women taking hormone replacement therapy; a few years of estrogen deficiency are necessary before gout becomes evident in this population).[150]

A family history of gout increases the risk of developing the disorder. The prevalence of gout increases with increasing serum urate concentration and age; with the aging of the American population, decreased renal function is becoming more prevalent, accompanied by a rise in the number of cases of gout.

Heavy alcohol consumption, obesity, fasting, medications (e.g., thiazide diuretics, levodopa, salicylates), renal insufficiency, hypertension, hypothyroidism, and hyperparathyroidism can all lead to decreased excretion of uric acid. Among the associated factors, age, duration of hyperuricemia, genetic predisposition, heavy alcohol consumption, obesity, thiazide drugs, and lead toxicity contribute the most to the conversion from asymptomatic hyperuricemia to acute gouty arthritis.[354]

A diet rich in purines (nitrogen-containing compounds found in foods such as shellfish, trout, sardines, anchovies, meat [especially organ meats], asparagus, beans, peas, spinach) can increase the risk of gout or make gout attacks more severe. Conversely, there is a lower prevalence of gout in vegetarians.[150]

In many cases of primary gout, the specific biochemical defect responsible for the hyperuricemia is unknown. A majority of cases probably result from an unexplained impairment in uric acid excretion by the kidneys. This impairment could result from decreased renal filtration, increased reabsorption, or decreased urate excretion by the renal tubules.

Structures involved. Uric acid is a substance that normally forms when the body breaks down cellular waste products called *purines*. In healthy people, uric acid dissolves in the blood, passes through the kidneys, and is then excreted through the urine. If the body produces more uric acid than the kidneys can process or if the kidneys are unable to handle normal levels of uric acid, then the acid level in the blood rises.

When the uric acid in the blood reaches high levels, it may precipitate out and accumulate in body tissues, forming supersaturated body fluids, including in the joints and kidneys. These crystals frequently collect on articular cartilage, epiphyseal bone, and periarticular structures. The crystal aggregates trigger an inflammatory response, resulting in local tissue necrosis and a proliferation of fibrous tissue secondary to an inflammatory foreign-body reaction.

Although the first metatarsophalangeal joint (i.e., the big toe) is a common site of pain, the ankle, instep, knee, wrist, elbow (olecranon bursa), and fingers can all be the site of the initial attack (Fig. 17.33).

Signs and symptoms. The disease occurs in four stages: asymptomatic hyperuricemia (defined as serum urate of more than 7 mg/dL), acute gouty arthritis, intercritical gout, and chronic tophaceous gout.[246] Many people who have elevated uric acid levels for prolonged periods never develop signs or symptoms.

The most common clinical presentation is the acute, monoarticular, inflammatory arthritis manifested by exquisite joint pain that occurs suddenly at night. Besides local, intense pain of quick onset, erythema, warmth, and extreme tenderness and hypersensitivity are typically present. Chills, fever, and tachycardia may accompany the joint complaints.

After recovering from the initial episode, the person enters an asymptomatic phase called the *intercritical period*. This period can last months or years despite persistent hyperuricemia and synovial fluid that contains monosodium urate crystals.[246]

The gouty attacks return suddenly with increasing frequency and severity and often in different joints. These attacks may be precipitated by trauma, surgery, alcohol consumption, or overindulgence in foods with high purine content. The arthritis can enter the chronic phase up to a decade after the initial attack, characterized by joint damage, functional loss, and disability. Deposits of monosodium urate crystals in soft tissue (tophi) and bone abnormalities are the hallmarks of chronic disease (Fig. 17.34).[354] Tophi can be located in tendons, ligaments, cartilage, subchondral bone, bursae, synovium, and subcutaneous tissue around the joints. Common sites of these hard, sometimes ulcerated masses that extrude chalky material include the helix of the ear, forearm, knee, and foot.[246]

Common tests and measures. Often termed "the great imitator," gout may masquerade as septic arthritis, RA, or neoplasm. The diagnosis can be delayed for weeks or months. A definitive diagnosis of gout is made when monosodium urate crystals (tophi) are found in synovial fluid, connective tissue, or articular cartilage.

Serum uric acid levels are elevated in approximately 10% of the affected population (more than 7 mg/dL); the presence of hyperuricemia alone does not equal a diagnosis of gout, nor does a normal serum level exclude its presence. The diagnosis is made most often on the basis of the triad of acute monoarticular arthritis, hyperuricemia, and prompt response to drug therapy.[246]

Bone abnormalities seen on imaging studies (e.g., calcification, overhanging edges of bone erosions with sclerotic margins but with normal bone density) may be present in a small number of affected individuals. These are usually late findings in the disease process, occurring most often in the chronic phase.

Common management. The goals of intervention are twofold: (1) to end acute attacks and prevent recurrent attacks and (2) to correct the hyperuricemia. NSAIDs are effective in treating the pain and inflammation of an acute attack. Occasionally intraarticular injection of corticosteroids is used to manage acute attacks. Allopurinol can prevent or lessen future gout attacks by slowing the rate at which the body makes uric acid in cases of excess uric acid production.

Other medications can be used to lower uric acid levels in the blood by increasing the amount of uric acid passed in the urine. These pharmacologic agents must be taken on a continuous basis to maintain a lower concentration of uric acid in the blood. Colchicine is another medication given during the acute phase but is less commonly used now because of its narrow therapeutic range and numerous side effects. Involved joints should also be rested, elevated, and protected (e.g., crutches, foot cradle, assistive devices, orthotics, proper shoe wear).

Once the acute attack has been relieved, the hyperuricemia may be treated, especially in the case of recurrent attacks of acute gouty arthritis or chronic gout. This requires lifelong management, and compliance is absolutely necessary. Dietary changes, weight loss, and moderation of alcohol intake are all

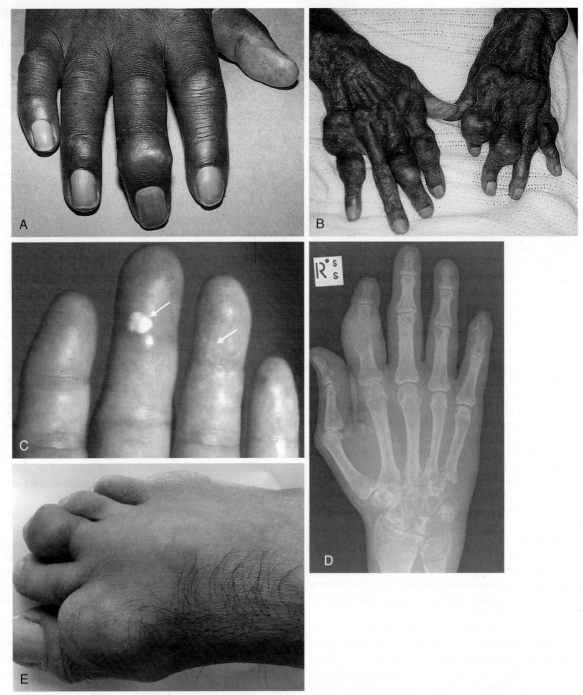

FIG. 17.33 (A) and (B) Tophaceous gout of the hands. The nodules are full of uric acid crystals. (C) Digit with white, tophaceous deposits beneath the skin. (D) Radiograph of the right hand of a patient with tophaceous gout. Note the soft tissue swelling surrounding the index finger proximal interphalangeal joint, with associated erosion and bone resorption. Well-corticated erosions are present through the hand and wrist. (E) Right foot with tophi over the first metatarsophalangeal joint and third distal interphalangeal joint. (A and B, From Roberts JR: Roberts and Hedges' clinical procedures in emergency medicine, ed 6, Philadelphia, 2014, Saunders. C, From Dalbeth N, Doyle AJ: Imaging of gout: an overview, Best Pract Res Clin Rheumatol 26: 823–838, 2012. D, From Falasca GF: Metabolic diseases: gout, Clin Dermatol 24:498–508, 2006. E, From Saeed RR, Mahwi TO: A case of acute gout in the background of chronic tophaceous gout caused by essential thrombocythemia, INJR 10:176, 2015.)

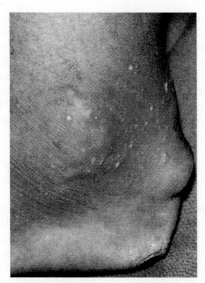

FIG. 17.34 Tophus, a chalky deposit of sodium urate present in the Achilles tendon and foot, occurs in cardiac transplant recipients who have an associated history of gout. These tophi form most often around the joints in cartilage, bone, bursae, and subcutaneous tissue, producing a chronic foreign-body inflammatory response. Tophi are not clinically significant for the therapist but indicate an underlying condition that requires medical attention. (From Howe S, Edwards NL: Controlling hyperuricemia and gout in cardiac transplant recipients, Musculoskelet Med 12:15–24, 1995.)

important. Controlling the hyperuricemia is the key to preventing this disease from becoming chronic and disabling.[244]

CONNECTIVE TISSUE

The final section of this chapter will cover systemic and isolated diseases and dysfunctions that affect the connective tissues in the musculoskeletal system. The section begins with a discussion of connective tissue disease and then moves to problems that occur with muscles. The section concludes with soft tissue injuries that are common in orthopedic practice and may involve a variety of tissues.

Connective Tissue Disease
Definition and Incidence
Sometimes people have features of more than one rheumatic disease, which has been called the overlap syndrome or mixed connective tissue disease. This category includes people who have overlapping features of SLE, scleroderma, or polymyositis. The incidence of this disease is unknown, but adults, particularly women, are predominantly affected. The designation *overlap connective tissue disease (OCTD)* became the preferred name for the disorder in people having features of different rheumatic diseases.

More advanced technology has brought about immunogenetic and serologic studies that demonstrate once again that mixed connective tissue disease (MCTD) is quite distinctive from other disorders, especially SLE and systemic sclerosis. There is now good evidence that the clinical and serologic features of OCTD are not just a haphazard association but represent a distinctive subset of connective tissue disease in which specific autoimmune response is relevant to clinical expression and to understanding the underlying pathogenesis.[210]

The cause of connective tissue disease is unknown, but hypotheses implicating modified self-antigens or infectious agents in the pathogenesis of OCTD have been advanced.[144] Persons with this condition often have hypergammaglobulinemia and test positive for rheumatoid factor, suggesting an immune injury.

There has been considerable controversy over the possible connection between silicone breast implants (and other silicone-containing devices, such as shunts and catheters) and the risk of connective tissue diseases. To date, there has been no convincing evidence of an association between breast implants in general, or silicone gel–filled breast implants specifically, and any of the individual connective tissue diseases or other autoimmune or rheumatic conditions.

Structures Involved
OCTD/MCTD combines features of SLE (rash, Raynaud's phenomenon, arthritis, arthralgias), scleroderma (swollen hands, esophageal hypomotility, pulmonary interstitial disease), polymyositis (inflammatory myositis), and, in most people, polyarthralgias; 75% have RA. Proximal muscle weakness with or without tenderness is common.

Pulmonary, cardiac, and renal involvement, as well as such findings as Sjögren's syndrome, Hashimoto's thyroiditis, fever, lymphadenopathy, splenomegaly, hepatomegaly, intestinal involvement, and persistent hoarseness, may occur. Neurologic abnormalities including organic mental syndrome, aseptic meningitis, seizures, multiple peripheral neuropathies, and cerebral infarction or hemorrhage occur in about 10% of people affected by this disorder. A trigeminal sensory neuropathy appears to be seen much more frequently in MCTD/OCTD than in other rheumatic diseases.

Signs and Symptoms
The diagnosis is considered when additional overlapping features are present in persons appearing to have SLE, scleroderma, polymyositis, RA, juvenile idiopathic arthritis, Sjögren's syndrome, vasculitis, idiopathic thrombocytopenic purpura, or lymphoma. High titers of serum antibodies to U1-RNP are a characteristic serologic finding seen much more often with OCTD/MCTD than with any other rheumatic disease.

Common Management
General medical management and drug therapy are similar to the approach used in SLE. Most persons are responsive to immunosuppression with corticosteroids, especially if administered early in the course of the disease. Mild disease often is controlled by salicylates, other NSAIDs, antimalarials, or very low doses of corticosteroids. High doses of steroids may be used in combination with cytotoxic drugs when the disease is progressive and widespread.

The overall mortality has been reported as 13%, with the mean disease duration varying from 6 to 12 years. Individuals who respond well to steroid therapy have a good prognosis. Pulmonary and cardiac complications (e.g., pulmonary hypertension) are the most common cause of death in MCTD.[127] Sustained remissions for several years in some people receiving little or no maintenance corticosteroid therapy have been observed.

Muscle
Polymyalgia Rheumatica

Definition and incidence. Polymyalgia rheumatica, literally "pain in many muscles" is a disorder marked by diffuse pain and stiffness that primarily affects the shoulder and pelvic girdle musculature. This condition is significant in that diagnosis is difficult and often delayed; severe disability can occur unless proper intervention is initiated. Polymyalgia rheumatica may be the first manifestation of a condition called giant cell arteritis, an endocrine disorder, malignancy, or an infection.[353]

The initial symptoms associated with polymyalgia rheumatica are often subtle and of gradual onset, resulting in a delay in the person's seeking care. The complaints also may be localized to one shoulder, leading to an initial diagnosis of bursitis. As the disease progresses, carrying out ADLs becomes increasingly difficult. Bed mobility and sit-to-stand transfers are among the functional activities affected.

Finally, a significant number (15% to 20%) of those with polymyalgia rheumatica also develop giant cell arteritis, a condition characterized by inflammation in the arteries of the head and neck. The risk related to the arteritis is blindness secondary to obstruction of the ciliary and ophthalmic arteries from inflammation-associated swelling.

Female gender, age, and race are the three primary risk factors associated with polymyalgia rheumatica. Women are affected twice as often as men, and the disease is rare before the age of 50 years; most cases occur after age 70 years. White women are more commonly affected than are women of other ethnicities. Polymyalgia rheumatica is a relatively common condition, with incidence estimated at 1 in 200 (one-half as common as RA).[320]

The cause of polymyalgia rheumatica is unknown, but experts suspect that genetic factors, infection, or an autoimmune malfunction may play a role.

Structures involved. Despite complaints of pain and stiffness in the muscles, polymyalgia rheumatica is not associated with any histologic abnormalities. Serum creatinine kinase levels, electromyograms, and muscle biopsy results are negative in this population. Rather, the aching and stiffness typical of this condition are caused by joint inflammation.

MRI studies have shown that subacromial and subdeltoid bursitis of the shoulders, iliopectineal bursitis, and hip synovitis are the predominant and most frequently observed lesions in active polymyalgia rheumatica. The inflammation of the bursae associated with glenohumeral synovitis, bicipital tenosynovitis, and hip synovitis may explain the diffuse discomfort and morning stiffness.[280]

Signs and symptoms. Polymyalgia rheumatica may begin gradually, taking days or weeks for symptoms to become fully evident, but more often it develops suddenly, and the person wakes up one morning feeling stiff and sore for no apparent reason. Getting out of bed in the morning can be the biggest challenge for individuals with polymyalgia rheumatica before initiating drug therapy.

Even though the initial muscle pain and stiffness may occur unilaterally, the symptoms are often bilateral and symmetric, affecting the neck, sternoclavicular joints, shoulders, hips, low back, and buttocks. Painful stiffness lasts more than 1 hour in the morning upon arising and is a hallmark feature of this disorder. Flulike symptoms such as fever, malaise, and weight loss are not uncommon.

Peripheral manifestations (e.g., wrists or metacarpophalangeal joints) are present in about one-half of all cases of polymyalgia rheumatica and include joint synovitis, diffuse swelling of the distal extremities with or without pitting edema, tenosynovitis, and carpal tunnel syndrome.[319] Many people are misdiagnosed with fibromyalgia, myositis, tendonitis, thyroid problems, or depression and spend months searching for answers and help before the correct diagnosis is made.

Despite the complaints of difficulties with bed mobility, sit-to-stand maneuvers, and accomplishing ADLs such as combing the hair or brushing the teeth, muscle weakness is not the problem. Pain and stiffness are the primary issues. Local tenderness of the involved muscles is noted with palpation. In addition, fever, malaise, unexplained weight loss, and depression may occur.

For those individuals with concomitant giant cell arteritis, additional symptoms of headache, jaw pain, scalp tenderness, fever, fatigue, weight loss, anemia, or blurred or double vision can occur.

Common tests and measures. Because there are no definitive tests to identify polymyalgia rheumatica, the diagnosis is often based on the presence of a constellation of findings and the person's rapid response to a trial of prednisone. In addition to the signs and symptoms listed, the person may be anemic and present with an elevated erythrocyte sedimentation rate (ESR; measure of viscosity), lowered hemoglobin and elevated platelet count (indicators of inflammation), and elevated C-reactive protein (indicator of current disease activity).

The current diagnostic criteria include as a requirement an ESR higher than 30 or 40 mm/hour. However, several reports have indicated that a large number of people with polymyalgia rheumatica (7% to 22%) have a normal or slightly increased ESR at the time of diagnosis, supporting the notion that an increased ESR should not be an absolute requirement for the diagnosis of polymyalgia rheumatica. This subset is characterized by younger age, less marked predominance of females, lower frequency of constitutional symptoms (e.g., weight loss, fever), and a longer diagnostic delay.[219]

MRI or ultrasonography of the joint or joints may facilitate diagnosis in anyone with typical proximal symptoms of polymyalgia rheumatica who also has normal ESR values.[36]

Common management. Untreated, polymyalgia rheumatica can result in significant disability. It is imperative that the individual be checked for giant cell arteritis, a frequently concurrent condition that can cause irreversible blindness.[387]

Treatment is with corticosteroids (e.g., prednisone); the response is dramatic. In fact, if dramatic improvement is not noted within 1 week of starting the prednisone, the diagnosis of polymyalgia rheumatica is questioned and the person must be reevaluated.

Most people require a maintenance dosage of prednisone for 6 months to 2 years that is gradually tapered to the lowest effective dose required to control symptoms. Treatment may take up to 5 years or longer before complete clinical remission occurs.[387] Methotrexate may be used for individuals who develop a dependency on corticosteroids.[353]

Polymyalgia rheumatica is not life threatening but it can limit daily activities, decrease restful sleep with nighttime awakenings and difficulty turning in bed, and decrease a sense of well-being and quality of life. With proper treatment, the prognosis is good, as the disease is self-limiting in many people with resolution within a period of 1½ to 2 years; however, recurrence can be as high as 30% in people who received treatment for 1 to 2 years.

When treating someone with a history of polymyalgia rheumatica, the PTA must be aware of the potential risk of giant cell or temporal arteritis. An adult older than age 65 years with sudden onset of temporal headaches, exquisite tenderness over the temporal artery, scalp sensitivity, or visual complaints should be seen by his or her physician immediately as this vasculitis is associated with stroke and blindness.

Because polymyalgia rheumatica has been shown to be an inflammatory response involving bursitis and tenosynovitis, therapy intervention can begin with this pathogenesis in mind. For example, the use of ultrasound as a deep heating agent in the presence of inflammation is not recommended for this type of problem.

Myopathy

Definition and incidence. Myopathy is a term used to describe nonspecific muscle weakness secondary to an identifiable disease or condition. The term *myositis* is also used to describe idiopathic inflammatory myopathies.

Many metabolic and hormonal diseases and autoimmune diseases can cause muscle weakness. Myopathies are usually classified as either hereditary or acquired (see Box 17.12). Myopathy may be associated with polymyositis or dermatomyositis.

The idiopathic inflammatory myopathies are thought to be immune-mediated processes that are triggered by environmental factors in genetically susceptible individuals.

Diabetes is associated with myopathy of three origins: vascular, neurogenic, and metabolic. Diabetes affects the small blood vessels and is associated with chronic hypoperfusion of muscles with blood. Diabetes also affects the peripheral nerves and causes neurogenic muscle atrophy and weakness. The disturbances of carbohydrate and lipid metabolism caused by insulin deficiency or insulin resistance adversely affect muscle function.

Acquired myopathy can also occur when tumors produce muscle weakness with or without inflammation. HIV-associated myopathies are less common now with improved medical intervention but may still be encountered by the PTA.

A new disorder called *critical illness myopathy* (CIM) has also been introduced. Disorders associated with prolonged stays in intensive care units (ICUs; e.g., acute respiratory illness, septic inflammatory response syndrome, acute respiratory distress syndrome) often result in excessive and prolonged weakness. CIM is a nonnecrotizing myopathy accompanied by fiber atrophy, fatty degeneration of muscle fibers, and fibrosis. As improvements in medical technology and medical management of individuals with severe illness continue to improve, the incidence of CIM is expected to rise.[307]

Use of systemic corticosteroids combined with prolonged exposure to neuromuscular blocking (paralytic) agents during the treatment of various critical illnesses in the ICU may be the key risk factor for this type of acute myopathy. Septic inflammatory response syndrome may be another risk factor.[307]

Structures involved. Myopathy is characterized by progressive proximal muscle weakness with varying degrees of pain and tenderness. Distal involvement is possible but is more common in myositis. During the early stages of disease, the muscles may be acutely inflamed and painful to move and touch. Muscle weakness and easy fatigability eventually compromise aerobic capacity and affect the person's ability to work, socialize, and complete ADLs.[137] Other symptoms of systemic illness may be present, including fever, fatigue, morning stiffness, and anorexia.

Signs and symptoms. Reduced muscle strength, endurance, and coordination accompanied by fatigue are commonly reported with myopathies. Myalgia occurs at rest and with exercise in half or more of all affected individuals in all stages of the disease. Left untreated, most cases of muscle weakness associated with inflammatory myopathies progress slowly over months and result in further decline of muscle strength and endurance.[4]

Common tests and measures. Determining the underlying cause for the myopathy is critical. Muscle biopsy, electromyography (EMG), and laboratory findings (measurement of muscle enzymes) are essential to ensure diagnostic accuracy, especially in the case of idiopathic myopathy. EMG can allow differentiation between myopathy and neuropathy and can localize the site of the neuropathic condition. The typical laboratory profile reveals mild to marked elevations in muscle enzymes, including creatine kinase and aldolase.

Some imaging techniques such as MRI and magnetic resonance spectroscopy of muscles can assess changes in local inflammatory activity.

Baseline measurement of muscle function using manual muscle testing assesses strength but not endurance, an important feature with this condition. Measurement of muscle endurance should be included in the physical therapy examination. A functional index to specifically test muscle impairment is under investigation but has not been finalized. Outcome measures that track activity limitation and participation restriction should also be used.[4]

Common management. Inflammatory myopathies may respond to pharmacologic treatment, especially corticosteroids but also immunosuppressives and antimalarial agents. Oral creatine supplements combined with exercise have proven effective for improving muscle function without adverse effects in adults with inflammatory myopathies.[48]

Effective therapy for noninflammatory myopathies remains lacking; antiinflammatory agents do not appear to be helpful in these cases. Presently there is no known pharmacologic treatment or prevention for critical illness myopathy (CIM). Medical management to minimize the risks is suggested.[307]

Prognosis is variable, with some people responding well to medical therapy and rehabilitation and others continuing to decline. Long-standing disability is not uncommon despite aggressive immunosuppressive treatment; the reasons for the persisting disability remain unknown.[4] Additionally, corticosteroid-related complications can have a significant impact.

Factors associated with poor survival include onset after age 45 years, delayed diagnosis and intervention, severe weakness and pharyngeal dysphagia, malignancy, myocardial involvement, and interstitial lung disease. CIM is reversible, but there is often considerable morbidity (e.g., persistent pain and weakness, HO with frozen joints).[184] ICU-acquired myopathy prolongs hospitalization because of the need for extensive rehabilitation. Even with rehabilitation, many affected individuals remain heavily dependent on others for personal care and ADLs.[217]

Acute care physical therapy. PTAs in the acute care setting frequently see the effects of bed rest, even without associated injury and after only as little as 1 week as disuse atrophy causes decrease in muscle mass. Often this occurs in the older adult population who have already experienced significant decline in muscle mass. CIM is also often accompanied by critical illness polyneuropathy (CIP), a disorder of the peripheral nerves triggered by the same events as CIM.[307]

Clients with the combination of these two conditions have difficulty weaning from the ventilator. Once the individual is alert and less sedated, weakness and atrophy of the limbs becomes more readily apparent. Severe flaccid tetraparesis may even be observed. Muscles innervated by the cranial nerves appear to be spared. Whereas CIP can affect all limbs and muscle groups, distal weakness and sensory changes are more common. CIM typically affects larger, more proximal muscle groups; sensation is not impaired.[307]

The PTA can use a handheld dynamometer to measure progress and improvement over the course of the treatment plan. Some experts suggest that a neuromuscular rehabilitation program should be started as soon as possible, including strength training and bracing as needed. Shorter sessions conducted more often may be needed during the initial phase of recovery.[149]

Recovery can be delayed by weeks to months. Regaining ambulatory status at 4 months postillness is achieved by approximately 50% of affected individuals.[183] The therapist is a key member of the rehabilitation team, recognizing the need for psychologic and emotional support to the client and the family. Understanding that the client is not just deconditioned and has a complex pathologic condition can help facilitate appropriate referrals to other disciplines (e.g., occupational therapy, psychology, social work, physiatry, speech pathology).[307]

Exercise. Early rehabilitation is important in the course of myopathy, with careful application of rest and exercise, focusing on rest during the active inflammatory phase and rebuilding of muscle strength during remission. During periods of severe inflammation, bed rest and passive ROM are recommended; active ROM exercises are contraindicated.

It is important to design a rehabilitation program according to the type, stage, and severity of myopathy. Muscle assessment and functional evaluation are prerequisites to determining an appropriate intervention program. In extremely acute cases, a tilt table may be necessary to reacclimate the cardiovascular system and assist with balance training for the individual who has been on bed rest.

The exercise program begins in the acute phase with stretching and passive ROM and progresses throughout the recovery process according to the person's tolerance to include isometric, isotonic, and low-intensity aerobic activities. Moist heat applied before stretching inflamed or sore muscles may be helpful. Performing exercises in a gravity-eliminated environment (aquatic program) or gravity-eliminated position may be necessary in the beginning.[137] Attention to the muscles of respiration and breathing assessment are also important, and anyone with cardiac involvement must be evaluated before initiating an aerobic program.

Concern about stressing the already inflamed muscles with a resultant increase in CPK level has traditionally prevented the use of strengthening exercises for anyone with inflammatory myopathies. But exercise itself can cause elevated serum creatine kinase levels in healthy individuals,[212] and studies have shown that people with stable active disease can perform isometric exercise without causing a sustained rise in CPK level.

Continued studies evaluating the effect of exercise training on inflammatory myopathies are under way; preliminary exercise guidelines are available.[138,140] Studies have shown improvement in adults with stable myopathies after a 12-week 20-minute home exercise program combined with a 15-minute walking program 5 days/week. Improvement was measured as reduced impairment and reduced activity limitation/participation restriction.[5]

Similar results have been reported for individuals with active myopathies performing an intensive resistive exercise program.[3,6] People in a variety of exercise programs—including stair climbing, stationary cycling, strength training, group exercise in a pool or at a gym, and outdoor walking using a wide range of frequency, intensity, and duration—have all shown improvement in fatigue and aerobic fitness, whereas serum creatine kinase levels remain unchanged.[4]

A home program including heat modalities, prescriptive exercise, and assistive devices helps the individual manage with functional disability. Upper extremity splinting and lower extremity bracing may be necessary to prevent contractures, prolong mobility, and enhance functional skills. A weak quadriceps mechanism combined with foot drop or a shuffling gait can contribute to increased falls, necessitating a muscle strength, balance, and fall assessment with appropriate intervention.

Client education about this condition is important and should include energy conservation and joint protection education. Serious side effects can accompany high-dose corticosteroid therapy, compounding the functional difficulties already present with the myopathy.

Myofascial Pain Syndrome

Definition and incidence. Myofascial pain syndrome (MPS) is an overuse or muscle stress syndrome marked by the presence of myofascial trigger points (TrP) within a taut band of muscle. These hyperirritable foci located in skeletal muscle or its fascial components were first described in 1952.[384] On palpation of these points, a characteristic pattern of local and referred pain is provoked. Referred pain may be provoked at quite a distance from the points of local tenderness.

TrPs may be either *active* (those that cause pain at rest or with activity of the involved muscle) or *latent* (not painful but causing movement restriction and weakness of the involved muscle with increased muscle tension and muscle shortening present). A latent TrP may become active in the presence of an acute, sudden overload of the muscle or a more chronic strain. A *satellite* TrP may develop in the same or other muscles within the referred pain pattern of the primary TrP or in synergistic muscles.

TrPs are separate and distinct from the tender points associated with fibromyalgia. TrPs appear to be a peripheral muscle phenomenon, whereas the widespread pain of fibromyalgia syndrome is a combination of both peripheral and central nervous system factors. Although it is possible to have both TrPs and tender points in the same person, usually the individual presents with a distinct clinical presentation of predominantly either MPS or fibromyalgia syndrome. The widespread tender points of fibromyalgia have a very different underlying physiology compared with the TrPs of MPS.

The cause of myofascial pain dysfunction is thought to be related to a sudden overload or overstretching of a muscle, direct-impact trauma, postural faults, psychologic stress, or chronic repetitive or sustained muscle activity.[348] TrPs can be the source of pain in other conditions such as tension headache.

People involved in occupations or recreation marked by repetitive or sustained activities or postures are at increased risk of developing this condition. Structural abnormalities or postural or mechanical stress could also place a chronic strain on certain muscle groups. Structural abnormalities that can predispose an individual to TrPs include significant leg length discrepancy, small hemipelvis, short upper arms in relation to torso height, and a foot with a relatively long second metatarsal compared with the first metatarsal.[348]

Other predisposing factors that can trigger activation of TrPs include overwork fatigue, chronic infection, impaired sleep, psychologic stress, and nerve entrapment (i.e., radiculopathy).[348,384] TrPs can be activated indirectly by other existing TrPs, visceral disease (e.g., myocardial infarction, peptic ulcer, renal colic, gallbladder disease), arthritic joints, joint dysfunctions, and emotional stress.[348]

Structures involved. Current evidence suggests that TrPs are the result of an established neuromuscular disease characterized by muscle tension and its sequelae.[288] Myofascial TrPs are most likely triggered by the performance of unaccustomed eccentric muscle activity. Eccentric movement of a muscle requires it to contract while being lengthened at the same time. A buildup of acetylcholine causes the muscle to remain tense and even activate nearby muscles in the referral zone to activate latent triggers, making them satellite myofascial TrPs.[99]

Spontaneous EMG activity in the TrP is greater than EMG activity in a noninvolved area of the same muscle, with a specific electrical discharge characteristic of a TrP identified. It appears that the electrical signal originates from the motor endplate rather than from the muscle spindle.[145]

The myofascial TrP mechanism is also closely related to spinal cord integration. When the input from nociceptors in an original receptive field persists (pain from an active TrP), central sensitization in the spinal cord may develop and the receptive field corresponding to the original dorsal horn neuron may be expanded (referred pain). Through this mechanism, a new (satellite) TrP may develop in the referred zone of the original TrP.[145]

Muscles protecting themselves against perceived trauma from overuse or repetitive contraction do not go into a protective spasm as was once thought but rather shorten and "shut off" as a means of guarding and self-protection. Energy requirements are reduced through this mechanism, and the body compensates by finding other muscles to do the task. It is hypothesized that the nervous system forgets to "turn the muscle back on" as identified by surface EMG studies.[130]

The muscle fiber shortening also impairs local circulation, which causes a loss of oxygen and nutrient supply to the region. This completes a vicious cycle; thus an energy crisis occurs, and taut bands form. It appears that these taut bands are necessary precursors for the development of TrPs based on the fact that taut bands frequently exist in pain-free individuals.[145]

Signs and symptoms. A taut, palpable myofascial band that is exquisitely tender on palpation with a characteristic and reproducible referred pain pattern (with sustained palpable pressure) is the hallmark of myofascial pain dysfunction. This clinical manifestation has also been described as a ropelike, nodular, or crepitant (crackling or grating) area within a muscle; there may be fibrotic tissue resembling a small pea present that exhibits a highly localized, exquisitely tender spot. Once present, the TrPs are self-sustained and self-perpetuating hyperirritable foci.

Pain referral patterns associated with TrPs are documented by several authors.[177,348,385] Besides the pain, myofascial pain dysfunction is manifested by a reduced ROM of joints under the control of the involved muscle and muscle weakness. The affected individual may be aware of numbness or paresthesia rather than pain, but there are no neurologic abnormalities, and the hypesthesia does not follow a radicular distribution.[281]

Systemic signs and symptoms are absent (unlike in fibromyalgia syndrome with its multiple presentation of various systemic manifestations), although a mild autonomic nervous system response to pain may result in nausea, diaphoresis, or change in blood pressure when TrPs are palpated. Related proprioceptive disturbances caused by TrPs may also include imbalance, dizziness, tinnitus, and distorted weight perception of lifted objects.[348]

Disturbances of motor function caused by TrPs include spasm of other muscles, weakness of the involved muscle function, loss of coordination by the involved muscle, and decreased work tolerance of the involved muscle. The weakness and loss of work tolerance are often misinterpreted as an indication for strengthening exercise, but if this is attempted without inactivating the responsible TrPs, the exercise is likely to encourage and further ingrain muscle substitution and further deconditioning of the involved muscle.[348]

Common tests and measures. The diagnosis is first made by clinical examination. Several diagnostic tests can help substantiate objectively the presence of characteristic TrP phenomena, including surface EMG, needle EMG, and ultrasound. There is limited consensus on the diagnostic criteria for TrPs associated with MPS. A literature review of criteria used to diagnose TrPs found no less than 19 different diagnostic criteria. The four most commonly applied criteria were a tender spot in a taut band of skeletal muscle, client pain recognition, predicted pain referral pattern, and local twitch response.[383]

Mechanical stimulation of the TrP—either by manual palpation or dry needling—frequently results in a local twitch response (a brief contraction of the palpable mass in response to a brisk rolling or snapping palpation of the band, a visible indication of an active TrP). The same stimulus also produces a jump sign characterized by vocalization or withdrawal (person jumps away from the examiner in response to pressure exerted on the TrP). These two signs are usually present, observable, and reproducible before effective intervention eliminates the TrP and the signs. Additionally, the examiner may palpate a distinct nodule in the center of the taut band that is tender, sometimes exquisitely tender.

There is also the possibility of a visceral–somatic cause of TrPs, such as occurs with myocardial infarction or enteric (abdominal) disease. Because of the referred nature of visceral pain, application of vapocoolant spray into the somatic reference zone can temporarily relieve the visceral pain with no real effect on the underlying visceral pathologic condition. Screening for medical disease is always necessary when evaluating muscle pain and myofascial TrPs.[348]

The PTA's knowledge of biomechanics, kinesiology, and mechanisms of injury is an important tool in identifying the cause that activated the TrPs and in recognizing current perpetuating factors. Perpetuating factors (Box 17.20) are often different from what caused activation of the TrPs and may include body positions, postural positions, skeletal asymmetries, and activities that increase mechanical stresses, causing reactivation of TrPs. After the TrP is inactivated (specific techniques are available for the PTA),[177,348,385] the muscle or muscles must be retrained, and full-stretch ROM must be restored in order to return to normal motor function (Box 17.21).[348]

Common management. Many techniques aimed at desensitizing TrPs have been employed, such as injections using dry needling, saline, or local anesthetics (performed by a physician or in some states by a qualified PT); application of ice

---

BOX 17.20   Perpetuating Factors in Myofascial Trigger Points

Mechanical Stress
- Leg length discrepancy
- Postural imbalance (e.g., shoulder protraction, forward head position)
- Movement impairment
- Pelvic upslip
- Muscle imbalance
- Overuse, repetitive muscle contraction, unaccustomed eccentric muscle activity[99]

Nutrition
- Vitamin deficiency of B_1, B_6, B_{12}, folic acid, vitamin D
- Mineral deficiency or imbalance (iron, calcium, potassium, magnesium)

Metabolic Conditions
- Hypothyroidism
- Hypoglycemia
- Allergies
- Visceral disease (e.g., peptic ulcer, renal colic, colitis, myocardial infarction)

Psychologic Factors
- Anxiety
- Depression
- Emotional stress and tension

Other
- Chronic viral infections
- Sleep disturbance
- Indirectly triggered by other existing trigger points

BOX 17.21   Myofascial Trigger Point Diagnosis and Treatment

Steps to Diagnosis of Myofascial Trigger Points
- Complete a past medical history
  - Assess for sudden onset from acute injury, trauma, overload stress, overstretching, or overshortening
  - Assess for gradual onset with chronic overload, microinjury, microtrauma, repetitive trauma
- Determine the biomechanics of the injury
- Determine the referred pain patterns
- Assess for limitations in joint and muscle range of motion
- Assess for muscle weakness of involved muscle or muscles
- Palpate for local tenderness with possible referred pain; palpate for taut band and nodularity of the affected muscle
- Assess for latent or satellite trigger points
- Complete examination (other orthopedic, neurologic, special, differential diagnostic tests including fibromyalgia tender point assessment)
- Complete evaluation
- Determine diagnosis, prognosis
- Perform intervention and reexamine

Guidelines in Myofascial Intervention
- Modalities to the affected muscle (e.g., moist heat, electrical stimulation, laser, ultrasound); begin teaching client how to recognize and avoid perpetuating factors
- Trigger point therapy, ischemic compression; instruct client in breathing and relaxation techniques; physician may perform dry needling or procaine injection; qualified physical therapists may perform dry needling (depending on state laws)
- Myofascial stretching; observe for positive stretch sign indicating need to decrease stretch while remaining within the muscle's therapeutic range; observe for pain from stretching the involved muscle, indicating need for vapocoolant or ice combined with stretching
- Persistent increased trigger point activity after treatment may require repeating above steps for a few sessions until referred pain pattern is significantly decreased and range of motion is 70% of normal before initiating muscle-strengthening sequence
- When the above steps are completed, add muscle-strengthening sequence; when joint and muscle ranges of motion are within functional levels and the client is pain free, proceed to the next step
- Proprioceptive training
- Home exercise program is ischemic pressure, massaging of the affected area, and sustained self-stretching with good breathing techniques emphasized
- Reexamination to modify or redirect intervention based on new clinical findings, client progress, or lack of client progress; assess for need for consultation with or referral to another provider

Data from Kostopoulos D, Rizopoulos K: Hands-on seminars: an intensive training on trigger point, myofascial and proprioceptive training, Astoria, NY, 2001; Kostopoulos D, Rizopoulos K, Kurman RJ, et al.: The manual of trigger point and myofascial therapy, Thorofare, NJ, 2001, Slack.

---

in the direction of prescribed patterns; laser; ultrasound; and sustained (ischemic) manual pressure to the TrP. High-power, pain-threshold, static ultrasound technique has been shown to resolve acute TrPs more rapidly than conventional methods of using ultrasound for this condition.[211,358] All of these techniques should be accompanied by sustained stretch of the involved muscle to desensitize the band.[348,385]

Ischemic compression is described as one that applies a steady pressure using the thumbs or four fingers on one or both hands inward toward the center and then is slowly released. Pressure application varies and may start from a few pounds and increase up to 10 lb, lasting from 30 to 45 seconds. On release, the skin blanches and then shows reactive hyperemia. The person should breathe deeply and slowly as pressure is progressively increased.

Non–ozone depleting vapocoolant spray (a topical skin refrigerant) may be used with the stretching procedures to facilitate pain relief and return of function. It is hypothesized that elongation of the muscle to its full normal length is the underlying mechanism that relieves pain caused by myofascial TrPs. Muscle lengthening utilizing postisometric relaxation may also be a successful technique.[197]

Additional rehabilitation to restore muscle strength and proprioception is required (see Box 17.21). The PTA may employ a variety of additional modalities in the treatment of TrPs, such as low-voltage electrical stimulation, ultrasound, moist heat, or laser. Some experts recommend nutritional counseling with supplementation of vitamins B_1, B_6, and B_{12}; folic acid; and vitamin C.

When ultrasound is used for treating TrPs, the continuous mode appears to be more effective than the intermittent mode. To avoid aggravating a highly irritable TrP, the ultrasound intensity should be gradually increased from 0.5 W/cm^2 until the client reports feeling warmth under the sound head. More specific details of ultrasound application for myofascial pain versus fibromyalgia are available.[204]

A home program of pressure followed by sustained stretch for the treatment of myofascial TrPs has been shown to be effective in reducing TrP sensitivity and pain intensity. It is important to instruct the person in how to apply a sustained stretch without initiating a protective spasm or guarding contraction.[123] This can be done by combining superficial heat or cold, ischemic pressure, breathing techniques, and slow stretching. Compliance regarding the stretching of the involved muscle is paramount to lasting success of treatment. The client can also apply sustained deep pressure over a TrP using a tennis ball or some other firm object. Stretching without applying pressure to minimize the nodules (TrPs) can have a rebound effect, making matters worse. The TrP must be released first before applying stretching alone.

It may be necessary to rely on medications to increase the pain threshold (e.g., antidepressants) or muscle relaxants to help loosen muscles first. Gentle stretching can be initiated, possibly in addition to or combined with surface electrode biofeedback.[130]

Helping the individual with active TrPs to achieve restful sleep is essential. Proper positioning, bed, and pillow (or other props) should be evaluated and discussed. Sleep disturbances caused by painful symptoms occur when body weight is compressing a TrP. This, in turn, increases pain sensitivity the next day. Active myofascial TrPs become more painful when the muscle is held in the shortened position or compressed for long periods.

Myofascial Compartment Syndrome

Definition and incidence. *Myofascial compartment syndromes* develop when increased interstitial pressure within a closed myofascial compartment compromises the functions of the nerves, muscles, and vessels within the compartment. Many clinical conditions predispose to the development of compartment syndromes, including fractures, severe contusions, crush injuries, excessive skeletal traction, and reperfusion injuries and trauma. Other risk factors may include burns, circumferential wraps or restrictive dressings, or a cast or other unyielding immobilizer. Ischemia and irreversible muscle loss can occur, resulting in functional disability (and even potential loss of limb) if the condition is left untreated.

Structures involved. Compartment syndromes may be acute or chronic and are most likely to occur within the "envelopes" of the lower leg, forearm, thigh, and foot where the fascia cannot give or expand.

Signs and symptoms. The earliest clinical symptom of impending compartment ischemia is pain out of proportion to that expected from the injury. The pain is described as deep, throbbing pressure. There may be sensory deficit or paresthesia within the region distal to the area of involvement.

Common tests and measures. In severe compartment syndromes, objective signs are visible, such as a swollen extremity with smooth, shiny, or red skin. The extremity is tense on palpation, and passive stretch increases the pain.[228]

Common management. Prompt surgical decompression is the standard intervention. After resolution of the acute symptoms, a specific program to regain mobility, strength, and endurance should be designed.

Rhabdomyolysis

Definition and incidence. Rhabdomyolysis is the rapid breakdown of skeletal muscle tissue due to mechanical, physical, or chemical traumatic injury (Box 17.22). The principal result is a large release of the creatine phosphokinase (CPK) enzymes and other cell byproducts into the blood system. Accumulation of muscle breakdown products can lead to acute renal failure.

Of particular note is the potential for muscle pain from statins (cholesterol-lowering medications) and rhabdomyolysis from high-dose statins.[60] Less than 5% of the adult population who take statins develop this problem. However, with more

---

> **BOX 17.22 Causes of Rhabdomyolysis**
>
> **Physical**
> * Prolonged high fever; hyperthermia
> * Electric current (electrical and lightning injuries)
> * Excessive physical exertion (push-ups, cycling, marathon running)
>
> **Mechanical**
> * Crush injury
> * Burns (including electrical injuries)
> * Compression (e.g., tourniquet left on too long)
> * Compartment syndrome
>
> **Chemical**
> * Medications (e.g., antibiotics, statins, first-generation H_1-receptor antagonists)
> * Herbal supplements containing ephedra (rare)
> * Excessive alcohol use
> * Electrolyte abnormalities
> * Infections
> * Endocrine disorders
> * Heritable muscle enzyme deficiencies
> * Mushroom poisoning (rare)

---

than 15 million Americans taking these drugs, the prevalence is on the rise.[326]

Underlying neuromuscular diseases may become clinically apparent during statin therapy and may predispose to myotoxicity.[16,46] Rhabdomyolysis also has been reported in performance athletes taking herbal supplements containing ephedra; there are similar reports of rhabdomyolysis in individuals using weight-loss herbal supplements.[215,359]

Strenuous exercise, including marathon running, biking, and exercises such as push-ups, sit-ups, or pull-ups, can result in damage to skeletal muscle cells, a process known as exertional rhabdomyolysis.[50] Acute excessive consumption of alcohol exacerbated by a hot environment and dehydration can also predispose individuals competing in athletic events to exercise-induced rhabdomyolysis.

Structures involved. The exact mechanism for statin-induced myopathy remains unknown. There may be a drug influence on deoxyribonucleic acid (DNA), an enzyme deficiency, or autoimmune reaction triggered by the drug.[46] The effect of the process is well known; specifically, when muscle proteins are released into the blood, one of these proteins (myoglobin) can precipitate in the kidneys and spill into the urine.

Massive skeletal muscle necrosis can also occur, further complicating the situation with reduced plasma volumes leading to shock and reduced blood flow to the kidneys resulting in acute renal failure. As the injured muscle leaks potassium, hyperkalemia may cause fatal disruptions in heart rhythm.

Signs and symptoms. The individual may report muscle pain (myalgia) and weakness ranging from mild to severe. The client may report a change in color of the urine, most often tea colored or the color of cola soft drinks. This may occur with military recruits or marathon runners who have been exercising in hot and humid weather, or who have taken analgesics, had a viral or bacterial infection, and/or have a preexisting condition.[50]

Common tests and measures. The diagnosis is typically made by history and clinical presentation and confirmed by laboratory studies when an abnormal renal function and elevated CPK are observed. A careful medication history is considered useful to distinguish the causes. Often the diagnosis is suspected when a urine dipstick test is positive for blood but no cells are seen on microscopic analysis. This suggests myoglobinuria and usually prompts a measurement of the serum CPK, which confirms the diagnosis.

Common management. Treatment is directed toward rehydration and correction of electrolyte imbalances by administering intravenous fluids, and in the case of renal failure, dialysis may be necessary. In most cases of rhabdomyolysis, especially in the case of exertional rhabdomyolysis, damage to skeletal muscle cells resolves without consequence. Clinically significant rhabdomyolysis is uncommon but, when present, can be life threatening.[326]

Soft Tissue

Soft Tissue Injuries

Soft tissue injuries, such as strains and sprains, lacerations, tendon ruptures, muscle injuries, dislocations, and subluxations, are described briefly in this section. For a more detailed description of these conditions, the reader is referred to the *Guidelines for Exercise Testing and Prescription* by the American College of Sports Medicine (ACSM)[9] or other appropriate orthopedic textbooks.

Definition and incidence. Strains refer to stretching or tearing of the musculotendinous unit; they may be partial or full tears. The musculotendinous junction is a region of highly folded basement membranes between the end of the muscle fiber and the tendon. These involutions maximize surface area for force transmission but contain a transition zone where the compliant muscle fibers become relatively noncompliant tendon, placing this junction at increased risk for injury.[32] A helpful mnemonic device to recall strain versus sprain is that the *t* in *strain* can be matched to the *t* in musculotendinous. A *sprain* is an injury of the ligamentous structures around a joint caused by abnormal or excessive joint motion.

Strains and sprains can be classified as mild, moderate, or severe (complete) tears or as injuries of first, second, or third degree depending on the severity of tissue damage. Stretching or minor tearing of a few fibers without loss of integrity is classified as *first degree* (mild), with only minor swelling and discomfort accompanied by no or only minimal loss of strength and restriction of movement.[162]

Second-degree (moderate) strain refers to partial tearing of tissue with clear loss in function (ability to contract). Pain, moderate disability, point tenderness, swelling, localized hemorrhaging, and slightly to moderately abnormal motion are typical.

A *third-degree* (severe) strain or sprain refers to complete loss of structural or biomechanical integrity extending across the entire cross section of the muscle and usually requires surgical repair. An alternate classification scheme uses three grades of injury (I, II, III). Common sites for this type of injury include the ankle, knee, and fingers.

Structures involved. The tendon is most vulnerable to injury (*tendinitis, tendon rupture*) when the attached muscle is maximally contracted or stressed and tension is applied quickly or obliquely. Tendinitis and spontaneous tendon ruptures have been reported to occur as a potential side effect of antibiotic treatment, especially with the use of fluoroquinolone antibiotics (e.g., drugs ending in "floxacin," such as ofloxacin, norfloxacin, levofloxacin). A growing number of people are experiencing tendinopathy as a result of quinolone antibiotics. The presentation of joint tenderness and swelling of apparently

unknown cause can occur up to 6 months or more after the administration of the drug. The PTA should be alert to this kind of presentation in anyone with a history of fluoroquinolone use with any of the following risk factors: older than age 60 years, previous history of tendinopathy, magnesium deficiency, hyperparathyroidism, diuretic use, peripheral vascular disease, RA, diabetes mellitus, or participation in strenuous sports activities.[104,330]

Reports suggest that fluoroquinolone-associated tendon disorders are more common in people older than age 60 years, especially those who are also taking oral corticosteroids.[391] Tendon injuries occur at a higher rate in kidney transplant recipients, possibly caused by medications. In such cases, care should be taken to avoid overloading tendons, because dramatic ruptures following even small trauma have been reported.[352]

Ligamentous injuries occur after a traumatic injury or from overuse of a particular joint. Ligamentous strains are classified into the three degrees described previously. Chronic ligamentous instability can lead to disruption of the entire joint.

The terms *subluxation* and *dislocation* relate to joint integrity. *Subluxation* is partial disruption of the anatomic relationship within a joint. Mobile joints are at the greatest risk for subluxation. These include the glenohumeral, acromioclavicular, sacroiliac, and atlantoaxial joints. *Dislocation* is the complete loss of joint integrity with loss of anatomic relationships. Often, significant ligamentous damage occurs or causes this type of injury. Dislocations most often occur at the glenohumeral joint. Joint dislocation can also be a late manifestation of chronic disease, such as rheumatoid arthritis (RA), paralysis, and neuromuscular disease. In the presence of a joint dislocation, the integrity of nerve and vascular tissue must be assessed. If compromise is suspected, timely reduction is essential to prevent serious complications.

Injured muscle is also at increased risk for complete rupture if the muscle is subjected to high tensile force. The clinical manifestations of soft tissue injuries are local pain, edema, increased local tissue temperature, ecchymosis, hypermobility or instability, and loss of function. Muscle contusion (bruising with intact skin) is common in contact sports and incites an inflammatory response, sometimes involving hematoma formation.

The PTA working with athletes at all levels (high school, collegiate, recreational, amateur, professional) and of all ages should be aware that performance-enhancing supplements can cause muscle damage despite their intended use to build muscle mass in order to increase strength or power. One example of this type of supplement is creatine (Cr), which is used to increase lean body mass in conjunction with a resistance training program. Potential side effects of creatine supplementation include muscle cramping, diarrhea and other GI symptoms, and dehydration.[294]

Signs and symptoms. Injuries to the tendon or muscle will present with isolated pain at the injury site and increased pain during contraction of the involved muscle. ROM may be impaired, usually as a protective mechanism to decrease disruption of the tissue. Soon after an injury, swelling, warmth, and edema will also be present.

Ligamentous injuries will also present with localized tenderness if the ligament is superficial. Disruption of the deeper ligaments, such as the anterior cruciate in the knee, will present as generalized pain and soreness. Joint ROM will be limited, but there should not be pain during isolated muscle contractions unless they move the joint. Swelling, warmth, and edema may also be present soon after the injury.

Subluxations and dislocations usually involve ligamentous injury and will present in much the same way. There may be an obvious change in the joint contour in a displaced dislocation, but many joints will reduce (go back into place) quickly.

Common tests and measures. Radiographs are commonly used to rule out any associated fractures for traumatic injuries. Avulsion fractures may be mistaken for a tendon tear if the bony insertion site is pulled loose. Third-degree ligament strains will demonstrate increased joint space on a radiograph, but the soft tissues are not visualized on the image. MRI is more helpful to visualize the extent of soft tissue damage but is more expensive and may be reserved for use after the initial swelling decreases and symptoms are more focused.

A complete history including any emergency medical management, imaging studies, and medications will help the PT plan the examination and determine a plan of care for the therapy team. Functional measures of muscle strength, joint ROM, and gait should be made within the client's tolerance. Some tests may be too painful to complete during the initial visit. Functional outcome and disability measures should be used to monitor the client's progress over time.

Common management. The inflammatory reaction from injured soft tissue may lead to structural adaptation of tissue, scarring, weakness, and inflexibilities that can cause structural deficits or functional adaptations. If, after an injury, the PTA notes quick onset of joint effusion and the joint feels hot to the touch and movement is extremely painful and limited, the joint needs to be examined by a physician to rule out hemarthrosis.

Immediate immobilization is required with serious (grade 2 or 3) soft tissue lesions to avoid excessive scar formation and prevent rerupture at the injury site. Further retraction of the ruptured muscle stumps and hematoma size can be minimized by placing the injured extremity to rest.[161] Immobilization appears to provide the new granulation tissue with the needed tensile strength to withstand the forces created by muscle contractions. Immobilization should not extend beyond the first few days following the injury.[162]

Early mobilization for the treatment of acute soft tissue injuries has proven effective, especially in treating injured athletes. Early mobilization has been shown to induce rapid and intensive capillary in-growth into the injured area with better repair of muscle fibers and more parallel orientation of the regenerating myofibers in comparison to immobilization. Early mobilization has the added benefit of improved biomechanical strength in muscle, which returns to the level of uninjured muscle more rapidly using active mobilization.[162]

The PTA can guide the injured individual in following a recovery protocol to enhance healing. Crutches may be advised with severe lower extremity muscle injuries, especially injuries where adequate early immobilization is difficult to achieve (e.g., groin area).[180] Movement during the first 3 to 7 days should be with care to avoid stretching the injured muscle.

Once the joint condition has stabilized, rehabilitation should address local muscle imbalances and adjacent joint hypomobility, which could increase mechanical stresses at the joint. Between 7 and 10 days, the PTA can gradually progress the individual in using the injured muscle more actively, using pain and tolerance as a guide to setting limits. All rehabilitation activities should begin with a warm-up of the injured muscle, as it has been shown to reduce muscle viscosity and relax muscles neurally.[266] Stimulated, warm muscles absorb more energy than unstimulated muscles and can better withstand loading. Combining a warm-up with stretching can improve the elasticity of injured muscle.[316]

Isometric training should be started first and progressed to isotonic training; isotonic strengthening begins without a resisting load/counterload, then one is progressively added. All exercises should be done within the limits of the client's pain. When the individual can complete isometric and isotonic exercises without pain, then isokinetic training with minimal load can begin.[162]

The effects of loading on the musculotendinous unit during rehabilitative exercise are increased tendon size, tensile strength, and enhanced collagen fiber organization of newly formed collagen. Restoring kinesthetic and proprioceptive awareness at the site of injury and restoring mobility and strength are also important elements of the rehabilitation program.

Injury prevention. Overuse injuries from repetitive stresses and microtrauma are common among children and adults, especially young athletes participating in organized sports. The PTA working with athletes from any sport can emphasize injury prevention by educating both the athletes and their parents and encouraging coaches to emphasize injury prevention.

Prevention begins with conditioning, especially at the beginning of the season for one-sport athletes who do not play year round. Training errors, variable skeletal and muscle growth rates, anatomic malalignment, and faulty equipment are just a few of the key factors that contribute to injury. For those individuals involved in multiple sports, volume and intensity of athletic involvement combined with inadequate time for recovery after injuries of any kind are key issues.[286]

Learning and practicing the basic skills (e.g., sliding into bases correctly, making a tackle in football, learning how to head-butt the ball in soccer) and understanding the fundamentals for each sport activity is essential. Many more injuries occur during practice than during actual competitive play, because this is where more time is spent. Early participation in organized sports at younger ages often results in overuse injuries, likely due to strength and flexibility imbalances.[286]

The PTA can help identify and correct such risk factors before they translate into injury. Early detection of risk factors and injuries can help minimize the severity of injury and reduce long-term consequences of soft tissue damage. Everyone should be encouraged to think about injury prevention during practices as well as during competitions.

REFERENCES/SUGGESTED READINGS

To enhance this text and add value for the reader, references and suggested readings are included on the companion Evolve site that accompanies this textbook. The reader can view the source and access it online whenever possible.

18

Introduction to Central Nervous System Disorders

CHAPTER OBJECTIVES

1. Review neuroanatomy and neurophysiology.
2. Consider the role of neurochemicals in neuropathology.
3. Orient to clinical manifestations of neuropathology.
4. Orient to the various types of diagnostic tests used in neurology.
5. Consider the types of interventions used in treating neurologic dysfunctions, including potential for recovery.
6. Orient to motor and cognitive learning theories.

OUTLINE

VOCAB BUILDERS

Agnosia	Asthenia	Macroglia
Alexia	Ataxia	Microglia
Allele	Diaschisis	Motor learning
Amines	Dysarthria	Neuropeptides
Amino acids	Dysdiadochokinesia	Neurotransmission
Aphasia	Dysmetria	Nystagmus
Apoptosis	Free radical	Oxidative stress
Apraxia	Glial cells	Proprioception

The central nervous system (CNS) controls and regulates all mental and physical functions. The nervous system is unparalleled among organ systems in terms of diversity of cellular constituents. It is composed of a network of neural tissue that includes both receptors and transmitters. There is a complex interaction among the areas that control different functions. A variety of neurons provide transmission of specific information throughout the nervous system. Disease or trauma of the CNS may affect the nervous system through damage to several types of tissues in a local area, such as in stroke, or it may cause dysfunction in one type of tissue throughout many areas of the CNS, such as in multiple sclerosis. Dysfunction of the neurons in an area of the brain can disrupt the complex organization of firing, resulting in abnormal perception of the environment, uncoordinated movement, loss of force production, and decreases in cognition.

Behavior, including thought and movement, is shaped by the interplay between genes and the environment. There are genes that control entry into the cell cycle where cells synthesize deoxyribonucleic acid (DNA) and undergo mitosis. Proliferation can be triggered by internal signals or in response to external growth factor stimulation. There is a complex spectrum of alterations produced by aging, disease, and neoplastic transformation. Neoplastic transformation, which is the basis of cancer, is characterized by mutations of genes regulating cell growth, differentiation, and death. A set of genes appears to inhibit cellular proliferation; these genes are the "brakes" of the cell cycle, and loss of these genes may lead to tumor growth.[15]

Inherited patterns of DNA expression appear to cause a predisposition for neurologic disease and affect the ability to repair damage from an insult in the nervous system. Genetic information is stored in the chromosomes within each individual cell in the body; about 80,000 genes are represented and arranged in a precise order. More than one-third of the genes are expressed as messenger ribonucleic acid (RNA) in the brain, more than in any other part of the body. An anomaly or alternative gene version is referred to as an *allele*. Single-gene mutations or alleles have been identified and can be associated with degenerative neurologic disease such as Huntington's disease. However, for most chronic disorders there appear to be multiple abnormalities, and it is clear that environmental conditions have an effect on how the abnormality manifests.[2]

Pathologic derangements of normal cellular processes are a way of looking at possible causes of disease. Diseases in which cells are lost are characterized as necrotic and apoptotic. Both necrosis and apoptosis underlie diseases as diverse as stroke, trauma, demyelinating disorders, infections, and neurodegenerative disorders.

PATHOGENESIS

Cellular Dysfunction

Neuronal cell death is a hallmark of many disorders of the nervous system through the processes of necrosis and apoptosis. When cell death is caused by necrosis, there is cellular swelling, fragmentation, and cell disintegration. Necrosis causes the internal structure of the cell to swell as water enters the cell through osmosis and the cell membranes rupture. Lymphocytes and polynuclear cells can cause inflammatory cells to surround the necrotic debris, resulting in release of cytotoxic compounds and destruction of neighboring cells. Excitotoxicity results from the inappropriate activation of excitatory *amino acid* receptors

leading to the entry of calcium ions into the cell. The calcium activates intracellular function. Damaged cells release excitotoxins that damage surrounding cells.[15]

Apoptosis is programmed cell death, or a type of cellular suicide, but apoptosis does not cause inflammatory responses. It is a more organized process with fragmentation of the cells and degradation of the DNA. It is common during the development of cells to eliminate the overproduction of one cell type. The biochemical pathway is present in all cells of the body and is used normally in the maturation and regulation of the nervous system with systematic removal of neurons from the brain. In apoptosis the cell is removed by macrophages and leaves no residual damage to other components of the CNS. If the cell sustains genetic damage through neurodegenerative disease or injury and cannot be repaired by the system, the cell dies. Damage to the CNS can cause excessive apoptosis through the process of trophic factor withdrawal, oxidative insults, metabolic compromise, overactivation of glutamate receptors, and exposure to bacterial toxins.[33] These processes are described in the next paragraphs.

The intensity of cellular injury determines whether the cell dies or is able to survive. Very severe injury leads to the passive process of necrosis, less severe but irreparable injury leads to the active process of apoptosis, and survivable injury leads to reactive changes such as gliosis or scarring.

Free radical formation is a byproduct of excitotoxicity. Free radicals are capable of destroying cellular components and triggering apoptosis. Free radicals are molecules with an odd number of electrons. The odd, or unpaired, electron is highly reactive as it seeks to pair with another free electron. Free radicals are generated during oxidative metabolism and energy production in the body. Free radicals are related to normal metabolism but can be the cause of oxidative stress in brain injury and disease.

Oxidative stress refers to cells and tissues that have been altered by exposure to oxidants. Oxidation of lipids, proteins, and DNA leads to tissue injury. Nitrogen monoxide (nitric oxide [NO]) is a free radical generated by NO synthase (NOS). This enzyme modulates physiologic responses, such as vasodilation or signaling, in the brain. Oxidative stress, rather than being the primary cause, appears to be a secondary complication in many progressive disorders, such as Alzheimer's disease, Parkinson's disease, and amyotrophic lateral sclerosis (ALS), as well as disorders of mental status. An enhanced antioxidant status is associated with reduced risk of several diseases.[40]

The blood–brain barrier is made from endothelial cells and its tight junctions, so that substances can pass only through the cell and not between cells. Drug entry into the CNS is determined by the drug's lipid solubility. Glucose and amino acids cross the endothelial cell barrier via protein transporters.

The ependymal cells line the ventricles and spinal canal and regulate metabolism between the channels of the extracellular space and the ventricles. Ependyma forms the basis of the cerebrospinal fluid barrier. There is movement of molecules through the extracellular space, with the possibility of long-range and relatively diffuse actions of neurotransmitters released into the extracellular space. This type of signaling is known as *volume transmission* and may have a major role in setting large-scale neuronal excitability or inhibition.[15]

Dysfunction within the nervous system can affect either or both of the two main classes of cells: the *glial cells* and the neurons. Stem cells create new glia and new neurons. The region immediately beneath the ependymal cell layer produces new cells at a very low rate in the adult compared with the number created during neurogenesis in early development. They migrate widely through the brain and conform phenotypically to the regions where they end up.

Glial Cells

Aside from neurons, *macroglia* and *microglia* are the two primary cell types located throughout the CNS. The macroglia are derived from a nerve cell lineage and are classified into three distinct subtypes: astrocytes, oligodendrocytes, and Schwann cells. These macroglia are the most populous cells of the CNS and support and maintain neuronal plasticity throughout the CNS. Glial cells are often implicated in the disease process that affects brain tissue.[25]

Microglia are the resident immune cells of the brain. Microglia also are interspersed throughout the brain and represent approximately 10% of the CNS population. Microglia differ from the macroglia because they are derived from a monocyte cell lineage. Microglia respond to CNS insult both by diffuse proliferation and by infiltration of CNS tissue. Microglia are pivotal in innate immune activation and function to modulate neuroinflammatory signals throughout the brain. In the absence of stimulus, microglia are dormant.

During an immune response, microglia are activated. Inflammatory cytokines produced within the CNS target neuronal substrates, triggering a response of fever, increased sleep, reduced appetite, and lethargy. Collectively, these behavioral symptoms of sickness are evolutionarily conserved and function to increase the metabolic demand for clearance of pathogens via the microglia.[19] Active microglia show macrophage-like activities, including scavenging, phagocytosis, antigen presentation, and inflammatory cytokine production. Microglia recruit and activate astrocytes to propagate these inflammatory signals further. Normally, these neuroinflammatory changes are transient and beneficial, with microglia returning to the dormant state after the resolution of the immune challenge. Aging, however, may provide a brain environment in which microglia activation is not resolved, leading to a heightened sensitivity to immune activation; this lack of resolution may contribute to the pathogenesis of neurologic disease.[50]

Activated microglia and monocytes coming in from the bloodstream can assume the form of macrophages, or giant multinucleated cells filled with ingested debris. Nearby neurons may be damaged by toxins released from activated macrophages and microglia.

Astrocytes are so named because they look like star cells. They are the most numerous cells in the brain and outnumber neurons by 10:1. Fig. 18.1 shows the relationship of the glial cell to the neuron. The glial cells provide support and structure for the CNS and play the role that connective tissue performs in other parts of the body. The glial cells are active in the system but are not involved in signaling information. The neurons communicate information to one another in order to process sensory information, program motor and emotional responses, and store information through memory.

In addition to their support function, the cells serve a nutritive function because they connect to the capillary wall and to the nerve cell. They may be responsible for the release of nerve growth factor. Astrocytes are permeable to potassium and therefore are involved in maintaining the correct potassium balance in the extracellular space. Astroglia have the ability to monitor and remove extracellular glutamate and other residual neuronal debris after brain injury and can seal off damaged brain tissue.[25,47] When the astroglial cells become dysfunctional as part of an injury or degenerative process, neuronal damage may be reinforced. Astroglial changes are widely recognized to be one of the earliest and most remarkable cellular responses to CNS injury.[38] Astrocyte swelling is a common pathologic finding

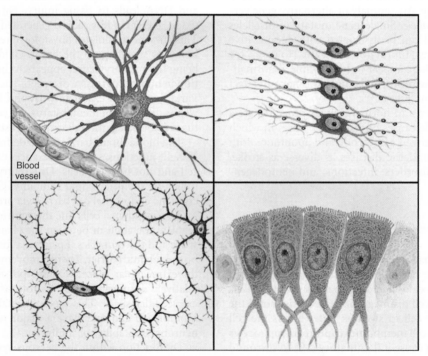

FIG. 18.1 The relationship of the glial cells (astrocytes, oligodendrocytes) to the neurons and capillaries. (Redrawn from Chipps E, Clanin N, Campbell V: Neurologic disorders, St Louis, 1992, Mosby.)

and is often seen at the interface with the vascular system. The swelling may be a factor in gliosis, a reaction of the glial cells that produces tissue that is laid down in a scarlike manner, producing glial scarring.[37] Astroglial cell tissue can be the site of neoplastic disorders that disrupt nerve cell function by compressing the neurons and blood supply in the surrounding area.

The two other glial cell types—the oligodendrocyte, a part of the CNS, and the Schwann cell found in the peripheral nervous system—are responsible for the production of the myelin sheath, which surrounds the axon. Demyelinating disorders that target the CNS, such as multiple sclerosis, are often the result of disrupted function of the oligodendrocyte.[1] Figs. 18.2 and 18.3 show the oligodendrocyte and describe the process of myelination.[37]

Pain was classically viewed as being mediated solely by neurons, as are other sensory phenomena. Spinal cord glia amplify pain and are activated by certain sensory signals arriving from the periphery. These glia express characteristics in common with immune cells in that they respond to viruses and bacteria, releasing proinflammatory cytokines, which create pathologic pain. Altering glial function has become a new approach to pain control.[58]

Nerve Cells

There are many mechanisms of communication between nerve cells related to the structure and function of each cell type. The location in the nervous system, the input cells, and the target cells will determine how a cell communicates. The cell body size and the shape and configuration of dendrites and axons will also affect the method of communication. However, almost all neurons will typically fire through a manner that can be described schematically.

Essentially, the chemical information encoded by a gene within one nerve cell is delivered to the appropriate postsynaptic genome through a series of molecular reactions.[51] Information is transferred via electrical signals that travel along the neuron and is carried to the next neuron through a series of biochemical events that will influence the behavior of the second-order neuron.

The cell body of the neuron is the metabolic center of the neuron and includes the nucleus, where the genetic material is located. The gene expressed in a cell directs the manufacture of proteins that determine the structure, function, and regulation of the neural circuits. Mutation, or changes in the structure of the DNA, can lead to the production of abnormal proteins that can be associated with vulnerability to neurologic disease. Abnormalities within the gene structure leading to predisposition to mutations can be inherited. Toxicity or abuse of drugs can also affect the ability of the DNA to replicate in a normal manner and can cause long-term dysfunction of the nervous system. Cell body inclusions are growths that occur within the cell body as a part of aging, such as Lewy bodies, but can also be a part of the disease process and can cause loss of function of the cell as a result of the obliteration of the nucleus of the cell.[40]

The cell body generates electrical activity through action potentials. A transient increase in sodium permeability is the molecular foundation of the action potential. The increase in sodium permeability causes this ion to be dominant and establishes the membrane potential as +40 mV, or action potential.

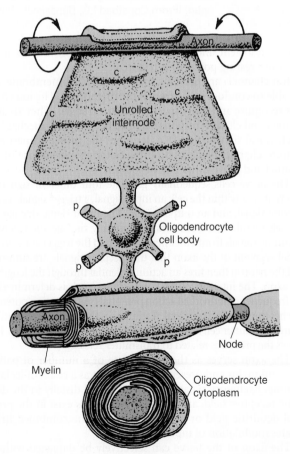

FIG. 18.3 Schematic diagram of the formation of myelin in the central nervous system (CNS). (Adapted from Krstié RV: Illustrated encyclopedia of human histology, Berlin, 1984, Springer-Verlag.)

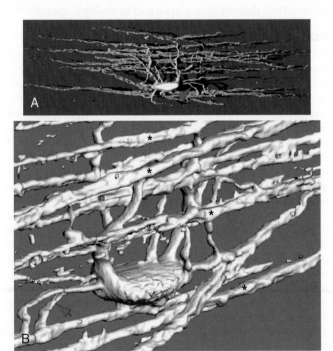

FIG. 18.2 (A) Single oligodendrocyte from a rat. (B) More magnified view showing the process as they emerge from the cell body. (From Vanderah TW, Gould DJ: Nolte's the human brain: an introduction to its functional anatomy, ed 7, Philadelphia, 2016, Elsevier. Courtesy Dr. Peter S. Eggli, Institute of Anatomy, University of Bern, Bern, Switzerland.)

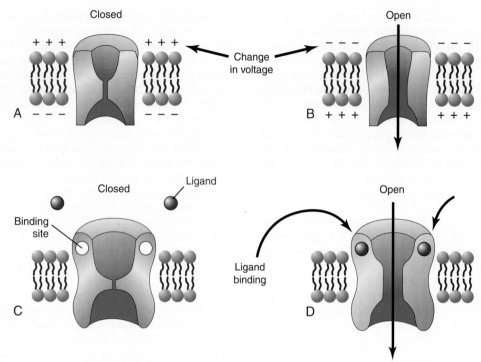

FIG. 18.4 Ion channels respond to the changes in voltage. (A) represents the closed state, and (B) represents the open state that allows neurotransmitters to gain entry into the cell. (C) and (D) represent the opening based on the ligand attaching to the protein that causes the channel to open. (From Copstead LC, Banaski JL: Pathophysiology, ed 5, St. Louis, 2013, Saunders.)

This is transient and soon closed as the potassium channels open and resting potential is restored.

Ion channels are proteins that span the cell membrane and are able to conduct ions through the membrane. The ion channels recognize and select specific ions for transfer. They are able to open and close in response to specific electrical, mechanical, or chemical signals. Fig. 18.4 describes the gating properties.[37] Sodium channel blockers bind the outer axonal surface of the channel and prevent the flux of sodium.

The nerve cells sequentially generate four different signals at different sites within the cell: an input signal, a trigger signal, a conducting signal, and an output signal. The input signal depolarizes the cell membrane. Dendrites are typically the site for receiving incoming signals from other neurons. It is in the trigger zone on the initial segment of the axon that the receptor signals are summed, and the neuron then fires an action potential through the length of the axon. The intensity of the conducting signals is determined by the frequency of individual action potentials. As the action potential reaches the neuron's terminal, it stimulates the release of a chemical neurotransmitter cell through the presynaptic terminals.[25] Fig. 18.5 shows the processes related to transmitter release.[37]

The axon serves as the entry route of a number of pathogens and toxins and presents a large target as a result of its large volume. Excitatory synapses are distributed distally in the dendritic receptive field, and inhibitory synapses exist in the proximal dendritic field or on the cell body. The combined firing creates modulation of input.

The axon of the nerve can selectively be damaged without destruction of the cell body, causing a decrease or loss of presynaptic activity. The stretch damage to the axon is responsible for the abnormal or delayed firing associated with damage to the brainstem in head trauma. Axonal spheroid formation is a reaction to injury resulting in formation of axon retraction balls and can be seen in radiation necrosis and traumatic brain injury. Axon degeneration plays a part in multiple sclerosis.[15]

Neurotransmission

By means of its axonal terminals, one neuron contacts and transmits information to the receptive surface of another neuron. The release of a neurotransmitter from the presynaptic terminal and the uptake of that substance in the postsynaptic receptor are known as a *synapse*. A simplified diagram is shown in Fig. 18.6. Virtually all communication between neurons occurs via chemicals. The chemical communication involved in this process is universally known as either *neurotransmission* or *neuromodulation*.[26] Changes in neurotransmitter substances in the space surrounding the neurons have been implicated in many nervous system disease processes.

Neurotransmitters are synthesized within each neuron, stored in presynaptic vesicles, and released from depolarized nerve terminals. They bind specifically to presynaptic or postsynaptic receptors, which recognize the neurotransmitter's chemical conformation. A single neuron can release several different neurotransmitter substances, and a single neuron can be selectively receptive to different types of neurotransmitters because of the differences in ion channels.[52] Activation of a receptor in response to neurotransmitter can cause changes in a variety of molecules. Modification, or modulation, of the system can take place presynaptically, postsynaptically, or within the cell body.

Changes in the target cell can cause abnormal responses to normal levels of transmitters. The amount of neurotransmitter released in the synaptic cleft is determined by the neuronal firing rate, the quantity of transmitter in the nerve terminal, and the cumulative regulatory actions of excitatory and inhibitory

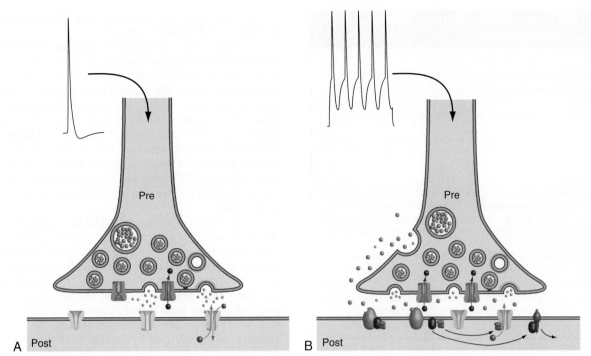

FIG. 18.5 (A) Depolarization of the terminal causes sodium influx and opening of the channels in the postsynaptic neuron. (B) Release of transmitters from large and small vesicles; the status of the postsynaptic proteins will affect the binding capability. (From Vanderah TW, Gould DJ: Nolte's the human brain: an introduction to its functional anatomy, ed 7, Philadelphia, 2016, Elsevier.)

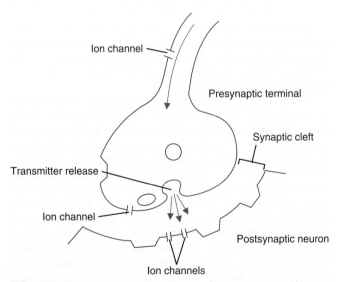

FIG. 18.6 Schematic representation of the postsynaptic neuron and the presynaptic terminal. Transmitter substances are synthesized in presynaptic terminals, released into the synaptic cleft, and occupied in the postsynaptic terminal.

neurotransmitters. These biochemical actions alter the electrical activity of the postsynaptic neurons.

One aspect of chemical transmission that is extremely important in signaling is the time course of transmitter in the synaptic cleft. The breakdown of a transmitter is an important variable and can change the concentration of the substance in the synaptic cleft.[21] Control of the neurotransmitter in the synaptic cleft is the basis for pharmacologic treatment in degenerative neurologic disease. Fig. 18.7

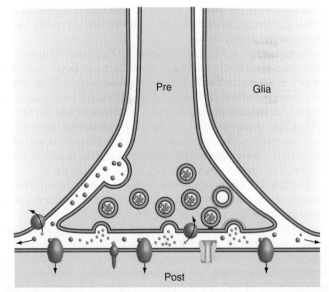

FIG. 18.7 The transmitter substances can be removed by (1) enzymatic inactivation of neurotransmitter, (2) reuptake of the neurotransmitter by the presynaptic terminal, (3) removal by the nearby glial cells, (4) uptake by the postsynaptic terminal, or (5) simply moving out of the synaptic space into adjoining spaces. (From Vanderah TW, Gould DJ: Nolte's the human brain: an introduction to its functional anatomy, ed 7, Philadelphia, 2016, Elsevier.)

diagrams the various ways that the substances in the synaptic cleft can be removed.[37]

An important concept for all neurotransmitters is that the final result of either hyperpolarization or depolarization

BOX 18.1 Neurotransmitters and Associated Responses

Amines

- Acetylcholine: production decreased in diseases such as Alzheimer's disease and myasthenia gravis
- Catecholamines
- Dopamine: decreased levels responsible for symptoms associated with parkinsonism
- Norepinephrine: related to cocaine or amphetamine
- Serotonin: involved in the control of mood and anxiety

Amino Acids

- GABA: increasing GABA activity decreases incidence of seizure activity
- Glutamate: degenerative diseases, such as Parkinson's, ALS, or Alzheimer's, may be related to increases in glutamate; increased levels contribute to the secondary damage associated with stroke and spinal cord injury
- Glycine: more active in the spinal cord than the cerebral cortex

Neuroactive Peptides[a]

- Enkephalins and β-endorphins: pain control achieved by use of drugs (opiates) that bind to endorphin and enkephalin receptors
- Substance P: involved in pain pathways

[a]Over 50 neuroactive peptides have been identified; these are most typical.

ALS, Amyotrophic lateral sclerosis; *GABA,* γ-aminobutyric acid.

depends on both the transmitter and its receptor. The concept of an inhibitory transmitter should be abandoned for the more accurate concept of an inhibitory interaction between neurotransmitter and receptor.

A wide range of substances makes up the neurotransmitter substances used by the nervous system. In some cases they can coexist in the same neuron. Box 18.1 lists some typical substances that can be used as neurotransmitters. These substances can be used by neurons in different ways, according to the function of the specific neuron. To be used as a neurotransmitter, these substances are packaged in vesicles within the neuron and respond to the particular enzymes that are specific to that neuron.[52]

Amino acids. One of the small-molecule neurotransmitters, glutamate, is an excitatory amino acid transmitter used throughout the brain and spinal column. It is an intermediate transmitter in cellular metabolism, so the presence of glutamate in a cell does not necessarily suggest neurologic activity. Glutamate functions with its receptors in an excitatory or depolarizing system at primary afferent nerve endings, the granule cells of the cerebellum, the dentate gyrus, and the corticostriatal and subthalamopallidal pathways important to basal ganglia function. When the levels of glutamate rise above normal, it can become neurotoxic and cause cell death. Glutamate opens ion channels to bring calcium into the cell. In the case of excess glutamate, too much calcium is allowed into the cell, and the calcium eventually destroys the cell. Excess glutamate can be an effect of neuronal injury, as in stroke, brain, or spinal cord injury.

It appears that the genes in the nerve cell body may trigger this excitotoxic mechanism, resulting in release of excess glutamate, which may lead to the degenerative processes associated with diseases such as ALS, Alzheimer's, Huntington's, and Parkinson's.[39] Part of the activation of seizure is caused

by glutamate receptors. Toxins or drug abuse can also trigger an excitotoxic level of glutamate.[51]

γ-Aminobutyric acid (GABA) is a tiny amino acid that serves both as a neurotransmitter and as an intermediate metabolite in the normal function of cells. GABA is synthesized from glutamate by way of the vitamin B_6–dependent enzyme glutamate decarboxylase. GABA is the major transmitter for brief inhibitory synapses. GABAergic cells have a dense representation within the basal ganglia.[20] Loss of GABAergic neurons that inhibit glutamate results in increased excitation. Glycine is another amino acid neurotransmitter and is the transmitter at some inhibitory CNS synapses. The distributions of GABA and glycine synapses overlap, but glycine is more prominent in the spinal cord.[37]

The N-methyl-D-aspartate (NMDA) receptor has a complex process using glutamate and glycine activation at the same time but also requiring membrane polarization to remove magnesium from inside the cell, so that the cell can allow sodium to be active within the cell. NMDA receptors are widely distributed throughout the neocortex, hippocampus, and anterior horn motor neurons. The NMDA response thus works when the membrane bearing the receptor has already been depolarized by another stimulus, so it prolongs or augments the initial depolarization. This activity supports the activities of learning and memorization. During cellular energy failure induced by ischemia, collapse of membrane potentials (depolarization) occurs, along with uncontrolled synaptic and transmembrane release of excitatory amino acids into the extracellular space. NMDA receptors will open and allow calcium into the intracellular space, causing damage to the mitochondria and limiting the production of adenosine triphosphate (ATP). Drugs that are NMDA receptor antagonists include ketamine and eliprodil. Antiepileptic drugs, such as felbamate and lamotrigine, block the glutamate and glycine activity at the NMDA receptors.[15]

Amines. Cholinergic neurons play two different roles in the nervous system. Acetylcholine was the first neurotransmitter discovered and has primary activity at the level of the peripheral nervous system. It is the transmitter released by the motor neurons at neuromuscular junctions and within the autonomic nervous system. The role of the cholinergic neurons in the CNS is quite different because it is involved with the regulation of the general level of activity. Cholinergic systems can be mapped to the medial cortex and to the areas responsible for information flow to the hypothalamus and amygdala through the reticular formation. They also constitute a major element of the autonomic nervous system as preganglionic neurons of sympathetic ganglia and postganglionic parasympathetic neurons. The cholinergic and biogenic *amine* systems appear to establish the activity set point of the cortex and basal ganglia rather than point-to-point neural firing.[15] Biogenic amines are synthesized from amino acid precursors, dopamine, serotonin, and norepinephrine. Two transmitters known as *catecholamines* are dopamine and norepinephrine.

Dopamine is synthesized in four major CNS pathways. The most important and most widely understood involves the nigrostriatal pathway of the basal ganglia. Dopaminergic function is decreased in individuals with Parkinson's disease and attention disorders affecting the frontal lobe. The synthetic pathway for dopamine is tyrosine to dopa to dopamine.

Norepinephrine is a neurotransmitter found in the hypothalamus and the locus ceruleus in the brainstem. It is synthesized from dopamine and therefore shares the same enzymes, including the rate-limiting tyrosine hydroxylase. Like dopamine, norepinephrine is removed from the synapse by active reuptake into the presynaptic cell and then is metabolized by two enzymes, monoamine oxidase (MAO) and catechol-*O*-methyltransferase (COMT).[20] Dopamine and norepinephrine are the primary neurotransmitters associated with the task of attending. Both need to be enhanced for sustained clinical benefit to be achieved.

The catecholamines appear to have an important role in working memory. The cholinergic system appears to be critical for the acquisition of long-term declarative memories. Cholinergic function decreases somewhat with age and greatly in individuals with Alzheimer's disease, and these changes may contribute importantly to corresponding reductions in declarative memory ability. Newer centrally acting cholinesterase inhibitors that can be administered orally and have been marketed for improvement of memory have been developed.

Serotonin has its main cell bodies in the dorsal raphe nucleus of the brainstem as well as the spinal cord, hippocampus, and cerebellum. In parallel to dopamine, it is synthesized by a two-step process, first with a rate-limiting enzyme and then with a general enzyme. The first step takes tryptophan to 5-hydroxytryptophan (5-HTP) with the rate-limiting enzyme tryptophan hydroxylase. The second step takes this intermediate to serotonin (5-hydroxytryptamine [5-HT]) by aromatic amino acid decarboxylase, which is the same enzyme involved in dopamine synthesis. There are several types of serotonin receptors spread throughout the brain. Serotonin is metabolized like the catecholamines by active reuptake into the presynaptic cell and then metabolism by MAO. Serotonin is removed from the synaptic cleft by reuptake pumps rather than by degradation. Tricyclic antidepressants work by inhibiting this reuptake.[15]

Neuropeptides. Neurons can secrete hormones, or *neuropeptides*, and most or all of them can function as neurotransmitters. Neuropeptides are metabolically difficult for cells to make and transport and can be effective at very low concentrations. Synthesis of neuropeptides begins in the nucleus of the cell, where the gene is transcribed into RNA. In the endoplasmic reticulum the RNA is translated into the neuropeptide transmitter. When they have been activated and used to produce a signal, a new supply must be produced in the cell body. Neuropeptides coexist in neurons with both amino acid and amine neurotransmitters. Neuroactive peptides are involved in modulating sensibility and emotions.

Gaseous neurotransmitters and others. NO and carbon monoxide (CO) are gases that can diffuse easily through neuronal membranes and can influence subsequent transmitter release. Astrocytes may be the target, mediating cell-to-cell communication between vessel endothelium and smooth muscle, and are critical in vasomotor control, inflammation, and neuronal communication. NO sets the functional state of adjacent cells and has a short half-life. NO released from endothelial cells acts on vascular smooth muscle, causing vasodilatation. NO released from inflammatory cells occurs in high concentrations and kills cells. NO may play a role in neurodegeneration, and acute elevations may contribute to damage in ischemia and trauma. NO synthesis is augmented by NMDA receptor activation by glutamate; therefore NO may synergize excitotoxicity.[26]

Neurotrophic factors are essential to maintenance and survival of neurons and their terminals but are produced by the body in a limited supply. Four major neurotrophins have been identified in humans: nerve growth factor, brain-derived

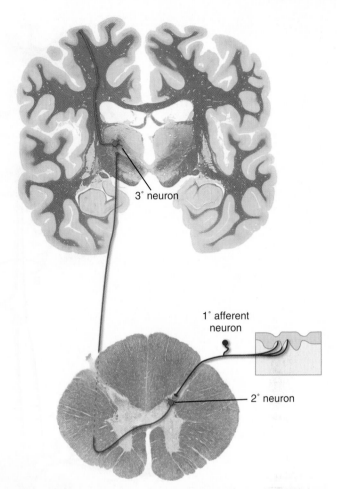

FIG. 18.8 The minimum sensory pathway from the periphery to the cerebral cortex. (From Vanderah TW, Gould DJ: Nolte's the human brain: an introduction to its functional anatomy, ed 7, Philadelphia, 2016, Elsevier.)

neurotrophic factor, neurotrophin 3, and neurotrophin 4/5. Neurotrophins interact with receptor cells to prolong the life of the neuron. Although this class of substances is also not fully understood, it is clear that it plays a role in the development of the nervous system. It appears to work by suppressing the pathway that leads to apoptosis.[25]

CLINICAL MANIFESTATIONS

Sensory Disturbances

The skin, muscles, and joints contain a variety of receptors that create electrical activity as described previously.[8,49] The electrical input is carried to the CNS through the *afferent axons* via the spinal cord. The cell bodies rest in the ganglion of the dorsal root that lies adjacent to the spinal cord. The afferent fibers are arranged somatotopically in the spinal column and ascend to the brainstem and the sensory cortex. Fig. 18.8 shows the simplified synapse.[37] A characteristic of the fibers that run in the dorsal column of the spinal cord is that they synapse at the level of the brainstem nuclei, where they cross over to the contralateral (opposite) hemisphere of the brain. This phenomenon is illustrated in Fig. 18.9.[37] When there is a disorder of the brain that affects the afferent system above the level of the brainstem, symptoms occur on the side contralateral to the lesion.[25,37]

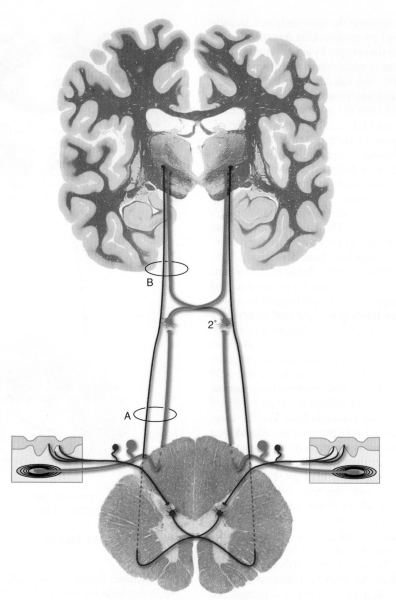

FIG. 18.9 (A) In the spinal cord a lesion would result in decreased touch on the same side of the lesion and decreased pain sensation on the contralateral side. (B) A lesion above the medulla would cause decreased touch and pain on the contralateral side. (From Vanderah TW, Gould DJ: Nolte's the human brain: an introduction to its functional anatomy, ed 7, Philadelphia, 2016, Elsevier.)

The brainstem receives information from specialized senses. For example, vestibular information is received via cranial nerve VIII and integrated through the brainstem nuclei, contributing to postural control and locomotion. Disorders of the afferent nerve, dorsal columns of the spinal cord, and brainstem result in changes in the sensory input available. This can manifest as lack of cutaneous sensation, numbness, tingling, paresthesias, or dysesthesias in the distribution of the nerves affected. Sensory input from the joints and muscles is known as *proprioception*. When this sensory function is lost or disturbed, the person will have difficulty maintaining the body in the appropriate position for the voluntary and involuntary movements necessary for most functional activities, especially those required for postural control. Movements become ataxic or uncoordinated because of the loss of feedback on position from the joints.[3]

The nervous system has several pain-control pathways available, some of which suppress and some of which facilitate the experience of pain. Modulation of noxious stimuli is directed by the reticular formation. Noxious stimuli can be experienced as more or less painful, depending on the individual's circumstances. If an individual is focused on a task during an injury, such as a soldier or athlete, the pain of the injury may be suppressed until the task is completed. When a lesion affects the midbrain areas that modulate and interpret sensory input, such as the thalamus, the result can cause exaggeration of sensory stimuli.

Disruption of the sensory input provided by the optic nerve is evident in some disorders of the brain and will result in loss of vision in some or all of a field of view. Visual-field cuts are common with stroke. Visual hallucinations can also be part of a CNS disorder when the optic radiations or occipital lobe is

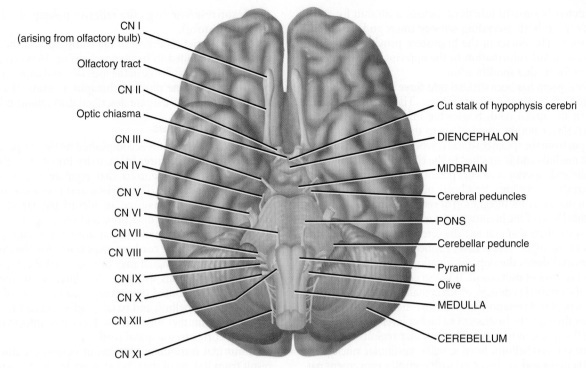

CN I
(arising from olfactory bulb)

Olfactory tract

CN II

Optic chiasma

CN III

CN IV

CN V

CN VI

CN VII

CN VIII

CN IX

CN X

CN XII

CN XI

Cut stalk of hypophysis cerebri

DIENCEPHALON

MIDBRAIN

Cerebral peduncles

PONS

Cerebellar peduncle

Pyramid

Olive

MEDULLA

CEREBELLUM

A

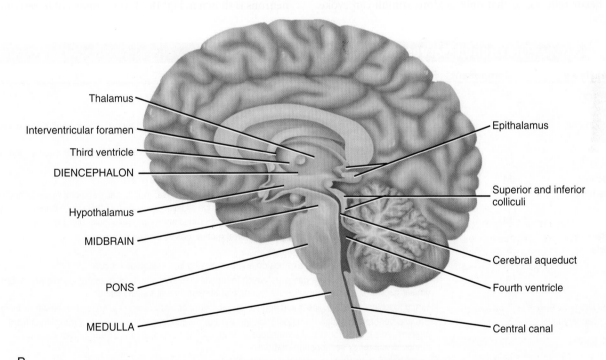

Thalamus

Interventricular foramen

Third ventricle

DIENCEPHALON

Hypothalamus

MIDBRAIN

PONS

MEDULLA

Epithalamus

Superior and inferior
colliculi

Cerebral aqueduct

Fourth ventricle

Central canal

B

FIG. 18.10 Inferior view of brain to show the cranial nerves (A) and brainstem (B). (From Liebgott B: The anatomical basis of dentistry, ed 3, St. Louis, 2011, Mosby.)

disrupted, which may also be caused by stroke or a degenerative disease such as multiple sclerosis.

Brainstem Dysfunction

The brainstem contains the lower motor neurons for the muscles of the head and does the initial processing of general afferent information concerning the head. The cranial nerves enter the system at the brainstem through the respective nuclei and provide sensation and motor control of the head and neck. An anatomic view of the cranial nerves and the relationship of the nuclei to central structures is provided in Fig. 18.10.[37] The sensory and motor functions of the cranial nerves are outlined in Table 18.1. A working knowledge of the attributes of the cranial nerves assists in the understanding of the level and impact of lesions within the CNS.

Distinctive brainstem functions include a conduit for spinal cord activity in both ascending sensory tracts and descending motor tracts. The nuclei in the brainstem provide relay functions to divert the information to the appropriate higher-level structures for further modification.

The brainstem has been divided into three major subdivisions related to a characteristic set of features. The medulla, attached directly to the spinal cord, houses the inferior olivary nucleus, which has direct output connections to the cerebellum and gets direct input from the spinal cord and cerebellum. The pons extends from the medulla and is attached to the cerebellum through both the middle and superior cerebellar peduncles, receiving major outflow from the cerebellum. Vestibular nuclei sit within the pons, making it the center for integration of vestibular input.

The third level of the brainstem, the midbrain, contains the red nucleus with fibers that connect the cerebellum to the thalamus. The substantia nigra, found here, connects to the basal ganglia structures and shares the dopamine pathway related to the initiation and control of movement. It is also connected to the cortex through the cerebral peduncle, which contains descending fibers.

The reticular formation is a diffuse network of neurons extending through the brainstem to higher levels and is important in influencing movement. The reticular regions are closely related to the cerebellum, basal ganglia, vestibular nuclei, and substantia nigra and are involved with complex movement patterns. It is through the reticular formation that there is inhibition of flexor reflexes, so that only noxious stimuli can evoke the flexor response (e.g., the reflexive pulling of a hand away from a hot stove).

This is a brief reflection of the complexity of the brainstem and is not intended to be comprehensive. However, it is clear that advanced knowledge of the interface and connections of the brainstem helps the physical therapist assistant (PTA) understand the functions that are described throughout this text.

Movement Disorders

Control of movement is accomplished by the cooperative effort of many brain structures.[8,49] Activity initiated in the cerebral cortex triggers interneurons that regulate interaction of the lower motor neurons. The parietal and premotor areas of the cerebral cortex are involved in identifying targets in space, determining a course of action, and creating the motor program. The cortex determines strategies for movement. The brainstem and spinal cord are responsible for the execution of the task. The same signal may be processed simultaneously by many different brain structures for different purposes, showing parallel distributed processing. Various areas of the brain, such as the cerebellum and basal ganglia, interact to establish a motor program that modifies the hierarchic information going from the cortex to the spinal cord.

Abnormal movement patterns in neurologic disorders can result from lesions of the CNS at many levels. A simplified representation of the typical synaptic flow of neurons and interneurons is shown in Fig. 18.11. It is important to recognize that

TABLE 18.1	The Cranial Nerves and Their Functions	
Cranial Nerve	**Component**	**Function**
I—Olfactory	S	Olfaction
II—Optic	S	Visual acuity
III—Oculomotor	M	Extraocular eye movements; innervation of inferior oblique muscle and medial, inferior, and superior rectus muscles of eye
	A	Innervation of ciliary ganglion, which regulates papillary constriction (papillary constrictor muscle) and accommodation to near vision (ciliary muscle)
IV—Trochlear	M	Extraocular eye movements; innervation of superior oblique muscle of eye
V—Trigeminal	S	Sensation (pain, temperature, discriminative touch) from face, nose, mouth, nasal and oral mucosa, anterior two-thirds of tongue, and meningeal sensation, through all three divisions (ophthalmic, maxillary, mandibular)
	M	Innervation of muscles of chewing and tensor tympani muscle through mandibular division only)
VI—Abducens	M	Extraocular eye movements; innervation of lateral rectus muscle of eye
VII—Facial	S	Taste from anterior two-thirds of tongue
	M	Innervation of muscles of facial expression and eye closing and stapedius muscle
	A	Innervation of pterygopalatine ganglion, which innervates lacrimal and nasal mucosal glands, and submandibular ganglion, which innervates submandibular and sublingual salivary glands
VIII—Vestibulocochlear	S	Hearing (cochlear division); linear and angular acceleration, or head position in space (vestibular division)
IX—Glossopharyngeal	S	Taste and general sensation from posterior one-third of tongue; sensation (epicritic, protopathic) from pharynx, soft palate, tonsils; chemoreception from carotid body and baroreception from carotid sinus (unconscious reflex sensory information)
	M	Innervation of pharyngeal muscles for swallowing
	A	Innervation of otic ganglion, which supplies parotid gland
X—Vagus	S	Visceral sensation (excluding pain) from heart, bronchi, trachea, larynx, pharynx, GI tract to level of descending colon; general sensation of external ear; taste from epiglottis
	M	Innervation of pharyngeal and laryngeal muscles and muscles at base of tongue
	A	Innervation of local visceral ganglia, which supply smooth muscles in respiratory, cardiovascular, and GI tract to level of descending colon
XI—Accessory	M	Innervation of trapezius and sternocleidomastoid muscles
XII—Hypoglossal	M	Innervation of muscles of tongue

A, Autonomic nervous system; *GI*, gastrointestinal; *M*, motor nervous system; *S*, sensory nervous system.
From Farber SD: Neurorehabilitation: a multisensory approach, Philadelphia, 1982, Saunders; and Gutman SA: Quick reference neuroscience for rehabilitation professionals, ed 2, Thorofare, NJ, 2008, Slack, Inc.

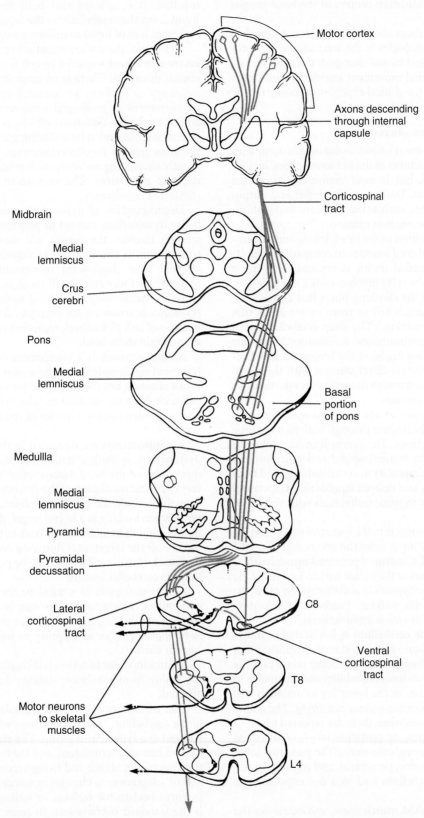

FIG. 18.11 Pathway of the motor system from the cortex to the skeletal muscle as it courses through the brainstem structures and spinal cord. (From Cramer GD, Darby SA: Clinical anatomy of the spine, spinal cord, and ANS, ed 3, St. Louis, 2014, Mosby.)

there are many synapses not represented here in the levels of the brainstem and central modulation centers of the basal ganglia and limbic lobes.

Damage at any level brings about the movement disorders that are related to the pathologies in the next chapters. Motor output is critically evaluated by the therapist; thus the knowledge of patterns of abnormal movement associated with disorders of the brain is part of the clinical expertise necessary for the physical therapist (PT) and PTA to practice.

Disorders of Coordinated Movement

Lack of coordinated movement known as *ataxia* can occur with damage to a variety of structures of the nervous system, including sensory neuropathies, but is most commonly associated with cerebellar dysfunction. Damage to the input and output structures of the cerebellum, such as the thalamus and vestibular nuclei, can also cause ataxic movements.

Input regarding the position of the head, trunk, and extremities comes from the spinal cord in order to compare the resulting activity with the intended motor command. This input comes in rapidly because the relay involves only a few synapses. The input comes through the climbing fibers that connect the inferior olive to the Purkinje's cell or from mossy fibers that relay the remaining information.[5] The deep cerebellar nuclei are the structures that communicate information from the Purkinje's cell to the various nuclei of the brainstem and thalamus.[25] The cerebellum has no direct synapse with the spinal cord but exerts its influence through the action on interneurons within the nuclei of the brainstem.

The medial region known as the *vestibulocerebellum* connects with the cortex and brainstem through both its ascending and its descending projections. The cerebellum has influence on movement through the vestibulospinal and reticulospinal tracts. Lesions result in the inability to coordinate eye and head movement, postural sway, and delayed equilibrium responses.[5] Postural tremor is present in some individuals with vestibulocerebellar lesions.

The spinocerebellum connects to the somatosensory tracts of the spinal cord. It receives input from the cortex regarding the ongoing motor command. Control of proximal musculature is achieved via the connections to the motor cortex. Lesions of the spinocerebellum can cause hypotonia and disruption of rhythmic patterns associated with walking. Precision of voluntary movements is lost when this area is dysfunctional.[35]

The anterior lobe of the cerebellum is implicated in disorders of gait with loss of balance noted in stance. Proprioception may give inaccurate cues because the cerebellar relays become disrupted. Long loop reflexes lose adaptability and are unable to trigger appropriate responses in the lower leg to maintain balance when the body sways or the surface is moving. The ability to modify reflexes is lost even when there are repeated trials.[55]

In the cerebrocerebellum, or posterior lobes, connections are made to the cortex through the pons. The posterior lobes are involved in complex motor, perceptual, and cognitive tasks. Lesions of the cerebrocerebellum lead to a decomposition of movement and timing.

Hypotonicity, or decreased muscle tone, can occur on the side of the lesion or bilaterally if the lesion is central and is seen primarily in the proximal muscle groups. The person with hypotonicity is unable to fixate the limb posturally, leading to incoordination with movement. *Asthenia,* or generalized weakness, is sometimes seen in the person with cerebellar lesions.

Hypotonicity and asthenia, however, do not always occur together. It is believed that both disorders represent loss of input from the cerebellum to the cerebral cortex, but they may represent loss of input to different areas of the cortex.

Dysmetria, the underestimation or overestimation of a necessary movement toward a target, is commonly seen with cerebellar disorders. There is an error in the production of force necessary to perform an intended movement. The initiation of movement is prolonged compared with normal, and the ability to change directions rapidly is impaired. The resulting overshoot and undershoot during movement are known as an *intention tremor. Dysdiadochokinesia,* the inability to perform rapidly alternating movements, is related to the inability to stop ongoing movement. The movement becomes slow, without rhythm or consistency.

Decomposition of movement is seen in persons with cerebellar dysfunction. Instead of performing a movement in one smooth motion, the person will move in distinct sequences to accomplish the motion. Multijoint movements are more affected than single-joint movements. Disruption in force and extent of movement will result in difficulty with grip control and maintaining static hold against resistance. When the resistance is removed, for example, the extremity will oscillate because of lack of feedback regarding position and force needed to maintain static hold.

Scanning speech is a component of cerebellar dysfunction representing complexity of the motor activity. Word selection is not affected, but the words are pronounced slowly and without melody, tone, or rhythm. This reflects the incoordination or hypotonicity of the muscles of the larynx in controlling the voice.

Eye movements are disrupted in the person with cerebellar dysfunction, in both a static head and eye position and with movement of the head. *Gaze-evoked nystagmus,* or nonvoluntary rhythmic oscillation of the eye, occurs when the cerebellum is unable to hold the gaze on an object, especially a lateral position. When looking at a lateral target, the eyes drift back toward midline and then immediately back to the target. Eyes flickering on and off the target, eyes fluttering around the target, or spastic bursts of eye oscillations may be present with brainstem or midline cerebellar lesions.

Ocular dysmetria is similar to the dysmetria seen in the extremities. This dysmetria is seen in cerebellar lesions when the eyes are moving from one target to another (known as *saccadic movement*) or attempting to follow a target (known as *smooth pursuit*).

Vestibuloocular function is disrupted in medial lesions, and the ability to maintain eye stability during head movement is affected.

Gait disturbance is another disorder related to dysfunction of the cerebellum. The gait becomes wide based and staggering without the typical arm swing. The step length is uneven, the step widths are inconsistent, and the feet are often lifted higher than necessary. Stance and swing become irregular, and there is loss of adaptation to changes in terrain. It becomes difficult to perform heel-to-toe walking or walking a straight line, which is the standard sobriety test. In some persons, there is a surprising ability to avoid a fall, although the standing balance is abnormal. When the person is able to perform compensatory movements of the upper body and limbs, falls can be avoided.[18]

The cerebellum plays a major role in *motor learning.* The cerebellum is vital in anticipatory, or feed-forward, activity and

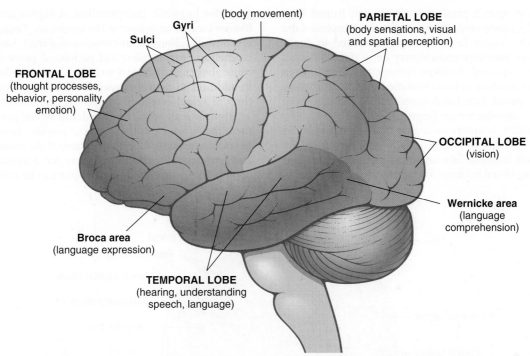

Gyri (body movement)

Sulci

PARIETAL LOBE
(body sensations, visual
and spatial perception)

FRONTAL LOBE
(thought processes,
behavior, personality,
emotion)

OCCIPITAL LOBE
(vision)

Wernicke area
(language
comprehension)

Broca area
(language expression)

TEMPORAL LOBE
(hearing, understanding
speech, language)

FIG. 18.12 Schematic representation of functional specialization in the cortex. (From Chabner DE: The language of medicine, ed 10, St Louis, 2014, Saunders.)

modification of response.[28] The cerebellum learns or memorizes small movements that are integrated into complex activity. During the acquisition phase of motor learning, the cerebellum is active.[23] Increased activity has also been noted during mental imagery or mental rehearsal of a motor program.[42] The cerebellum is active during cognitive and emotional processes, and lesions can cause difficulty in shifting attention from one sensory or thought domain to another.

Deficits of Higher Brain Function

The cortex has a great deal to do with the abilities and activities that are a part of the highest development in humans, including language and abstract thinking. Perception, movement, and adaptive response to the outside world depend on an intact cerebral cortex. As with other parts of the CNS, it is subdivided for ease of understanding the separate functions, although the structure and function are full of overlap. Fig. 18.12 represents some of the functional specialization of the brain. Fig. 18.13 describes the lobar relationship to the cerebellum and brainstem.

The *frontal lobe* is the largest single area of the brain, constituting nearly one-third of the brain's cortical surface. It is phylogenetically the youngest area of the brain and has major connections with all other areas of the brain. The frontal lobe is responsible for the highest levels of cognitive processing, control of emotion, and behavior. An individual's personality is established as a frontal lobe function, and one of the most disturbing deficits seen with lesions affecting the frontal lobe is change from the person's premorbid personality. A person's character and temperament are changed by damage to the frontal lobe. Slow processing of information, lack of judgment based on known consequences, withdrawal, and irritability can be the result of an insult to the frontal lobe. Lack of inhibition and apathy are common clinical problems related to frontal lobe damage. The person with a frontal lobe disorder may lack

insight into the deficits, and therefore behavior can be difficult to control.

The *right hemisphere syndrome* represents the inability to orient the body within external space and generate the appropriate motor responses. Hemineglect is one of the most common deficits seen with right hemisphere lesions. The individual does not respond to sensory stimuli on the left side of the body and does not respond to the environment surrounding the left side. Hemineglect is evident in the involved extremities and trunk during mobility and self-care activities. The ability to draw in two and three dimensions is lost along with other drawing skills, such as perspective and accurate copying. Spatial disorientation can result, with the person losing familiarity with the environment and becoming lost in areas that should be familiar. Inability to read and follow a map can be an indication of right hemisphere deficit.[13]

Disorders of emotional adjustment often follow a lesion in the right hemisphere. These disorders are primarily in the affective domain of interpersonal relationships and socialization. Cortical control of the limbic system is believed to be responsible, but the exact mechanism of control of more complex emotional behavior is not completely understood at this time. There appears to be hemispheric lateralization of emotions with suggestions that the right hemisphere is the dominant hemisphere in controlling emotions.

Language is one of the higher functions of the brain that is affected in many disorders of the CNS. Speech is a more elementary capacity than language and refers to the mechanical act of uttering words using the neuromuscular structures responsible for articulation. *Dysarthria,* a disturbance in articulation, and *anarthria,* the lack of ability to produce speech, are disorders of speech, not language. One common language disorder is *expressive aphasia,* a deficit in speech production or language output, accompanied by a deficit in communication, in which speech comes out as garbled or inappropriate words.

Localization of speech production in the left frontal lobe and impaired language comprehension in the temporal lobe demonstrate how higher functions can be related to brain regions. However, language control may be in different areas for different persons, and therefore damage to the same area of the brain may produce aphasia in some individuals whereas others may be spared. Left hand–dominant people may have right hemisphere dominance for language.[29]

Alexia is another symptom of higher brain dysfunction. It is the acquired inability to read. Alexia is typically caused by lesions in the left occipital lobe and the corpus callosum that prevent incoming visual information from reaching the angular gyrus for linguistic interpretation. *Agraphia* can be caused by lesions located anywhere in the cerebrum. Because writing is a motor skill, lesions of the corticospinal tract, basal ganglia, and cerebellum; myopathies; and peripheral nerve injuries can all cause abnormal or clumsy writing. These disorders may be seen in addition to neurobehavioral syndromes. Typically the features of agraphia tend to parallel the characteristics of aphasia.

Apraxia is an acquired disorder of skilled purposeful movement that is not a result of paresis, akinesia, ataxia, sensory loss, or comprehension. *Ideomotor apraxia* is the most common type and represents the inability to carry out a motor act on verbal command. Ideomotor apraxia appears to be caused by a lesion

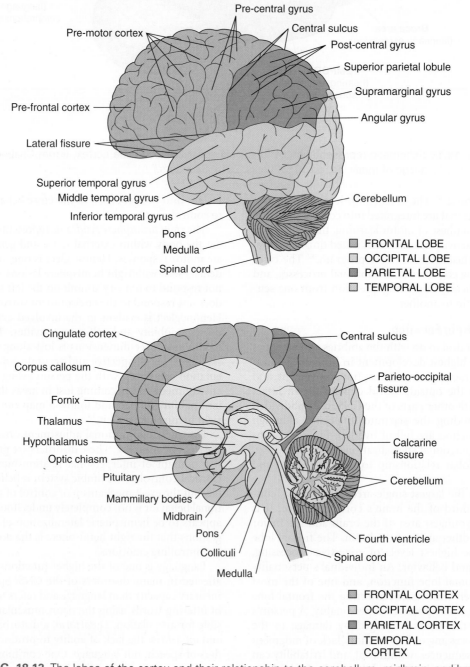

FIG. 18.13 The lobes of the cortex and their relationship to the cerebellum, midbrain, and brainstem. (Redrawn from Farber SD: Neurorehabilitation: a multisensory approach, Philadelphia, 1982, Saunders.)

in the arcuate fasciculus. The anterior connection from the left parietal lobe may be disrupted, preventing the motor system from receiving the command to act. A lesion in the left premotor area can cause apraxia by directly interrupting the motor act. Damage to the anterior corpus callosum can lead to apraxia that is evident in the left hand only. *Ideational apraxia* is failure to perform a sequential act even though each part of the act can be performed individually. The lesion causing ideational apraxia appears to be in the left parietal lobe, as in hemiparesis, or in the frontal lobe, as in Alzheimer's disease. The syndrome is seen as well with diffuse cortical damage associated with degenerative dementia.

Agnosia is the inability to recognize an object; the previously acquired meaning of an object is no longer attached to it. Agnosia is associated with lesions of the sensory cortices involved with seeing, hearing, and feeling and with the loss of one sensory modality. It is difficult to assess because the person is often easily able to compensate. Although the ability to recognize an object by vision is gone, the ability to recognize that same object by hearing or feeling is retained.

Altered States of Consciousness

Alteration of consciousness is not considered an independent disease entity but a reflection of some underlying disease or abnormal state of brain function. The human brain possesses a mechanism that allows a waking and sleeping state (arousal), as well as a separate ability to focus awareness on relevant environmental stimuli (attention).[13,34] To achieve a state of consciousness the cerebral cortex must be activated by the ascending reticular formation fibers in the brainstem. The fibers extend to the thalamus, limbic system, and cortex. The upper part of this system acts as an "on-off" switch for consciousness and controls the sleep–wake cycle. The lower part controls respiration.

Disturbances of arousal and attention can range from coma after brainstem injury to confusional states caused by drug intoxication. Metabolic or systemic disorders generally cause depressed consciousness without focal neurologic findings.[54] CNS disorders may or may not have concomitant focal signs. Table 18.2 compares metabolic and drug-induced coma with coma caused by space-occupying lesions.

Clinical disorders of arousal may result in hyperaroused states and can appear as restlessness, agitation, or delirium. This is presumably a result of the loss of hemispheric inhibition of brainstem function. Hypoarousal can be described on a spectrum ranging from drowsiness to stupor and coma. Stupor is a state of unresponsiveness that requires vigorous stimulation to bring about arousal. Coma is a state of unarousable unresponsiveness. Small and restricted lesions of the brainstem can result in stupor and coma. Massive bilateral hemispheric lesions are necessary to cause coma.

Damage to the cerebral cortex can be caused by loss of blood flow, subarachnoid hemorrhage, anesthetic toxicity, hypoglycemia, hypothermia, or status epilepticus. If the link to the brainstem is destroyed, the person will remain in a persistent vegetative state (PVS). Although the person may make random movements and the eyes may open, mentation remains absent. Akinetic mutism, similar to PVS, reflects damage to the mediofrontal lobe and results in lack of motivation to perform any motor or mental activity (abulia). In the *locked-in syndrome*, there is damage to the pons resulting most often from thrombosis of the basilar artery. This is a remarkable impairment, involving no mental deficit at all but resulting in inability to move anything but the eyes. It is in essence the opposite of PVS.

Supratentorial lesions that cause increased pressure, such as hemorrhage, cerebral edema, or neoplasm, can cause coma by producing tentorial herniation and subsequent compression of the brainstem. There is usually a hemiparesis with a dilated pupil on the side of the lesion because of central compression involving the third cranial nerve by the herniation.

In infratentorial lesions, brainstem damage can be related to drugs, hemorrhage, infarction, or compression from the posterior fossa. Disruption of ocular movements is an early sign of brainstem involvement.[59] There is loss of the pupillary reaction to light while the corneal reflex remains intact.

Brain death relates to destruction of both the upper and lower parts of the reticular formation in the brainstem, which will eventually lead to death. Cortical electrical activity and spinal reflexes may be preserved, but these are of no consequence because they are unable to be used for thought or movement.

Attention is more difficult to relate to specific brain structure than arousal. However, the acute confusional state is one of the most common neurologic disorders encountered. Although there is not a clear understanding of the mechanism of attention from the neuroanatomic perspective, there appears to be a major role played by the parietal and frontal lobes. Frontal and prefrontal areas of the brain are responsible for mental control,

TABLE 18.2	**Characteristics of Comas**	
Manifestations	**Metabolic and Drug-Induced Comas**	**Comas from Space-Occupying Lesions**
Onset	Behavioral changes, decreased attention and arousal	Usually severe headache, focal seizures
Pain response	Present and equal	May be different on each side
Reflexes	Intact deep tendon reflexes, equal responses	Deep tendon reflexes may be unequal; positive Babinski's sign (UMN lesion)
Pupillary reaction	Bilateral normal response	May be unequal
Size of pupil	May be at midpoint with anticholinergics; pinpoint from opiates; dilated from anoxia	Midbrain lesion—midpoint Pons lesion—pinpoint Herniation to brainstem—large
Corneal reflex	Bilateral, intact	Unequal, may be absent
Eye movement	Spontaneous movement without intention; no reaction to VOR testing	May have paresis of lateral gaze with CN III compression
Decorticate or decerebrate posturing	Absent; movement is normal	Posturing may be present depending on level of lesion
Extremity movement	Equal movement on both sides	Paresis may be unilateral

CN III, Third cranial (oculomotor) nerve; *UMN*, upper motor neuron; *VOR*, vestibuloocular reflex.

TABLE 18.3   Correlation of Anatomic Site to Disorders of Memory and Other Neurologic Findings

Anatomic Site of Damage	Memory Finding	Other Neurologic and Medical Findings
Frontal lobe	Lateralized deficit in working memory Right spatial defects, left verbal defects, impaired recall with spared recognition	Personality change Perseveration Chorea, dystonia Bradykinesia, tremor, rigidity
Basal forebrain	Declarative memory deficit	
Ventromedial cortex	Frontal lobe–type declarative memory deficit	Upper visual field defects
Hippocampus and parahippocampal cortex	Bilateral lesions yield global amnesia, unilateral lesions show lateralization of deficit—left, verbal deficit; right, spatial deficit	Myoclonus Depressed level of consciousness Cortical blindness Autonomations
Fornix	Global amnesia	
Mammillary bodies	Declarative memory deficit	Confabulation, ataxia, nystagmus, signs of alcohol withdrawal
Dorsal and medial dorsal nucleus thalamus	Declarative memory deficit	Confabulation
Anterior thalamus	Declarative memory deficit	
Lateral temporal cortex	Deficit in autobiographic memory	

concentration, vigilance, and performance of meaningful activity. Cognition and emotional control are established by extensive white matter connections between the frontal lobes and the remainder of the cerebrum.[44] Diseases that affect the white matter, such as multiple sclerosis, can affect the level of attention without decreasing arousal. Psychiatric disease has an effect on both arousal and attention.[34] The acute confusional state may be the result of a number of causes. Intoxicants, metabolic disorders, infections, epilepsy, blood flow disorders, traumatic injuries, and neoplasms can all be responsible for a change in orientation or attention.

Memory Problems

Memory is associated with various areas of the brain, and a particular area may be responsible for different aspects of memory. The hippocampus, the thalamus, and the basal forebrain are critical to the performance of recent memory (Table 18.3). Fig. 18.14 shows the relationship of learning strategies and brain regions. For immediate auditory memory, left and right temporal–parietal cortices mediate auditory verbal and nonverbal material. Neurogenesis has been observed in the dentate gyrus of the hippocampus throughout the lives of many species, including humans. Not all newly generated hippocampal neurons survive, but hippocampal-dependent memory tasks can enhance the survival of these neurons.[20] Inflammatory cytokines reduce hippocampal neurogenesis and impair the ability to maintain long-term potentiation in the hippocampus, which is a critical physiologic process involved in memory consolidation.[19]

Working memory, the ability to hold information in short-term storage while permitting other cognitive operations to take place, appears to depend on the prefrontal cortex. Keeping a spatial location in mind may involve a right frontal area that directs the maintenance of that information in a right parietal area, whereas keeping a word in mind may involve a left frontal area that directs the maintenance of that information in a left temporal or parietal area. Specific basal ganglia and cerebellar areas appear to support the working memory capacity of particular frontal regions.

Disorders of recent memory, known as *amnesia,* are a significant neurobehavioral phenomenon and common in persons after traumatic brain injury. *Declarative memory* is retention of facts and events of a prior experience or the memory of what

has occurred and is related to explicit learning. *Procedural memory* describes the learning of skills and habits, or how something is done. Implicit learning is based on procedural memory. The relationship to memory and relearning motor skills is discussed in Special Implications for the PTA 18.1 Motor Learning Strategies in this chapter.

Anterograde amnesia is the failure of new learning or formation of new memory. *Retrograde amnesia* is the loss of ability to recall events. The inability to acquire new learning is often accompanied by *confabulation,* the fabrication of information in response to questioning. *Traumatic amnesia* refers to an individual's inability to recall significant aspects of his or her traumatic experience. Traumatic memories are reported to be fragmented, compartmentalized, and disintegrated, suggesting that the hippocampus still may have a role to play in the phenomenon of traumatic amnesia. Dysregulation in the hippocampal system has the potential to generate narratives of traumatic events that are spotty and unreliable.

Neuromodulators, such as norepinephrine, have the potential to affect hippocampal functioning in a more dynamic fashion. The locus ceruleus, located in the brainstem, for example, projects directly to the hippocampus and modulates its functioning through norepinephrine release. The effects of such a network are unclear, although the implications are that stress-related memory alterations might occur on a split-second basis, and deficient or extreme locus ceruleus input may disrupt normal hippocampal processing severely. Given that the hippocampus plays a role in integrating input from diverse sources when encoding memory, disruptions in its functioning may lead to memories that seem fragmented and nonlinear. Over time, fragments of the memory may become consolidated, vivid, and easily recalled, whereas other fragments rarely are accessed.[27]

The role of stress in neurologic disease often is overlooked. Several chronic neurologic disease states, such as Alzheimer's disease, are associated with elevated secretion of stress hormones, in particular cortisol, which results from overactivity of the hypothalamic–pituitary–adrenal (HPA) axis. The stress or perceived threat activates the hypothalamus, triggering release of hormones that cause increased adrenal output of cortisol.[43] Stress also can trigger or exacerbate symptom onset and perhaps progression of chronic illness such as Parkinson's disease.

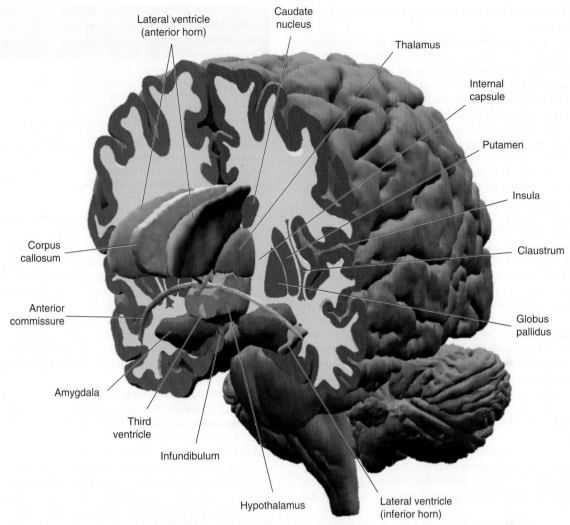

FIG. 18.14 Anatomic correlates for explicit and implicit learning. (From Vanderah TW, Gould DJ: Nolte's the human brain: an introduction to its functional anatomy, ed 7, Philadelphia, 2016, Elsevier.)

Stress hormones also can mitigate the impact of acute neurotrauma; for example, there is a positive correlation between cortisol levels and mortality after head injury. Thus neurologic disease states can occur within a context of elevated glucocorticoids, which may have profound influences on recovery and neuroplasticity. In addition, abnormal regulation of glucocorticoid release is associated with many affective disorders, such as depression and posttraumatic stress disorder (PTSD), that are overrepresented in populations with neurologic disease; Parkinson's disease is a prime example. Acute and sustained glucocorticoid release also can precipitate changes in peripheral and central immune signaling, resulting in cytokine profiles that may be deleterious for functional recovery in the face of neurologic challenge.[22]

Accumulation of risk is another concept that plays a pivotal role in the life-course model of chronic diseases. *Allostasis* is defined as the ability to achieve stability through change. The price of this accommodation to stress has been defined as the *allostatic load*. It follows that acute stress (the "fight, flight, or freeze" response) and chronic stress resulting from the cumulative load of minor day-to-day stresses can add to the allostatic load and have long-term consequences. Subacute stress is

defined as an accumulation of stressful life events over a duration of months and includes emotional factors, such as hostility and anger, as well as affective disorders such as major depression and anxiety disorders. Chronic stressors include low social support, work stress, marital stress, and caregiver strain, and chronic stress manifests as feelings of fatigue, lack of energy, irritability, and demoralization.

The link between chronic psychologic distress and adverse behavior, such as overeating, may be centrally mediated. Normally glucocorticoids help end acute stress responses by exerting negative feedback on the HPA axis. The combination of chronic stress and high glucocorticoid levels seems to stimulate a preferential desire to ingest sweet and fatty foods, presumably by affecting dopaminergic transmission in areas of the brain associated with motivation and reward.[16]

Brain areas associated with reward are linked with those that sense physical pain. Chronic pain can cause depression, and depression can increase pain. Most individuals who have depression also have physical symptoms. Studies using functional magnetic resonance imaging have shown that social rejection lights up brain areas that are also key regions in the response to physical pain. The area of the anterior cingulate cortex that is activated by visceral pain also is activated in cases of social rejection.

Disturbances of neurologic function can result in behavioral disturbances that mimic disturbances of mental function in psychiatric disorders. *Delusions,* or fixed false beliefs, have been reported in a great variety of neurologic conditions and appear to be associated with the limbic system. Paranoid delusions are common in disorders of the medial temporal lobe or a combination of the frontal and right parietal lobes. *Hallucinations* are sensory experiences without external stimulation. Visual hallucinations generally suggest neurologic involvement; auditory hallucinations imply psychiatric disease. Midbrain lesions in the cerebral peduncles can cause hallucinations involving animals. Temporal lesions can cause recurrent auditory experiences.[13]

Rapid eye movement (REM) sleep behavior disorder is characterized by loss of muscular atonia and prominent motor behaviors during REM sleep. Sleep behavior disorder can cause sleep disruption. The disorder is strongly associated with neurodegenerative diseases such as multiple-system atrophy, Parkinson's disease, dementia with Lewy bodies, and progressive supranuclear palsy. The symptoms of sleep behavior disorder precede other symptoms of these neurodegenerative disorders by several years. Furthermore, several recent studies have shown that sleep behavior disorder is associated with abnormalities of electroencephalographic activity, cerebral blood flow, and cognitive, perceptual, and autonomic functions. Sleep behavior disorder might be a stage in the development of neurodegenerative disorder. Box 18.2 lists the areas of the brain that play a role in sleep behavior.[17]

Lesions of the hemispheres or lobes may cause loss of the functions that each hemisphere controls. Because diseases and damage caused by trauma will often affect one area of the brain, the associated syndromes for the main areas of the brain are described.[31]

Autonomic Nervous System

The term *autonomic nervous system* was introduced to describe the system of nerves that controls the unstriated tissue, the cardiac muscle, and the glandular tissue of mammals involved in the control of autonomic function. The autonomic CNS neurons are located at many levels from the cerebral cortex to the spinal cord. Efferent autonomic pathways are organized in two major outflows: the sympathetic and parasympathetic. Finally, the enteric nervous system, which is considered a separate and independent division of the autonomic nervous system, is located in the walls of the gut. The schematic diagram of the autonomic nervous system is shown in Fig. 18.15.

Neurons in the cerebral cortex, basal forebrain, hypothalamus, midbrain, pons, and medulla participate in autonomic control. The central autonomic network integrates visceral, humoral, and environmental information to produce coordinated autonomic, neuroendocrine, and behavioral responses to external or internal stimuli. A coordinated response is generated through interconnections among the amygdala and the neocortex, forebrain, hypothalamus, and autonomic and somatic motor nuclei of the brainstem. The insular and medial prefrontal cortices (paralimbic areas) and nuclei of the amygdala are the higher centers involved in the processing of visceral information and the initiation of integrated autonomic responses. The central nucleus of the amygdala projects to the hypothalamus, periaqueductal gray (PAG) matter, and autonomic nuclei

---

> ## BOX 18.2 Rapid Eye Movement Sleep Behavior Disorder and Related Brainstem Structures
>
> - Substantia nigra (midbrain, dopaminergic)
> - Locus coeruleus (brainstem, noradrenergic)
> - Pedunculopontine nucleus (pons, cerebellum)
> - Dorsal vagus nucleus
> - Dorsal raphe nucleus (involved in serotonin pathways)
> - Gigantocellular reticular nucleus (control of arousal)

Modified from Gagnon JF, Postuma RB, Mazza S, et al.: Rapid-eye-movement sleep behaviour disorder and neurodegenerative diseases, Lancet Neurol 5:424–432, 2006.

of the brainstem to integrate autonomic, endocrine, and motor responses to emotionally relevant stimuli.

The hypothalamus integrates the autonomic and endocrine responses that are critical for homeostasis. The PAG matter of the midbrain is the site of integrated autonomic, behavioral, and antinociceptive stress responses. It is organized into separate columns that control specific patterns of response to stress. The lateral PAG matter mediates sympathoexcitation, opioid-independent analgesia, and motor responses consistent with the fight-or-flight reaction. The ventrolateral PAG matter produces sympathoinhibition, opioid-dependent analgesia, and motor inhibition.

Neurons in the medulla are critical for the control of cardiovascular, respiratory, and gastrointestinal functions. The medullary nucleus of the solitary tract is the first relay station for the arterial baroreceptors and chemoreceptors, as well as cardiopulmonary and gastrointestinal afferents.

Preganglionic sympathetic neurons are organized into different functional units that control blood flow to the skin and muscles, secretion of sweat glands, skin hair follicles, systemic blood flow, and the function of viscera. Selectivity is refined by the release of different neurotransmitters. Acetylcholine is the neurotransmitter of the sympathetic and parasympathetic preganglionic neurons. The main postganglionic sympathetic neurotransmitter is norepinephrine.

Visceral afferents transmit conscious sensations (e.g., gut distention and cardiac ischemia) and unconscious visceral sensations (e.g., blood pressure and chemical composition of the blood). Their most important function is to initiate autonomic reflexes at the local, ganglion, spinal, and supraspinal levels. Visceral sensation is carried primarily by the spinothalamic and spinoreticular pathways, which transmit visceral pain and sexual sensations. Brainstem visceral afferents are carried by the vagus and glossopharyngeal nerves. Brainstem visceral afferents are important in complex automatic motor acts such as swallowing, vomiting, and coughing.[20]

Traumatic spinal cord injury, particularly injury above the T5 level, is associated with severe and disabling cardiovascular, gastrointestinal, bladder, and sexual dysfunction. Affected individuals have both supine and orthostatic hypotension and are at risk for developing bradycardia and cardiac arrest during tracheal suction or other maneuvers that activate the vagovagal reflexes.

Pure autonomic failure with no other neurologic deficits is rare. More often, autonomic failure occurs in combination with other neurologic disorders, such as Parkinson's disease, and multiple system atrophy. In such individuals it is important for the examiner to inquire about abnormalities in gait, changes in

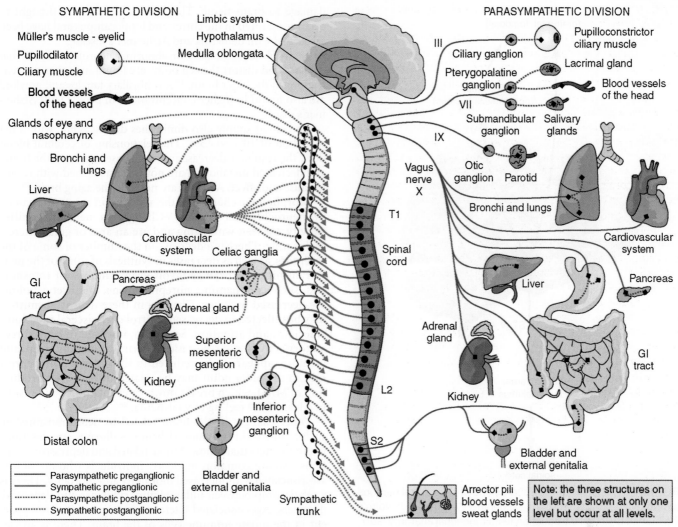

FIG. 18.15 Sympathetic (A) and parasympathetic (B) divisions of the autonomic nervous system: efferent systems. (From Bertorini TE: Neuromuscular disorders: treatment and management, Philadelphia, 2011, Saunders.)

facial expression, the presence of dysarthria, difficulty in swallowing, and balance problems. Autonomic failure also occurs in individuals with some peripheral neuropathies such as those associated with diabetes. Because autonomic failure may be caused by lesions at different levels of the nervous system, a history of secondary trauma, cerebrovascular disease, tumors, infections, or demyelinating diseases should be established. In addition, because the most frequent type of autonomic dysfunction encountered in medical practice is pharmacologic, there should be a thorough review of medication use, especially antihypertensive and psychotropic drugs.

Some conditions may be confused with autonomic failure, including neurally mediated syncope, which is referred to as *vasovagal, vasodepressor,* or *reflex syncope.* This condition is caused by a paroxysmal reversal of the normal pattern of autonomic activation that maintains blood pressure in the standing position; these individuals do not have autonomic failure. A detailed history is important to differentiate this disorder. In contrast to individuals with chronic autonomic failure in whom syncope appears as a gradual fading of vision and loss of awareness, individuals with neurally mediated syncope often have signs and symptoms of autonomic overactivity such as

diaphoresis and nausea before the event. This distinction and the episodic nature of neurally mediated syncope should be part of a thorough clinical history.

The complexity of the nervous system cannot be overstated. The information provided in this overview of the components of the CNS is meant to illuminate the many facets of the system that can be affected by pathologic processes. Fig. 18.16 shows the relationship of the areas that have been described here.[37] Familiarity with this relationship is the basis for attempting to understand the pathologies that will be considered in the next chapters. To understand pathology, one must have a good working knowledge of brain structure and function. The Whole Brain Atlas website provides dynamic images of the brain, integrating imaging techniques that link anatomy and pathology.[60]

Aging and the Central Nervous System

Senescence, or aging, results from changes in DNA, RNA, and proteins. Errors in the duplication of DNA increase with age because of random damage over time. There may be a specific genetic program for senescence. Fibroblasts from an older individual double fewer times than those of an embryo.

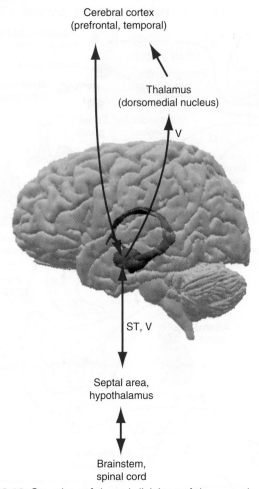

Cerebral cortex
(prefrontal, temporal)

Thalamus
(dorsomedial nucleus)

V

ST, V

Septal area,
hypothalamus

Brainstem,
spinal cord

FIG. 18.16 Overview of the subdivisions of the central nervous system (CNS). (Adapted from Vanderah TW, Gould DJ: Nolte's the human brain: an introduction to its functional anatomy, ed 7, Philadelphia, 2016, Elsevier.)

Age-related reduction in adult brain weight represents loss of brain tissue. There is highly selective atrophy of brain tissue in the aging CNS. It is not clear how much of the change represents actual loss of nerve cells, because the changes in vascular tissue and glial cells may account for some of the loss. Simple loss of cells is common. Nerve cell shrinking, causing possible changes in functional efficiency, may be a more important effect of old age than cell loss. Nerve conduction velocity decreases with age in both the motor and sensory systems. By the eighth decade there is an average loss of 15% of the velocity in the myelinated fibers.[30]

The inner structure of the nerve cell changes with aging. The presence of lipofuscin, or wear-and-tear pigment, a pigmented lipid found in the cytoplasm, may interfere with normal cell function via pressure on the cell nucleus. The pigmented nuclei of the brainstem catecholaminergic neurotransmitter accumulate with age. Damage to an axon close to the neuronal cell body results in changes in the area of the cell body and is referred to as an *axonal reaction*. The mechanism and relationship to dysfunction are still not clearly understood. The deposition of amyloid-β protein, creating plaques in the cerebral cortex, is found in many but not all older people. Neuritic, or senile, plaques are found outside the neuron and are filled with degenerating axons, dendrites, astrocytes, and amyloid. They represent damage to brain tissue. The neuritic plaques are thought to occur most often in the cortex and hippocampus and have been associated with dementia and Alzheimer's disease.[14]

Neurofibrillary tangles, or abnormal neurologic fibers that displace and distort the cell body, are found in higher concentrations in the older brain. Neurofibrillary tangles and amyloid are also found in higher concentrations in people with Alzheimer's disease.

The blood supply also diminishes during aging, with a net reduction of 10% to 15%. The relationship of cerebral blood flow, the resultant decrease in the glucose supply to the brain, and decreased metabolism are not well established with regard to cause and effect. All three are noted in the aging brain.[40]

Morphologic changes in the aging brain are accompanied by neurochemical changes. Changes in neurotransmitter activity are seen with aging and are an area of great interest at this time. There is a decrease in the number of some of the receptors, as well as decreases in synthesis of some of the neurotransmitters. Enzymes involved in synthesis of transmitters, such as dopamine, norepinephrine, and acetylcholine, are decreased with age. Changes in these neurotransmitters may be reflected in decreased control over visceral functions, emotions, and attention. Serotonin, involved in central regulatory activities of respiration, thermoregulation, sleep, and memory, appears to be reduced in the older brain. Depression in the older adult may be related to increased production of MAO, which breaks down catecholamines and results in a loss of the feeling of well-being.[26]

Other changes in the brain related to neurotransmission, such as in Parkinson's and Alzheimer's diseases, are described in the chapters that follow. Mood-related and depressive symptoms also are common in elderly individuals who are ill and are associated with increased morbidity and mortality. There is a relationship between inflammatory cytokines and depressive disorders. Age-associated alterations in immunity are apparent in the innate immune cells of the brain. There is an elevated inflammatory profile in the aging brain consisting of an increased population of reactive glia. A potential consequence of a reactive glial cell population in the brain is an exaggerated inflammatory response to innate immune activation. Even in the absence of detectable disease, the glial population undergoes an age-related transformation that creates a more sensitive brain environment.

An amplified and prolonged inflammatory response in the aged brain promotes protracted behavioral and cognitive impairments, and the behavioral consequences of illness and infection in the elderly, if prolonged, can have deleterious effects on mental health. There is an increased prevalence of delirium in elderly individuals who visit the emergency department as a result of infections unrelated to the CNS. Viral or bacterial pneumonia in the aged frequently manifests clinically as delirium, even in the absence of classic pneumonia symptoms.[19]

The central mechanisms that are involved in the control of balance do not appear to change excessively with age but are more likely to be affected by degenerative neurologic diseases such as Parkinson's or Alzheimer's disease. Age-related changes in the peripheral vestibular system include a decrease in hair cell receptors that begins at the age of 30 years and a loss of the vestibular receptor ganglion cells by age 55 to 60 years. The myelinated nerve cells of the vestibular system show up to a 40% loss. Partial loss of vestibular function in the older population can lead to complaints of dizziness, with less ability of the nervous system to accommodate the loss compared with younger persons.

In addition to vestibular losses, there is concomitant loss of other sensory inputs relating to balance and mobility: vision and somatosensation. Maintaining equilibrium, or balance, requires a multimodal system integrating vestibular, visual, and somatosensory signals. The integration of these signals in the CNS coordinates multiple output responses: eye movement, postural correction, motor skill, and conscious awareness of spatial orientation. There are longer response latencies and delayed reaction times. Vision changes include loss of acuity, decreased peripheral fields, and loss of depth perception. The loss of input from this combination is slow, with compensation developing through the years.[11]

Eventually a loss of functional reserve, or redundant function, that is normally present in virtually all physiologic systems is seen with aging. There is an apparent decrease in the ability to integrate conflicting sensory information to determine appropriate postural responses. Changes occur as well in motor output that may contribute to the loss of balance and mobility.[10] Although the response patterns are the same in young and old people, with responses being activated in the stretched ankle muscle and radiating up to the thigh, in some older people this response is disrupted, with the proximal muscles being activated before the distal muscles. In the older person there appears to be more cocontraction of muscles around the ankle as a result of perturbation.[48]

Neurologic disease is more prevalent in older persons, as is the risk of neurologic sequelae as a result of intracranial hemorrhage, subdural hematoma, and neoplasms. Awareness of the signs and symptoms of these disorders is essential. The PTA may be the person able to identify a disease or the potential for a disorder that may manifest during a treatment session.

DIAGNOSIS

Clinical Localization

Clinical localization is the first step to differential diagnosis for an individual with neurologic disease. Coupling the time course of the illness with the clinical localization is the essence of neurology. The history of the onset and nature of the symptoms is critical to establish the diagnosis related to the neurologic disorder. In many cases, based on the history and symptoms the clinician is able to generate a hypothesis regarding the site in the nervous system that has been affected and the nature of the lesion. A complete history of the nature of the symptoms is also critical to determining which diagnostic tools will provide the most accurate differential diagnosis and best determine the cause.

The examination of the client with neurologic dysfunction often begins with mental status changes. Alterations of consciousness and disturbances of higher brain function give the clinician clues about the nature of the disease process and the location of damage within the brain[54] (Table 18.4).

Motor and sensory changes will also reflect the type, level, and extent of damage to the system in the case of both disease and trauma. Understanding the typical motor and sensory changes associated with a particular disease or disorder leads the evaluation. For example, knowing that ALS involves both upper and lower motor signs may help the clinician when this otherwise perplexing condition is seen in the clinic. Understanding the functional deficits related to each condition can also lead the clinician to a diagnosis. Gait disorders are often representative of the level or location of damage within the nervous system.

The diagnosis of neurologic disorders remains a clinical specialty, although the use of sophisticated imaging and measurement of neural function have provided insight into the pathologic state of the nervous system. The following sections give examples of diagnostic tests currently performed.

Computed Tomography

Computed tomography (CT) scans allows a snapshot of the CNS, and damage within tissue can be identified. Disorders affecting blood flow, multiple sclerosis, neoplasm, and infection can be identified with these scans. CT is an excellent study to evaluate for acute intracranial hemorrhage, particularly in the subarachnoid space. Active bleeding may be detected in either epidural or subdural hemorrhages as a relative lucency, which is commonly referred to as the "swirl sign." Edema from excitotoxic damage associated with infarct or diffuse anoxia can be seen representing intracellular fluid, and vasogenic edema is the abnormal accumulation of extracellular fluid in the white matter that looks like fingers following the white matter tracts. Evaluation of ventricular size can be done by CT. Enlargement of the temporal horns out of proportion to the lateral ventricular bodies is helpful in recognizing early hydrocephalus. CT can be helpful to follow ventricular size after shunting.

CT is very useful for detecting intracranial calcifications such as those seen in congenital infections, vascular lesions, and metabolic disease. The location and distribution of calcifications is helpful in differentiating these various causes. The identification of calcification in a neoplasm aids in differential diagnosis.[20]

Magnetic Resonance Imaging

Magnetic resonance imaging (MRI) signal patterns are recognizable with common diseases such as cerebral edema, neoplasm, abscess, infarcts, or demyelinating processes. MRI is the study of choice to evaluate all lesions in the brain and spine. CT, however, is more sensitive than MRI for the evaluation of calcifications and subtle fractures and remains pivotal in the diagnosis of acute subarachnoid hemorrhage. In addition, MRI cannot be performed in individuals who have intraorbital foreign bodies, pacemakers, or non–MRI-compatible implants, such as artificial heart valves, vascular clips, cochlear implants, or ventilators. MRI is the modality of choice for detecting congenital malformations. Infection of the spine is better evaluated by MRI.

Functional Magnetic Resonance Imaging

Functional magnetic resonance imaging (fMRI) is based on blood oxygenation level–dependent (BOLD) imaging of the brain and provides functional data regarding cerebral activation during any given task (e.g., motor, visual, or cognitive). This method allows for a quantitative nonclinical method for assessing changes in cerebral function as related to cerebral activities (i.e., performance of physical or cognitive tasks). The BOLD fMRI technique allows for detection of minute changes in cerebral oxygenation. fMRI studies of various pathways of the brain, including the language, memory, and visual pathways, will enhance our ability to connect activity to changes in the brain. For example, frontal and lateral three-dimensional (3D) fMRI renderings show functional activity in the occipital lobe secondary to a visual stimulus.

TABLE 18.4	Useful Studies in the Evaluation of Disorders of Level of Consciousness			
Syndrome	Neuroimaging	Electrophysiology	Fluid and Tissue Analysis	Neuropsychologic Tests
Bilateral cortical dysfunction; confusion and delirium	Usually normal; may show atrophy; rarely bilateral chronic subdural hematoma or evidence of herpes simplex encephalitis; dural enhancement in meningitis, especially neoplastic meningitides	Diffuse slowing; often, frontally predominant intermittent rhythmic delta activity (FIRDA); in herpes simplex encephalitis, periodic lateralized epileptiform activity (PLEDS)	Blood or urine analyses may reveal cause; CSF may show evidence of infection or neoplastic cells	In mild cases, difficulty with attention (e.g., trailmaking tests); in more severe cases, formal testing is not possible
Diencephalic dysfunction	Lesion(s) in or displacement of diencephalon; also displays mass displacing the diencephalon	Usually, diffuse slowing; rarely, FIRDA; in displacement syndromes, effect of the mass producing displacement (e.g., focal delta activity, loss of faster rhythms)	Usually not helpful	Usually not obtained
Midbrain dysfunction	Lesion(s) in the midbrain or displacing it	Usually, diffuse slowing; alpha coma; evoked response testing may demonstrate failure of conduction above the lesion	Rarely, platelet or coagulation abnormalities	Usually not performed
Pontine dysfunction	Lesion(s) producing syndrome; thrombosis of basilar artery	EEG: usually normal; evoked responses usually normal	Rarely, platelet or coagulation abnormalities	Usually not performed
Medullary dysfunction	Lesion(s) producing dysfunction	EEG: normal; brainstem auditory and somatosensory evoked responses may show conduction abnormalities	Rarely, platelet or coagulation abnormalities	Usually not performed
Herniation syndromes	Lesion(s) producing herniation; appearance of perimesencephalic cistern	Findings related to cause	Findings related to cause	Usually not performed
Locked-in syndrome	Infarction of basis pontis	EEG and evoked potential studies: normal	Findings related to cause	Usually not performed
Death by brain criteria	Absence of intracranial blood flow above the foramen magnum	EEG: electrocerebral silence; evoked potential studies may show peripheral components (e.g., wave I of brainstem auditory evoked response) but no central conduction	Absence of hypnosedative drugs	Not done
Psychogenic unresponsiveness	Normal	Normal	Normal	Helpful after patient "awakens"

CSF, Cerebrospinal fluid; EEG, electroencephalogram.
From Goetz CG: Textbook of clinical neurology, ed 2, Philadelphia, 2003, Saunders.

Positron Emission Tomography

Positron emission tomography (PET) and single-photon emission CT (SPECT) scanning can show cellular activity via regional blood flow in the brain and are now used to monitor changes in the brain with functional activity. Both techniques can be used to depict the regional density of a number of neurotransmitters, allowing researchers to better understand the role of different parts of the brain during activity.

Electroencephalography

Cerebral ischemia produces neuronal dysfunction, leading to slowing of frequencies or reduced amplitude in the electroencephalogram (EEG) tracing. These changes may be generalized (global ischemia) or regional (focal ischemia). The depth of ischemia is associated with the severity of EEG changes. Electroencephalography cannot be used to assess the whole cerebral cortex, however, and is less reliable at assessing subcortical structures.

Brainstem Auditory Evoked Potentials

Potentials generated in the auditory nerve and in different regions of the auditory pathways in the brainstem can be recorded. The attention of the subject is not required. Because the brainstem auditory evoked potential (BAEP) is of very low voltage, 1000 to 2000 responses are generally recorded so that

the BAEP can be extracted by averaging from the background noise. Wave III probably arises in the region of the superior olive, whereas waves IV and V arise in the midbrain and inferior colliculus. Waves VI and VII are of uncertain origin and little clinical utility because of their inconsistency in normal subjects. The most consistent components are waves I, III, and V, and it is to these that attention is directed when BAEPs are evaluated for clinical purposes.

The BAEP is an important means of evaluating function of cranial nerve VIII and the central auditory pathways in the brainstem. In infants, young children, and adults who are unable to cooperate for behavioral testing, BAEPs can be used to evaluate hearing. The wave V component of the response is generated by auditory stimuli that are too weak to generate other components. The BAEP is also useful in assessing the integrity of the brainstem. The presence of normal BAEPs in comatose individuals suggests either that the coma is a result of bihemispheric disease or that it relates to metabolic or toxic factors; abnormal BAEPs in this context imply brainstem pathology and a poorer prognosis than otherwise. When coma is caused by brainstem pathology, the BAEP findings help in localizing the lesion.

BAEPs have been used to detect subclinical brainstem pathology in individuals with suspected multiple sclerosis. However, the yield in this circumstance is less than with the visual or somatosensory evoked potentials, possibly because the auditory

TABLE 18.5	**Neuroimaging Applications in Diagnosis and Therapy**				
Technique	Diffuse or Multifocal Cerebral	Focal Cerebral	Subcortical	Brainstem	Spinal Cord
Plain film	Neoplasm Metabolic Congenital	Neoplasm	Not useful	Not useful	Trauma Neoplasm Degenerative
CT	Hemorrhage Calcification Infarct Neoplasm Inflammation Vascular	Hemorrhage Calcification Infarct Neoplasm Inflammation Vascular	Hemorrhage Calcification Infarct Neoplasm Inflammation Vascular	Hemorrhage Calcification Infarct Neoplasm Inflammation Vascular	Hemorrhage Calcification Neoplasm Inflammation
MRI	Neoplasm Inflammation Hemorrhage Vascular White matter disease Congenital Infarct	Neoplasm Inflammation Hemorrhage Vascular White matter disease Congenital Infarct	Neoplasm Inflammation Hemorrhage Vascular White matter disease Infarct	Neoplasm Inflammatory Hemorrhage Vascular White matter disease Infarct	Neoplasm Inflammatory Hemorrhage Vascular White matter disease Infarct
Myelography	Not useful	Not useful	Not useful	Not useful	Degenerative Neoplasm Hematoma Inflammatory Vascular Congenital
Angiography	Mass effect Vasculopathy Atherosclerosis	AVM tumor Aneurysm Atherosclerosis	AVM tumor Aneurysm Atherosclerosis	AVM tumor Aneurysm Atherosclerosis	AVM
Ultrasonography	Hemorrhage Neonatal Congenital Neoplasm Infection Vascular	Hemorrhage Neonatal Congenital Neoplasm Infection Vascular	Hemorrhage Neonatal Congenital Neoplasm	Congenital Neoplasm	Congenital Neoplasm
PET-SPECT	Vascular Neoplasm Infection Degenerative Trauma	Vascular Neoplasm Infection Degenerative Trauma	Vascular Neoplasm Infection Degenerative Trauma	Not useful	Not useful

AVM, Arteriovenous malformation; *CT,* computed tomography; *MRI,* magnetic resonance imaging; *PET-SPECT,* positron emission tomography–single-photon emission computed tomography. From Goetz CG: Textbook of clinical neurology, ed 3, Philadelphia, 2007, Saunders.

pathway is relatively short or is more likely to be spared. Cerebral ischemia results in delay in the arrival of or reduction in amplitude of evoked responses.[20]

Transcranial Doppler Ultrasonography

Transcranial Doppler ultrasonography uniquely measures local blood flow velocity in the proximal portions of large intracranial arteries. Hemodynamic compromise is inferred when there is reduction in mean flow velocities or when there is slow flow acceleration. In addition, transcranial Doppler ultrasonography can detect cerebral microembolic signals, reflecting the presence of gaseous or particulate matter in the cerebral artery. Solid, fat, gas, or air materials in flowing blood are larger and of different composition and thus have different acoustic impedance than surrounding red blood cells. Thus the Doppler ultrasound beam is both reflected and scattered at the interface between the embolus and blood, resulting in an increased intensity of the received Doppler signal. A completely accurate and reliable characterization of embolus size and composition, however, is not yet possible with current technology.

Near-Infrared Spectroscopy

In brain tissue, the venous oxygen saturation predominates (70% to 80%), and cerebral oximetry relies on this fact. Near-infrared spectroscopy (NIRS) uses light optical spectroscopy in the near-infrared range to evaluate brain oxygen saturation by measuring regional cerebral venous oxygen saturation. Table 18.5 describes the use of various imaging techniques correlated to anatomic site.

TREATMENT

Treatment is based on an understanding of the level and type of neuronal dysfunction. Treatment of neurologic disorders has been a frustrating science in the past, but with better understanding of the cellular processes and changes related to disease, treatment holds more promise.

Methods to Control Central Nervous System Damage

Damage or disease of the nervous system often results in changes in the production and uptake of neurotransmitters. Many important drugs that alter nervous system function act by selective interaction with neurotransmitter receptors. Drugs that act at synapses either enhance or block the action of these neurotransmitters. Most neurotransmitters with a prominent role in brain function produce very brief receptor-mediated actions at specific groups of synapses. A few neurotransmitters are more prolonged and act more widely throughout the extracellular space. The combined action of both a briefly acting and a more enduring neurotransmitter produces a modulation of postsynaptic neuronal activity. Pharmacologic strategies are currently aimed at modulation of neurotransmitter synthesis, release, reuptake, and degradation.[24] Some drugs mediate inhibition of neurotransmitter release by acting at presynaptic receptors. Opiates are one group of drugs that act by the inhibition of neurotransmitter release. Drugs used to control excessive tone in specific muscle groups often work by inhibiting neurotransmitter release. Anesthetic drugs modify the actions of neurotransmitter receptors by changing the membranes of cells on or within which the receptors are located.

Drug therapy can stimulate neurotransmitter release. Drugs aimed at maintaining neurotransmitter activity in the synaptic cleft can be useful in neuromuscular junction diseases. Another way to regulate the level of neurotransmitters is to influence the rate of chemical degradation. Drugs can inhibit the breakdown of certain elements that may be broken down by natural processes such as oxidation. One action of these drugs is to prolong the efficacy of released neurotransmitters by inhibiting their degradation.[56] An example of this process is the regulation of dopamine. Dopamine activity can be increased by four mechanisms:

- Increased synthesis
- Increased release
- Prolongation of neurotransmitter activity
- Direct receptor stimulation

Synthesis of the neurotransmitter can be increased by giving dopa because it is the product beyond the rate-limiting enzyme and there is ordinarily an abundant amount of aromatic amino acid decarboxylase in the CNS. When dopa is combined with a peripherally active decarboxylase inhibitor, more dopa is delivered across the blood–brain barrier and can be used to synthesize central dopamine. Drugs such as cocaine, amphetamine, and methylphenidate can increase release.

The normal metabolism of dopamine involves reuptake of dopamine into the presynaptic cell, with subsequent metabolism by two enzymes, MAO and COMT. Prolongation of dopamine activity can be effected by blocking reuptake or altering enzyme activity. Amantadine and possibly some tricyclic antidepressant medications operate on the dopaminergic system through blockade of reuptake. MAO inhibitors and COMT inhibitors for human use also increase dopaminergic activity. Finally, direct activation of the dopamine receptors on the striatal cell can be induced by agonists such as bromocriptine, pergolide, and other drugs. It is important to note that orally administered dopamine itself has no place in altering CNS dopamine levels because, being a positively charged molecule, it cannot cross the blood–brain barrier.[20]

Other drugs protect the cell membrane in the presence of toxins that act on the membrane—for example, the toxic effects of the free radicals produced in brain tissue after hypoxia, ischemia, and seizures. Damage to the neuron occurs when the free radical is allowed to penetrate the membrane.[41] The best defense is to prevent penetration. Antioxidant therapies are being examined for a variety of neurodegenerative disorders and the sequelae of stroke and spinal cord injury. It is believed that the toxicity of glutamate can be blocked by various antioxidants. Vitamin E, a free radical scavenger, is an antioxidant that has been tested widely. However, it does not pass easily through the blood–brain barrier, and as a fat-soluble vitamin it can be toxic in large doses. Estrogen can work as an antioxidant through intrinsic neurotrophic activities. Ongoing studies are looking at the natural substances that have been noted, as well as at manufactured substances that will provide antioxidant or free radical scavenging. There is great hope that substances that will slow down the destruction related to oxidative stress will prove to be curative for progressive diseases of the CNS, as well as other degenerative processes associated with connective tissue, neoplasm, and aging.[7] Specific drugs used for primary neurologic disorders are described in the next chapters.

Exciting new advancements in the field of molecular genetics have begun to identify novel candidate genes that may be involved in many inherited or acquired neurologic disorders. The basic principle of gene therapy is to transfer exogenous genes into specific cell types within the human body to correct a pathologic disorder. Currently gene therapies are based on simple nucleic acid sequences or derived from unique viruses. Researchers have attempted to use the power of viruses to essentially hijack cells for gene expression of appropriate therapeutic molecules.

Stem cells are unspecialized living cells that have the capacity to renew themselves for long periods through cell division. Under certain physiologic or experimental conditions, they can be induced to become cells with special functions such as the beating cells of the heart muscle or the insulin-producing cells of the pancreas. *Embryonic stem cells* are derived from embryos that develop from eggs that have been fertilized in vitro and then donated for research purposes with the informed consent of the donors. The embryos from which human embryonic stem cells are derived are typically 4 or 5 days old and consist of a hollow microscopic collection of cells called the *blastocyst*. An *adult stem cell* is an undifferentiated cell found among differentiated cells in a tissue or organ. The primary roles of adult stem cells in a living organism are to maintain and repair the tissue in which they are found. Some researchers now use the term *somatic stem cell* instead of adult stem cell. Unlike embryonic stem cells, which are defined by their origin, the origin of adult stem cells in mature tissues is unknown. A single adult stem cell could have the ability to generate a line of genetically identical cells, or *clones.*[2]

There is evidence for the impact of immune system dysfunction in these diseases despite the blood–brain barrier protection of the CNS from the direct effects of autoimmune responses. Identification of immune system elements is leading researchers toward an understanding of the role of the immune system in diseases such as multiple sclerosis, ALS, Parkinson's disease, and Alzheimer's disease.

Use of catheters to deliver drugs directly into the cerebrospinal fluid or brain tissue has enhanced the ability to deliver drugs that act directly on the neuron. Although the catheters have been made more sophisticated and can deliver the drugs in measured doses, complications of administration and uneven levels of absorption continue to be limiting factors.

Treatment of Nonneural Dysfunction

Many drugs used to treat neurologic disorders influence non-neuronal tissue, including cerebral blood vessels and glia. Cerebral edema can increase the permeability of the blood–brain barrier, causing an increase in fluid within the brain. The resulting compression of brain tissue can be life-threatening. Drugs such as mannitol that control cerebral edema or drugs that provide diuresis can help preserve neuronal function. In demyelinating disease, antiinflammatory and immunosuppressive drugs are used to preserve the function of the glial cells that produce the myelin sheath.

For some of the viruses that invade the CNS there is replication of cells in nonneural tissue. Use of drugs that inhibit RNA or DNA synthesis can prevent viral replication without disrupting neuronal integrity. Acyclovir, used in the treatment of herpes encephalitis, is an example of this type of drug.

In infants and children there is an altered drug metabolism that should be considered whenever administering drugs that act on the nervous system. Concomitant illness and fever will further alter drug metabolism. An immature blood–brain barrier can also affect the absorption of drugs into brain tissue. When anticonvulsants are administered, close monitoring of blood levels is necessary.

PROGNOSIS

Prognosis is the keystone to management of neurologic disorders because it links diagnosis to outcomes and identifies the need for treatment. Prognostic studies can also identify whether available treatment is ineffective. In addition, these studies can indicate which diseases have an important impact on function or disability.[32]

Disability resulting from neurologic disease and trauma can be extensive, and care of these clients often requires use of limited resources: time and money. With the tremendous advances made in the emergent medical care of trauma victims and people with significant neurologic disease, the number of people living with neurologic disorders is increasing at a steady rate.[6]

Permanent or progressive impairments can be demoralizing to clients and their families. Clients must reorganize their perspectives in order to learn alternative ways of regaining as much control as possible over life activities. Success builds a sense of efficacy, and failure undermines self-worth. Tackling challenges in successive attainable steps will lead to further competencies in associated tasks. When individuals see others with similar disabilities perform successfully, they may have increased confidence in their own abilities. The persuasion of health care providers and caregivers can boost effort but must be realistic. Perceived self-efficacy can influence the course of health outcomes and functional status. The prognosis for an individual should take into consideration both the social and the cognitive status of the individual in relation to the diagnosis.[4]

The economic evaluation of health care reflects the complexity of the disease treatment process and the value of health effects. Policy makers are demanding information about the economic outcomes of diseases and their treatments. Research methodologies oriented toward cost-of-illness and cost–benefit analyses have emerged. Clinicians should be involved in this analysis to maintain perspective, especially in catastrophic and degenerative processes.[28]

Several chronic neurologic disease states, such as Alzheimer's disease, are associated with elevated secretion of stress hormones such as cortisol. Stress also can trigger or exacerbate symptom onset and perhaps progression of chronic illness such as Parkinson's disease. Stress hormones also can mitigate the impact of acute neurotrauma; for example, there is a positive correlation between cortisol levels and mortality after head injury. Thus neurologic disease states can occur within a context of elevated glucocorticoids, which may have profound influences on recovery and neuroplasticity. In addition, abnormal regulation of glucocorticoid release is associated with many affective disorders, such as depression and PTSD, that are overrepresented in populations with neurologic disease. Release of glucocorticoids, however, also can occur in anticipation of adverse events, which is a mechanism particularly relevant to neurologists and psychoneuroimmunologists. Anticipatory release of glucocorticoids occurs in the absence of a frank physical stimulus, keyed by memories or instinctive predispositions.

Measures of health-related quality of life address the impact of health on physical, social, and psychologic aspects of life. The particular scale may address issues related to a specific population or may be sensitive to a clinical intervention. The PTA should be familiar with the measurement tools typically used during intervention for a condition or disease. As much as possible, these tools are described in the appropriate chapter in this section.[6]

Physiologic Basis for the Recovery of Function

After injury to the nervous system, there are changes in the structure and function of the neurons. In some instances the changes can lead to further damage, whereas other changes facilitate recovery.

Diaschisis, or neural shock, occurs when there is injury to a nerve and disruption of the neural pathway that extends a distance from the site of injury. When the neurons distal to the injury regain function, which may be soon after the injury, partial function may return.

Injury may be secondary to either swelling of the axon or edema in the surrounding tissue that blocks *synaptic activity* in the injured neurons, as well as that in the surrounding area. With reduction of the edema, function may return. This is the reason that medications that reduce edema are often given in the context of diffuse brain swelling.

When there is a loss of presynaptic function in one area, the postsynaptic target cells for that area may become more sensitive to neurotransmitters that are now produced in lower concentrations. The compensatory mechanism is known as *denervation supersensitivity. Regenerative synaptogenesis* occurs when injured axons begin sprouting. *Collateral sprouting* is the process of neighboring axons sprouting to connect with sites that were previously innervated by the injured axon.

Suppression of a response to a stimulus is considered habituation, whereas sensitization is an increased response to a stimulus, usually related to noxious stimuli or pain. Adaptation is the ability to modify a motor response based on changes in the sensory environment or input received.

Long-term potentiation occurs when a weak input and a strong input arrive at a dendrite at the same time. The weak stimulus is enhanced by the strong stimulus. With repeated activation of combined stimuli, there is an increase in the presynaptic transmitter associated with the stimulus. After the long-term potentiation has been established, the weak input will elicit a stronger response than it did initially.[29]

The characteristics of a lesion will have a profound effect on recovery from a brain injury. Small lesions of the brainstem may in fact be as devastating as large lesions of the cerebral cortex. Cerebellar damage can affect both learning and memory of movements. Lesions that occur gradually appear to cause less disruption of function than lesions that occur all at once such as with strokes. Advanced age will adversely affect the return of function. Studies show that a person's prior level of activity and environment will affect the rate and extent of recovery. An enriched environment will positively affect recovery when it is available either before the insult or during the recovery period.

Redistribution of cortical mapping is seen after a lesion in the brain.[9] The changes may involve unmasking of previously nonfunctional synaptic connections from adjacent areas, or the ability of the neighboring inputs may take over. It is clear that both sensory and motor maps in the cortex are constantly changing according to input from the environment. In addition, the brain appears to increase use of ipsilateral pathways after a lesion that affects one side of the brain.

Recovery of function by strict definition is the return to original processes for an activity. When alternative processes are used to complete the task, it is considered compensation. Neural modifiability may be seen as a change in the organization of connections among neurons and is often referred to as *plasticity*. Some of the recovery after CNS damage is considered spontaneous. Forced recovery is the result of specific interventions that create change in the neural structure.[48] Constraint-induced training makes use of this action.

Physiologic studies suggest that motor relearning and recovery of function may be accomplished through the same neural mechanisms and reflect the plasticity of the brain. Learning alters our capability to perform the appropriate motor act by changing both the effectiveness of the neural pathways used and the anatomic connections.

Learning involves storage of memory and can occur in all parts of the brain with both parallel and hierarchic processing. The area of representation within the brain becomes specialized for both inputs and outputs. Areas of the brain used during the early phase of learning movement are different from those used once a skill is learned. Initially, more areas of the brain are active, because skill develops both the number of neurons firing and location of activity change. The use of sensory input is increased in the early stages of learning. The prefrontal areas are also more active in the learning phase and become less active during automatic movements.[9] The stimuli repeatedly excite cortical neuron populations, and the neurons progressively grow in number. Repetition will lead to greater specificity, and the responses become stronger. With skill acquisition, sensory feedback appears to be less critical.

Control of learning comes from many areas of the CNS working together. The area involved may depend on a number of variables associated with the type of learning taking place and is influenced by the environment. The cortex is involved in learning through sensorimotor integration. It is postulated that there are widely distributed groups of neurons acting as a cortical engram, composed of multiple functional groupings. Thus when an activity is repeated and stored in memory, the engrams are available to trigger groups of cells that fire synchronously

during movement. The engrams appear to influence the precision, speed, and accuracy of movement.[29]

The limbic system is critical to the learning phase because it generates need-directed motor activity and communicates the intent to the rest of the brain. The limbic system is a critical part of the neural representation necessary for memory that includes the cortex and thalamus.

The cerebellum appears to be active during procedural learning. A possible mechanism is through the influence of the climbing fibers on the mossy fibers with eventual change in the output fibers, the Purkinje's fibers.[53] The lateral cerebellum affects cognition through its relationship to the frontal areas active during cognitive processes.[42]

The basal ganglia appear to be highly involved in the cognitive aspects of motor behavior, although the level of contribution remains unclear. Habit formation appears to be associated with functions of the basal ganglia, and the control of internally generated movement here appears to be a part of the motor learning continuum.[29]

18.1 Special Implications for the PTA: Motor Learning Strategies The PTA should recognize the impairments that contribute to abnormal motor control. Force production, speed of motion, coordination of movement, and cognition are often affected in neurologic disorders. Identification and modification of environments that can alter responses should be made early in the management process. Difficulty with bowel and bladder control can affect progress with recovery and should be managed with either physical or medical means. Treatment of nonneural tissue changes secondary to weakness or changes in tone should be addressed in the intervention. Substitution devices, assistive devices, and environmental changes should be considered when it is clear that the client will not recover from specific impairments. Reintegration into social and personal roles is of prime importance to the client with neurologic dysfunction. Functional status is the critical outcome marker, and PTAs are able to positively influence outcomes in this area.

The recovery of function after central nervous system (CNS) injury involves the reacquisition of complex tasks. Inherent in the recovery of function that has been lost secondary to a neurologic insult is the process of motor relearning, which can be defined as the process of acquisition or modification of movement.[11,48] Clients with a neurologic deficit must learn appropriate strategies to move through the environment. Motor learning is a modification of behavior by experience. Memory is the retention of these modifications; therefore memory plays a critical role in motor learning.[31]

Theories underlying the relationship of motor control, motor learning, memory, and recovery of function are varied, and research continues toward increasing our understanding of that relationship.[12,36,45,48] Various types of motor learning are recognized today and incorporated into the programs established for individuals with brain injury.

Two forms of associative learning based on an association between two different stimuli are classical and operant conditioning. *Classical conditioning* is a form of learning in which a conditioned stimulus produces a greater response by association with a strong stimulus. The consequences related to the pairing of the stimuli can be predicted. An example is Pavlov's dogs salivating in response to the bell that had previously been associated with feeding. Using verbal feedback in a practice session and then withdrawing or fading the input can be a form of classical conditioning. In *operant conditioning* a consequence is predicted associated with a behavior. A change in behavior will elicit a given response. Biofeedback is a form of operant conditioning. Both classical conditioning and operant conditioning appear to be under the control of the same cellular mechanisms.

Procedural learning results from the repetition of a movement that results in its automatic performance without much mental concentration. The rules of the movement, or the efficiencies of control, are learned and can be performed repeatedly in the same manner. Procedural learning results in implicit knowledge and is considered to be noncognitive, mediated through the striatum. In a treatment environment, there is emphasis on procedural learning in a variety of environments so that the rules of the task can be demonstrated with more than one set of constraints. This concept is demonstrated when the client learns movement strategies for a transfer in one environment and then learns the movement through experience in another context and environment.[46]

Declarative learning requires attention and thought that can be expressed and communicated consciously. Declarative learning results in explicit knowledge and is mediated through the medial temporal lobe. It involves describing or thinking of the components of a movement before execution and then performing the task. This concept can be demonstrated by the use of mental imaging before performance of an activity. In the clinic a client may go through the actions required for a transfer before beginning the task.[29]

Memory for motor behaviors is developed through different forms of learning and involves different brain regions. Memory associated with fear or other emotional stimuli is thought to involve the amygdala. Memory established through operant conditioning requires the striatum and cerebellum. Memory acquired through classical conditioning and habituation involves changes in the sensory and motor systems included in the learning. Input to the brain is processed into short-term working memory before it is transformed into more permanent long-term storage.[20]

Motor learning, or the precision of movement, takes place as the client determines the optimal strategy of movement to perform a motor task. There are defined stages of motor learning involved in skill acquisition. The *cognitive stage* is the first stage and requires a great deal of thought, experimentation, and intervention. Performance is variable, as is seen in the first attempts to walk after brain injury. In the cognitive stage, the treatment environment is highly structured to allow clients to think and focus on a task. Feedback is given more frequently and may involve more sensory systems. Problem solving is focused on the movement strategies necessary to complete the task. The task may be broken down at this time to work on component parts of the total movement and practiced with repetition.[43,45]

The second stage of skill acquisition is the *associative stage*, represented by refining of the skill. Fewer errors of performance are experienced, and the motor programs elicited are more consistent and efficient. Feedback can be given in a summary format, often after a few trials. The individual will use trial and error to fine-tune the movement.

The final stage is the *autonomous stage,* in which the movement is efficient and the need for attention to the activity is decreased. The motor program has been integrated by the basal ganglia, and each component is initiated with little thought. This activity can now be performed in conjunction with another activity.

The need for feedback during each stage is different. The PTA can enhance treatment by providing the correct amount of feedback for the client attempting to perform a task. For a skill to be acquired, learning principles that promote associative and automatic phases need to be incorporated in the intervention. This appears to be related to the practice conditions. It is clear that repetition is required at every stage. Initially, blocked or serial practice is used until the learner understands the dynamics of the task. When cognition is limited, it may be better to keep to a blocked practice schedule longer. For a skill to become learned or transferred to other activities, random practice is more effective. Part-task training can be beneficial if the task can naturally be broken down into component parts that create the whole movement when put back together.

For maximal effectiveness, CNS injury should be treated as soon as possible. As we learn more about the role of individual parts of the brain in relation to function and learning, the location of the injury should drive the intervention. The interaction between the client with neurologic dysfunction and the PTA is critical for optimal motor learning to take place. To elicit the highest level of function within the motor system and allow insight regarding the program, goal-directed activities must be included.[57,61]

Comorbid impairments should always be considered, as well as the individual's prior health status, age, motivation, and established life practices. In every case, it is important to remember that the focus of intervention should be not so much on the disease that the person has as on the person who has the disease.

REFERENCES/SUGGESTED READINGS

To enhance this text and add value for the reader, references and suggested readings are included on the companion Evolve site that accompanies this textbook. The reader can view the source and access it online whenever possible.

19

Infectious Disorders of the Central Nervous System

VOCAB BUILDERS

Decerebrate posturing	Encephalitis	Meningitis
Decorticate posturing	Kernig's sign	West Nile virus

Infection of the central nervous system (CNS) is relatively rare because many protective responses limit the access of harmful organisms to the nervous tissue. However, when neurologic infections occur they are a major cause of mortality and morbidity. Although bacteria and virus are the most common causes, infections may also be caused by parasites and fungi. Bacterial infections are generally more serious and life threatening than viral infections.[11,16]

Despite protective mechanisms, once there is access to the brain, infectious processes can produce a wide range of neuropathologic conditions.[28] Depending on the causative agent, these CNS infections can result in abscesses, infectious intracranial aneurysms,[23] and meningitis.[27]

There are a number of ways that infectious agents can enter the CNS. The cerebrospinal fluid (CSF) can be contaminated when the meninges are penetrated. This is often a result of trauma or a neurosurgical procedure.[7] Damage or fracture of nasal structures can also lead to infection in the CSF. Similarly, infections of the inner ear can spread to the brain via the CSF.[24] Bacterial endocarditis can lead to infected emboli traveling to the CNS.[23] Bacteria that colonize in the nasopharynx, especially in young children, can spread to the CNS. Enteroviruses as well as viruses transmitted by rodents and mosquitoes present additional avenues for CNS viral infections.[5] Treatment for central nervous system infections will depend on the type of infection, where it is in the body, and how quickly the infection manifests.

MENINGITIS

Definition

There are many types of *meningitis*. The most common form is viral meningitis, whereas the most severe form is bacterial meningitis. By definition meningitis is inflammation of the meninges of the brain and spinal cord. All three layers of the meningeal membranes, dura mater, arachnoid, and pia mater, can be involved. The relationship of the meninges to the brain tissue is shown in Fig. 19.1. The pia mater and arachnoid become congested with inflammation. The inflammation and congestion can produce thrombosis in the cortical veins and scarring in the affected areas. Thrombosis presents an increased chance of infarction, and scar tissue can restrict the flow of CSF, especially around the base of the brain. This restriction of CSF can result

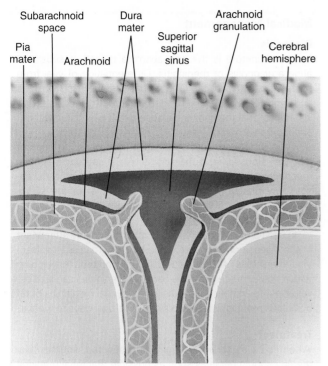

FIG. 19.1 The meninges, showing the relationship of the dura, arachnoid, subarachnoid space, pia, and brain tissue. (From Lundy-Ekman L: Neuroscience: fundamentals for rehabilitation, ed 4, St Louis, 2013, Saunders.)

in hydrocephalus or a subarachnoid cyst. Stretch or pressure on the meninges will cause the cardinal sign of headache.[1]

Incidence

The estimated incidence of meningitis is two to six per 100,000 adults per year in developed countries and is up to 10 times higher in less-developed countries.[32] According to the National Meningitis Association, there are approximately 3000 new cases of meningitis in the United States each year, with adolescents and young adults accounting for 30% of these cases; 83% of adolescent meningitis is preventable with vaccination.[19] Worldwide, there are some areas that are more susceptible to meningitis; these are primarily tropical and developing countries. Additionally, there is a meningitis belt in sub-Saharan Africa, where the incidence is five to 10 times higher than in the developed world. Although it has been reported that there is a genetically determined deficiency that increases susceptibility and risk, this accounts for only a small portion of those who develop the infection.[14,25]

Etiologic and Risk Factors

Vaccines developed in the past 15 years to protect against *Haemophilus influenzae* type B (Hib) infection have dramatically decreased the incidence of meningitis in young children in countries where there is access to the vaccine. There is a second period of increased susceptibility during late adolescence through early college years. As a result, the Centers for Communicable Disease issued a recommendation for routine meningococcal vaccination for adolescents and those college freshmen who will be living in dormitories.[19] Susceptibility to meningitis in adulthood is primarily related to weakened immune systems, including those with human

immunodeficiency virus (HIV)[11,16]; these remain at high risk for developing meningitis.

Pathogenesis

The process of infection is complex. Immune responses destroy organisms at the site of the infection and in the blood. Bacteria and viruses are removed from the blood. However, infection can be carried by blood products or other fluids and can cause changes in the cerebral capillary endothelium. The blood–brain barrier then fails to prevent entry of infectious organisms into the brain or CSF.

Once there is penetration of the blood–brain barrier and infectious agents move into the CSF and parenchyma of the brain, there is less immune protection than in the rest of the body. The CSF has about 1/200 the amount of antibody as blood, and the number of white blood cells is very low compared with the blood. The brain lacks a lymphatic system to fight infection.[10]

During infection and inflammation, the level of leukocytes in the brain increases. Cytokines, chemokines, macrophages, and microglia respond to viral and bacterial infections. The blood vessels leak these cells along with fluid and white blood cells into the meninges. This causes damage to the surrounding brain tissue by the release of cytotoxic free radicals and excitatory amino acids such as glutamate. The resultant inflammation can block CSF, resulting in hydrocephalus, edema, and increased intracranial pressure. Vasculitis can lead to infarction and decreases in cerebral blood flow, causing a drop in the glucose level of the CSF.[6,25] Drugs that scavenge for free radicals and the use of *N*-methyl-D-aspartate receptor blockers can help reduce tissue injury.[28]

Aseptic (Viral) Meningitis

Viral infection is the most common cause of inflammation of the CNS. Viral meningitis is an acute febrile illness with signs and symptoms of meningeal irritation, usually with a lymphocytic pleocytosis of the CSF. Enteroviruses are the major cause of viral meningitis, occurring in 40% of cases in 30- to 60-year-old individuals. The second most common cause of viral meningitis is herpes simplex virus 2, which is detected in approximately 20% of individuals with meningitis. Epstein–Barr virus (EBV) can also be responsible and is more often seen in late adolescence and early adulthood. Systemic lupus erythematosus (SLE), a disorder of connective tissue, can also cause aseptic meningitis. Sarcoid tumors and other intracranial tumors or cysts can lead to aseptic meningitis through rupture.[3] Often the meningitis occurs days or weeks after the exposure.

Certain drugs or chemicals can cause aseptic meningitis. The drugs most commonly involved are nonsteroidal antiinflammatory medications. Chemicals can also cause direct meningeal irritation; this is often related to surgical procedures in which there is exposure to the chemical.

Tuberculous Meningitis

Tuberculous meningitis is an infection caused by *Mycobacterium tuberculosis*, which enters the body by inhalation.[11,30] CNS involvement includes abscess or spinal cord disease. A computed tomographic (CT) image of a tuberculoma is seen in Fig. 19.2. Tuberculous brain abscesses may produce mass effect and edema. CSF may demonstrate formation of multiple cysts with lymphocytes and an elevated protein level. Infected bacilli enter the subarachnoid space, causing diffuse meningitis.[18]

Bacterial Meningitis

The organisms generally responsible for bacterial meningitis are those found in mucosal surfaces in the upper respiratory

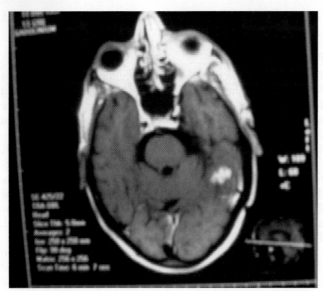

FIG. 19.2 Computed tomography of the brain showing a left hemisphere tuberculoma in a diabetic patient who presented with a seizure. (From Myers JN: Miliary, central nervous system, and genitourinary tuberculosis, Dis Mon 53:22–31, 2007.)

tract. However, bacteria in the birth canal can be transferred from the mother to the infant during birth. Group B streptococcus, *Escherichia coli*, and *Listeria monocytogenes* are bacteria that can cause infection in the neonate. As maternal antibodies decline in the neonate, the susceptibility to Hib, pneumococcus, and meningococcus increases, especially in the second half of the first year of life. On the other end of the spectrum, *Streptococcus pneumoniae* and *Neisseria meningitis* are the most common bacteria causing infection in the adult and geriatric populations.[22,25]

In bacterial meningitis, inflammation initially is confined to the subarachnoid space and then spreads to the adjacent brain parenchyma. Vasculitis starts in the small subarachnoid vessels. Thrombotic obstruction of vessels and decreased cerebral perfusion pressure can lead to focal ischemic lesions. Veins are more frequently affected than arteries, probably because of their thinner vessel walls and the slower blood flow. Damage to the nerve cell bodies causes the production of amyloid-β precursor protein that is carried through the axon and accumulates within terminal axonal swellings. This axonal pathology contributes to neurologic sequelae seen after bacterial meningitis.[20]

Clinical Manifestations

Early features of meningitis include fever, vomiting, and headache associated with a stiff and painful neck. There is often pain in the lumbar area and the posterior aspects of the thigh. There is a positive *Kernig's sign*, pain with combined hip flexion and knee extension. As the inflammation progresses, flexion of the neck will produce flexion of the hips and knees. This is known as a positive Brudzinski's sign.[26] The positions for Kernig's and Brudzinski's tests are shown in Fig. 19.3. If the infection remains undetected or untreated, the brainstem centers may be affected. The individual may then experience vomiting, papilledema (swelling and protrusion of the optic disk), seizures, and coma. Focal neurologic signs, including cranial nerve palsies and deafness, can also be seen when the brainstem is affected.

Medical Management

Diagnosis

Lumbar puncture is the only absolute means of substantiating a diagnosis of meningitis. Differentiation of viral from bacterial infection of the CNS is made on the basis of signs and symptoms and CSF changes.[22] Prompt diagnosis is critical in bacterial meningitis because death can occur without antibiotic treatment.

Other diagnostic testing includes radiographs to rule out fracture, sinusitis, and mastoiditis. A CT scan or magnetic resonance imaging (MRI) will reveal evidence of brain abscess or infarction that may be responsible for the symptoms. Fig. 19.2 shows evidence of abnormal MRI with tuberculous meningitis.

In addition to laboratory testing, the time course after onset of the disease often indicates the type of organism involved. Viral meningitis is hyperacute, with symptoms developing within hours. Acute pyogenic bacterial meningitis can also develop in 4 to 24 hours. Individuals with fungal meningitis or tuberculous meningitis develop symptoms over days to weeks.

Treatment

When acute bacterial meningitis is suspected, antimicrobial therapy should begin as soon as possible. Bacterial meningitis is a neurologic emergency; progression to more severe disease reduces the likelihood of a full recovery. Targeted antimicrobial therapy can begin in adults following a positive CSF Gram stain result. Antibiotic therapy should not be delayed pending the results of Gram stain or other diagnostic tests. Antimicrobial therapy should be modified as soon as the pathogen has been isolated. Duration of therapy depends on individual responses.[28]

Suspected bacterial meningitis in a child or infant is considered a medical emergency. The general picture involves fever, decreased feeding, vomiting, bulging fontanel (in infants), seizures, and a high-pitched cry. In neonates with meningitis caused by gram-negative bacilli, the duration of therapy should be determined in part by repeated lumbar punctures documenting CSF sterilization. If there is no response after 48 hours of appropriate therapy, repeated CSF analysis may be necessary. Any complications of bacterial meningitis usually occur within the first 2 or 3 days of treatment, hence outpatient management requires close follow-up. Criteria for outpatient therapy are inpatient antimicrobial therapy for 6 or more days; no fever for at least 24 to 48 hours; no significant neurologic dysfunction, focal findings, or seizure activity; stable or improving condition; ability to take fluids by mouth. There should be an established plan for physician and nurse visits, laboratory monitoring, and emergencies. Seizures can be controlled with antiseizure medications. As the infection is controlled, the seizures are resolved, so a short course is all that is usually necessary.[28]

The addition of dexamethasone can reduce the subarachnoid space inflammatory response that is related to morbidity and mortality and may therefore alleviate many of the pathologic consequences of bacterial meningitis related to cerebral edema or cerebral vasculitis. Change in cerebral blood flow, increase in intracranial pressure, and neuronal injury can be controlled by judicious steroid use.

Usual treatment for viral meningitis focuses on the symptoms. Medication is given for the headache and nausea. The prognosis in viral meningitis is excellent, and most individuals recover within 1 to 2 weeks. Treatment of acute episodes of herpes meningitis with acyclovir has been shown to decrease the duration and severity of symptoms.

Tuberculous meningitis is managed with medications given to treat the tuberculosis. In addition, adjunctive therapy with corticosteroids may reduce mortality and decrease neurologic sequelae in severe meningitis. Guidelines for the diagnosis and treatment of bacterial meningitis from the Infectious Diseases Society of America can be found at http://www.idsociety.org/Organ_System/# Central Nervous System (CNS).[28]

Prognosis

Mortality ranges from 5% to 25% depending on the infecting bacteria and the health and age of the person infected. At least one neurologic complication, such as impairment of consciousness, seizures, or focal neurologic abnormalities, typically develops in 75% of individuals with bacterial meningitis. Systemic complications, cardiorespiratory failure, or sepsis are also common and found about 40% of the time. Hyponatremia (low sodium ion levels in blood) occurs about 30% of the time, with an average duration of 3 days, and can be well managed by fluid restriction.

Cranial nerve palsies occur about 30% of the time, with hearing impairment during hospitalization a common complaint, but more than half of the patients have full return of hearing. The severity of hearing loss presents as mild one-third of the time, moderate one-third, and profound in another third. When there is hearing loss, it is more likely to be bilateral than unilateral.[32]

In children, long-term neurologic consequences of bacterial meningitis include developmental impairment, hearing loss, blindness, hydrocephalus, hypothalamic dysfunction, hemiparesis, and tetraparesis. There is a 30% mortality rate, with increasing death rates with individuals older than age 60 years. Most death occurs within 2 weeks, as a result of both systemic and neurologic complications. Aseptic or viral meningitis is usually self-limiting, and there is not the same degree of neurologic sequelae. Mortality rates for tuberculous meningitis range from 20% to 50%, and survivors may be left with neurologic sequelae similar to those seen in acute bacterial meningitis.[14,15] With better understanding of the role of cytokines, therapies targeting these processes are under study and show promise. These therapies may help to further control damage to the nervous system during the infectious or inflammatory process.[6]

ENCEPHALITIS

Definition

Encephalitis is an acute inflammatory disease of the parenchyma, or tissue of the brain, caused by direct viral invasion or hypersensitivity initiated by a virus. Encephalitis is characterized by inflammation primarily in the gray matter of the CNS. Neuronal death can result in cerebral edema. There can also be damage to the vascular system and inflammation of the arachnoid and pia mater.[2] Viruses carried by mosquitoes or ticks are responsible for most of the worldwide known cases of primary CNS infection. In many cases, such as *West Nile virus* and herpes simplex virus, the individual can develop either encephalitis or meningitis. This is reflected in the different levels of impairment that may be experienced after exposure.

Incidence

It is difficult to determine the true incidence of encephalitis because of lack of standardization of reporting. Arboviruses (viruses carried by ticks and mosquitoes) are the most common forms of episodic encephalitis, yet only 10% of those bitten develop encephalitis. One cause of encephalitis is the West Nile virus. Before 1994, outbreaks of West Nile virus were sporadic and occurred primarily in the Mediterranean region, Africa, and Eastern Europe. Since 1994, outbreaks have occurred with a higher incidence of severe human disease, particularly affecting the nervous system. By 2002, incidence was four to 14 per 100,000 population in the Midwest. Fig. 19.4 illustrates the spread of the virus through the United States. The virus has caused meningitis, encephalitis, and poliomyelitis, resulting in significant morbidity and mortality.[17] Up to 20% of infected people suffer permanent neurologic damage, and 2% die.[4]

Etiologic and Risk Factors

In almost two-thirds of cases of viral encephalitis, the cause cannot be identified. Viral infection may cause encephalitis as a primary manifestation or as a secondary complication.

Acute viral encephalitides—such as eastern and western equine encephalitis, St Louis encephalitis, and California virus encephalitis, and the most recent outbreak of West Nile virus—depend on mosquitos for transmission and tend to occur in the mid- to late summer. The eastern variety is the least common but most deadly. It occurs in outbreaks along the entire East Coast of the United States. It is rapidly progressive with

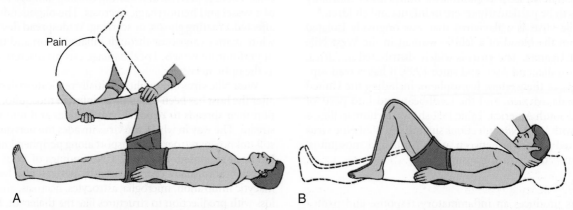

FIG. 19.3 Assessing a client with meningeal irritation. (A) Kernig's sign. (B) Brudzinski's sign. (From Monahan FD, Sands JK, Neighbors M, et al. (eds): Phipp's medical-surgical nursing: health and illness perspectives, ed 8, St. Louis, Mosby, 2007.)

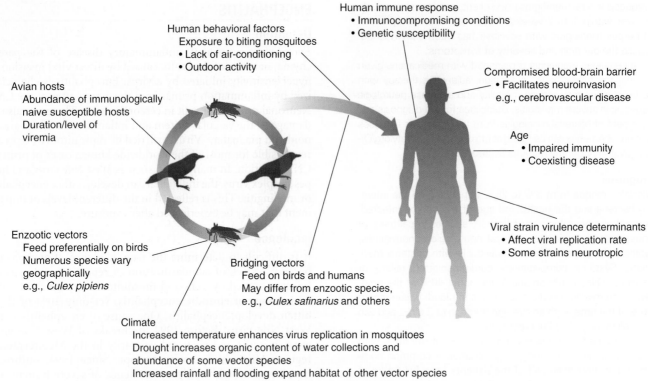

FIG. 19.4 West Nile virus transmission cycle and examples of modifying climatologic, vertebrate, mosquito, and human factors on infection and illness. (From Bennett JE, Dolin R, Blaser MJ, editors: Mandell, Douglas, and Bennett's principles and practice of infectious diseases, ed 8, 2015, Saunders.)

TABLE 19.1 **Human Illness from West Nile Virus Infections Reported in the United States, 2009 to 2015**

	2009	2010	2011	2012	2013	2014	2015
Cases	72	1021	712	5674	2469	2205	2175
Neuroinvasive disease (%)	54.0	62.0	68.0	51.0	51.0	61.0	67.0
Deaths	32	57	43	286	119	97	146

From The Centers for Disease Control and Prevention: West Nile virus disease cases and deaths reported to CDC by year and clinical presentation, 1999-2015, as of July 15, 2016.

lesions in the basal ganglia. It carries high mortality and morbidity rates. The western version has a much lower mortality but appears to be particularly severe in infants and children.[8]

West Nile virus is a flavivirus that was originally isolated in 1937 from the blood of a febrile woman in the West Nile province of Uganda. The virus is widely distributed in Africa, Europe, Australia, and Asia, and since 1999, it has spread rapidly throughout the western hemisphere, including the United States, Canada, Mexico, and the Caribbean and into parts of Central and South America. Table 19.1 shows the human illness associated with West Nile infections since 2009. West Nile virus is transmitted primarily between avian hosts and mosquitos. Fig. 19.4 shows the cycle of transmission.

Pathogenesis

Encephalitis produces an inflammatory response and pathologic changes in the brain. Ballooning of infected cells and degeneration of the cellular nuclei can lead to cell death. Plasma membranes are destroyed, and cells form multinucleated giant cells. There is perivascular cuffing causing damage to the lining of a vessel and hemorrhagic necrosis. The oligodendrocytes are affected, creating gliosis, or scarring. Widespread destruction of white matter can occur through inflammation and thrombosis of perforating vessels. Focal damage can hit discrete areas such as the optic nerve.[12]

West Nile virus is thought to initially replicate in dendritic cells after the host has been bitten by an infected mosquito. The infection then spreads to regional lymph nodes and into the bloodstream. The way in which the virus invades the nervous system is still unknown; retrograde transport along peripheral nerve axons has been proposed. Histologic CNS findings of West Nile virus infection are usually characterized by perivascular lymphoplasmacytic infiltration, microglia, astrocytes, necrosis, and neuronal loss with predilection to structures like the thalamus, brainstem, and cerebellar Purkinje's cells. These variable anatomic involvements explain different clinical presentations.[13]

Herpes simplex virus is found in neonatal infants and appears to arise from maternal genital infection with the virus. It is acquired as the baby passes through the birth canal. Fifty percent of those who contract herpes simplex virus will develop CNS disease, whereas others may only develop skin, eye, and mouth disease. Herpes simplex encephalitis is found after the age of 3 months and is often a latent infection found in the gray matter of the temporal lobe and surrounding structures of the limbic system and the frontal lobe. It is the most common cause of sporadic nonepidemic encephalitis in the United States. Possible genetic factors are undergoing study.[1]

Encephalomyelitis can result from viral infections such as measles, mumps, rubella, or varicella. Mumps is usually benign and self-limited, but it can trigger encephalitis and other CNS complications such as acute hydrocephalus, ataxia, transverse myelitis, and deafness.[29] Vaccines that contain neuronal antigens have been known to precede these infections, particularly for rabies or smallpox. When there is an illness at the time of vaccination, the risk of developing infection increases. Neurologic problems typically occur within 3 weeks of the illness or vaccination.[3]

EBV and hepatitis A have been associated with CNS disorders of an infectious nature. Acute toxic encephalitis occurs during the course of a system infection with a common virus. Parasites, bacteria, and toxic drug reactions can lead to infection of the brain and cause encephalitis or encephalopathy.

Clinical Manifestations

Signs and symptoms of encephalitis depend on the etiologic agent, but in general, headache, nausea, and vomiting are followed by altered consciousness. If the person becomes comatose, the coma may persist for days or weeks. Agitation can be associated with the degree of infection and may be associated with abnormal sensory processing. Depending on the area of the brain involved, there may be focal neurologic signs, with hemiparesis, aphasia, ataxia, or disorders of limb movement. There can be symptoms of meningeal irritation with stiffness of the back and neck. With herpes simplex encephalitis, there can be repeated seizure activity, hallucinations, and disturbance of memory, reflecting involvement of the temporal lobe.[24]

Although many individuals infected with West Nile virus are asymptomatic, symptoms develop in 20% to 40% of people with West Nile virus infection. The incubation period is 2 to 14 days before symptom onset. Most complaints are of flulike symptoms. West Nile virus is characterized by fever, headache, malaise, myalgia, fatigue, skin rash, lymphadenopathy, vomiting, and diarrhea. Kernig's and Brudzinski's signs may be found on physical examination. Less than 1% of infected individuals develop severe neuroinvasive diseases. West Nile meningitis usually presents with fever and signs of meningeal irritation such as headache, stiff neck, nuchal rigidity, and photophobia. Box 19.1 lists the findings that are most critical to watch for to determine potential for high level of disability or death. In addition, West Nile virus can present as acute flaccid paralysis. Fig. 19.5 shows the pattern of weakness found in some individuals with this form of West Nile virus infection. The lesion of spinal anterior horns results in a paralysis similar to polio and reaches a plateau within hours. Deep tendon reflex can be diminished in severely paralyzed limbs. Reports of substantial muscle ache in the lower back and bowel and bladder dysfunction are common. There is minimal or no sensory disturbance.[13,31]

BOX 19.1   Clinical Characteristics of Nonfatal and Fatal Hospitalized West Nile Virus–Infected Patients

Signs and Symptoms Most Likely Related to Death
- Fever >38° C (>100.4° F)
- Headache
- Mental status changes
- Nausea
- Vomiting
- Chills
- Muscle weakness
- Confusion
- Fatigue
- Lethargy
- Abdominal pain

Underlying Conditions that Have Potential to Increase Risk of Complications
- Diabetes
- Hypertension
- Chronic obstructive pulmonary disease
- Dementia
- Coronary artery disease
- Alcoholism
- Asthma
- Cancer
- Immunosuppression

Other Common Signs and Symptoms
- Decreased appetite
- Diarrhea
- Myalgia
- Malaise
- Neck stiffness
- Skin rash
- Shortness of breath
- Cough
- Dizziness
- Increased sleepiness
- Balance problems
- Photophobia
- Back pain
- Joint pain (arthralgia)
- Tremor
- Weight loss
- Slurred speech
- Neck pain
- Sore throat
- Seizures
- Blurred vision
- Coma
- Numbness
- Flaccid paralysis
- Lymphadenopathy
- Paresthesias

From Mazurek JM: The epidemiology and early clinical features of West Nile virus infection, Am J Emerg Med 23:536–543, 2005.

Encephalitic lesions appear to alter sleep patterns as sequelae of brain-immune interactions. Responses of the immune system to invading pathogens are detected by the CNS, which responds by orchestrating complex changes in behavior and physiology. Sleep is one of the behaviors altered in response to immune challenge. Cytokines may play an active role in infectious challenge by regulating sleep.[21]

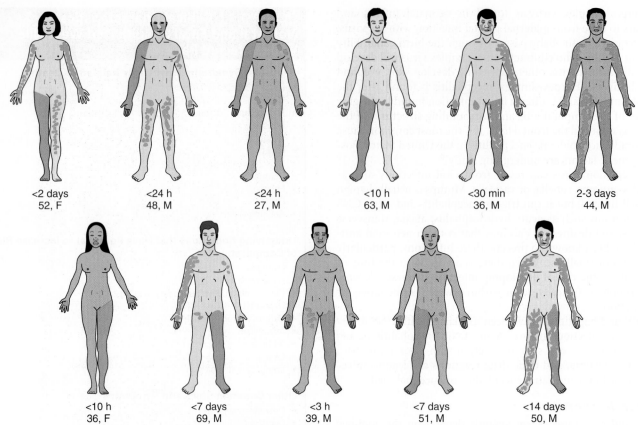

| <2 days | <24 h | <24 h | <10 h | <30 min | 2-3 days |
| 52, F | 48, M | 27, M | 63, M | 36, M | 44, M |

| <10 h | <7 days | <3 h | <7 days | <14 days |
| 36, F | 69, M | 39, M | 51, M | 50, M |

FIG. 19.5 Clinical features induced by West Nile virus paralysis in 11 representative individuals. Weak limbs at the peak of paralysis are darkened. Degree of darkness corresponds to the severity of weakness. Duration of weakness, age, and sex are noted. (Redrawn from Kramer LD: West Nile virus, Lancet Neurol 6:171-181, 2007.)

Medical Management

Diagnosis

Differential diagnosis of the types of infections of the brain has improved with the use of MRI and polymerase chain reaction assay to diagnosis herpes simplex encephalitis. The electroencephalogram will show seizure activity in the temporal lobe in herpes simplex. In general, lumbar puncture is abnormal, with increased proteins. The glucose level, however, may be normal or moderately increased. CT scans do not show much until the damage is extensive. MRI shows cerebral edema and vascular damage earlier in the process and leads to earlier detection.[1] In West Nile virus, lesions can sometimes be seen in the white matter, pons, substantia nigra, and thalamus. An important MRI finding is the focal abnormal signal intensity within the anterior horns; the level of abnormal spinal MRI findings corresponds to the paralysis. Change can be seen in the spinal roots, possibly a result of axonal degeneration secondary to spinal motor neuron loss or Wallerian degeneration in the spinal roots. Fig. 19.6 shows the imaging studies of individuals with West Nile virus.

Treatment

Treatment varies with the infectious agent. No antiviral treatment is available for encephalitis except for that caused by the herpes simplex virus. Acyclovir appears to improve the outcome in herpes simplex encephalitis.

There is no specific regime currently available for treatment of flavivirus infections. Close monitoring of the symptoms is critical, especially with the complication of cerebral edema, which may require surgical decompression, hyperventilation, or administration of mannitol. The use of corticosteroids is controversial because of the potential suppression of antibody protection within the CNS. Because no effective therapy is known, only supportive care is now available.

Prognosis

The prognosis depends on the infectious agent. The rate of recovery can range from 10% to 50% even in individuals who may have been very ill at the onset. Individuals with mumps meningoencephalitis and Venezuelan equine encephalitis have an excellent prognosis. Other encephalitides—such as western equine, St Louis, and California encephalitis and West Nile virus—have a moderate to good rate of survival. With the use of medication, herpes simplex encephalitis has a moderately good outcome (20% mortality); neurologic sequelae are common in 50% of persons.[2,8] Recovery for paralysis is remarkably variable. The variation may be caused by different degrees of motor neuron or motor unit loss.[13]

Some recovery is complete within weeks, but outcome is highly variable. The severity of the original illness does not always predict the final outcome. Permanent cerebral problems are more likely to occur in infants. Young children will take longer to recover than adults with similar infections.

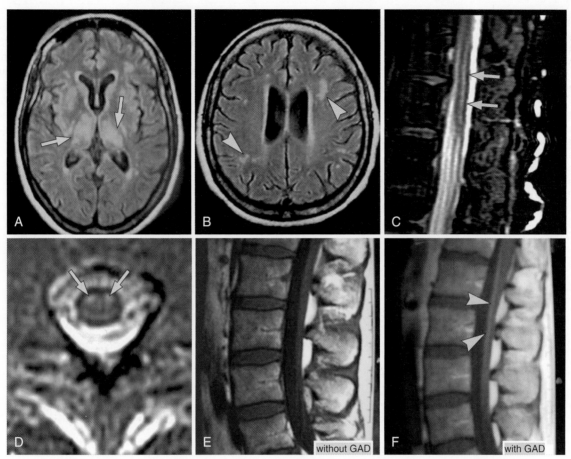

FIG. 19.6 Abnormal magnetic resonance imaging (MRI) findings in patients with West Nile virus. (A) Image of the brain from a 57-year-old woman with encephalitis shows abnormal signals in bilateral thalamus and weighted MRI in other areas of basal ganglion. (B) Focal white matter lesions are also seen. (C) Sagittal T2-weighted MRI of the lumbar spinal cord shows abnormal signal intensity *(arrows)* conspicuous within the cord. (D) Transverse view of the cord at the midlumbar level; abnormal signal intensity *(arrows)* is confined to the anterior horns. (E) T1-weighted lumbar spine MRI from a patient with both meningitis and acute flaccid paralysis shows no discernible abnormality; however, after giving gadolinium contrast, spinal roots are significantly enhanced (F). (A, B, E, and F, From Kramer LD: West Nile virus, Lancet Neurol 6:171–181, 2007; C and D, From Li J, Loeb JA, Shy ME, et al.: Asymmetric flaccid paralysis: a neuromuscular presentation of West Nile virus infection, Ann Neurol 53:703–710, 2003.)

19.1 Special Implications for the PTA: Infectious Disorders of the Central Nervous System The physical therapist assistant (PTA) must understand and observe all isolation procedures. Often the treatment of these clients begins in the intensive care unit. Monitoring vital signs throughout the treatment session may be necessary when the client is in the acute stage. The client may demonstrate symptoms that are similar to many noninfectious brain disorders. The clinical picture may represent the diffuse disorders typical of brain trauma, or there may be only focal neurologic symptoms that may appear similar to stroke or neoplasm.[26]

Initially, when the inflammatory response is greatest, there may be a profound alteration of consciousness. The PTA should be familiar with the scales used to monitor levels of consciousness such as the Glasgow Coma Scale. The client may be agitated, with difficulty in processing sensory input resulting in increased sensitivity to sound and light. Cognitive and perceptual disorders with memory deficits probably represent the involvement of the brain in the area of the ventricles.[24] It is essential that the PTA understand the behavioral changes that accompany diffuse brain disorders.

Sensory dysfunction should be thoroughly evaluated by the physical therapist before the PTA begins working with the client. If the client has a history of instability of heart rate, blood pressure, or respiration, these should be monitored during the evaluation of sensation, because sensory input may aggravate responses in some individuals. Cutaneous sensation may be affected in different distributions, depending on whether the damage is diffuse or deep in one area of the brain. Distorted or absent sensory input can affect mobility and functional status in a dramatic way.

Movement disorders also reflect the nature and depth of the insult to the brain. Abnormal posturing of the client in the acute phase may be noted, and abnormal postural reflexes may be present. *Decorticate posturing* (indicated by rigidity, flexion of the arms, clenched fists, and extended legs) and *decerebrate posturing* (rigid extension of the arms and legs, downward pointing of the toes, and backward arching of the head) are often seen in the early stages of these brain disorders. Positioning and range-of-motion exercises are critical in the early phases because the stiffness of the back and neck can exacerbate the pain. Often, maintaining a darkened environment during treatment will decrease the complaints of headache. Understanding motor learning strategies is important, because movement often must be relearned in the context of residual damage or agitated behaviors.

When interacting with the client and family, it is important to be familiar with the acute, subacute, and chronic prognosis related to the type of infection causing the brain injury. Knowing there may be a good outcome will be encouraging during the acute and devastating onset of the infections. Neurologic recovery will continue for many years if the brain remains stimulated as a course of appropriate physical rehabilitation.[24]

During the late summer season, the PTA should be aware of the manifestations of mosquito or tick-borne illnesses. Changes in clients that are consistent with infections should be monitored and a referral made to the appropriate health care provider when necessary.

REFERENCES/SUGGESTED READINGS

To enhance this text and add value for the reader, references and suggested readings are included on the companion Evolve site that accompanies this textbook. The reader can view the source and access it online whenever possible.

20

Degenerative Diseases of the Central Nervous System

CHAPTER OBJECTIVES

1. Review neuroanatomy and physiology as it relates to degenerative pathogenesis.
2. Discuss the role of neurotransmission in movement and cognition.
3. Discuss the different clinical manifestations of upper versus lower motor neuron disease.
4. Discuss the similar clinical manifestations seen across the neuropathologic spectrum.
5. Outline the role of the physical therapist assistant in the continuum of care for people with amyotrophic lateral sclerosis, Alzheimer's disease, dystonia, Huntington's chorea, multiple sclerosis, and Parkinson's disease.

OUTLINE

VOCAB BUILDERS

Akinesia
Anomia
Aspiration
Bradykinesia
Chorea

Dementia
Dystonia
Fasciculation
Festination
Pseudobulbar

Rigidity
Saccades
Sclerosis
Spasticity
Tremor

Degenerative diseases of the central nervous system (CNS) can affect gray matter, white matter, or both. The neurodegenerative disorders are characterized by loss of functionally related groups of neurons. The pattern of neuronal loss is selective, affecting one or more groups of neurons while leaving others intact. The cause of the neuronal loss is unknown but is clearly multifactorial. The diseases appear to arise without any clear inciting event in individuals without previous neurologic deficits. The clinical symptoms produced depend on which neuronal populations are lost. Degenerative changes in gray matter diseases interfere with the function of the neuronal cell bodies and synapses. The diseases can affect the cortex, the gray matter of the spinal cord, or both. The most common factor in this group of diseases is the slow deterioration of body functions controlled by the brain and spinal cord.

The neuropathologic findings observed in the degenerative diseases reflect changes in different components. In some disorders there are intracellular abnormalities such as Lewy bodies and neurofibrillary tangles, whereas in others, there is primary loss of neurons.[27] Some degenerative diseases have prominent involvement of the cerebral cortex, such as Alzheimer's disease (AD); others are more restricted to subcortical areas and may present with movement disorders such as *tremors* and dyskinesias, such as Parkinson's disease (PD). Demyelination has a major impact on other disorders such as multiple sclerosis (MS). Through genetic and molecular studies of these diseases, it is becoming clearer that there are many shared features across the disorders.

Cellular stress is a major component of neurodegenerative disease. When the cell is stressed, the proteins that form filaments and microtubules creating the cytoskeleton can collapse and form perinuclear bundles or clumps of protein aggregates. If the stress experienced by the cell is not lethal, the cell adapts and manufactures several proteins that may restore functional activity of partially denatured proteins. If the proteins cannot be restored, then a process begins to destroy the proteins. If the proteins do not fully degrade, they become clumped together to form intracellular inclusions. The inclusions in neurodegenerative disorders are examples of such aggregates. The aggregated proteins are generally cytotoxic, but the mechanisms by which protein aggregation is linked to cell death may be different in these various diseases. The histologic characteristics of the inclusions often form the diagnostic hallmarks of these different diseases.

Disorders of movement associated with gray matter destruction are reflected in functional loss and decreased fractionation of movement. Dementia can be present and always represents a pathologic process; dementia, despite popular belief, is not part of normal aging. The majority of the degenerative diseases that affect the basal ganglia are associated with involuntary movements. Disruption of smooth coordination of muscles can be seen in diseases affecting the cerebellum and brainstem. Many of the disorders appear later in life and mimic the normal deterioration of the nervous system that comes with aging.

The cost of care for people with degenerative neurologic disease is significant because of the protracted time of disability before death and the extent of the disability. Although medical science has made tremendous progress in the past few years, degenerative disorders continue to be a challenge to health care providers and a burden to modern society.

AMYOTROPHIC LATERAL SCLEROSIS

Overview and Definition

Amyotrophic lateral sclerosis (ALS) is a disorder that is generally recognized as an adult-onset progressive motor neuron disease but is also a complex disease process underlying a multisystem illness. It is the most physically devastating of the neurodegenerative diseases. ALS is a progressive disease of unknown cause, characterized by degeneration and scarring of the motor neurons in the lateral aspect of the spinal cord, brainstem, and cerebral cortex, giving rise to the terms *lateral* and *sclerosis* in identifying the disease. Peripheral nerve changes result in muscle fiber atrophy or amyotrophy. The resulting weakness causes profound limitation of movement.[100] Executive dysfunction, characterized by deficiencies in attention, language comprehension, planning, and abstract reasoning, represents cortical involvement.

Incidence

The incidence of ALS between 2010 and 2011 has been reported at about 4 per 100,000, diagnosed each year.[116] In the western and southern Pacific the incidence continues to be much higher than the global average.[109] Electrodiagnostic equipment for testing may not be available in an area, so there may be greater numbers than are currently identified.

Etiologic and Risk Factors

Approximately 90% of ALS cases occur sporadically and are clinically manifested in the fifth decade or later. The cause is unknown. There have been clusters of ALS noted in which there have been three or four individuals living or working in close proximity or individuals participating in the same sport, and military service appears to hold a possible risk for ALS. Chronic intoxication with heavy metals, such as lead or mercury, has been suggested as an etiologic agent, but there still does not seem to be a clear cause. ALS occurs predominantly in men, although bulbar onset occurs more often in women. There may be an increased incidence in white males, with a lower rate reported in Mexico, Poland, and Italy.[100] There appears to be little evidence of active poliovirus in persons with ALS. In fact, there are very few postpolio individuals who develop ALS, and it is postulated that polio may protect against developing ALS. There is an increased incidence of cancer in individuals with motor neuron disease.[25]

Familial ALS (FALS) is an inherited autosomal trait. It occurs in 5% to 10% of all ALS cases. The identification of at least one additional family member with ALS in successive generations is essential for the diagnosis of FALS. Most FALS is inherited in an autosomal dominant pattern and is characterized by an early onset. Family linkage may be missed if there was a death of a family member before the usual age of onset. Copper and zinc superoxide dismutase (SOD1) gene mutation may account for about 15% of cases of FALS. SOD1 genetic testing can be used for genetic counseling in families in which SOD1 mutations are already established.

Clinical Manifestations

Cognitive impairments are noted in up to 50% of individuals with ALS. With careful assessment, these deficiencies can be noted early on. Executive function deficits can be found in visual attention, working memory, cognitive flexibility, problem solving, and visuoperceptual skills. Verbal fluency declines before dysarthria develops. The cognitive deficits are caused by changes in frontal lobe function and may be related to frontotemporal dementia. Bulbar onset is more predictive of cognitive impairment than limb onset. Pseudobulbar affect, resulting in emotional lability, emotional outbursts, and pathologic laughing or crying, is not related to a psychologic or psychiatric condition and is not a part of the frontotemporal dementia.

The motor control manifestations of ALS vary depending on whether upper or lower motor neurons are predominantly involved. With lower motor neuron cell death and early denervation, the first evidence of the disease typically is insidiously developing asymmetric weakness, usually of the distal aspect of one limb progressing to weakness of the contiguous muscles. Extensor muscles become weaker than flexor muscles, especially in the hands. Cervical extensor weakness develops and can lead to drooping of the head and pain associated with overstretched muscles. Increased lumbar lordosis occurs as part of the compensatory strategy to attempt to right the head and bring the eyes level.

The neurons innervating muscles controlling articulation, chewing, and swallowing originate in the medulla, or the "bulb," and any weaknesses in the muscles are considered bulbar signs. In the lower motor or flaccid component, facial muscles are affected. Inability to hold the eye closed against pressure is a standard test. Weakness around the mouth develops, and air leaks out. The movement of the tongue is decreased, and atrophy is present. Fasciculations in the tongue are present with lower motor neuron dysfunction. Dysarthria associated with lower motor neuron involvement is reflected by the inability to shout or sing, a hoarse or whispering quality of the voice, and nasal tone. Manipulating food inside the mouth becomes difficult. Eventually, weak swallowing may trigger reflex coughing.

Individuals with ALS complain of drooling because of the absence of automatic swallowing, which is made worse by the forward head position. Breathing becomes difficult, and accessory breathing replaces diaphragmatic breathing. Respiratory distress can occur when sleeping, especially on the back.

Deformities of the extremities are common, especially because weakness causes shortening of the extensor muscles. Clawhand develops as the weakness of lumbricals and interossei hinders metacarpal flexion and tenodesis flexes the distal joints. Fig. 20.1 shows the hand of an individual with ALS.

Weakness caused by denervation is associated with progressive wasting and atrophy of muscles. Cramping with volitional movement in the early morning is often reported, with complaints of stiffness. Muscle cramps indicate lower motor neuron dysfunction. It may be related to hyperexcitability of distal motor axons. Early in the disease there are fasciculations, or spontaneous twitching of muscle fibers. *Fasciculation*s are the result of spontaneous contractions of a group of muscle fibers belonging to a single motor unit. The impulse for the fasciculation appears to arise from hyperexcitable distal motor axons. This is random in time and in muscles affected. It should be noted that both muscle cramping and fasciculations are found in healthy adults and should never be taken alone as a concern for the development of ALS.

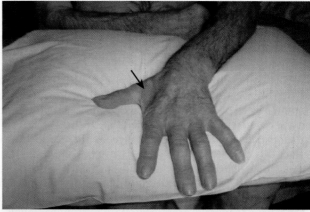
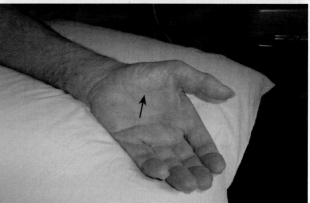

FIG. 20.1 Wasting of hand muscles in amyotrophic lateral sclerosis *(arrows)*. (From Eisen A: Amyotrophic lateral sclerosis: a 40-year personal perspective, J Clin Neurosci 16(4):505–512, 2009.)

Upper motor neuron symptoms are characterized by loss of inhibition and the resulting lack of dexterity and spasticity. Muscle strength is decreased along an upper motor neuron pattern. Extensor muscles of the upper extremity and flexor muscles of the lower extremity are weakened, because spasticity develops as the result of loss of brainstem control of the vestibulospinal and reticular formation control. As in other upper motor lesions, spasticity can limit the ability to accurately assess muscle strength.

Spastic bulbar palsy occurs when upper motor neurons and the corticobulbar fibers controlling speech, mastication, and swallowing are affected. This is termed *pseudobulbar palsy* and differs from the palsy associated with lower motor neuron loss in the brainstem. Pseudobulbar affect may manifest as inappropriate laughter, irritability, anger, and tearfulness.

The tendon, or muscle stretch, reflexes become hyperactive based on the loss of the Ia inhibitory reflex. This also extends to the development of clonus, in which manual quick stretch of a muscle induces repeated rhythmic muscle contraction. Babinski's sign is positive, characterized by extension of the great toe, often accompanied by fanning of the other toes in response to stroking the outer edge of the ipsilateral sole upward from the heel with a blunt object. If there is enough wasting of the dorsiflexors, the response may appear to be flexor despite upper motor neuron involvement.

It is characteristic of ALS that, regardless of whether the initial disease involves upper or lower motor neurons, both categories are eventually implicated. In most people with ALS, Babinski's and Hoffmann's signs are present or the tendon jerks are disproportionately active.[126] Throughout the course of the disease, eye movements and sensory, bowel, and bladder functions are preserved.

ALS is characterized by differing areas of CNS involvement and has been categorized in terms of four major groups of symptoms listed next.[59,90] Fig. 20.2 shows the levels of dysfunction associated with the terms that describe them.

1. *Pseudobulbar palsy* reflects damage in the corticobulbar tract.
2. *Progressive bulbar palsy* is a result of cranial nerve nuclei involvement. There is weakness of the muscles involved in swallowing, chewing, and facial gestures. Fasciculations of the tongue are usually prominent. With early bulbar involvement, there can be difficulty with respiration before weakness of the limbs. Dysarthria and exaggeration of the expression of emotion, or pseudobulbar affect, indicate involvement of the corticobulbar tract. The oculomotor system is usually not involved, and eye movement remains normal.
3. *Primary lateral sclerosis* results in neuronal loss in the cortex. Signs of corticospinal tract involvement include hyperactivity of tendon reflexes, with spasticity causing difficulty with active movement. Weakness and spasticity of specific muscles represent the level and progression of the disease along the corticospinal tracts. There is no muscle atrophy, and fasciculations are not present. This form of ALS is rare.
4. In *progressive spinal muscular atrophy*, there is progressive loss of motor neurons in the anterior horns of the spinal cord, often beginning in the cervical area. There is progressive weakness, wasting, and fasciculations involving the small muscles of the hands. Other levels of the spinal cord can be the site of the initial disease process, with symptoms reflecting the level involved. These areas of weakness can be present without evidence of higher level corticospinal involvement, such as spasticity.

ALS with probable upper motor neuron signs is a condition in which there are no overt upper motor neuron signs, but involvement of the corticospinal tracts is indicated by the incongruous presence of active tendon reflexes in limbs with weak, wasted, and twitching muscles. Upper and lower limbs are usually affected first, with progression to facial symptoms and respiratory failure.

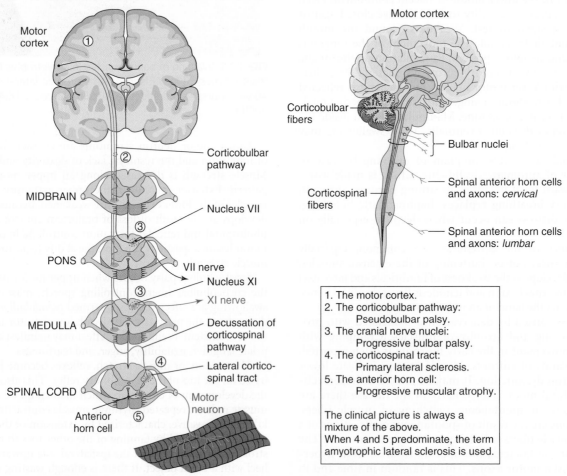

1. The motor cortex.
2. The corticobulbar pathway: Pseudobulbar palsy.
3. The cranial nerve nuclei: Progressive bulbar palsy.
4. The corticospinal tract: Primary lateral sclerosis.
5. The anterior horn cell: Progressive muscular atrophy.

The clinical picture is always a mixture of the above.
When 4 and 5 predominate, the term amyotrophic lateral sclerosis is used.

FIG. 20.2 Areas of damage in the central and peripheral nervous system as a result of amyotrophic lateral sclerosis. (Redrawn from Lindsay KW, Bone I, Fuller G: Neurology and neurosurgery illustrated, ed 5, Edinburgh, 2010, Churchill Livingstone. Insert redrawn from Pryse-Phillips WM, Murray TJ: Essential neurology: a concise textbook, New York, 1992, Medical Examination Publisher.)

Medical Management

Diagnosis

Diagnosis is predominantly made by the combination of clinical presentation and electromyogram (EMG). The time to diagnosis differs, typically according to the first presenting symptoms. With upper limb onset the time to diagnosis is approximately 15 months, with lower extremity onset it is 21 months, and with bulbar involvement as the first sign it is approximately 17 months.[24] Box 20.1 describes diagnostic criteria.

The symptoms are generally first reported to a primary care physician, and it appears that there is a greater delay in reaching the diagnosis in such cases than when the initial symptoms are reported to a neurologist. Often in the early cases and those that are progressing slowly, there may be minimal abnormality on the first EMG, and the changes that lead to diagnosis may not appear for 6 to 12 months. In electrodiagnosis, rapidly progressive ALS shows different changes on the EMG compared with slowly progressive ALS. It is believed that some of these differences comes from the adaptation and sprouting that occur early in the process. This adaptation cannot be sustained as the disease progresses.[84]

EMG studies include the muscles of the extremities and trunk and are selected based on the propensity for weakness in ALS. EMG criteria for the diagnosis of ALS include the presence of fibrillations, positive waveforms, fasciculations, and motor unit potential changes in multiple nerve root distributions in at least three limbs and the paraspinal muscles. These changes occur without change in sensory response.[101]

In 1990 the World Federation of Neurology El Escorial criteria for the diagnosis of ALS were established, and four categories of ALS were outlined (Box 20.2). Suspected ALS is characterized by lower motor neuron signs alone in two or more regions to which might be added upper motor neuron signs on the basis of the clinical examination. Possible ALS is defined as upper and/or lower motor neuron signs in only one region, possibly with a grouping of upper or lower motor neuron signs in other regions. Exclusion of structural lesions would be attempted. Probable ALS is considered if there are upper and lower motor neuron signs in two regions, and the upper motor neuron signs are above the lower motor neuron signs. Structural lesions must definitely be ruled out by neuronal imaging studies. Definite ALS requires lower motor neuron signs to be present in addition to upper motor neuron signs in three CNS regions concomitantly with upper or lower motor neuron signs in other regions with structural lesions excluded. Definite EMG signs of lower motor neuron degeneration require the presence of evidence of acute denervation with fibrillations or positive sharp waves and chronic denervation represented by large-amplitude and long-duration motor unit potentials as well as reduced recruitment in each muscle.[24]

There are several disorders that resemble ALS that are treatable. ALS must be differentiated from other conditions that produce a combination of upper and lower motor neuron lesions. Lymphoma and Lyme disease can cause diffuse lower motor axonal neuropathy. Disorders of the cervical cord, such as skull base deformities, syringomyelia, cord tumors, and cervical spondylosis, must be ruled out.[12] Box 20.3 describes disorders that can mimic ALS.

Weight loss may suggest carcinoma, and investigations should be undertaken to rule out underlying malignancy if there is any atypical feature on examination or investigation, such as marked slowing of motor nerve conduction velocities. Most other mimics can be excluded by history, such as hereditary neuropathy, prior gastrectomy, polio, or electrical injury. Dyspnea may suggest chronic obstructive pulmonary disease or heart failure. Thorough examination will reveal hyperthyroidism or acromegaly. Laboratory tests will reveal lead

---

BOX 20.2 World Federation of Neurology El Escorial Criteria for Diagnosis of Amyotrophic Lateral Sclerosis

Weakness/Atrophy/Hyperreflexia/Plasticity EMG/NCV/Neuroimaging

Suspected ALS	Possible ALS	Probable ALS	Definite ALS
LMN signs in more than two regions	UMN + LMN signs in one region	UMN + LMN signs in two regions	UMN + LMN signs in three regions
UMN signs in more than one region	UMN + LMN signs in more than two regions	UMN + LMN signs in more than two regions	UMN + LMN signs in more than three regions
	Add LMN signs to UMN regions	Add LMN signs to UMN regions	(Discern from ALS plus, ALS LAUS, ALS mimics)
	Add LMN signs to UMN regions	Add LMN signs to UMN regions	Exclude structural lesions (exclude other causes)
	Exclude structural lesions (exclude other causes)	Exclude structural lesions (exclude other causes)	

EMG, Electromyography; *LAUS,* laboratory abnormalities of uncertain significance; *LMN,* lower motor neuron; *NCV,* nerve conduction velocity; *UMN,* upper motor neuron; ( ), proposal to add this category to diagnostic criteria for ALS, WFN El Escorial Revisited.

Data from Brooks BR: Introduction: defining optimal management in ALS: from first symptoms to announcement, Neurology 53(suppl 5):S1–S3, 1999.

BOX 20.1 Abnormal Diagnostic Findings in Amyotrophic Lateral Sclerosis

- Clinical features of weakness, atrophy, and fatigue
- Electromyography shows fibrillations and fasciculations
- Unstable motor units (in rapidly progressing amyotrophic lateral sclerosis [ALS])
- Increased duration/amplitudes (in slowly progressing ALS)
- Low-amplitude polyphasic motor unit potentials
- Muscle biopsy shows denervation atrophy
- Muscle enzymes, such as creatine phosphokinase, elevated
- Cerebrospinal fluid normal
- No changes on myelogram

BOX 20.3 Disorders that Can Mimic Amyotrophic Lateral Sclerosis

- Myasthenia gravis
- Cervical myelopathy
- Multifocal motor neuropathy
- Hypoparathyroidism
- Inclusion body myositis
- Bulbospinal neuronopathy
- Lymphoma
- Radiation-induced effects

or other metal poisoning. ALS symptoms may mimic nonneurologic diseases, and neurologic signs may be missed.[9]

Treatment and Pharmacology

A medication or combination of medications that targets more than one pathogenic pathway may slow disease progression in an additive or synergistic fashion. Riluzole, a Food and Drug Administration (FDA)–approved drug for ALS, has a broad range of pharmacologic effects, including inhibition of glutamate release, postsynaptic glutamate receptor activation, and voltage-sensitive sodium channel inactivation. It appears to be neuroprotective and slows the disease course by approximately 10% to 15%, but it is not curative. Myotrophin (insulin-like growth factor I) appears to affect motor dysfunction by promoting the survival of motor neurons and regeneration of motor nerves. Drug resistance can develop with prolonged periods of medication. Specific targets for therapy are not well defined, and issues of dose, duration, and bioavailability in the diseased state are unknown. Furthermore, the timing of drug initiation is an important factor in determining the response to therapy, which is based on the ratio of reversible and irreversible injury at any time point in the disease.

Although no medication can stop the disease, much can be done in the form of symptomatic therapy. Health care providers should emphasize the value of maintaining the highest level of function throughout the course of the disease, providing education and support to prepare for the rapid decline in function. Symptomatic measures may include the use of anticholinergic drugs to control drooling and baclofen or diazepam to control spasticity. Dextromethorphan, a drug long used for cough suppression, has been effective in controlling the tearfulness that comes with pseudobulbar involvement.[137]

Maintenance of nutrition is a significant problem because of the difficulty chewing and swallowing. Weakness of jaw movement, loss of tongue mobility, and difficulty in lip closure, in addition to impairment of the swallowing reflex, are common. This may lead to respiratory complications from *aspiration*. By modifying the consistency and texture of food and fluids, the risk of aspiration is reduced.[6]

There is a shift in the care of individuals with ALS toward the use of multidisciplinary ALS clinics to provide coordinated care. Survival has been found to be longer for individuals with bulbar symptoms, the use of aids and appliances was greater, and the mental quality of life was better for the individuals with ALS treated at the multidisciplinary clinics than for individuals who do not receive specialty clinic care. With focused care, up to 80% of individuals with ALS can die at home.[47]

Prognosis

The course of ALS is relentlessly progressive. It appears that earlier onset (before age 50 years) has a longer course. Death from the adult-onset sporadic type usually occurs within 2 to 5 years, resulting mainly from pneumonia caused by respiratory compromise. Generally, those with bulbar palsy have a more rapid course than those with primary lateral sclerosis in whom the prognosis is markedly better. Respiratory failure and inability to eat are part of the final stages of ALS. Nasogastric tube feeding and use of a respirator may be options to prolong the life of the client. Individual and family wishes concerning these procedures should be discussed as early as possible in the course of the disease, because some clients may experience a rapid decline in function at any time.

20.1 Special Implications for the PTA: **Amyotrophic Lateral Sclerosis** The ALS-Specific Quality of Life Instrument is based on the McGill Quality of Life Questionnaire, modified by changes in format and by adding questions on religiousness and spirituality. A 59-item tool with a completion time averaging 15 minutes, it is a practical tool for the assessment of overall quality of life in individuals with ALS and appears to be valid and useful across large samples. Validation studies of a shortened version are now under way.[133]

The ALS Functional Rating Scale (ALSFRS-R), which can be found at and downloaded from www.alsconnection.com/ALSFRS.asp, is a functional scale that can be used to follow the progression of ALS. Six months are needed to detect changes in the ALSFRS-R score because of variability, due principally to differing rates of progression among patients.[58]

The relationship between verbal associative fluency, verbal abstract reasoning, and judgment in ALS can be evaluated using a 20-minute screening evaluation. Deficiencies in these measures were found in 20% to 35% of patients with limb-onset ALS and in 37% to 60% of patients with bulbar-onset ALS. This simple screen identifies deficits that affect discussions of treatment interventions and end-of-life issues.

Muscle strength declines in an overall linear progression throughout the course of the disease. Staging of ALS helps the physical therapist (PT) and physical therapist assistant (PTA) to determine the most effective intervention based on the current functional status and on the predicted progression of the disease. Table 20.1 describes interventions associated with the various stages of the disease.

The rate of loss is stable within a broad range after the first year, but during the first year there is fluctuation of strength that may be caused by the potential for adaptation within the CNS. At this point, the goal of therapy is to maintain general physical activity and muscular tone. Regular exercise in moderation can help

TABLE 20.1 Exercise and Rehabilitation Programs for Clients with Amyotrophic Lateral Sclerosis

Stage	Treatment
Phase I (Independent)	
Stage I	

Patient characteristics
  Mild weakness
  Clumsiness
  Ambulatory
  Independent in ADLs
	• Continue normal activities or increase activities if sedentary to prevent disuse atrophy
	• Begin program of ROM exercises (stretching, yoga, tai chi)
	• Add strengthening program of gentle resistance exercises to all musculature with caution not to cause overwork fatigue
	• Provide psychologic support as needed

Stage II	

Patient characteristics
  Moderate, selective weakness
  Slightly decreased independence in ADLs
    Difficulty climbing stairs
    Difficulty raising arms
    Difficulty buttoning clothing
  Ambulatory
	• Continue stretching to avoid contractures
	• Continue cautious strengthening of muscles with MMT grades above F+ (3+); monitor for overwork fatigue
	• Consider orthotic support (i.e., AFOs, wrist, thumb splints)
	• Use adaptive equipment to facilitate ADLs

TABLE 20.1 Exercise and Rehabilitation Programs for Clients with Amyotrophic Lateral Sclerosis—cont'd

Stage	Treatment
Stage III Patient characteristics (see Stage II)	• Continue stage II program as tolerated; caution not to fatigue to point of decreasing patient's ADLs independence • Keep patient physically independent as long as possible through pleasurable activities, walking • Encourage deep-breathing exercises, chest stretching, postural drainage if needed • Prescribe standard or motorized wheelchair with modifications to allow eventual reclining back with head rest, elevating legs
Phase II (Practically Independent)	
Stage IV Patient characteristics (see Stage II)	• Active assisted passive ROM exercises to the weakly supported joint—caution to support, rotate shoulder during abduction and joint accessory motions • Encourage isometric contractions of all musculature to tolerance • Try arm slings, overhead slings, or wheelchair arm supports • Motorize chair if patient wants to be independently mobile; adapt controls as needed
Stage V Patient characteristics Severe lower extremity weakness Moderate to severe upper extremity weakness Wheelchair dependent Increasingly dependent in ADLs Possible skin breakdown secondary to poor mobility	• Encourage family to learn proper transfer, positioning principles, turning techniques • Encourage modifications at home to aid patient's mobility and independence • Electric hospital bed with antipressure mattress • If patient elects HMV, adapt chair to hold respiratory unit
Phase III (Dependent)	
Stage VI Patient characteristics Bedridden Completely dependent in ADLs	• For dysphagia: soft diet, long spoons, tube feeding, percutaneous gastrostomy • To decrease flow of accumulated saliva: medication, suction, surgery • For dysarthria: palatal lifts, electronic speech amplification, eye pointing • For breathing difficulty: clear airway, tracheostomy, respiratory if HMV elected • Medications to decrease impact of dyspnea

ADLs, Activities of daily living; *AFOs*, ankle-foot orthoses; *HMV*, home mechanical ventilation; *MMT*, manual muscle test; *ROM*, range of motion.
Modified from Sinaki M: Exercise and rehabilitation measures in amyotrophic lateral sclerosis. In Yase Y, Tsubaki T, editors: Amyotrophic lateral sclerosis: recent advances in research and treatment, Amsterdam, 1988, Elsevier.

alleviate fatigue and have a beneficial effect on the client's general well-being.[17] Complaints of diffuse pain will start in the early stages, related to joint stiffness and decreases in muscle control in the limbs or trunk.

Spasticity contributes to complaints of weakness. Consistent slow stretching that decreases tone may be of benefit. The Ashworth scale can be used to measure the degree of spasticity. Cramps, which can be a source of pain, also respond to a daily stretching routine.

Changes in gait are significant, and gait analysis is necessary to assess the need for assistive devices. Falls caused by weakness are a major problem. Ankle dorsiflexion is lost before loss of strength in plantar flexion. Hamstring strength appears to correlate with walking, and the decrease parallels the loss of walking ability. Isometric muscle strength as a percentage of normal shows a dramatic decrease late in the course of the disease when fewer muscle fibers are available. This is when the greatest functional losses are noted. A surprisingly small amount of muscle activity is necessary across the joints to allow normal function of a joint. Some movement and joint stability are maintained until the degeneration causes atrophy of muscle activity to less than 20% of normal. The weakness and wasting often produce painful subluxation of the scapulohumeral joint, and the arm should be supported.[2] Contractures should be routinely stretched, taking care to support the joints, because there is minimal control of muscle activity in the late stages. Complaints of pain may begin when the client is unable to shift weight in bed or in sitting. Changing the reclining angle of the bed or wheelchair or the position of the legs will give some relief. Caregivers need to be educated in this aspect of care.

Braces, other assistive devices, and motorized scooters or wheelchairs help to maintain mobility and freedom. Many upper extremity devices are available to maintain joint alignment at rest, to make daily activities easier to perform, and to support mobility when it is lost. Braces for the lower extremity can extend the time of upright walking, and braces for the back and neck can assist with head and trunk control. Pain is often a complaint brought to the PTA. Thermal modalities and transcutaneous electrical nerve stimulation can help the pain associated with muscle shortening, joint stiffness, and muscle cramping.

Evaluation of the home environment, providing rails, hoists, or supports; eliminating stairs where possible; and advising on helpful devices for feeding, shaving, and dressing is essential as the individual becomes limited to household mobility. Posture for activities of daily living (ADLs) may be improved with a collar, a brace, or spring-loaded splints. Special beds can be leased or borrowed. Family and friends may organize a roster of people to sleep over, sparing the spouse from waking every 3 hours to turn the patient. The legs should be elevated and elastic stockings used if leg swelling is a problem. Avoid using diuretics for leg swelling.

Frustration and boredom are common. Family and volunteers can be mobilized from neighborhood groups, such as church or social groups, to visit to talk, listen, play cards, turn pages or read, or just to be there for a while.

Sexual frustration is common and is not often discussed. The clinician should do so freely and without embarrassment with both the patient and spouse; the problems are mainly matters of method. The partner may need counseling to understand that he or she needs to take the active role and to learn effective techniques that overcome weakness and muscle spasms.

Respiratory changes cause the most disability and eventually lead to death. Respiratory distress is a mechanical problem because of lack of muscle support. From the earliest stages of care of the client with ALS, prevention of respiratory complications should be emphasized. Early evidence of respiratory involvement may be shortness of breath, poor cough reflex, and headache. Some clients can be taught to use their abdominal muscles to increase inspiration and expiration when the muscles of the diaphragm and intercostal muscles become weak. Swallowing becomes difficult and should be evaluated by a speech pathologist. Pseudobulbar affect causing uncontrolled laughing or crying decreases the capacity to regulate breathing and increases risk of shortness of breath. Aspiration is common, and techniques to control this can be taught. Mechanical ventilation is an option to prolong the ability to breathe. Individuals with a relatively slow disease progression, and those with spinal onset, might benefit more from treatment with noninvasive ventilation than patients with rapid disease progression or bulbar onset. Noninvasive positive pressure ventilation has been shown to improve patient quality of life, despite progression of ALS, and without increasing the caregiver burden or stress.[64] In addition, suction, intermittent positive pressure breathing, and postural drainage appear to be useful in maintaining bronchial hygiene. Only 5% of individuals choose long-term, invasive ventilation because of the restriction of activity, caregiver involvement, and overall cost.[83] Communication becomes limited, again because of loss of oral muscle control and breath support. Communication strategies can be taught, and augmentative equipment is available. In all cases, the individual becomes dependent over time. In the terminal stages, the comfort of the patient is the therapeutic goal.

As patients with ALS weaken, the decisions facing the patient progress from issues of morbidity to mortality. Traditionally, the neurologist and other therapeutic support staff have deferred to the wishes of the patient and family members in determining level of support in response to progressive physical decline. Impairments in judgment have potentially significant clinical implications that should be considered by health care providers and caregivers when discussing treatment interventions and end-of-life issues with these patients.[53]

All patients with ALS and their families have to come to grips with the many end-of-life decisions that confront them. These include the need to get the many events in life in order, come to terms with relationships, and decide how forthcoming disabilities will be handled. Decisions regarding care at home versus in a nursing facility should be made as early as possible. Information about advance directives, living wills, and power of attorney should be available. Patients may raise the question of suicide or assisted suicide, and the caregivers should be comfortable not only talking about these issues but also calling on others who may have more expertise and experience in discussing these issues. It makes things more difficult for the patient and family if the caregivers avoid these sensitive areas and talk only about the disease and medical management. Psychologic and emotional support for the individual and the family is critical. A direct and informative approach is appreciated; giving false hope should be avoided.

ALZHEIMER'S DISEASE, ALZHEIMER'S DEMENTIA, AND VARIANTS

Overview and Definition

The two terms *Alzheimer's disease* and *Alzheimer's dementia* are related but not synonymous. AD is the disease process that ultimately results in Alzheimer's dementia. Alzheimer's dementia has a characteristic cognitive pattern. In some individuals, early in the disease course AD may cause memory loss of insufficient severity to warrant the designation of dementia. In other individuals, AD may follow an atypical course with progressive aphasia or progressive apraxia rather than a typical Alzheimer's dementia.

Dementia is a term for a decline in intellectual functioning severe enough to interfere with a person's relationships and ability to perform daily activities. A significant decline in memory is a hallmark of dementia but is not the only characteristic. Age-associated memory impairment, or benign senescent forgetfulness, is a decline in short-term memory that does not progress to other mental or intellectual impairments. Other causes of dementia must be carefully ruled out, and there are syndromes that mimic AD in relationship to the dementia but have different neurologic causes. Listed here are a few of the other dementias that cause change in cognitive status.

Pick's Disease

Much less common and sometimes clinically indistinguishable from AD, Pick's disease is characterized by cortical atrophy involving predominantly the frontal and temporal regions with sparing of the posterior two-thirds. Loss of frontal inhibition of socially unacceptable and previously suppressed behavior emerges early in the disease, often overshadowing the memory disturbance. The inclusions are known as Pick bodies. The neurons balloon in the area of involved tissue, but there are no plaques or tangles as seen in AD.

Lewy Body Dementia

This disorder exhibits highly variable clinical and neuropathologic overlap with AD and PD. It is characterized by initial parkinsonism unresponsive to standard medications, progressing to deterioration of cognition. Cellular changes include presence of the Lewy bodies found in PD and neurofibrillary tangles, senile plaques, and granulovacuolar degeneration similar to those in AD.

Corticobasal ganglionic degeneration is characterized by a striking asymmetric gait and speed apraxia, "alien hand" syndrome, rigidity, myoclonus, and cortical sensory loss. Dementia is usually a late manifestation of the disease.

Frontotemporal Dementia

This term is used to describe the various progressive disorders that have a predilection for the frontal lobes. The cellular neuropathology is variable, and in some cases it seems to be the frontal lobe manifestations of AD, Pick's disease, and Lewy body dementia.

AD is the most common cause of dementia overall. It is one of the principal causes of disability and decreased quality of life among older adults.[2] Progress in clinical knowledge of AD has led to more reliable diagnostic criteria and accuracy; the earliest manifestations and even the presymptomatic phases of the disease may soon be identifiable.

Incidence and Etiologic and Risk Factors

There are approximately 5 million people with AD in the United States and 25 million affected around the world. The prevalence of AD rises with each decade of age. The known prevalence is 6% in people older than age 65 years, 20% in people older than age 80 years, and more than 95% in those age 95 years or older.[153] Because life expectancy continues to rise, so does the potential for more individuals to be afflicted. It is believed that many individuals with the symptoms go undiagnosed and untreated. The cause of AD remains unknown, but there appears to be a relationship among genetic predisposition; the abnormal processing of a normal cellular substance, amyloid; and advanced age.[73] Lifetime risk of developing AD is estimated to be between 12% and 17%. Twin studies show evidence that in identical twins one may develop AD whereas the other remains dementia free. People with a family history of the disease are at higher than average risk for AD. Researchers are identifying important genetic factors, notably the apolipo-protein E ε4 (ApoE4) gene.

The same genes may have different effects depending on the ethnic population. Dietary and other cultural factors that increase the risk for hypertension and unhealthy cholesterol levels may also play a role. For example, a study of Japanese men showed that their risk increased if they emigrated to America; the disease is much less common in West Africa than in African Americans, whose risk is the same as or higher than that of white Americans.

Some studies have reported an association between AD and systolic hypertension (the higher and first number in blood pressure measurement). Furthermore, some studies report a lower risk for AD in individuals whose blood pressure was reduced. Nevertheless, although hypertension is strongly linked to memory and mental difficulties, stronger evidence is needed to prove any causal relationship between hypertension and AD.

There has been research suggesting an association between high cholesterol levels and AD in some people. A number of recent studies support the link between AD and cholesterol by suggesting that certain cholesterol-lowering drugs known as statins may be protective against AD. The ApoE genotype is linked with both atherosclerosis and AD because it reflects abnormal cholesterol transport.[151]

Box 20.4 outlines some of the key risk factors as well as possible protective factors related to AD.

Pathogenesis

Like other degenerative conditions, AD has no single identified cause. The loss of neurons is thought to be caused by the breakdown of several processes necessary for sustaining brain cells.

AD is characterized by disruptions in multiple major neurotransmitters, of which cholinergic abnormalities are the most prominent. Acetylcholine is an important neurotransmitter in areas of the brain involved in memory formation, and loss of acetylcholine activity correlates with the severity of AD. The reduction in the number of acetylcholine receptors precedes other pathologic changes, and these receptors

---

BOX 20.4 Key Risk Factors and Protective Factors for Alzheimer's Disease

- Primary risk factors: age; family history; genetic markers such as apolipoprotein E ε4 gene; trisomy 21; mutations in presenilin 1 and 2; female gender after age 80 years; cardiovascular risk factors such as hypertension, diabetes, obesity, and hypercholesterolemia
- Possible risk factors: head injury, depression, progression of Parkinson-like signs in older adults, lower thyroid-stimulating hormone level within the normal range, hyperhomocysteinemia, folate deficiency, hyperinsulinemia, low educational attainment
- Possible protective factors: apolipoprotein E ε2 gene; regular fish consumption; regular consumption of omega-3 fatty acids; high educational level; regular exercise; nonsteroidal antiinflammatory drug therapy; moderate alcohol intake; adequate intake of vitamins C, E, B6, and B12, and folate

From Desai AK: Diagnosis and treatment of Alzheimer's disease, Neurology 64(12 suppl 3):S34–S39, 2005.

---

are reduced significantly in late AD, particularly in the basal forebrain. There is selective loss of nicotinic receptor subtypes in the hippocampus and cortex. Presynaptic nicotinic receptors control the release of neurotransmitters important for memory and mood, such as acetylcholine, glutamate, serotonin, and norepinephrine. There is still some question whether this plays a primary role in the disease or is a secondary reaction.

Synaptic loss is the best pathologic correlate of cognitive decline, and synaptic dysfunction is evident long before synapses and neurons are lost. Once synaptic function stops, despite the number of surviving neurons, there may be little chance of changing the disease process.

Clinical Manifestations

The early symptoms of AD may be overlooked because they resemble signs of natural aging. Still, older adults who begin to notice a persistent mild memory loss for recent events may have a condition called mild cognitive impairment (MCI). MCI is now believed to be a significant sign of early-stage AD in older people. Studies now suggest that older individuals who experience such mild memory abnormalities convert to AD at a rate of about 10% to 15% per year.

Disorders of function are found in the person with AD that correlate with the level of damage in the various components of the cortex as described earlier. Visuospatial deficits are an early clinical finding. Navigating the environment, cooking, and fixing or manipulating mechanical objects in the home are all visuospatial tasks that often are impaired in the first stages of AD. Drawing is abnormal; the ability to draw a three-dimensional object is often lost. The loss of ability to solve mathematical problems and handle money is typical in the early stages of AD. Judgment is impaired, and safety in driving is diminished.

Subtle personality changes occur in AD, such as indifference, egocentricity, impulsivity, and irritability. People with AD become withdrawn and anxious. Memory is affected, and this is seen as inability to recall current events. Studies show that particular memory subsystems are relatively more or less vulnerable to diffuse cortical pathologies.[28] People with AD seem to retain higher capacity in implicit memory than was originally thought. AD causes loss of older memories, and recall of events from early life disappears. Language declines in a characteristic progression. Word-finding difficulty is first, followed by inability to remember names (*anomia*), and finally diminished comprehension. Social situations become difficult, and mood swings are common.[95] Between 40% and 60% of individuals with late-onset AD suffer from psychotic symptoms, which may include hallucinations, delusions, and dramatic verbal, emotional or physical outbursts. This is a severe form of AD, with a genetic basis, that has a more rapid and aggressive course. Table 20.2 describes the difference between normal aging and AD.

Major depression is uncommon, but many persons with AD have periods of depressed mood associated with feelings of inadequacy and hopelessness. AD-associated depression is often more modifiable by environmental manipulation than depressions not associated with AD. As AD progresses, delusions, agitation, and even violence may occur.

Abnormal motor signs are common, related to the area of the brain that is involved, and perhaps because of the type of neurotransmitter dysfunction. A relationship between the

TABLE 20.2 Differences between Normal Signs of Aging and Dementia

Normal	Dementia
Early Signs of Alzheimer's Disease	
Memory and Concentration	
Periodic minor memory lapses or forgetfulness of part of an experience	Misplacement of important items
	Confusion about how to perform simple tasks
Occasional lapses in attention or lapses in attention or concentration	Trouble with simple arithmetic problems
	Difficulty making routine decisions
	Confusion about month or season
Mood and Behavior	
Temporary sadness or anxiety based on appropriate and specific cause	Unpredictable mood changes
	Increasing loss of outside interests
Changing interests	Depression, anger, or confusion in response to change
Increasingly cautious behavior	Denial of symptoms
Later Signs of Alzheimer's Disease	
Language and Speech	
Unimpaired language skills	Difficulty completing sentences or finding the right words
	Inability to understand the meaning of words
	Reduced and/or irrelevant conversation
Movement/Coordination	
Increasing caution in movement	Visibly impaired movement or coordination, including slowing of movements, halting gait, and reduced sense of balance
Slower reaction times	
Other Symptoms	
Normal sense of smell; no abnormal weight changes in either men or women	Impaired sense of smell
	Severe weight loss, particularly in female patients

Data from Alzheimer's Disease: Early warning signs and diagnostic resources, The Junior League of NYC, Inc. 1988.

motor impairments and levels of function can be seen. Presence of tremor appears to be associated with increased risk for cognitive decline, presence of bradykinesia with increased risk for functional decline, and presence of postural-gait impairments with increased risk for institutionalization and death. This may reflect a need for assistance with mobility and number of falls. See 20.2 Special Implications for the PTA: Alzheimer's Disease later in the chapter.

Disorders of sleep, eating, and sexual behavior are common. The electroencephalogram shows more awake time in bed, longer latencies to rapid eye movement sleep, and losses in slow-wave sleep.[97]

Medical Management

Diagnosis

The most important diagnostic step in evaluating dementias is to determine whether a chronic encephalopathy results from a potentially reversible cause. Interaction of multiple medications can also trigger dementia and should be assessed.

A decline from previous levels of functioning and impairment in multiple cognitive domains beyond memory are critical in establishing dementia. Determining the rate of change is useful, because abrupt changes are not consistent with AD.[18] The progression is usually continuous and does not fluctuate or improve. Information obtained from family members or caregivers can provide data when there seems to be lack of insight from the client. The Functional Activities Questionnaire is a useful informant-based measure.

Clinical screening tests, such as the Short Test of Mental Status, the Mini-Mental State Examination (MMSE), and Mattis Dementia Rating Scale provide a baseline for monitoring the course of cognitive impairment over time and document multiple cognitive impairments.[2]

A clock drawing test is also a good test for AD. The individual is given a piece of paper with a circle on it and is first asked to write the numbers in the face of a clock and then to show 10 minutes after 11. The score is based on spacing between the numbers and the positions of the hands.

Neuropsychologic tests can accurately predict the probability of conversion to incident AD after 5 or 10 years.[48,143] Clues on physical examination include a variety of findings that may be common in elderly individuals but are not part of the typical picture of AD, such as ataxia, hyperreflexia, and tremulousness.

Depression can be difficult to distinguish from dementia, and it can coexist with dementia. Changes in memory, attention, and the ability to make and perform plans suggest depression, the most common psychiatric illness in older persons. Marked visuospatial or language impairment suggests a dementing process. Depression scales can be used to determine levels of depression.

Ruling out a partially or completely reversible dementia by performing a blood count, chest radiography, and general neurologic examination is critical in the diagnostic evaluation of a person with suspected AD. Autoimmune and paraneoplastic serologic studies may be helpful in such individuals as well.

Use of neuroimaging can be beneficial in the diagnosis of AD. Both magnetic resonance imaging (MRI) and computed tomography (CT) can identify the changes in brain size that are associated with AD. Diagnostic criteria are based on the measurement of medial temporal lobe atrophy or on the volumetric measurement of the entorhinal cortex and hippocampus.[15] The brain demonstrates atrophy with normal aging, so this is not the only diagnostic test.

Single-photon emission computed tomography (SPECT) can be used to determine brain activity, especially in areas in which information is processed for memory functions. This may be used in the future to predict potential for development of AD.

Researchers are looking at different components of the human brain cell to identify molecular changes in DNA and RNA seen in individuals with dementia and AD. Approaches are widespread, because it is clear that the disease is multifactorial. The National Institute on Aging (NIA) held a consensus conference in 1998 with the creation of an NIA Reagan profile that requires that neuropathologic assessment include assessment of both plaques and neurofibrillary tangles.

Treatment and Pharmacology

There is currently no cure for AD. Current treatment focuses on establishing an early accurate clinical diagnosis, early institution of cholinesterase inhibitors and/or N-methyl-D-aspartate receptor–targeted therapy. Treating medical comorbidities and dementia-related complications, ensuring that appropriate services are provided, addressing the long-term well-being of caregivers, and treating behavioral and psychologic symptoms with appropriate nonpharmacologic and pharmacologic interventions also are important.[89]

Current drugs approved for treatment of AD have modest symptomatic benefits but do not have profound disease-modifying effects. Disease-modification approaches including neuroprotection are now the most active area of investigation, with focus on antiamyloid treatment. Oxidative stress and cell cycle–related abnormalities are early events in AD, occurring before any cytopathology can be identified, and together may create disease pathogenesis. Therefore antioxidants are an AD prevention strategy under investigation. Inflammation and activation of microglia is a relatively early pathogenic event that precedes the process of neuron destruction in AD. Therefore despite the early negative results of clinical trials with nonsteroidal antiinflammatory drugs for the treatment of AD, these and other antiinflammatory agents may still have a role in reducing the risk for AD. Modulation of cardiovascular risk factors may also reduce the risk for AD. Although hormone replacement therapy with estrogen showed no benefit and even a potential deleterious effect in individuals with AD, estrogen may still have a role in reducing the risk for AD if given early in menopause and when neurons are in a healthy state. Other neurodegenerative processes, such as excitotoxicity and apoptosis, may also have a pathophysiologic role in AD and are now under study. Medications currently in use are outlined in Box 20.5.

Treatment oriented at preventing the breakdown of tau, or the formation of plaques, is being tested now and shows promise. The treatment of those persons identified as at high risk may someday be protective gene therapy. Future drug therapies may be targeted at specific cognitive modules.

Management of the client with AD is a challenge to health providers and to the family who become caregivers. Manipulation of the environment can be effective. It is difficult to manage aggressive behavior in the home, and long-term care in a facility with a special Alzheimer's unit is often the most appropriate place for that client.

A management model for AD that incorporates a diagnostic protocol to identify and assess people with possible dementia and care management addressing individual function, caregiver support, medical treatment, psychosocial needs, nutritional needs, and advance directives planning is critical. To improve end-of-life care for people with AD, any treatment model should also incorporate patient-centered care and palliative care from the initial diagnosis of AD through its terminal stages. Short-term intensive counseling can significantly reduce the long-term risk for depression among those who care for spouses or partners with AD.[42]

In many individuals with AD, treating comorbid conditions such as depression, hearing or vision impairment, congestive heart failure, symptomatic urinary tract infection, or hypothyroidism may produce a greater benefit than focusing treatment only on AD. Cardiovascular disease may influence the expression and clinical manifestations of the disease.

There is compelling evidence for the important role of regular physical activity.[92] Exercise training combined with behavioral management techniques can improve physical health and depression in individuals with AD. Leisure-time physical activity at midlife is associated with a decreased risk of dementia and AD later in life. Regular physical activity may reduce the risk or delay the onset of dementia and AD, especially among genetically susceptible individuals.[125]

Diet in midlife shows potential for neuroprotection, and findings can be generalized to a combination of the consumption of a diet low in fat, high in omega-3 oils, and high in dark vegetables and fruits; use of soy (for women only); supplementation with vitamin C, coenzyme Q10, and folate; and moderate alcohol intake. It appears that no single item creates the protection, but the foods and supplements may work together to lower risk.

Prognosis

AD is the fourth leading cause of death in adults. The period from onset to death typically is 7 to 11 years. Initially, deficits in higher cortical function are the most noticeable. Motor signs may reflect a higher burden or a different type or a more biologically detrimental localization of neuropathology. The association of different aspects of motor signs with different outcomes may reflect varying underlying neurotransmitter systems being affected. For example, in PD, tremor and bradykinesia have been viewed as representing more purely dopaminergic manifestations, whereas posture, balance, and gait disorders may be mediated by other neurotransmitter systems in addition to dopamine. Changes caused by the dementia may advance relentlessly over

---

BOX 20.5 Common Medications Used in Alzheimer's Disease

- **Donepezil** (Aricept) has only modest benefits, but it does help slow loss of function and reduce caregiver burden. It works equally in patients with and without apolipoprotein E ε4. It may even have some advantage for patients with moderate to severe Alzheimer's disease (AD).
- **Rivastigmine** (Exelon) targets two enzymes (the major one, acetylcholinesterase, and butyrylcholinesterase). This agent may be particularly beneficial for patients with rapidly progressing disease. This drug has slowed or slightly improved disease status even in patients with advanced disease. (Rivastigmine may cause significantly more side effects than donepezil, including nausea, vomiting, and headache.)
- **Galantamine** (Razadyne). Galantamine not only protects the cholinergic system but also acts on nicotine receptors, which are also depleted in AD. It improves daily living, behavior, and mental functioning, including in patients with mild to advanced-moderate AD and those with a mix of AD and vascular dementia. Some studies have suggested that the effects of galantamine may persist for a year or longer and even strengthen over time.
- **Tacrine** (Cognex) has only modest benefits and has no benefits for patients who carry the apolipoprotein E ε4 gene. In high dosages, it can also injure the liver. Generally, newer cholinergic-protective drugs that do not pose as great a risk for the liver are now used for AD.
- **Memantine** (Namenda), targeted at the N-methyl-D-aspartate receptor, is used for moderate to severe AD.
- **Selegiline** (Eldepryl) is used for treatment of Parkinson's disease, and it appears to increase the time before advancement to the next stage of disability.

many years, creating not only deep emotional and psychologic distress but also practical problems related to caregiving that can overwhelm affected families. During the middle stages of the disease, the client often develops behavioral and motor problems. Finally, the client becomes mute and unable to comprehend. Death is often secondary to dehydration or infection.

20.2 Special Implications for the PTA: Alzheimer's Disease

Cognitive decline consistent with the diagnosis of primary degenerative dementia is a unique clinical syndrome with characteristic phenomena and progression. The Global Deterioration Scale can be used for the assessment of primary degenerative dementia and delineation of its stages.[121]

Use of a comprehensive cognitive stimulation program in AD patients enhances neuroplasticity, reduces cognitive loss, and helps the patient to stretch functional independence through better cognitive performance. Remarkable effects have been observed also in the areas of mood and behavior. Behavioral disturbances influence caregiver burden and institutionalization as well as being associated with patient and caregiver distress. Increase in social attention and interaction has been noted to improve mood and behavior in demented elderly. Important mood benefits have been reported from stimulation programs predominantly aimed at cognition.[110]

Cognitive rehabilitation programs can minimize demands on executive control systems in favor of structured tasks that are designed to exploit implicit memory. Appropriate feedback is critical because there is increased agitation and anxiety when mistakes are recognized. Nonverbal cues can be helpful when language is the source of confusion. Moving through parts of a task with guidance can facilitate understanding and promote confidence to proceed. When the experience is more pleasurable, the response is improved, because the stress of the task may be reduced.

The client with AD has generalized weakness and abnormality of movement. Movements become more stereotyped and rigid. Postural reflexes are diminished, and the incidence of falls increases. Falls occur in approximately 30% of clients with AD, which may be attributable to their lack of perception of where their bodies are in space and their inability to move adequately around objects. Having the client move in a space that has few obstacles appears to decrease the number of falls. The use of increased lighting, especially in the early evening, will decrease the agitation often referred to as *sundowning*.[155]

The PTA often sees a client with AD in a structured living environment, because many people become difficult to maintain at home. Movement and exercise can provide the client with an activity that he or she can succeed in as well as maintaining mobility, good breathing patterns, and endurance. Restlessness and wandering are typical of the client with AD, and a structured exercise program appears to decrease restlessness. Daytime exercise can also help control nighttime pacing and the resulting daytime drowsiness. Some residential programs have set up areas that the client can access without wandering out of the facility. The use of these areas may decrease agitation and allow individuals to pace safely.[19]

Group therapy with simple exercises that use images rather than commands is most effective. Storytelling integrated into the exercise program helps to stimulate thinking as well as movement. Clients need to be able to attend to an activity for at least 5 minutes, and the group therapy session must not provide more stimulation than clients are able to tolerate. Exercises should be short and simple and done in the same order each day. Repetition and reassurance can help keep clients engaged. The exercise program should

include group interaction with physical touching, such as holding hands or working in pairs. Use of exercise bands, balls to kick and throw, and light weights works well.[16,91]

In working with the individual with AD, knowing something about him or her may enable the PTA to use words and terms that are more familiar. Approach to the person should be slow and from the front. Always identify yourself and use the person's name before intervention begins. Identifying pain during activity is important, because pain may be involved in aggressive behavior. Use of modalities to decrease the client's pain may result in improved behavior. The Alzheimer's discomfort rating scale is useful.[68]

Intervention should be based on the individual's stage of progression. In the early stages, work on high-level balance and gait activities will help to maintain mobility and balance. Strength gains have been reported to be significant in older persons in a strengthening program, and strength is an important component of balance. Maintaining range of motion (ROM), especially in the trunk and distal extremities, will help to maintain function. Caregiver training is important for consistent follow-through with activities and provision of appropriate cues. When assistance is needed for mobility, caregiver training on transfers, contracture management, and assistance with gait is included in the intervention.

Choosing the appropriate orthotic, assistive device, and wheelchair can be a challenge as dementia develops. Walkers have been designed for the AD client to use on flat surfaces with appropriate support and safety.

The PTA should be familiar with the warning signs of AD. Because the disease mimics other signs of old age, the symptoms may go unreported. It is often the spouse who asks questions regarding the possibility of the client's developing AD. Information regarding the types of symptoms related to the disease can be helpful to the family in deciding whether more evaluation is needed. The Alzheimer's Association's 10 warning signs of AD are listed in Box 20.6.

BOX 20.6 Ten Warning Signs of Alzheimer's Disease

1. Recent memory loss that affects job performance. People with Alzheimer's disease (AD) will forget things often and may repeat the same question, forgetting the earlier answer.
2. Difficulty performing familiar tasks. The person may make a meal and then forget to serve it, forgetting even that he or she made it.
3. Problems with simple language: forgetting simple words or using them inappropriately.
4. Disorientation. The person with AD may get lost on his or her own block.
5. Decreased judgment; for example, the person may sometimes forget that he or she is responsible for a child's care.
6. Abstract thinking difficulties, for example, forgetting what numbers are for when balancing a checkbook.
7. Misplacing things, such as putting an iron in the freezer.
8. Changes in mood or behavior: getting angry easily and crying often.
9. Personality changes: becoming irritable, suspicious, or fearful.
10. Loss of initiative: not wanting to get involved in activities he or she previously enjoyed.

Adapted from Alzheimer's Association, 919 N. Michigan Ave., Suite 100, Chicago, IL 60611-1676.

DYSTONIA

Definition and Overview

Dystonia is a neurologic syndrome dominated by involuntary, sustained muscle contractions frequently causing twisting and repetitive movements. These abnormal postures are often exacerbated when the person performs active voluntary movements.

Traditionally, dystonia was classified according to type, including primary (idiopathic or of unknown cause) or secondary (occurring as a result of injury or other brain illness). These classifications are still reported in the literature, but the current classification scheme for dystonia now describes the disorder in each person according to three separate categories: age of onset, distribution of symptoms, and etiology. A second type of classification is by body involvement. In focal dystonia one body area is affected, in segmental dystonia two or more body areas are involved, and generalized dystonia is wider spread. There has been some confusion in the literature regarding the name *cervical dystonia*. This neurologically based movement disorder affecting the head and neck is a separate entity from spasmodic torticollis. Torticollis is a musculoskeletal phenomenon treated as an orthopedic condition.

Incidence

An estimated 250,000 persons are afflicted with dystonia in North America. About 1.1 in 100,000 persons per year develop dystonia, with a female to male ratio of 1.6:1.[46] The Mayo Clinic in Rochester, MN, found 3.4 cases of primary generalized dystonia and 29.5 cases of focal dystonia per 100,000.[108] Focal dystonia is estimated to be six times more common than other well-known neuromuscular disorders such as muscular dystrophy, Huntington's disease (HD), and ALS.

The average age of onset of idiopathic dystonia is 8 years. For focal dystonias, the age of onset is between 30 and 50 years.

Etiologic Factors

Idiopathic, or primary, dystonia is the most common diagnosis, accounting for two-thirds of all cases. A genetic basis on the DYT1 gene locus is responsible for causing primary torsion dystonia.[21] It appears that persons with generalized dystonia carry a different gene than those with focal dystonias.[49] Another inherited dystonia is dopa-responsive dystonia, or Segawa's dystonia.

Secondary dystonia is the result of small areas of brain damage or scarring of the CNS. The changes have been attributed to drugs, infections, tumors, and demyelinating processes as well as acute trauma, such as caused by auto accidents. Box 20.7 lists the major causes of secondary dystonia.

Focal dystonias involving hand function are particularly common among those in certain occupational groups, such as keyboard operators and musicians. Writer's cramp is also a focal dystonia. Focal dystonia related to occupational cramps may be a result of abnormal or repetitive biomechanics. Focal dystonia involving the hand may also occur as part of a peripheral nerve disorder.

Drug-induced extrapyramidal symptoms may include dystonia as a common side effect associated with antipsychotic drugs (neuroleptics). This results in various acute and chronic manifestations of neuroleptic-induced dystonia (e.g., blepharospasm [difficulty in opening the eyelids], torticollis or retrocollis [involuntary extension of the neck]).[70] The fact that β-blocking agents are effective in reducing symptoms in these cases points to the possibility that neuroleptic drugs increase the activity of β-adrenergic transmitters.

Clinical Manifestations

Cervical dystonia is the most common focal dystonia and is characterized by rotation of the neck, lateral flexion, and flexion and extension occurring in various combinations. The condition is usually painful, is disruptive to functional activity, and leads to osteoarthritis and hypertrophy of the sternocleidomastoid muscle if remission does not occur. Dystonia-induced cervical fracture has been reported.

Writer's or occupational cramp is a form of dystonia that can be particularly disabling, resulting in deterioration of handwriting or fine motor control. The fingers and wrist flex excessively, causing the hand to grasp a pen tightly and press unnecessarily hard on the paper. Another type of cramp results in extension of the fingers, making it difficult to hold a pen. Tremor or myoclonic jerks may occur while writing or trying to play a musical instrument. Lower extremity dystonia is common, including dystonic movements in the foot and toes.

Blepharospasm is uncontrolled blinking or closure of the eyelids for seconds to hours. In oromandibular dystonia, face and jaw muscles contract, causing grimaces or facial distortions, and dysphonia affects the speech muscles of the throat, causing strained, forced, or breathy speech.

Involvement of the respiratory muscles has been considered unusual but may in fact be underestimated, either because it is not conspicuous or because the problem is improperly attributed to another cause. Clinical manifestations of respiratory involvement may include involuntary deep and loud inspirations combined with dystonia, breathing arrests, or broken speech caused by deep inspirations when speaking or reading aloud.[86]

Dystonia usually is present continually throughout the day whenever the affected body part is used. In more severe cases, the dystonia can appear at rest. The symptoms may begin in one area only with a particular movement. For example, it may be apparent when walking forward but not when walking backward or the foot may turn under after walking or other exercise, causing the person to walk on the lateral border of the foot.

BOX 20.7 **Causes of Secondary or Symptomatic Dystonia**

- Drugs, including neuroleptics, dopamine agonists, anticonvulsants, antimalarial drugs
- Intramedullary lesions of the cervical cord
- After hemiplegia: often a delayed reaction to stroke
- Focal brain lesions: vascular malformation, tumor, abscess
- Demyelinating lesions, such as with multiple sclerosis
- Traumatic brain injury with lesion to contralateral basal ganglia or thalamus
- Encephalitis
- Environmental toxins: manganese, carbon monoxide, methanol
- Hypoparathyroidism
- Degenerative disease: Parkinson's disease, Huntington's disease, Wilson's disease, progressive supranuclear palsy, multiple system atrophy
- Cerebral palsy

Medical Management

Diagnosis

Dystonia is a clinical diagnosis except for those cases that have a genetic basis. Testing for genetic forms of dystonia appears to be most appropriate for people younger than age 26 years.[77] Otherwise, there is no definitive test for dystonia, and the diagnosis of idiopathic dystonia is often delayed 1 year or more. The clinical presentation of dystonic movements, such as head deviation or neck pain, may be the first diagnostic sign. The person usually has a normal perinatal and developmental history. EMG studies show sustained simultaneous contractions of agonists and antagonists. Determining that there is no evidence for symptomatic, or secondary, dystonia is essential in the diagnosis of idiopathic dystonia (see Box 20.7).

Treatment and Pharmacology

Treatment remains symptomatic and includes drug therapy, including botulinum toxin type A (BTX) injections, physical and occupational therapy, and sometimes surgery.

Anticholinergics such as trihexyphenidyl (Artane) have been the most widely used medications to decrease acetylcholine and correct a cholinergic imbalance in the basal ganglia. Side effects of these drugs vary, with blurred vision, dry mouth, confusion, voiding, sleeping difficulties, and personality changes observed.

Baclofen and other muscles relaxants are used occasionally for relief.

Botulinum toxin, injected intramuscularly, has emerged as a safe and effective symptomatic treatment for a number of conditions associated with excessive muscle activity, particularly focal dystonias involving a limited number of muscles. These injections are effective in improving postural deviation and pain in about 80% to 90% of people with cervical dystonias.[71,72] Injection directly into the actively contracting muscles blocks the neuromuscular junction by acting presynaptically to reduce the release of acetylcholine, producing a chemical denervation. Muscle weakness can result from this treatment. Response occurs in 3 to 7 days and lasts 3 to 4 months. Dysphagia is the most serious side effect but can be decreased in incidence and severity by injecting lower doses, particularly into the sternocleidomastoid. The need to continue indefinitely with repeat injections approximately every 3 months is a major drawback.

Surgery may be considered only when other treatments are no longer effective, although surgical intervention may also lose its effect over time, providing only temporary symptomatic relief. Surgeries to interrupt the pathways or foci responsible for the abnormal movements can be effective. Thalamotomy is the destruction of a portion of the thalamus. Pallidotomy is a destructive operation on the globus pallidus. Pallidus stimulation is achieved by placing an electric stimulator in the globus pallidus. Rhizotomy involves the surgical resection of the anterior cervical spinal nerve roots and is used along with selective peripheral denervation, or removal of the nerves at the point in which they enter the contracting muscles.

Prognosis

Age of onset is the best predictor of prognosis. If dystonia starts in childhood and affects other members of the family, it tends to get progressively worse over the years.

If the condition starts in childhood and is secondary to cerebral palsy or other brain injury close to the time of birth, the dystonia tends to remain static for many years. In one-third of cases of adult-onset focal dystonia there is progression to segmental dystonia, although there is less than a 20% chance that the disease will progress to generalized dystonia.

Spontaneous remission occurs in 30% of cases within the first year, but the majority of clients show steady progression of their focal dystonia, with maximal disability occurring after 5 years. Neck pain, occurring in 70% to 80% of clients, contributes significantly to disability. Cervical dystonia has important psychosocial consequences, because many people with this condition withdraw from their jobs and social activities.[150]

20.3 Special Implications for the PTA: Dystonia The Toronto Western Spasmodic Torticollis Rating Scale[38] is a commonly used impairment and disability scale for rating the severity of cervical dystonia. The Barry–Albright Dystonia Scale[8] is used for secondary dystonia. ROM, pain, and descriptions of active motion as well as limitations in functional activities are also useful measurements. Outcomes can be measured with life satisfaction scales, such as the SF-36.[20]

The PTA should address all aspects of functional ability with the client who has been affected by dystonia, including stress management, energy conservation, adaptive equipment, mobility, and splinting.[29]

Sensory processing abnormalities, as discussed under Pathogenesis with Clinical Manifestations, may be involved in the abnormal movements of dystonia. In owl monkeys who developed dystonic movements of the hand and particularly the fingers in response to a high number of repetitive movements of the forearm and hand,[31] the sensory cortex reorganized by decreasing the representation (dedifferentiation) of the hand and fingers. The cortical thalamic reorganization occurred after the monkeys began experiencing dystonia of the hand secondary to overuse. Later research by the same laboratory demonstrated recovery of the cortical representation and redifferentiation using sensory stimulation therapy rather than motor retraining. These studies suggest that treatment approaches should focus on sensory retraining, and particularly active interpretation of sensory stimuli. A case series using sensory retraining demonstrated success with this method in humans who had writer's cramp, which is a focal dystonia.[30] A recent literature review[29] of effective therapies for focal hand dystonia reported support for sensory retraining, motor sensory retuning, and limb immobilization. There was less support for modalities, stretching, and strengthening. However, Tassorelli et al.[140] reported success using physical therapy of stretching, strengthening, postural control and balance exercises along with surface EMG biofeedback in a study comparing outcomes of two groups: one receiving BTX only and the other receiving BTX and physical therapy. The group given physical therapy and BTX showed significantly better outcomes than the BTX-only group. Surface EMG feedback is effective in reducing symptoms in persons with focal hand dystonia.[30,82] Trials using surface EMG for hand dystonia demonstrated results in as few as five sessions.[39] Theoretically, visual input provides an alternate, nondysfunctional route for sensory input to reach the motor output system through the surface EMG visual feedback.[82] The primary motor cortex, which is responsible for initiating motor tasks, receives highly processed visual information from cortical areas other than the somatosensory cortex (i.e., parietal lobe, basal ganglia). These pathways may be able to override the malfunctioning input systems.[82]

Task-oriented treatment, rather than more traditional strengthening and stretching exercises, has a better potential for improving function. Having clients do highly skilled tasks in treatment that are challenging and stimulating will improve learning. A combination of treatments often is most effective. For example, a client with right lower extremity dystonia of 8 years' duration used a combination of surface EMG feedback on the anterior tibialis and gastrocnemius during stepping to targets and using the foot to identify and manipulate small objects to normalize motion. BTX injections into the hip flexor and gastrocnemius were done later to assist in reducing the abnormal hip flexor component of walking. The outcome was a normal gait pattern.

In some cases of dystonia, splinting has been effective for improving function. In cases in which the foot or feet turn in, insoles placed in the shoes to build up the outer border of the foot may help to put the foot in a neutral position and produce a more normal gait pattern. The use of a cervical collar has been tried by some with good results, but it may be that the sensory information to the skin accounts for this success rather than the mechanical support provided. If the collar minimizes pain or provides a more functional midline position, there may be some merit in its use. Otherwise, if it only works as a sensory trick, a piece of cloth wrapped around the neck may accomplish the same effect. The person who uses a cervical collar should be taught to do task-oriented exercises outside the collar to minimize weakness in the noninvolved muscles, for example, reading letters placed on the side opposite head rotation while the body stays facing forward.

When the jaw, tongue, or lips are involved, gentle pressure on the lips or teeth may lessen spasm. Exerting slight pressure against the jaw on the side to which the head is rotated may decrease or inhibit muscle spasm, although this is an immediate and short-term reaction. Guidelines for chewing and swallowing may be helpful for the client with oromandibular dystonia.

Swimming therapy can be especially helpful in reducing discomfort and facilitating movement.

Aggressive strengthening and ROM treatments may increase the symptoms of dystonia; any treatment should be performed within the client's tolerance and without increasing the manifestations of the dystonia. Because dystonia originates in the CNS, passive techniques such as massage provide only temporary relief from symptoms and do not affect the underlying movement disorder. Likewise, focal dystonia does not respond to facilitatory or inhibitory techniques used for modulating spasticity. When relief of spasm allows the client to assume a more normal or correct posture, underlying tight soft tissues may benefit from short-term use of physical therapy modalities and soft tissue mobilization to restore full ROM.[29,140]

HUNTINGTON'S DISEASE

Overview and Definition

Huntington's disease (HD) is a progressive hereditary disorder characterized by abnormalities of movement, personality disturbances, and dementia. Known also as Huntington's chorea, it is most often associated with choreic movement that is brief, purposeless, involuntary, and random. However, the disease course involves more than just a movement disorder, and hence the name Huntington's disease. HD is a disorder of the CNS and is classified as a neurologic disorder, but because it is a condition with effects that are complex, management requires a multidisciplinary approach.[61,156]

Incidence and Etiologic and Risk Factors

The prevalence of HD in North America ranges from 4 to 8 per 100,000. It is estimated that there are 25,000 cases in the United States. HD may begin at any time after infancy but usually starts in middle age. Twenty-five percent of persons with HD have disease of late onset, which is defined as onset of motor symptoms after age 50 years. There is almost always a history of an affected parent. There is a 50% risk in each child of an affected adult.[6] Transmission of the juvenile form of HD (onset before age 20 years) appears to be primarily from the father. With adult onset, there is more equal transmission from both parents.

HD is an autosomal dominant disease with the IT15 or HD genetic marker found on the tip of chromosome 4. In a subset of cases, the Junctophilin 3 gene is responsible for the HD genotype. All the people who inherit the gene will develop symptoms of the disease if they do not die prematurely. Because there is no cure for HD, there is an ethical dilemma associated with testing. Studies are under way to determine the psychiatric and social problems that may result from the knowledge that one will develop HD.[54]

Pathogenesis

Although the cause remains unknown, pathologic findings show a consistent pattern of tissue changes in the brain. The ventricles are enlarged as a result of atrophy of the adjacent basal ganglia, specifically the caudate nucleus and putamen (collectively the striatum; Fig. 20.3). This is caused by extensive loss of small- and medium-sized neurons. The volume of the brain can decrease by as much as 20%. Caudate atrophy correlates with a measured decline in MMSE scores but not with

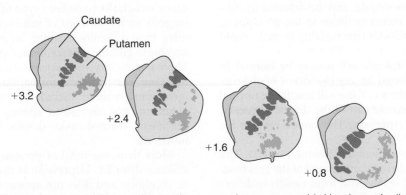

FIG. 20.3 Atrophy seen in the caudate and putamen in a person with Huntington's disease. As the disease progresses there is a change in the caudate at the interface with the ventricle. The outline becomes more and more concave, representing the progressive atrophy.

the severity or duration of neurologic symptoms. It is the atrophy of the putamen that correlates with neurologic symptoms. The atrophy of the cortices appears to occur at the same rate as that of the striatum. White matter degeneration in the frontal cortex appears to be associated with the course of the disease. Slower disease progression appears to be correlated with more white matter changes. The more aggressive progressive disease is related to less white matter and more striatal damage. Other subtle changes occur in the cortex and cerebellum, including both loss of neurons and production of glial cells that inhibit neural transmission.[60]

As with other progressive diseases, there is selective vulnerability of neurons in a particular region with preservation of others. In the early and middle stages of HD, neurons projecting from the striatum to the substantia nigra are depleted. This reduces the amount of neurotransmitters, including GABA, acetylcholine, and metenkephalin. This leaves relatively higher concentrations of other neurotransmitters, such as dopamine and norepinephrine. The normal balance of inhibition and excitation responses in the complex organization of the basal ganglia and thalamus that allows for smooth, controlled movement is disrupted. The result is an excess of dopamine and excessive excitation of the thalamocortical pathway. This may explain the excessive abnormal involuntary movements described as chorea.[9,119,156]

In the later stages of HD, there is a loss of the direct inhibitory substance that causes more inhibition of the thalamocortical output with resultant rigidity and bradykinesia, or slowness of movement. By the late stages of HD, virtually all the caudate nucleus projection neurons are affected. The mechanism of neuronal loss is not known. One hypothesis is that an excitotoxin causes the cell death noted in the basal ganglia.[118]

Clinical Manifestations
Movement Disorders

Many individuals with suspected early HD will show almost no neurologic abnormality on routine examination other than minor choreic movements. The movements may be suppressed during the examination because they can often be integrated into a purposeful movement, such as raising the hand to the head as if to smooth the hair. Early in the course the involuntary movements may appear to be no more than an exaggeration of normal restlessness, usually involving the upper limbs and face. The chorea is increased by mental concentration, emotional stimuli, performance of complex motor tasks, and walking. Problems with voluntary movement may be detected by asking for rapid tongue movements or finger-to-thumb tapping, or testing for dysdiadochokinesia (the inability to make rapid alternating movements).

Assessment of muscle strength will usually be normal in early cases but may be affected by any significant bradykinesia or general motor disturbance. Tone will usually be normal initially, but rigidity will become part of the clinical picture in many cases as the disease progresses. The tendon reflexes are usually normal.

Abnormalities in eye movement are common in HD. The ability to execute a saccade (a rapid movement of the eyes from one target to another to move the visual focus rapidly to different objects) is disturbed. There is often a decrease in the velocity of eye movement, an undershooting of the target, or latency in initiation of movement. Gaze fixation abnormalities have been noted, that is, inability to fix on a light source without the intrusion of small saccadic movements. Smooth pursuit, or tracking of the eye to follow a moving object, is interrupted by the same small, jerky saccadic movements. There is often an inability to suppress reflex saccades to a visual stimulus, which leads to visual distractibility.

The term *chorea* is derived from the Greek word for dance, and gait abnormalities are common in HD. When chorea is a predominant sign, persons walk with a wide-based, staggering gait. Those persons with bradykinesia and hypertonicity may walk with a slow, stiff, unsteady gait.

Dysarthria, reflected as a decrease in the rate and rhythm of speech, may be mild in the early course with an increase to the point in which speech may be unintelligible. In addition to the mechanical problems, neuron loss disrupts linguistic abilities, resulting in reduced vocabulary and syntactic errors. Some persons become mute at a stage before motor disability is severe.

Abnormalities of swallowing, or dysphagia, can cause choking and asphyxia. Dysphagia may involve multiple abnormalities of ingestion, including inappropriate food choices, abnormal rate of eating, poor bolus formation, and inadequate respiratory control.

Cachexia, or the wasting of muscle with weight loss, is found despite an adequate diet. This appears to be independent of the hyperkinesia and is found in persons with rigidity as well.

Sleep disorders become a progressive problem throughout the course of HD. An increased latent period before sleep and increased periods of wakefulness are common in moderately affected persons. Sleep reversal—daytime somnolence and nighttime restlessness—is seen in severely affected persons and is probably related to the dementia. Choreic movements are reduced during the deepest part of sleep.

Urinary incontinence is often a problem. This could be related to dementia, depression, decreased mobility, or hyperreflexia of the muscles that control urine output. There can be a concomitant increase in the incidence of urinary tract infections.

Neuropsychologic and Psychiatric Disorders

Early mental disturbances in persons with HD include personality and behavioral changes, such as irritability, apathy, depression, decreased work performance, violence, impulsivity, and emotional lability.[104] Intellectual decline usually follows the personality changes. The neuropsychologic profile characteristically includes a type of memory disturbance that suggests an impairment of information retrieval. Individuals often have difficulty recalling information on command but are able to give the correct answer in a multiple-choice format. There is difficulty with organization, planning, and sequencing, even when all the information is provided. Other prominent abnormalities include visuospatial deficits, impaired judgment, and ideomotor apraxia (the inability to perform previously learned tasks despite intact elementary motor function).

More than one-third of persons with HD will develop an affective disorder. Depression is the most common psychiatric condition and does not appear to be simply a reaction to a fatal illness. Evidence for this is the fact that mood disorders are not randomly distributed but occur in subsets of families with HD.[54]

Medical Management

Diagnosis

The clinical diagnosis of HD depends on recognition of patterns of symptoms given in the client's history and clinical signs, and the family history. Difficulties in diagnosis arise when the family history appears negative. Some families deny the presence of cognitive or psychiatric disease. Understanding of the clinical signs must take into account the fact that signs change during the course of the illness. Different patterns may be observed depending on the age of onset.[61]

MRI demonstrates atrophy of the striatum that is most easily appreciated as enlargement of the frontal horn of the lateral ventricles. Fig. 20.4 shows this change in brain structure. This is not of great diagnostic value unless it is very pronounced, given the normal reduction in brain mass with age and the occurrence of atrophy in other disorders that might be confused with HD. Positron emission tomography (PET) will also show atrophy, but its value as a diagnostic tool has the same limitations as MRI.

In addition to genetic linkage analysis, which requires testing of family members, it is now possible to evaluate the DNA of an individual to identify specific components that are diagnostic for HD. This eliminates the need to compare DNA of affected family members, but there are still problems with this method, because there is a small percentage of affected individuals who do not display the characteristics on the specific gene and there are nonaffected individuals who carry the gene.

Recognition of HD in older persons is critical to establish the genetic link for future generations. Often the diagnosis is overlooked in favor of the label of senile chorea, because there are minimal changes in behavior and cognition. The differential diagnosis of HD in the older population includes various degenerative, systemic, and drug-related conditions. An individual treated with neuroleptics for a psychiatric presentation of HD, for example, may go on to develop movement disorders, and these may be confused with the typical side effects of the medication.[106]

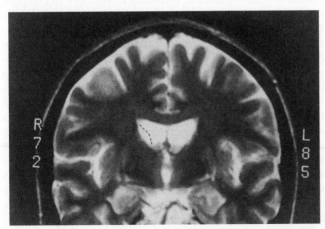

FIG. 20.4 Magnetic resonance scan showing the degeneration of the caudate in a person with Huntington's disease (HD). The *dotted lines* show where the tissue would be in a person without HD. (From Ramsey R: Neuroradiology, ed 3, Philadelphia, 1994, Saunders.)

Treatment and Pharmacology

Management of HD requires a team approach, including medical and social services. Education of clients and their families about the implications of the disease is important. Genetic, psychologic, and social counseling are started as soon as the diagnosis is confirmed. Organizations designed to help families with HD are often of great help.

Medical treatment is symptomatic. The most useful drugs for the symptomatic relief of chorea are anticonvulsants or antipsychotic agents that block dopamine neurotransmission. They can also help with the emotional outbursts, paranoia, psychosis, and irritability seen in HD. Drug therapy for chorea should be held in reserve if the abnormal movements are slight. There is a high incidence of side effects with the drugs, including acute dystonias, pseudoparkinsonism, and akathisia, which is characterized by uncontrollable physical restlessness. The most serious effect is chronic tardive dyskinesia resulting in involuntary movement of the face, tongue, and lips. Another adverse reaction is neuroleptic malignant hyperpyrexic syndrome, characterized by fever and rigidity.

The dopaminergic stabilizer pridopidine shows some effect on voluntary motor function with most effect related to eye movements, hand coordination, dystonia, gait, and balance problems.[44,52]

Tetrabenazine, now available in the United States, was recently approved by the FDA for the treatment of chorea associated with HD. It is a reversible inhibitor of the vesicle monoamine transporter type 2, and it inhibits primarily dopamine and to a lesser degree serotonin and norepinephrine. Side effects include parkinsonism and depression.

Surgical procedures to remove the medial globus pallidus, thought to be overexcited by neuronal loss in the striatum, have been tried with mixed results. Implantation of adrenal medullary grafts has not been encouraging; the improvement appears to be transient.

Prognosis

It is characteristic of the disease that younger people, with onset of symptoms at ages 15 to 40 years, will experience a more severe form of the disease than older people, with onset in their fifties and sixties. The advance of the disease is slow, with death occurring on average 15 to 20 years after onset. Survival into the eighties is not uncommon, and persons living to past age 90 years have been recorded. Age at onset and age at death frequently show a familial correlation.

Increasing disability from involuntary movements and mental changes often results in death from intercurrent infection. Suicide accounts for approximately 6% of deaths, and 25% of persons with HD attempt suicide at least once.

20.4 Special Implications for the PTA: Huntington's Disease
Education of the client and family about movement disorders, including gait and safety in mobility, is the basis for therapeutic intervention. Clients with HD do fall, but it is surprising that mobility is maintained despite the seemingly precarious arrangements of the limbs and trunk. As the disease progresses, postural stability becomes impaired and axial chorea may throw the client off balance. In clients whose bradykinesia is predominant, there is a propensity to freeze, especially in confined spaces, and this may precipitate falls.

Apraxia, the inability to perform skilled or purposeful movements, may become severe. This impairment may lead to significant disability in performance of ADLs. The client may lose the ability to dress and do self-care activities such as grooming, regardless of cues provided by caregivers.

Positioning to prevent soft tissue deformities and safety in transfers should be taught according to the current movement disorder identified. Both the PTA and the family should understand that these techniques may need to be changed as the movement disorder progresses. The PTA should be aware that it is possible that chorea and bradykinesia are manifested in the patient at the same time because of the progressive neuronal loss in the basal ganglia described earlier.

The ability to intervene with neurotherapeutic techniques, including motor learning, may be limited in the face of the concomitant decline in mental function as the motor system impairments progress.

? MULTIPLE SCLEROSIS

Overview and Definition

Multiple sclerosis (MS) is a major cause of disability in young adults. The name is descriptive of the sclerotic plaques disseminated throughout the CNS that are the hallmark of the disease. There are multiple lesions found throughout the brain and spinal cord. These lesions slow or block neural transmission, resulting in weakness, sensory loss, visual dysfunction, and other symptoms. The course of MS is highly variable. Complications of MS may affect multiple body systems and require profound adjustments in lifestyle and expectations for clients and their families; therefore, a multidisciplinary approach is necessary to optimize clinical care.

MS is a chronic illness that may be manifested in multiple forms and courses. There are four generally recognized subtypes. Relapsing-remitting MS is characterized by relapses or attacks, which are periods of neurologic dysfunction lasting days to months and followed by full or partial recovery. By convention, new symptoms must last at least 24 hours and be separated from other symptoms by at least 30 days to qualify as a new attack. The hallmark is that there is a stable course between relapses. This is the most common pattern, seen in about 85% of newly diagnosed individuals. Secondary progressive MS describes an initial pattern of relapse and remission that changes into a steadily progressive pattern over time in more than 50% of the relapsing individuals. Sometimes there are continued relapses during this phase. This conversion generally occurs 5 to 10 years after the initial onset of relapsing symptoms. Primary progressive MS is a steady decline in neurologic function from the outset with episodes of minimal recovery. The most common clinical presentation of primary progressive MS is myelopathy, a gradual, progressive weakening and wasting of muscles, which is typically seen in persons with onset past the age of 40 years. Progressive-relapsing MS is a progressive disease from the onset with clear exacerbations. This is considered the rarest form of MS.

Incidence

Marked differences in the prevalence of MS exist among different populations and ethnic groups. MS is a disease of temperate climates. Highest known prevalence occurs in the Orkney Islands, off Scotland. MS is also common in

Scandinavia and elsewhere in northern Europe. There are more than 2 million persons affected worldwide; the incidence is 12 per 100,000 persons. In the United States it is estimated that 450,000 people are affected, with about 10,000 new cases per year. Caucasians of northern European descent have significantly higher rates of the disease than other racial groups. MS is extremely rare in Japan and virtually unknown in Africa, but Japanese Americans and African Americans show an increased prevalence.[123] African Americans with MS have a greater likelihood of developing opticospinal MS and transverse myelitis and have a more aggressive disease course than white Americans.[62]

MS rarely begins before adolescence; it rises steadily in incidence from the teens to age 35 years and declines gradually thereafter. Similar to many other autoimmune diseases, MS has a predilection for women, with a female to male ratio of 2.5 : 1. Men have a slightly later age of onset and more severe clinical outcomes than women. Men with MS transmit the disease to their children (independently of the child's sex) more often than do women who have MS.[34] Relapse rates may decline 70% in the third trimester of pregnancy, most likely because of circulating levels of estriol. These facts suggest a complex hormonal modulation of the immune system.

Etiologic and Risk Factors

There is a clear genetic component in the risk of developing MS.[35] When one parent is affected, and especially if that parent developed MS at an early age, such as before 20 years, a child has a fivefold higher risk of developing MS.[128] The human leukocyte antigen (HLA) region on chromosome 6 has been identified as one genetic determinant for MS, but this contributes only a small fraction to the genetic basis of MS.[38] Refinement of the genetic linkage map is in progress. The linkages are complex and may involve multiple weak links that are difficult to identify using current research methods. In Scotland, where risk of developing MS is high, there is an increase in the incidence of HLA-DR2 allele in the population that has a proven correlation to MS. The presence of HLA-DR2 is associated with a nearly twofold increase in the likelihood of having a second attack of MS within 5 years. The severity and course of MS may also be associated with different genes. A variety of genes have been associated with the disease, including interleukin-1b receptor, interleukin-1 receptor antagonist, and immunoglobulin Fc receptor.

Coexisting autoimmune disorders are seen in a majority of individuals, such as Hashimoto's disease, psoriasis, inflammatory bowel disease, and rheumatoid arthritis. Families with a history of MS have autoimmune disorders in greater than 65% of first-degree relatives. Hashimoto's disease, psoriasis, and inflammatory bowel disease are the most common disorders also occurring in family members. The presence of various immune disorders in families with several members with MS suggests that the disease might arise on a background of a generalized susceptibility to autoimmune disorders. A distinct MS phenotype, defined by its association with other autoimmune diseases, segregates with specific genotypes that could underlie the common susceptibility.

Viral infection often precipitates an attack of MS. In fact, it is the only natural event that has been shown unequivocally to increase the risk of a new attack of MS. Less than 10% of infections are followed by relapses, but more than one-third of the relapses are proceeded by infection.[38] The possibility that infections, especially viral infections, actually may cause MS has been investigated for many years. Numerous candidate viruses and a smaller number of bacteria have been proposed and then rejected. Most recently, human herpesvirus 6 and the bacterium *Chlamydia pneumoniae* have been touted as environmental triggers of MS. Research attempting to clarify these issues continues. Vitamin D intake appears to have a protective effect on the risk of developing MS.

Clinical Manifestations

In most individuals, MS is characterized by progressive disability over time, but the amount of accumulated disability varies widely. A benign course may affect up to 20% of individuals and is characterized by an abrupt onset with one or a few relapses followed by complete or nearly complete remitting periods. These individuals experience little or no permanent disability and remain relatively symptom free. This is a designation that can only be made with certainty in retrospect, because there are no perfect prognostic markers. More recent MRI scan data suggest that even in individuals with benign MS there is likely significant progression of lesions.

Each individual's CNS appears to have a different threshold for producing symptoms and signs reflecting the affected regions of the CNS. This threshold, or the capacity of the individual's brain to adapt to the lesions, will determine the severity of the clinical manifestations.

Optic neuritis is often the first manifestation of MS. The optic nerve is an extension of the cerebral cortex, virtually a tract of the CNS, and is therefore subject to the effects of demyelination with the syndrome of optic neuritis. Optic neuritis typically presents as a unilateral, painful decrease or loss of vision. It is commonly associated with visual field defects, decreased color vision, and reduced clarity of vision.[55] Individuals with optic neuritis must be carefully evaluated for an ocular mobility abnormality to determine the possibility of a second anatomically distinct lesion, because the symptoms of blurring may be caused by an eye movement disorder.[78]

Early-onset MS is associated with lesions within the spinal cord. The spinal cord may be abnormal when the brain MRI is normal. However, an abnormal spinal cord is found more than half the time when there are nine or more brain lesions. Approximately 80% to 85% of individuals present with a relapsing-remitting course, with symptoms and signs evolving over days and typically improving over weeks.[134]

Sensory changes are most often the initial complaint. This is often a paresthesia or dysesthesia noted in one extremity or in the head and face. Visual blurring, diplopia, weakness, and balance problems also may be early signs. Often these symptoms are transient and not even reported. It is usually when there is a pattern or the symptoms are unchanging that the person seeks medical attention. Dorsal column symptoms include paresthesias (tingling, pricking) and hypoesthesia (diminished sensitivity). These may begin in an extremity and ascend over hours or several days to include the rest of the leg or arm, the perineum, the trunk, and perhaps other extremities. Other sensory complaints include a feeling of swelling, of wetness, or that the body part is tightly wrapped. Involvement of a cord level is diagnostically helpful in distinguishing this attack from a peripheral neuropathologic incident. Other positive dorsal column signs are loss of vibration, position, and two-point discrimination. Sensory complaints are often not substantiated by objective findings, especially if the symptoms are mild or the remission has already begun before the individual is examined. For example, the feeling of numbness may not result in a loss of response to pinprick.

The single most common and most disabling symptom of MS is fatigue.[56] Fatigue is typically present in midafternoon and may take the form of increased motor weakness with effort, mental fatigue, and sleepiness. MS-related fatigue presents as an overwhelming feeling of tiredness in those who have done little and are not depressed. People who are depressed, whether they have or do not have MS, often do not sleep properly, eat properly, or feel well. They may describe this as fatigue, but the treatment revolves around the treatment of depression. Deconditioning and lack of endurance may lead to fatigue.

Neuromuscular or short-circuiting fatigue is common. The demyelinated nerve fires again and again until it shorts when it is called upon to do a repetitive task. Thus progressive resistive exercises often result in a feeling of increased fatigue and weakness rather than a feeling of increased strength. Short breaks with energy conservation can make this fatigue less prominent.

Spasticity, velocity-dependent stiffness about a joint, is an extremely common problem with MS, occurring in 90% of all cases. It can vary from nonexistent to severe, even in the same person, and from moment to moment, making its management challenging. It seems to be the result of disequilibrium in the ascending and descending excitatory and inhibitory pathways in the brain and spinal cord. GABA and other neurotransmitters are involved. Often those who have significant spasticity use their spasticity to walk, transfer, and manage their daily living. Treatment becomes an issue only if the spasticity is causing discomfort, pain, or problems with daily living. Pain, either from an injury or from a bladder infection, exacerbates spasticity. Thus the management of spasticity begins with the removal of noxious stimuli. In some individuals, spasticity can be intractable. The high doses of medications necessitated by this circumstance sedate and cause disability on their own. Spasms may accompany the spasticity and usually are more severe and frequent at night. They often interrupt the sleep cycle, even in those who do not recognize their awakenings. This may lead to severe fatigue the next day; thus minimizing nocturnal spasms is important. Associated signs of upper motor neuron syndrome may include clonus, spontaneous extensor or flexor spasms, positive Babinski's sign, and loss of precise autonomic control.[94,99,129]

Weakness in MS usually is a result of decreased neuromuscular impulses secondary to demyelination and axonal loss. As discussed previously, progressive resistive exercises may contribute to fatigue and give the appearance of increasing weakness. Signs of muscle weakness secondary to damage of the motor cortex and tracts reflect the loss of orderly recruitment and rate modulation of motor neurons. Muscle activation patterns and agonist–antagonist relationships are disturbed.

Heat, either from increased ambient temperature or from fever, often increases weakness. This may be the result of a conduction block. Cooling often allows more efficient conduction and improved strength if there is appropriate innervation.

Involvement at the level of the brainstem reflects lesions of cranial nerves III through XII at the root, nuclear, or bulbar level. Trigeminal neuralgia (also called tic douloureux) is a shocklike pain in the face. Although not a common finding, it is highly characteristic of MS in a young person. Spasm or weakness of facial muscles can also be seen. Dysarthria, abnormal speech resulting from poor control of the muscles of speech, and dysphagia, including signs of gurgling, coughing, weight loss, pneumonia, choking, or a weak voice, can present in brainstem involvement.

There can also be gaze palsies, the loss of active control of eye movement, and nystagmus (involuntary rhythmic tremor of the eye). Intranuclear ophthalmoplegia is the most common gaze palsy, resulting in lateral gaze paralysis, and is caused by demyelination of the pontine medial longitudinal fasciculus, an area of the brain's white matter involved in the control of eye movement. Other lesions in the brainstem and reticular formation can cause other palsies, resulting in difficulty with conjugate gaze and ipsilateral gaze palsy. Idiopathic nystagmus that improves over time also can be caused by lesions in the vestibular nuclei or cerebellum.

Other abnormalities of ocular mobility, such as instability of fixation or inability to suppress the vestibuloocular response, are related to lesions involving brainstem nuclei and tracts. Vertigo, the sensation of spinning, may appear suddenly and in dramatic fashion with gait unsteadiness and vomiting. In MS this reflects a brainstem rather than end organ vestibular disorder; a careful look at associated brainstem symptoms will help to distinguish the cause.

Coordination (ataxia) problems often accompany tremor and are among the most difficult symptoms to manage. Compensatory techniques taught via exercises can be helpful but rarely enough to satisfy. Cerebellar syndrome deficits may be symmetric, with all four limbs involved, or asymmetric, with only one side affected. Manifestations include ataxia, hypotonia, and truncal weakness, causing postural and movement disorders. Dysarthria of cerebellar origin (scanning speech, producing abnormalities in the rhythm of speech) is common. Cerebellar signs are often associated with the progressive phases of the illness.[145]

Pain is surprisingly common in MS, occurring in 50% of individuals. The pain usually is a burning neuropathic type. It may be disturbing, and pain medicine offers little if any relief. The distribution of the pain may not follow any recognizable neurologic distribution. It can be paroxysmal in nature but often is fairly constant, with nocturnal worsening when the body is at rest in bed. Another clinical symptom is Lhermitte's sign, a momentary electricity-like sensation evoked by neck flexion or cough.

Depression is a primary symptom of MS because of actual changes in the brain and its chemistry. It can occur as a direct result of the MS plaques or as a reaction to the diagnosis or disability. Depression may lead to greater disability than that caused by the level of neurologic impairment. Medication use for other symptoms may contribute to the cognitive problems with sedation and confusion; thus, these must be reviewed regularly in those who have dulled cognition. Depression may be an additive culprit and is treatable if recognized. There is no question that reactive (exogenous) depression occurs frequently in MS and is amenable to counseling and other nonpharmacologic techniques, but the brain disease seen in MS clearly leads to chemical (endogenous) depression in many. Cognitive decline is of significance in up to 50% of persons with MS.[132] Memory loss is the most common cognitive

problem, and there commonly are a variety of slowed response types. The suicide rate for MS seems greater than that for many other neurologic diseases, some of which have a worse perceived prognosis.

Bladder and bowel symptoms are common and usually occur when the spinal cord is involved. Bladder urgency, frequency, and incontinence associated with an overactive bladder are often seen early in the disease and generally precede incontinence. Bladder issues are prominent in those who have MS. The bladder can present itself with frequency, urgency, hesitancy, and incontinence with differing mechanisms. Most frequent is the small, failure-to-store bladder characterized by a low postvoid residual. This can be measured by catheterization or ultrasound. It often has uncontrollable contractions.

More problematic from a management point of view is the large, failure-to-empty bladder. It overfills with residuals from 200 to 900 mL and presents with the same symptomatology despite looking different anatomically and physiologically. Frequently, there is a dyssynergia between the bladder and the urinary sphincter, causing similar symptoms from yet another mechanism. Residual urine after emptying, with subsequent overflow incontinence and heightened risk of urinary tract infections, is a problem for 50% of persons with MS, especially later in the course of the disease. This may require intermittent or chronic catheterization, or use of the Credé method (manual pressure on the bladder to express urine).[14] Neurogenic disorders may also impair bowel function, resulting in incontinence or constipation.

Bowel function is affected less than bladder function but can be problematic. Irritable bowel is a common associated problem, and regulating the bowel often means changing treatments, depending on the circumstances. It is better to be slightly constipated than slightly loose.[129]

Sexual expression may require special attention in MS. Relationships remain of utmost importance and need to be stressed, without diminishing the importance of the actual sexual performance in the face of disability. In men, erectile dysfunction is frequent. Occasionally, penile prostheses may be placed. This is less common today because of alternative treatment options. Female sexual expression may be diminished by vaginal dryness or decreased or altered sensation in the vaginal area.

Unique symptoms in MS are called paroxysmal because they come in bouts. Sometimes they are sensory in nature and may be painful. Trigeminal neuralgia is a common example of this type of painful, paroxysmal symptom. This lancinating, electrical sensation along the distribution of a branch of the trigeminal nerve can be terribly disabling. It may be a stand-alone problem in some individuals but also is a symptom associated with MS. Periodic electrical sensation down the spine with the bending of the neck is called Lhermitte's sign, another paroxysmal sensory symptom. These types of sensations occasionally may be felt in other parts of the body. Often the paroxysmal symptoms are motor in nature. They may be twitching of an eyelid or myokymia in the facial muscles. They may manifest as a true spasm of an arm in an extended or, occasionally, flexed position lasting for seconds. They can occur frequently, several times an hour. The spasm may occur with speech as a paroxysmal dysarthria or speech arrest. All of these can be disconcerting to the individual and the clinician.

Medical Management

Diagnosis

No clinical sign or diagnostic test is unique to MS, but a typical clinical syndrome with typical MRI of the brain or spinal cord and exclusion of other similar illnesses can result in a correct diagnosis very rapidly. MRI of the brain and spinal cord is critical to the diagnosis of MS. It is, however, important to first exclude other potentially treatable causes of the presenting symptoms before making a diagnosis of MS. Box 20.8 shows some examples of differential diseases for which screening should be done. The corpus callosum is usually involved in MS, whereas this is not as common in hypoxic-ischemic diseases. This is because this structure receives a unique double blood supply, and with short arterioles, perfusion deficits may be less likely to result in injury.

The whole spinal cord can be imaged with high resolution and phased-array coils, showing abnormalities in 80% to 90% of individuals with MS, usually without accompanying neurologic symptoms or signs. Hypoxic-ischemic disease does not present with spinal cord abnormalities. Incidental spinal cord lesions do not occur with aging and are rarely reported in other immune-mediated disorders. Most individuals with early MS have lesions within the spinal cord, but imaging may not be performed, so they may not be isolated. Spinal cord lesions tend to increase as the number of brain lesions rises; this is associated with higher risk for a second attack and a diagnosis of clinical MS. Ultimately, abnormal brain MRI scans are present in more than 90% of individuals with clinically definite MS. Normal brain MRI scans may represent disease that is relatively restricted to the spinal cord.

Reductions in nerve fiber density are seen in the spinal cord, including in otherwise normal-appearing tissue, and are likely related to permanent disability. Axonal loss can be profound in later stages of disease.

Fig. 20.5 shows the plaques seen on MRI. The lesions do not always correlate with the clinical signs, and there can be evidence of focal lesions in the absence of disease. In fact, the vast majority of enhancing lesions are considered to be asymptomatic when they first appear on the brain scan. However, there is a correlation between periods of clinical worsening of the disease and increases in the total number of lesions, the number of new lesions, and the total area of enhancement on MRI.[22] Thus a single brain MRI scan after a first event is highly prognostic of development of clinically definite MS.[111] Fig. 20.6 shows an example of aggressive MS over 2 years revealed in MRI imaging.

Contrast enhancement in CT and MRI suggests inflammation but is more accurately a measure of leakage of moderate-size molecules across the damaged tight junctions of the CNS endothelium. The enhancement pattern (size, shape, solid versus ring) may be variable within and more so between individuals, which reflects a heterogeneous pathology. Ring enhancement, for example, may suggest a more severe pathology. Fig. 20.7 demonstrates the development of a T2-weighted hyperintense lesion by serial MRI. The correlation between the pattern of enhancement, the underlying pathology, and the clinical course in given individuals may not be straightforward. Monitoring serial MRI studies with enhancement helps to identify agents that may be active against the early inflammatory stage of MS.[136]

BOX 20.8   Differential Diagnosis of Multiple Sclerosis

Other Inflammatory Demyelinating Central Nervous System Conditions

- Acute disseminated encephalomyelitis
- Neuromyelitis optica

Systemic or Organ-Specific Inflammatory Diseases

- Systemic lupus erythematosus
- Sjögren's syndrome

Inflammatory Bowel Disease

- Vasculitis
- Periarteritis nodosa
- Primary central nervous system angiitis
- Susac's syndrome
- Eales' disease
- Granulomatous diseases
- Sarcoidosis

Infectious Disorders

- Lyme neuroborreliosis
- Syphilis
- Viral myelitis
- Progressive multifocal leukoencephalitis
- Subacute sclerosing panencephalitis

Cerebrovascular Disorders

- Multiple emboli
- Hypercoagulable states

- Sneddon's syndrome
- Neoplasms
- Metastasis
- Lymphoma
- Paraneoplastic syndromes

Metabolic Disorders

- Vitamin B_{12} deficiency
- Vitamin E deficiency
- Central (or extra) pontine myelinolysis
- Leukodystrophies (especially adrenomyeloneuropathy)
- Leber's hereditary optic neuropathy

Structural Lesions

- Spinal cord compression
- Chiari malformation
- Syringomyelia/syringobulbia
- Foramen magnum lesions
- Spinal arteriovenous malformation/dural fistula

Degenerative Diseases

- Hereditary spastic paraparesis
- Spinocerebellar degeneration
- Olivopontocerebellar atrophy

Psychiatric Disorders

- Conversion reactions
- Malingering

From Goetz CG: Textbook of clinical neurology, ed 3, Philadelphia, 2007, Saunders.

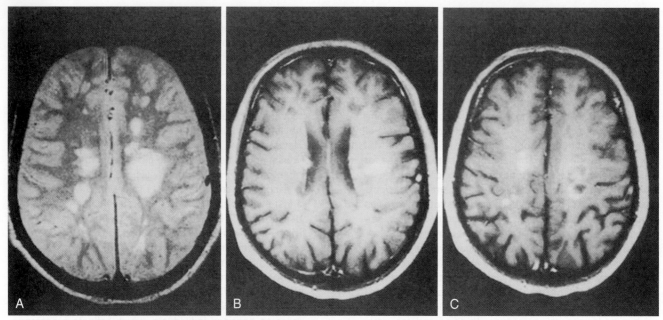

FIG. 20.5 (A) Typical scattered, variably sized plaques in the brain associated with the diagnosis of multiple sclerosis (MS). (B) Contrast-enhanced magnetic resonance imaging reveals scattered area of solid and ring-shaped enhancement. (C) Note the atrophy, greater than would be expected for the person's age, a common finding in MS. (From Ramsey R: *Neuroradiology*, Philadelphia, 1994, Saunders.)

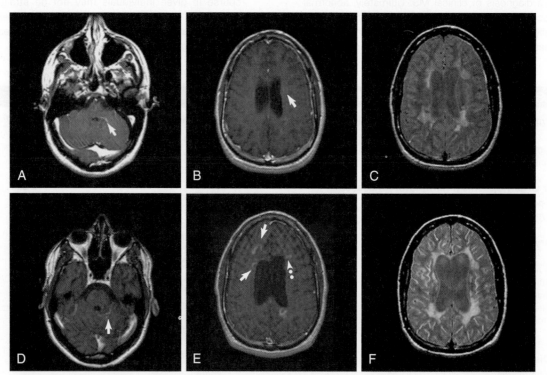

FIG. 20.6 Aggressive multiple sclerosis over 2 years. Disease was initially relapsing-remitting but converted relatively quickly to secondary progressive MS. *Top row:* Contrast-enhanced left pons (A) and left frontal-parietal white matter (B), both showing a relatively rare edge enhancement pattern *(arrows).* Typical confluent T2 hyperintensities and mild-moderate volume loss based on lateral ventricle size (C). *Bottom row:* Two years later magnetic resonance image shows different edge-enhancing lesions *(arrows)* in posterior fossa (D) and both edge enhancement *(arrows)* and ring enhancement *(dotted arrow)* in deep white matter along the lateral ventricles (E). Progressive volume loss based on moderately large lateral ventricles and more extensive confluent T2 hyperintensity is seen in F. (From Simon JH: Update on multiple sclerosis, *Radiol Clin North Am* 44(1):79–100, 2006.)

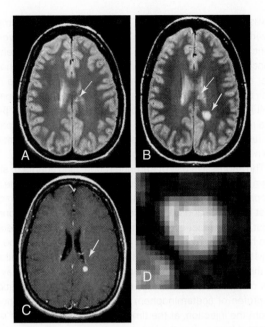

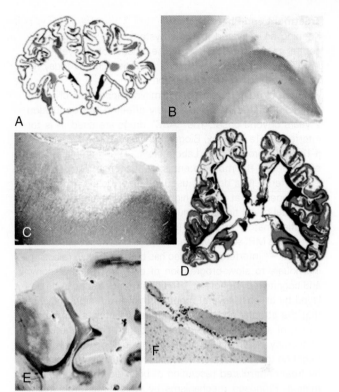

FIG. 20.7 Development of a T2 hyperintense lesion by serial magnetic resonance imaging. (A) Case of relapsing multiple sclerosis with low T2 hyperintense lesion burden, including chronic lesions in the corpus callosum *(arrow)*. (B) One month later, a new T2 hyperintense lesion develops in the left parietooccipital white matter *(solid arrow)*, whereas the corpus callosum lesions remain stable *(dotted arrow)*. (C) Corresponding enhancement in acute lesion *(arrow)* from blood-brain barrier breakdown and concurrent inflammation. (D) Exploded view of the new lesion showing the complex structure, centrally hyperintense, most likely from mixed pathology including demyelination, matrix including glial change, and, importantly, axonal degeneration. The intermediate black ring may be a zone of macrophage infiltration, and the outer ring is likely from edema. (From Simon JH: Update on multiple sclerosis, Radiol Clin North Am 44(1):79–100, 2006.)

FIG. 20.8 Cortical plaques in progressive forms of multiple sclerosis (MS). Cortical demyelination and diffuse white matter inflammation are hallmarks of primary progressive MS (PPMS) and secondary progressive MS (SPMS). (A and D) Schematic lesion maps based on whole hemispheric sections from two archival cases of progressive MS. Case A (PPMS): A 37-year-old man with a history of gradually progressive hemiparesis (left greater than right), sphincter dysfunction, and dysarthria, requiring use of a wheelchair within 6 years of disease onset. Patient died at age 72 years of aspiration pneumonia and acute myocardial infarction. Case D (SPMS): A 33-year-old woman initially presenting with diplopia and hemiataxia that partially resolved following a short course of corticosteroids. Subsequent course characterized by gradually progressive dysarthria, dysphagia, ophthalmoplegia, and limb and gait ataxia, requiring use of a wheelchair within 7 years of disease onset. She also developed a focal seizure disorder 4 years before death and died at age 46 years of aspiration pneumonia. (B and C) Subpial cortical demyelination is demonstrated in Case A at low (B) and high (C) magnification. (E) Extensive subpial demyelination involving multiple gyri is illustrated in Case D at low magnification. (F) Meningeal inflammation may be prominent, often in close proximity to areas with subpial cortical demyelination. Proteolipid protein immunocytochemistry; *green,* focal demyelinated plaques in the white matter; *orange,* cortical demyelination; *blue,* demyelinated lesions in the deep gray matter. (From Pirko I: Gray matter involvement in multiple sclerosis, Neurology 68:634–642, 2007.)

Individuals with MS have significant atrophy of both white matter and gray matter. It is considered an important measure in MS because in most cases it likely reflects irreversible injury, much of which is from axon loss, but with additional contributions from myelin loss and structural changes from astrogliosis. The demyelinated cortex contains apoptotic neurons. Cortical demyelination could affect neurons, dendrites, and axons, which may lead to disease progression. The cerebral cortex may be affected by tissue loss and atrophy, particularly in areas adjacent to severe white matter pathology. Neurons in such lesions may show signs of retrograde damage as described earlier. Fig. 20.8 shows changes related to progressive forms of MS.

Whole-brain atrophy reflects the destructive aspects of the disease. The data linking brain atrophy to clinical impairments suggest that irreversible tissue destruction is a major determinant of disease progression, whereas white matter lesion activity has less correlation. The strongest correlations between MRI measures and disability may be those provided by atrophy measures. Confounding factors must be considered when assessing whether loss of brain volume directly indicates tissue atrophy. Secondary progressive disease causes significantly more atrophy of both white matter and

gray matter and a significantly higher lesion load than relapsing-remitting disease.[141] Primary progressive disorders show decreased numbers and volume of enhancing lesions, related to the less intense inflammation. Spinal cord pathology has been hypothesized to be an important factor in disease progression in primary progressive MS but is not always predictive (see Fig. 20.8).

Treatment and Pharmacology

Keeping an activated immune system from getting to the central myelinated fibers slows the process of demyelination in MS. Therefore the principle of treatment in MS today revolves around immune modulation.

Current drug therapy can diminish approximately one-third of the attacks in the actively affected MS population 2 years beyond onset. The "ABC" drugs are used. A is for interferon β-1a (Avonex, Biogen Idec), and B is for interferon β-1b (Betaseron, Berlex Laboratories). The higher the dose of interferon, the more potent is the response. Rebif, another interferon β-1a drug, is used in higher doses. It is given subcutaneously at a 46% higher dose three times weekly, for a total of 4.4 times as much drug as Avonex. The potent antiinflammatory effects of interferons have a dramatic effect on the MRI scans, with a decrease in contrast-enhancing lesions.[85,88] Interferon β-1a also has been shown in relapsing individuals to slow progression of disability, brain atrophy, and cognitive dysfunction.[74] The treatment effect can be delayed by at least several months. This delay might indicate that the atrophy occurring in the first months is the culmination of a cascade of events that began before the onset of therapy. Alternatively, the ongoing loss of brain volume might be the result of "pseudoatrophy," such as that caused by treatment-related resolution of brain edema and inflammation. Proposed mechanisms by which interferon might limit brain atrophy include increasing nerve growth factors, limiting immune-mediated destructive inflammation, and limiting toxic mechanisms such as pathologic iron deposition.[98] Thus, the question remains as to whether controlling acute relapses and inflammation will ultimately be adequate. Other factors may have an influence on demyelination and axon injury.[107]

The C drug, glatiramer acetate (Copaxone, Teva Pharmaceutical Industries) is a polypeptide that appears to fool the immune system. It seems to decrease the attack by blocking immune cells headed toward myelin, preventing damage. It also has a partial and delayed but significant effect of limiting the rate of brain atrophy in relapsing-remitting MS. Glatiramer acetate has gained wide acceptance as one option for the treatment of relapsing-remitting MS because there is less occurrence of the flulike symptoms that are associated with the interferons. Although its precise immunologic mechanisms continue to be investigated, current views suggest that its principal effect may be mediated by a shift from a proinflammatory cell bias to an antiinflammatory cell bias. Ongoing studies are exploring the possibility that glatiramer acetate confers neuroprotection and are seeking novel ways to use the agent alone or in combination with other medications.[96]

Mitoxantrone (Novantrone, Immunex) is used to modify relapsing and secondary progressive MS. It is the only drug approved for treatment of secondary progressive MS. It presumably works by depression of T-cell counts and removal of activated T cells from the immune repertoire. Because of potential side effects, its use is limited at present to individuals whose MS is clearly advancing in spite of aggressive ABC therapy or who already are in a secondary progressive phase. The ABC drugs have not yet been found conclusively to be helpful in secondary progressive disease, and no drugs have been found effective in primary progressive disease.[135]

Natalizumab (Tysabri) is a monoclonal antibody that prevents immune cells from moving from the blood to the CNS. It was originally approved by the FDA based on a dramatic lowering of relapse rate and a 50% reduction in the development of a sustained increase in disability. This treatment is a once-monthly intravenous infusion. Unfortunately, shortly after approval of the treatment by the FDA, there were two fatal cases of progressive multifocal leukoencephalopathy (PML) when it was used in conjunction with interferon β-1a. As a result, the distribution of natalizumab was halted, pending further evaluation. Studies continue, and it may emerge again for use in treating MS, perhaps as a monotherapy.[149]

The aggressive use of immune-modulating agents to slow down the actual disease process has contributed to the development of a whole new set of symptoms that the clinician must recognize and manage. Interferon initiation often brings about a fever reaction, which may be disabling to the person who has MS. It often is recommended that interferon be administered in the evening before going to bed. This allows for the impact of the fever during the night, when it may be less disabling to activities of living. Antipyretic medications (ibuprofen or acetaminophen) may be administered 4 hours before the injection, at the time of injection, and then, if necessary, 4 hours after the injection.

Fingolimod (FTY720) is a new oral immunomodulating agent under evaluation for the treatment of relapsing MS. Its final effect is also to reduce the normal circulation and trafficking of leukocytes. It also nears the 50% mark for decreasing the mean cumulative number of lesions. A phase III trial is under way to definitively assess clinical efficacy. Encephalopathy is a risk, and fingolimod is also associated with an initial reduction in the heart rate.[76]

Despite the time and effort given to slow the disease, the bulk of current intervention is devoted to symptomatic management. Improvement in the ability to control symptoms through therapy and medications can enhance quality of life in the individual with MS. Amantadine, pemoline, modafinil, and other medicines can reduce fatigue. Depression and sleep disorders may contribute to fatigue and must be recognized and treated appropriately. Centrally acting and peripherally acting muscle relaxants, such as baclofen (Lioresal), tizanidine, and dantrolene, decrease hypertonicity and leg spasms. Anticonvulsants and antidepressant medicines are used to treat pain. Intrathecal baclofen pumps reduce severe spasticity. Oxybutynin and tolterodine diminish bladder hyperactivity. Focal injections of BTX can be helpful in decreasing muscle spasticity.[1] Repetitive transcranial magnetic stimulation may improve spasticity in MS. The antiepileptic agents and antidepressant treatments often are effective in modulating the painful symptoms. Gabapentin in relatively high doses often is necessary for the desired effect. Spasms occurring during the day usually are handled best by the addition of the antiepileptic medications, including gabapentin and topiramate.

Amitriptyline is helpful, especially at night, because it can sedate and provide pain relief. Clonazepam, given at bedtime, can aid in sleep initiation and decrease spasms with minimum side effects. Diazepam has a similar effect. Dose escalation should be avoided. Dopamine agonists and dopamine itself also decrease nocturnal spasms reasonably effectively at low dosages.

All of these treatments require adjustment from time to time to maintain some relief. All medications currently available to control symptoms of MS have potential side effects and therefore must be used judiciously. Careful monitoring of systems affected by MS is essential to medical management.[127]

Both corticosteroids (prednisone, cortisone, and methylprednisolone) and adrenocorticotrophic hormone are known to shorten the recovery period after an acute MS attack. There appears to be no consensus about the optimal form, dosage, route, or duration of corticosteroid therapy, but there is now a consensus statement from the American Academy of Neurology regarding treatment of acute optic neuritis with methylprednisolone. Oral prednisone should not be used. Corticosteroids can alter almost every aspect of the immune system. Corticosteroid-induced restoration of the blood-brain barrier, which becomes less effective during active demyelination or plaque formation, has an antiedema benefit and may prevent circulating toxins, viruses, or immunoactive cells from entering the CNS. Decreased activity of the macrophages and lymphocytes results in less damage to the myelin in response to steroid therapy.[54] Individuals with severe demyelination who do not respond to corticosteroids may improve with plasma exchange.[79,154]

Based on the rapid advances in our understanding of the immunopathogenesis of MS, a variety of experimental approaches presently are under study. These include the hormonal agent estriol, matrix metalloproteinase inhibitors, statin drugs, adhesion molecule antibodies, T-cell peptides, combination therapies (especially ABC drugs with other types of agents), intravenous immunoglobulin, and stem cell transplantation. All these are preventive and not restorative of previously damaged CNS function. Growth factors that enhance CNS remyelination are being studied as a method to restore the loss of oligodendrocytes in MS.[114] Findings of neural stem cells in the adult CNS and the potential of blood-derived stem cells to become neural cells offer the possibility of transplanting cells into the CNS that will restore function. Studies on intense immunosuppression with bone marrow transplantation (autologous and stem cell) continue, but results are not positive enough to recommend its use.

Prognosis

The average frequency of attacks of MS is approximately 1 per year. The attacks vary in severity; therefore close observation is required to reliably track the attack frequency. Attacks tend to be most common in the early years of MS and become less frequent in later years, regardless of the disability. The risk for rapid development of moderate disability may be greater in persons in whom the frequency of attacks is higher than average.

Multiple factors may predict a severe course, such as motor and cerebellar symptoms, disability after the first attack, and short time interval between attacks. Numerous relapses within the first year negatively influence the clinical course. Conversely, sensory symptoms, infrequent attacks, full neurologic recovery after a relapse, and a low level of disability after 5 to 7 years may be associated with an improved prognosis.

Burden of disease on MRI scans may be the strongest predictor of clinical outcomes. Over 14 years, there was no significant disability accrued in individuals with normal MRI findings at the time of diagnosis, whereas MRI scans with greater than 10 lesions predicted that individuals would require a cane for walking within that same time frame.

A change in lesion load within the first year also is a negative predictor of outcome. Late-onset MS is not necessarily associated with a worse outcome. Progression of primary progressive and relapsing MS differed little between late-onset and early adult–onset disease. The individuals with late-onset disease were older when reaching an Expanded Disability Status Scale score of 6.[146]

Because disability is often significant in individuals with MS, lifestyle changes are frequently necessary. Movement impairment is frequently associated with MS, and difficulty in walking is a major disability. If MS is untreated, 15 years after diagnosis 50% of individuals with MS will require the use of an assistive device to walk, and at 20 years 50% will be wheelchair bound. About one-fourth of persons with MS will require human assistance with ADLs.[78]

It is the coexistence of physical and cognitive impairments together with emotional and social issues in a disease with an uncertain course that makes MS rehabilitation unique and challenging. Individual rehabilitation improves functional independence but has only limited success in improving the level of neurologic impairment. Severely disabled people derive as much as or more benefit than those who are less disabled, but cognitive problems and ataxia tend to be refractory. Cost and utility are significantly correlated with functional capacity.[81] There is now good evidence that exercise can improve fitness and function for those with mild MS and helps to maintain function for those with moderate to severe disability. Several different forms of exercise have been investigated. For most individuals, aerobic exercise that incorporates a degree of balance training and socialization is most effective. Time constraints, access, impairment level, personal preferences, motivations, and funding sources influence the prescription for exercise and other components of rehabilitation. Just as immunomodulatory drugs must be taken on a continual basis and be adjusted as the disease progresses, so should rehabilitation be viewed as an ongoing process to maintain and restore maximum function and quality of life.[26]

Life expectancy is reduced by a modest amount in MS; the risk of dying of MS is strongly associated with severe disability. The death rate in persons who are unable to stand or walk is more than four times that in persons the same age without MS. In mildly disabled individuals, the death rate is approximately 1.5 times that of the age-matched population. Persons with more frequent initial episodes with rapidly developing disability have a poorer long-term outcome. Individuals with primary progressive disease also have decreased life expectancy. Suicide is more than seven times more common than in age-matched controls, and depression must be treated aggressively.

20.5 Special Implications for the PTA: Multiple Sclerosis
Because MS is typically progressive, it is expected that individuals will need to access the medical community with greater needs over time. Maintaining function in the household and community is a typical rehabilitation goal. Although people with MS are advised to be as active as possible in all ways of life, there is no consensus on the best method to attain that goal. Activity performed in accordance with individual strength and abilities (avoiding exhaustion) will help to prevent or diminish the complications leading to disability. Skin breakdown following sensory loss and immobility is

BOX 20.9 Kurtzke Expanded Disability Status Scale

0.0 Normal neurologic examination
1.0 No disability, minimal symptoms
1.5 No disability, minimal signs in more than one functional level
2.0 Slightly greater disability in one functional system
2.5 Slightly greater disability in two functional systems
3.0 Moderate disability in one functional system; fully ambulatory
3.5 Fully ambulatory but with moderate disability in one functional system and more than minimal disability in several others
4.0 Fully ambulatory without aid, self-sufficient, up and about 12 h/day despite relatively severe disability; able to walk about 500 m without aid or rest
4.5 Fully ambulatory without aid, up and about much of the day, able to work a full day; may otherwise have some limitation of full activity or require minimal assistance; characterized by relatively severe disability; able to walk about 300 m without aid or rest
5.0 Ambulatory for about 200 m without aid or rest; disability severe enough to impair full daily activities (e.g., to work a full day without special provisions)
5.5 Ambulatory for about 100 m without aid or rest; disability severe enough to preclude full daily activities

6.0 Intermittent or unilateral constant assistance (cane, crutch, brace) required to walk about 100 m with or without resting
6.5 Constant bilateral assistance (canes, crutches, braces) required to walk about 20 m without resting
7.0 Unable to walk beyond approximately 5 m with aid; essentially restricted to a wheelchair; wheels self in standard wheelchair and transfers alone; up and about in wheelchair 12 h/day
7.5 Unable to take more than a few steps; restricted to wheelchair; may need aid in transfer; wheels self but cannot be in standard wheelchair a full day; may require motorized wheelchair
8.0 Essentially restricted to bed or chair or perambulated in wheelchair but may be out of bed much of the day; retains many self-care functions; generally has effective use of arms
8.5 Essentially restricted to bed much of the day; has some effective use of arm or arms; retains some self-care functions
9.0 Helpless bed patient; can communicate and eat
9.5 Totally helpless bed patient; unable to communicate effectively, eat, or swallow
10.0 Death from multiple sclerosis

Modified from Kurtzke J: Rating neurological impairment in multiple sclerosis: an expanded disability status scale (EDSS), Neurology 33:1444, 1983.

a common problem that can be controlled by appropriate skin care and positioning.

Fatigue and weakness are the complaints most often taken to a PTA. The Modified Fatigue Index is a self-report scale to monitor changes in the level of fatigue. This can be helpful for PTAs to measure changes associated with interventions or to describe changes in function following a relapse.

The replacement of oral spasticity medications with intrathecal baclofen has become more routine, and the therapy team should be involved in the dosing and management. Any spasticity the individual is having during ADLs may be altered. Thus transferring techniques may require a different approach. The perception of strength that may be given by stiffness may disappear, giving the perception of weakness.

In establishing a training program for endurance and strengthening, careful consideration of the neurologic changes is critical.[64] Careful monitoring of exercise appears to be necessary because of impaired cardiopulmonary systems. Individuals with MS have poor exercise tolerance as a result of respiratory muscle dysfunction.[73] Repetitive submaximal strength training appears to be of benefit to most people, with an increase in both peak torque generated and a decrease in the reported perception of fatigue.[139] Changes achieved in strength and endurance are probably the result of the normal physiologic changes that are associated with this type of training. Clients demonstrating increased reflex activity with exertion will need a longer time to recover after fatigue and may notice increased extensor tone and difficulty with flexion. Use of cooling vests to lower core temperature during exercise can be beneficial to those who have heat intolerance. It is important to realize that for most people with MS, fatigue will exacerbate symptoms.[33]

Establishing individually designed fitness programs is an important role of the PT and PTA. Models for such programs can lead the PTA in the appropriate direction and provide protocols taking into consideration the common concerns associated with MS.[80]

Understanding movement disorders common to lesions in specific brain regions and the spinal column is essential for the PTA. Analysis of movement is the most critical skill necessary to determine sensory

and motor deficits that may be contributing to loss of postural control and mobility. The PTA must be able to identify the specific impairments to maintain the appropriate stretching and strengthening exercises. A successful exercise program depends on a number of factors essential to motor learning, including practice, adequate feedback, and knowledge of results. The client with MS is often restricted in practice by neurologic fatigue and by impairments that disrupt sensory feedback, attention, memory, and motivation. The PTA will need to carefully identify the client's resources and abilities and capitalize on them to minimize the level of disability.[112]

A common disability scale used by rehabilitation professionals and researchers working with patients with MS is the Kurtzke Expanded Disability Status Scale (Box 20.9). It is used to monitor changes in disability levels and has value in determining prognosis. PTAs working with this patient population should become adept at using this tool.[63]

The day-to-day variation in MS makes determination of an appropriate training program challenging. Use of both impairment and disability scales will assist in monitoring changes. The scales show the relative improvement after intervention or overall decline regardless of intervention. The scales are useful in tracking the disease process for both the client and the health care provider. PTAs making decisions regarding the need for adaptive equipment can use the scales to establish trends in the course of the disease.

PARKINSONISM AND PARKINSON'S DISEASE

Overview and Definition

Atrophy of the brain leading to degeneration of neurons in the basal ganglia can be caused by a variety of disorders that are not well understood. These include striatonigral degeneration, Shy–Drager syndrome, progressive supranuclear palsy, olivopontocerebellar atrophy, corticobasal ganglionic degeneration, and diffuse Lewy body disease. Parkinsonian features can be manifested as a part of other diseases affecting the CNS, such as atherosclerosis, ALS, and HD.[152]

PD, or idiopathic parkinsonism, is a chronic progressive disease of the motor component of the CNS, characterized by rigidity, tremor, bradykinesia, and postural instability. The disease is thought to result from a complex interaction between multiple predisposing genes and environmental effects, although these interactions are still poorly understood. PD is still regarded as a sporadic neurodegenerative disorder, characterized by the loss of midbrain dopamine neurons and presence of Lewy body inclusions.

Incidence

Parkinsonism, including PD, affects more than 800,000 adults in the United States, with prevalence rates of 350 per 100,000. Approximately 42% of parkinsonism is related to PD. The lifetime risk of developing parkinsonism is 7.5% according to a Mayo study. There appears to be a higher rate among white Americans and Europeans compared with black Africans. African Americans and Chinese in Taiwan have higher rates of disease than their counterparts in West Africa or China.[13] PD becomes increasingly common with advancing age, affecting more than 1 person in every 100 older than age 75 years. A possible explanation of the correlation between age and prevalence may be the age-related neuronal vulnerability. Because of the increase in life expectancy, the aging of the baby boomers, and the precision of diagnosis, the incidence of PD is expected to rise. It is estimated that there will be more than 1.5 million persons living with PD in the United States and close to 40 million worldwide by the year 2020. The majority of cases begin between the ages of 50 and 79 years. Approximately 10% will develop initial symptoms before the age of 40 years.[87]

Etiologic and Risk Factors

An increasing number of chromosomal features linked to familial parkinsonism have been found, notably PARK1 to PARK11. Among these, seven genes have been identified, four causing autosomal dominant parkinsonism (synuclein, UCHL1, NURR1, LRRK2) and three causing autosomal recessive disease (DJ1, PINK1, parkin). These provide insights into the molecular pathogenesis of the disease, but genetic testing for these mutations is of little clinical relevance. The chance of identifying parkin mutations is less than 5% in sporadic cases with onset at younger than age 45 years. The probability is much greater in those with onset at younger than age 30 years and in those with an affected sibling. Confirmation of this recessive form of disease might be helpful in genetic counseling, because it renders transmission to the subsequent generation very unlikely.[41] Given the late onset of typical PD, it is likely that by the time individuals become symptomatic, many first-degree relatives are deceased from other causes.

Many potential exposures have been cited as possible risk factors for PD. Three major groups include toxic exposures, infection exposures, and a heterogenic group of miscellaneous exposures. Some toxic agents such as carbon monoxide, manganese, cyanide, and methanol can damage the basal ganglia and produce parkinsonian symptoms. A rapidly developing Parkinson-like disease has been linked to the use of 1-methyl-4-phenyl-1,2,3,6-tetrahydropyridine (MPTP), a synthetic narcotic related to heroin. Some neuroleptics can produce a parkinsonian syndrome. In drug-induced parkinsonism, the symptoms can usually be reversed by withdrawal of the drug.

The link to infection exposure remains unresolved, despite years of study. There may still be a possibility that infection

plays a role, based on observations of serum antibody titers for measles virus, rubella virus, herpes simplex virus types 1 and 2, and cytomegalovirus in persons with PD. Pesticides and herbicides may be environmental causes and are likely to produce between 2% and 25% increased risk. If some individuals are determined to be particularly susceptible to low environmental exposure, then pesticides may pose a more serious risk. In every age group, men are more likely than women to develop parkinsonism. This finding is not completely understood, but perhaps hormones may protect women, whereas men may be exposed to more environmental toxins according to their occupational choices. Long-term exposure to either manganese or copper has been linked to an increased incidence of parkinsonism.

More years of formal education appear to increase the risk of PD. Physicians are at significantly increased risk of PD when occupational data are used. In contrast, four occupational groups show a significantly decreased risk of PD according to one source: construction and extractive workers (miners, oil well drillers), production workers (machine operators, fabricators), metalworkers, and engineers.[57]

There is a relatively well-established relationship between PD and a history of smoking. Individuals with a history of smoking seem to have a lower risk of developing PD.

High levels of physical exercise may lower PD risk. The risk of PD appears to be lower among women who report strenuous exercise during early adulthood. Physical exercise can promote secretion of growth factors in the CNS that in turn may contribute to the survival and neuroplasticity of dopaminergic neurons. Moreover, exercise decreases the ratio between dopamine transporter and vesicular monoamine transporter; a decrease in this ratio may lower the susceptibility of dopaminergic neurons to neurotoxins and reduce dopamine oxidation. Finally, physical exercise may activate the dopaminergic system and increase dopamine availability in the striatum. Any of these or other mechanisms may be responsible for the beneficial effects of forced exercise in animal experiments; however, the relevance of these short-term animal findings to possible neuroprotective effects of leisure physical exercise in human PD pathogenesis remains to be established. In the rat model of PD, forced exercise before chemically induced parkinsonism caused a significant increase of glial-derived neurotrophic factor that has neuroprotective effects for dopaminergic neurons.[36]

Clinical Manifestations

Movement disorder is the hallmark of parkinsonism, although other symptoms are evident and may actually precede the impairment of movement. The ability to move is not lost, but there is a problem with movement activation and loss of reflexive or automatic movement. Movement becomes reliant on cortical control. The ability to perform known tasks, such as walking, changing direction, writing, and basic ADLs, is diminished. The considerable variation among individuals in the clinical manifestations and the level of deterioration in movement over time can be explained by the complex mechanism of dysfunction.[45]

The tremor of PD, the most common initial manifestation, often appears unilaterally and may be confined to one upper limb for months or even years. It is first seen as a rhythmic, back-and-forth motion of the thumb and finger, referred to as the pill-rolling tremor. It is most obvious when the arm is at rest or during stressful periods. The tremor starts unilaterally but can eventually spread to all four limbs as well as neck and facial muscles. Tension or exertion will cause the tremor to increase, and it will disappear during sleep. Tremor does not usually impact the functioning of the individual.

Rigidity is an increased response to muscle stretch that appears in both antagonist and agonist muscle groups. Rigidity, like tremor, usually appears unilaterally and proximally in an upper limb and then spreads to the other extremities and trunk. One of the earliest signs of rigidity is the loss of associated movements of the arms when walking. Rigidity is identified when another person is trying to passively move the extremity and there is a jerky response, known as cogwheel rigidity, or a slow and sustained resistance, known as lead-pipe rigidity. Rigidity does not appear to have a direct effect on volitional movement. Axial rigidity usually limits rotation and extension of the trunk and spine. Reduced variability and less adaptation of movement between thoracic rotation and pelvic motion appears early in the onset of PD. This rigidity can decrease the ability to make adjustments of the extremities during functional tasks, such as transfers, reaching, and bed mobility as well as gait.

Bradykinesia is the slowness of movement seen in parkinsonism. Impairment of the normal mechanisms that scale the output of agonist muscles causes the inability to produce, modulate, and terminate quick movements. Persons diagnosed with PD show relatively small EMG bursts in agonist muscles and move the legs in a series of small steps rather than in a single movement. Bradykinesia results from disruption of the neurotransmitter from the internal globus pallidus to the motor cortical regions known as the supplementary motor area and the primary motor cortex.

The slowing of lip and tongue movements during talking causes a garbled speech pattern. There is loss of fine motor skills with the gradual development of small, cramped writing, or micrographia. Parkinsonism is accompanied often by diminished efficiency of pursuit eye movements, so that small accelerations of eye movement (*saccades*) are required to catch up with a moving target, which causes smooth pursuit eye movements to be jerky instead of smooth. Eye movement in the vertical plane may be reduced.

Akinesia is a disorder of movement initiation and is seen in parkinsonism as a paucity of natural and automatic movements, such as crossing the legs or folding the arms. Small gestures associated with expression are reduced. The face is masklike, with infrequent blinking and lack of expression. Freezing, or gait akinesia, is the sudden cessation of movement in the middle of an action sequence, as if the foot is stuck to the floor. Sometimes it is the environment that seems to trigger freezing, such as when the individual walks through a doorway or over a change in surface like stepping from a carpet to a hard floor. Freezing most often affects walking, but it can affect speech, arm movements, and blinking. It is uncommon in the early phase but increases over time.[50,102]

The gait pattern in parkinsonism is highly stereotyped and characterized by impoverished movement. ROM in the joints of the lower extremity is often limited. Trunk and pelvic movement is diminished, resulting in a decreased step length and reciprocal arm swing. The gait is narrow based and shuffling. The speed is decreased. Persons with plantar flexion contractures will toe-walk, and this further narrows the available base of support. In gait, there is a loss of heel strike, reduced toe elevation, reduced movement at the knee joints, loss of dynamic vertical force, reversal of ankle flexion–extension movement, and loss of backward-directed shear force.[120] Festination is

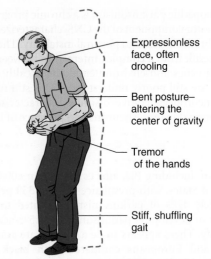

FIG. 20.9 Typical posture that results from Parkinson's disease.

Expressionless face, often drooling

Bent posture—altering the center of gravity

Tremor of the hands

Stiff, shuffling gait

BOX 20.10 **Causes of Balance Impairment in Parkinson's Disease**

- Loss of postural reflexes
- Visuospatial deficits
- Retropulsion
- Start hesitation
- Freezing
- Festinating gait
- Orthostatic hypotension
- True vertigo

---

common when attempting to stop or change direction; the stride becomes smaller but more rapid, and instead of stopping, the individual actually increases speed and is usually stopped by running into something or by falling. Preparatory postural responses to move from a bipedal to single-limb stance are frequently absent for induced steps, which may increase instability during first step.[126] There is reduced ability to adapt to changes of environments or to perform new tasks.

The posture in PD is characterized by flexion of the neck, trunk, hips, and knees (Fig. 20.9). Kyphosis, or extensive flexion of the spine, is the most common postural deformity. Scoliosis, an abnormal lateral curvature of the spine, can result from the unequal distribution of rigidity in posture. Persistent posturing of a forward head and trunk tends to pull the center of gravity forward. This may result in a tendency to keep weight shifted posteriorly to compensate. Postural instability is also associated with abnormal patterns of postural responses, including excessive antagonist activity that results in coactivation of distal and proximal muscles. Adapting to changing support conditions is less efficient in individuals with PD.[103] The ability to sequence motor activity appears to have an impact on postural correction. Abnormal control of the center of mass results in decreased limits of stability.[66] Lateral postural stability is compromised by lack of trunk flexibility. During posterior perturbations, lack of stability appears to be the result of a lack of appropriate knee flexion. Box 20.10 outlines some of the contributions to imbalance seen in individuals with parkinsonism.

Performing dual tasks causes more slowing in individuals who have parkinsonism. Smooth performance of sequential motor tasks is broken down into distinct components. Changing the "set" for an activity is more difficult for the individual with parkinsonism when the context or environment requires a sudden change in activity.

Olfactory function is diminished along with impaired color vision and visual perception.[148] Spatial organization is often disturbed, resulting in difficulty with orientation to the environment. The inability to distinguish self-movement from movement in the environment can contribute to abnormal balance reactions.[23] There is an increased dependence on visual information for motor control. There is strong visual dependency for balance, resulting in the inability to choose a balance strategy based on vestibular information even when the visual surround is unavailable for visual stability.[19]

Most people with PD experience weakness and fatigue once the disease becomes generalized. The person has difficulty sustaining activity and experiences increasing weakness and lethargy as the day progresses. Repetitive motor acts may start out strong but decrease in strength as the activity progresses. This compounds bradykinesia and increases immobility.

Nonmotor symptoms, such as those related to autonomic dysfunction, are common and potentially disabling manifestations of the disease. Loss of neurons in the sympathetic ganglia may cause autonomic dysfunction. This results in excessive sweating, excessive salivation, incontinence, and disabling orthostatic hypotension.[43] There is a greasy appearance to the skin of the face and occasional drooling because of loss of the swallowing movements that normally dispose of saliva. Olfactory dysfunction is an early sign of PD in most individuals, and it overlaps with multiple system atrophy and progressive supranuclear palsy.

Rapid eye movement sleep behavior disorders result in lack of the normal muscle atonia and jerking of body and limbs causing disrupted sleep. Restless leg syndrome appears to be associated, mostly because of the similarities in treatment response. Abnormal sleep patterns may also contribute to the daily fatigue.

Fatigue is related to other nonmotor features such as depression and excessive daytime sleepiness. In more than half of the individuals, mental fatigue is persistent and seems to be an independent symptom that develops parallel to the progressive neurodegenerative disorder of PD.[4]

Many persons with PD experience pain that is poorly localized but is generally described as cramping in the axial muscles or the limbs. Paresthesias are reported by many persons, including tingling, numbness, and abnormal temperature sensation.

Dementia and intellectual changes occur in almost 50% of persons with PD. Development of dementia is associated with more rapid progression of disability and potential for need for assisted living. Bradyphrenia, a slowing of thought processes, with lack of concentration and attention may also occur. Coexisting AD, organic brain disease, and vascular compromise may also contribute to the dementia.[115]

Depression is common and is probably related to the dopamine depletion. Loss of serotonin in the brainstem and limbic lobes has been found using PET studies. Behavioral changes, such as apathy, lack of ambition, indecisiveness, and anhedonia, are common and may be related to depression. Depressive episodes or panic attacks can precede the onset of motor symptoms.

Although reduced motor activity by itself would not seem to be a functional disorder, many of the small automatic muscular adjustments are important for successfully performing functional activities. For example, in attempting to rise from a chair a person may fail to make the small initial adjustments of legs

Stage	Character of Disability
I	Minimal or absent; unilateral if present
II	Minimal bilateral or midline involvement; balance not impaired
III	Impaired righting reflexes; unsteadiness when turning or rising from chair; some activities restricted but patient can live independently and continue some forms of employment
IV	All symptoms present and severe; standing and walking possible only with assistance
V	Confined to bed or wheelchair

TABLE 20.3 Hoehn and Yahr Classification of Disability

Modified from Hoehn MM, Yahr MD: Parkinsonism: onset, progression and mortality, Neurology 17:427, 1967.

that are crucial to standing up and fail to be able to get from sitting to standing without assistance.

The person with PD typically becomes deconditioned. Rapid heart rate and difficulty breathing are common. Vital capacity is reduced as the kyphosis increases and the intercostal muscles develop rigidity.[117] Respiratory complications are the leading cause of death. The Hoehn and Yahr classification (Table 20.3) is a common scale used to define the level of disability associated with PD.

Medical Management

Diagnosis

The classic triad of the major signs of PD is made up of tremor, rigidity, and akinesia.[141] The combination of asymmetry of symptoms and signs, the presence of a resting tremor, and a good response to levodopa best differentiates PD from parkinsonism caused by other causes. Diagnostic problems may occur in mild cases. Other movement disorders that do not fall under the category of parkinsonism need to be recognized by clinicians to establish a differential diagnosis. See Box 20.11 for features of parkinsonism due to causes other than PD.

Depression, with its associated expressionless face, poorly modulated voice, and reduction in voluntary activity, may be difficult to distinguish from mild parkinsonism. Olfaction is frequently impaired in PD, suggesting that deficiencies in smell may be a potentially useful test to distinguish PD from related disorders.

CT or MRI is not helpful in diagnosis of PD but can identify other causes of symptoms, such as Wilson's disease, or mass effects causing disruption of the basal ganglia function, such as stroke or hydrocephalus.

Functional imaging through PET is highly sensitive to regional changes in brain metabolism and receptor binding associated with movement disorders. SPECT shows differences in the posterior putamen, contralateral to the predominantly affected limb. Asymmetric scan findings have been observed in individuals with mild, newly recognized symptoms. Unilateral disease produces a significant difference in striatal uptake between the ipsilateral and contralateral sides in both the caudate and putamen nuclei. One explanation is that there is a preceding unequal functional reactivity of the basal ganglia, which results in an asymmetric clinical response.

Altropane (a close cousin of cocaine), a component of radioactive technetium 99m, is a compound that can measure

BOX 20.11 Parkinsonism Versus Parkinson's Disease

Parkinson's Disease
- Rigidity
- Tremor
- Akinesia
- Depression
- Expressionless face
- Poor voice quality
- Reduction in voluntary activity

Multisystem Atrophy: Striatonigral Degeneration, Sporadic Olivopontocerebellar Atrophy, Shy–Drager Syndrome
- Orthostatic hypotension, sexual impotence, bladder dysfunction
- Cerebellar dysfunction
- Myoclonus of face and hands
- Neck flexion
- Mottled, cold hands
- Dysarthria
- Good response to levodopa initially for a small percentage; dyskinesia and cranial dystonia associated with use of levodopa

Progressive Supranuclear Palsy
- Vertical ophthalmoplegia
- Oculomotor dysfunction
- Axial rigidity greater than limb rigidity
- Early falls
- Speech and swallowing disturbances

- Cognitive or behavioral changes
- Hypertension
- Poor response to levodopa

Corticobasal Degeneration
- Apraxia, cortical sensory changes, alien limb phenomenon
- Asymmetric rigidity
- Limb dystonia
- Myoclonus
- Negligible response to levodopa

Vascular Parkinsonism
- Dysfunction in lower extremities
- Gait disturbances
- Additional focal signs of midbrain lesion
- Poor response to levodopa

Dementia with Lewy Bodies
- Early dementia
- Rigidity more prominent than bradykinesia or tremor
- Hallucination
- Fluctuating cognitive status
- Falls
- Motor features may respond to levodopa but with psychiatric side effects

Modified from Lang AE, Lozano AM: Parkinson's disease, N Engl J Med 339:1044–1053, 1998.

the concentration of dopamine transporters imaged by SPECT. This may lead to a diagnosis of PD based on identifying decreasing levels in the brains of persons when only mild symptoms appear.

Assessing progression of PD using clinical rating scales such as the United Parkinson's Disease Rating Scale is a common way to track progression. However, the progression may be masked by medication and, because of the multitude of symptoms that may change at different rates, it is hard to determine a change in the course of the disease.

Treatment and Pharmacology

The current therapeutic approach to PD is symptomatic; major studies to determine possible therapeutic neuroprotection are under way, but no single intervention has proven to be disease modifying. Drug therapy is adapted to the person's needs, which may vary with the stage of the disease and the predominant manifestations.[5] When mobility becomes affected to the degree that walking and self-care activities become difficult, medications improve the control of movement. As the disease progresses over time, the effectiveness of medication changes, leaving the individual with a shorter "on" time during which symptoms are reduced and more rigidity during "off" times when symptoms are active. Long-term use of medication can also increase the dyskinesia or chorea-like movement resulting from the change in activity in the basal ganglia. Side effects can become more problematic as the dosages needed to control symptoms are increased. The management of these medications becomes the focus of intervention.[51]

Levodopa (L-dopa), which is taken up by remaining dopaminergic neurons in the basal ganglia and converted to dopamine, improves most of the major features of parkinsonism, including bradykinesia. Initially it leads to nearly complete

reversal of symptoms, with effects lasting up to 2 weeks, which is known as a long-duration levodopa response. As the disease progresses, the length of the effect becomes shorter, it takes longer for the effect to be noticed after dosing, and symptoms increase during the end of the dose period. Eventually there is dose failure or lack of any effect at all. Levodopa can cause dyskinesias that produce chorea, athetosis, dystonia, tics, and myoclonus. Predictable fluctuations include a wearing-off effect and early-morning akinesia. The duration of effect of each dose becomes shorter and will often match the drug's half-life of less than 2 hours. Although levodopa is the most effective drug for PD, the time to start taking it is controversial. Early use may contribute to greater activity levels and employability but cause more disability at later stages when the effect fluctuates and ultimately decreases. Protein in food uses the same mechanism as levodopa for crossing the blood-brain barrier. When levodopa is given with protein, the protein blocks the ability of the levodopa to cross the blood-brain barrier. This is usually managed by having the individual eat most of the daily protein in the evening, when immobility will cause the least inconvenience. Caffeine administered before levodopa may improve its pharmacokinetics in some individuals with parkinsonian symptoms.[40] Infusion of levodopa directly into the intestines gives a more stable response but is expensive and invasive. Levodopa should be avoided in persons with malignant melanoma and in persons with active peptic ulcers, which may bleed.

Carbidopa inhibits the breakdown of levodopa and is often used in combination with levodopa. It reduces the amount of levodopa required daily for beneficial effects and is often combined with levodopa in a single preparation (Sinemet).

Catechol-O-methyl transferase inhibitors are reported to provide smoother and more sustained levels of levodopa to the brain. Of these, entacapone and tolcapone reduce the off time and allow for decreased dosing of levodopa.[113] Liver function must be monitored regularly with the use of tolcapone. Tolcapone must be used with levodopa but can decrease the amount of levodopa needed.

Dopamine agonists act directly on dopamine receptors. Bromocriptine seems to be the best tolerated, and its use in parkinsonism is associated with a lower incidence of response fluctuations. It is often given in combination with levodopa and carbidopa. Pramipexole or ropinirole can be used either to delay starting levodopa or to decrease the amount needed. Transdermal application of dopamine agonists can be provided with rotigotine and lisuride.

Selegiline (Eldepryl) and rasagiline have been used to inhibit the monoamine oxidase type B (MAO-B) enzyme in the basal ganglia (MAO-B inactivates dopamine). It was thought that selegiline also may be able to delay the neuronal degeneration, but studies do not support that claim.[37]

Persons with mild symptoms but no disability may be helped by amantadine, which is also effective for the dyskinesia that develops later in the course of the disease. Coadministration of levodopa and amantadine controls dyskinesia without disrupting the effect of levodopa.

In the striatum the low level of dopamine is accompanied by increased cholinergic transmission. Accordingly, motor functions in individuals are improved by anticholinergic drugs. The side effects of the anticholinergic medications, including sedation, confusion, and psychosis, limit their usefulness, especially with advancing age. MAO-B inhibitors have replaced the use of anticholinergics in treatment of PD.[32]

Antioxidants have been studied for neuroprotection, such as coenzyme Q10, which helps stabilize mitochondria and appears to decrease the worsening of symptoms. Trophic factors, antiinflammatories, antiapoptotics, and antioxidants have been identified by the National Institutes of Health for further study for control of neuronal death.

Deep brain stimulation uses a pacemaker-like device surgically implanted with electrodes in the nuclei of choice and a pulse generator implanted in the chest. The generator is controlled externally through a magnetic field. When a tremor begins, the client activates the low-voltage, high-frequency generator by passing a magnet over it. Stimulation through the electrodes can be applied to the internal globus pallidus and the subthalamic nucleus or thalamus. Thalamic stimulation is most effective for tremor, with less effect on dyskinesia and rigidity. Electrode implantation in the globus pallidus appears to have good initial effect; however, there is a chance of psychosis and punding activity over time. Most centers are now stimulating the subthalamic nucleus bilaterally, but the individual's profile leads the decision. Preoperative response to levodopa predicts better outcome after deep brain stimulation of the subthalamic nucleus. The ability to perform ADLs is improved, and there is typically improved sleep time. Apathy and abulia can occur over time; this may be related to withdrawal of levodopa. There can be an increase in sadness or the opposite response with excessive hilarity that may be related to stimulation of the surrounding area or change in subthalamic limbic activity. Edema around the electrode may contribute to the psychotropic effects. The implant is believed to last approximately 5 years and can be removed if another more effective type of treatment is found.[8] Bilateral subthalamic stimulation, alone or in combination with levodopa, causes improvement in axial signs for posture and postural stability.

Although there is little evidence for drug effect on postural stability and gait disorders, researchers in motor control are making progress in identifying the nature of the abnormal responses both inside and outside of the basal ganglia.[131] (See 20.6 Special Implications for the PTA: Parkinson's Disease later in the chapter.) Based on the strong evidence that relates prior exercise and activity status to risk of PD, and the recent knowledge gained about neuroplasticity in the brain, it is likely that changes in postural control may come through interventions that drive neuroplastic changes.

Although orthostatic hypotension affects less than 20% of individuals with parkinsonism, it can limit activity. Use of midodrine, fludrocortisone, and etilefrine can be helpful in maintaining normal blood pressure. Supine hypertension may result and must be monitored. Urinary dysfunction is treated via antimuscarinic agents or β-agonists. Anticholinergics or scopolamine patches may be helpful for drooling, and the use of intraparotid injection of BTX can help. Constipation is common and may precede the motor symptoms in PD; it is usually managed by fluids, fiber, stool softeners, and exercise.

Depression is found in more than 40% of individuals with PD. Medication interactions must be looked at carefully. Use of serotonin uptake inhibitors may interact with selegiline. Tricyclics can be useful, but the central effects must be monitored more carefully than in the healthy younger population.

Respiratory complications, which are the leading cause of death, can be prevented to some extent with an early aggressive aerobic exercise program, followed by regular moderate activity as the disease progresses. Control of breathing can be facilitated using verbal and tactile stimuli and should be integrated into any intervention.

Behavioral abnormalities can be associated with high doses of dopaminergic replacement therapy, including the phenomenon of punding, characterized by fascination with technical equipment and excessive sorting of objects, grooming, hoarding, or use of a computer. This may be related to the impaired frontal lobe function and a result of psychomotor stimulation. Other abnormalities in reward-seeking behavior related to dopamine are hypersexuality and excessive gambling. Reducing the level of medication is helpful, and some neuroleptics such as clozapine will lessen symptoms of psychosis.

Experimental therapeutics targeted at improving dopaminergic drugs to increase selectivity for various receptor subtypes and at controlling the uptake of dopamine are currently under study. Improved plasma stability is achieved through transdermal application, which bypasses the fluctuations in gastric release. Studies are aimed at potential substances that evoke antiparkinsonism through neurotransmitter systems outside of dopamine. Pharmacologic manipulation of glutamate and GABA neurotransmission includes the drug istradefylline, which is currently undergoing a phase III study.[13] Cell transplantation of grafted dopaminergic neurons in PD continues to hold promise. The striatum (caudate and putamen) are primary targets for the implants. Individual selection, cell-handling variation in surgical techniques, and immunosuppression currently make it difficult to determine success. Graft-induced dyskinesia much like that associated with long-term levodopa use appears in some recipients. It is not clear which individual will develop the dyskinesia, and at this time there is no medication for controlling the abnormal movements. Fetal stem cells remain the most successful;

however, alternative types are being studied. There is hope for cells derived from the individual's own body, but the response has been less than hoped for and the current graft survival is low. Rejection of the graft continues to limit effects, and immunosuppression has to be considered as a possible long-term adjunctive therapy with grafts.[147]

Prognosis

Generally, all the clinical manifestations in PD worsen progressively, although not to the same extent. Tremor as a presenting symptom may be used to predict a more benign course and longer therapeutic benefit to levodopa. In individuals with newly diagnosed PD, older age at onset and rigidity/hypokinesia as an initial symptom can be used to predict a more rapid rate of motor progression.[138]

The presence of associated comorbidities, stroke, auditory deficits, and visual impairments as well as male sex may be used to predict faster rate of motor progression. Older age at onset and initial hypokinesia/rigidity may be used to predict earlier development of cognitive decline and dementia. Older age at onset, dementia, and decreased dopamine responsiveness may be used to predict earlier nursing home placement as well as decreased survival. Lack of mobility, loss of balance reactions, and weakness result in more falls than in an age-matched normal population. Osteoporosis can result from prolonged inactivity and may be present secondary to advanced age at onset. Falls more often lead to fractures because of the prevalence of osteoporosis. Fracture healing may be delayed. Posture and gait abnormalities are the most difficult to control in advanced cases.

PD does not significantly reduce life span in most persons who develop the generalized form between ages 50 and 60 years. However, because there is progressive neuronal loss despite the response to treatment, deterioration continues until death occurs, often from infection or other conditions associated with debilitation.

Because the onset of disease is typically in the fifth or sixth decade of life and is progressive despite medication, the economic cost of the disease can be quite high because of loss of income, cost of drugs, assistive devices, and assisted living. Pain, fatigue, and depression also adversely affect the quality of life compared with that of age-matched normal subjects.[130]

20.6 Special Implications for the PTA: Parkinson's Disease

There are clearly various and separate components of the movement disorders related to parkinsonism, especially in PD. As we become better able to identify the relationship between specific impairment and the resulting function, intervention by the PTA will have more impact on the ability to participate in typical activities. Each individual's needs and goals must be addressed and programs modified as the movement disorders change as the disease progresses.[26,39,42,122] Skills are learned most effectively when they are practiced repeatedly in relation to meaningful goals.

Spinal flexibility or axial mobility contributes to function. It can impact the ability to perform many of the components of tasks, including functional reach.[11,130]

External temporal constraints and input can provide individuals with PD a means of organizing the timing and speed of their movements that compensates for their loss of internal cueing. Speed of arm movement in persons with PD can be increased by external cues that require faster movement to reach a moving target

compared with self-selected fastest speed to reach a nonmoving target.[93]

Cognitive impairment may impact the ability of individuals with PD to learn new motor skills.[10,65] Pathways leading to and from the frontal cortex, limbic lobe, and hippocampus are affected in PD. Learning strategies and environments that best eliminate stress need to be identified.

Tasks involving a similar movement of each hand do not appear to pose as many problems for individuals with PD as those that require different movements for each hand.[75] The ability to sequence the muscles in the upper extremity when it is necessary to perform complex movements with disparate postures appears to be under the control of the basal ganglia. The ability to perform tasks under this constraint may be appropriate as a screening tool to determine progression of disease in persons with PD.[47] Therapy that incorporates cueing and feedback appears to have most effect.[60] Dual task performance and motor planning generally diminishes with the complexity of the task. Studies are now under way looking at the training of breaking tasks down into manageable steps.

The movement disorders resulting in postural instability predispose people with PD to increased falls. Strategies to improve postural stability show promise, with better understanding of the control mechanisms within and parallel to basal ganglia function.[67] The changes that occur over time related to both the disease process and aging can affect the ability to respond to interventions addressing postural control and balance.[105] Integration of sensory input through the thalamus and basal ganglia has been identified, and better understanding of the mechanisms and pathways implicated will no doubt provide new interventions.[65,103]

The use of rhythmic auditory stimulation in persons with PD leads to an increase in gait velocity, cadence, and stride length associated with an increase in the EMG activity around the ankle.[142] Complexity of task appears to be related to gait. Individuals with moderate disability associated with PD experience considerable difficulty when they are require to walk while attending to complex visuomotor tasks involving the upper limbs.[18] Visual cueing for improved gait appears to have the most effect on stride length and decreases time spent in double stance during walking.[7] Walking speed, arm swing amplitude, and step length can be increased by verbal instructional sets, using cognitive strategies.[7] Gait training strategies and goals will vary according the progression of the disease.[102]

Managing the home environment is critical, because most falls occur at home. The training of a caregiver to give the appropriate verbal and visual cues can be beneficial.[69] Use of grab bars can be valuable, especially if there is a bathtub, because stepping over the edge requires significant weight shift. Recognizing areas that may induce freezing (doorways, narrow spaces) may decrease the fall risk in those areas. Keeping a diary of falls can be helpful.

Strategies mentioned earlier can work by means of bypassing the basal ganglia and making use of the supplementary motor area. External feedback can be effective in improving movement when it cannot be controlled from internal organization. Use of virtual reality has been shown to be effective in persons with parkinsonism. Until the time that it is readily available, techniques used by persons with PD to trigger movement or to "unfreeze" are used by most individuals with PD. Typical tactics are included in Box 20.12.

Intervention strategies have been established and can be used to establish programs. Clinical trials with randomized approaches are under way to provide evidence of interventions addressing the movement disorders discussed here. This will assist PTAs the most when the components studied can be extrapolated into functional tasks.

Disease-modifying aspects of exercise show strong promise. Future research may look at the complexity of the motor skills and degree of protection. With evidence for exercise benefit within this population, it should also be recognized by the PTA that submaximal responses to exercise testing occur in PD, with higher heart rate and increased oxygen consumption.[75]

BOX 20.12 **Methods to Improve Movement Noted by Individuals with Parkinsonism**

- Walking sideways
- Rocking the body to generate weight shift
- Stamping feet, shaking legs
- Self-talk
- Stepping over objects, such as the handle of a cane, lines on the floor, or laser pointer
- Quick head movements
- Music
- Clapping
- Snapping fingers
- Virtual reality

Modified from Stern GM, Lander CM, Lees AJ: Akinetic freezing and trick movements in Parkinson's disease, J Neural Transm Suppl 16:137–141, 1980.

Secondary Parkinson's Syndrome

Parkinsonian syndromes, also called *atypical parkinsonism* or *Parkinson's plus syndromes,* are a family of neurodegenerative disorders that result from neuronal loss in different components of the basal ganglia, such as the brain system, of which the dopaminergic midbrain neurons affected in PD are a part. All of these disorders can be difficult to differentiate from PD early in the course of the illness. These disorders have distinctive clinical features, which may emerge only after the onset of parkinsonism. Important clinical clues that one of these disorders is present are symmetric onset of parkinsonism, absence of typical resting tremor, early autonomic dysfunction, prominent dystonia, significant early cognitive impairment, and prominent early falls.[3]

Iatrogenic parkinsonism or drug-induced parkinsonism results from the use of pharmacologic agents that block dopamine effects or interfere with dopamine metabolism. The most common causes of drug-induced parkinsonism are dopamine antagonist antipsychotic medications. The risk of drug-induced parkinsonism is reduced significantly with newer atypical antipsychotic agents. Another group of drugs that can cause drug-induced parkinsonism is older (non–serotonin antagonist) dopamine antagonist antiemetics. Agents interfering with dopamine production or synaptic vesicular storage can cause drug-induced parkinsonism. These include methyl-para-tyrosine, methyldopa, and reserpine. Flunarizine and cinnarizine, when they are used as vestibular suppressants or cerebral vasodilators, can cause parkinsonism. Sodium valproate may cause tremor that can progress to parkinsonism. Features of iatrogenic parkinsonism are bilateral onset and predominant bradykinesia with increased involvement in the arm compared with the legs in the younger population, but it is more consistent with PD in older individuals. If drug-induced parkinsonism is suspected, the suspected offending agent is withdrawn, and the individual should improve. With dopamine antagonists or reserpine, improvements can occur within days to weeks after medication withdrawal, but there is sometimes a prolonged latency of months before marked improvement occurs.

Vascular parkinsonism involves primarily the lower extremities. It is associated with lacunar infarcts and probably represents small infarcts in the basal ganglia or corticobasilar pathways. A stroke in the region of the striatum (caudate and putamen) and hemiparesis of the arm is common. Systemic lupus erythematosus may also cause cerebral vasculitis. Vascular parkinsonism presents typically with start hesitation, a broad-based shuffling gait (rather than the narrow-based gait associated with PD), and frequent falls. Depending on the level of damage and the cause, the response to levodopa will vary.

Infectious causes of parkinsonism are suspected when the symptoms develop during the acute or recovery phase of an illness with fever. Cases of parkinsonism have been reported as a result of West Nile virus infection and have historically been associated with encephalitis. HIV infection can cause parkinsonism via the viral damage in encephalopathy or opportunistic infections.

Toxicity, often related to manganese accumulation in the substantia nigra, can cause parkinsonism and dystonia, which is seen in miners, factory workers making dry cell batteries, and those exposed to some fungicides.

Disorders with Parkinsonian Characteristics
Benign Essential Tremor

Benign essential tremor is not associated with any underlying cause, is common after the age of 50 years, and is usually hereditary. This tremor is of a different character, and there is a lack of other neurologic signs.

Progressive Supranuclear Palsy

Progressive supranuclear palsy has symptoms of bradykinesia, rigidity, and postural instability similar to those of PD and is frequently misdiagnosed as PD. Neurofibrillary tangles are the main pathology in progressive supranuclear palsy; oligodendrocytes are also affected. Postural instability is the most pronounced symptom, with falls that are not associated with obstacles or change in surface. Gait freezing and apraxia are common. Dysarthria and dysphagia are on a continuum, with dysphagia typically occurring later than 2 years after onset. Loss of upward gaze, saccades, and smooth pursuit eye tracking progresses over time. Inhibition of eyelid opening and closure, or blepharospasm, can cause functional blindness. Inability to perform vestibuloocular reflex cancellation is lost. There is apathy, intellectual slowing, and impairment of executive function progress, and there can be pseudobulbar laughter or crying. The autonomic nervous system maintains near-normal function.

Levodopa and deep brain stimulation are effective for the movement disorder, and BTX can help to improve blepharospasm.

Multiple System Atrophy

There is extreme clinical variability within the multiple system atrophy group of disorders that is primarily familial but can be sporadic. Neuronal atrophy is seen to a variable degree in the brainstem, cerebellum, spinal cord, and peripheral nerves. The differential pathology is associated with gliosis and cytoplasmic inclusion in the glia. Multiple system atrophy typically has its onset in the fifth to seventh decade, and parkinsonism is the primary condition; however, there is more evidence of cerebellar involvement, and autonomic dysfunction is greater and more disabling that that found in PD. Levodopa is used in the treatment, but with less success than when it is used in PD. Cerebellar and autonomic nervous system dysfunction respond poorly to anticholinergics. Large European studies are under way to examine pathogenesis and intervention strategies.

Olivopontocerebellar Atrophy

Olivopontocerebellar atrophy is one of the most common and variable of the non-PD parkinsonian conditions. Neuronal loss with gross atrophy is concentrated in the pons, medullary olives, and cerebellum. Ataxia, rigidity, spasticity, and oculomotor movement disturbances are present in variable degrees and combinations. The intracytoplasmic inclusions are predominantly oligodendrocytic, and there is modest tau and synuclein immunoreactivity.

Wilson's Disease

Wilson's disease, or progressive hepatolenticular degeneration, is rare but also represents degeneration of the basal ganglia and is related to excess deposition of copper. Cysts or cavities form in the basal ganglia with necrosis. The lateral ventricles can be enlarged with associated brain atrophy. This can be imaged using MRI, PET, or SPECT studies. Cerebellar and brainstem damage is common, and there can be spheroid bodies in the cerebral cortex. The symptoms of Wilson's disease go far beyond movement disorder mimicking PD and include profound affective disorders. Ophthalmologic signs of brownish or greenish rings in the periphery of the cornea are a hallmark sign. The disorder is treated via copper chelating.

Restless Leg Syndrome

Restless leg syndrome is reported as the desire to move the extremities associated with paresthesia, motor restlessness with worsening of symptoms at rest (typically at night), and relief with activity or sensory stimulation. It is familial in 60% of cases, and the effect is related to reduced iron stores in the substantia nigra. There is no loss of dopaminergic neurons as is seen in PD, but the dysfunction lies within the presynaptic and postsynaptic junction of dopaminergic neurons. Levodopa is the traditional treatment, and it is effective when movement is the most problematic symptom. Opioids such as methadone can help when dopamine agents are not effective. For the individual with pain or dysesthesia, neuroleptics can be of benefit.

REFERENCES/SUGGESTED READINGS

To enhance this text and add value for the reader, references and suggested readings are included on the companion Evolve site that accompanies this textbook. The reader can view the source and access it online whenever possible.

21

Stroke

CHAPTER OBJECTIVES

1. Discuss the differences between types of cerebrovascular accidents.
2. Outline and discuss multiple signs and symptoms of stroke.
3. Recognize the clinical manifestations of stroke dependent on location of lesion and be able to list multiple therapeutic interventions used for each.
4. Outline the role of the physical therapist assistant in the care of a person following stroke.

OUTLINE

VOCAB BUILDERS

Anticoagulation
Constraint-induced training
Hemorrhagic

Ischemic
Ischemic penumbra
Orthosis

Parenchyma
Pusher syndrome
Statins

STROKE

Overview and Definition

Stroke, or cerebrovascular accident, is the result of an interruption of blood supply to the brain, either through hemorrhage or ischemia. It is the third most common cause of death in the United States and a leading cause of serious long-term disability, with estimated health care costs totaling $62.7 billion annually.[10]

Transient ischemic attack (TIA), often referred to as a ministroke, presents in a similar manner as a stroke, with focal neurologic symptoms that completely resolve within 1 to 24 hours. Approximately a third of those who experience a TIA will have a stroke in the future.[10] Because a TIA is considered a warning for future strokes, it is prudent to determine and treat the underlying etiology. Recurrent strokes are common. Approximately 25% of people who have recovered from a stroke will have

another within 5 years. The risk of death and severe disability increases with each subsequent stroke.[10]

Cerebrovascular disease, the primary cause of stroke, is caused by one of several pathologic processes involving the blood vessels of the brain. The damage may be intrinsic to the vessel, or the stroke may originate remotely, such as when an embolus from the heart or extracranial circulation lodges in an intracranial vessel. The stroke may result from the rupture of a vessel in the subarachnoid space or intracerebral tissue. Fig. 21.1 shows the effects of different types of stroke on brain tissue.[74]

Incidence

Every 40 seconds someone in the United States will have a stroke, resulting in approximately 795,000 strokes a year, with 610,000 of those being new strokes. Every 3 to 4 minutes, someone in the United States dies from a stroke.[12] This equates to approximately 137,000 deaths each year.[11]

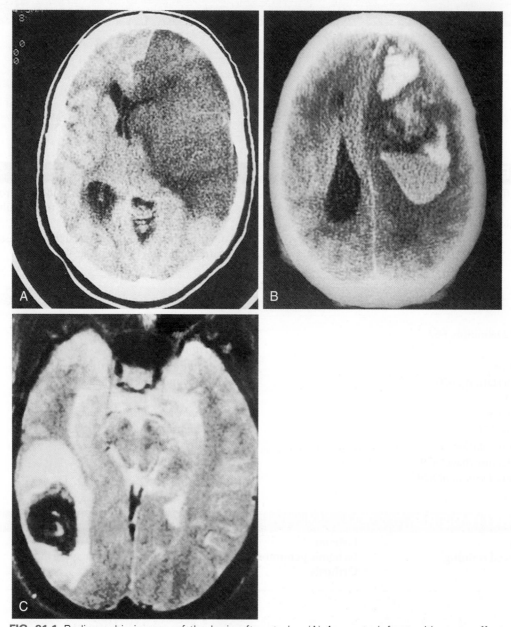

FIG. 21.1 Radiographic images of the brain after stroke. (A) An acute infarct with mass effect and compression of the ventricle. (B) An acute intracerebral hemorrhage in the hemisphere. (C) Amyloid angiopathy with acute hemorrhage; the edema surrounding the area results in a slight mass effect on the midbrain. (From Ramsey R: Neuroradiology, Philadelphia, 1994, Saunders.)

Although strokes can occur at any age, risk increases with age. The risk doubles for every decade after age 55 years, with two-thirds of all strokes occurring in people older than age 65 years. Men have a higher risk for strokes, yet more women die of strokes. The risk of stroke also varies with race and ethnicity. The incidence of stroke is double in African Americans compared with white Americans. Between the ages of 45 and 55 years, African Americans have a four to five times greater death rate from strokes than whites. However, after the age of 55 years, the risk of death equalizes. Hispanics and Native Americans have similar incident and mortality rates as white Americans. Within the United States, the southeastern states have the highest stroke and mortality rate, with North Carolina, South Carolina, and Georgia having the greatest mortality rates in all of the United States. The increased risk may be from geographic, environmental, and/or lifestyle factors, including higher rates of cigarette smoking and high-fat diets.[10]

Interestingly, strokes occur more often in the spring.[53] There are several stroke types with different etiologies and risk factors; therefore, management is driven by the stroke subtype. Fig. 21.2 shows the prevalence of stroke types.

Risk Factors

Risk factors for stroke can be divided into those that are modifiable and those that are not. Among the nonmodifiable risk factors (age, race, and sex), age constitutes the greatest risk. Additionally, risk of stroke increases when there is either a maternal or paternal family history of stroke.[38] Fig. 21.3 shows the interaction of genetics, disease, and environment.[15]

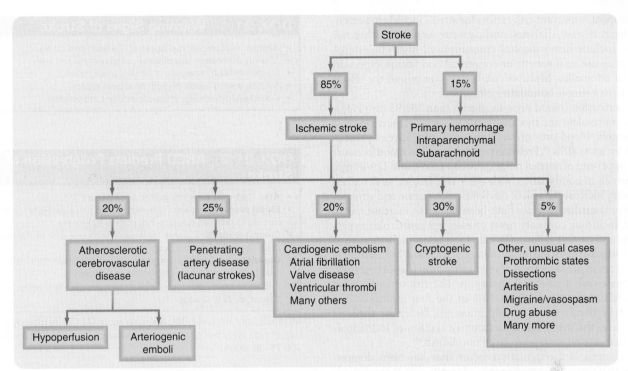

FIG. 21.2 Percentage of strokes caused by different etiologies. (From Townsend CM: Sabiston textbook of surgery, ed 17, Philadelphia, 2004, Saunders.)

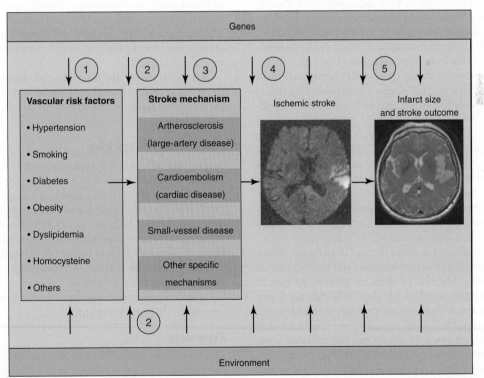

FIG. 21.3 Genetic factors and ischemic stroke. Genetic factors may affect stroke risk at various levels. They could act through conventional risk factors *(1)*, interact with conventional and environmental risk factors *(2)*, or contribute directly to an established stroke mechanism such as atherosclerosis or small-vessel disease *(3)*. Genetic factors could further affect the latency to stroke *(4)* or infarct size and stroke outcome *(5)*. Similarly, environmental factors and interactions between genes and the environment could occur at various levels. (From Dichgans M: Genetics of ischaemic stroke, Lancet Neurol 6:149–161, 2007.)

The most important risk factors for stroke include hypertension, heart disease, diabetes, and cigarette smoking. Other risk factors include heavy alcohol consumption, high cholesterol, illicit drug use, and genetic or congenital conditions, especially vascular anomalies. Multiple risk factors compound the effects more than a simple cumulative effect.[10]

Hypertension (blood pressure greater than 160/95 mm Hg) is the most prevalent and modifiable risk factor for stroke. Decreasing diastolic blood pressure by 5 to 6 mm Hg decreases risk of stroke by up to 40%.[18] Prehypertension describes blood pressure at the upper end of normal range (between 120/80 and 129/89 mm Hg), which in combination with other risk factors, as described later, may increase the risk of cardiovascular disease and stroke.

Various cardiac diseases have been shown to increase risk of stroke, including coronary heart disease, left ventricular hypertrophy, and cardiac failure. Cardiac valve abnormalities such as mitral stenosis and mitral annular calcification are moderate risk factors as are structural abnormalities, such as patent foramen ovale and atrial septal aneurysm. The risk of stroke after myocardial infarction (MI) is 30% in the first month.[74] Further, atrial fibrillation is an important risk factor for stroke.[63] It increases the stroke risk by a factor of six; 8% of individuals older than age 80 years have atrial fibrillation.[85]

Fibrinogen is a coagulation factor that has been demonstrated to be associated with increased stroke risk. It plays a crucial role in platelet aggregation. Platelets initiate thrombosis by attracting fibrin and other clot-forming substances. Conditions associated with increased fibrin deposition or increased blood viscosity include rheumatic heart disease, endocarditis (growth of bacteria on one of the heart valves), atherosclerosis (formation of plaque on the inner lining of arterial walls), polycythemia (abnormal increase in number of circulating blood cells), and thrombocytosis (abnormal increase in number of platelets).

Diabetes mellitus has long been established as a risk factor for stroke. It is known to cause large artery atherosclerosis, increased cholesterol levels, and plaque formation. The ability of the cerebral arterioles to vasodilate is reduced in long-standing type 2 diabetes.[35]

Cholesterol has been considered a part of the stroke risk profile.[71] High total cholesterol levels create increased risk of *ischemic* stroke. Younger individuals and those with low high-density lipoprotein levels are at greater risk; higher levels of high-density lipoprotein cholesterol are associated with decreased risk of ischemic stroke. Low-density lipoprotein cholesterol levels currently are believed to be predictors of coronary artery disease associated with carotid athrerosclerosis.[75]

Cigarette smoking almost doubles the risk of ischemic stroke because of the promotion of atherosclerosis and the increase in blood-clotting factors. The risk of stroke is directly related to the number of cigarettes smoked per day. This risk decreases with smoking cessation, with a major reduction in risk seen in 2 to 4 years postcessation.[10]

High alcohol consumption increases the risk of both *hemorrhagic* and ischemic strokes. Heavy alcohol consumption depletes platelet levels and compromises blood viscosity and clotting, leading to hemorrhagic strokes. The rebound effect of heaving or binge drinking occurs when the alcohol is purged from the body, resulting in increased platelet levels and blood viscosity, which precipitates ischemic strokes. However, small, daily alcohol consumption has been associated with lower risks of ischemic strokes; this may be caused by alcohol decreasing the clotting ability of platelets.[10]

BOX 21.1 **Warning Signs of Stroke**

- Sudden weakness or numbness of the face, arm, or leg
- Sudden dimness or loss of vision, particularly in one eye
- Sudden difficulty speaking or understanding speech
- Sudden severe headache with no known cause
- Unexplained dizziness, unsteadiness, or sudden falls

BOX 21.2 **ABCD Predicts Progression of Stroke**

- **Age:** 1 point for being older than age 60 years
- **Blood pressure:** 1 point for systolic blood pressure higher than 140 mm Hg or diastolic pressure higher than 90 mm Hg
- **Clinical features:** 2 points for weakness on one side of the body; 1 point for speech trouble but no weakness
- **Duration:** 2 points for symptoms lasting longer than 60 minutes and 1 point for symptoms lasting less than 60 minutes
- Predictive value for stroke within 7 days: 0 to 4, 4% chance; 5, 12% chance; 6, 32% chance

Modified from Rothwell PM: A simple score (ABCD) to identify individuals at high early risk of stroke after transient ischaemic attack, Lancet 366:29–36, 2005.

Cocaine and crack cocaine reduces cerebral blood flow up to 30%, causes vasoconstriction, and inhibits vascular relaxation, leading to narrowing of the arteries. It also causes cardiac arrhythmias and increased heart rate, leading to the formation of blood clots. Amphetamines, heroin, and anabolic steroids are vasoconstrictors and are suspected to increase the risk of stroke. Marijuana use may also be a risk factor because of its effect on alternating blood pressure, which may result in damage to the vascular system.[10]

Recognition of the multiple risk factors that can interact to increase the probability of stroke is important. Use of risk profiles can assist in the ability to predict stroke in a single individual.[86]

Clinical Manifestations

Symptoms of a stroke typically occur suddenly. They may include weakness or numbness in the upper extremities, lower extremities, or face, particularly on one side; confusion; difficulty speaking or understanding language; difficulty seeing; dizziness; loss of balance; or sudden severe headache.[10] Early warning signs are listed in Box 21.1. Specific clinical manifestations are typically related to specific types of stroke and are discussed later in the chapter. Although the risk factors and early warning signs have been well publicized, often individuals at highest risk ignore warning signs and may not seek out medical attention when the symptoms occur.

Prognosis

The University of Oxford ABCD scale can be used to determine the chance of progression to a stroke with greater consequences (Box 21.2). Risk of a second stroke varies between 3% and 5% in 5 years and is related to the concomitant cardiac and vascular disorders. The recurrence rate of stroke is highest in the first 30 days after the first stroke and remains higher for 1 year. Men have 30% to 80% higher rates of recurrence than do women.[64]

Mortality associated with stroke has decreased in the past 20 years in all age groups. However, the mortality rate after stroke

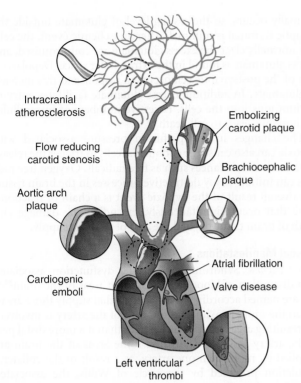

FIG. 21.4 Cardiogenic and arterial atherosclerotic sources for stroke. (From Townsend CM, Beauchamp RD, Evers BM, et al., editors: Sabiston textbook of surgery, ed 18, Philadelphia, 2008, Saunders.)

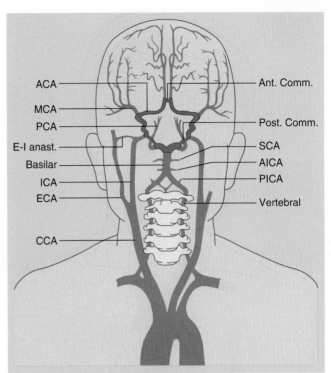

FIG. 21.5 Extracranial and intracranial arterial supply to the brain. Vessels forming the circle of Willis are highlighted. *ACA,* anterior cerebral artery; *AICA,* anterior inferior cerebellar artery; *Ant. Comm.,* anterior communicating artery; *CCA,* common carotid artery; *ECA,* external carotid artery; *E-I anast.,* extracranial-intracranial anastomosis; *ICA,* internal carotid artery; *MCA,* middle cerebral artery; *PCA,* posterior cerebral artery; *PICA,* posterior inferior cerebellar artery; *Post. Comm.,* posterior communicating artery; *SCA,* superior cerebellar artery. (Redrawn from Lord R: Surgery of occlusive cerebrovascular disease, St Louis, 1986, Mosby.)

is higher in African Americans and appears to be increasing. Further, stroke still remains the number one cause of disability in the adult population.[28]

Concomitant diseases of aging such as arthritis, diabetes, osteoporosis, and decreased plasticity of the nervous system associated with aging often make the recovery from stroke a challenge. Medical complications occur in up to 85% of stroke survivors and present potential barriers to optimal recovery. Infections occur in almost 25% of stroke survivors, primarily in the urinary tract and chest. Incidence of deep vein thrombosis and pulmonary emboli is increased. Falls resulting from impaired mobility are also prevalent, with serious injury reported in 5% of falls. Approximately 75% of stroke survivors will have a fall within the first 6 months after stroke. Pain and depression are reported in more than 30% of stroke survivors.[44] These impairments can affect the individual's functional abilities and societal interactions.

Ischemic Stroke

Pathogenesis

Occlusion of major arteries. The most common causes of ischemic stroke are occlusion of a major vessel caused by thrombosis or embolism. The most common source of embolitic occlusion is from the heart as a result of atherothrombotic disease. Atrial fibrillation is believed to cause thrombus formation in the fibrillating atrium. Left ventricular MI can also be a source of emboli, especially in the first few weeks following the event when thrombus formation is most prevalent.[66] Mitral valve prolapse or congenital septal defects are also sources of emboli. Formation of emboli during or after coronary artery surgery or intracardiac surgery is a well-recognized complication.

Further, embolism arising from an atherothrombotic lesion in the carotid or vertebrobasilar system may lead to stroke. Other causes of emboli may be thrombus in the pulmonary vein, fat emboli in the blood, and tumor emboli from a neoplastic process.[19] Sources of emboli are shown in Fig. 21.4.

Changes in the collateral pathways of the circle of Willis are apparent in response to internal carotid artery obstruction that may provide some protection against neurologic damage associated with occlusion. The anterior circle of Willis and the posterior communicating artery show increased diameter in some individuals when the internal carotid artery is blocked. Fig. 21.5 shows the distribution of the circle of Willis.

Secondary vascular responses. When a cerebral artery is occluded, the formation of thromboemboli likely begins in the distal vessels of that artery. These presumed microvascular occlusions progressively increase in number and continue to impair blood flow in the brain. Cell death surrounding the area of blocked blood flow may be caused by the effects of swelling of the cellular support structures of the nervous system. Fig. 21.6 shows how the emboli can affect the brain tissue. The formation of fibrin in the gray matter surrounding the occluded vessel also may contribute to the lack of reperfusion of microvessels. Other factors include bleeding into the brain tissue, increased platelet aggregation, endothelial cells swelling in the walls of the vessels, and vasospasm.[25,54]

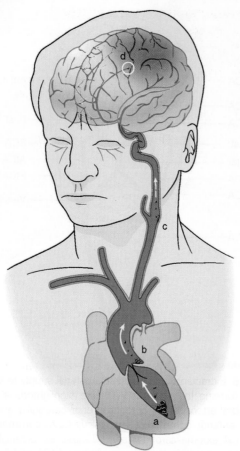

FIG. 21.6 Examples of potential sources of embolism: cardiac mural thrombus *(a)*; vegetation on heart valve *(b)*; and emboli from carotid plaque *(c)*. Also shown is an infarcted cortex from an embolism *(d)* in the area supplied by the terminal anterior cerebral artery. (From Caplan LR: Caplan's stroke: a clinical approach, ed 4, Philadelphia, 2009, Saunders.)

Secondary neuronal damage. The tissue of the brain, or the *parenchyma*, is highly vulnerable to an interruption in its blood supply. When the cerebral blood flow falls below 20 mL/100 mg of tissue per minute, neuronal functioning is impaired. Neuronal death, or infarction, occurs when the brain receives less than 8 to 10 mL/100 mg/min. Frequently, in an acute infarction, a portion of the affected brain receives no blood, while a surrounding area receives sufficient blood from collateral circulation to maintain viability but not to sustain function. This territory has been termed the *ischemic penumbra*.[77] Although the major injury to the neurons in the brain is caused by hypoxia and ischemia, further damage to the brain tissue and neurons occurs as a secondary response. There is a characteristic uncoupling between cerebral blood flow and metabolism in the area of infarction. There is decreased cerebral perfusion relative to the necessary oxygen requirements, which affects cerebral metabolism. If blood flow to this ischemic area is restored before irreversible damage occurs, then the tissue will likely recover and resume normal function.

These changes caused by a hypoxic-ischemic event are thought to also affect the neurotransmitters. Glutamate, a neurotransmitter, is normally present throughout the central nervous system gray matter and is stored in synaptic terminals. When it is released into the extracellular space, rapid uptake

normally occurs, so the resting level of glutamate outside the synaptic terminal is minimal. After an ischemic event, the cells that normally clear the excess glutamate are compromised, and excess glutamate is found in the extracellular space. Depolarization of the postsynaptic cell occurs in response to this increase in glutamate. In addition, excess glutamate facilitates entry of calcium ions into the cells. Excessive numbers of intracellular calcium ions leads to cell death.[48]

The changes in the perfusion pressure associated with hypoxia can also cause the endothelial cells to trigger the release of neurotoxic substances such as free radicals. Oxygen free radicals can initiate many destructive processes in the brain tissue. The overall result of the hypoxic event is a chain of reactions, some that occur simultaneously, extending the damage and death of brain tissue beyond the area of vascular supply.

Clinical Manifestations

Syndromes. Syndromes reflect the dysfunction associated with disruption of blood flow in specific areas of the brain[39,47] and are named according to the arteries that supply those areas. When the more proximal component of the artery is involved, the resulting area of hypoxia is greater than if a more distal part of the artery is affected. Because some areas of the brain are supplied by more than one artery, as a result of the collateral circulation provided by the circle of Willis, the associated clinical syndromes are not as extensive.

Middle cerebral artery syndrome. If the entire middle cerebral artery is occluded at its stem, the clinical findings are contralateral *hemiplegia* and *hemianesthesia.* If the dominant hemisphere is affected, *global aphasia*, or the loss of fluency, ability to name objects, comprehend auditory information, and repeat language, results.

Partial syndromes include (1) brachial syndrome, or weakness of the upper extremity, and (2) frontal opercular syndrome, or facial weakness with motor aphasia with or without arm weakness. A combination of sensory disturbance, motor weakness, and motor aphasia suggests that large portions of the frontal and parietal cortices have been affected.

If Wernicke's aphasia occurs without weakness, the inferior division of the middle cerebral artery supplying the temporal cortex of the dominant hemisphere has been occluded. Jargon speech and an inability to comprehend written and oral language are prominent features. Hemiplegia or spatial agnosia without weakness indicates that the inferior division of the middle cerebral artery in the nondominant hemisphere is involved. Fig. 21.7 represents the area of the middle cerebral artery.

Anterior cerebral artery syndrome. Infarction in the territory of the anterior cerebral artery is uncommon and is more often the result of embolism than atherothrombosis. Collateral flow is able to compensate for most occlusion of the artery so that dysfunction is minimal. Contralateral hemiparesis and sensory loss are usually seen with the lower extremity more involved. Profound *abulia* and a delay in verbal and motor response are common. Akinetic mutism also can result in significant disability. Fig. 21.8 represents the area of blood flow of the anterior cerebral artery.

Internal carotid artery syndrome. The clinical picture of internal carotid occlusion varies depending on whether the cause of ischemia is thrombus, embolus, or low flow. The cortex supplied by the middle cerebral territory is affected most often. Occasionally, the origins of both the anterior and middle cerebral arteries are occluded at the top of the carotid

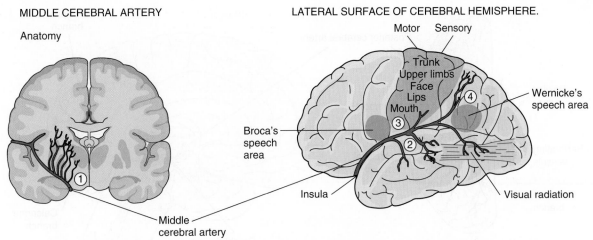

FIG. 21.7 The middle cerebral artery is the largest branch of the internal carotid artery and the most common site of emboli. Its deep branches feed the internal capsule and basal ganglia. On the lateral surface, the branches feed areas of the parietal, frontal, and temporal lobes. (Redrawn from Lindsay KW, Bone I, Fuller G: Neurology and neurosurgery illustrated, ed 5, Edinburgh, Churchill Livingstone, 2010.)

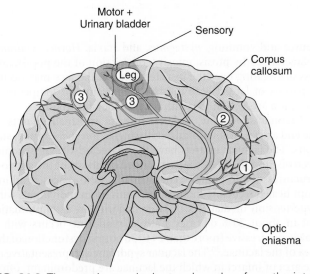

FIG. 21.8 The anterior cerebral artery branches from the internal carotid. Deep branches supply the internal capsule and basal ganglia. Superficial branches supply the frontal and parietal lobes. (Redrawn from Lindsay KW, Bone I, Fuller G: Neurology and neurosurgery illustrated, ed 5, Edinburgh, Churchill Livingstone, 2010.)

artery. Symptoms consistent with both syndromes result. With a competent circle of Willis producing adequate collateral circulation, the occlusion can be asymptomatic.

Posterior cerebral artery syndrome. If the proximal posterior cerebral artery is occluded, the areas of the brain that are affected are the subthalamus, medial thalamus, and ipsilateral cerebral peduncle and midbrain. Signs include thalamic syndrome, including abnormal sensation of pain, temperature, proprioception, and touch. Sensations may be exaggerated and light pressure may be interpreted as painful stimuli. This may develop into intractable, searing pain, which can be incapacitating. Perseverations and superimposition of unrelated information, apathy, and amnesia result from occlusion in its anterior distribution. With paramedian involvement, the most

frequent features are disinhibition syndromes with personality changes, loss of self-activation, amnesia, and, in the case of extensive lesions, thalamic dementia; this pattern may often be difficult to distinguish from primary psychiatric disorders. After inferolateral lesion, executive dysfunction may develop. Cognitive dysfunction with neglect and aphasia are present after a posterior lesion.[8]

If the posterior cerebral artery is completely occluded at its origin, hemiplegia results. Contralateral ataxia, oculomotor palsy, hemiballismus, paresis of upward gaze, drowsiness, and abulia are other problems associated with occlusion of the posterior cerebral artery. If the posterior cerebral stem is occluded, coma and decerebrate rigidity may result.

Peripheral supply of the posterior cerebral artery includes the temporal and occipital lobes. Occlusion of this component of the artery often affects the occipital lobe with homonymous hemianopsia, in which the visual field defect is on the side opposite to the lesion. Cortical blindness is one of the visual disturbances that are seen with an infarct in this region.

Medial temporal lobe involvement (including the hippocampus) can cause an acute disturbance in memory, particularly if it occurs in the dominant hemisphere. However, because memory is represented on both sides of the brain, if one area is affected the intact side can compensate to a considerable extent. If the dominant hemisphere is affected and the infarct extends to the corpus callosum, the individual may demonstrate alexia without agraphia, or impairment of reading without the impairment of writing. Agnosia, or difficulty in identification or recognition, of faces, objects, mathematical symbols, and colors, may occur. Anomia, impaired ability to identify objects by name, and visual hallucinations can occur with peripheral posterior cerebral infarction. Fig. 21.9 represents the area of blood flow of the posterior cerebral artery.

Vertebral and posterior inferior cerebellar artery syndrome. Blood supply to the brainstem, medulla, and cerebellum is provided by the vertebral and posterior cerebellar arteries. Collateral circulation is provided by the bilateral component of the vertebral artery so that ischemia often is not manifested in the presence of atherothrombosis.

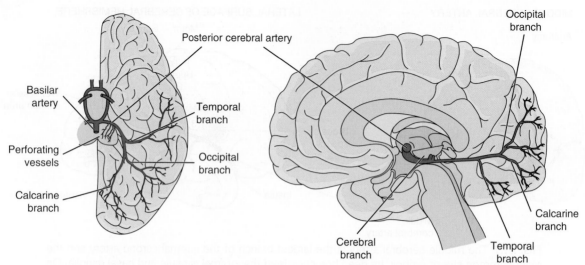

FIG. 21.9 The posterior cerebral arteries branch from the basilar artery. The small perforating branches supply the midbrain structures and posterior thalamus. The temporal branch supplies the temporal lobe, and the occipital and calcarine supply the occipital lobe, including the visual cortex. (Redrawn from Lindsay KW, Bone I, Fuller G: Neurology and neurosurgery illustrated, ed 5, Edinburgh, Churchill Livingstone, 2010.)

When infarction ensues, the lateral medulla and the posteroinferior cerebellum are affected, resulting in Wallenberg syndrome, which is characterized by vertigo, nausea, hoarseness, and dysphagia (difficulty swallowing). Other symptoms include ipsilateral ataxia, ptosis, and sensory impairment in the ipsilateral face and contralateral trunk and extremities. These individuals complain of numbness, burning, and cold in the face and limbs that are aggravated by a cold environment.[37] A medial medullary infarction results in contralateral hemiparesis of the arm and leg, sparing the face. In more extensive infarcts, loss of joint position sense and ipsilateral tongue weakness can occur.

The edema associated with cerebellar infarction can cause sudden respiratory arrest from raised intracranial pressure (ICP) in the posterior fossa. Gait unsteadiness, dizziness, nausea, and vomiting may be the only early symptoms. Fig. 21.10 shows the area of distribution of the superior cerebellar, anterior inferior cerebellar, and posteroinferior cerebellar arteries.

Basilar artery syndrome. Although atherothrombotic lesions can occur anywhere along the basilar trunk, they occur most often in the proximal basilar and distal vertebral area. Ischemia as a result of occlusion of the basilar artery can affect the brainstem, including the corticospinal tracts, corticobulbar tracts, medial and superior cerebellar peduncles, spinothalamic tracts, and cranial nerve nuclei.

If the basilar artery is occluded, the brainstem symptoms are bilateral. When a branch of the basilar artery is occluded, the symptoms are unilateral, involving the sensory and motor aspects of the cranial nerves.

Superior cerebellar artery syndrome. Occlusion of the superior cerebellar artery results in severe ipsilateral cerebellar ataxia, nausea and vomiting, and *dysarthria*. Loss of pain and temperature in the contralateral extremities, torso, and face also occurs. *Dysmetria* affecting the ipsilateral upper extremity is common.

Anterior inferior cerebellar artery syndrome. Principal symptoms include ipsilateral deafness, facial weakness, vertigo,

nausea and vomiting, *nystagmus,* and ataxia. *Horner syndrome* characterized by ptosis, miosis (constriction of the pupil), and loss of sweating over the ipsilateral side of the face may occur. A paresis of lateral gaze may be seen. Pain and temperature sensation are lost on the contralateral side of the body.

Lacunar syndrome. Lacunar infarcts are small infarcts of the end arteries found in the basal ganglia, internal capsule, and pons. The lacunar infarcts have the characteristics of ischemic necrosis, and the cysts are surrounded by gliosis of the support structures of the brain.[33] These small, cystic spaces resulting from healed ischemic infarcts are common in individuals with hypertension or diabetes. A large majority are asymptomatic, but in about 20% of cases a stroke syndrome occurs with a slowly progressive (more than 24 to 36 hours) dysfunction of the area of the lacunae.[50] The lacunar syndrome is representative of the area of infarct in which the lacunae are predominant, often in the deep structures of the brain, and have their effect often on white matter. If the posterior limb of the internal capsule is affected, a pure motor deficit may result; in the anterior limb of the internal capsule, weakness of the face and dysarthria may occur. If the posterolateral thalamus is affected, there is a pure sensory stroke. When the lacunae occur predominantly in the pons, ataxia, clumsiness, and weakness may be seen. Fig. 21.11 shows the areas of predilection for lacunae to develop.

Medical Management

Diagnosis
Because embolic and thrombotic strokes present differently, it is important to obtain a thorough history of the neurologic event, including timing, pattern of onset, and course. An embolic stroke occurs rapidly, with no warning. A more progressive and uneven onset is typical with thrombosis. The presenting symptoms will help to determine the location of the lesion.

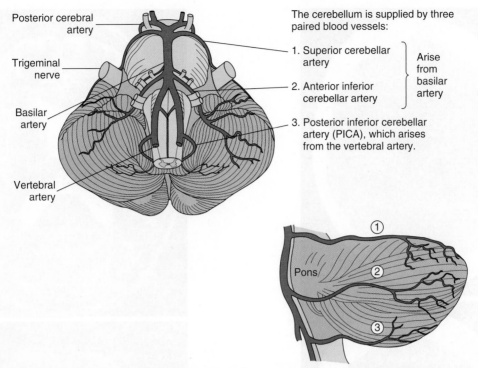

FIG. 21.10 A lesion in the cerebellar territory will produce both cerebellar and brainstem signs and symptoms. (Redrawn from Lindsay KW, Bone I, Fuller G: Neurology and neurosurgery illustrated, ed 5, Edinburgh, Churchill Livingstone, 2010.)

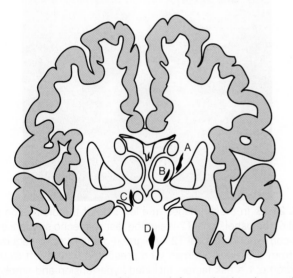

FIG. 21.11 Usual sites of lacunar infarcts in the deep white matter. *A,* Internal capsule/putamen; *B,* thalamus; *C,* mesencephalon; *D,* Pons. (From Pryse-Phillips W, Murray TJ: Essential neurology: a concise textbook, ed 4, New York, 1992, Medical Examination Publishing.)

Neuroimaging of the brain has become a standard procedure in the diagnosis of stroke. Computed tomographic (CT) scan is the fastest, most convenient, and widely available test to use for the diagnosis and early treatment of acute stroke. It can confirm the diagnosis and rule out other pathologies and extent of the lesion. Fig. 21.12 shows how an acute stroke looks on CT scan. In ischemic stroke, CT scans reveal the area of decreased density and loss of gray/white matter differentiation resulting from edema. However, CT scans may be normal in the acute stage of an embolic stroke.[58] Images of lacunae and be seen in Fig. 21.13. Magnetic resonance imaging (MRI) allows for the identification of an ischemic event within 2 to 6 hours of onset and is widely accepted as the method of diagnostic choice. It provides an indication of the brain tissue's physiologic response to ischemia and can document the evolution of stroke.[65]

Positron emission tomographic (PET) imaging has been of great benefit in advancing the understanding of the pathophysiology of cerebrovascular disorders. PET imaging allows for the detection of stroke earlier and with higher sensitivity than anatomic imaging with either MRI or CT. Further, PET imaging has been useful in evaluating the extent of the functional damage because areas not immediately affected by the infarct may show hypometabolism or decreased blood flow (Fig. 21.14).[51]

Cerebral angiography can be used in the absence of CT or MRI but is an invasive procedure and used only when other forms of imaging are not appropriate.

Treatment and Pharmacology

Treatment of individuals with ischemic stroke consists of managing the stroke and preventing further embolic strokes. Cerebral perfusion, or the blood flow around the area of the stroke, is the main concern when the cause is embolic. Managing blood pressure is critical. The goal is not to try to normalize the pressure but to bring it down from dangerously high levels, but it must be high enough to perfuse the brain tissue. Blood pressure should not be lowered unless it is as high as 230/120 mm Hg. If the blood pressure is low, raising it is appropriate in the first few hours after the stroke. An excessive rise in blood pressure may cause an increase in edema. When clinically stable, individuals with blood pres-

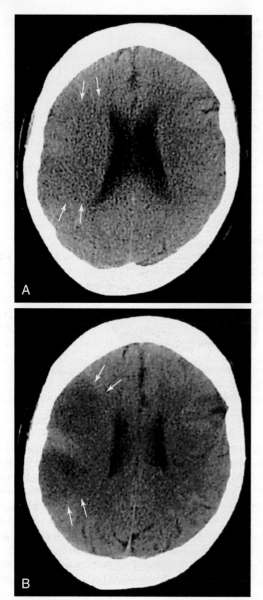

FIG. 21.12 (A) Computed tomographic (CT) scan taken 2 hours 50 minutes after large right middle cerebral artery occlusion. There are subtle, ultraearly ischemic changes, including loss of the gray-white interface *(arrows)* and subtle evidence of sulcal effacement. (B) CT scan of the same patient approximately 8 hours after symptom onset shows acute hypodensity *(arrows)* and more prominent sulcal effacement. (From Marx JA: Rosen's emergency medicine: concepts and clinical practice, ed 8, Philadelphia, 2014, Saunders.)

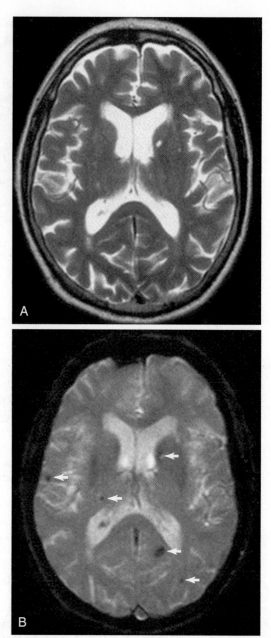

FIG. 21.13 In these images, the left side of the brain is on the right of the panel. Axial T2-weighted fast spin-echo sequence (A) and corresponding axial T2*-weighted gradient echo sequence (B) from a 57-year-old man who presented with a left lacunar syndrome; his risk factors included hypertension and smoking. The T2-weighted fast spin-echo sequence shows several hyperintense foci in the cerebral white matter and basal ganglia but no microbleeds. The T2*-weighted gradient echo image shows several areas of focal signal loss consistent with microbleeds *(arrows)* in the right frontal lobe, right thalamus, left parietal lobe, and left caudate nucleus. (From Werring DJ, Coward LJ, Losseff NA, et al.: Cerebral microbleeds are common in ischemic stroke but rare in TIA, Neurology 65:1914–1918, 2005.)

sure higher than 140/90 mm Hg should be given medication to lower blood pressure. Unless contraindicated, use of diuretics and β-blockers should be the medication of choice.[52]

Emboli that lodge in the artery stem can cause edema. If not controlled, the edema can spread and create pressure in the area of the cerebellum and brainstem. Even a small amount of edema in the cerebellum can cause respiratory arrest from compression of the brainstem and lead to coma and death. It is the most common fatal complication. Water restriction and agents that raise the serum osmolarity should be considered with the onset of significant edema.

Thrombolytic and antithrombotic agents form the cornerstone of ischemic stroke treatment and prevention.[2] Recombinant tissue plasminogen activator (t-PA) is used for the emergent care of embolic stroke. It activates plasminogen to form plasmin, which actively digests fibrin strands, and is

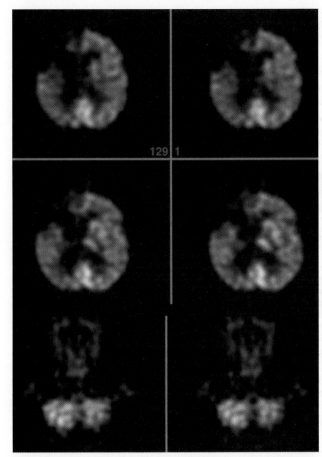

FIG. 21.14 Fluorodeoxyglucose positron emission tomographic scan of a patient after embolic stroke in the distribution of the right anterior cerebral artery. There is severely decreased metabolism in the right frontal lobe extending to the midline. There is also crossed cerebellar diaschisis with decreased metabolism in the left cerebellum. (From Newburg AB, Alavi A: The role of PET imaging in the management of patients with central nervous system disorders, Radiol Clin North Am 43:49–65, 2005.)

effective in dissolving the thrombosis or blood clot responsible for the blockage. By promoting early recanalization of occluded vessels and early reperfusion of ischemic fields, there is potential to salvage penumbral neuronal tissue. If it is received within 3 hours after the initial stroke, the person is 30% more likely to recover from the stroke. The greatest risk factor is the chance of hemorrhage and the inappropriate use in a stroke that is hemorrhagic in origin. It must be determined on CT that the stroke is purely embolic; guidelines are established by the National Institute of Neurologic Disorders and Stroke study.[21] Several prognostic factors must be considered for selecting candidates for intravenous thrombolysis. Younger age, absence of cardiac disease or diabetes, lower blood pressure on admission, lower neurologic score, absence of early ischemic parenchymal changes, large artery thrombus visible on baseline brain CT, and a developed collateral circulation are all factors associated with a more favorable outcome. Risk factors for developing brain hemorrhage include time to treatment, dose of thrombolytics, blood pressure level, severity of neurologic deficit, and severity of ischemia. Along with hemorrhage, potential complications of thrombolysis include reperfusion injury, arterial

reocclusion, and secondary embolization caused by thrombus fragmentation. Following t-PA, blood pressure should be closely monitored and kept at less than 180/105 mm Hg, and antithrombotic agents should be avoided for 24 hours.

Intracranial clot retrieval is now possible with the mechanical embolus removal in cerebral ischemia (MERCI) retrieval system (Concentric Medical, Inc., Mountain View, CA). When outcomes using MERCI were compared with those in individuals who were treated and those who were not, good outcomes occurred in 49% versus 10%, respectively, and mortality rate was 25% versus 52%, respectively. The retriever device goes in as a straight wire that turns into a corkscrew when it comes out of the guide catheter that is screwed into the clot; a balloon is pumped proximal to the clot to prevent antegrade flow. The clot is then pulled out. Most stroke centers are now offering this system with trials done up to 8 hours after symptom onset when used with very large clots.[69]

Prophylaxis Pharmacology
Anticoagulation

Anticoagulation therapy has played a prominent role in the prevention of acute infarction for several decades, and current research supports its use in high-risk individuals. Large, randomized trials have also highlighted the effectiveness and safety of early and continuous antiplatelet therapy in reducing atherothrombotic stroke recurrence. These trials have shown the benefit of four different agents: (1) aspirin, (2) ticlopidine, (3) clopidogrel, and (4) dipyridamole.[55]

Antiplatelets, such as aspirin, are used to decrease risk of a second MI and may reduce the chance of stroke after MI. Further, aspirin has become the antiplatelet standard for individuals with acute ischemic stroke who are not receiving thrombolysis. There are, however, several other antiplatelet agents such as ticlopidine, clopidogrel, and aspirin-dipyridamole that have been shown to be more effective.[17]

Anticoagulation medications should not be used with high blood pressure or other risk factors of hemorrhagic stroke.[34] However, heparin can be used prophylactically against deep venous thrombosis and pulmonary embolism.

Although aspirin has been used to decrease the risk of MI, warfarin sodium (Coumadin, Panwarfin) appears to be about twice as effective as aspirin in the prevention of stroke in individuals with atrial fibrillation. Use of warfarin after MI has shown reduced stroke risk overall but increases the chance for hemorrhagic stroke. Persons older than age 75 years have the highest risk of stroke and can benefit from anticoagulation. The risk of bleeding increases with age, and the ability to determine the risk-benefit ratio is complex.[57] Fig. 21.15 shows an algorithm for treatment options in stroke.

Lipid-Lowering Agents

Cholesterol-lowering agents such as *statins* decrease the risk of stroke after MI. Studies show that the antistroke effects may be separate from the lipid-lowering properties through changes in the endothelium, inflammatory response, plaque stabilization, and thrombus formation. Several organizations, including the United States Food and Drug Administration (FDA), American Heart Association, and American Academy of Neurology, have endorsed the use of statins for stroke prevention.[68]

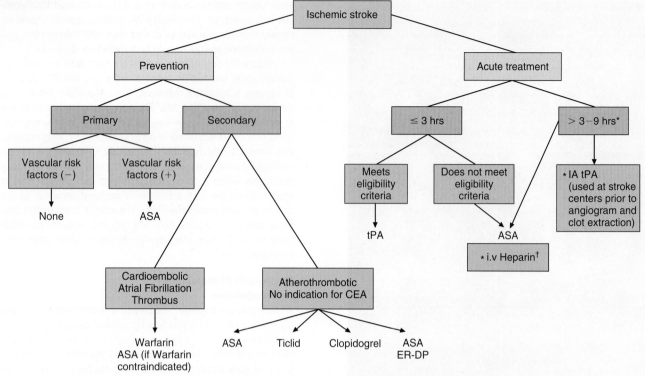

FIG. 21.15 Prevention and treatment of ischemic stroke. *Experimental or ongoing trials. †Used in clinical practice for specific stroke syndromes. *ASA,* Aspirin; *ER-DP,* extended-release dipyridamole; *IA tPA,* intraarterial tissue plasminogen activator; *Ticlid,* ticlopidine. (Modified from Ocava LC: Antithrombotic and thrombolytic therapy for ischemic stroke, Clin Geriatr Med 22:135–154, 2006.)

Neuroprotection

Medications aimed at creating neuroprotection to decrease the amount of cell death secondary to excitotoxicity are being developed, and clinical studies are underway.[20] Approaches directed at presynaptic reduction of glutamate release may control the damage caused by excess extracellular glutamate. Reducing the amplification of excitotoxic calcium ion release also may help control cell death. In this category are endogenous growth factors, which may improve recovery from calcium overload and appear to improve outcome after focal brain ischemia.[20]

A tetracycline derivative, minocycline, reduces inflammation and appears to protect against focal cerebral ischemia after stroke. It is most effective when started before ischemia develops but can be effective after the onset of ischemia. It has no therapeutic effect on astrogliosis but may provide some protection from glutamate toxicity.[87] Timing is critical in the administration of these drugs. The window of opportunity may be 2 to 6 hours after infarction. These antiexcitotoxic therapies may be suitable for either hemorrhagic or ischemic stroke and someday may be given by paramedics before full neurologic evaluation.[80]

Nerve Growth

Animal studies show positive results when stem cells have been implanted into the brain. However, the ability to repair damaged tissue and reform neural connections is limited when vast amounts of parenchyma are lost. Enhancement of neural processes, reformation of cortical tissue, and promotion of connectivity all appear to be possible.

Surgical Intervention

Carotid endarterectomy is the treatment of choice for low-flow or embolic TIA in individuals younger than age 80 years[3] or when stenosis is greater than 70% at the origin of the internal carotid artery. Because women have arteries that are 10% smaller than men to begin with, the absolute size of the artery becomes significantly smaller with 70% occlusion. Therefore this equation may need to be looked at differently in women.

Control of Symptoms

Pharmacotherapy for spasticity in stroke is controversial. Stroke survivors may use spasticity to overcome the effects of weakness when attempting to use the involved side for functional activities. This action may be diminished if the client takes medication to reduce spasticity. Antispasmodic medications include baclofen and benzodiazepines, which work at the level of the spinal cord, and dantrolene, which works on the muscle fibers.

Botulinum toxin (botox) injections allow more discrete targeting of spastic muscles. However, the effects of botox are temporary, usually lasting for approximately 3 to 6 months. According to a recent FDA press release, botox has not been shown to be effective for lower extremity spasticity. Further, patients may experience systemic side effects such as nausea, fatigue, and muscle weakness; in some cases, symptoms similar to botulism occurred, including life-threatening difficulty in breathing and swallowing.[22]

Urinary incontinence can be a disabling sequela of stroke. Urge incontinence is treated with behavioral therapy and anticholinergics. An areflexic bladder can be managed with self-catheterization or use of a Foley catheter.

Depression after stroke is common and does not appear to be related to the area of lesion. It responds to treatment and should be guided by the other concomitant medical conditions and the side effects of the particular medication. Use of tricyclic antidepressants shows improvement within 3 to 6 weeks and should be continued for a minimum of 6 months.[29]

Prognosis

The prognosis for survival after cerebral infarction is better than after intracerebral or subarachnoid hemorrhage (SAH). Loss of consciousness after an ischemic stroke implies a poorer prognosis. Individuals with ischemic stroke are at risk for other strokes or MIs. The risk factors and type of damage related to the stroke syndrome relate to degree of disability and mortality.

Recovery from stroke is the fastest in the first few weeks after onset, with the most measurable neurologic recovery (approximately 90%) in the first 3 months.[56] However, movement patterns, speed, and control of movement can continue to be influenced by intervention up to 5 or more years after stroke. (See 21.1 Special Implications for the PTA: Stroke Rehabilitation, later in this chapter.)

Intracerebral Hemorrhage
Overview and Definition

Intracerebral hemorrhage (ICH) is bleeding from an arterial source into brain parenchyma and is regarded as the most deadly of stroke subtypes. Primary ICH describes spontaneous bleeding in the absence of a readily identifiable precipitant and is usually attributable to microvascular disease associated with hypertension or aging. Secondary ICH occurs most often in association with trauma, impaired coagulation, toxin exposure, or an anatomic lesion. Chronic hypertension causes fibrinoid necrosis in the penetrating and subcortical arteries, weakening of the arterial walls, and formation of small aneurysmal outpouchings, or microaneurysms, that predispose an individual to spontaneous ICH. Acute rises in blood pressure and blood flow can also precipitate ICH even in the absence of preexisting severe hypertension. A ruptured vascular malformation is the second most common cause of ICH.

Bleeding is limited by the resistance of tissue pressure in the surrounding brain structures. If a hematoma is large, distortion of structures and increased ICP cause headache, vomiting, and decreased alertness. Because the cranial cavity is a closed system, enlargement of a hematoma or development of severe edema may shift brain tissues into another compartment, or herniate, and cause deterioration in the clinical condition.

Incidence

The incidence of ICH is low among persons younger than age 45 years, increasing dramatically after the age of 65 years. In one study, the incidence of ICH doubled with each advancing decade until age 80 years, after which the incidence became 25 times higher.[64] ICH tends to occur more frequently in men. In the United States African Americans are more likely to have an ICH than are whites. Worldwide rates are higher in Asian populations than in Western populations. ICH is a major cause of morbidity and death and accounts for 10%

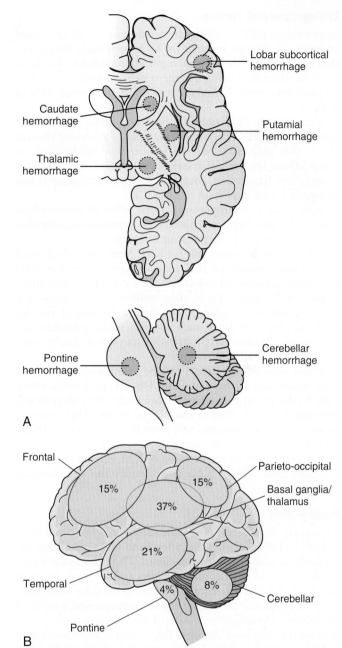

FIG. 21.16 (A) Horizontal cerebral section *(top)* and sagittal brainstem section *(bottom)* showing the most common sites of intracranial hemorrhage (ICH). (B) Sites of predilection of ICH. (A, Redrawn from Caplan LR: Caplan's stroke: a clinical approach, ed 4, Philadelphia, 2009, Saunders; B, redrawn from Lindsay KW, Bone I, Fuller G: Neurology and neurosurgery illustrated, ed 5, Edinburgh, Churchill Livingstone, 2010.)

to 15% of all strokes in whites and about 30% of strokes in African Americans and individuals of Asian origin. Fig. 21.16 represents the areas most likely to be involved in ICH and occurrences.

Spontaneous ICH can also occur in association with the use of anticoagulants, primary or metastatic brain tumors or granulomas, and the use of sympathomimetic drugs. Aneurysms rarely bleed only into the brain, but when they do, they cause a local hematoma near the brain surface.

Etiologic and Risk Factors

Spontaneous ICH usually is from an anomaly of the vessel structure or changes brought on by hypertension. Hypertension represents the single most important modifiable risk factor for ICH. Abnormal changes in the vessels as a result of cerebral amyloid angiopathy (CAA) account for approximately 10% of ICHs.[23]

Excessive use of alcohol has been associated with massive spontaneous ICH. Alcohol has a number of acute and chronic effects that may contribute to hemorrhagic stroke, such as direct effects on cerebral vessels, hypertension, and impaired coagulation. In addition, cocaine and amphetamine use is also recognized as an important cause of ICH.

ICH is the most important adverse effect of thrombolytic therapy. Hemorrhage from fibrinolytic agents can occur within 12 to 24 hours.[67] Long-term anticoagulant therapy is associated with an increased risk for ICH. Many individuals with anticoagulant-associated ICH are also hypertensive; therefore, the extent of increased risk is difficult to clearly identify independently.[63] Further, use of other medications in conjunction with thrombolytic therapy may place individuals at risk for ICH. A number of drugs, such as nonsteroidal antiinflammatory agents, nitrates, and propranolol, may affect platelet function and contribute to bleeding.[88]

Other possible risk factors include liver disease, prior ischemic stroke, and cigarette smoking. Obesity, sickle cell anemia, mitral valve prolapse, patent foramen ovale, and polycythemia have also been identified as possible risk factors. More research in this area is ongoing and will provide more insight into the relation of chronic disease and lifestyle to ICH.

Pregnancy may increase the risk of ICH. Eclampsia accounts for more than 40% of ICHs in pregnancy and is a common cause of death.

Pathogenesis

Changes in the cerebral microvasculature of hypertensive individuals include processes that affect both the contents and the walls of the blood vessels of the brain. These changes are seen in small cerebral arteries and arterioles and are more severe in the distal and small penetrating vessels in the deep white matter. Smooth muscle cells in the vessels are progressively replaced by collagen (hyalinization). Altered permeability of the vessel wall leads to fibrinoid changes. This results in accumulation of protein material and fat deposits, and the vessel wall becomes prone to leakage or rupture.[83]

Individuals with hypertension also have a substantial reduction in the percentage of smooth muscle in the vessel wall. This decreased smooth muscle mass most likely represents structural weakening, resulting in rupture and hemorrhage. Necrosis of the endothelium may be a result of vessel ischemia brought about by the changes in the smooth muscle and thickening of the vessels walls, which increases the metabolic requirements and impedes the flow of oxygen to the outermost part of the vessel wall.

CAA is characterized by protein fibrils in the arterioles and small cerebral arteries. Amyloid replaces smooth muscle in the media, separating the elastic membranes. Lymphocytic infiltrates, hyaline arteriole degeneration, and fibrinoid necrosis are characteristic changes in the vessel wall. The parenchymal changes seen in CAA reflect the consequences of the vascular pathology and direct deposition of amyloid in the brain tissue. Brains with evidence of CAA frequently demonstrate periventricular demyelination, believed to be caused by ischemia from amyloid deposition in the vessels supplying the deep white matter.[24,29]

In drug-related ICH, some underlying vascular pathologic lesion may be present, such as an arteriovenous malformation (AVM) or chronic vasculitis. The ICH occurs as a result of a sudden increase in blood pressure triggered by the drug. The proposed mechanism for the increased incidence of ICH in the individual with increased alcohol ingestion is decreased circulating levels of clotting factors produced by the liver. Thrombocytopenia, which is often associated with alcoholism, may underlie or potentiate hemorrhage.[26]

Hemorrhagic transformation, or conversion of an ischemic cerebral infarction, refers to secondary bleeding. It is believed to occur either with early reperfusion or the development of collateral circulation.

When hemorrhage occurs, it spreads along a path of least resistance, primarily following the fiber tracts of the white matter. In the presence of a hematoma, gray matter, because of its dense cell structure, is more likely to be compressed than infiltrated. Edema forms in the brain tissue surrounding the hematoma. Blood is reabsorbed by macrophages at the periphery of the hemorrhage, leaving a cavity surrounded by necrotic tissue. This process usually takes weeks to months.[82]

Clinical Manifestations

Neurologic symptoms occur gradually in most cases, representing the expansion of the hematoma. In some cases (approximately 30%), onset is sudden, which is also characteristic of an ischemic stroke. The earliest signs relate to the area of the brain in which bleeding occurs. For example, a hematoma in the left putamen and internal capsule would first cause weakness of the right limbs; a cerebellar hematoma would cause gait ataxia. As the hematomas enlarge, the focal symptoms increase. If the hematoma becomes large enough to raise ICP, headache, vomiting, and decreased alertness develop. Some hematomas remain small and the only symptoms relate to the focal collection of blood. Once the condition is stabilized, the symptoms improve in parallel with the resorption of the hematoma.

Although headache is an important symptom of ICH, it is present in severe form in only 30% to 40% of cases. Headache is most common as a sign of superficial and large hemorrhages.

The incidence of seizure correlates with the location of the hemorrhage. Cerebral cortex hemorrhage causes the most prevalent seizure activity. Two-thirds of the seizures are generalized and one-third is focal.

Syndromes. Syndromes associated with ICH are representative of the area of bleed and reflect brain activity of the particular site. Table 21.1 gives typical signs in individuals with ICHs at various sites.

Putamen. Approximately 50% to 80% of hemorrhages occur in the putamen. The result is contralateral sensorimotor deficit resulting from its proximity to the internal capsule. Smaller hemorrhages that affect more isolated areas of the putamen can produce a variety of symptoms, such as pure motor weakness, expressive aphasia, receptive aphasia, and abulia. Pupillary abnormalities, visual field loss, and oculomotor deficits are common. Headache and vomiting occur in about 25% of cases.

TABLE 21.1 Signs in Patients with Intracerebral Hemorrhages at Various Sites

Location	Motor/Sensory	Eye Movements	Pupils	Other Signs
Putamen or internal capsule	Contralateral hemiparesis and hemi-sensory loss	Ipsilateral conjugate deviation	Normal	Left: aphasia
				Right: left-sided neglect
Thalamus	Contralateral hemisensory loss	Down and in upgaze palsy	Small; react poorly	Somnolence, decreased alertness; left: aphasia
Lobar				
Frontal	Contralateral limb weakness	Ipsilateral conjugate gaze	Normal	Abulia
Temporal	None	None		Hemianopia
				Left: aphasia
Occipital	None	None		Hemianopia
Parietal	Slight contralateral hemiparesis and hemisensory loss			Hemianopia; left: aphasia; right: left neglect; poor drawing and copying
Caudate	None or slight contralateral hemiparesis	None	Normal	Abulia, agitation, poor memory
Pons	Quadriparesis	Bilateral horizontal gaze paresis, ocular bobbing	Small; reactive	Coma
Cerebellar	Gait ataxia, ipsilateral limb hypotonia	Ipsilateral gaze or cranial nerve VI paresis	Small	Vomiting, inability to walk, tilt when sitting

Thalamus. Sensory losses, or dysesthesias, are common with thalamic hemorrhage. Some motor deficits occur secondary to internal capsular involvement. Oculomotor dysfunction may also be present, and constriction (miosis) of the pupil is observed in 50% of cases. In dominant hemisphere thalamic lesions, aphasia, disorientation, and memory disturbances may be seen. With nondominant lesions, apraxia may be evident. Midline thalamic hematomas are associated with alterations in the level of consciousness during the acute phase followed by prefrontal signs, such as change in personality, speaking to oneself, memory disturbance, and impaired learning.

Cerebellum. A hallmark of cerebellar hemorrhage is ataxia. Additional symptoms may include nausea and vomiting, dizziness with nystagmus and vertigo, and dysarthria. Brainstem signs, such as facial paresis, can be present with a hemorrhage that extends to the brainstem. The signs of cerebellar hemorrhage should be carefully monitored, because the progression to compression of vital structures in the region of the fourth ventricle and medulla can be rapid and can produce life-threatening changes.

Pons. Brainstem hemorrhages commonly arise in the midline of the pons, leading to coma, quadriparesis, and nonreactive pupils with absent horizontal eye movement.

Caudate. Caudate hemorrhages can rupture into the ventricles and therefore have a presentation like that of a SAH. Headache, vomiting, and loss of consciousness may occur. The internal capsule may be involved, causing sensorimotor involvement.

Internal capsule. Internal capsule hemorrhages often result in a pure motor, pure sensory, or sensorimotor stroke with ataxia.

Lobar. Lobar hematomas are centered in the immediate subcortical white matter. Symptoms are lobe specific (see the section on Ischemic Stroke, Clinical Manifestations in this chapter). Seizures are more common with lobar hemorrhages than with deeper bleeds.

Medical Management

Diagnosis

The availability of CT allows for prompt diagnosis of ICH. It accurately documents the size and location of the hematoma, the presence and extent of any mass effect, and the presence of hydrocephalus and intraventricular hemorrhage. CT scans should be performed immediately in individuals suspected of having an ICH. Follow-up CT scans are requested when there is a change in clinical signs or state of alertness to monitor changes in the size of the lesion and ventricular system and to detect important pressure shifts. In patients with substance abuse, increased sympathetic outflow caused by the hemorrhage may lead to an increase in dysrhythmias. Dysrhythmias also may signal impending brainstem compression from an expanding hemorrhage.

MRI can provide multiplanar views and can discriminate subtle tissue changes and rapidly flowing blood. The differential diagnosis for ICH is similar to that of ischemic stroke and includes migraine, seizure, tumor, abscess, hypertensive encephalopathy, and trauma.

Treatment and Pharmacology

The acute reduction of elevated blood pressure is advisable and is most readily accomplished with rapid-acting, potent antihypertensive medication along with effective control of increased ICP, which exacerbates blood pressure elevation.[36] A major issue in the management of ICH is control of edema.

The frequency of ICH may increase with the use of long-term anticoagulation therapy. Treatment with vitamin K is useful to correct an elevated prothrombin time; however, it takes 12 to 24 hours to have an effect. Fresh-frozen plasma immediately restores diminished clotting factors.

An individual with a potential ICH requires rapid assessment and intensive care management. The prehospital management is similar to that for ischemic stroke. The circumstances surrounding the event and other concomitant medical conditions also should be ascertained. An evaluation of the initial level of consciousness, Glasgow Coma Scale, any gross focal deficits, difficulty with speech, clumsiness, gait disturbance, or facial asymmetry should be noted.

Supportive care involving attention to airway management and perfusion is of the highest priority. Individuals with hemorrhagic stroke are more likely to have an altered level of consciousness that may progress rapidly to unresponsiveness, requiring emergent endotracheal intubation.

Hyperventilation and diuretics, such as mannitol, move fluid from the intracranial compartment, reducing cerebral edema. Although this effect may be temporarily helpful in the acute setting, the brain tissue reequilibrates, and rebound swelling can occur and worsen the individual's clinical status. These agents also can cause dehydration and lead to hypotension. Other experimental modalities include barbiturate coma and hypothermia. Seizure activity can cause neuronal injury, elevations in ICP, and destabilization of an already critically ill individual. Seizure prophylaxis should be considered for individuals with ICH, especially individuals with lobar hemorrhage.

Selected individuals with sizable lobar hemorrhage and progressive neurologic deterioration may benefit from surgical drainage. Surgery is more efficacious in individuals with cerebellar hemorrhage. The clinical course in cerebellar hemorrhage is notoriously unpredictable. Individuals with minimal findings may deteriorate suddenly to coma and death with little warning. For this reason, most neurosurgeons consider emergent surgery for individuals with cerebellar hemorrhage within 48 hours of onset.

Prognosis

Although the overall mortality from ICH is high, functional recovery among survivors is also high. The older the individual, the less complete is the expected recovery. The most important predictor of mortality is hemorrhage size; survival also depends on the location of the hemorrhage and the rapidity of hematoma development. Individuals who are comatose at onset or who have a wide spectrum of neurologic deficits tend to do poorly compared with those who remain alert and have focal neurologic symptoms. Individuals with small hematomas located deep and near midline structures often develop secondary herniation and have a high mortality rate. Survivors of these ICHs invariably have severe neurologic deficits. In individuals with medium-sized hematomas, most survive with some residual neurologic signs. Survival for individuals with hemorrhage in the posterior fossa is more dependent on location of hemorrhage than size. Midline pontine hemorrhage is often fatal, whereas lateral hemorrhages carry a better prognosis.

Subarachnoid Hemorrhage
Overview and Definition

SAH can begin with the sudden onset of a headache with searing pain; sometimes the headache begins with exertion. SAH results in frank blood in the subarachnoid space between the arachnoid and the pia mater, which are contiguous membranes that surround the brain tissue. SAH can be spontaneous, is often seen in persons with normal blood pressure, and results in a sudden, severe headache. One percent to 4% of all individuals presenting to the emergency department with a headache have an SAH.

Etiologic and Risk Factors

Aneurysm and vascular malformations are responsible for most SAHs. SAH can also result from trauma, developmental defects, neoplasm, or infections that cause rupture into the subarachnoid space. Hypertension may be seen in 32% and fever in 5% of cases. Vascular malformations are responsible for approximately 6% of hemorrhages into the subarachnoid space. Included in vascular malformations are venous malformation, AVM, and cavernous malformation. The highest incidence of SAH is in women older than age 70 years. However, individuals with hemorrhage resulting from an aneurysm tend to be younger than those with hemorrhage secondary to hypertension. Risk factors for SAH include smoking, excessive alcohol consumption, and hypertension. First-degree relatives of persons who have experienced an SAH have a threefold to sevenfold increased risk of an SAH.

Clinical Manifestations

Forty percent of individuals who have SAH present with a headache. The headache results from a minor aneurysm leak that precedes rupture by days or weeks. Individuals who experience a headache typically report the headache as the only symptom and have a normal physical examination

Common associated symptoms include nausea and vomiting (75%), syncope (36%), neck pain (24%), coma (17%), confusion (16%), lethargy (12%), and seizures (7%). Physical examination in individuals who have SAH can have variable findings. For example, nuchal rigidity may take several hours to develop and is present in only 35% to 52% of individuals. Thirty-six percent have a normal level of consciousness, whereas 28% are somnolent or confused. Focal motor weakness is detected in only 10%, and cranial nerve palsies are seen in 9%. Often noted initially is cessation of physical and intellectual activity, vomiting, and alteration of consciousness. Drowsiness, restlessness, and agitation are especially common. Severe focal neurologic signs such as hemiplegia and hemianopia are absent at onset unless the aneurysm also bleeds into the brain.

Medical Management

Diagnosis

Up to 38% of individuals who have an SAH are misdiagnosed initially. Misdiagnosis of SAH is associated with increased morbidity and mortality. The most common misdiagnoses for SAH are viral meningitis, migraine, and headache of uncertain etiology. Often individuals have subtle presentations and normal neurologic examinations. It is important to realize that the headache of SAH may occur in any location, may be mild, may resolve spontaneously, or may be relieved by analgesics. Prominent vomiting may lead to a misdiagnosis of viral syndrome, gastroenteritis, influenza, or viral meningitis.

A CT scan is the diagnostic modality of choice in individuals suspected of having SAH. The sensitivity of CT for SAH is approximately 90% to 95%. However, the longer the duration is from onset of symptoms, the lower the sensitivity of CT for SAH. Therefore a lumbar puncture should be performed in all individuals suspected of having an SAH when the CT scan is negative or inadequate.

Treatment

Once the diagnosis of SAH is made, prompt neurosurgical consultation is necessary. The treatment of individuals with

SAH involves the prevention and management of the relatively common secondary complications of SAH: rebleeding, vasospasm, hydrocephalus, hyponatremia, and seizures. About half of individuals with SAH have vasospasm; this problem may resolve or progress to cerebral infarction. Angiographic vasospasm has a typical temporal course: onset between 3 and 5 days after hemorrhage, maximal narrowing at 5 to 14 days, and gradual resolution over 2 to 4 weeks. However, 15% to 20% of individuals with vasospasm die despite maximal therapy. Effective measures to decrease the risk of delayed cerebral ischemia are liberal fluids, avoidance of antihypertensive drugs, and administration of the calcium antagonist nimodipine.

Prognosis

Mortality rate from SAH is high in elderly persons. Functional outcomes are poor, and few individuals age 75 years or older are able to live independently at discharge. Early aggressive surgical treatment of elderly individuals admitted in good condition may lead to better outcomes. Seizure-like episodes occur in 25% of individuals after SAH.

If the resulting hematoma is less than 3 cm, the prognosis is good. Evacuation of hematomas that are larger should include resection of the causative aneurysm. Prompt removal may result in dramatic and early improvement of neurologic function. Repeat hemorrhage is more likely to occur if the hematoma is evacuated without treatment of the ruptured aneurysm.[57,70]

Types of Subarachnoid Hemorrhage

Berry aneurysm is a congenital abnormal distention of a local vessel that occurs at a bifurcation, in which the medial layer of the vessel is the weakest. About 90% of SAHs are caused by berry aneurysms. Aneurysms are probably caused by a combination of congenital defects in the vascular wall and degenerative changes. They usually occur at branching sites on the large arteries of the circle of Willis. When an aneurysm ruptures, blood is released under arterial pressure into the subarachnoid space and quickly spreads through the cerebrospinal fluid around the brain and spinal cord. Fig. 21.17 shows the typical formations of berry aneurysms.

Venous malformations are composed entirely of veins, which are usually thickened and hyalinized, with minimal elastic tissue or smooth muscle. Normal brain parenchyma is interspersed among the vessels. Fifty percent of malformations are venous malformation, with the risk of hemorrhage estimated at 20% per year. Individuals with a cerebellar venous malformation have the greatest risk of hemorrhage. Occasionally, seizures may be associated with venous malformations. Headaches and focal neurologic deficits are manifested according to the area of the brain that is disrupted.

Treatment

Spontaneous rupture of a venous malformation is not common, and the resulting bleed is often not of great consequence. Surgical resection of the hematoma may be necessary if it is significantly extensive. With evacuation of the hematoma, the malformation is most often left intact.

Arteriovenous malformation is characterized by direct artery-to-vein communication without an intervening capillary bed. AVMs are the result of abnormal fetal development at approximately 3 weeks' gestation. More than 90% of AVMs occur in the cerebral hemispheres.

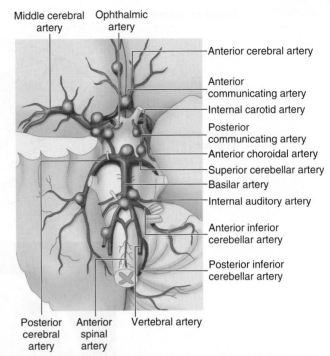

FIG. 21.17 Berry aneurysms typically develop at the bifurcations of arteries on the undersurface of the brain. (From Goldman L, Schafer AI: Goldman-Cecil Medicine, ed 25, Philadelphia, 2016, Saunders; courtesy Dr. Justin Zivin.)

Angiography is the definitive diagnostic procedure for an AVM. It should be suspected as a cause of hemorrhage in persons younger than 40 years, especially if they have normal blood pressure. Fig. 21.18 represents the vascular disorder and its appearance on imaging.[59]

Approximately 10% of individuals die of an AVM hemorrhage. In the first year following the hemorrhage, the chance of recurrence is 6%, increasing to 7% if there is a concomitant aneurysm.[5]

Neuroradiologic embolization, stereotactic radiotherapy, and surgery are the current treatments for AVM. These techniques are used alone or in combination depending on the size and site of the lesion. Vasospasm after surgery is a side effect, and it appears that surgeries in the posterior circulation are better tolerated than those in the anterior circulation.[42]

Cavernous malformations consist of a cluster of dilated, abnormal vessels that may be found in area of the brain. Cavernous malformations represent approximately 10% of vascular malformations. Multiple malformations can occur in the same person. There is some evidence suggesting a predisposition for cavernous malformations is related to the 7th chromosome.[76] The majority of individuals recover from a cavernous malformation hemorrhage, and the risk of repeat bleeding is low. Surgery is the treatment of choice for malformations that have hemorrhaged and are in an accessible part of the brain.

Subdural Hemorrhage

A subdural hemorrhage, or hematoma, is most often the result of tearing of the bridging veins between the brain surface and

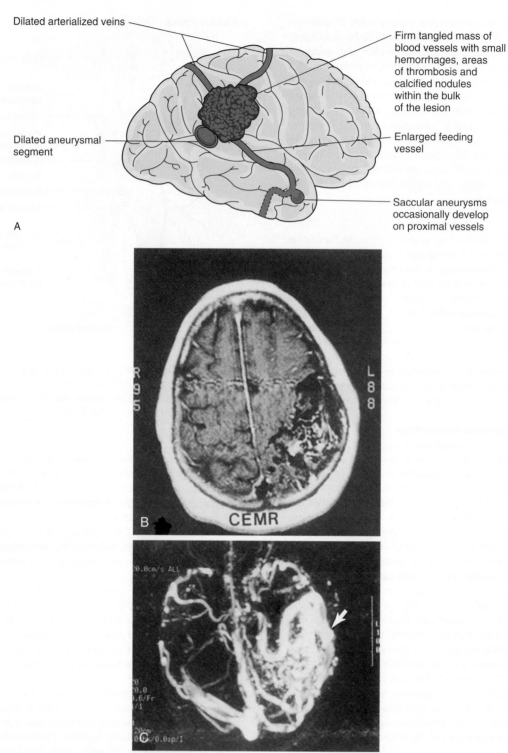

FIG. 21.18 (A) Typical deformation of blood vessels and brain tissue in relation to an arteriovenous malformation (AVM). The AVM as seen with magnetic resonance imaging (B) and magnetic resonance angiography (C). *Arrow* points to enlarged vessel in periphery of AVM. (A, Redrawn from Lindsay KW, Bone I, Fuller G: Neurology and neurosurgery illustrated, ed 5, Edinburgh, Churchill Livingstone, 2010; B and C, from Ramsey R: Neuroradiology, Philadelphia, 1994, Saunders.)

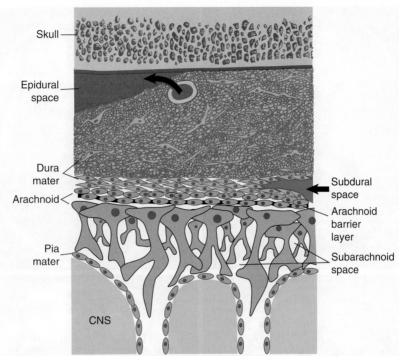

FIG. 21.19 Actual spaces and potential spaces in the cranial meninges. Epidural space between dura and skull can be opened up by blood from a ruptured meningeal artery. Subdural space may be opened up by blood from a vein that tears as it crosses the arachnoid to enter a dural sinus. (From Vanderah TW, Gould DJ: Nolte's the human brain: an introduction to its functional anatomy, ed 7, Philadelphia, 2016, Elsevier.)

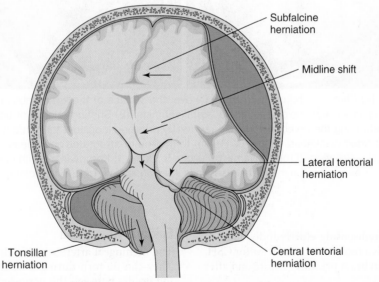

FIG. 21.20 Compression of brain tissue with herniation into adjacent structures produced by the subdural hemorrhage. (Redrawn from Lindsay KW, Bone I, Fuller G: Neurology and neurosurgery illustrated, ed 5, Edinburgh, Churchill Livingstone, 2010.)

dural sinus. It results in accumulation of blood in the dural space. If it is a small amount, the body can reabsorb the fluid; if the blood is of great enough volume, as can occur with trauma, it becomes a space-occupying lesion. The lesion is reflected in the area of the hemorrhage and the result can be herniation of the cortex into the adjoining spaces (Figs. 21.19 and 21.20).

Chronic subdural hematoma (CSH) is defined as a subdural hemorrhage that is more than 20 days old. The peak incidence for CSH occurs in the sixth and seventh decades, with up to 80% occurring in elderly men. In elderly persons, CSH often is caused by minor trauma, especially falls. In the majority of cases there is no underlying brain injury. Fragility of the bridging veins and cerebral atrophy allow increased movement of

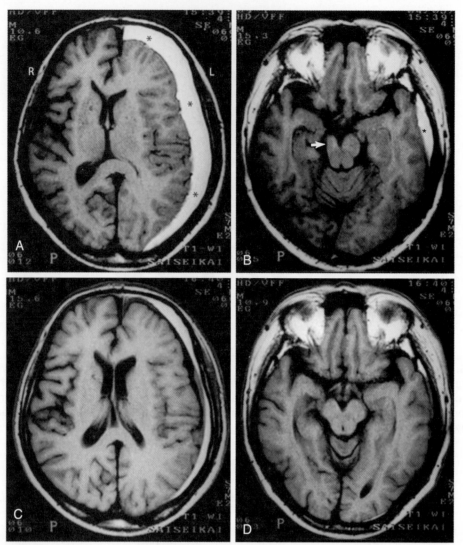

FIG. 21.21 (A) Chronic subdural hematoma (*) over the surface of the left cerebral hemisphere, compressing its subarachnoid spaces and lateral ventricle. (B) Shifting midline structures to the right and deforming the cerebral peduncle *(arrow)* by pressing it against the tentorium cerebelli, causing left-sided weakness. (C and D) Return to midline of structures and release of pressure after surgical evacuation. (From Itoyama Y, Fujioka S, Ushio Y: Kernohan's notch in chronic subdural hematoma: findings on magnetic resonance imaging: case report, J Neurosurg 82:645–646, 1995.)

the brain within the skull, predisposing elderly individuals to CSH. Anticoagulant therapy is a recognized risk factor for CSH. Fig. 21.21 shows the change in brain pressures before and after removal of a CSH.[81]

Elderly individuals who have CSH typically present with a complaint of headache and/or changes in mental status. Mild generalized headache is present in up to 90% of individuals who have CSH. Any elderly individual who has a headache, especially with a change in mental or functional status, should be evaluated for CSH.

Epidural Hematoma

The meningeal arteries run in the periosteal layer of the dura. They can be torn during a traumatic skull injury, and bleeding occurs between the periosteum and the skull, resulting in an epidural hematoma. The damage comes from compression of the brain. Because there is potential for extensive pooling of blood, this is considered a medical emergency and should be evacuated immediately to prevent compression on the posterior structures, which may cause death. Fig. 21.22 presents an MRI showing an epidural hematoma.

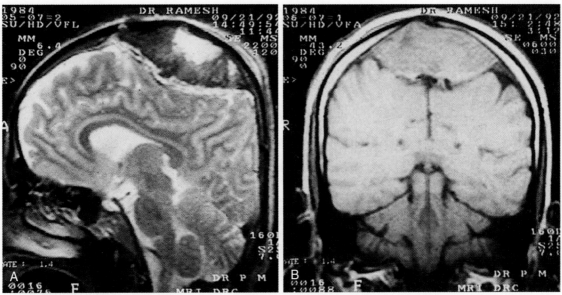

FIG. 21.22 Epidural hematoma seen on magnetic resonance image. (A) Sagittal view. (B) Coronal view. (From Ramesh VG, Sivakumar S: Extradural hematoma at the vertex: a case report, Surg Neurol 43:138, 1995.)

BOX 21.3   Movement Problems Associated with Stroke

- Decreased force production
- Sensory impairments
- Abnormal synergistic organization of movement
- Altered temporal sequencing of muscle contractions
- Impaired regulation of force control
- Delayed responses
- Abnormal muscle tone
- Loss of range of motion
- Altered biomechanical alignment

21.1 Special Implications for the PTA: Stroke Rehabilitation

Disability resulting from stroke is a major problem for the stroke survivor, the family, and health care providers. A team of professionals is necessary to address the multitude of problems present after stroke. Physical therapist assistants (PTAs) play a key role in this team. Evidence supports the correlation between therapeutic intervention and decreased levels of disability. Although certain characteristics of stroke have been discussed, the effects of stroke remain highly individualized. Each individual must be managed according to the particular impairments and disability that remains after the stroke.[9]

Movement typically is altered after stroke. This can be a result of a number of impairments that reflect damage in specific areas of the brain. Reflex patterns can be altered, which may limit postural reactions and hence balance. Patterns of muscle activation are often disrupted, which disrupt efficient motor control and also contribute to balance deficiencies.[41,46] Box 21.3 gives examples of typical motor impairments after stroke.

Assessment

Although there is a degree of spontaneous recovery after stroke, some impairments persist over time. Identification of impairments and functional limitations that may lead to disabilities is essential to provide effective therapeutic interventions. An understanding of the typical characteristics of the different stroke syndromes is helpful in establishing appropriate strategies for intervention. Fig. 21.23 represents areas of brain damage and associated clinical signs.

Discrete differences exist according to the side of hemispheric lesion. Right hemisphere lesions tend to cause impairments related to spatial awareness and processing along with poor judgment and short-term memory problems.[6] *Pusher syndrome,* pushing toward the hemiparetic side, is often observed with right hemispheric lesions.[62] Left hemisphere lesions typically result in impairments related to calibrating movements, language, and sequencing movements, resulting in slow cautious movements.[6] Despite these differences, there does not appear to be an overall difference in functional level as measured by instrumental activities of daily living. However, patients with pusher syndrome typically take longer to reach a level of independent daily activities and ambulation.[62]

Intervention

Skill acquisition for recovery of function is the main goal in movement retraining. Although problem solving is critical for improving skill, impairments of motor control such as decreased force production, increased tone, and poor control of degrees of freedom in movement must be adequately addressed. Motor learning also depends on neural plasticity and the neural network affected in the pathogenesis of stroke.[5,40]

Constraint-induced training with the affected limb is effective and is being used in a variety of formats. Increased dexterity and function are possible even after extended time poststroke.[78]

Positive results have been associated with the electrical stimulation orthoses and robotics for upper extremity movement and functional use.[1] Virtual reality applications are being developed with a focus on attention, executive function, memory, and spatial ability. Functional training for activities such as crossing the street, driving, preparing meals, and navigating by wheelchair are possible with virtual reality.[60] Conductive education has been used with adult stroke patients in Europe and Canada with good success.

Fall prevention is always a primary goal for the individual who sustained a stroke. Falls are frequent and in more than 5% of cases result in significant injury. They more commonly occur during the transition from sit to stand. Evidence shows that people who fall take more time to rise and to sit down, with increased sway in the mediolateral directions.[13,31]

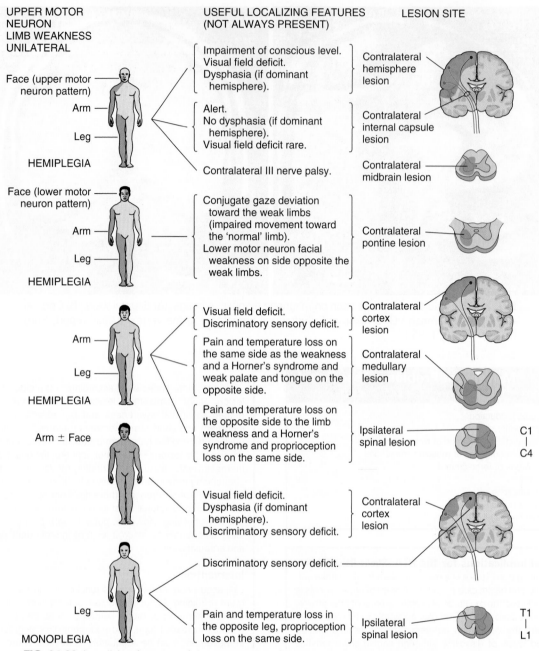

UPPER MOTOR
NEURON
LIMB WEAKNESS
UNILATERAL

Face (upper motor neuron pattern)

Arm

Leg

HEMIPLEGIA

USEFUL LOCALIZING FEATURES
(NOT ALWAYS PRESENT)

Impairment of conscious level.
Visual field deficit.
Dysphasia (if dominant hemisphere).

Alert.
No dysphasia (if dominant hemisphere).
Visual field deficit rare.

Contralateral III nerve palsy.

LESION SITE

Contralateral hemisphere lesion

Contralateral internal capsule lesion

Contralateral midbrain lesion

Face (lower motor neuron pattern)

Arm

Leg

HEMIPLEGIA

Conjugate gaze deviation toward the weak limbs (impaired movement toward the 'normal' limb).
Lower motor neuron facial weakness on side opposite the weak limbs.

Contralateral pontine lesion

Arm

Leg

HEMIPLEGIA

Visual field deficit.
Discriminatory sensory deficit.

Contralateral cortex lesion

Pain and temperature loss on the same side as the weakness and a Horner's syndrome and weak palate and tongue on the opposite side.

Contralateral medullary lesion

Arm ± Face

Pain and temperature loss on the opposite side to the limb weakness and a Horner's syndrome and proprioception loss on the same side.

Ipsilateral spinal lesion

C1
|
C4

Visual field deficit.
Dysphasia (if dominant hemisphere).
Discriminatory sensory deficit.

Contralateral cortex lesion

Discriminatory sensory deficit.

Leg

MONOPLEGIA

Pain and temperature loss in the opposite leg, proprioception loss on the same side.

Ipsilateral spinal lesion

T1
|
L1

FIG. 21.23 Localizing features of damage to specific areas of the brain and spinal cord. (Redrawn from Lindsay KW, Bone I, Fuller G: Neurology and neurosurgery illustrated, ed 5, Edinburgh, Churchill Livingstone, 2010.)

Obtaining a functional and normal-looking gait has long been the goal of PTAs and stroke survivors. Research continues in this area.[50,73] Treadmill training[45] has been shown to be effective and perhaps more effective than conventional gait training for improving some gait parameters, such as stride length and single limb stance. Treadmill training with partial body weight support shows functional changes over typical terrain, with more normal movement of the affected limb during both stance and swing.[30,79] Computer-assisted gait training results in increased stride length and speed of walking.[72,73] Balance retraining with center of pressure feedback provides more even distribution and control of center of gravity.[66]

Although a therapeutic goal is often to move clients out of assistive devices, studies show that for some components of gait the *orthosis* or assistive device still provides better control. Rigid ankle braces resulted in longer relative single-stance duration, improved swing symmetry, and ankle excursions. The decreased activity in the anterior tibialis continues to be a drawback.[32] Use of a cane improves weight shift to prepare for the next step and results in decreased circumduction.[43]

Control of spasticity and contractures through positioning, range-of-motion exercise, stretching, and splinting has long been a part of the rehabilitation process. In the past, PTAs avoided strengthening hypertonic or spastic muscles for fear of increasing tone; however, it has been shown that strengthening activities in a spastic muscle can be performed without increasing the spasticity.[7]

Cardiovascular endurance training is indicated for the stroke survivor and should be incorporated into rehabilitation programs. Treadmill training has been shown to reduce the energy expenditure and cardiovascular demands of gait within the stroke population.[49] Research is ongoing to establish the parameters of cardiovascular training within the limits created by neurologic deficits.

Based on the theory of motor learning, the ability to learn a new motor program or a different way of moving does not follow a specific time frame following brain damage.[4] Potential for adaptation based on learning goes beyond the time frame of spontaneous recovery.[84]

Failure to maintain functional gains after the course of therapy is a concern for all individuals involved in poststroke rehabilitation. Functional exercise done on a regular basis has been shown to have a positive impact on recovery.[16] Early and consistent involvement of the family or primary caretakers is paramount, as is the follow-through of a home management program of activity and exercise. Compliance of stroke survivors and caregivers continues to be low despite efforts toward better education.[61] The functional consequence of fatigue in physical, professional, and social activities should be considered.[27]

The clinician and family should watch for symptoms related to angina, peripheral vascular disease, and deep vein thrombosis that may arise after stroke. Osteoporotic bone loss has been demonstrated with immobility of the upper extremity, especially in women, and should be addressed as a part of a standard protocol.[14]

REFERENCES/SUGGESTED READINGS

To enhance this text and add value for the reader, references and suggested readings are included on the companion Evolve site that accompanies this textbook. The reader can view the source and access it online whenever possible.

Traumatic Brain Injury

VOCAB BUILDERS

Cheyne–Stokes
Coma
Community reentry
Concussion

Gliding contusion
Posttraumatic amnesia
Rancho Los Amigos Scale
Retrograde amnesia

Somatosensory
Wallerian degeneration

TRAUMATIC BRAIN INJURY

Overview and Definition

Traumatic brain injury (TBI) results from an external physical force with the potential to cause mild to complex alterations of brain function. Outcomes are variable, depending on the extent of the injury, other injuries sustained, and management of the injury. Almost half of those sustaining a closed head injury die on site. For survivors, appropriate management improves outcome. For those with complex injuries resulting in persistent morbidity, long-term rehabilitation is expected.[37]

Initial injuries typically present with a diminished or altered state of consciousness. Impairment of cognition and physical function are common and may be temporary or permanent. Changes are also seen in behavior and emotional control. Functional disability and/or psychologic maladjustment can be persistent. Many persons who sustain a TBI are left with lifelong disabilities that keep them from returning to their preinjury lifestyles. Initial predictions of outcomes are difficult as differences in recovery are seen in people who appear to have identical injuries.

One of the great medical challenges in the management of TBI is the need to balance cerebral perfusion and intracranial pressure (ICP). This balancing act can affect ventilation, renal function, and overall perfusion. For this reason, integration of care is critical on all levels, from understanding the pathophysiologic principles to treatment through interdisciplinary communication.[11]

Incidence and Risk Factors

More than 30% of all injury-related deaths are due to TBI. Each year 1.7 million people sustain a TBI, resulting in 52,000 deaths and 275,000 hospitalizations, whereas 75% of all TBIs are concussions or other mild forms of injury.[9] Falls are the leading cause of head trauma, with the highest percentage (almost 61%) seen in those older than age 65 years, followed by children 0 to 14 years of age (slightly more than 50%). The second leading cause of TBI is motor vehicle accidents, followed by assaults, with percentages varying by age group.[9] The incidence of penetrating TBI from gunshot wounds is increasing, and in some urban communities it is now the most common type of injury seen.[21] Brain injury due to firearms is associated most often with attempted suicide.[33]

Men are twice as likely to sustain a TBI as are women. African Americans, American Indians, and Alaska Natives have a higher rate of hospitalization due to TBI than their white counterparts, whereas mortality rates are highest among African Americans.[34] Alcohol use and abuse are frequently associated with brain trauma; 50% of people admitted into hospitals with head trauma are intoxicated at the time. Brain injury may be two to four times higher in alcoholics than in the general population.[26]

Although TBI accounts for a disproportionate share of morbidity and mortality, there was been a significant decline in mortality from the 1970s to the 1990s. This improvement paralleled an understanding of the secondary injury process and an appreciation that neurologic damage not only occurs at the moment of insult but also evolves over the ensuing hours and days as a result of biochemical and molecular derangements.

TBI peaks at three different age ranges. The first peak occurs in early childhood at age 1 to 2 years and is related most often to child abuse. The second occurs in late adolescence to early adulthood between ages 15 and 24 years and may be related to risk-taking behaviors. One of the most widespread causes of head injury among this age group is bicycling. The risk of sustaining a severe head injury while bicycling can be reduced by 88% by wearing an appropriate helmet.[3] The third peak in TBI occurs in the elderly population and is related most often to falls. This group is the most likely to be hospitalized, and approximately 7% will die while hospitalized.[2] Approximately 300,000 sports-related concussions occur annually. Actual incidence may be higher as there is the potential to underreport concussion symptoms by athletes. Although a single concussion does not necessarily lead to long-term neuropsychologic or cognitive complications, multiple concussions can cause long-term neuropsychologic abnormalities, particularly in executive functioning and information-processing speed. Those athletes who have had previous concussions are more likely to have future concussions with longer recovery time.[17]

Of the severely brain injured, approximately 60% of adults and 92% of children are injured in a motor vehicle accident. Pedestrians injured by automobiles represent some of the most seriously injured individuals in trauma. The elderly make up a significant percentage of pedestrians who have been struck by a motor vehicle and they have significantly increased mortality rates, with a majority of deaths occurring at the scene or at the emergency department.[2]

Etiologic Factors

TBIs can come from open head injury or closed head injury. With an open head injury, the skull has been penetrated and the meninges have been breached, leaving the brain exposed. Penetrating missile injuries create localized, focal lesions that, when not fatal, cause limited damage to the brain. It is not the size of a missile but its velocity that generally determines the extent of damage. Penetrating injury also causes vascular injury,

including disruption or the formation of aneurysms or pseudo-aneurysms.[37] Fig. 22.1 shows the kind of damage that can occur from a gunshot wound.

A closed head injury occurs in the absence of a skull fracture, but when the soft tissue of the brain is forced into contact with the hard, bony skull. The initial blow occurs under the point of impact, known as a coup injury. Then, as the brain decelerates against the contralateral skull, injury occurs to tissue on the opposite side, contrecoup. Such contrecoup injury is frequently worse than the injury underlying the impact.

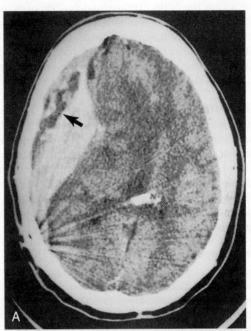

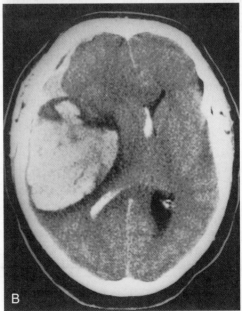

FIG. 22.1 Gunshot wound resulting in both intracerebral and epidural hemorrhage. (A) The bullet is shown on computed tomographic scan resting in a midline position with streaking effect of fragments also seen. The *arrow* points to area of decreased density thought to be epidural bleeding. (B) Large intracerebral hemorrhage is noted with blood present in the ventricle. (From Ramsey R: Neuroradiology, Philadelphia, 1994, Saunders.)

Actual loss of consciousness does not always occur, although there is generally an altered state of consciousness. Mild closed head injuries can occur after a severe neck injury without the head actually striking any surface. The symptoms are worse when there is a rotational component to the head injury in addition to the back-and-forth jarring.[20] Both diffuse injury and rupture of veins can result in subdural and subarachnoid hemorrhage. Rotational forces are the most likely forces to cause diffuse axonal injury, including damage to brainstem structures, such as the reticular activating system.

Severe head injuries result from significant bruising and bleeding within the brain. Approximately 25% of people with a normal initial computed tomographic (CT) scan will develop late hemorrhages. Contusions are usually more severe in persons with skull fracture than in those without fracture. Although contusion is the hallmark of TBI, severe or even fatal damage to the brain can occur without contusion.[5]

Pathogenesis

Primary damage is the result of forces exerted on the brain at the time of injury. Secondary damage refers to changes in brain function that result from the brain's reaction to trauma or other system failure. Causes of secondary damage include brain swelling and impaired cerebral perfusion (Fig. 22.2). Diffuse brain injury includes axonal injury, hypoxic damage, and edema. Multiple small hemorrhages may occur and are predictive of a poor outcome.[10]

Vascular Changes

Focal brain injuries usually result in cerebral contusions. Vascular damage is sustained at the moment of impact and leads to infarction within the cortical gray matter. Glial elements encapsulate the infarction, ultimately creating a residual cystic cavity.[29] Contusions typically occur at the poles and on the inferior surfaces of the frontal and temporal lobes. Occipital blows are more likely to produce contusions than are frontal or lateral blows. Areas where the cranial vault is irregular, such as on the anterior poles, undersurface of the temporal lobes, and undersurface of the frontal lobes, are commonly injured. With fracture of the cranial vault, there may be damage to the superficial epidural vessels and, particularly in the case of falls, there can be

rupture of the bridging vessels between hemispheres.[43] Fig. 22.3 shows CT scan images of changes seen after TBI.

TBI can be associated with other forms of vascular change. *Gliding contusions,* or hemorrhagic lesions in the cortex, may be the result of movement of the cortical gray matter in relation to the underlying white matter, causing shear strains to damage the penetrating vessels found at the gray and white matter interface.[60] Fig. 22.4 shows the effects of shearing injury as seen on CT scan. Subarachnoid hemorrhage is common as a result of the rupture of vessels within the subarachnoid space. This may trigger vasospasm that can lead to reduced regional blood flow. Injury to the vessels within the white matter can also cause significant neurologic consequences, especially if it is in the area of the basal ganglia.[29]

The increase in blood volume is considered to be the most important cause of increased ICP after head trauma. There can be bleeding into the epidural compartment, creating a mass effect that can displace the brain and increase ICP. The shear and tensile forces of traumatic injury can also create a subdural hematoma. Acute hydrocephalus occurs when blood accumulates in the ventricular system, expanding the size of the ventricles and causing increased pressure on brain tissue by

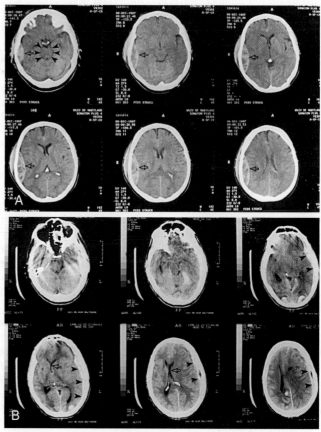

FIG. 22.3 Computed tomographic scans of two patients with closed head injury. (A) This patient has a right temporal epidural hematoma *(arrows).* The mesencephalic cisterns are patent in the top left, indicating a lack of brainstem compression despite mass *(arrowheads).* (B) This patient has suffered an acute left subdural hematoma *(arrowheads)* with midline shift *(arrows).* (From Townsend CM, Beauchamp RD, Evers BM, et al., editors: Sabiston textbook of surgery, ed 18, Philadelphia, 2008, Saunders.)

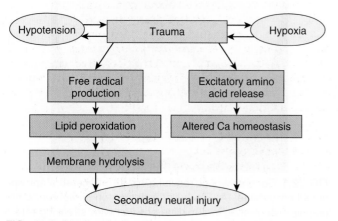

FIG. 22.2 Biochemical and molecular substrates of the secondary injury cascade. (Redrawn from Salcman M: Current techniques in neurosurgery, ed 2, Philadelphia, 1993, Current Medicine.)

compressing the brain between the skull and the fluid-filled ventricles.[19] Vascular volume can increase if venous outflow is blocked or cerebral blood flow (CBF) increases passively because of loss of autoregulation. Cerebrospinal fluid (CSF) volume increases may be the result of blockage of outflow pathways or interference with reabsorption. When the volume of one compartment changes slowly, compensatory decreases in the volume of other compartments may prevent a rise in ICP. When the volume change is rapid or the compensatory mechanisms are exhausted or dysfunctional, the ICP goes up.[11]

The overall result of these vascular changes is the decreased ability of the cerebral vessels to maintain homeostasis in the face of changing blood pressure or blood gas composition. Initially, within the first few hours after severe injury, there is decreased CBF both globally and at the impact site, which can induce ischemia. Within 24 hours, the blood flow can be at normal or above-normal levels.[29]

The impairment of autoregulation of circulation in the presence of moderate to severe head injury allows blood flow to the brain to become dependent on the systemic arterial pressure. Elevated blood pressure can result in hyperemia and decreased blood pressure can cause hypoperfusion. Impaired vascular responsiveness results in abnormal arteriole vasoconstriction in the presence of carbon dioxide.

Posttraumatic aneurysms of the intracavernous internal carotid artery can be associated with delayed and sometimes lethal massive epistaxis, nosebleed. This can be a result of basal skull fractures in the region of the carotid canal or cavernous sinus and/or orbital fractures and compromise of the optical nerves. Knowledge of these risk factors and early diagnosis can minimize the high mortality risk. Fig. 22.5 demonstrates this relationship. It can take from days to years for the artery weakening to develop, with an average time of 3 weeks. Because of the close anatomic relationship of the intracavernous portion of the internal cerebral artery (ICA) to the oculomotor, optic, abducens, trochlear, and trigeminal nerves, these structures may also be damaged during the aneurysm development, resulting in effects such as blindness, facial numbness, and/or oculomotor palsy.[22]

There appears to be a change in the endothelium of the blood vessels following brain injury. In the normal brain, neurotransmitters such as acetylcholine induce dilation, causing relaxation of the smooth muscle in the vessel wall. In the injured brain, this reaction can be missing, resulting in abnormal vasoconstriction.[18] Additional changes at the level of the endothelium result in a disturbed blood-brain barrier in the injured brain. This results in leakage of serum proteins and neurotransmitters into the parenchyma, causing edema.

Parenchymal Changes

Axonal injury is a consistent feature of the traumatic event. Shear and tensile forces most likely disrupt the axolemma, which impairs transport of proteins from the cell body and

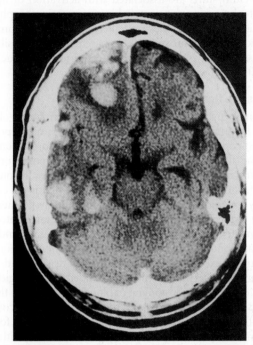

FIG. 22.4 Contusion with shearing injury. Computed tomographic scan shows multiple rounded areas of blood density with surrounding edema. Many of these areas are at the junction of gray and white matter consistent with shear injury. (From Ramsey R: Neuroradiology, Philadelphia, 1994, Saunders.)

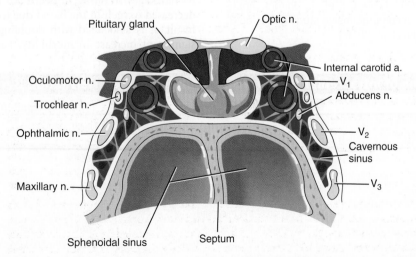

FIG. 22.5 Diagram showing the close proximity of the intracavernous internal carotid artery and the sphenoid sinus. (From Waldman SD: Pain management: expert consult: online and print, ed 2, Philadelphia 2011, Saunders.)

causes swelling of the axon. The distal axon segment detaches and undergoes *Wallerian degeneration.* The myelin sheath pulls away from the axon. These axonal changes are seen throughout the brain regardless of site of impact. The damage is different from that of stroke or tumor, which produces a more complete but local deafferentation. Typically, with diffuse axonal injury, there remain intact axons interspersed with the damaged axons. There is evidence of the potential for recovery of function based on the possible sprouting of undamaged axons to reoccupy the areas left vacant by degenerating axons. Secondary cell death by necrosis of the cellular membrane can be a result of edema. Apoptosis, or programmed destruction from within the cell, can result in cell death that occurs days, weeks, or months after injury.[44]

Study of excitotoxicity related to diffuse brain injury shows that the increase in extracellular neurotransmitters, resulting

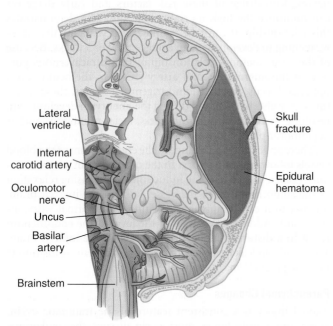

FIG. 22.6 Anterior view of transtentorial herniation caused by large epidural hematoma. Skull fracture overlies hematoma. (From Tintinalli J, Stapczynski J, Ma OJ, et al., editors: Tintinalli's emergency medicine: a comprehensive study guide, ed 8, New York, McGraw-Hill Education, 2016.)

Labels on figure:
- Lateral ventricle
- Internal carotid artery
- Oculomotor nerve
- Uncus
- Basilar artery
- Brainstem
- Skull fracture
- Epidural hematoma

in increased potassium, causes a massive depolarization of the injured brain. There is a complex interaction of the various amino acids and neurotransmitters, which may affect the postsynaptic functions, resulting in secondary dysfunction of the neural mechanisms of the brain. The excitatory neurotransmitter glutamate appears to rise to abnormal amounts following brain injury. Glutamate is neurotoxic when concentrations increase.

Free radicals are generated by TBI. Extensive membrane depolarization, induced by trauma, allows for a nonselective opening of the voltage-sensitive calcium channels and an abnormal accumulation of calcium within neurons and glia. Such calcium shifts are associated with activation of lipolytic and proteolytic enzymes, protein kinases, protein phosphatases, dissolution of microtubules, and altered gene expression.[21]

Frank blood that moves into the parenchyma is possible and can cause extensive damage and infection of the tissue, especially with open wounds.

Compressive Damage

Intracranial hypertension can produce herniation. During trauma, the brain may shift from its normal symmetric position. The most common herniation is the lateral tentorial membrane separating the cerebral hemispheres from the posterior fossa. This shift may cause compression of the brainstem, the pituitary, or other delicate brain structures. Because the brainstem controls the body's major visceral functions, brainstem involvement may result in paralysis or death. In less severe situations, autonomic nervous system changes may include changes in pulse and respiratory rates and regularity, temperature elevations, blood pressure changes, excessive sweating, salivation, tearing, and sebum secretion. Because the brain is surrounded by the rigid skull, swelling of the brain, or pooling of blood, pushes tissue through openings in the base of the skull or through the other compartments of the brain, resulting in herniation through the foramen magnum. Fig. 22.6 shows the herniation possible with brain injury with epidural bleeding. Table 22.1 lists the possible signs of intracranial hypertension and associated herniation syndromes.

Hypoxia. Hypotension (systolic blood pressure less than 90 mm Hg) occurring between injury and resuscitation occurs in one-third of severe TBI victims. It can be caused by blockages resulting in decreased blood in the brain or by decreased oxygen in the blood due to concomitant pulmonary insult. It is associated with doubling of mortality rate and a significant increase in morbidity. Early hypotension is also a

TABLE 22.1	Signs of Intracranial Hypertension and Associated Herniation Syndromes	
Sign	**Mechanism**	**Type of Herniation**
Coma	Compression of midbrain tegmentum	Uncal, central
Pupillary dilation	Compression of ipsilateral third nerve	Uncal
Miosis	Compression of the midbrain	Central
Lateral gaze palsy	Stretching of the sixth nerves	Central
Hemiparesis[a]	Compression of contralateral cerebral peduncle against tentorium	Uncal
Decerebrate posturing	Compression of the midbrain	Central, uncal
Hypertension, bradycardia	Compression of the medulla	Central, uncal, cerebellar (tonsillar)
Abnormal breathing patterns	Compression of the pons or medulla	Central, uncal, cerebellar (tonsillar)
Posterior cerebral artery infarction	Vascular compression	Uncal
Anterior cerebral artery infarction	Vascular compression	Subfalcine (cingulate)

[a]Hemiparesis will occur ipsilateral to the hemispheric lesion (false-localizing sign).

strong predictor of poor outcome and can lead to intracranial hypertension in later stages.[45]

Hypertension. Intracranial hypertension can interfere with perfusion by lowering the cerebral perfusion pressure (CPP). Under normal circumstances, cerebral pressure autoregulation maintains CBF constant over a CPP range of approximately 50 to 150 mm Hg. Following trauma, this relationship may be partially or totally disrupted; the brain can weather limited changes in CPP without notable alterations of CBF.

Cerebral perfusion pressure. Although there is no definitive evidence of the ideal CPP following TBI, the general consensus is that a critical threshold is 70 to 80 mm Hg. Mortality rates increase by 20% for each 10-mm Hg loss of CPP. When CPP has been maintained at 70 mm Hg there has been a 35% reduction in mortality rates.[53] CPP = mean arterial pressure (MAP) − intracranial pressure (ICP). MAP = 1/3*systolic blood pressure + 2/3*diastolic blood pressure.

Clinical Manifestations
Signs and Symptoms
Mild TBI is termed a *concussion.* Concussions are infrequently associated with structural brain injury and rarely lead to significant long-term sequelae. Moderate TBI may be associated with significant structural injury, such as hemorrhage or contusion, but death is uncommon. Severe TBI generally results in some form of cognitive and/or physical disability or in death, especially with very low Glasgow Coma Scale (GCS) scores.[21]

Concussion. In minor head injury, or concussion, the loss of consciousness lasts a relatively short time, or there may be no loss of consciousness. The postconcussion syndrome is a distinct entity that occurs within the first 7 to 10 days following the concussion and typically resolves within 3 months. These symptoms may vary and resemble those associated with concussion.[39] Symptoms usually associated with concussion are dizziness, disorientation, nausea, and headache. The client may be irritable or distractible and have difficulty with reading and memory. There may be complaints of headache, fatigue, personality changes, and decreased control of emotions.

The symptoms generally reflect both the focal and the diffuse nature of the damage. Changes to neurons, axons, neurotransmitter metabolism, neuroendocrine system (pituitary gland), CBF, and reticular activating system are common. The shearing effects and coup/countercoup can be responsible for dysfunction in frontal and temporal lobes. A right-sided cortical lesion could cause problems of visual–spatial processing, whereas a left-sided lesion could result in verbal processing deficits. Damage in the area of the amygdala may lead to heightened arousal, which enhances sensory information processing and is linked to emotional responses. The function of the amygdala is essential to the learning process and understanding of the consequences of action. Divided attention deficit, a reduction in information processing capacity, speed, or amount of information that can be processed, is associated with acceleration and deceleration head injury. This may be related to the diffuse white matter lesion, brainstem dysfunction, or a disruption in the frontal-limbic reticular activating system.[16] Neuropsychologic testing has shown significant cognitive disability following a concussion, including a reduction in information processing speed, attention, reaction time, and memory for new information.[21] Although cognitive impairment has been shown to resolve within about 7 days for most concussions, cognitive impairment has been shown to persist, particularly for athletes suffering multiple concussions.

Migraine headaches with and without aura can develop in the hours to weeks after a mild concussion. Immediately after mild TBI in sports such as soccer, football, rugby, and boxing, children, adolescents, and young adults may have a first-time migraine with aura. This syndrome may be triggered multiple times after additional mild TBI and has been termed *footballer's migraine.* Cluster headaches can also develop after mild TBI.[21]

Nonspecific psychologic symptoms such as personality change, irritability, anxiety, and depression are reported by more than one-half of individuals within 3 months of mild TBI. Fatigue and disruption of sleep patterns are also often reported. Posttraumatic stress disorder, which has many symptoms similar to those of the postconcussion syndrome, may occur after mild TBI.

In 2012 the American Physical Therapy Association and the House of Delegates implemented a position that recognizes physical therapists as being a part of the multidisciplinary team of licensed health care providers that can provide concussion management. A physical therapist assistant is able to work directly under the supervision of a PT that has been trained in examining, evaluating, and managing a person suspected of having a concussion. The PTA would be involved in providing education and monitoring of prevention in minimizing the risk of re-injure while performing therapeutic interventions that would reduce pain, restore strength, and return the person to prior level of activity/sport.[1a] (See Box 22.3 later in the chapter for an outline in physical therapy interventions.)

Levels of consciousness. Altered level of consciousness is a state that can occur with both diffuse and focal head injuries. This can be a result of diffuse bilateral cerebral hemispheric damage or a smaller lesion that affects the brainstem. In many cases, it is probably a combination. In moderate or severe head injury, unconsciousness can be prolonged or persistent. Arousal is associated with wakefulness and depends on an intact reticular formation and upper brainstem.

Coma is regarded as the lowest level of consciousness and is characterized as being unable to obey commands, utter words, open the eyes, or being in a state of unresponsiveness. This is indicative of advanced brain failure, with bilateral cerebral hemispheric or direct involvement of the brainstem. Coma rarely lasts longer than 4 weeks. The GCS is the most widely used instrument for determining level of consciousness; it is used to determine current status and potential for improvement (Box 22.1).

Some individuals may continue to exhibit a reduced level of consciousness, a condition referred to as *persistent vegetative state,* or postcomatose unawareness, characterized by a wakeful, reduced responsiveness with no evident cerebral cortical function. The individual exhibits eye opening with sleep–wake cycles and tracking of the eyes, controlled at a subcortical level. The vegetative state (VS) is notable for preserved arousal mechanisms associated with a complete lack of self- or environmental awareness. There is no purposeful movement and the individual remains mute. The VS can result from diffuse cerebral hypoxia or from severe, diffuse white matter impact damage. The brainstem is usually relatively intact.[4]

Locked-in syndrome consists of quadriplegia with preserved awareness and arousal. It is caused by injury to the ventral pons.[21] It spares vertical eye movements and can be seen with disordered breathing patterns associated with injury to brainstem respiratory centers.

Respiratory impairments. *Cheyne–Stokes breathing* is a rhythmic pattern of alternating rapid breathing and momentary stopping of breathing. It often presents in individuals with hemispheric lesions that are bilateral or can be the result of lesions in the diencephalon. *Hyperventilation* is seen in individuals with pontine or midbrain lesions. *Apneustic breathing* is characterized by a prolonged pause at the end of inspiration and indicates lesions of the mid- and caudal portions of the pons. *Ataxic breathing,* seen with damage to the medulla, is irregular in both rate and tidal volume.

Cognitive and behavioral impairments. Cognitive impairments include problems with attention, memory, concentration, and executive functions. Residual cognitive and behavioral deficits often remain despite a return to full consciousness. Deficits—including disorders of learning, memory, and complex information processing and loss of abstract thinking and complex problem solving—reflect the frontal lobe pathology associated with TBI. Loss of executive functions is observed and there is often confusion and disorientation in addition to difficulty in problem solving, delayed processing, and lack of initiation. Mood disturbances include depression and anxiety. Symptoms are related to the area of the brain injured.

When the damage is in the orbitofrontal area, behavior may be excessive and disinhibited. Inappropriate social and interpersonal behaviors, including inappropriate sexual behavior, occur with lesions in this area. Septal area lesions result in irritability and rage. Damage to the cortical bulbar pathways (i.e., those connecting the cerebral cortex to the brainstem) can result in emotional lability, including euphoria, involuntary laughing, or crying that is not associated with negative emotions.

Cognitive deficits are not always directly observable, but the observable behavior provides information regarding the ability to integrate cognitive processes. The observable behavior of a person with a brain injury is directly related to the integrity of cognitive function. The behaviors reflect the inability to adjust to the environment. Typical behaviors include erratic wandering; motor, sensory, and verbal perseveration; imitation of gestures; restlessness; refusal to cooperate; and striking out in response to stimulus or in random fashion. Often the individual will attempt to run away from the institution or home. Deficits in attention are also common. Clients show impulsiveness, hyperactivity, and difficulty sustaining attention. Behavioral changes can be present without cognitive or physical deficits.[52] Box 22.2 describes some of the typical cognitive characteristics and the resulting behavioral disturbances seen in persons after TBI. A useful tool to assess behaviors as a function of cognitive recovery is the *Rancho Los Amigos Scale* (Table 22.2). Table 22.3 includes some of the behavioral disturbances and their manifestations in people with TBI.

BOX 22.1 Glasgow Coma Scale

Eye Opening Response

Spontaneous—open with blinking at baseline: **4 points**
To verbal stimuli, command, speech: **3 points**
To pain only (not applied to face): **2 points**
No response: **1 point**

Verbal Response

Oriented: **5 points**
Confused conversation, but able to answer questions: **4 points**
Inappropriate words: **3 points**
Incomprehensible speech: **2 points**
No response: **1 point**

Motor Response

Obeys commands for movement: **6 points**
Purposeful movement to painful stimulus: **5 points**
Withdraws in response to pain: **4 points**
Flexion in response to pain (decorticate posturing): **3 points**
Extension response in response to pain (decerebrate posturing): **2 points**
No response: **1 point**

References

Teasdale G, Jennett B: Assessment of coma and impaired consciousness, Lancet 2:81–84, 1974.
Teasdale G, Jennett B: Assessment and prognosis of coma after head injury, Acta Neurochir 34:45–55, 1976.

Categorization

Coma: No eye opening, no ability to follow commands, no word verbalizations (3-8)

Head Injury Classification

Severe Head Injury—GCS score of 8 or less
Moderate Head Injury—GCS score of 9 to 12
Mild Head Injury—GCS score of 13 to 15

Adapted from: Advanced Trauma Life Support: Course for Physicians, American College of Surgeons, 1993. http://www.cdc.gov/masstrauma/resources/gcs.pdf. Accessed October 3, 2016.

BOX 22.2 Cognitive Characteristics and Behavioral Disturbances Associated with Frontal Lobe System Pathology

Cognitive Characteristics

- Loss of verbal fluency
- Loss of nonverbal or visual design fluency
- Decreased modulation of attention; specificity of attention
- Increased distractibility and pull toward interfering stimuli
- Slowed speed of cognitive processing
- Decreased ability to monitor and self-correct performance
- General intellectual functions may be within expectations
- Mental inflexibility and inability to shift cognitive set (the way a person thinks)
- Poor abstract reasoning and complex problem solving
- Inability to apply novel strategies in problem solving
- Loss of concrete thinking

Behavioral Disturbances

- Disordered planning and anticipation of events
- Lack of inhibition regarding social behaviors
- Psychomotor agitation
- Sexual inappropriateness
- Euphoria and inappropriate jocularity
- Irritability, emotional lability, depression
- Abulia, apathy, indifference, flat affect
- Paucity of spontaneous movement and gesture
- Motor, sensory, verbal perseveration
- Confabulation
- Echopraxis or imitation of gestures
- Anosognosia or explicit denial of illness or deficit
- Anosodiaphoria or lack of genuine concern about a deficit

Modified from Vomoto JM: Neuropsychological assessment and rehabilitation after brain injury. In Berrol S, editor: Physical medicine and rehabilitation clinics of North America: Traumatic brain injury, 3(2):303, 1992.

TABLE 22.2 Rancho Los Amigos Scale for Levels of Cognitive Functioning

Level	Behaviors Typically Demonstrated
I	No response: Client appears to be in a deep sleep and is completely unresponsive to any stimuli.
II	Generalized response: Client reacts inconsistently and nonpurposefully to stimuli in a nonspecific manner. Responses are limited and are often the same regardless of stimulus presented. Responses may be physiologic changes, gross body movements, or vocalization.
III	Localized response: Client reacts specifically but inconsistently to stimuli. Responses are directly related to the type of stimulus presented. May follow simple commands in an inconsistent, delayed manner, such as closing eyes or squeezing hand.
IV	Confused—agitated: Client is in heightened state of activity. Behavior is bizarre and nonpurposeful relative to immediate environment. Does not discriminate among persons or objects; is unable to cooperate directly with treatment efforts. Verbalizations frequently are incoherent or inappropriate to the environment; confabulation may be present. Gross attention to environment is very brief; selective attention is often nonexistent. Client lacks short-term and long-term recall.
V	Confused—inappropriate: Client is able to respond to simple commands fairly consistently. However, with increased complexity of commands or lack of any external structure, responses are nonpurposeful, random, or fragmented. Demonstrates gross attention to the environment, but is highly distractible and lacks ability to focus attention on a specific task. With structure, may be able to converse on a social-automatic level for short periods of time. Verbalization is often inappropriate and confabulatory. Memory is severely impaired, often shows inappropriate use of objects; may perform previously learned tasks with structure but is unable to learn new information.
VI	Confused—appropriate: Client shows goal-directed behavior but is dependent on external input for direction. Follows simple directions consistently and shows carryover for relearned tasks with little or no carryover for new tasks. Responses may be incorrect because of memory problems but appropriate to the situation; past memories show more depth and detail than recent memory.
VII	Automatic—appropriate: Client appears appropriate and oriented within hospital and home settings; goes through daily routine automatically, but frequently robotlike with minimal to absent confusion; has shallow recall of activities. Shows carryover for new learning, but at a decreased rate. With structure is able to initiate social or recreational activities; judgment remains impaired.
VIII	Purposeful—appropriate: Client is able to recall and integrate past and recent events and is aware of and responsive to environment. Shows carryover for new learning and needs no supervision once activities are learned. May continue to show a decreased ability relative to premorbid abilities, abstract reasoning, tolerance for stress, and judgment in emergencies or unusual circumstances.

Modified from Hagen C, Malkmus D, Durham P: Levels of cognitive functioning. In Rehabilitation of the head injured adult: comprehensive physical management, Downey, CA, 1979, Professional Staff Association of Rancho Los Amigos Hospital.

Impairment of memory is common with head injury. *Retrograde amnesia* is the partial or total loss of ability to recall events that have occurred during the period immediately preceding head injury. *Posttraumatic amnesia* is the time lapse between the injury and the point at which functional memory returns.[7] During this time there may be improvement in automatic activities, but there is no carryover of tasks requiring memory or learning. The duration of posttraumatic amnesia is considered a clinical indicator of the severity of the injury.[40]

Anterograde memory is the ability to form new memory. Loss of anterograde memory is common and manifests as decreased attention or inaccurate perception. The capacity for anterograde memory is frequently the last function to return following recovery from loss of consciousness.

Memory disturbance is common with concussion and minor head injury. Memory function is disbursed throughout the brain, and there appears to be a lack of ability to use semantic organizational strategy to remember something by associating it with relevant cues. Commonly there is difficulty identifying nonverbal stimuli, reproducing visual stimuli, and recalling verbal material. Complaints of memory problems are associated with poor performance on tests of speed, reaction time, attention tasks, and complex perceptual–motor abilities. Language deficits are often seen as word- and name-finding problems. However, recovery of language function appears to surpass that of memory in individuals with minor head injury.[16]

TBI is associated with several neuropsychiatric disturbances that can range from subtle deficits to severe disturbances including cognitive deficits, mood and anxiety disorders, psychosis, and behavioral problems. More than 50% of individuals with TBI develop psychiatric sequelae.[42]

Pain. Pain is a common complaint after brain injury, with complex interaction on both physical and neuropsychologic function. Head and neck pain is common with whiplash, and there is an increased incidence of physical trauma associated with the severity of head injury. Pain can cause a persistent distraction that pulls the individual's attention away from activity and can decrease the ability to concentrate. It can affect the ability to sleep, which leads to daytime lethargy, and it contributes to emotional reactions such as anxiety and depression.[47]

Neuropathic pain can result from the aberrant *somatosensory* processing in the peripheral or central nervous system, most common with damage in the area of the thalamus. Myofascial pain is common with trigger points, stiffness, and weakness. Fibromyalgia can develop, as it is related to sleep disturbances, anxiety, and depression. Another component of pain is suffering, in which the intensity is dependent on the person's mood, life experience, and level of social support. The result can lead to a condition that mimics chronic pain syndrome. Managing this syndrome in the individual with brain injury can be challenging.[16]

Cranial Nerve Damage

Focal damage in the brainstem can be reflected in the loss of cranial nerve function. The following are signs of specific cranial nerve deficits.[24,48] Table 22.4 lists brainstem reflexes, including the corresponding afferent/efferent cranial nerve pathways, observed in the comatose individual.

Although the olfactory nerve is well protected, shearing of the fibers to the extent of damage occurs in about 7% of brain injuries. In about 50% of those cases, this is a temporary condition.

The most vulnerable component of the optic nerve in people is the portion of the nerve located within the optic canal. Damage to this portion can result in monocular blindness, a dilated pupil with an absent direct pupillary response, and a brisk consensual response to light. Partial visual defects may also be noted.

TABLE 22.3   A Typology of Behavioral Disturbances After Traumatic Brain Injury

Symptom	Description
Behavioral Excesses	
Inappropriate abrupt physical action	Responds to a situation too quickly without thinking about the adequacy or consequences of the behavior: doing before thinking. Does not include verbal interruptions.
Tangential verbal output	Expresses one thought after another in disconnected or unrelated sequences: rambling speech, unable to get to the point.
Excessive verbal output	Provides too much information; content may be overly detailed or redundant; may be unaware of conversational turn exchange signals or unable to terminate conversation.
Verbal interruptions	Inserts comments that disrupt the flow of conversation or the task at hand; may force other person to relinquish conversational turn before completing the thought.
Inappropriate topic selection	Poor discrimination of appropriate topics for the social context. Revealing statements about personal matters, relationships, feelings that are inappropriate for the social context or level of relationship: excessive self-disclosure.
Inappropriate word choice	Use of profanity or emotionally charged words that are inappropriate for the social context. Overly explicit descriptions and explanations.
Physical proximity violation	Positions body within a spatial proximity of another person that is inappropriate for the level of relationship or social context: violating personal space.
Sexual inappropriateness	Acts with intent to develop intimate or sexual contacts or relationships inappropriate for the level of relationship or in violation of social mores (e.g., with adolescent minors); conversation contains sexual innuendos or lewd comments. May misinterpret others' expression of friendship as sexual advances, and responds as above.
Poor social judgment	Unaware of or does not apply rules governing social behavior; does not consider personal safety or safety of others in social context: rude, immature, coarse, tactless. Violates rules of etiquette.
Irritability	Feelings of annoyance or impatience; may accompany restlessness; easily provoked but generally does not escalate into an anger outburst. Tends to be a constant state, usually neither improving nor worsening by a significant degree.
Lability of affect	Magnitude of affect displayed is disproportionate to the antecedent event or social context and does not necessarily reflect the true nature or extent of feelings.
Anxious affect and rumination	Feelings of worry, tenseness, fearfulness, uncertainty about the future. Complains or oververbalizes concern over trivia.
Angry transition—verbal	An escalation of verbal output, where pitch, volume, or speaking rate increases, dysfluency occurs, aggressive content is delivered. Still within the realm of appropriate. A building-up phase before an outburst.
Angry transition—behavioral	Facial flush; posture threatening; personal space may be violated, body positions exaggerated; agitation behavior is evident, such as hair pulling, wringing of hands, clutching the fist.
Anger outburst—verbal	Explosive speech, screaming, abusive language, forceful or harmful content, self-deprecating content, or threats toward another person.
Anger outburst—behavioral	Hitting objects, striking out, exaggerated motions, forceful actions.
Behavioral Deficits	
Absence of or decrease in self-directed action	Decrease in spontaneous behaviors, requires prompts for behavioral action.
Depressed mood	Downcast facial expression, tearfulness, verbalizations of sadness, hopelessness, helplessness, low self-esteem; paucity of interest in pleasant events.
Restricted affect	Display of affect less than proportional to the event; face expressionless; voice monotonous; movement fails to reflect stated feelings.

Modified from Vomoto JM: Neuropsychological assessment and rehabilitation after brain injury. In Berrol S, editor: Physical medicine and rehabilitation clinics of North America: Traumatic brain injury, 3(2):307, 1992.

TABLE 22.4   Brainstem Reflexes in the Comatose Patient

	Examination Technique	Normal Response	Afferent Pathway	Brainstem	Efferent Pathway
Pupils	Response to light	Direct and consensual pupillary constriction	Retina, optic nerve, chiasm, optic tract	Edinger–Westphal nucleus (midbrain)	Oculomotor nerve, sympathetic fibers
Oculocephalic	Turn head from side to side	Eyes move conjugately in direction opposite to head	Semicircular canals, vestibular nerve	Vestibular nucleus; medial longitudinal fasciculus; parapontine reticular formation (pons)	Oculomotor and abducens nerves
Vestibulo- oculo- cephalic	Irrigate external auditory canal with cold water	Nystagmus with fast component beating away from stimulus	Semicircular canals, vestibular nerve	Vestibular nucleus; medial longitudinal fasciculus; parapontine reticular formation (pons)	Oculomotor and abducens nerves
Corneal reflex	Stimulation of cornea	Eyelid closure	Trigeminal nerve	Trigeminal and facial nuclei (pons)	Facial nerve
Cough reflex	Stimulation of carina	Cough	Glossopharyngeal and vagus nerves	Medullary "cough center"	Glossopharyngeal and vagus nerves
Gag reflex	Stimulation of soft palate	Symmetric elevation of soft palate	Glossopharyngeal and vagus nerves	Medulla	Glossopharyngeal and vagus nerves

The oculomotor nerve works in conjunction with the trochlear and abducens nerves to move the eyeball to maintain gaze stability and scanning. Damage is often due to direct insult to the musculature, but it can also be due to cerebral herniation. This nerve is damaged in less than 3% of people with head injury.

The fourth cranial nerve, (i.e., the trochlear nerve) is the least frequently injured. Damage is usually in the form of contusion or stretching, resulting in a vertical diplopia. The prognosis for recovery in fourth nerve palsy is poor because the nerve is so slender that it is often avulsed by the trauma.

Trigeminal nerve injury after head trauma results in anesthesia of a portion of the nose, eyebrow, and forehead.

The abducens nerve is often injured when the head is crushed in an anteroposterior plane with resultant lateral expansion and distortion of the skull. It can also be damaged in fractures of the petrous bone. Vertical movement of the brainstem may severely stretch the sixth nerve as it leaves the pons. There can also be damage in relation to the third and fourth nerves in the orbital fissure. There is failure of the eye to abduct when the head is passively turned away from the side of the lesion. Abnormal wandering movements are present in midbrain lesions, and they usually disappear when the person regains consciousness.

Trauma to the facial nerve is common, with injury to the temporal bone, or swelling of the nerve, or external compression. Symptoms of facial nerve palsy include loss of tear production, saliva secretion, and taste in the anterior two-thirds of the tongue. Muscles controlling facial expressions become weak.

Hearing and vestibular dysfunction occur in brain injuries. Transverse fractures of the temporal bone may cause disruption of the auditory and vestibular end organs or transient eighth nerve dysfunction. A blow to the head creates a pressure wave that is transmitted through the petrous bone to the cochlea, resulting in hair cell damage and degeneration of cochlear nerves.

The glossopharyngeal, vagus, spinal accessory, and hypoglossal cranial nerves pass through the jugular foramen at the base of the skull. The twelfth nerve passes through the hypoglossal foramen nearby. Injury is most often from a missile wound, but fractures of the occipital condyle can also produce lower cranial nerve palsies. Symptoms include cardiac irregularities, excessive salivation, loss of sensation and gag reflex of the palate, loss of taste on the posterior third of the tongue, hoarse voice, dysphagia, and deviation of the tongue to the side of the lesion.

Motor Deficits

Abnormalities of movement include monoplegia, hemiplegia, tetraplegia, and abnormal reflexes. Muscle tone is typically altered. Initially, there can be *flaccidity,* which is gradually replaced by increased tone, spasticity, and/or rigidity. *Decorticate posturing* is also common initially and reflects the loss of cortical control. The individual presents with increased flexor tone and posturing in the upper extremities and increased extensor tone and posturing in the lower extremities. *Decerebrate posturing,* or increased extensor tone and posturing in both the upper and lower extremities, reflects injury at the pons resulting in the loss of inhibitory control of the cortex and basal ganglia.[3,36]

The specific manifestations of paresis may include loss of selective motor control, abnormal balance reactions, and sensory loss. Cerebellar and basal ganglia dysfunction can result in ataxia, dysmetria, and tremor or bradykinesia.

Direct trauma to subcortical and substantia nigral neurons can result in movement disorders occurring shortly after an injury. Movement disorders occurring months following the injury have been hypothesized to be related to sprouting, remyelination, inflammatory changes, oxidative reactions, and central synaptic reorganization. Peripheral trauma that precedes the development of a movement disorder may alter sensory input, leading to central cortical and subcortical reorganization.

Heterotopic Ossification

Another complication associated with brain injury is the formation of *heterotopic ossification* (HO), or abnormal bone growth around a joint. The cause and pathogenesis of HO is unknown, but bone scans show evidence of increased uptake and elevation of alkaline phosphatase.

The onset of HO is usually 4 to 12 weeks after the injury, and it first appears as a loss of range of motion. Local tenderness and a palpable mass can be detected, along with erythema, swelling, and pain with movement. HO in the hip area can mimic deep vein thrombosis. Peripheral nerve compression will sometimes develop, especially if the HO is in the elbow. HO can also result in vascular compression and possible lymphedema.[56]

Medical Complications

Multiple medical complications can occur after TBI. Cardiovascular effects of TBI include neurogenic hypertension and cardiac dysrhythmias. Respiratory complications such as neurogenic pulmonary edema, aspiration pneumonia, and pulmonary emboli usually caused by deep venous thrombosis are common. Other complications include disseminated intravascular coagulation, hyponatremia, diabetes insipidus, and stress gastritis. Iatrogenic infections are common.

Medical Management

Diagnosis

The diagnosis of brain injury starts at the level of concussion, with the American Academy of Neurology guidelines including three levels of concussion. In general, people who have lost consciousness for 2 minutes or more following head injury should be observed medically from the time of the impact. Athletic injury, falls, and minor auto accidents can result in concussions that are often not reported to health care providers. Given the possibility of developing *second impact syndrome,* cumulative damage from multiple concussions that can lead to long-term brain damage and disability, every possible concussion should be reported and maintained as part of an individual's medical record.

Athletes should undergo formal neuropsychologic evaluations when injury is suspected because this may unmask subtle continued deficits compared with baseline testing. Such deficits have been shown to correlate with duration of symptoms. This has become an increasingly important tool in concussion evaluation. Postural stability testing may also be undertaken for adjunctive data in determination of concussion severity.

Current imaging with CT or magnetic resonance imaging (MRI) does not permit quantification of neural injury that occurs after a traumatic brain concussion. Proton magnetic resonance spectroscopic imaging can be used to assess the neurochemical damage derived from a cerebral concussion. The ability to identify postconcussive individuals who are in a vulnerable cellular state is important as there can be a catastrophic deterioration in individuals even with a simple head injury. The combination of metabolic data, physiologic data, and clinical observations satisfactorily addresses the complete recovery from concussion.[38]

When a person sustains a severe head injury, the GCS is used to assess level of consciousness (see Box 22.1). Using this scale, three aspects of coma are observed independently: eye opening, best motor response, and verbal response. A score of 8 or less indicates coma.

Oculomotor and pupillary signs are valuable in assisting with the diagnosis, localizing brainstem damage, and determining the depth of coma. Pupillary examination should document size and reactivity to light. Greater than 1 mm difference in size or asymmetry should be considered abnormal. Once the baseline neurologic status has been determined, repeated evaluations are critical to monitor improvement, provide prognostic data, or detect deterioration, which should be addressed immediately. Symptoms of focal neurologic deficits, lethargy, or skull fractures should be monitored. A mental status examination is important in all head-injured individuals. Subtle abnormalities may be a guide to significant intracranial injury.

Diagnostic imaging can provide significant information that can guide the intervention and allow a more accurate prognosis. CT is the primary imaging modality for the initial diagnosis and management of the head-injured person. CT scanning of the head reveals the presence of hemorrhage, swelling, or infarction. In individuals with traumatic coma, patterns on CT that have been associated with worse neurologic outcome include lesions in the brainstem, encroachment of the basal cisterns, and diffuse axonal injury (Fig. 22.7).[54] An initially normal CT scan, however, is no assurance that hemorrhagic lesions will not occur. Approximately 10% to 15% of individuals with clinically severe TBI have a normal CT scan. In such situations, the possibility of extracranial or intracranial vascular disruptions may exist, and angiography should be considered.[21]

Diffuse axonal injury (DAI) is a frequent CT and pathologic correlate of severe TBI, accounting for about 50% of primary brain injuries. DAI is usually associated with a poor outcome. It is readily identifiable on CT as multiple hemorrhages, typically in the deep white matter and corpus callosum and occasionally in the brainstem. DAI may also occur as a result of mild TBI and may culminate in subtle types of cognitive deficits.[21]

Clinical examination is of no diagnostic value in predicting head CT scan findings and should not be used as a means of avoiding head CT scans in pediatric practice. If clinical examination alone is used to evaluate children with loss of consciousness or amnesia and minor TBI, intracranial injuries will be missed. Because of possible implications for learning, return to athletic activity, parent education, and potential medical-legal issues, a head CT scan should be considered as part of the evaluation in all children with observed loss of consciousness or amnesia. Warning signs that may indicate the need for urgent intervention include any vomiting, restlessness, any GCS score decrease, severe headache, confusion, and focal temporal blow.[13] MRI is complementary to CT and is used in conjunction with—not as a replacement for—CT.

Lesions in the posterior fossa, as well as shear injury, are better demonstrated on MRI than on CT. MRI can also detect small hemorrhages, or intraventricular hemorrhages, which can lead to the diagnosis of increasing ICP, a significant risk in brain injury.[28]

MRI offers a sensitive window of detection for neuropathology from mild TBI. MRI is more sensitive than CT to DAI. Anatomic distribution of tissue damage and precise indications of the volume of lesions seen on MRI can predict recovery of the brain in the subacute phase. Prediction of outcome should not be based on CT scanning or MRI alone.[25] Positron emission tomography can be used to identify both structural and functional consequences and is especially valuable for mild head injury.[31]

Electrophysiologic tests that have been used for predicting coma outcomes include somatosensory evoked potentials, transcranial motor evoked potentials, brainstem auditory evoked potentials, and event-related potentials. Visual, auditory, and somatosensory evoked potentials make it possible to observe changes in a lesion, and therefore may aid in prognosis, but are not routinely used in isolation.

Neuropsychologic evaluation is valuable in identifying the extent of the cognitive deficits. The evaluation consists of a series of cognitive challenges given to the individual, including assessment of sensorimotor status, attention span, memory, language, sequencing, problem solving, and verbal and spatial integration tasks. Comparisons of normal and brain-injured persons have been well documented. Previous tests of intellectual function, including IQ tests and achievement tests, can be helpful for comparison, especially in mildly brain-injured clients. Cognitive impairment is the primary contributor to disability with moderate to severe brain

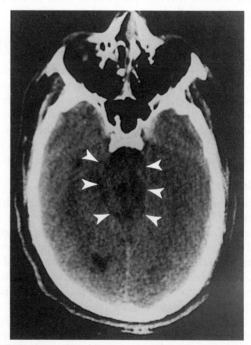

FIG. 22.7 Computed tomographic scan of the head in a patient with a closed head injury. Severe compression of mesencephalic cisterns is seen, indicating midbrain compression. (From Townsend CM: Sabiston textbook of surgery, ed 17, Philadelphia, 2004, Saunders.)

injury.[30] Examination of language and cognitive problems can include neuropsychologic testing with naming tests, aphasia examinations, as well as tests of auditory comprehension and speed of comprehension.

Approximately 5% to 10% of individuals with severe TBI have an associated spine and/or spinal cord injury. Initial head injury evaluation and management thus require simultaneous evaluation and management for potential spinal injuries. The majority of individuals with severe TBI have multisystem injury. Possibility of other significant and potentially life-threatening injuries should be evaluated and the proper treatment priorities accordingly established.

Treatment and Pharmacology

Acute

Treatment of TBI requires coordinated care and services from the onset of injury through the person's lifetime. Fig. 22.8 represents the levels of care that are utilized in the course of treatment. Note that primary prevention is the first step, and it is only when prevention is not provided that the client must begin the acute medical phase.

Prehospital management of a person with a severe head injury includes rapid triage, resuscitation, and efficient transport. Survival and medical management with the goal of stabilization and prevention of secondary complications are the primary medical focus. Hypoxia is a frequent secondary insult; often the upper airway is obstructed, and clearing the airway is the first treatment administered. Intubation and ventilation are critical, with positive-pressure breathing techniques supplemented by 100% oxygen and early intervention.[28] Hypotension (systolic blood pressure less than 90 mm Hg) and hypoxia (Pao_2 less than 60 mm Hg) should be avoided if possible and corrected if present.

Emergency department treatment includes determination of head injury severity, identification of persons at risk of deterioration, and control of hypoxia and hypotension. Prevention of secondary brain damage caused by edema, increased ICP, or bleeding should be addressed. Close clinical observation remains the best tool for neurologic monitoring in the early stages of head injury.

Surgical intervention is critical in the presence of hemorrhage to prevent neurologic compromise and can improve both short- and long-term outcomes. Brain herniations can result with hematomas. In some cases, the individual may be lucid after the injury and then, in the presence of undetected hematoma, lapse into coma and die.

Injury to the dural sinus can occur with a depressed fracture over a major sinus and requires evacuation. Decompression of the skull, often using burr holes, is warranted in the presence of significant cerebral edema or subdural hematoma. Decompressive craniectomy for intractable brain swelling is an older treatment that has recently received renewed attention. A number of operations have been developed for or applied to decompression of the brain at risk for the sequelae of uncontrollable intracranial hypertension.

Individuals with a Glasgow Coma Score (GCS) score of less than 8, or individuals whose neurologic status cannot be assessed because of administration of sedative drugs or neuromuscular blocking agents, should be monitored for ICP increases. The institution of ICP monitoring remains somewhat controversial; however, ICP monitors provide the most reliable guide to treatment of the underlying brain injury. Elevation of ICP more than 20 mm Hg is a significant predictor of a poor outcome. Monitoring of ICP can be accomplished in a number of ways. The ventriculostomy catheter allows monitoring and drainage of CSF but it is the most invasive method and is associated with risk of infection. The epidural catheter,

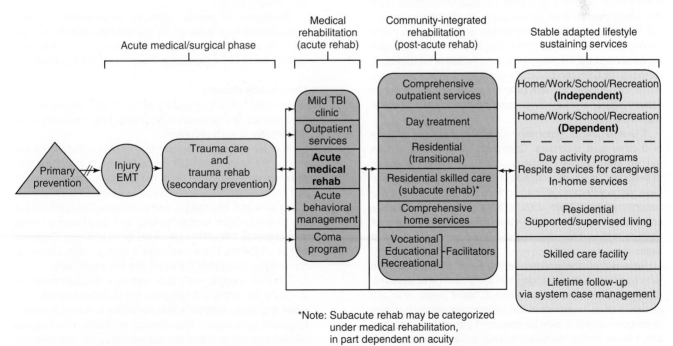

*Note: Subacute rehab may be categorized under medical rehabilitation, in part dependent on acuity

FIG. 22.8 System of care for the person with traumatic brain injury showing the components that should be considered in each phase. (Redrawn from Horn LJ: Systems of care for the person with traumatic brain injury, *Phys Med Rehab Clin North Am* 3:475–493, 1992.)

hollow subarachnoid bolt, and subarachnoid fiberoptic catheter are other options. All must be surgically placed. The noninvasive Doppler waveform can also provide information regarding ICP. If an ICP monitor is in place, the drainage of CSF may have significant therapeutic benefits.

Although there is no definitive evidence of the ideal cerebral perfusion pressure (CPP) following traumatic brain injury, the general consensus is a critical threshold of 70 to 80 mm Hg. Mortality rates increase by 20% for each 10 mm Hg loss of CPP. When CPP has been maintained at 70 mm Hg there has been a 35% reduction in mortality rates.[53]

CPP is determined by subtracting the ICP value from mean arterial blood pressure and represents the pressure driving CBF (cerebral blood flow). (MAP = 1/3*systolic blood pressure + 2/3*diastolic blood pressure.)

Thus CPP and CBF can be positively affected by either lowering ICP or elevating systemic blood pressure. It is generally believed that active attempts to maintain CPP above 70 mm Hg improve outcome; however, there are no systematic scientific studies to validate this.[21]

Cerebral fluid volume can be reduced pharmacologically. Mannitol is used to control blood volume. Hyperventilation has been used as a mechanism for controlling cerebral blood volume by increasing in blood Pco_2, resulting in vasoconstriction of the central vessels and reduced CBF. This must be considered a short-term procedure to be used judiciously because the cerebral vasoconstriction induced may produce ischemia. There remains debate on its usefulness in light of the possibility for a worse outcome.[40] High-dose barbiturate therapy is generally reserved for those situations in which ICP changes becomes resistant to other available therapies.

Blood pressure control is important in clients with brain injury, and systolic blood pressure should be kept at a minimum of 90 mm Hg. If fluid management cannot keep the blood pressure at an adequate level, then vasopressor drugs are used. Phenylephrine is effective at maintaining stability. CSF can also play a role in ICP. This can be controlled by the use of hypertonic saline or mannitol. Removal of CSF can be accomplished by ventriculoscopy. In clinical studies, the use of mild hypothermia appears to reduce neuronal injury by decreasing the amount of glutamate released.

Management of secondary injury is as critical in TBI as it is in other brain disorders. Controlling the presence of free radicals and cerebral edema are critical in the management of secondary injury associated with TBI. Vitamin E appears to have some effect on managing free radicals. Although glucocorticoids have been used to treat cerebral edema, there appears to be little long-term effect.[15] However, they are still used to reduce brain swelling and neuronal injury in select cases.[49]

Because of the intense sympathetic stimulation seen with head injury, hypertension and tachycardia are prevalent. Cushing's phenomenon, or a rise in blood pressure in the presence of an acute rise in ICP (most often caused by brainstem compression), may be present. Moderate increases in blood pressure can be tolerated, but extreme hypertension should be treated because it could lead to increased blood volume.[28]

Subacute

In addition to attempting to maintain homeostasis in the brain, management of the other sequela of brain injury is important. Spasticity is controlled by the administration of baclofen, diazepam, or dantrolene. These medications must be used carefully because of their side effects, which include increased weakness, lethargy, and drowsiness. Intrathecal baclofen can be used selectively to decrease tone with a baclofen pump, and the overall side effects are decreased. Abnormal muscle tone can also be controlled by nerve and motor point blocks or by the administration of botulinum toxin directly into the muscle belly.[28]

Control of seizures is provided by the use of medication such as divalproex sodium (Depakote). If the thalamus is affected, there can be abnormal sensations or intractable pain. The use of antiseizure medications is effective but carries high side effects and is often not tolerated by the individual whose system is already compromised. Attempts to control aggressive behavior through use of carbamazepine (Tegretol) and propranolol (Inderal) have had limited success. The nontricyclic antidepressants seem to be the most effective when the person is depressed.[23]

Rehabilitation

Rehabilitation and return to optimal function are the goals once the injured person's medical status is stabilized. Highly skilled, specially trained interdisciplinary teams provide an organized approach to the complex deficits encountered after head injury. Rehabilitation management of the individual is dependent on the cognitive and behavioral level of function of the individual. The Rancho Los Amigos Scale (see Table 22.2), which assesses components of cerebral function, is widely used. Treatment protocols are established according to the level at which the individual is functioning.

Psychotherapy is critical in posttraumatic stress disorder and can be helpful to establish coping mechanisms to address the cognitive deficits and problem solving in relationship to daily activity.

Restoration of mobility, self-care, employment, and recreational activities depends on the level of sensorimotor impairment as well as cognitive status. See 22.1 Special Implications for the PTA: Traumatic Brain Injury, in this chapter.

Community Reentry

Community reentry programs enhance the transition from rehabilitation unit to independent living. Therapists play a significant role in such programs.

In order to return to a lifestyle that may include work and school, the person with TBI needs to learn how to cope with the multiple demands on his or her attention. The person with TBI will have difficulty with executive functions such as organizing time and information, self-monitoring, and self-correcting. Self-motivation is often lacking, and structuring is necessary to ensure follow-through on assigned activities. Extensive use of checklists and environmental cues is helpful when attempting to reintegrate the client into the community.

The PTA working with brain-injured individuals must understand the interaction between the deficits related to cognitive and social behaviors and the ability to learn to move.[58] Cognitive rehabilitation and physical rehabilitation are closely related. Functional outcomes are limited by the cognitive status, and the understanding of the techniques that foster behavioral modification and learning in the head injured should be used by the PTA while motor skill acquisition is being attempted.[52] For information regarding working on mobility in individuals with focal brain injury, see 22.1 Special Implications for the PTA: Traumatic Brain Injury in this chapter.

The lack of motivation associated with TBI becomes a challenge for the PTA. Lack of internal initiation and decreased ability to learn may persist despite cues from the external environment. The first step in establishing motivation is to determine goals that are meaningful to the client, even though they may seem to be unrealistic. Alterations in attention span can be detrimental to progress in therapy. Reducing distracting stimuli can be helpful initially; distractions can be reintroduced as the ability to manage multiple stimuli improves. In most cases, the family of the survivor needs help understanding their family member's social and behavioral changes.[51]

Individuals with higher level physical skills and moderate- or low-level cognition skills are often the most difficult to reintegrate into the family and society. Therefore they may have higher levels of disability remaining after rehabilitation. Generally it is the cognitive functions that make one more successful in society. Aggressive counseling should start as soon as the behavioral and cognitive impairments are identified. Neuropsychologists and counselors can suggest interventions that help with cognitive functions, especially techniques to deal with memory loss, decreased attention span, and inappropriate behavior. Significant deficits in motor skills but higher levels of cognitive skills generally lead to a higher quality of life.

Prognosis

Because of the complex nature of the injury, predicting outcomes in brain injury is difficult at best. However, there are some indicators that can be considered broadly.[55] For those individuals who sustain a concussion, the probability of having persistent symptoms and neuropsychologic deficits is the same whether an individual is only dazed or loses consciousness for less than 1 hour. The effects of repeated concussions are cumulative because the ability of the brain to accommodate the damage is compromised by previous trauma. Individuals with moderate TBI usually experience both cognitive and physical disabilities and typically require rehabilitation services after acute hospitalization. Nevertheless, the incidence of severe long-term disability is small.[21]

Injury severity is one of the main factors determining outcome. The depth of impaired responsiveness and the duration of altered consciousness have been related to outcome.[32,57] In addition, the duration of posttraumatic amnesia has been used as a predictor of severity of the head injury. Other aspects of neurologic functioning are predictive of outcome. Loss of pupillary light reflexes following head injury reflects significant damage to the brainstem and is indicative of a poor prognosis. Oculomotor deficits often signal concomitant cerebral damage resulting in severe cognitive deficits. The degree of hypoxemia and hypotension encountered in the early stages can also have an effect on the long-term prognosis.[50]

CT has increased the ability to predict outcome in the head-injured person with a lesion of the brain parenchyma, intracranial hematoma, subdural hematoma, or massive hemispheric swelling. Acute hemispheric swelling with an extracerebral hematoma is associated with the worst prognosis. Unilateral brain contusion and DAI also carry a poor prognosis. A midline shift of brain structures, absent or compressed basal cisterns (indicating rising ICP), and subarachnoid hemorrhage will increase the risk of death or remaining in a VS.[54]

Epilepsy occurring within 7 days is often related to severe injury, depressed fracture, or intracranial hemorrhage. Posttraumatic epilepsy may emerge months or years following brain trauma and is more common after severe brain injury. Late epilepsy occurs most often as grand mal seizures or temporal lobe seizures.[26]

Dementia has been long recognized as a sequela of multiple head injuries in boxing, as evidenced by the term *punch drunk*. Neuropathologic studies of brains of boxers with dementia demonstrate β-amyloid protein–containing diffuse plaques and neurofibrillary tangles, which are pathologic features of Alzheimer's disease.

Neuropsychologic dysfunction appears greater in people older than age 30 years and those with less education. Social outcomes may be related to the premorbid status of the individual. History of substance abuse, low educational level, and psychiatric disorders can also limit success. Social and family problems are common and can cause isolation and poor quality of life.[35]

Cognitive deficits that affect motivation, attention, emotion, memory, or learning will slow progress. Lack of social skills has been reported to affect an individual's ability to reintegrate into the community. Often it becomes difficult to sustain relationships that were stable before the injury. Working with professionals who recognize these deficits and are trained to treat them will improve the chances of increasing quality of life after head injury.

TRAUMATIC BRAIN INJURY IN CHILDREN

TBI is one of the leading causes of death and disability in children of all ages.[41] Nonaccidental injury is a common cause of head injury in infants and toddlers and is often the result of the battered child syndrome. The head injury is often caused by shaking or striking the child.

Although the pathology of the brain injury in the child reflects damage similar to that in the adult, there are differences. Infants typically have tears in the white matter of the temporal and orbitofrontal lobes. The infant will more often sustain a subdural or epidural hemorrhage than an older child but is less likely to have skull fracture because of the pliancy of the skull.

Drowning is the third leading cause of death in children age 1 to 4 years. Peak incidences occur in 1- to 4-year-olds and in adolescent boys. Boys are three times more likely to be injured. Rapid resuscitation leads to better outcomes. As in adults, the motor activity return and pupillary light response are prognosticators of outcome.

Early management of the infant or child with TBI follows that of the adult, with some difference in the child's ability to tolerate the medications used. Late seizures are less common with children than with adults, so the need to be maintained on seizure medication is less.

Rehabilitation goals for the child are similar to those of the adult, although play is used during therapy. Orthotic and assistive devices are used frequently but for a shorter time than for adults. Agitation is common and is often difficult for the parents and siblings to handle. Aggression, decreased attention span, hyperactivity, and socially inappropriate behavior are seen. These children often require a great deal of behavior modification.

Community reintegration can be as difficult for the child as it is for the adult. Schools are better prepared to handle cognitive delays than abnormal behaviors. Cognitive status may return in one area and remain defective in another. Attention and memory deficits may produce the greatest obstacles to learning.

22.1 Special Implications for the PTA: Traumatic Brain Injury Rehabilitation for individuals with brain injury involves the PTA at many different levels and in different settings (Box 22.3). Understanding the deficits common in acute injury and the natural recovery patterns of the brain dependent on the site and type of injury is paramount for the PTA treating head injury.

Often the PTA will be involved in a dedicated head injury unit or in a community reentry program. Even in a more general setting, the PTA is often responsible for intervention with individuals sustaining head injury, often acutely, or when an individual has been through a rehabilitation setting and is referred for follow-up based on residual deficits. Provision of therapy in the long-term care setting involves care for individuals in a persistent VS or with behavioral deficits precluding independent living.[8]

Acute Management

In the acute care setting, the therapist is responsible for the evaluation of neurologic function in conjunction with physicians and nurses. One role may be consistent monitoring of cranial nerve function. In addition, the PTA is involved in monitoring reflexive and voluntary motor behaviors. The treatment plan often includes pulmonary care, positioning, range-of-motion exercises, and relaxation techniques. Movement facilitation begins early in the treatment and continues throughout rehabilitation in many cases. Because treatment starts while the individual is still in the intensive care unit, a discussion of life-sustaining equipment follows.

Chest tubes are common with a pneumothorax or hemothorax. The drainage tube should be kept below the level of the chest at all times. Upper extremity movement should be monitored so as not to interfere with the tube. Nasogastric tube feeding is also common initially, and when a tube is in place, the head of the bed should be placed at 30 degrees to avoid aspiration. It is important that cerebral venous blood volume be controlled in head injury. Maintaining the head at a 20- to 40-degree tilt will usually provide adequate drainage. Lines such as central venous pressure catheters, pulmonary or arterial lines, and ICP monitors can be compromised during movement, and often the movement will trigger an alarm that can be upsetting for the client and family. Close communication with the nursing staff will give the PTA confidence in moving the person in the intensive care setting.

Pulmonary management is another critical area. Normal levels of partial pressure oxygen are between 80 and 100 mm Hg. Normal oxygen saturation is between 95% and 100%. Techniques such as percussion, vibration, and suctioning are used to keep the airway clear but must be done with caution and may be contraindicated in the presence of increased ICP. Monitoring blood gases and oxygen saturation is critical in some clients, because movement may alter these values. Weaning from the ventilator is an individual endeavor. Some clients are able to continue to incorporate activity during weaning, but for others it may mean a decrease in tolerance to movement.[27]

Management of decreased range of motion from spasticity or HO is another focus of intervention. Joint contractures develop as secondary problems. Serial casting and dynamic splinting are used to maintain joint motion in the presence of spasticity, rigidity, or HO.[5] Managing excessive muscle and reflex activity through movement and positioning begins in the acute phase and often must still be addressed in the rehabilitative phase.

BOX 22.3 Physical Therapy Interventions after Concussion Provided by a PT/PTA Team

Rest and Recovery

A period of rest helps the brain heal and helps symptoms clear up, as quickly as possible. The physical therapist will prescribe the rest and recovery program most appropriate for the patient's condition.

Restore Strength and Activity Tolerance

The physical and mental rest required after a concussion can result in muscle weakness, and a decrease in physical endurance. The physical therapist will design a therapeutic exercise program at the appropriate time and closely monitor symptoms.

Eliminate Dizziness and Improve Balance

If there is dizziness or difficulty with balance following a concussion, a type of physical therapy called vestibular physical therapy may help. A qualified vestibular physical therapist may be able to help reduce or stop dizziness or balance problems after a concussion by applying special treatments or instructing in specific exercises.

Reduce and Eliminate Headaches

The physical therapist will assess the different possible causes of the headaches and use specific treatments and exercises to reduce and eliminate them. Treatment may include stretches, strength and motion exercises, eye exercises, specialized massage, and the use of modalities such as electrical stimulation.

Return to Normal Activity/Sport

As symptoms ease and the patient is able to regain normal strength and endurance without symptoms returning, the physical therapist will gradually add normal activities back into the daily routine. The physical therapist will instruct in how to avoid overloading the brain and nervous system, as the activity level is increased. Overloading the brain during activity after a concussion interferes with the healing of the brain tissue and can make symptoms return.

Modified from original article, Concussion, in MoveForwardPT.com, ©American Physical Therapy Association 2016, available at: http://www.moveforwardpt.com/symptomsconditionsdetail.aspx?cid=4f2ebb00-f1c0-4691-b2ab-742df8dffb99.

Similar concepts apply to decisions for wheelchair seating and positioning in the nonambulatory individual. Prevention of secondary joint disorders and pain is facilitated by provision of support in the anatomically proper position. Materials and equipment that are lightweight and provide total contact offer the most comfortable support.[12]

Swallowing deficits and related problems with respiration or coughing occur in approximately one-third of persons with head injury. Head, neck, and trunk control affect the ability to swallow. Intervention to address lack of strength and mobility of the perioral structures often starts in the acute phase.[59]

Loss of motor function and control often persists and is seen in more than 50% of individuals with head injury 6 months after onset. Diffuse damage to the central white matter tracts and midbrain with loss of integration of reflexes can have a devastating effect on function.

Long-Term Management

All three of the mechanisms that can lead to dizziness and imbalance can be affected after TBI (i.e., vestibular, visual, somatosensory). Intervention can be effective if the appropriate program is established. Visual stimulation is often disorienting, and the client prefers to maintain an environment without peripheral visual stimulus. This individual typically has difficulty reading and avoids situations with florescent lighting. Often the individual is hypervigilant in regard to the vestibular input as the vestibular system is easily overstimulated. This individual frequently has a sensation of moving when at rest. This can be an indication of maladaptation of the vestibular system. Therapy and other techniques, such as putting weights on the shoulders or pressing down on the top of the head, can increase the somatosensory input and help to decrease the sensitivity to vestibular input.

The individual with TBI typically will have complex movement disorders related to force production, timing, reaction time, and fatigue. In addition, sensory disturbances are significant. Together these impairments make learning new tasks difficult, and a lack of motivation can further limit progress. The PTA should understand, however, that with repetition of appropriate and task-specific activities, these individuals can make significant gains in all areas.

REFERENCES/SUGGESTED READINGS

To enhance this text and add value for the reader, references and suggested readings are included on the companion Evolve site that accompanies this textbook. The reader can view the source and access it online whenever possible.

Traumatic Spinal Cord Injury

CHAPTER OBJECTIVES

1. Become familiar with the mechanisms of injury for spinal cord injuries.
2. Define the terms primary and secondary with regard to spinal cord injury.
3. Recognize the clinical manifestations of spinal cord syndromes.
4. Review innervations by spinal cord level for dermatomes and myotomes.
5. Recognize the signs of autonomic dysreflexia.
6. Orient to typical approaches to rehabilitative care and the role of the physical therapist assistant following spinal cord injury.

OUTLINE

VOCAB BUILDERS

Autonomic dysreflexia
Complete lesion
Dysesthesia

Incomplete lesion
Paraplegia

Syringomyelia
Tetraplegia

SPINAL CORD INJURY

Spinal cord injury (SCI) is a catastrophic event of low incidence and high cost. It occurs most often in highly active persons. SCI rarely occurs in isolation, with more than 75% of these individuals having some other systemic injury. In 10% to 15%, there is an associated head injury. Because of the frequency of associated head trauma, any patient with a severe head injury should be presumed to have a spinal cord injury until proven otherwise.[29]

Incidence and Risk Factors

Males account for more than 80% of all cases of traumatic SCI. Historically, spinal cord injuries occurred in younger males;

however, the mean age of SCI increased in the 1990s and is now recorded as the early thirties.[11,12] It is estimated that there are approximately 30 to 40 cases per 1 million persons on an annual basis, with an additional six to eight deaths per 1 million occurring before hospitalization, although this number is decreasing The number of individuals living with SCI is approximately 300,000, with approximately 12,000 new cases each year.[63]

The primary cause of SCI is motor vehicle accidents, accounting for 38% of SCIs. The next most common cause is due to falls, followed by acts of violence and recreational sporting injuries. The number of SCIs due to sports has declined; however, those due to falls have remained proportionally the same. The number of injuries due to acts of violence peaked in the 1990s, and saw a slight decline after 2005.[63]

Sports-related accidents resulting in SCI are most prevalent in diving, and in contact sports such as football and wrestling, high-speed sports such as snow skiing and surfing, and sports in which injuries can involve a fall from a height, such as a trampoline or a horse. Fig. 23.1 shows a breakdown of the typical incidence of injury types.

According to the Foundation for Spinal Cord Injury Care, Prevention and Cure, at discharge, 30.1% of individuals have an incomplete tetraplegia, 25.6% have complete *paraplegia*, 20.4% have complete tetraplegia, and 18.5% incomplete paraplegia. Complete neurologic recovery by discharge occurs in less than 1% of individuals with SCI. The percentage of incomplete tetraplegia has increased slightly since 1994, whereas complete paraplegia has decreased slightly.[63]

The incidence of traumatic SCI in small children is low, representing less than 10% of the traumatic SCI population. In children, SCI is most often related to an automobile accident.

Definition and Etiologic Factors

SCI is classified as concussion, contusion, or laceration. A *concussion* is an injury caused by a blow or violent shaking and results in temporary loss of function, similar to the cerebral concussion associated with head injury. In *contusion* injury, the glial tissue and spinal cord surface remain intact. There may be a loss of central gray and white matter, creating a cavity surrounded by a rim of intact white matter at the periphery of the spinal cord. *Laceration* or *maceration* of the cord occurs with more severe injuries in which the glia is disrupted, and the spinal cord tissue may be torn. This can result in complete transection of the cord. Gunshot wounds, knife wounds, and puncture injuries fall into this category.

Hemorrhages into the dura are common, although they rarely become large enough to compromise the spinal cord. Subarachnoid hemorrhages, caused by contusion and laceration of the cord, are frequent and can cause further compression of the cord.

The mechanism of injury influences the type and degree of the spinal cord lesion. Approximately 50% of injuries come from excessive flexion of the spinal column; approximately one-third of these injuries results in complete spinal cord lesions.[18] Fig. 23.2 shows the flexion damage that is referred to as the hangman's fracture, related to excessive flexion. Fig. 23.3 shows how extension forces can cause SCI. When there is displacement of the vertebral column, vascular changes may ensue. Fig. 23.4 illustrates this phenomenon. Fig. 23.5 illustrates damage

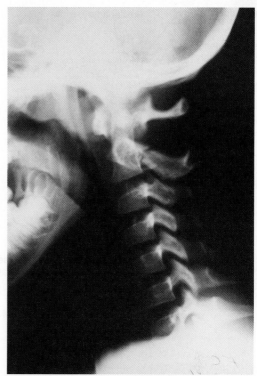

FIG. 23.2 Fracture of C2 (hangman's fracture). (From Green NB, Swiontkowski MF, editors: Skeletal trauma in children, ed 3, Philadelphia, 2003, Saunders.)

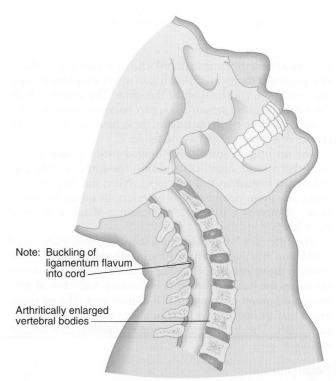

Note: Buckling of ligamentum flavum into cord

Arthritically enlarged vertebral bodies

FIG. 23.3 Patients subjected to extension forces can sustain cervical spinal cord injury as a result of compression of the spinal cord between the posterior hypertrophic ligamentum flavum and the arthritically enlarged anterior vertebral bodies. (From Marx JA, Hockberger RS, Walls RM: Rosen's emergency medicine: concepts and clinical practice, ed 8, Philadelphia, 2014, Saunders.)

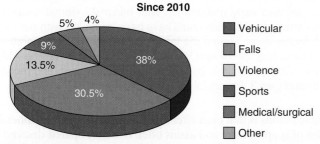

Since 2010

- 38% Vehicular
- 30.5% Falls
- 13.5% Violence
- 9% Sports
- 5% Medical/surgical
- 4% Other

FIG. 23.1 Etiology of spinal cord injury. (From National Spinal Cord Injury Statistical Center, Facts and Figures at a Glance. Birmingham, AL, University of Alabama at Birmingham, 2016.)

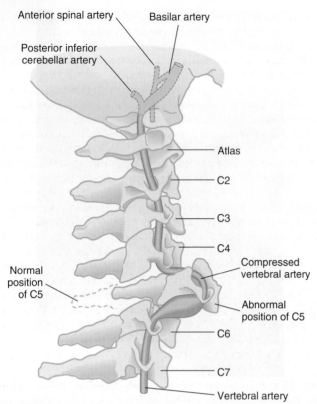

FIG. 23.4 Mechanism of vascular injury of the spinal cord resulting from cervical vertebral injury. (From Marx JA, Hockberger RS, Walls RM: Rosen's emergency medicine: concepts and clinical practice, ed 8, Philadelphia, 2014, Saunders.)

that often results to the spinal cord when it is violently displaced or compressed momentarily during an injury with forceful flexion, extension, and rotation of the spine. The vertebral body can burst and cause pressure or scatter bone fragments into the spinal cord. With crush fractures of the vertebrae, there is a 75% chance of a complete spinal cord lesion.

The majority of spinal cord–injured patients have at least one other system injury. Occasionally, these injuries take precedence in evaluation and treatment. When one level of bony injury has been identified, it is necessary to survey the entire spine, as there is a 10% to 15% incidence of spinal injury at other levels.[29]

The difference between a complete and an incomplete spinal cord lesion may depend on the survival of a small fraction of the axons in the spinal cord. Evidence of axonal conduction across the lesion site has been found in individuals with clinical neurologic diagnoses of complete SCI at that level. The surviving axons may be injured and therefore have a decreased response to stimuli. The injured axon conducts slowly and fatigues rapidly.[76]

Pathogenesis

The pathophysiology of SCI may be divided into phases. *Primary injury* refers to the structural damage occurring instantly after the traumatic event. Trauma to the spinal cord results in primary destruction of neurons at the level of the injury by disruption of the membrane, hemorrhage, and vascular damage. More extensive primary injury may occur, however, if an injured spine is not adequately immobilized. A critical aspect of

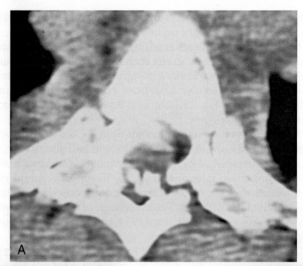

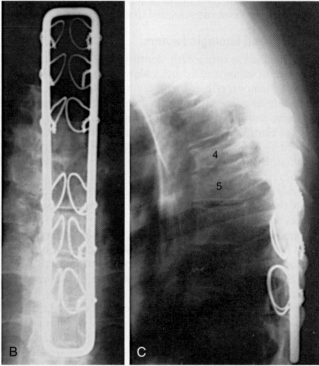

FIG. 23.5 A T4–T5 fracture-dislocation resulted in a complete spinal cord injury in a 30-year-old man. (A) A computed tomographic scan through the injured level demonstrates marked displacement and comminution at T4–T5, with multiple bone fragments within the canal. (B) A postoperative anteroposterior radiograph shows stabilization with a Luque rectangle and sublaminar wires. This instrumentation provided rigid fixation and allowed early mobilization with minimal external support. The strength of fixation could have been improved with the use of double wires around the lamina bilaterally. (C) Postoperative lateral radiograph. (From Browner BD, Jupiter JB, Levine AM, et al.: Skeletal trauma: basic science, management, and reconstruction, ed 3, Philadelphia, 2003, Saunders.)

these lesions is that even after severe injuries, a small peripheral rim of spared tissue and axons often remains. Spared descending systems play an important role in recovery. In paraplegia, the amount of spared rim correlates with the level of locomotor function.[5,68]

Secondary injury refers to a pathophysiologic cascade initiated shortly after injury. In the first 18 hours after injury, there is necrotic death of axons that were directly disrupted by the trauma. However, in the ensuing days and weeks, there is further progression of tissue injury both superiorly and inferiorly from the lesion. The immune system likely plays a major role during this phase. It appears that immune cells, such as monocytes and macrophages, emit chemical signals, such as cytokines and chemokines, which trigger apoptosis, or programmed cell death. This breakdown of cell function can occur away from the lesion site, often as far away as four spinal segments.[17]

Furthermore, ischemia, hypoxia, edema, and various harmful biochemical events contribute to further damage. The spread of damage is thought to be due to initiation of biochemical events leading to necrosis and excitotoxic damage and can continue for hours, days, or weeks.[3] Fig. 23.6 shows the changes that can result from SCI.

Because it is extremely rare for the primary injury to cause transection of the spinal cord, it is very important to focus attention on these secondary injury process.

Electrolyte disturbances following SCI include increased intracellular calcium, increased extracellular potassium, and increased sodium permeability. The route of calcium entry rather than the amount may be the critical component. The influx of calcium ions in the neuronal cell can then lead to activation of various secondary processes resulting in cellular death. Excitatory neurotransmitter accumulation, arachidonic acid release, endogenous opiate activation, and prostaglandin production can cause damage as part of the postinjury cascade of events that results in ischemia, edema formation, membrane destruction, cell death, and eventually permanent neurologic deficits.[29]

Blood Flow Changes

Ischemia is a prominent feature of post-SCI events. Damage to blood vessels results in microhemorrhage in the central gray matter, which spreads radially and axially. The resulting hypoxic and ischemic events deprive gray and white matter of oxygen and nutrients necessary for neural cell survival and function. Within 2 hours of injury, there is a significant reduction in spinal cord blood flow. Swelling rapidly occurs at the injury level and increases pressure on the cord. Ischemia in the area of injury may also be due to the presence of norepinephrine, serotonin, histamine, and prostaglandins, all of which cause vasoconstriction. The ischemia may be compounded by loss of the normal autoregulatory response of the spinal cord vasculature.

Ischemia and necrosis occur primarily in the gray matter, presumably because of the richer blood supply. Macrophages enter the lesion and begin to digest the necrotic debris. Axonal swelling and increased permeability of blood vessels result in a visibly swollen spinal cord.[74] Glial cells become active after about 6 days, and astrocytic fibers form scarlike tissue that lines the cavities created by the necrosis.

Autoregulation of circulation is disabled at the injury site. The changes in blood flow may reflect rather than cause secondary injury.[33]

Edema

Edema formation is another feature of the secondary injury process. Edema develops first at the injury site and subsequently spreads into adjacent and sometimes distant segments of the cord. The relationship between this edema and worsening of neurologic function is not well understood. Fig. 23.7 illustrates the relationship of mechanisms of damage leading to cell death.

Demyelination

Demyelination results in reduced rate of firing in the injured spinal cord. The demyelination is due to direct trauma to the oligodendroglial cells that produce myelin. The myelin sheath becomes thin between the nodes. Loss of a single segment of myelin renders an axon dysfunctional; therefore, a large subset of axons crossing the lesion eventually become nonfunctional despite the axon's remaining physically intact.

Changes in white matter begin with Wallerian degeneration in the ascending posterior columns above the level of the lesion and in the descending corticospinal tracts. Wallerian degeneration may be triggered by microglial activation and by the destruction of the oligodendrocytes via the release of cytokines or other neurotropic factors.[41] The immune system appears also to trigger the

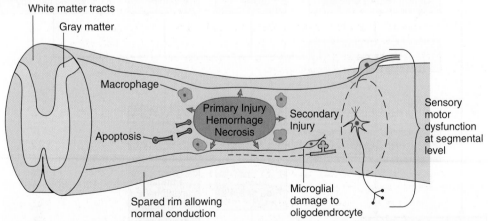

FIG. 23.6 Spinal cord contusion lesions are characterized by a primary area created by hemorrhage of blood vessels causing necrosis of cells. This area eventually spreads because of secondary injury associated with apoptosis (programmed cell death), macrophages acting as immune mediators, and microglia causing damage to oligodendrocytes. The secondary damage may continue for days to weeks and move along the segmental levels, causing sensory and motor dysfunction. The spared rim may allow normal processing and preservation of function.

release of nerve growth factor, which can be neuroprotective to some cells whereas it is toxic to other cells in the spinal cord.

A prominent feature of subchronic SCI is the maturation of a scar around the lesion. This scar tissue forms a cellular and molecular barrier to axonal regeneration. By the chronic injury phase, the scar is well formed and consists of several cell types, such as the reactive astrocytes, fibroblasts, Schwann cells, microglia, and macrophages that have invaded the scar.

Gray Matter

Typically, the loss of central gray matter is confined to between one and one and one-half segmental levels of the spinal cord, causing central cavitation. The result is either (1) a fluid-filled cyst or syrinx (see later) or (2) a collapse of the cord around the loss of tissue in an hourglass shape, with the minimal diameter located at the spinal segment of the original injury.

Dural Scarring

Scarring of the dura mater can cause a permanent connection of the cord to the overlying dura. Normally the cord is freely mobile within the spinal canal; however, dural scarring results in restricted motion, which produces unusual forces on the cord when the neck is bent or with normal breathing or the cardiac cycle. These forces can produce microscopic injury, which may limit optimal regeneration and recovery.

Neural Function

Substantial reduction of neural activity limits the body's ability to maintain the cellular functions of the spinal cord circuitry. It is believed that the injured central nervous system (CNS) undergoes accelerated aging, with abnormal cell production and impairments in mechanisms of cellular repair. The cellular mechanisms important for regeneration may be lost as a part of this process.

Syringomyelia

One type of pathologic condition that can appear over time in the spinal cord related to trauma is *syringomyelia*. It is a clinical syndrome that results from cystic cavitation and gliosis of the spinal cord. This is reported to occur in close to 2% of persons with paraplegia and in 0.2% of quadriplegic individuals. In the chronic spinal cord lesion, the cysts may continue to develop, become tubular in shape, like that of a syrinx, and extend over several spinal levels (Fig. 23.8). Posttraumatic syringomyelia can develop up to 30 years after the initial lesion, but most commonly occurs within 4 to 9 years after trauma. One mechanism of syrinx formation is an initial hematomyelia followed by resorption and formation of a cyst cavity.[29]

In some cases, there are multiple cavities. The cavity may occupy almost the entire cross-sectional area of the cord, compressing the posterior columns. As the cyst develops, usually below the level of the initial lesion, there can be significant pain as a result of the compromise of the central spinal cord structures.[70] The spinothalamic tracts are involved, which can result in the sharp pain that is often the first presenting symptom. There can be lower motor neuron dysfunction, causing weakness, atrophy, and loss of reflex activity. Sensory loss is common, and the sympathetic nervous system can become involved.[46]

The thoracic area of the spine is the most common site for the syrinx to develop, with descending and ascending fibers running in the walls of the cavitated lesions. The syringomyelia may be responsible for the spasms, phantom sensations, reflex changes, and autonomic visceral phenomena that may occur.[41] Anything that blocks the free flow of cerebrospinal fluid (CSF) can cause pressure to build up in the syrinx, causing expansion and possible rupture, damaging normal spinal cord tissue, and injuring nerve cells. Many people with posttraumatic syringomyelia do not develop any symptoms until midlife or later.[31]

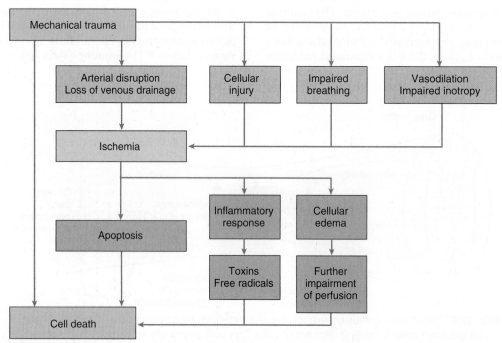

FIG. 23.7 Mechanisms of spinal cord injury. Mechanical trauma to the spinal cord is exacerbated by systemic hypoperfusion or hypoxia. (Redrawn from Dutton RP: Anesthetic management of spinal cord injury: Clinical practice and future initiatives, Int Anesthesiol Clin Summer 40:103–120, 2002.)

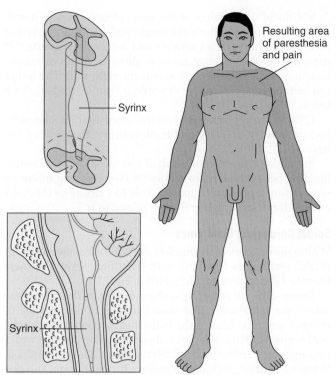

FIG. 23.8 The syrinx formed in the late stages of spinal cord injury as a part of syringomyelia.

Syringomyelia can be a very disabling condition. As previously stated, spasms, phantom sensations, and autonomic visceral (organ) changes can occur. Further, sexual dysfunction, muscle spasticity, and loss of bowel or bladder control may also develop. Along with the initial symptom of sharp pain, muscle atrophy, stiffness, and weakness of the neck, back, shoulders, arms, or legs, along with loss of reflexes, are also common. Symptoms may be distributed like a cape over the shoulders and back. Headaches and loss of sensation (pinprick and temperature) in the hands may also be reported. The symptoms may only occur on one side of the body, depending on where the syrinx develops.

Clinical Manifestations
Level of Injury

SCIs are named according to the level of neurologic impairment. Injury of the cord in the cervical region creates *tetraplegia*, or paralysis of all four limbs. In addition to the limbs, the trunk and muscles of respiration are involved. Damage in the thoracic or lumbar region will result in paraplegia or paraparesis involving only the lower extremities and generally the lower trunk.

Differences may exist in the motor versus sensory levels identified. Standards for the assessment and classification have been established by the American Spinal Injury Association (ASIA). These standards are widely accepted and are presented in Fig. 23.9. The sensory examination consists of testing 28 dermatomes on each side of the body using pinprick and light

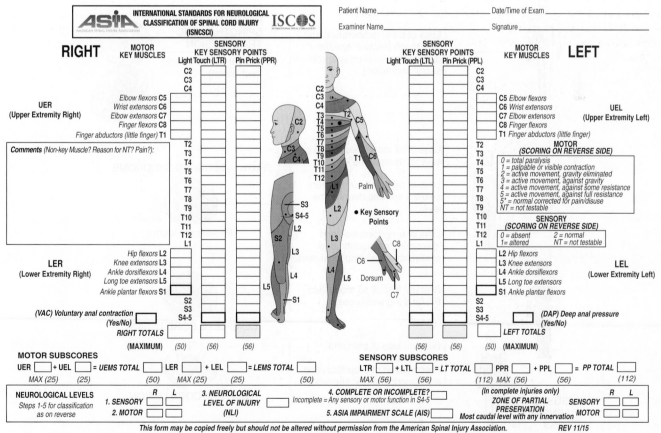

FIG. 23.9 International Standards for Neurologic Classification of SCI (ISNCSCI) Exam. (From the American Spinal Injury Association: International standards for neurological classification of spinal cord injury, revised 2011, Atlanta, GA. Revised 2011, updated 2015.)

touch. Sensation is scored for left and right dermatomes as follows: 0 = absent, 1 = impaired, 2 = normal. Sensation of the external anal sphincter is tested as yes or no.[21,26]

Identification of motor impairment is more problematic, given the dual innervation of many muscles. The strength of a given muscle is a reflection of the functioning of two or more cord segments. Loss of innervation from a spinal cord level results in weakness of the dual innervated muscle. The level of motor innervation is determined by the most distal key muscle with a muscle grade of 3 or better, with the segment above being a grade 5.[22]

Volitional contraction of the anal sphincter is also noted. The level of injury reflects the most caudal level of the spinal cord that exhibits intact sensory and motor functioning.[21,26] Asymmetric damage may result in different levels of neurologic impairment on the left versus the right side. The lesion can be then reported as, for example, a right C5 and a left C6 lesion.

Lesions are reported as *complete* when there is complete loss of sensory and motor function below the level of the lesion.

Incomplete lesions are the partial loss of sensory and motor function below the level of the injury. The resulting motor or sensory function is called *sparing*. Box 23.1 describes the ASIA method for describing impairment related to SCI.

Spinal Cord Injury Syndromes

Within the category of incomplete spinal cord lesions are recognizable syndromes that have been identified. Several of these identified syndromes are illustrated in Fig. 23.10.

Brown–Séquard syndrome is characterized by damage to one side of the spinal cord. The most common causes are stab or gunshot wounds. Loss of the entire hemisection of the spinal cord is rare; the natural lesion is always irregular. There is weakness ipsilateral to the lesion. Lateral column damage results in abnormal reflexes, including a positive Babinski's sign, and clonus. Often there is ipsilateral spasticity in the muscles innervated below the lesion. As a result of dorsal column damage,

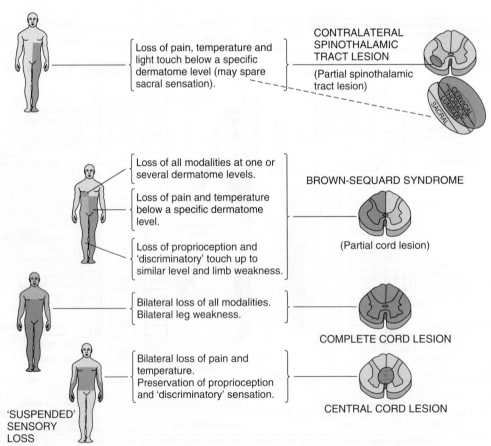

FIG. 23.10 Spinal cord syndromes. Patterns of sensory loss and weakness. (Redrawn from Lindsey KW, Bone I, Fuller G, et al., editors: Neurology and neurosurgery illustrated, ed 5, Edinburgh, 2010, Churchill Livingstone.)

there is loss of proprioception, kinesthesia, and vibratory sense. On the contralateral (opposite) side, there is pain and temperature loss starting a few levels below the lesion. The lateral spinothalamic tract ascends on the same side for several segments before crossing, giving rise to the discrepancy between the level and contralateral signs.

Anterior cord syndrome is frequently associated with flexion injuries and often results from loss of supply from the anterior spinal artery. Damage to the anterior and anterolateral aspect of the cord results in bilateral loss of motor function as well as loss of pain and temperature sensation due to the interruption of the anterior and lateral spinothalamic tracts and corticospinal tract.

Central cord syndrome is a result of damage to the central aspect of the spinal cord, often caused by hyperextension injuries in the cervical region. There is characteristically more severe neurologic involvement in the upper extremities than in the lower extremities. Peripherally located fibers are not affected, and therefore function is retained in the thoracic, lumbar, and sacral regions, including the bowel, bladder, and genitalia.

Posterior cord syndrome is extremely rare. There is loss of proprioception below the level of the lesion preservation of motor function, pain, and light touch sensation. The individual with a posterior cord syndrome typically has a wide-based steppage gait.

Conus medullaris syndrome and *cauda equina syndrome* reflect damage at the base of the spinal cord and generally result in lower limb paralysis, reflexive bowel, or both.

Changes in Muscle Tone

Paralysis of the voluntary musculature is the most obvious effect of SCI. Damage can involve the descending motor tracts, anterior horn cells, or spinal nerves, and it is often seen in combinations of these. Spinal shock is the loss of sensory, motor, and automatic control below the level of the lesion that occurs immediately after the trauma but resolves within a few weeks after injury.[25]

When the descending tracts are involved, immediate flaccidity is present and reflexes are absent at and below the level of injury. This is followed by autonomic symptoms, including sweating and reflex incontinence of bladder and rectum. Within weeks, there is a gradual increase in the resting tone of the muscles innervated below the lesion and reflexes reappear.

Spasticity is an inevitable consequence of spinal cord lesions. There is an essential or basic spasticity, which may be of some benefit to the individual when emptying the bladder or flexing the hip and knee. Excess spasticity is due to afferent stimuli. Spasticity can be made worse by the presence of constipation, infection, fracture, or a pressure sore below the level of the lesion, and it can be exacerbated by a sudden change in temperature or by physical or emotional stress. Typically the flaccid condition lasts longer. Spasticity occurs later in a cervical injury compared with a thoracic injury.[38,42]

Autonomic Nervous System Changes

Autonomic dysreflexia (AD) can occur with a lesion above T5 and is the result of impaired function of the autonomic nervous system (ANS) caused by simultaneous sympathetic and parasympathetic activity. The ANS regulates body functions such as heart rate, blood pressure, and gland activity. Noxious stimuli, such as elevated blood pressure, overextended bladder or bowel, or other visceral stimuli, will typically elicit a sympathetic

response, resulting in vasoconstriction and an increase in blood pressure. In the non–spinal cord–injured individual, the descending sympathetic output compensates for this increase in blood pressure by causing vasodilation to bring blood pressure to a more normal level. Following SCI, sensory nerves below the level of the injury continue to transmit excitatory impulses, causing similar vasoconstriction and increased blood pressure. With the lack of sympathetic inhibitory output below the lesion, however, the blood pressure keeps rising unchecked. Secretions of neurotransmitters, such as norepinephrine, epinephrine, and dopamine, support this sympathetic response. Control of this situation occurs at the brainstem level, leading to parasympathetic stimulation via the vagus nerve, which will slow the heart rate (bradycardia). However, this response is not strong enough to overcome the extreme vasoconstriction. The vasoconstriction continues above the level of the lesion and results in profuse sweating and skin flushing. A severe pounding headache follows, with sweating and chills without fever. The increase in blood pressure makes the person susceptible to subarachnoid hemorrhage, renal or retinal hemorrhage, and seizure or myocardial infarction. AD should be handled as a medical emergency.[1,26] See Box 23.2 for signs and triggers of AD.[77]

Loss of thermoregulation below the level of the spinal cord lesion is a result of the disruption of the autonomic pathways from the hypothalamus, resulting in subnormal body temperature in a normal ambient environment. Vasoconstriction, the ability to shiver, and the ability to sweat are lost. The body

---

BOX 23.2 Signs and Triggers of Autonomic Dysreflexia

Signs

- Sudden and significant (>20 mm Hg) increase in both systolic and diastolic blood pressure above normal (normal blood pressure when the lesion is above T6 is 90–110 mm Hg systolic and 50–60 mm Hg diastolic)
- Onset of a sudden throbbing or pounding headache
- Sweating and flushing of the face, neck, or shoulders
- Goose bumps above the level of the lesion
- Blurred vision
- Visual field changes
- Nasal congestion
- Increased anxiety and apprehension without cause
- Changes in heart rhythm, such as arrhythmias, fibrillation, premature ventricular contractions

Triggers

- Full bladder
- Full or impacted bowel
- Scrotal compression
- Kidney stones
- Gastritis
- Contractions of labor and delivery
- Onset of menses
- Deep vein thrombosis
- Pulmonary embolus
- Pressure ulcers
- Insect bites
- Bruises caused by sharp objects
- Tight and constrictive clothing or apparatus
- Changes in temperature
- Pain or irritation below the level of the lesion

Adapted from Zabel RJ, Forest BH: Autonomic dysreflexia: an acute care emergency, Acute Care Perspect 7:9–14, 1999.

temperature then is greatly influenced by the external environment, and sensory feedback from the head and neck must be used to assist in regulating body temperature. The higher the lesion is, the more severe the problem becomes.

Skeletal Changes

Joint ankylosis caused by heterotopic ossification, or ectopic bone formation in the soft tissue, can limit range of motion, cause pain, and impair seating and posture. It often develops near the large joints, such as the anterior area of the hip, knee, shoulder, and elbow. It is always found below the level of the lesion, and it begins to develop within the first year after injury. The initial symptoms are soft tissue swelling, pain, redness, and increased temperature in the affected area. Other skeletal changes include alterations in bony alignment secondary to muscle imbalances caused by unopposed contractions. For example, scoliosis can develop over time due to lack of paraspinal support, as is evidenced in Fig. 23.11.

Pain

Individuals with SCI must deal with a number of secondary complications in addition to any disability caused by the injury itself. Pain, weakness, and fatigue appear to be most common and most closely linked to individual's social and mental health functioning.[40] The number of reported pain sites increases with time, regardless of level or completeness of injury. Although physical independence, mobility, and social integration remain relatively stable despite increasing numbers of pain sites, increases in depressive symptoms are associated with increased pain. Smokers with SCI report more pain sites than their non-smoking counterparts.[58]

Pain caused by irritation of the nerve root is common, especially in cauda equina injury. *Dysesthesia*, impairment of

sensation usually perceived as pain, can occur in areas with sensory loss and is often described as burning, pins and needles, or tingling. Disturbances of proprioception are related, and the person feels that a limb is in a different position than it is.

Musculoskeletal pain can result from faulty posture and overuse of limbs. Joint, ligament, and tendon deterioration is common, and secondary injury from muscle imbalances can occur.

Fatigue

Complaints of fatigue, noted to be higher than in the general population, may be associated with changes in several systems. ANS changes with inadequate sweating and thermoregulation can cause activity intolerance. Psychologic well-being is associated with fatigue; depression and decreased community mobility can be predicted by increasing complaints of fatigue.

Respiratory Complications

Respiratory complications associated with spinal cord lesions can be life threatening. Pulmonary complications are a common cause of death in both the acute and chronic phases. Spinal shock and poor management of edema can reduce vital capacity.

Lesions above C4 result in paralysis of muscles of inspiration and generally require artificial ventilation because of loss of the phrenic nerve innervation. Pulmonary complications with lesions at C5 through T12 arise as a result of loss of innervation of the muscles of expiration, the abdominal and intercostal muscles. The position of the diaphragm is compromised, and the abdominal musculature is unable to exert pressure during forced expiration. Paralysis of the external oblique muscles also inhibits the person's ability to cough and expel secretions.

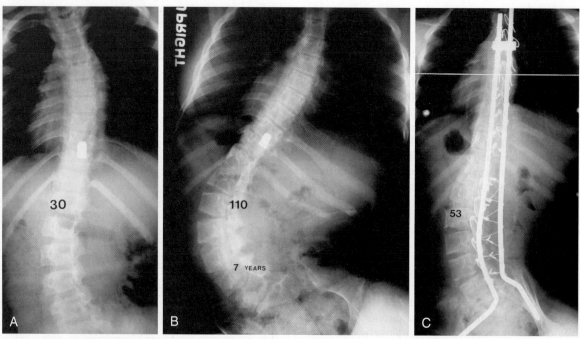

FIG. 23.11 Progressive paralytic scoliosis after gunshot wound. (A) Initial curve of 30 degrees. (B) Seven years later, curve is 110 degrees. (C) After fusion and segmental instrumentation, correction to 53 degrees. (From Canale ST, Beaty, JH: Campbell's operative orthopedics, ed 12, Philadelphia, 2013, Mosby.)

An altered breathing pattern develops in conjunction with the loss of the diaphragmatic muscle, the intercostal muscles, and the accessory muscles of inspiration. The upper chest wall flattens and the abdominal wall expands, leading to musculoskeletal changes in the trunk.

Aspiration and pneumonia occur frequently in individuals with SCI, particularly in individuals with high-level injuries, *complete lesions,* and advanced age. Pneumonia is the most common cause of death, especially in the period immediately after the injury. With no other complications, proper rehabilitation, and stable respiration, the death rate from pneumonia matches that in the general population.[57]

Cardiovascular Conditions

Cardiovascular conditions, including deep vein thrombosis and pulmonary embolism, are associated with SCI because of increased coagulation ability of blood and decreased venous return. This may be associated with sympathetic dysfunction and unopposed vagal action. For long-term SCI, morbidity and mortality from cardiovascular causes now exceeds that caused by renal and pulmonary conditions, the primary causes of mortality in previous decades. Risk of cardiovascular involvement comes from a greater prevalence of obesity, lipid disorders, metabolic syndrome, and diabetes. Daily energy expenditure is significantly lower in individuals with SCI, not only because of a lack of motor function, but also because of a lack of accessibility and fewer opportunities to engage in physical activity. Autonomic dysfunction caused by SCI is also associated with several conditions that contribute to heightened cardiovascular risk, including abnormalities in blood pressure, heart rate variability, arrhythmias, and a blunted cardiovascular response to exercise that can limit the capacity to perform physical activity.[53]

Metabolic Conditions

Persons with SCI are prone to abnormal carbohydrate metabolism and are found to develop hyperinsulinemia and insulin resistance. During the acute phase of SCI, there is significant weight loss, especially with tetraplegia, associated with increased metabolic demands, muscle atrophy, and a negative nitrogen and calcium balance. Over time, there is usually an increase in body fat in proportion to lean tissue in the person with chronic SCI.

Further, soon after SCI, bones start losing minerals, becoming less dense. This may be due to alteration of the ANS and circulation. Inactivity and lack of weight bearing also foster the development of osteoporosis. It is believed that individuals with SCI may have an earlier onset and a greater extent of osteoporosis.

Pressure Ulcers

Pressure ulcers are a frequent complication of SCI. They arise primarily because of the pressure associated with lack of mobility resulting in pressure over areas of a bony prominence. Individuals with complete lesions and sensory loss are at greater risk for developing pressure sores. In addition, moisture, poor nutrition, acute illness, and cigarette smoking predispose the skin to breakdown. Persons who do not follow through on self-care requirements because of depression, lack of motivation, substance abuse, or alcoholism are also prone to develop more and deeper pressure ulcers. Initially, the sacrum, heel, and scapula are the most common sites of ulcer formation because of time spent in bed. As the individual begins to use a chair for mobility, the trochanter and ischium become common sites of pressure ulcers.[72]

Bowel and Bladder Control

Bowel and bladder control is always affected in the person with SCI. The spinal center for urination is the conus medullaris. Primary reflex control originates from the sacral segment. During the stage of spinal shock, the urinary bladder is flaccid. All muscle tone and bladder reflexes are absent. Lesions above the conus medullaris will cause a reflex neurogenic bladder, reflected by spasticity, voiding difficulties, detrusor muscle hypertrophy, and urethral reflux. Lesions at the conus medullaris cause nonreflex bladders, resulting in flaccidity and decreased tone of the perineal muscles and urethral sphincter. Bowel patterns mimic bladder responses in their response to spinal shock; reflex bowel occurs in lesions above the conus medullaris, and nonreflex bowel is caused by damage to the conus and cauda equina.[45] Fig. 23.12 shows bladder reflex pathways.

Urinary tract infection is the most frequent secondary medical complication seen in persons with SCI. This persists despite improved catheter materials and design and use of antibiotics. In concert with this is the increased concentration of calcium in the urinary system, which leads to formation of kidney stones. Calculi in the kidney are a complication found more frequently in individuals using an indwelling catheter.[14]

Sexuality

Sexual response is directly related to the level and completeness of injury. Sexual function relies on nervous pathways similar to those of the bladder and bowel and is similarly altered. There are two types of responses: reflexogenic, or a response to external stimulation seen in persons with upper motor neuron lesions, and psychogenic, a response that occurs through cognitive activity such as fantasy, associated with lower motor neuron lesions. Men with higher-level lesions can often achieve a reflexive erection but typically do not ejaculate. Those with lower lesions can more easily ejaculate, but achieving an erection is more difficult. With cauda equina lesions, erection and ejaculation are not usually possible. Bladder and bowel concerns during sexual activity are not strong enough to deter the majority of the population from engaging in sexual activity. In addition, the occurrence of autonomic dysreflexia during typical bladder or bowel care is a significant variable predicting the occurrence and distress of AD during sexual activity.[2] In women, menses are typically interrupted for approximately 3 to 6 months; when restored, they can be another cause of AD. Fertility and pregnancy are uninterrupted, but the pregnancy must be observed closely, especially in the last trimester. Labor may begin without the woman's knowledge because of loss of sensation. Labor may initiate AD.[60]

Sleep Disorders

The prevalence of obstructive sleep apnea–hypopnea syndrome (OSAHS) is high after cervical cord injury. OSAHS is characterized by repeated oxygen desaturation. OSAHS should be suspected especially in individuals with daytime sleepiness, obesity, and frequent awakenings during sleep.[47] The changes in heart rhythm associated with OSAHS include sinusal arrhythmia, severe bradycardia, and ventricular and supraventricular tachycardia. The risk of sudden death, particularly of cardiovascular cause, is well known.[16]

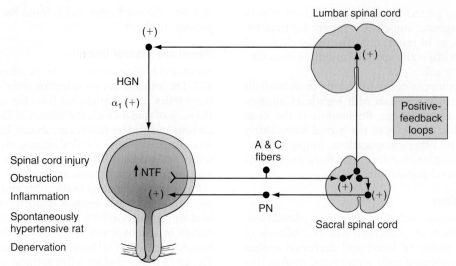

FIG. 23.12 Possible mechanisms underlying spasticity in bladder reflex pathways induced by various pathologic conditions. Bladders from rats with chronic spinal cord injury exhibit increased level of neurotrophic factors (NTFs), such as nerve growth factor. NTFs can increase the excitability of C-fiber bladder afferent neurons and alter reflex mechanisms in parasympathetic excitatory pathways in the pelvic nerve (PN) as well as in sympathetic pathways in the hypogastric nerve (HGN). These reflex circuits are organized in the spinal cord as positive-feedback loops that induce involuntary bladder activity. (From Wein AJ, Kavoussi LR, Partin AW, et al., editors: Campbell-Walsh urology, ed 11, Philadelphia, 2016, Elsevier.)

Medical Management

Diagnosis

Delayed recognition of SCI is a significant problem in emergent care of traumatic injuries, occurring in more than 20% of cases.

Lateral film studies with plain radiographs are a rapid and effective way of evaluating cervical SCI, with the ability to detect approximately 85% of such injuries. When the open-mouth odontoid view and supine anteroposterior view are added, the accuracy rises to almost 100%. Any area that is inadequately demonstrated in the three-view spinal series is examined by computed tomography (CT). Flexion–extension studies are used primarily to evaluate instability caused by occult ligamentous injury and should not be done if there is any neurologic, bony, or soft tissue injury. CT demonstrates soft tissue structures and allows visualization of the bony limits of the spinal canal in the axial plane. CT is superior to other diagnostic procedures in demonstrating impingement on the neuronal canal.[19]

Fig. 23.13 shows a Jefferson fracture seen on x-ray and magnetic resonance imaging (MRI) scan. Fig. 23.14 compares fractures at time of injury and after stabilization. Myelography is indicated for optimal visualization of compression of the spinal cord after trauma. Myelography alone is rarely indicated, and it is used in conjunction with CT. In many cases, MRI has replaced myelography.

In acute SCI, MRI is sometimes problematic because of its limited use around ferromagnetic objects such as respirators, oxygen tanks, and traction devices. When these obstacles do not exist, the extent of spinal cord damage and the possibility of disk herniation can be more readily assessed by MRI. The presence of intradural or extradural hematoma can often be demonstrated on MRI. MRI is useful in excluding spinal cord contusion or hemorrhage in persons with neurologic deficits and normal CT scans and plain films.[21]

Treatment and Pharmacology

Interventions at several levels are required to improve mortality, morbidity, and quality of life. This begins with early surgical stabilization and with pharmacologic treatments aimed at blocking excitotoxicity and apoptosis. Prevention of the delayed wave of cell death that occurs in the weeks following injury is critical at the secondary level. Once injury is complete, the focus shifts to promoting regeneration. Pharmacologic treatments and transplantation are paired with the appropriate physical activity to optimize regeneration. It is now clear that spontaneous regeneration can be facilitated, and there is potential for optimizing regeneration even long after the injury and possibly extending throughout the remaining life span.

Emergent Care

The emergent phase of care is crucial for the person with traumatic SCI. It can make the difference between living the rest of life with a disability or recovering with only temporary neurologic deficits. An incomplete injury can be made worse by mishandling and can be made better by prompt attention to critical procedures. Box 23.3 describes guidelines for essential trauma care.[11,29]

Assessment of the likelihood of SCI includes understanding the mechanics of the trauma and obtaining vital signs to determine whether the individual is in neurogenic shock. Movement of the distal components of the body reflects the intactness of the spinal cord. In the case of a cervical injury, paradoxical respiration or abdominal breathing may be present, and immediate immobilization should be instituted. Use of a rigid collar and spinal board can help to prevent movement of the spinal column. Oxygen and medication should

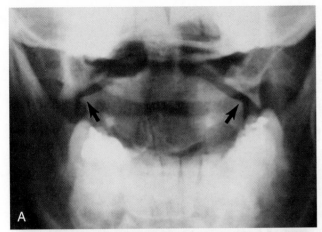

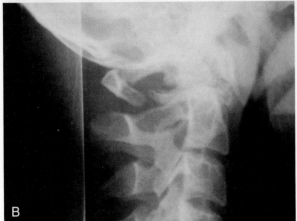

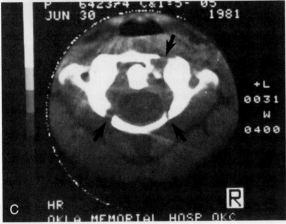

FIG. 23.13 Fracture of C1 (Jefferson fracture). (A) Anteroposterior view showing lateral displacement of the lateral mass and articulating facets of C1 on C2. (B) Oblique view illustrating disruption of the posterior aspect of the ring of C1. (C) Computed tomographic scan revealing the true extent of the injury. (From Green NE, Swiotkowski MF, editors: Skeletal trauma in children, ed 3, Philadelphia, 2003, Saunders. Courtesy of Dr. Teresa Stacy.)

be given to control the hyperperfusion and swelling of the spinal cord. Transport should be swift, with care taken to avoid physical jarring caused by an uneven road surface and sudden stops.[12,75]

Monitoring in the critical care phase includes cardiac and neurologic status. Orthopedic management may begin at this phase and includes closed and open reduction of the vertebrae and decompression of the spinal cord. Insertion of a halo is common in treatment of cervical injuries, and a halo can be used without surgical intervention. In the more than 50% of individuals with SCI requiring surgery, fusion and internal fixation is the most common procedure performed. The goal is to restore spinal alignment, establish spinal stability, and prevent further neurologic deterioration, enhancing recovery. Blood pressure dysregulation in persons with SCI may reflect increased vascular nitrous oxide. Treatment of hypotension using nitrous oxide inhibition has been shown to be effective in this population.[69]

Pharmacologic control of edema, blood flow, and secondary neurologic sequelae shows promise in current studies. Corticosteroids such as methylprednisolone have shown good results in large doses, but the side effects must be considered. MRI findings suggest that methylprednisolone therapy in the acute phase of SCI may decrease the extent of intramedullary spinal cord hemorrhage.[48] Although the concern about steroids continues, methylprednisolone should be administered to individuals with incomplete cervical SCI according to the Second National Acute Spinal Cord Injury Study protocol.[67]

Drugs that block opiate receptors appear to protect the spinal cord by decreasing endotoxic and hemorrhagic shock. Preservation of spinal cord function can be achieved by modulation of the neurotransmitters that are produced when there is injury to the nervous system.[73]

When considering the appropriate type and dose of medication to be given to a person with an acute SCI, the degree of SCI must be assessed accurately. A moderate injury may require a different set of extracellular substances than that required in the secondary damage management for a severe injury.[33]

Management of Complications

Management of complications of SCI is critical. High cervical injuries require immediate placement of ventilation equipment and maintenance of pulmonary hygiene. Therapy consists of intermittent positive pressure breathing (IPPB), bronchodilators, and mucolytics. Prevention of pulmonary infection is critical in SCI.

In electrophrenic respiration, the phrenic nerve is implanted with a single electrode, and the client carries a transmitter to activate the lung. This works well in persons with high cervical lesions and sparing of C3 to C5 anterior horn cells. This method of respiration more closely mimics normal physiology than does IPPB.[12]

Loss of ANS control affects the function of the cardiovascular system. Acute management of blood pressure is critical. The autonomic lesion predisposes persons with high spinal cord lesions to abnormal cardiovascular responses to vasoactive agents.

Treatment of spasticity includes use of muscle relaxants and spasmolytic agents.[59] Compared with oral baclofen, intrathecal baclofen infusion does not affect respiratory function and results in improved sleep continuity. Intrathecal baclofen infusion in therapeutic doses acts at the spinal level rather than at the supraspinal level.[9] Sustained-release fampridine is effective in individuals with chronic SCI.[13] One of the things that should be considered in the use of these medications is the fact that baclofen profoundly inhibits cell

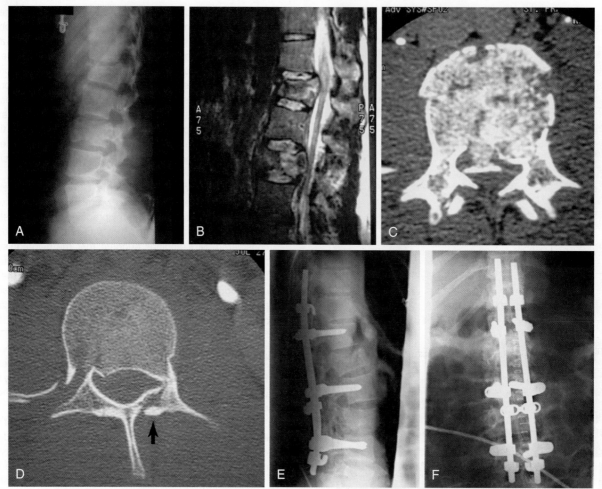

FIG. 23.14 A 21-year-old man involved in a motor vehicle accident sustained a burst fracture of L1 and L3. The patient had an incomplete spinal cord injury. (A) A preoperative lateral view shows loss of height predominately at L1. (B) A sagittal-cut magnetic resonance image shows compression at both L1 and L3. (C) An axial-cut computed tomographic (CT) scan at L3 shows a retropulsed fragment filling half the canal. (D) An axial CT scan at L1 shows a fracture of the lamina and retropulsion of a fragment into canal. (E) This injury was stabilized with Isola instrumentation combining both pedicle screws and laminar hooks. Sagittal alignment was maintained. (F) Postoperative anteroposterior radiograph showing a cross-connection added for additional stability. (From Browner BD, Jupiter JB, Levine AM, et al.: Skeletal trauma: basic science, management, and reconstruction, ed 3, Philadelphia, 2003, Saunders.)

BOX 23.3   Essential Trauma Care Services Endorsed by IATSIC as the "Rights of the Injured"

- Obstructed airways are opened and maintained before hypoxia leads to death or permanent disability.
- Impaired breathing is supported until the injured person is able to breathe adequately without assistance.
- Pneumothorax and hemothorax are promptly recognized and relieved.
- Bleeding (external or internal) is promptly stopped.
- Shock is recognized and treated with intravenous fluid replacement before irreversible consequences occur.
- The consequences of traumatic brain injury are lessened by timely decompression of space-occupying lesions and by prevention of secondary brain injury.

- Intestinal and other abdominal injuries are promptly recognized and repaired.
- Potentially disabling extremity injuries are corrected.
- Potentially unstable spinal cord injuries are recognized and managed appropriately, including early immobilization.
- The consequences to the individual of injuries that result in physical impairment are minimized by appropriate rehabilitative services.
- Medications for these services and for the minimization of pain are readily available when needed.

IATSIC, International Association for Trauma Surgery and Intensive Care.
From Mock C, Lormand JD, Goosen J, et al.: Guidelines for essential trauma care, Geneva, 2004, World Health Organization; with permission.

proliferation, survival, and differentiation, particularly myelination. Baclofen produces an irreversible loss of function. Baclofen is not an extremely effective oral agent, and there is now evidence that it can harm by inhibiting regeneration and recovery. Current research has shown that patterned activity, such as functional electrical stimulation (FES) bicycling (three times per week for 1 hour each time) may be a better way to control spasticity than medications.[7] Peripheral nerve blocks, such as botulinum toxin (Botox), provide a temporary reduction of spasticity. If there is long-term, severe spasticity, the contractile potential of the muscle can be modified by surgery. Therefore spasticity-related interventions need to be aimed at what matters most to the individual. It is critical for clinicians to understand individuals' experiences to make accurate assessments, effectively evaluate treatment interventions, and select appropriate management strategies.[50,51]

Suburothelial injection of botulinum A toxin can effectively inhibit the occurrence of neurogenic detrusor overactivity, providing increased bladder capacity and improved incontinence grade in individuals with SCI. The therapeutic effect declines gradually after 3 months, and all symptoms return within 6 months.

Pain Management

Despite the fact that SCI causes loss of sensation, there is often significant pain that develops over time. Pain in SCI is classified in many different ways associated with intrinsic or neurogenic dysfunction, such as pain associated with syringomyelia or central cord pain, peripheral nerve pain, and musculoskeletal or mechanical pain. Psychogenic pain is also addressed in some classifications.

Management of neurogenic pain in SCI is by systemic or local drug therapy and by neuroaugmentative and neurodestructive intervention. The pharmacologic approach includes nonsteroidal analgesics, opioids, antidepressants, and anticonvulsants.[37] Pregabalin (Lyrica) is associated with relief of central neuropathic pain and with reduction in pain-related sleep interference and significant improvement in sleep problems. Action on centrally located calcium channels may be important in the effectiveness of pregabalin in managing central neuropathic pain.

Neuroaugmentative procedures include transcutaneous electrical nerve stimulation (TENS), epidural spinal stimulation, and central thalamic stimulation. Neurodestructive procedures include both chemical and surgical destruction of nervous structures. Procedures may include deafferentation, interruption of ascending pain systems, or destruction of cells in the dorsal horn.

Diffuse, chronic, and dysesthetic pain following SCI has been described by several authors using different terms. Dysesthetic pain syndrome is difficult to treat. This pain is distinguished by its quality and is usually described using words such as *burning, stabbing, crushing, pressing,* or *pounding,* referred to as allesthesia and allodynia, and can be called the "central Tinel" sign. Light touch or tapping over areas rostral to the level of injury can be painful, and pain can be triggered by nonnoxious stimuli such as movement of the bed. It can also be triggered by noxious stimuli, such as smoking or gastrointestinal disturbances.[71]

Decompressive surgery is performed in individuals with spinal cord syringomyelia, depending on which area is affected. Surgery to create a pseudomeningomyelocele, an arti-ficial CSF reservoir, performed to normalize the CSF flow, has been shown to be effective. By draining the cyst, it is possible to prevent the cyst from reexpanding. Draining the fluid can relieve pain, headache, and a sensation of tightness in the head or neck. In a dural graft procedure, the space around the spinal cord is enlarged to allow free flow of fluid and reduce pressure.

Strategies for Spinal Cord Repair

Nervous system repair is now feasible, and there is much research related to various strategies. A small degree of regeneration can result in recovery of function. A substantial loss of spinal cord tissue does not preclude function based on corticospinal tracts. There are two main regenerative approaches that are currently being studied: (1) optimizing spontaneous regeneration to restore function, and (2) transplanting stem cells. At this time there is no treatment that can clearly aid regeneration, but given the following information, primarily based on animal studies, it is likely that it will be developed in the near future.[7]

Embryonic stem cells are true stem cells that show unlimited capacity for self-renewal. In contrast, adult stem cells are progenitor cells or cells that are immature or undifferentiated. Their capacity for unlimited self-renewal and plasticity has not been as comprehensively demonstrated. Most progenitor cells are dormant or possess little activity in the tissue in which they reside. They exhibit slow growth, and their main role is to replace cells lost by normal attrition. Upon tissue damage or injury, progenitor cells can be activated by growth factors or cytokines, leading to increased cell division important for the repair process. Progenitor cells participate in the normal maintenance of the CNS. These mechanisms include production and replacement of cells lost to normal aging and cell turnover.

Critical components of optimal care following SCI are protection of neural tissue and limitation of secondary damage, facilitation of axonal regrowth, and control of factors that inhibit intrinsic neural repair. Because the consequences of SCI are complex, it is most likely that a hierarchy of intervention strategies will be needed to restore suprasegmental control leading to the recovery of function in the spinal cord.[8,34] The phases of injury and the neurophysiologic events will create both limitations and advantages related to potential treatments. For example, progenitor cells transplanted during the acute injury phase are vulnerable to the same set of cell death mechanisms predominant during the secondary phase of acute injury. Understanding the function of growth-inhibiting factors within the adult CNS may lead to control of the neural destruction after SCI.[9]

Improving regeneration of axons after SCI has been attempted by transplantation of various cell types. Success has been achieved in creating and sustaining function in both neurons and glial cells in some but not all areas of the CNS.[49]

Astrocytes can express molecules that are both growth permissive and growth inhibitory at the same time. Reactive astrocytes appear to create an inhibitory environment within the injured spinal cord and form an astroglial scar that acts as a physical and chemical barrier to axonal regeneration. Maintaining an environment to support the growth of axons may involve the selective removal of astrocytes from the site of injury.[20,65] In contrast, glial restricted precursors–derived astrocytes may promote axonal regeneration via suppression of astrogliosis, realignment of host tissues, and delaying of expression of inhibitory proteoglycans. The glia, not neurons, are the critical elements in preventing growth and in restoring it. Neurons retain the power to grow, and their sprouts only await the provision of a suitable glial pathway to be able to advance across the lesion.

Inflammatory reactions in the CNS have a dual nature; they may be neuroprotective as well as neurotoxic. Studies illustrate that the nervous and immune systems have overlapping rules of organization and intercellular communication. As a result, both systems express a host of common cytokines and neurotrophic factors that regulate cell survival and function. These shared mediators enable the two systems to engage in cross-talk and may provide a molecular explanation for neuroprotective effects of inflammation.

Remyelination of bare axons after nervous system injury can be promoted by injecting endogenous stem cells that can be mobilized to become oligodendrocytes.[36] Schwann cells have been used to facilitate a permissive environment for the injured spinal cord to regenerate. Previous experiments have shown compressive mechanical stress to be important in stimulating the regenerative behavior of Schwann cells. Transplantation of highly permissive Schwann cell–enriched peripheral nerve grafts may enhance regeneration in SCI.[24] Fig. 23.15 demonstrates the neuroprotective processes that may be integral within the immunomodulation.

Peripheral nerves may be able to provide an axonal bridge across the longer areas of spinal cord damage. This can be accomplished by activating nerve impulses from implanted nerves placed at the distal end of the transected cord that bridge the transection and connect to neurons in the gray matter. It is possible that inferior-to-superior nerve bridging can produce return of function, just as superior-to-inferior nerve bridging does. This is related to the concept that axons have a "relentless compulsion" to grow until they participate in return of function. Regeneration-associated genes are allied with developing neurons, and as a response to CNS injury, are considered an important element for biochemical therapies driving regeneration of the axon.[26] Electrical stim-

ulation may provide an avenue for accelerated axonal outgrowth from the proximal nerve stump. (See 23.1 Special Implications for the PTA: Traumatic Spinal Cord Injury at the end of this chapter.)

Stem Cell Transplantation

Transplantation of stem cells is being studied extensively in relation to the treatment of SCI. Processes include producing regenerative growth factors, expressing substances capable of breaking down scar tissue and modulating the immune system's response to injury. It appears that there will be potential for reprogramming the host microenvironment; for example, embryonic stem cell transplantation reduces macrophage influx by more than 50%.

An immature CNS does not produce the same inhibitory effect on axon growth as the mature CNS does. After spinal cord lesions and transplantation of spinal cord tissue, there is extensive growth of descending axons into the transplants. A transplant of fetal spinal cord tissue may serve as a bridge to permit the regrowth of axons from spinal and supraspinal levels across the site of SCI.[6] Transplants combined with neurotrophin treatment appear to have an additive effect compared with each intervention individually. Transplants and exogenous application of neurotrophic factors regulate cellular programs associated with regrowth and increase the extent of axonal regrowth with a favorable environment.[5]

Human umbilical cord blood stem cells hold great promise for therapeutic repair after SCI. Human embryonic stem cells may offer a renewable source of a wide range of cell types for use in research and cell-based therapies to treat disease. Cografted neural stem cells and NT-3 gene–modified Schwann cells promote the recovery of transected SCI and are a potential therapy for SCI.[18,32]

Prognosis

The prognosis for recovery and repair depends on the phase of the injury and the age of the individual, with the best potential related to a younger age. The chronic consequences of SCI are related to maintenance as well as plasticity and repair. More than 90% of persons admitted to an acute care

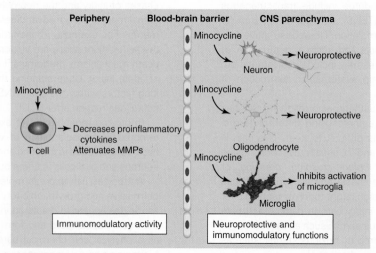

FIG. 23.15 Peripheral and central functions of minocycline. Minocycline has immunomodulatory activity in the periphery and both immunomodulatory and neuroprotective capacity within the central nervous system. (From Yong VW, Wells J, Giuliani F, et al.: The promise of minocycline in neurology. Lancet Neurol 3:744–751, 2004.)

hospital for treatment of SCI are ultimately discharged home. Morbidity and mortality during the first 4 weeks following SCI are most often related to paralysis of the respiratory muscles. The presence of proteinuria is associated with increased mortality in the chronic SCI population.[31]

Long-term urinary tract infection continues to be a cause of death, but control of sepsis has improved markedly since 1970. This is primarily because of improvement in bladder training, antibiotic treatment, control of fluid intake, and surgery for obstruction of the lower urinary tract. Another common cause of death is respiratory disease, and this is the leading cause of death among high cervical injury clients. Pneumonia continues at a rate higher than in the general population, with pulmonary edema associated with injuries above T6. Heart disease is common, including myocardial infarction, cardiac arrest, myocarditis, and pulmonary embolism. However, the mortality rate is not much higher than that in the general population and is improving with increased pharmacologic control and improved medical knowledge of the cardiovascular changes accompanying SCI.

Most motor recovery occurs during the first 6 months, and strength can continue to increase with appropriate facilitation. The muscles graded 1 to 3 in the zone of partial preservation have potential to recover motor function. Overall, more than one-half of the SCI population will have return of some neurologic function. Compression fractures have the most favorable prognosis for return of function; crush fractures having the least chance for return of function.[41] Skeletal complications are related to the deformity and degenerative changes associated with nonuse of extremities. These can lead to pain and further neurologic compromise.

Prognosis related to mobility is a concern to most persons, especially those with thoracic-level injury. Preservation of axonal integrity and regrowth of neural tissue will have a significant effect on the recovery of mobility after SCI. Nervous system recovery and improved functional status is part of current and ongoing research in the rehabilitation field.

People with SCI experience significant problems in a number of areas of life, resulting in ongoing stress related to pain, spasticity, difficulty in sex life, lack of income, and associated worries. These problems do not appear to be highly correlated with aging, suggesting that they will not necessarily become more problematic, nor are they likely to self-remediate.[44]

? 23.1 Special Implications for the PTA: Traumatic Spinal Cord Injury Rehabilitation to enhance the function and lifestyle of SCI clients has traditionally been aimed at helping clients achieve the ability to perform most daily tasks. The goal is to reach the point where the disability is no longer the major focus of clients' lives. Included are psychosocial adjustment, physical skills, health maintenance, and vocational adjustments. One goal of rehabilitation is to involve clients in all aspects of rehabilitation, provide the information and environment to foster independence, and have clients work as partners with the clinicians. Rehabilitation involves setting outcome goals related to changes in future lifestyle. Clients must sort through what they must give up, what they will have to do differently, and what they can still enjoy.

Among young adults, 40% to 50% of people with traumatic SCI are unmarried at the time of the incident. Available caregiver support is more limited, and external support systems will need to be established. For older individuals sustaining SCI, there are more

---

BOX 23.4 Safety Parameters to Be Addressed in Future Mobility Studies

- What are the ventilator settings at which mobilization should be withheld?
- Fever is known to increase oxygen consumption—should mobilization be withheld in febrile patients?
- Is there a dose of norepinephrine that predicts harm if mobilization occurs?
- How soon after respiratory failure or shock should mobilization be implemented?
- How should the appropriate mode and intensity of mobilization be selected?
- What is appropriate action if a decrease in oxygenation or blood pressure occurs?

---

preexisting medical conditions, more secondary medical complications, and more need for long-term care.[29]

It is critical throughout the rehabilitation process that the therapist be prepared for the systemic and neurologic changes that could be life threatening, such as orthostatic hypotension and AD.

Guidelines for management of these conditions as defined by the Consortium for Spinal Cord Medicine begin with monitoring blood pressure and pulse rate. Identification and elimination of the causal factor and notification of the occurrence to other team members are critical.[77] Refer to Box 23.2 for symptoms and triggers of AD.

Physical therapist assistants (PTAs) are concerned with mobilization of the client, beginning in intensive care. Emphasis here is on respiratory management. Postural drainage, Trendelenburg and reverse Trendelenburg positioning, and assisted coughing must be initiated. Monitoring of arterial blood gas level and oxygen saturation at rest and during activity is critical. Box 23.4 outlines the considerations that should be included in determining the most appropriate parameters regarding mobility in clients at this level. An active program to increase strength and excursion of the diaphragm and other innervated accessory muscles of respiration, such as the sternocleidomastoid and trapezius muscles, is critical for pulmonary health. Included in the early program are range of motion, the beginning of a strength and endurance program, and education of both the client and family about the process of therapy. The goal of early intervention is to prevent secondary sequelae, such as pressure sores or contractures, that would interfere with the rehabilitation process and to begin to prepare the musculoskeletal system for a different method of mobility.[55]

Orthotic management of the unstable spinal column is often necessary, and the PTA should be familiar with the types of orthotic devices used. Fig. 23.16 illustrates several orthoses used with different levels of spinal cord lesions.[56,57]

As Box 23.5 demonstrates, the level of the lesion will determine the degree to which independence can be expected in certain activities. The development of wheelchair skills includes transfers, propelling the wheelchair, motorized wheelchair propulsion, management of the wheelchair components, and, most important, weight shifts in the chair to prevent skin breakdown. Adaptations within the environment are necessary for the client with weak upper extremities or poor hand control.

In determining the training program for a client with SCI, there must first be an assessment of physical capabilities and skills. When possible, the client should be taught to maintain range of motion of the extremities independently. Adequate hamstring length is critical for performance of transfers and independent dressing.[43,62]

While working with clients on seated stability and functional movement, clinicians should be encouraged to incorporate bilateral reach tasks, as these have the strongest relationship to performance of activities of daily living (ADLs).[64] Seventy-five percent of individuals with SCI sustain at least one fall per year. Even though most injuries are minor, there is potential for fracture and reduced

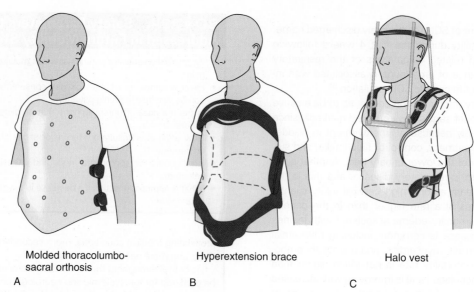

Molded thoracolumbo-
sacral orthosis

Hyperextension brace

Halo vest

A   B   C

FIG. 23.16 (A) Molded thoracolumbosacral orthosis, designed to control extension and rotary movements. (B) Hyperextension brace, which restricts flexion in the thoracic area. (C) Halo vest, which restricts upper thoracic and cervical motion.

BOX 23.5 Disabilities Associated with Level of Injury

C1–C5 Quadriplegia

- Dressing
  Dependent in all dressing activities
- Bathing
  Dependent in all bathing activities
- Communication
  Independent with assistive devices for verbal communication (C1–C3)
  Independent verbal communication (C4–C5)
  Assistive devices necessary for keyboarding, writing, page turning, and use of telephone

C6–C8 Quadriplegia

- Dressing
  Independent with assistive device in bed (C7) or wheelchair (C8)
  Minimal assistance with lower body dressing in bed
  Moderate assistance undressing lower body in bed
  Able to dress and undress in wheelchair with assistive devices (C8)
- Bathing
  Minimal assistance for upper body bathing and drying
  Moderate assistance for lower body drying (C6)
  Independent with assistive devices (C7–C8)
  Assistive devices (tub chair necessary for tub or shower)
- Communication
  Independent in verbal communication
  Assistive devices necessary for keyboarding, writing, and use of telephone
  Setup required (C6)

T1 and Below Paraplegia

- Dressing
  Independent with use of assistive device
- Bathing
  Independent with use of assistive device (tub bench or cushion on bottom of tub)
- Communication
  Independent

Data from Umphred DA, Burton G, Lazaro RT, et al., editors: Umphred's neurological rehabilitation, ed 6, St. Louis, 2013, Mosby.

community mobility. Factors perceived to contribute to falls most often were decreased strength in the trunk and lower extremities, loss of balance, and hazards in the environment.[10]

Rehabilitation traditionally focused on social reintegration is now giving way to inclusion of restoration of function by means of regeneration.[6] An approach known as activity-based rehabilitation (ABR) is a noninvasive approach to enhance recovery and optimize spontaneous regeneration by inducing regular activity in the injured nervous system. The activity-based hypothesis implies that nervous system injury produces a complex secondary phase of progressive deterioration in the integrity of neural circuitry. It is believed that the cellular events that occur during development are similar to the processes that promote regeneration. ABR is based on the theory that patterned neural activity assists the system in optimizing cellular regeneration.

ABR therapy includes the use of FES to drive mobility in the extremities. FES can be used for muscle strengthening during the recovery period. Muscles are strengthened by cyclic, isotonic FES activation increasing muscle force, bulk, and fatigue resistance. FES may also increase sensory awareness and muscles for augmentation of voluntary control. Supported standing and limited distances of ambulation can be part of a program to improve respiratory control. Loading of the joints can be achieved with the use of stimulation in multiple sites to achieve cocontraction necessary for standing. Another important effect of ABR is the reduction of complications. The severe complications that accompany immobility include infections, skin breakdown, spasticity, pathologic fractures, deep vein thrombosis, pain, and AD.

Electrical stimulation reverses the natural recruitment order of muscle fibers, resulting in excessive fatigue compared with a natural contraction. Attempts to minimize fatigue related to FES have led to use of units that are fired by feedback on voluntary muscle activity or control stimulation through weight shifting. The FES is intended to enhance the contraction as the extremity moves through the cycle. Stimulation of the common peroneal nerve can facilitate the flexor swing, and stimulation of the upper portion of the hamstring and gluteus can facilitate the stance phase. Stimulation of the lower portion of the hamstring and quadriceps can support correction of knee hyperextension (genu recurvatum).[23] Neuroprostheses via surgically implanted FES device are rehabilitative tools with the potential to increase independence. The muscles stimulated include the vastus lateralis, gluteus maximus, semimembranosus, and erector spinae. The implanted standing neuroprosthesis appears to be a clinically acceptable and effective means of providing the ability to exercise, stand, and transfer to selected individuals with paraplegia or low quadriplegia through the coordinated activation of the paralyzed lower limb musculature. FES is not intended to create mobility when there is no potential for walking but is a tool to augment natural recovery that would lead to walking with crutches rather than wheelchair mobility. FES is used to augment walking.

Computer-controlled surface stimulation of three muscle groups in each leg (quadriceps, hamstrings, and gluteal muscles) allows paralyzed individuals to rotate the wheels of a bicycle under their own muscle power despite lack of volitional control of muscles. FES ergometry is the only method by which paralyzed individuals are able to obtain the benefits of exercise. An hour of FES ergometry is the equivalent of 6000 steps. Such patterned stimulation activates the lumbar gait central program generator, sending a normal pattern of neural activity up the cord. In addition to providing the benefits of physical reconditioning, FES ergometry is done to replicate normal levels of patterned neural activity in the spinal cord below the lesion level in an effort to optimize spontaneous regeneration. Home-based, self-administered neuromuscular electrical stimulation resistance exercise therapy consisting of 80 contractions per week improves arterial health after SCI, which may reduce the risk of future cardiovascular disease.[66]

Evidence now indicates hope for more sparing of descending tracts at the level of the lesion. Even minimal sparing of white matter has a profound impact on recovery of function.[4] The potential for training motor responses associated with reflexes below the level of the lesion has been identified. Walking is typically a priority concern for many clients with SCI, especially those with paraplegia. Interventions such as body weight–supported treadmill training have shown potential for improved locomotion.[6] Walking and balancing abilities are related, and balance reactions must be integrated into overground carryover. Partial body support treadmill training and supported overground walking are used with dorsiflexion assisted through FES and noxious stimulation driving flexor responses.[27,52] Studies of these techniques are finding that the context specificity of training affects the outcomes, and future studies are directed toward discovering the most efficient and effective interventions to produce walking and the associated health benefits.

Deficits in upper extremity function in individuals with tetraplegia are primarily due to the loss of motor pathways. Detrimental cortical reorganization, however, may create further loss of function. An intensive training intervention may induce both functional and neurophysiologic changes by driving cortical reorganization.[35]

FES-assisted hand movement can enable clients with tetraplegia to perform most of their simple ADLs.

Exercise is critical to the individual with SCI to maintain cardiac fitness levels. There are numerous reports of strategies for exercises.[3] Circuit resistance training (CRT) improves muscle strength, endurance, and anaerobic power in individuals with paraplegia while significantly reducing their shoulder pain.[54] Skeletal muscle atrophy is associated with accumulation of greater intramuscular fat in thigh muscle groups in SCI and continues to increase over time in incomplete SCI.[30] There is a link between adiposity (accumulation of fat in adipose tissue) and defining characteristics of metabolic syndrome. Adiposity is related to dyslipidemia, vascular inflammation, hypertension, and insulin resistance.[28] There is persistent adaptive capability within chronically paralyzed muscles. Preventing musculoskeletal adaptations after SCI may be more effective than reversing changes in the chronic condition.[61]

Being independent of personal assistance in ambulation is related to lower levels of pain interference with life activity and work performance and less use of prescription medication to treat pain. Pain interference appears to be more problematic for those who are partially ambulatory than for individuals who are independent in ambulation.[58]

Age, employment status, motor level and completeness of injury, and ambulatory mode (use of hand-propelled or motorized wheelchair, use of crutches or canes, or walking independently) are independently associated with health-related quality-of-life (HRQoL) scores. Chronic cough, chronic phlegm, persistent wheeze, dyspnea with ADLs, and lower forced expiratory volume and forced vital capacity are each associated with a lower HRQoL.[15,39]

The importance of specific staff qualities, the need for a vision of future life possibilities, the importance of peers, the necessity for relevant program content, and the importance of the ability to reconnect the past to the future has been documented by individuals with SCI. If rehabilitation services are to be evidence based, relevant, and effective in meeting the needs of people with SCI, they must be informed by the perspectives of people with SCI. The most important dimension of rehabilitation for people with SCI is the caliber and vision of the rehabilitation staff.

REFERENCES/SUGGESTED READINGS

To enhance this text and add value for the reader, references and suggested readings are included on the companion Evolve site that accompanies this textbook. The reader can view the source and access it online whenever possible.

Cerebral Palsy

1. Define "cerebral palsy" as a diagnosis.
2. Review the clinical manifestations of cerebral palsy.
3. Review expected outcomes for the condition.
4. Be able to create an overview of therapeutic management of cerebral palsy throughout the lifespan as both a primary and secondary diagnosis.

OUTLINE

VOCAB BUILDERS

Ankle-foot orthosis (AFO)
Ataxia
Athetosis
Choreoathetosis

Contracture
Dynamic ankle-foot orthosis (DAFO)
Dorsal rhizotomy
Dystonia

Hydrocephalus
Microcephalus
Supramalleolar orthosis (SMO)
Spasticity

CEREBRAL PALSY

Overview

Cerebral palsy (CP) is a nonprogressive lesion of the brain occurring before 2 years of age resulting in a disorder of posture and voluntary movement. CP may be accompanied by impairment of speech, vision, hearing, and perceptual function. Common comorbidities include visual and hearing deficits, seizure disorders, hydrocephalus, microcephaly, scoliosis, hip dislocation, and cognitive limitations.

Classification

CP is often classified by the type of muscle tone, distribution of limb involvement, or functional skills. The types of muscle tone include hypotonia/low tone; hypertonia/high tone, spasticity; ataxia; and choreoathetosis or dystonia. *Choreoathetosis* is characterized by involuntary distal writhing movements *(athetosis)* and poorly graded proximal voluntary movement (chorea).

Spasticity is graded most commonly by using the modified Ashworth scale or the Tardieu scale and is characterized by a velocity-dependent resistance to passive stretch.[10]

Dystonia is characterized by sustained muscle contraction resulting in sustained end-range posture.

Ataxia is characterized by diametric movement patterns. The patterns of motor involvement and distribution are described in Table 24.1.

Spastic CP—particularly quadriplegia (also called tetraplegia) and spastic diplegia, accounts for the majority of cases. Hemiplegia, ataxia, dystonia, and choreoathetoid CP affect a relatively smaller number of children. New cases of choreoathetoid CP have become rare in the United States and Canada as a result of improved prenatal care.

Functional skills can also be used to classify individuals with CP. The Gross Motor Function Classification System (GMFCS) provides a five-level system to classify motor involvement of children with CP on the basis of their functional status and their need for assistive technology and wheeled mobility (Box 24.1). The GMFCS provides a means of objectively grading age-related developmental skill.[30,32]

Level I includes children with neuromotor impairments whose functional limitations are less than what is typically associated with CP. It also includes children who have traditionally been diagnosed as having "minimal brain dysfunction" or "cerebral palsy of minimal severity." The distinctions between levels I and II therefore are not as pronounced as the distinctions between the other levels, particularly for infants younger than age 2 years.[30,32]

The descriptions of the five levels are broad and not intended to describe all aspects of the function of individual children. The focus is on determining which level best represents the child's present abilities and limitations in motor function. Emphasis is on the child's usual performance in home, school, and community settings.[30]

TABLE 24.1 Classification of Cerebral Palsy

Type	Distribution or Description
Spastic	
Monoplegia	Only one limb affected
Diplegia	Involves trunk and lower extremities; upper extremities to a lesser degree
Hemiplegia	Primarily one total side involved; upper extremity usually more than the lower extremity
Quadriplegia (tetraplegia)	Involvement of all four limbs, head, and trunk
Ataxia	Irregularity of muscular action manifested by dysmetria; may be pure or combined with other forms
Dyskinesia (choreoathetosis)	Impairment of the power of voluntary movement; poor control of proximal movement (chorea) alternating with repetitive, involuntary, slow, writhing movements (athetosis); movements increase with emotional stress and around adolescence; often associated with rigidity or spastic quadriplegia or diplegia
Hypotonia	Abnormally reduced tension or muscle tone; accompanied by variable degrees of weakness

BOX 24.1 Gross Motor Function Classification System for Cerebral Palsy (GMFCS)

The GMFCS is based on self-initiated movement with emphasis on sitting (truncal control) and walking. The focus is on determining which level best represents the child's present abilities and limitations in motor function. User instructions and more information are available online at http://canchild.ca/system/tenon/assets/attachments/000/000/058/original/GMFCS-ER_English.pdf.

Before Second Birthday

Level I

Infants move in and out of sitting and floor sit with both hands free to manipulate objects. Infants crawl on hands and knees, pull to stand, and take steps holding onto furniture. Infants walk between 18 months and 2 years of age without the need for any mobility device.

Level II

Infants maintain floor sitting but may need to use their hands for support to maintain balance. Infants creep on their stomachs or crawl on hands and knees. Infants may pull to stand and take steps holding onto furniture.

Level III

Infants maintain floor sitting when the low back is supported. Infants roll and creep forward on their stomachs.

Level IV

Infants have head control but trunk support is required for floor sitting. Infants can roll to supine and may roll to prone.

Level V

Physical impairments limit voluntary control of movement. Infants are unable to maintain antigravity head and trunk postures in prone and sitting positions. Infants require adult assistance to roll.

Between Second and Fourth Birthdays

Level I

Children floor sit with both hands free to manipulate objects. Movements in and out of floor sitting and standing are performed without adult assistance. Children walk as the preferred method of mobility without the need for any assistive mobility device.

Level II

Children floor sit but may have difficulty with balance when both hands are free to manipulate objects. Movements in and out of sitting are performed without adult assistance. Children pull to stand on a stable surface. Children crawl on hands and knees with a reciprocal pattern, cruise holding onto furniture, and walk using an assistive mobility device as preferred methods of mobility.

Level III

Children maintain floor sitting often by "W-sitting" (sitting between flexed and internally rotated hips and knees) and may require adult assistance to assume sitting. Children creep on their stomachs or crawl on hands and knees (often without reciprocal leg movements) as their primary methods of self-mobility. Children may pull to stand on a stable surface and cruise short distances. Children may walk short distances indoors using an assistive mobility device and adult assistance for steering and turning.

Level IV

Children floor sit when placed but are unable to maintain alignment and balance without use of their hands for support. Children frequently require adaptive equipment for sitting and standing. Self-mobility for short distances (within a room) is achieved through rolling, creeping on stomach, or crawling on hands and knees without reciprocal leg movement.

Level V

Physical impairments restrict voluntary control of movement and the ability to maintain antigravity head and trunk postures. All areas of motor function are limited. Functional limitations in sitting and standing are not fully compensated for through the use of adaptive equipment and assistive technology. At level V, children have no means of independent mobility and are transported. Some children achieve self-mobility using a power wheelchair with extensive adaptations.

Between Fourth and Sixth Birthdays

Level I

Children get into and out of, and sit in, a chair without the need for hand support. Children move from the floor and from chair sitting to standing without the need for objects for support. Children walk indoors and outdoors, and climb stairs. Emerging ability to run and jump.

Level II

Children sit in a chair with both hands free to manipulate objects. Children move from the floor to standing and from chair sitting to standing but often require a stable surface to push or pull up on with their arms. Children walk without the need for any assistive mobility device indoors and for short distances on level surfaces outdoors. Children climb stairs holding onto a railing but are unable to run or jump.

Level III

Children sit on a regular chair but may require pelvic or trunk support to maximize hand function. Children move in and out of chair sitting using a stable surface to push or pull up on with their arms. Children walk with an assistive mobility device on level surfaces and climb stairs with assistance from an adult. Children frequently are transported when traveling for long distances or outdoors on uneven terrain.

Level IV

Children sit on a chair but need adaptive seating for trunk control and to maximize hand function. Children move in and out of chair sitting with assistance from an adult or a stable surface to push or pull up on with their arms. Children may at best walk short distances with a walker and

BOX 24.1　Gross Motor Function Classification System for Cerebral Palsy (GMFCS)—Cont'd

adult supervision but have difficulty turning and maintaining balance on uneven surfaces. Children are transported in the community. Children may achieve self-mobility using a power wheelchair.

Level V

Physical impairments restrict voluntary control of movement and the ability to maintain antigravity head and trunk postures. All areas of motor function are limited. Functional limitations in sitting and standing are not fully compensated for through the use of adaptive equipment and assistive technology. At level V, children have no means of independent mobility and are transported. Some children achieve self-mobility using a power wheelchair with extensive adaptations.

Between Sixth and Twelfth Birthdays

Level I

Children walk indoors and outdoors and climb stairs without limitations. Children perform gross motor skills including running and jumping but speed, balance, and coordination are reduced.

Level II

Children walk indoors and outdoors, and climb stairs holding onto a railing but experience limitations walking on uneven surfaces and inclines, and walking in crowds or confined spaces. Children have at best only minimal ability to perform gross motor skills such as running and jumping.

Level III

Children walk indoors and outdoors on a level surface with an assistive mobility device. Children may climb stairs holding onto a railing. Depending on upper limb function, children propel a wheelchair manually or are transported when traveling for long distances or outdoors on uneven terrain.

Level IV

Children may maintain levels of function achieved before age 6 or rely more on wheeled mobility at home, school, and in the community. Children may achieve self-mobility using a power wheelchair.

Level V

Physical impairments restrict voluntary control of movement and the ability to maintain antigravity head and trunk postures. All areas of motor function are limited. Functional limitations in sitting and standing are not fully compensated for through the use of adaptive equipment and assistive technology. At level V, children have no means of independent mobility and are transported. Some children achieve self-mobility using a power wheelchair with extensive adaptations.

Between Twelfth and Eighteenth Birthdays

Level I

Youth walk at home, school, outdoors, and in the community. Youth are able to walk up and down curbs without physical assistance and stairs without the use of a railing. Youth perform gross motor skills such as running and jumping but speed, balance, and coordination are limited. Youth may participate in physical activities and sports depending on personal choices and environmental factors.

Level II

Youth walk in most settings. Environmental factors (such as uneven terrain, inclines, long distances, time demands, weather, and peer acceptability) and personal preference influence mobility choices. At school or work, youth may walk using a handheld mobility device for safety. Outdoors and in the community, youth may use wheeled mobility when traveling long distances. Youth walk up and down stairs holding a railing or with physical assistance if there is no railing. Limitations in performance of gross motor skills may necessitate adaptations to enable participation in physical activities and sports.

Level III

Youth are capable of walking using a hand-held mobility device. Compared with individuals in other levels, youth in Level III demonstrate more variability in methods of mobility depending on physical ability and environmental and personal factors. When seated, youth may require a seat belt for pelvic alignment and balance. Sit-to-stand and floor-to-stand transfers require physical assistance from a person or support surface. At school, youth may self-propel a manual wheelchair or use powered mobility.

Outdoors and in the community, youth are transported in a wheelchair or use powered mobility. Youth may walk up and down stairs holding onto a railing with supervision or physical assistance. Limitations in walking may necessitate adaptations to enable participation in physical activities and sports including self-propelling a manual wheelchair or powered mobility.

Level IV

Youth use wheeled mobility in most settings. Youth require adaptive seating for pelvic and trunk control. Physical assistance from one or two persons is required for transfers. Youth may support weight with their legs to assist with standing transfers.

Indoors, youth may walk short distances with physical assistance, use wheeled mobility, or, when positioned, use a body support walker. Youth are physically capable of operating a powered wheelchair. When a powered wheelchair is not feasible or available, youth are transported in a manual wheelchair. Limitations in mobility necessitate adaptations to enable participation in physical activities and sports, including physical assistance and/or powered mobility.

Level V

Youth are transported in a manual wheelchair in all settings. Youth are limited in their ability to maintain antigravity head and trunk postures and control arm and leg movements. Assistive technology is used to improve head alignment, seating, standing, and mobility but limitations are not fully compensated by equipment. Physical assistance from one or two persons or a mechanical lift is required for transfers. Youth may achieve self-mobility using powered mobility with extensive adaptations for seating and control access. Limitations in mobility necessitate adaptations to enable participation in physical activities and sports including physical assistance and using powered mobility.

Distinctions Between Levels I and II

Compared with children at level I, children at level II have limitations in the case of performing movement transitions, walking outdoors and in the community, the need for assistive mobility devices when beginning to walk, quality of movement, and the ability to perform gross motor skills such as running or jumping.

Distinctions Between Levels II and III

Differences are seen in the degree of achievement of functional mobility. Children at level III need assistive mobility devices and frequently orthoses to walk, whereas children at level II do not require assistive mobility devices after age 4.

Distinctions Between Levels III and IV

Differences in sitting ability and mobility exist, even allowing for extensive use of technology. Children at level III sit independently, have independent floor mobility, and walk with assistive mobility devices. Children at level IV function in sitting (usually supported) but independent mobility is very limited. Children at level IV are more likely to be transported or use power mobility.

Distinctions Between Levels IV and V

Children at level V lack independence even in basic antigravity postural control. Self-mobility is achieved only if the child can learn how to operate an electronically powered wheelchair.

Adapted from Palisano R, Rosenbaum P, Walter S, et al.: Development and reliability of a system to classify gross motor function in children with cerebral palsy. Dev Med Child Neurol 39(4):214-223, 1997.

The levels are described on time line bands including before second birthday, between second and fourth birthdays, between fourth and sixth birthdays, between sixth and twelfth birthdays and was expanded to include 12- to 18-year-olds. Distinctions between adjacent levels are outlined in Box 24.1.

Incidence and Etiologic and Risk Factors

The reported incidence of CP ranges from 1.5 to 4.7 cases per 1000 births in the United States.[27] Despite the increased use of fertility drugs, survival of infants in multiple births, and survival of extremely low-birth-weight infants, the incidence of neurodisabilities, including CP, has remained constant among surviving premature infants.[25,33] In fact, incidence may have begun to show some recent decline,[22] although the prevalence has increased because of the improved survival rates.

The cause of CP may be unknown and is often multifactorial. In children of normal birth weight who have disabilities associated with CP, 80% of the disabilities are a result of factors occurring before birth and 20% are attributed to factors occurring around the birth or in the first 4 weeks of life.

In children of low birth weight who develop disabilities associated with CP, uncertainty remains as to when the brain damage occurred. Any prenatal, perinatal, or postnatal condition that results in cerebral anoxia, hemorrhage, or damage to the brain can cause CP (Table 24.2). CP is the second most common neurologic impairment in childhood (intellectual disability is the first).[48]

Pathogenesis

No consistent or uniform pathology is associated with CP. Several types of neuropathic lesions have been identified on the basis of autopsy: (1) hemorrhage below the lining of the ventricles, (2) hypoxia causing encephalopathy, and (3) malformations of the central nervous system.[54]

Until recently, intraventricular hemorrhage (IVH) was the most common form of brain injury in the premature infant. In recent years the incidence of IVH has declined from an incidence of 49% in very-low-birth-weight infants to 20% in the same population.[35]

Hypoxic injury can occur in the full-term infant; however, this represents only a small portion of infants with CP. It often occurs in the presence of bradycardia, intrauterine growth retardation, and preeclampsia and may also be facilitated by the presence of infection.[5]

Hypoxic–ischemic injury is known to disrupt the normal metabolic processes, starving the cells of oxygen because of poor perfusion and poor oxygen delivery to the cells. Eventually, insufficient energy is all that is available for powering the sodium–potassium pump in the cell membrane, and the ionic gradients across the cell membranes break down.

Focal injury to the brain can also result from hemorrhage and ischemia, with the resulting collection of blood creating injury from direct mechanical pressure on the tissue and secondary ischemia. In the premature infant, hemorrhage of the germinal matrix–nervous system is a common cause of CP and can result in venous infarction with a resulting cystic lesion in that portion of the brain.[52]

Children who develop CP fail to demonstrate normal central nervous system (CNS) maturation after a CNS injury. Persistence of immature layers of the primary motor cortex is often present, and many of the other layers demonstrate abnormalities, particularly those with projections to the pyramidal tract.[2]

Clinical Manifestations

Although the neurologic manifestations of CP are nonprogressive, the motor impairments change with growth and maturation and may become more apparent as the affected child grows. Clinical manifestations of motor impairments associated with CP may include alterations of muscle tone, delayed postural reactions, persistence of primitive reflexes (Fig. 24.1), delayed motor development, and abnormal motor performance, including a delay in movement onset, poor timing of force generation, poor force production, inability to maintain antigravity postural control, decreased speed of movement, and increased cocontraction.[15]

Persistence of primitive reflexes and impaired motor function can affect the head, neck, trunk, and extremities and impair sucking and swallowing, resulting in feeding difficulties, a major focus of occupational and speech therapists (Fig. 24.2).

Associated disabilities may include cognitive impairments such as mental retardation, learning disabilities, and seizure disorders; sensory impairments in vision and/or hearing; and constipation or bowel and bladder incontinence with their associated problems.[28,34]

TABLE 24.2	**Risk Factors for Cerebral Palsy**	
Prenatal	**Perinatal**	**Postnatal**
Maternal infection	Prematurity	Neonatal infection (meningitis, encephalitis)
• Rubella	Obstetric complications	Environmental toxins
• Cytomegalovirus	• Mechanical birth trauma	Trauma
• Herpes simplex	• Breech delivery	Kernicterus
• Toxoplasmosis	• Forceps delivery	Brain tumor
Maternal diabetes	• Twin or multiple births	Anoxia (e.g., near drowning, assault)
Rh incompatibility	Prolapsed umbilical cord or umbilical cord flow	Cerebrovascular accident
Toxemia (undiagnosed or untreated)	abnormalities	Neonatal hypoglycemia
Maternal malnutrition	Low birth weight (<1750 g)	Acidosis
Maternal thyroid disorders	Small for gestational age (SGA)	
Maternal seizures	Low Apgar scores (≤4 at 5 min)	
Maternal radiation	Placenta previa (intrauterine bleeding)	
Abnormal placental attachment	Abruptio placentae	
Congenital anomalies of the brain		
Coagulation factor abnormalities		
Factor V Leiden mutation		
Antiphospholipid antibodies		

Microcephalus and *hydrocephalus* are also common findings, with the latter being the result of increased intracranial pressure. Behavioral signs of increased intracranial pressure accompanying hydrocephalus may include extreme irritability, vomiting, and eventually delay in reaching developmental milestones, resulting from pressure-induced damage as discussed earlier.

Musculoskeletal problems of altered muscle tone, muscle weakness, and joint restrictions are common and can result in functional and orthopedic impairments. For example, the abnormal pull of the spastic iliopsoas and adductor muscles are the initiating deforming force in hip dislocations (Fig. 24.3).

When spasticity and *contracture* of the iliopsoas occur, the medial joint capsule is compressed and the femoral head is pushed laterally. As lateral drift of the femoral head occurs, the iliopsoas insertion on the lesser trochanter becomes the center of rotation. Acetabular development ceases when the femoral head is completely displaced laterally, and further hip flexion pushes the head posteriorly to complete the dislocation (Fig. 24.4).[9]

Joint restrictions associated with CP are a result of a decrease in the number of sarcomeres[44] per muscle fiber. Muscles also demonstrate an increased variation in fiber size and type[37] with both hypertrophy and atrophy present, possibly representing an ongoing dynamic process. Increases in fat and fibrous tissue and a decrease in blood flow have been identified.[36] In this process, bone grows faster than muscle, resulting in a disadvantageous length-tension relationship of the muscle and an increased risk of subsequent contracture.[43] A characteristic decrease in muscle mass also results in decreased muscle power and endurance.

Changes in muscle tone affect a person's ability to control movement, resulting in poor selective control of muscles, poor regulation of activity and muscle groups, decreased ability to learn unique movements, inappropriate sequencing of movements, and delayed anticipatory postural response (Table 24.3). Most often, the timing and sequence of muscle activity are also affected.

A significant number of children with a diagnosis of spastic CP present with low muscle tone early in the first year of life and later develop spasticity. They often have insufficient flexor skills to position themselves against gravity for activities such as lifting the head, reaching, and kicking. The child will attempt to develop alternative strategies to complete the tasks. If control is not available, these strategies result in postures that allow completion of a particular sequence but do not allow for subsequent movement and transitions.

Examples of such situations are a wide-based sitting posture that allows the child to maintain sitting but decreases the ability to turn and rotate in and out of the position. Pulling to stand with the arms only (without using the lower extremities) is another example of an alternative strategy used by children with CP. If practiced and repeated over time, these abnormal movements become habitual and are difficult to change.

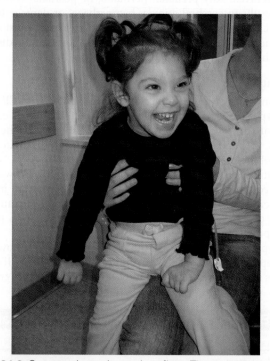

FIG. 24.2 Symmetric tonic neck reflex. The same 4-year-old with quadriplegic cerebral palsy as in Fig. 24.1 demonstrates another primitive reflex known as the symmetric tonic neck reflex (STNR). When the head and neck are extended, the arms extend; flexion usually predominates in the lower extremities. Flexion of the head and neck causes flexion in the upper extremities and extension in the lower extremities (not shown). In the normal infant the asymmetric tonic neck reflex and STNR are typically integrated by 6 to 8 months. Integration of the STNR allows voluntary flexion of both arms and legs needed to sit comfortably. Before 6 to 8 months, these reflexes can be observed in developing infants but when present are not obligatory (i.e., the person can voluntarily move out of the position). (Courtesy Allan Glanzman, Children's Seashore House of the Children's Hospital of Philadelphia.)

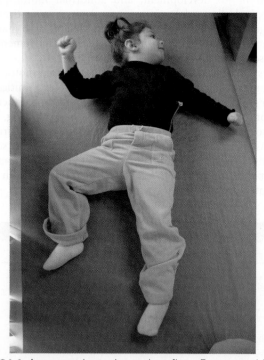

FIG. 24.1 Asymmetric tonic neck reflex. Four-year-old with quadriplegic cerebral palsy demonstrating the asymmetric tonic neck reflex. This primitive reflex contributes to an obligatory change in body posture resulting from a change in head position. With head turning to one side, the arm and leg on the same side extend while the arm and leg on the opposite side flex. This posture resembles a fencing position. (Courtesy Allan Glanzman, Children's Seashore House of the Children's Hospital of Philadelphia.)

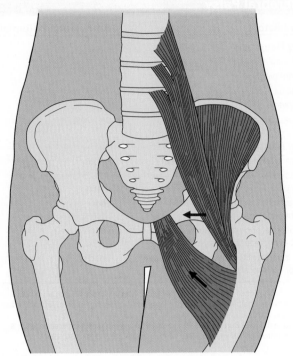

FIG. 24.3 Spastic iliopsoas and adductor muscles are the initiating deforming force in acquired spastic hip dislocation.

TABLE 24.3 Effects of Changes in Muscle Tone	
Effects of Moderate Hypertonia	**Effects of Moderate Hypotonia**
Decreased movement: gross motor delays	Decreased movement: gross motor delays
Tightness/contractures of hip and knee flexors, lower extremity adductors	Possible lower extremity external rotation tightness gastrocnemius, and soleus (heel cords)
Weak trunk; unstable kyphotic sitting	Truncal kyphosis
Flexed, adducted, pronated upper extremity (severe cases)	Compensatory widened lower extremity base of support in prone position, creeping, sitting, standing, and walking
Significant upper extremity compensations (pulling up with arms, using arms for sitting balance)	Delayed ambulation
Standing and ambulation usually require assistance (splinting, walking aids)	Unstable (pronated) feet
Usually at least one orthopedic (surgical) intervention required by age 5 years, often secondary to hip subluxation	Future difficulties with hopping, jumping, skipping, and higher level balance skills
Adaptive equipment required by age 5 years (e.g., stander, wheelchair or stroller, adaptive chair, walker)	

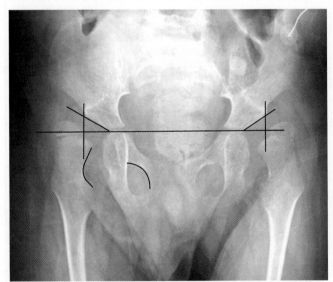

FIG. 24.4 Anteroposterior radiograph of a young child with spastic quadriplegia and subsequent hip dysplasia with subluxation on the left. Note that a line drawn vertically down from the outermost edge of the acetabulum would bisect the head of the femur. Failure of the acetabulum to deepen with weight bearing resulting in hip dysplasia and subluxation occur as a result of the inability to weight bear and abnormal muscular forces pulling on the bone. (Courtesy Allan Glanzman, Children's Seashore House of the Children's Hospital of Philadelphia.)

Medical Management

Diagnosis

Observation, a good history, and a neurologic examination will provide the physician with the information necessary to make an accurate and early diagnosis. The diagnostic studies performed depend on clinical findings. For example, electroencephalography (EEG) is indicated when seizures are present or suspected; hip radiographic films are indicated to rule out hip dislocations and should be followed over time, particularly in the presence of spasticity.

Blood or urine screening tests may be used to rule out certain metabolic diseases, and a thorough workup should be undertaken if a history reveals a progressive course of positive family history. A computed tomographic (CT) or magnetic resonance imaging (MRI) scan can provide information on the location of the insult.

Treatment

Comprehensive and cooperative planning with an interdisciplinary team including physicians, therapists, nurses, special educators, psychologists, social workers, nutritionists, and family members is essential.

Some of the most common medical management strategies include pharmacologic intervention, neurosurgical intervention, and orthopedic surgery. Skeletal muscle relaxants, including baclofen, diazepam, dantrolene, and botulinum toxin, can be used to assist in controlling increased spasticity and can be administered orally, intrathecally, or directly to muscles through injection at the motor point.

Intrathecal administration of baclofen uses an implantable infusion pump to deliver medication to the spinal cord without the associated sedation found with oral administration. After the pump is implanted, the dosage can be titrated to the optimal level for each person. Any attempts to control excess muscle tone should always be paired with functional goals to take advantage of the modulated tone.[1,3]

Motor point blocks can also be used to control spasticity and can be paired with serial casting to increase muscle length. Muscles such as the gastrocnemius, hip adductors, or hamstrings are injected with a botulinum toxin to create a temporary denervation and to decrease tone and increase movement.[12,46]

The type A botulinum toxin (Botox) is injected directly into the muscle at the motor point and is used to block the neuromuscular junction by acting to reduce the release of acetylcholine. Muscle weakness and decrease in muscle spasm occur in 3 to 7 days and gradually reappear in 4 to 6 months.

Successful use of botulinum toxin type A in the upper extremity and at lower doses has been reported.[20,21,42] The effects of these injections will wear off anywhere from several weeks to several months later.

Dorsal rhizotomy, surgically identifying the posterior roots of the spinal cord and selectively resecting some of them to reduce spasticity, has been used during the past decade. This is usually performed at the L2 to L5 spinal levels for clients with spastic diplegia or mildly increased tone who are independent ambulators but who have abnormalities of posture and gait.[51] A rhizotomy may also be used effectively for clients with severe positioning difficulties such as severe quadriplegia. This procedure may reduce muscle tone enough to facilitate personal hygiene and provide improved sitting and comfort.

Orthopedic surgery may include muscle lengthening or releases to address contracture, muscle transfers to increase control or decrease excessive muscle pull, or bone procedures to correct bony deformity, hip dislocation, or scoliosis.

Orthotic intervention may be used to maintain flexibility, support or stabilize a joint, or improve alignment. The ultimate goal is to delay the development of fixed contractures and improve function.

Prognosis

Little information is available about the causes of death of people with disabilities resulting from CP. In the United States no national registry of names of people with CP is available, and cause of death is not usually listed on a death certificate even if the CP was a meaningful contributing factor to the cause of death. Currently available data indicate that common causes of death in this population are related to infection, aspiration, respiratory compromise, and heart disease.[47]

Most children with mild to moderate CP have normal life spans, but there is some increased mortality in the early years (before age 4 years) and then again with advancing age (50 years and older). In those individuals with quadriplegic CP, the excess death rate declines during childhood and adulthood only to climb again after the age of 50 years, as is noted in the more mildly involved population.[41]

Ambulation potential may be predicted based on achievement of motor milestones (Table 24.4). Independent sitting before age 2 years is a positive indicator of future ambulation.[53] If it is going to occur, ambulation usually takes place by 8 years of age.

TABLE 24.4   Predictors of Ambulation for Cerebral Palsy

Predictors	Ambulation Potential
By Diagnosis	
Monoplegia	100%
Hemiplegia	100%[a]
Ataxia	100%
Diplegia	60%[a]–90%
Spastic quadriplegia	0%–70%
By Motor Function	
Sits independently by age 2 years	Good[b]
Sits independently by age 3–4 years	50% community ambulation
Presence of primitive reflexes beyond age 2 years	Poor
Absence of postural reactions beyond age 2 years	Poor
Independently crawled symmetrically or reciprocally by age 2.5 years	Good[b]

[a]From Pallas Alonso CR, de La Cruz Bértolo J, Medina López MC, et al.: Cerebral palsy and age of sitting and walking in very low birth weight infants, An Esp Pediatr 53:48–52, 2000.
[b]da Paz Júnior AC, Burnett SM, Braga LW: Walking prognosis in cerebral palsy: a 22-year retrospective analysis, Dev Med Child Neurol 36:130–134, 1994.

24.1 Special Implications for the PTA: Cerebral Palsy

In addition to the treatment options discussed in the previous section, physical therapist assistants (PTAs) are exploring a more focused and proactive approach of activity-based intervention through intense activity training protocols, lifestyle modifications, and mobility-enhancing devices. Increased motor activity has been shown to lead to better physical and mental health and improve various aspects of cognitive performance.[17]

Activity-based programs for individuals with CP focus on maximizing physical function while preventing secondary musculoskeletal impairments; foster cognitive, social, and emotional development; and potentially promote or enhance neural recovery.[17]

With new research information about the role of neural recovery in damaged nervous systems, therapists can expect to see continued changes in philosophy and intervention approaches with this unique population. Focus will continue with early intervention but include other phases through the life span. As attention is directed toward establishing, enhancing, and maintaining neural pathways, we may see changes in how CP is approached.

Family-Centered Care

When designing a therapy program for a child with CP, the therapist should take a broad view of the child's needs and consider the interactive effects that the child's family environment creates on the goals that have been developed. To provide family-centered care, the PTA must do the following[49]:

- Spend enough time with the family
- Listen carefully to the parents
- Make the parents feel like partners in the child's care
- Be sensitive to the family's values and customs
- Provide the specific information that the parents need

The strengths and weaknesses of each family need to be assessed and considered when designing a given child's program, and consideration must be given to what the impact of carrying out the program will be on the family and, as a result, on the child.

If the cost (emotional, social, financial) is too great, the family may choose to abandon the intervention. As a result, the child may lose ground in terms of altered musculoskeletal alignment and decreased function, and the family must bear the emotional impact.

If the therapy program matches with the family's cultural expectations, ability to participate, and emotional and financial resources, then a partnership with the family can develop that will most benefit the child in the long run. Expecting from family members only what they can succeed at and providing support and education where it is needed to help the family grow and care for the child with special needs will create the best therapeutic environment to allow the child to thrive.

There is often a fine line between balancing the natural history of the condition with the family's commitment and understanding in maximizing the child's quality of life. In addition, families make choices in terms of providing for the child with CP. Often these choices must take into consideration other family members, expectations of themselves, expectations of the child, and, as mentioned, cultural and ethnic beliefs that may not match up with the health care professional's defined goals and plans for intervention.

Early Intervention (IDEA Part C)

A general review of intervention studies shows that children benefit from early intervention compared with those children not involved in specific programmed activities. Programming focused on cognitive outcomes has relatively stronger support[6] than programming aimed at solely motor outcomes.[23] The potential for improvement is better for children younger than age 9 months but not older than age 2 years at a minimum frequency of intervention of two times per week.[8]

Early and accurate identification of CP provides the most likely opportunity for facilitation of optimal motor development.[40] Many motor milestone checklists are available from which a comparison with the normal can be made.[24] In fact, the gross motor function of children with CP and outcomes of intervention have often been evaluated using measures on children without motor impairment.

A more meaningful approach would be to make management decisions and evaluate intervention outcomes based on expectations for children with CP of the same age and gross motor function.[32] This type of evaluation can be made by using assessment tools specifically designed to evaluate the child with CP (e.g., Gross Motor Function Assessment,[38] Gross Motor Function Classification System[30,32]). An assessment of management practices with guidelines for the management of clients with CP is available,[16] as is a model for the acquisition of basic motor abilities and intervention implications.[7]

A significant number of children with a diagnosis of spastic CP present with low muscle tone early in the first year of life and later develop spasticity. They often have insufficient flexor skills to position themselves against gravity for activities such as lifting the head, reaching, or kicking. The child will attempt to develop alternative strategies to complete the tasks. If control is not available, these strategies result in postures that allow completion of a particular sequence but do not allow for subsequent movement and transitions.

Examples of such situations are a wide-based sitting posture that allows the child to maintain sitting but decreases the ability to turn and rotate in and out of the position. Pulling to stand with the arms only (without using the lower extremities) is another example of an alternative strategy used by children with CP. If practiced and repeated over time, these abnormal movements become habitual and are difficult to change.

Postoperative Concerns

After orthopedic surgery, the PTA can assist in reducing muscle spasms that increase postoperative pain by moving and turning the child carefully and slowly; however, adequate postoperative pain management should include medication prescribed by the surgeon.

In the case of postoperative casting, the PTA can instruct the family to wash and dry the skin at the edge of the cast frequently, inspecting often for signs of skin breakdown. Repositioning and ventilation under the cast with a cool-air blow dryer can also assist in preventing skin breakdown. A flashlight can be used daily to inspect beneath the cast.

Surgical procedures may expose areas of underlying muscle weakness and instability. It is critical that an intensive therapy intervention program begin after surgery to assist with strengthening and improving functional performance.

Assistive Technology

Properly prescribed assistive technology is vital in allowing the child with CP the least restrictive access to both the physical and social environment and is a critical part of the overall management of the child with CP. Assistive technology includes any device used to increase, maintain, or improve the functional ability of a person with a disability (Fig. 24.5).

This equipment can be either low tech (such as standers, positioning equipment, communication boards, or wheelchairs) or high tech (such as switch toys, power wheelchairs, or computer-based communication systems) as long as it is provided with a functional goal (Fig. 24.6).

Quality of life has become a new focus in the management of all clients seeking health care services. Mobility impairment limits can negatively affect overall development, including social, cognitive, emotional, and physical development. An increased emphasis on

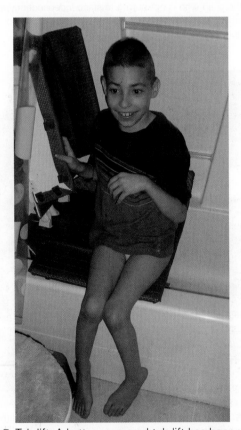

FIG. 24.5 Tub lift. A battery-powered tub lift has been very successful with this child, who has spastic quadriplegic cerebral palsy. With help, he transfers from the toilet next to the tub to the tub seat. With assistance, he swings his legs into the tub, and then can independently operate the unit to lower (and later elevate) himself. (Courtesy Tamara Kittelson-Aldred, Specialty Occupational Therapy PLLC, Missoula, MT. Used with permission.)

powered mobility to increase voluntary activity, function, and independence has contributed to improved quality of life for many individuals with CP (Fig. 24.7).

For children who are dependent for mobility, power mobility can be an option and can be successful in children as young as 2 years of age with corresponding cognitive skills.[13,14,45] These systems can be controlled with a standard joystick or adapted for control with a variety of input systems.

These systems allow control with the head—either by a switch array or by proportional control, control through the use of individual switches, or control by a single switch through a scanning program (Fig. 24.8). When computer access is educationally appropriate, the same wheelchair-based control system can be adapted to operate the computer. Use of mobility and speech-generating (communication) devices is encouraged earlier and with children at all levels of motor disability, including those with severe involvement. Differences in clinical practice and debate continue over providing an external means of mobility in favor of promoting more voluntary activity. Additionally, as the child ages, communication becomes a greater priority compared with all other functional skills. Proper positioning is critical to the child with CP, both from a functional perspective and to help prevent the soft tissue limitations that can develop over time. Appropriate positioning has been shown to encourage smoother and faster reach, decrease extensor tone, increase vital capacity, and improve performance on cognitive testing.[29]

In addition to proper wheelchair position, time out of the chair is necessary to counteract the flexed posture of the body. A daily standing program can be initiated between 12 and 18 months of age in the child who is not pulling to stand independently to maintain flexibility and provide the normal weight-bearing forces across the hip joint.

Standing helps orient children to the upright position, assists with visual perception, and can aid in digestion and elimination. Therapists hear anecdotal reports of decreased constipation and urinary tract infections in response to standing (Fig. 24.9). Standing also provides relief from pressure and can be used for prolonged muscle

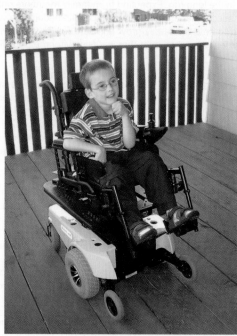

FIG. 24.7 Power wheelchair. This 4-year-old child with cerebral palsy receives a new power wheelchair with a seat elevator to enable him to reach age-appropriate items on countertops and tabletops. Trunk supports and footplates help with alignment. The joystick on the left allows him to navigate independently. (Courtesy Tamara Kittelson-Aldred, Specialty Occupational Therapy PLLC, Missoula, MT. Used with permission.)

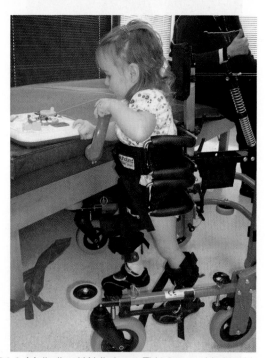

FIG. 24.6 Mulholland Walkabout. This 3-year-old girl with spastic quadriplegia can propel this wheeled upright walker through space to explore her environment and play where she wants to. Although she may not become a functional ambulator, the use of this equipment is developmentally appropriate. She could be a candidate for independent wheelchair mobility, but her parents have deferred this decision for now. (Courtesy Tamara Kittelson-Aldred, Specialty Occupational Therapy PLLC, Missoula, MT. Used with permission.)

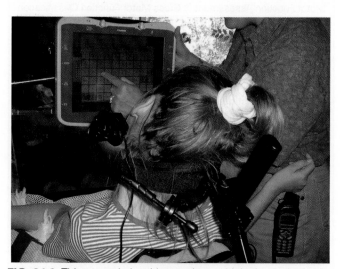

FIG. 24.8 This young lady with spastic quadriplegic cerebral palsy uses a DynaVox speech-generating device with a Tash Microlite switch on the left. By moving her head, she is able to hit the switch with her cheek to stop the electronic scan where she wants it to create a message. Stealth neck rest provides suboccipital head support. (Courtesy Tamara Kittelson-Aldred, Specialty Occupational Therapy PLLC, Missoula, MT. Used with permission.)

stretching, especially in the older or larger child. Standing activities can be embedded into the child and family's daily routine.

Positioning for feeding for the child with CP is often critical for his or her ultimate success and safety at this task. The child's head and neck posture, pelvic posture, and inclination with respect to gravity are important considerations. A team approach using the skills of the physical and occupational therapist in conjunction with those of the speech therapist is essential in designing a program to optimize the child's oral motor skills (Fig. 24.10).

For children with expressive communication deficits, sign language, communication boards, and a variety of high-tech communication systems with voice output are available to augment spoken communication and can also be linked with wheelchair-based control systems in the power wheelchair user.

When evaluating a person for assistive technology, consideration should be given both to the individual's unique abilities and challenges and to the environment in which the equipment will be used. The products should provide the person the greatest degree of functional independence in all the environmental situations encountered. The barriers in each environment may vary, and thus the solutions by necessity may be different in different environments.

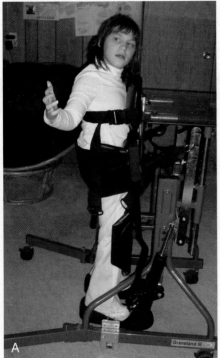

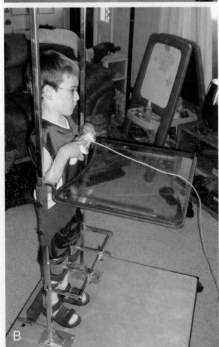

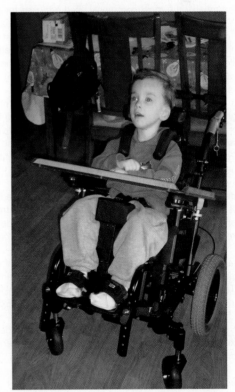

FIG. 24.9 Standing frame. Many different types and styles of standers are available with a variety of adaptive features. (A) Young girl with spastic hemiplegia from a birth injury/infection drives her power chair up to the stander. With assistance, she is able to get a seat sling under her buttocks to lift her up to standing. The sling is significant because it allows the parent to avoid lifting her into the stander. Shoe holders guide the placement of her feet. (B) This standing frame offers an additional fun feature: the ability to operate a PlayStation. (Courtesy Tamara Kittelson-Aldred, Specialty Occupational Therapy PLLC, Missoula, MT. Used with permission.)

FIG. 24.10 Young boy with schizencephaly and cerebral palsy with severe involvement has a planar seating system with postural components. A tilt-in-space feature and deep ischial ledge formed in the seat keep his pelvis aligned and hips back. Hip flexion is combined with the medial thigh support between his legs to keep his knees apart and allow him to relax. Shoulder pad retractors are a feature added when it was discovered that downward pressure and anterior support at the shoulders improved head control for this child. (Courtesy Tamara Kittelson-Aldred, Specialty Occupational Therapy PLLC, Missoula, MT. Used with permission.)

Manual Passive Range-of-Motion Exercise

It is generally accepted that manual straight-plane passive range-of-motion (ROM) exercise for children with a chronic neurologic disorder such as CP is not, by itself, the best way to meet the physiologic requirements necessary to stretch a muscle. However, passive trunk rotation has been found to be useful in assisting with general flexibility and modulation of increased tone for persons with spastic quadriplegia. Additionally, ROM that incorporates a diagonal or rotational component can be beneficial to decrease tone and improve range.

Instead, splinting or positioning that offers a low-load prolonged stretch for longer than 30 minutes or that is used throughout the day is recommended. For example, splints such as lower extremity *ankle-foot orthosis (AFOs)* to maintain ankle dorsi and plantar flexion ROM or supported standing to control lower extremity flexion contractures and assist with hip development and stability may be implemented. However, manual passive ROM exercise is not without its applications and is best combined with a well thought-out positioning and splinting program.

Other interventions used by therapists to improve ROM and facilitate motor development or improve function include relaxation techniques such as neutral warmth or acupressure points, serial or tone casts therapy ball activities, aquatic programs, hippotherapy, and manual therapy techniques.

Orthoses

AFOs are probably the most commonly used orthoses for children with CP. A rigid polypropylene AFO is used to provide medial–lateral stability to the foot and ankle while at the same time assisting with foot clearance during gait. The AFO can be set at + 3 degrees of dorsiflexion to facilitate the increased ankle dorsiflexion necessary for the swing phase of gait or to decrease genu recurvatum through ground reaction forces.

Hinged AFOs may be recommended once a child is moving in the upright position, especially when the child is beginning to walk, squat, or move up and down stairs, both to allow active ankle motion and to allow normal tibial progression during the stance phase of gait. A more flexible plastic may be used in the lighter child to provide more dynamic use of the foot musculature. In this case the term *dynamic ankle-foot orthosis (DAFO)* is used.

In some cases, dorsiflexion assist hinges may be used, either with a plantar flexion stop or in the more mild cases with free plantar flexion. Care must be taken to choose the correct degree of hinge strength or an adjustable hinge so as not to create a crouched posture.

A *supramalleolar orthosis (SMO)* provides medial–lateral stability for the foot and ankle while allowing free plantar flexion and dorsiflexion. The SMO can be used when decreased active ankle dorsiflexion and excessive genu recurvatum are not problems. Extending the SMO proximally to the malleoli provides important support, whereas support distal to the malleoli usually shifts the deformity in a proximal direction. General guidelines and recommendations for foot and ankle splinting can be found in Table 24.5 (Fig. 24.11).

Adolescents with Cerebral Palsy[31]

Therapy staff are encouraged to include the older child or teens in problem solving to help them become more self-sufficient, assuming more responsibility during this developmental phase despite their limitations in physical capability. Providing adolescents the opportunity to participate in planning and decision making is important for transition planning.

This may include decisions about assistive technology, environmental modifications, health and fitness, and prevention of secondary musculoskeletal impairments. Likewise, the therapist can work closely with those individuals interested in participating in recreation and sports activities.

Client-centered assessment of strengths and needs identifying self-care, productivity, and leisure activities is possible and has been reported with this population.[31] PTAs can be instrumental in connecting teens with each other. Many teens and young adults with CP have never met or encountered another person with CP. It

TABLE 24.5 General Foot and Ankle Splinting Guidelines

Splints	Status	Application
Solid AFO neutral to + 3 degrees DF	Nonambulators, beginning standers	1. Less than 3 degrees of DF 2. *Genu recurvatum* associated with decreased ankle DF or weakness 3. Need for medial–lateral stability 4. Nighttime/positional stretching
AFO with 90 degrees posterior stop and free DF (hinged AFO)	Clients with some, but limited, functional mobility	Applications 1–4 above, but need more passive DF during movement, such as ambulation, squatting, steps, and sit to stand
Floor reaction AFO (set dorsiflexion depending on weight line in standing)	Crouch gait Full passive knee extension in standing	For clients with decreased ability to maintain knee extension during standing and ambulation
SMO	Standers/ambulators with pronation at the ankles	1. Need medial–lateral ankle stability 2. Would like opportunity to use active plantar flexion 3. Decreased DF not a problem during gait

AFO, Ankle-foot orthosis; *DF,* dorsiflexion; *SMO,* supramalleolar orthosis.

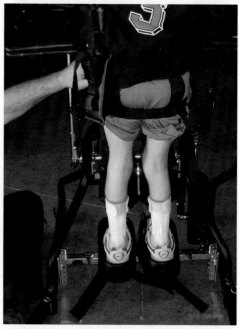

FIG. 24.11 Orthoses. Ankle-foot orthoses as seen from behind this client in a standing frame are used for foot alignment and inhibition of tone associated with spastic quadriplegia. (Courtesy Tamara Kittelson-Aldred, Specialty Occupational Therapy PLLC, Missoula, MT. Used with permission.)

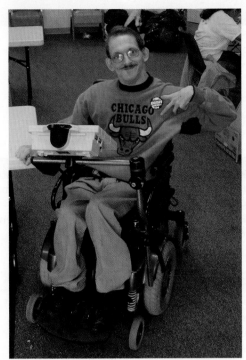

FIG. 24.12 Adult with cerebral palsy. This 33-year-old man with athetoid cerebral palsy uses a speech-generating (communication) device and power chair; the joystick to operate the chair is under the client's right hand. The communication device can be folded and moved out to the side to allow for transfers. The chair has power tilt for independent position changes and pressure relief. Ankle huggers wrapped around the ankles keep his legs from flailing. A neoprene chest harness was added later to help provide external stability and increase control of his movements (not shown). This individual has clearly communicated how much he likes having the chest support, saying he feels much more in control of his body with it on. Straps and supports are fashioned with buckles, because Velcro is not strong enough to hold this client. The additional supports help reduce athetoid movements and improve function. (Courtesy Tamara Kittelson-Aldred, Specialty Occupational Therapy PLLC, Missoula, MT. Used with permission.)

is important for young people with CP to connect to each other and discuss the trials and tribulations of growing up with CP.

Adults with Cerebral Palsy

Therapy staff must also recognize and address the ongoing and unique needs of adults with CP (Fig. 24.12). With improved understanding of CP and its associated long-term complications and with improved health care, increased longevity has brought a new area of concern for children with CP living into adulthood: effects of the aging process. Decline of already impaired muscle strength and elasticity and bone density can lead to loss of ambulatory status.[11]

Group homes, independent living centers, and sheltered workshops are now making it possible for many nonambulatory adults with disabilities to function independently or semiindependently. Regular daily living assistance is required by adults with spastic quadriplegia, especially in the area of lifts and transfers.

Degenerative arthritis, severe joint contractures, and other orthopedic deformities present the most common and challenging problems in this population (Fig. 24.13). Moderate to intense pain is a

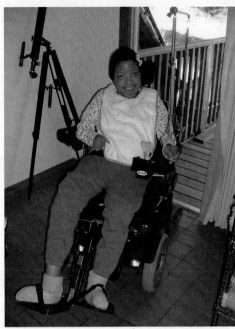

FIG. 24.13 Adult with cerebral palsy. Adults with moderate to severe effects of cerebral palsy can face some difficult physical challenges. This 21-year-old woman has a power chair with seat elevator, power tilt in space, and power elevating leg rests she can operate herself. Each leg rest can be raised or lowered separately to her comfort. This client changed her lower extremity position frequently to manage pain related to spasticity and immobility. A spring upper extremity assist on the left helps keep her hand on a modified joystick to allow her to independently control her chair. (Courtesy Tamara Kittelson-Aldred, Specialty Occupational Therapy PLLC, Missoula, MT. Used with permission.)

significant problem for the majority of adults with CP, accompanied by depressive symptoms interfering with activities.[19,39]

Management strategies for older children and adults are different by virtue of their ability to participate and understand the aims of therapy. Therapy to maintain functional skills through the adolescent growth spurt, when weight gain, weakness, and atrophy often result in a decline in function, is essential. Aerobic training may prevent deterioration in body composition and muscle strength.[50]

Strengthening has become an integral part of therapy programs for individuals with CP and is especially helpful in this population. Measuring isokinetic strength is considered reliable in this population and should be used in rehabilitation protocols.[4] Isokinetic strengthening three times a week for 8 weeks can improve muscle strength and gross motor skills[26,50] and increase cadence[18] for those people who remain ambulatory into adulthood. A traditional upper extremity strengthening program of six to 10 repetitions three times a week for 8 weeks has been useful in improving speed and endurance in independent wheelchair propulsion.

REFERENCES/SUGGESTED READINGS

To enhance this text and add value for the reader, references and suggested readings are included on the companion Evolve site that accompanies this textbook. The reader can view the source and access it online whenever possible.

The Peripheral Nervous System

OUTLINE

VOCAB BUILDERS

Axolemma	Mononeuropathy	Polyneuropathy
Axonotmesis	Myelinopathy	Polyradiculitis
Diabetic neuropathy	Neurapraxia	Radiculoneuropathy
Endoneurium	Neurotmesis	Segmental demyelination
Epineurium	Perineurium	

The peripheral nervous system (PNS) includes somatic motor and sensory components of cranial and spinal nerves arising from neurons whose cell bodies are located within the brainstem and spinal cord or lie in dorsal root ganglia. In addition, peripheral aspects of the autonomic nervous system (ANS) also contribute to axons found in peripheral nerves. Axons from the three components extend from the cell bodies to form peripheral nerves. Disorders of the PNS can be broadly divided into neuropathies, in which the pathology is confined to the nerve, and myopathies, in which the pathology occurs in muscle. Disorders of the PNS can be subdivided further according to site of anatomic involvement.[46]

Signs and symptoms of PNS involvement relate to the motor and sensory systems, as well as the ANS. Motor involvement, termed *lower motor neuron* (LMN) *involvement*, occurs when any of the following sites is affected:

- Cell body of the alpha motor neuron (anterior horn cell) located within the spinal cord or brainstem
- Axons that arise from the anterior horn cell that form spinal and peripheral nerves and cranial nerves

- Motor endplate of the axon
- Muscle fibers innervated by the motor nerve axon

Sensory fibers of the PNS will show involvement if a lesion occurs in the dorsal root ganglion in which the cell body is located or in the nerve root proximal to the ganglia, or distally in fibers of the peripheral nerve (Fig. 25.1). Similarly, when the ANS preganglionic or postganglionic motor fibers are involved, involuntary motor function of the organs will be affected, and when sensory ANS fibers are affected, unconscious sensory functions (such as baroreceptors signaling arterial pressure, receptors within organs signaling irritants, distention, hypoxia, and so forth) will have transmission into the central nervous system (CNS) altered.

STRUCTURE

Nerves in the PNS are supported and covered by three connective tissue coverings that act like a tube surrounding the nerve. The innermost covering is the *endoneurium*, which surrounds each individual axon. The middle layer, or *perineurium*, envelopes groups, or fascicles, of axons and is responsible for maintaining the blood-nerve barrier. The outermost layer, or *epineurium,* surrounds the entire nerve and provides cushioning for the entire nerve.[130] The surface of an axon is formed by a phospholipid membrane called the *axolemma.* Lying

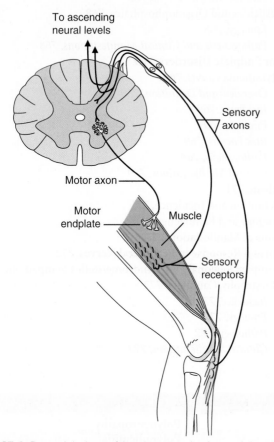

FIG. 25.1 Potential sites of involvement in the peripheral nervous system. Motor: motor neuron cell body, axon, motor endplate, muscle fiber. Sensory: cell body in ganglion, axon, sensory receptor.

between the axolemma and the endoneurium are Schwann cells (Fig. 25.2). Throughout life, axonal-Schwann cell molecular signaling occurs. In large-diameter axons (greater than 1 µm), the Schwann cell receives a signal to wrap its membrane around the axon, thus creating myelin. In small-diameter axons, the Schwann cell merely envelops and supports nonmyelinated fibers. Myelin not only provides electrical insulation essential for rapid saltatory conduction of the axon potential but also affects axonal properties. The presence of myelin causes sodium channels to cluster at the nodes of Ranvier, reinforcing efficient saltatory conduction.[96] In the smallest axons, Schwann cells do not make myelin but do provide support for these unmyelinated fibers, whose action potentials are conducted by local circuit conduction (Table 25.1). Within a peripheral nerve, only about 25% of the fibers are myelinated.[51]

Normal propagation of the action potential also requires sufficient energy, supplied by a vascular plexus interlaced between connective tissue layers. Each peripheral nerve receives an artery that penetrates the epineurium; this artery's branches extend into the perineurium as arterioles, and branches from the arterioles enter the endoneurium as capillaries. Vessels supplying peripheral nerves appear coiled when a limb is in a shortened position but uncoiled after movement so that neural vascular supply is not impaired with a limb's normal excursion. This rich vascular supply makes peripheral nerves relatively resistant to ischemia.[154]

PERIPHERAL NERVOUS SYSTEM CHANGES WITH AGING

Changes that occur in the PNS may be considered as one component of a continuum that relates to normal growth and development, or the changes may represent a combination of pathologic processes superimposed on the normal aging process. Because of the difficulty of studying human peripheral nerves in vivo, experimental animals have been used to assess the effects of aging.

Age does not affect the size or number of fascicles, but the perineurium and epineurium do thicken with age and the

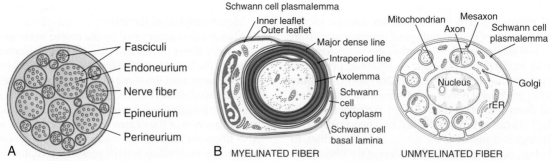

FIG. 25.2 (A) Cross section of a peripheral nerve showing connective tissue coverings. Externally, the nerve is enveloped by the epineurium; internally, individual axons are surrounded by endoneurium. The perineurium surrounds groups of axons (fascicles). (B) Although the majority of the fibers are unmyelinated, they are still associated with supporting Schwann cells. In myelinated fibers *(left),* each Schwann cell forms a myelin internode whose borders are formed by the nodes of Ranvier. Schwann cell sheath supporting unmyelinated fibers *(right).* (A, From Wildsmith JAW: Peripheral nerve and local anesthetic drugs, Br J Anaesth 58:692, 1986. B, From Haines DE: Fundamental neuroscience for basic and clinical applications, ed 4, Philadelphia, 2013, Saunders.)

endoneurium often becomes fibrosed with increased collagen. Even with these changes, the cross-sectional area decreases slightly with age because there are reduced numbers of unmyelinated and myelinated fibers. Ventral root fibers controlling motion are more affected than dorsal root fibers controlling sensation. Blood vessels to nerves may become atherosclerotic with aging, and occlusion may contribute to loss of nerve fibers. The prevalence of peripheral neuropathies seen in older people has been attributed to this vascular pathology.

Decreases in protein production are hypothesized to cause myelin deterioration.[161] When individual myelinated fibers are examined, shorter internodes are seen, suggesting that a demyelinating–remyelinating process occurs with aging. This structural alteration in peripheral nerve myelination may be reflected in diminished appreciation of vibratory sense.

ANS dysfunction is more common in the elderly. This dysfunction may be related to the changes seen in the nervous system in the elderly. Cell bodies show chromatolysis, as well as an accumulation of lipofuscins, representing a diminished ability of the cell to rid itself of toxins. Loss of cell bodies has been observed in the sympathetic ganglia, along with a loss of unmyelinated fibers in peripheral nerves. Sympathetic control of dermal vasculature shows an age-related decline that leads to a diminished wound repair efficiency. In an aging animal model, transcutaneous electrical nerve stimulation (TENS) improved the vascular response. Peripheral activity of sympathetic nerves were affected by the low-frequency electrical stimulation.[76]

When the motor endplate is examined, age-related changes have occurred, but these changes are seen as early as the third decade of life and are not reported in all muscles. When sensory receptors have been evaluated, density and morphology have been found to be altered in the elderly. Altered axonal myelination creates slowing of nerve conduction velocities (NCVs) in the elderly. In addition, the loss of fibers decreases the amplitude of the potential. Simultaneous with the decreased protein production is a decrease in intraaxonal transport by cytoskeletal elements in the peripheral nerve. Electromyographic (EMG) studies of elderly people without evidence of neurologic disorders of the PNS show loss of motor units, as well as signs of reinnervation. Morphologic changes observed in people older than age 60 years are manifested by decreased strength and sensory changes.[107]

Healthy elderly, with no evidence of neurologic disease, may provide a clinical history suggestive of peripheral neuropathy. This includes numbness and tingling in the hands and feet along with mild, diffuse weakness, especially in the distal muscles of the hand. Sensory alterations may lead to poor balance and gait instability. On examination, sensory thresholds are increased.

The cause of an aging neuropathy can be attributed to a combination of factors. First, loss of both motor and sensory cell bodies; second, a dying-back condition, suggesting neurons can metabolically support a limited number of fibers or receptors, similar to that seen in other systemic neuropathies; and last, over the course of a lifetime, chronic compression of the peripheral nerves or repetitive trauma may have damaged the nerves. All these factors, combined with coexisting medical conditions, atherosclerosis, and nutritional deficiencies, may create this neuropathy of aging.

When the aging PNS is damaged, wallerian degeneration is delayed and regeneration takes longer because secretion of trophic factors is slower than in younger individuals. Density of regenerating axons is less. In a partial nerve injury, collateral sprouting is reduced, further limiting recovery of function.[161]

RESPONSE TO INJURY

Peripheral nerve damage occurs by any one of several causal conditions: heredity, trauma, infections, toxins, and metabolism.[26] When either motor or sensory nerves are affected, there is a limited response to injury, regardless of the cause. Either fibers demyelinate or fibers degenerate. Segmental demyelination occurs when nerves are subject to external compression or disease. Degeneration occurs in any peripheral nerve disorder that directly affects the axon, including physical injury (crush, stretch, or laceration), as well as disease.

Loss of myelin, typically in segments, leaves the axon intact but bare where the myelin is lost. This is called *segmental demyelination*. More severe involvement causes axonal degeneration, distal to the lesion (termed *anterograde,* or *wallerian, degeneration*[14,72]), which begins immediately after involvement and is completed over a period of a few weeks. Neuropathic diseases that affect the axon or its cell body causing axonal degeneration typically affect the longest nerve fibers first (a length-dependent process), with signs and symptoms beginning distally and spreading proximally as the disease progresses. Because nerves in the legs are longer, the feet and lower legs are involved long before the fingers and hands. Those conditions that affect only myelin cause segmental demyelination in both sensory and motor fibers. Thus disruption of the conduction of the action potential from proprioceptors and mechanoreceptors causes sensory changes. Those neuropathies that affect myelin cause demyelination of motor nerves to muscle and preganglionic fibers of the ANS create weakness, proprioceptive and tactile changes, and autonomic involvement by disrupting conduction of the action potential.

CLASSIFICATION OF NERVE INJURY

Traumatic injury to peripheral nerves from mechanical involvement secondary to compression, ischemia, and stretching can be classified using one of two systems based on the structural and functional changes that occur. Seddon[138] initially divided nerve injury into three categories: neurapraxia, axonotmesis, and neurotmesis (Fig. 25.3). Sunderland[151] divided this classification into five categories, based on axonal and connective tissue covering involvement.

TABLE 25.1	**Relationship of Myelin Thickness, Conduction Velocity, and Sensory and Motor Fibers**		
Myelin	**Conduction Velocity**	**Sensory Fibers**	**Motor Fibers**
Very thick	Very fast	Proprioception (muscle spindle and Golgi tendon organ)	To skeletal muscle fibers (alpha)
Thick	Fast	Touch, pressure	To muscle spindle (gamma)
Thin	Slower	Touch, temperature	To ANS ganglia
None	Slow	Pain	From ANS ganglia to smooth muscle

ANS, Autonomic nervous system.

Neurapraxia involves segmental demyelination, which slows or blocks conduction of the action potential at the point of demyelination in a myelinated nerve. Neurapraxias often occur after nerve compression that induces mild ischemia in nerve fibers. When segmental demyelination occurs because of disease, the response may be termed a *myelinopathy*. Conduction of the action potential is normal above and below the point of compression, and because the axon remains intact, muscle does not atrophy. *Axonotmesis* occurs when the axon has been damaged, but the connective tissue coverings that support and protect the nerve remain intact. Prolonged compression that produces an area of infarction and necrosis causes an axonotmesis. In the presence of disease, wallerian degeneration creates an axonopathy, which is analogous to an axonotmesis. *Neurotmesis,* the most severe axonal loss, is the complete severance of the axon, as well as the disruption of its supporting connective tissue coverings (endoneurium, perineurium, and/or epineurium) at the site of injury. Neurotmesis is caused by gunshot or stab wounds or avulsion injuries that disrupt a section of the nerve or entire nerve. When axonal continuity is lost (either axonotmesis or neurotmesis), axons distal to the lesion degenerate (wallerian degeneration). Because muscle fibers innervated by the axon depend on the nerve cell body as a source of nourishment or trophic control, when axons degenerate, muscle fibers rapidly atrophy (Table 25.2).

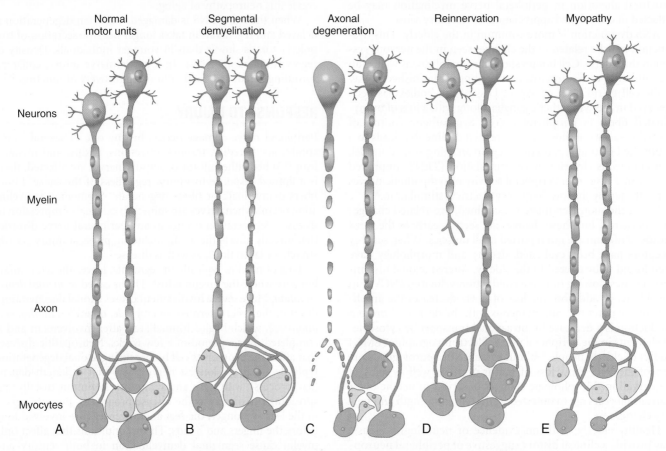

FIG. 25.3 Types of nerve involvement and recovery that occur in peripheral nerves. (A) Two adjacent normal myelinated nerves. (B) Segmental demyelination. Several internodes of myelin have demyelinated, but the axon remains intact. The repair process for segmental demyelination occurs rapidly because Schwann cells divide and remyelinate the bare portion of the axon. Shorter internodal distance occurs with remyelination, thus nerve conduction velocity may not return to normal, even though muscle contracts normally. (C) Axonal degeneration. The axon and myelin have degenerated, but the connective tissue covering remains intact in an axonotmesis. In neurotmesis, the connective tissue covering is disrupted at the lesion site. Signs of chromatolysis occur in the cell body after axonotmesis and neurotmesis. Note that muscle atrophies rapidly because it has lost the trophic influence from the nerve cell body. (D) The repair process for axonotmesis and neurotmesis is more complex. Growth cones from the proximal axon must cross the lesion site and regrow down the connective tissue channels and reestablish a motor endplate or sensory connection before remyelination occurs. In partial nerve injuries, while the injury axon is regrowing, adjacent motor units sprout collateral fibers, leading to expansion of the size of this *(red)* motor unit. (E) In myopathic conditions, scattered muscle fibers in adjacent motor units are small (degenerating or regenerating), whereas the neurons and axons are normal. (From Kumar V, Abbas A, Aster J: Robbins and Cotran pathologic basis of disease, ed 9, Philadelphia, 2015, Saunders.)

If segmental demyelination has occurred, molecular signaling to the remaining Schwann cells causes them to begin dividing mitotically. Newborn Schwann cells move to envelope the denuded segment of nerve, and once these cells are in place, they will begin to form myelin (Fig. 25.3B). The potential for regeneration after axonal/wallerian degeneration is possible as long as the nerve cell body remains viable; new axons can sprout from the proximal end of damaged axons (Fig. 25.3C). However, successful functional regeneration requires that the proximal and distal ends of the connective tissue tube are aligned. This occurs in an axonotmesis because the connective tissue coverings remain intact. In a neurotmesis, without surgical intervention, recovery is less likely because the proximal end of the endoneurium is not approximated to the distal endoneurium. Without surgery, axonal sprouts often enter nearby soft tissue and form a neuroma, or axonal regrowth occurs down the incorrect endoneurial tube, rendering reinnervation nonfunctional.[161] Once the axon has established a distal contact either with muscle or sensory receptor, remyelination will begin. When partial axonal degeneration occurs, adjacent noninvolved axons will produce collateral sprouts that will innervate muscle fibers before the damaged axons have time to grow and reinnervate those muscle fibers. This results in an enlarged motor unit for the neuron that has collateral sprouts (Fig. 25.3D). Numerous reports in the literature link various molecular factors to nerve regeneration and healing following repair.[115,153]

CLASSIFICATION OF NEUROPATHY

Neuropathies include a wide variety of causes and can be classified in many ways, including the rate of onset, type and size of nerve fibers involved, distribution pattern, or pathology (Table 25.3). For example, when a single peripheral nerve is affected, the result is a *mononeuropathy,* which is commonly a result of trauma. The term *polyneuropathy* indicates involvement of several peripheral nerves. A *radiculoneuropathy* indicates involvement of the nerve root as it emerges from the spinal cord, and *polyradiculitis* indicates involvement of several nerve roots and occurs when infections create an inflammatory response.

In addition to involvement of the peripheral nerve, the motor endplate or muscle itself may be involved in a peripheral disorder. Involvement of muscle, termed *myopathy,* follows a different clinical pattern than nerve. When muscle is involved, the disorder typically is reflected by proximal weakness, wasting, and hypotonia without sensory impairments.[169]

TABLE 25.2 Relationship of Nerve and Muscle Responses to Disease and Trauma

Level of Severity	Response to Disease	Response to Trauma	Response of Muscle
Mild	Myelinopathy (segmental demyelination)	Neurapraxia (segmental demyelination)	Paresis/paralysis, no atrophy
Severe	Axonopathy (wallerian degeneration)	Axonotmesis (wallerian degeneration)	Paresis/paralysis with atrophy
Severe	—	Neurotmesis (wallerian degeneration)	Paresis/paralysis with atrophy

TABLE 25.3 Causes of Peripheral Neuropathies and Myopathies and Their Effects

Cause	INVOLVEMENT[a]					
	Axonal Degeneration	Demyelination	Motor Endplate	Muscle	Motor	Sensory
Charcot–Marie–Tooth disease	X	X			X	X
Mechanical compression/entrapment						
Neurapraxia		X			X	X
Axonotmesis	X				X	X
Neurotmesis	X				X	X
Postpolio syndrome	X				X	
Diabetes mellitus	X	X			X	X
Alcohol	X	X			X	X
Guillain–Barré syndrome	X	X			X	X
Toxins						
Lead	X				X	X
Organophosphate	X	X			X	X
Myasthenia gravis			X		X	
Botulism			X		X	
Muscular dystrophy				X	X	
Inflammatory myopathy				X	X	
Steroid-induced myopathy				X	X	
Overuse myopathy				X	X	
Aging	X	X	X	X	X	X
AIDS/HIV (including associated vasculitis)	X	X			X	X
Vitamin B$_{12}$ deficiency	X	X				X
Chronic renal failure	X				X	X

[a]The Xs indicate the most common types of involvement for each cause.
AIDS, Acquired immunodeficiency syndrome; *HIV,* human immunodeficiency virus.

SIGNS AND SYMPTOMS OF PERIPHERAL DYSFUNCTION

The presence of signs and symptoms aid in the localization of the level or levels of involvement. Loss of sensory function will follow a peripheral nerve distribution if that is the anatomic region involved, or it will follow a dermatomal pattern when the spinal nerve or dorsal root ganglia (cell body) has been affected (Fig. 25.4).

Similarly, when a peripheral nerve has motor involvement, paresis or paralysis will occur in muscles innervated by that nerve distal to the lesion. When spinal motor nerves are involved, weakness occurs in all the muscles receiving axons from that spinal level (a myotomal pattern). Individuals with only peripheral nerve involvement will have no signs or symptoms of CNS dysfunction.

Although differences occur in symptom evolution and in progression and severity of a neuropathy, a classic pattern of involvement would occur as follows. Involvement of sensory fibers is reflected by distal sensory deficits with the longest nerves in the body involved first. The first noticeable features of neuropathies are often sensory and consist of tingling, prickling, burning, or bandlike *dysesthesias* and *paresthesias* in the feet. When more than one nerve is involved, the sensory loss follows a glove-and-stocking distribution that is attributed to the dying-back of the longest fibers in all nerves from distal to proximal (Fig. 25.5).

The most common symptoms of motor nerve involvement include distal weakness and abnormalities of tone (hypotonicity or flaccidity). When clients are asked to walk on their heels or toes, weakness of dorsiflexors or plantar flexors, respectively, becomes apparent. Deep tendon reflexes (DTRs) are diminished or absent, and distal-most DTRs will be affected first.

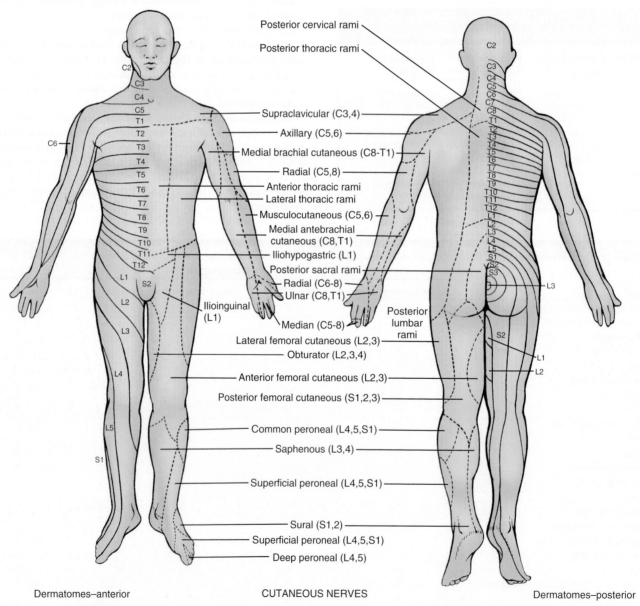

Dermatomes–anterior   CUTANEOUS NERVES   Dermatomes–posterior

FIG. 25.4 Dermatomal (right side of body, anterior and posterior) and peripheral sensory nerve (left side of body, anterior and posterior) patterns. (From Auerbach PS: *Wilderness medicine*, ed 5, St Louis, 2007, Mosby.)

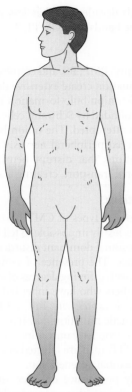

FIG. 25.5 A stocking-glove pattern of sensory loss occurs in polyneuropathy. A gradient of greater distal loss tapering to less proximal involvement is seen.

In the presence of axonal degeneration, rapid atrophy occurs, along with electrophysiologic changes (Tables 25.4 and 25.5). Prolonged paralysis gives rise to secondary complications such as contracture formation and edema.

In addition to weakness and hypotonia, a diagnosis of any one of the muscle diseases may be associated with muscle tenderness or cramping. Classically, the motor involvement in a myopathy is opposite to that of a neuropathy. *In a myopathy, the weakness tends to be proximal; in a neuropathy, motor symptoms tend to first occur distally.*

Finally, because the nerve fibers from the ANS are also located in peripheral nerves, they, too, are subject to the effects of trauma or disease. Preganglionic fibers are myelinated and can be affected by segmental demyelination. In the presence of axonal degeneration, changes will occur in vascular control and sweating. For example, when a person has sustained a laceration of the median nerve in the region of the hand that lacks innervation, autonomic involvement creates smooth skin that does not sweat or wrinkle, or when a neuropathy has a systemic metabolic cause, the person may develop hypotension with cardiac irregularities.[26]

PATHOGENESIS AND DIAGNOSIS OF PERIPHERAL DYSFUNCTION

Trauma, inherited disorders, environmental toxins, and nutritional disorders may affect the myelin (myelinopathy), axon (axonopathy), or cell body of a peripheral nerve. The anatomic region or regions affected determine the severity of the involvement and the amount of function lost (see Table 25.2). Although

TABLE 25.4   Normal Nerve Conduction Velocities and Distal Latencies[a]

Nerve	Motor Conduction Velocity (m/s)	Motor Distal Latency (ms)	Motor Amplitude (mV)	Sensory Conduction Velocity (m/s)	Sensory Distal Latency (ms)	Sensory Amplitude (µV)
Median	63.5 ± 6.2	3.49 ± 0.34	7.0 ± 2.7	56.2 + 5.8	2.84 ± 0.34	38.5 ± 15.6
Ulnar	61.0 ± 5.5	2.59 ± 0.39	5.5 ± 1.9	54.8 ± 5.3	2.54 ± 0.29	35.0 ± 14.7
Tibial	48.5 ± 3.6	3.96 ± 1.00	5.1 ± 2.2			
Peroneal	52 ± 6.2	3.77 ± 0.86	5.1 ± 2.3			

NORMAL F WAVE VALUES

Nerve	Stimulation Site	F Wave Latency to Recording Site (ms)
Median	Elbow	22.8 ± 1.9
Ulnar	Above elbow	23.1 ± 1.7
Peroneal	Above knee	39.9 ± 3.2
Tibial	Knee	39.6 ± 4.4

[a]Generally, in the upper extremities, nerve conduction velocity for motor fibers averages about 60 m/s. Investigators have reported values ranging from 45 to 75 m/s. In the lower extremity, the normal range for motor nerve conduction is in the 40- to 50-m/s range. Distal latency is the time value, reported in milliseconds, that it takes for an evoked potential to be propagated along the nerve and recorded from either the muscle (motor) or the skin (sensory).
Adapted from Dyck PJ, Thomas PK, editors: Peripheral neuropathy, ed 3, Philadelphia, 1993, Saunders.

TABLE 25.5   Relationship of Electromyographic Findings to Innervation

Condition	Normal Innervation	Segmental Demyelination	Axonal/Wallerian degeneration	Myopathy
Insertion	Normal insertional noise	Normal insertional noise	Increased insertional noise	Increased insertional noise
At rest	Quiet	Quiet	Spontaneous (abnormal) potentials: fibrillation potential, positive sharp wave potential	Quiet, except end stage: fibrillation potentials
Minimal contraction	Normal motor unit potential	Affected fibers: no motor unit potential	Affected fibers: no motor unit potential	Low amplitude, polyphasic potential
Maximal contraction	Complete interference pattern	Nerve partially affected: decreased interference pattern	Nerve partially affected: decreased interference pattern; nerve completely affected: no interference pattern	Low amplitude full interference pattern, accomplished with increased frequency of firing and with moderate effort

the phenotype of peripheral dysfunction (i.e., physical characteristics/traits) remains unchanged, much of the recent research in pathophysiology of these disorders has delved into genetic and molecular causes and consequences for what occurs. Findings in these areas may allow development of treatments aimed at altering cellular problems.

Because the nervous system is the means of signaling from the CNS to the muscle, conduction of the action potential is affected in neuropathies and myopathies. In most disorders, electrophysiologic studies are used to determine where and how the nerve or muscle may be affected.

HEREDITARY NEUROPATHIES

Hereditary neuropathies were once considered rare, genetically determined disorders; however, recent studies reflect, in some cases, that these represent 43% of undiagnosed neuropathies.[152] Hereditary neuropathies can be divided into two broad categories: those in which neuropathy is the primary disorder and those in which neuropathy is part of a greater multisystem disorder.[9] This section concentrates on the first group, which includes Charcot–Marie–Tooth (CMT) disease and its related hereditary polyneuropathies.

Charcot–Marie–Tooth Disease

CMT disease, also known as hereditary motor and sensory neuropathy or peroneal muscular atrophy, is the most common inherited disorder affecting motor and sensory nerves. It was originally described by three neurologists, Jean Martin Charcot, Pierre Marie, and Howard Henry Tooth, in the 1880s. Initially the disorder involves the fibular (peroneal) nerve and affects muscles in the foot and lower leg. It later progresses to the muscles of the forearms and hands, making activities like buttoning or writing difficult. CMT is a genetically heterogeneous group of disorders with the same clinical phenotype, characterized by distal limb muscle wasting and weakness, usually with skeletal deformities, distal sensory loss, and abnormalities of DTRs.[117]

Incidence

Of the neuropathies, CMT is relatively common; it is estimated that one in 2500 persons in the United States has some form of CMT. Onset may occur in childhood or adulthood.[107]

Etiology

CMT is a genetically heterogeneous neuropathy that is inherited as autosomal dominant, autosomal recessive, or an X-linked pattern.[167] Over 50 loci defects on chromosomes have been identified though deoxyribonucleic acid (DNA) testing.[9,111,144] These chromosomal defects create either duplication, deletion, or point mutations in the genetic code for proteins that are involved in the process of myelination. CMT1 is the most common autosomal dominant pattern and is subdivided into three forms: CMT1A, 1B, and 1C. CMT1A accounts for 70% of all CMT1 cases and is caused by a DNA duplication on chromosome 17 for peripheral myelin protein 22 (PMP22), creating segmental demyelination of the fibular (peroneal) nerve.[127] A less common form, CMT2, has had chromosomal abnormalities mapped to chromosomes 1, 8, and X. On chromosome 1, CMT2 is associated with a mutation in human myelin protein zero (P0), which has been associated recently with axonal dysfunction. This second form of CMT is associated with axonal degeneration. CMT2 has an onset that varies between the

second and seventh decades and has less involvement in the small muscles of the hands than CMT1.[24]

Pathology

Mutations in proteins (PMP, P0, and connexin) associated with Schwann cell myelination create extensive demyelination along with a hypertrophic onion bulb formation in which demyelinated axons are surrounded by Schwann cells and their processes as remyelination is attempted. The onion bulb formation creates palpable, enlarged peripheral nerves. CMT2 is associated with genetic mutations that disrupt neurofilament assembly and thus affect axonal transport, creating axonal involvement.[9]

Clinical Manifestations

Although the two major types of CMT have differing chromosomal etiologies, it is nearly impossible to tell CMT1 from CMT2 clinically. In all autosomal dominant disorders, there are degrees of genetic dominance. The presence of symptoms is not all or none but is graded, with differing degrees of signs and symptoms among family members who have inherited the defective gene. This is termed *variable expressivity*. In CMT1 some members of a family with the genetic mutation may have greater signs of the disorder than others, who have only minor involvement.[94] In the X-linked form of CMT, men are affected and have signs of both demyelination and axonal degeneration.

CMT is a slowly progressive disorder and although CMT1 begins in childhood, the actual onset may be difficult to determine. Clinical signs of CMT include distally symmetric muscle weakness, atrophy, and diminished DTRs. Feet have pes cavus (high arch) deformities and hammer toes (Fig. 25.6). Because of the muscles affected, the client will have weakness of the dorsiflexors and evertors (peroneal musculature) and will ambulate with a foot drop (steppage) gait pattern. As CMT progresses, involvement will be seen distally in the upper extremities. Weakness and wasting of the intrinsic muscles of the hand occurs, followed by progressive wasting in the forearms. Because CMT1 demyelinates peripheral nerves, proprioception is lost in the feet and ankles, and cutaneous sensation is diminished in the foot and lower legs. Sensory loss is minimal in CMT2. Sensory symptoms can include tingling and burning in the feet and legs, as well as impaired proprioception.[173]

As muscle atrophy progresses below the knee, the appearance of the client's legs takes on the shape of an inverted champagne bottle because normal muscle bulk is maintained above the knees.

Medical Management

Diagnosis

CMT is diagnosed by history and clinical examination, hereditary picture, electrophysiologic studies, and nerve biopsy. Most recently, because of the sensitivity and specificity of genetic studies, the diagnosis of CMT can be confirmed using gel electrophoresis to detect duplication, deletions, or sequence variations in genes.[9] Although CMT1 produces demyelination, electrophysiologic testing reveals underlying axonal degeneration. Slowed motor nerve conduction does not have a linear correlation with the clinical severity of the disease.[82]

Both motor and sensory NCVs will be slowed in CMT1[93] but are normal or only slightly slowed in CMT2. Abnormalities of electrophysiologic studies in CMT2 will be a decreased amplitude of the potential, indicating axonal loss. The nerve

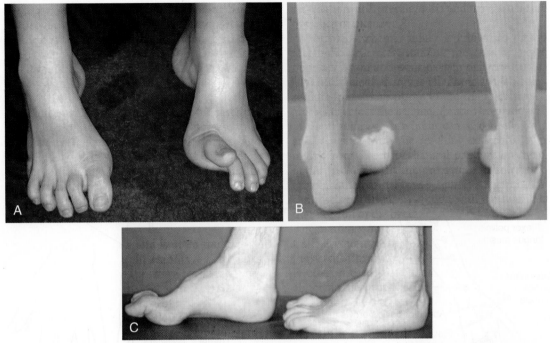

FIG. 25.6 Pes cavus foot deformity in Charcot–Marie–Tooth disease. (A) Clawing of left great toe. (B) Left foot varus deformity. (C) Cavus deformity with hammer toes. (A, Reproduced with permission from Charcot–Marie–Tooth UK. B and C, From Wicart P. Cavus foot, from neonates to adolescents. Orthop Traumatol Surg Res 98(7): 813–828, 2012.)

biopsy is abnormal and will demonstrate either a demyelinating or axonal degenerative process.

Treatment

Because CMT is an inherited disorder, there is no specific treatment to alter its course. Treatment is symptomatic to ensure that function is maintained in a safe manner. Foot drop and hand deformities can be helped by orthotic devices. Because the possibility of skin ulceration exists when tactile sensation and proprioception are affected, skin care precautions should be followed when total contact orthoses are used. To prevent contractures clients should be instructed in range-of-motion (ROM) exercises. Whether strengthening exercises can be used to counteract the effects of CMT has not been addressed; however, the long-term effects would be of little benefit in the presence of ongoing axonal degeneration. In a study examining the effects of weakness in CMT, results have found that individuals with CMT tend to be obese and have poor exercise tolerance. It is unknown whether exercise interventions can improve body composition and function.[17]

Studies using animal models have reported that antiprogesterone therapy combined with ascorbic acid has a positive effect on CMT1A. Although stem cell and gene therapies have been considered, the most promising treatments are pharmacologic therapies targeting the genetic mutation.[111]

Prognosis

CMT is a slowly progressive disorder; if unmanaged, contracture formation resulting from weakness will create further gait abnormalities, with clients reporting an increased number of falls. In the upper extremities, clients may develop problems with writing and handling objects. Individuals with CMT should be cautioned that some medications have been reported to cause an exacerbation of CMT. A database of the drugs that should be avoided is maintained by CMT North America. Among the identified medications are several anticancer drugs, including vincristine, cisplatin, carboplatin, and taxoids.[168]

25.1 Special Implications for the PTA: Charcot–Marie–Tooth Disease The goal in this progressive disorder is to minimize deformity and maximize function. As with other peripheral neuropathies in which muscle imbalances arise, for CMT, the physical therapist assistant (PTA) should anticipate that deformities will arise from the imbalance between the tibialis anterior and peroneus longus and the tibialis posterior and peroneus brevis, which leads to a pes cavus and varus deformity, respectively. This weakness may be combined with diminished or lost proprioception and some degree of cutaneous involvement that can lead to an unsteady gait. These problems should be addressed with stretching, ROM exercises, and bracing to improve ambulation. Along with an orthotic checkout and gait training, appropriate skin care should be taught to the client when total contact orthoses are used. When the individual has developed rigid deformities, a triple arthrodesis is the option to salvage remaining function.[113]

MECHANICAL INJURIES: COMPRESSION AND ENTRAPMENT SYNDROMES

The proximity of peripheral nerves to bony, muscular, and vascular structures can cause entrapment neuropathies characterized by changes in sensation and motor function, resulting from chronic neural compression. Another mechanical injury occurs as a result of traction on a nerve. As tension exceeds 10% to 20% of the axon's resting length, the axon's internal slack within fascicles is eliminated and structural damage occurs.[142]

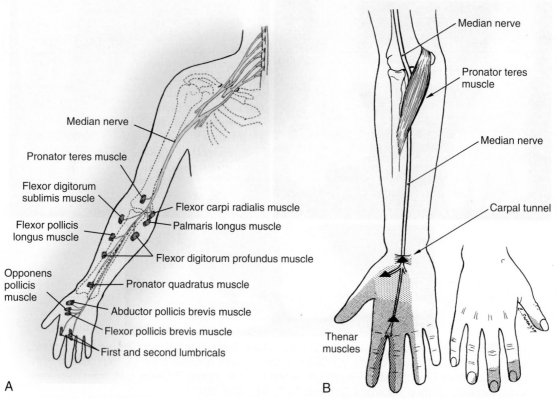

FIG. 25.7 (A) Median nerve course and motor innervation. (B) The point of compression of the median nerve as it passes through the carpal tunnel. The lightly stippled area shows the sensory supply of the palmar cutaneous branch, which arises proximal to the carpal tunnel and thus is spared in carpal tunnel syndrome. The densely stippled zone represents the cutaneous sensory area of the median nerve distal to the carpal tunnel. (A, From Canale ST, Beaty JH: Campbell's operative orthopedics, ed 12, Philadelphia, Mosby, 2013. B, From Noble J: Textbook of primary care medicine, ed 3, St Louis, 2001, Mosby.)

Carpal Tunnel Syndrome

Carpal tunnel syndrome (CTS) is the most common entrapment neuropathy in the United States. It results from compression of the median nerve within the carpal tunnel at the wrist. It is characterized by general signs and symptoms of neuropathies: pain, tingling, numbness, paresthesia (Fig. 25.7), and later, muscular weakness in the distribution of the median nerve.

Incidence

Incidence in the United States is nearly 3.5 cases per 1000 individuals per year, and prevalence is estimated at 2.1%. As a condition, it produces one of the largest number of lost workdays among occupations. Nearly 70% of all CTS cases occur in women. Approximately 500,000 surgeries annually are performed for CTS. The incidence of surgery peaks in women between the ages of 45 and 55 years and in men older than 65 years.

Etiology

Although CTS is associated with occupational activities, any disorder that increases the volume of the contents of the carpal tunnel or that decreases the volume of the carpal tunnel will create a sustained rise in pressure within the tunnel that impinges on the median nerve. This includes synovial proliferation in rheumatoid arthritis, edema from local and systemic infections, congestive heart failure, pregnancy, and tumors.

Callus formation after fracture, as well as malalignment of fractures, may reduce the volume of the canal. CTS is also more than 2.5 times more likely in obese individuals (body mass index >29).[39] Although some investigators[159] have hypothesized that a compressive lesion located more proximally (thoracic outlet syndrome [TOS] or cervical radiculopathy) on a nerve may predispose it to further injury (CTS), more recent examinations of clients with CTS have refuted this "double crush" hypothesis.[83,159]

Risk Factors

Also at risk for developing CTS are people with rheumatoid tenosynovitis, edema, pregnancy, hypothyroidism, and post-Colles' fractures (Box 25.1).[77,149] Although CTS has been reported in several occupations, because of the quality of the research, the convincing link between work and CTS is now questioned.[39] In examining occupational studies, the literature identifies studies that report greatest incidence of CTS in frozen-food workers and butchers. These support a positive association between a combination of factors: force and repetition and/or force and posture. Although the job of a computer operator has been linked to CTS, when symptoms of paresthesia are rigorously assessed, CTS and other musculoskeletal pain disorders associated with long-term keyboarding can be as alleviated with 5-minute breaks every hour.[149] Patients older than age 63 years have a different pattern of risk factors for CTS than

BOX 25.1 Causes of Carpal Tunnel Syndrome

Neuromusculoskeletal
- Amyloidosis
- Anatomic sequelae of medical or surgical procedures
- Basal joint (thumb) arthritis
- Cervical disk lesions
- Cervical spondylosis
- Congenital anatomic differences
- Cumulative trauma disorders
- Peripheral neuropathy
- Poor posture (may also be associated with TOS)
- Repetitive strain injuries
- Tendinitis
- Trigger points
- Tenosynovitis
- TOS
- Wrist trauma (e.g., Colles' fracture)

Systemic
- Alcohol
- Arthritis (rheumatoid, gout, polymyalgia rheumatica)
- Leukemia (tissue infiltration)
- Liver disease
- Medications
- Nonsteroidal antiinflammatory drugs
- Oral contraceptives
- Statins
- Alendronate (Fosamax)
- Multiple myeloma (amyloidosis deposits)
- Obesity
- Pregnancy
- Scleroderma
- Use of oral contraceptives
- Hemochromatosis
- Vitamin deficiency (especially vitamin B_6)

Endocrine
- Acromegaly
- Diabetes mellitus
- Hormonal imbalance (menopause; posthysterectomy)
- Hyperparathyroidism
- Hyperthyroidism (Graves' disease)
- Hypocalcemia
- Hypothyroidism (myxedema)
- Gout (deposits of tophi and calcium)

Infectious disease
- Atypical mycobacterium
- Histoplasmosis
- Rubella
- Sporotrichosis

TOS, Thoracic outlet syndrome.
From Goodman CC, Snyder TEK: Differential diagnosis for physical therapists: screening for referral, Philadelphia, 2007, Saunders.

---

younger patients. This suggests that CTS in the elderly population may have different underlying pathogenetic mechanisms.[10]

Pathogenesis

In the carpal tunnel, where there are 10 structures in a constrained compartment, normal tissue pressures are 7 to 8 mm Hg (Fig. 25.8). In CTS, these pressures rise above 30 mm Hg, when wrist flexion or extension occurs. Pressures go as high as 90 mm Hg when the wrist is fully flexed and up to 79.5 mm Hg when the wrist is extended.[39] Pressure this great produces ischemia in the nerve. Ischemia accounts for the nocturnal symptoms or those that occur with wrist flexion. Unrelieved compression creates an initial neurapraxia with segmental demyelination of axons. Because the axons have lost their myelin padding they are more vulnerable, so unrelieved compression can create an axonotmesis in which axon continuity is lost and wallerian degeneration occurs.

Clinical Manifestations

Persons with CTS experience sensory symptoms in the median nerve distribution (see Fig. 25.7). Pain may be located distally in the forearm or wrist and radiate into the thumb, index, and middle fingers. It may also radiate into the arm, shoulder, and neck. Comparing self-reported symptoms recorded on the Katz hand diagram allows symptoms to be assessed as classic, probable, possible, or unlikely to be CTS.[25] Nocturnal pain is the hallmark of CTS. Even in the early stages of CTS most people will report being awakened by painful numbness in the middle of the night. Sensory symptoms usually precede motor symptoms. Diminished two-point discrimination, diminished ability to perceive vibration, and elevation of threshold in Semmes–Weinstein monofilament testing routinely occur. Thenar weakness is seen in advanced cases. In nearly half of all cases, symptoms occur bilaterally. If CTS goes untreated, symptoms escalate into persistent pain with atrophy of the thenar musculature and the person will have a loss of grip strength. The combined loss of grip strength, inability to pinch, and sensory loss causes clumsiness in the hands.[27] Because conditions that impinge nerve fibers in the neck (radiculopathy) or in the thoracic outlet also cause sensory symptoms that are referred to the hand, it is important to ascertain that the symptoms are related to CTS (see Box 25.1).

Medical Management

Diagnosis

The diagnosis of CTS is considered in any person with hand or wrist pain, numbness, and weakness and must be distinguished from a cervical radiculopathy or ulnar neuropathy.[27] Diagnosis is determined by history, physical examination, and specialized tests. Provocation tests are used to replicate CTS symptoms. Phalen's test, in which the wrist is flexed to 90 degrees for 1 minute (Fig. 25.9A); Tinel's test, or wrist percussion over the carpal tunnel (Fig. 25.9B); and the carpal compression test (pressure is applied by the examiner by pressing his or her thumbs at the wrist over the flexor retinaculum) are all deemed positive when pain, numbness, and paresthesia are produced. The flick sign is a positive indicator of CTS when the client demonstrates what he or she does to relieve symptoms. Ask "What do you do with your hand(s) when your symptoms are the worst?" and the client demonstrates a flicking movement of the hand that looks similar to the motion seen in shaking a thermometer.[25] When tests available to diagnose CTS have been compared with the gold standard of NCV, varying degrees of reliability have been reported. Most recently, Tinel's test has sensitivity of 0.90 and specificity of 0.81, and Phalen's test to reproduce symptoms only has a sensitivity of 0.85 and specificity of 0.79.[84]

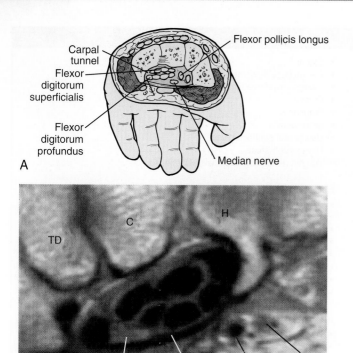

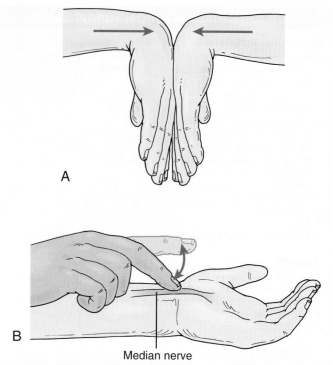

FIG. 25.8 (A) Cross-section of the carpal tunnel at the wrist. Contents of the tunnel include the tendon of the flexor pollicis longus, the four tendons of the flexor digitorum profundus, the four tendons of the flexor digitorum superficialis, and the median nerve. (B) Carpal tunnel. *C*, capitate; *fr*, flexor retinaculum; *H*, hamate; *mn*, median nerve; *TD*, trapezoid; *ua*, ulnar artery; *un*, ulnar nerve. (A, From Magee DJ: Orthopedic physical assessment, ed 6, St Louis, Saunders, 2014. B, From Yu JS, Habib PA: Normal MR imaging anatomy of the wrist and hand, Radiol Clin North Am 44:569–581, 2006.)

FIG. 25.9 (A) Phalen's test. Patients maximally flex both wrists and hold the position for 1 to 2 minutes. If symptoms of numbness or paresthesia within the median nerve distribution are reproduced, the test is positive. (B) Tinel's sign in carpal tunnel syndrome. (Redrawn from Brotzman SB, Manske RC, eds: Clinical orthopedic rehabilitation, ed 3, Philadelphia, 2011, Mosby.)

The criterion standard to confirm CTS is NCV testing. Distal motor and sensory latencies and sensory NCV across the carpal tunnel are most frequently administered. Changes in the sensory conduction across the wrist are reportedly the most sensitive indicator of CTS.[170] A modified NCV technique, termed *inching*, has been shown to provide greater sensitivity and specificity for precise localization of anatomic entrapment for carpal tunnel.[140] Although NCV testing generally provides the benchmark for CTS, a negative NCV study alone does not exclude the possibility of CTS. There are other imaging methods that are helpful in diagnosing CTS. Although magnetic resonance imaging (MRI) has also been found effective in identifying anomalies in the carpal tunnel, including altered tendon position, altered nerve position, swelling of the median nerve, and thickening of the tendon sheath to aid in establishing the diagnosis of CTS,[5] controversy exists over its use in diagnosis[171] because of its variable sensitivity and specificity.[176] Some believe that ultrasonography is more helpful in estimating the severity of symptoms and nerve conduction deficit.[37,75,86]

Treatment

There is no universally accepted treatment for CTS. Although many studies have been conducted over the years, there are few well-controlled investigations that demonstrate the most effective treatment intervention. Thus many approaches are used for symptom management.[44] For clients with mild symptoms, demonstrated by only subjective and objective sensory symptoms, conservative management is generally instituted. Medical management of mild symptoms includes steroid injection into the carpal canal to provide initial relief of symptoms. Early management also addresses ergonomic measures and modification of the client's occupation. Alternative computer keyboards have been evaluated and three configurations are reported to promote a more neutral wrist position than use of a regular keyboard.[100] Wearing of wrist splints to immobilize the wrist near neutral to minimize carpal tunnel pressures and client education are also instituted. These conservative approaches provide symptom relief up to 6 months.[54] However, the long-term use of antiinflammatory medications and immobilization demonstrated a cure rate of only 18%. Relapse was noted within 1 year. Most recently, injection of methylprednisolone proximal to the tunnel has resulted in symptom relief for 77% of those treated when reassessed after 1 month. Fifty percent of those treated reported prolonged relief (at least 1 year) after injection.[24]

Surgical intervention is advocated for persons without resolution of symptoms following a traditional conservative approach for 2 to 3 months. Surgery is also indicated in untreated persons whose symptoms have lasted longer than 1 year and who demonstrate both motor and sensory NCV involvement or in persons with denervation as evidenced by fibrillation potentials on EMG. Release of the transverse carpal ligament is commonly performed and is usually successful. Complications fall into two categories: errors in diagnosis or surgical technique. Newer surgical techniques (flexor tenosynovectomy with transverse carpal ligament division, endoscopic release of the ligament, and neurolysis of the median nerve) are performed through limited incisions and require less exposure and less manipulation of the nerve than the classic open techniques. Seventy-six percent of the surgical cases experience return of normal two-point discrimination and up to 70% have normal muscle strength return.[72] However, a systematic review of surgical procedures has identified that newer procedures are no more effective than traditional approaches. In offering symptom relief, conflicting evidence exists about whether endoscopic release allows earlier return to work than open tunnel release.[137] After surgery, nerve and tendon gliding techniques are advocated to reduce scarring, adhesions, and subsequent formation of fibrotic tissue.[159]

Prognosis

Prognosis relates directly to the severity of the nerve entrapment at diagnosis, clinical cause, and mode of treatment.

Sciatica

Incidence and Etiology

Sciatica is a radiculopathy occurring most often in individuals between the ages of 40 and 60 years in which the nerve root is affected, most typically by compression. Of those developing lumbosacral radiculopathy, 10% to 25% develop symptoms that last more than 6 weeks. Less commonly, sciatica may occur in the presence of abscess, blood clots, or tumors. It may be mistaken for intermittent claudication or low back pain without diskogenic involvement and is one of the most common conditions managed in primary care settings.

Pathogenesis

The epidural space is innervated by a meningeal branch of the spinal nerve, the recurrent sinuvertebral nerve. Arising from the dorsal root ganglion, this nerve enters through the intervertebral foramen, divides into ascending and descending branches to blood vessels, and supplies the posterior longitudinal ligament, the superficial annulus fibrosis, anterior dura mater, and dural sleeve.[101] In animal studies, the sinovertebral nerve responded to high-threshold mechanical stimuli. Conduction velocity for fibers in the nerve corresponded to types III and IV, which lead researchers to correlate nerve function with nociception.[139] Herniation of the intervertebral disk can impinge on the nerve root or structures innervated by the recurrent sinuvertebral nerve to cause pain.

Clinical Manifestations

In addition to low back pain, when sensory fibers are affected, pain will radiate into one or both legs. One of the reasons the motor and sensory nerves are affected so easily in a radiculopathy is that the pressure occurs in an area in which CNS connective tissue coverings meet the protective tissue coverings of the peripheral nerve, leaving that region of the nerve "at risk."[71] Coughing, sitting, and sneezing worsens the pain. Both clinical and experimental studies have shown that adjacent nerve roots may be affected when the lumbar disk herniates. Inflammatory chemical mediators released into the epidural space affect nearby nerve roots, without any direct compression of those roots.[112]

Medical Management

Diagnosis

Both radiologic tests and electrophysiologic studies are ordered. Various specific tests have been reported to provide reliable results. MRI is preferred to computed tomography (CT) scanning for lumbar spine imaging; however, because 60% of people without back symptoms have disk bulging on MRI, protrusion and bulges may not correlate with symptoms.[7] A screening EMG examination of only four muscles in the leg identified more than 89% of surgically confirmed cases.[32] Others have noted that the H-reflex has provided better predictive value than standard motor and sensory nerve conduction radiculopathies.[2] Radiologic studies and electrophysiologic testing are not sufficient alone to distinguish sciatica.

Treatment

The effectiveness of medications has been reported as disappointing. Selective epidural injection of steroids at target nerve roots through the intervertebral foramina has offered short-term benefit for pain relief, as has the use of nonsteroidal antiinflammatory drugs (NSAIDs).[21] Also unclear are the long-term effects of chemonucleolysis, which has been reported to be less effective than diskectomy.[49]

Prognosis

Subjects who were evaluated 1 year after diskectomy had recovery in unmyelinated and small myelinated fibers; the function of larger myelinated fibers did not improve. This provides a physiologic rationale for residual motor and sensory involvement.[112]

25.2 Special Implications for the PTA: Sciatica For those PTAs using the visual analog scale (VAS) to assess pain in sciatica, a range of minimal clinically relevant change has been reported. Using a 100-mm VAS, Todd et al.[158] reported that a 13-mm change is needed to discriminate a crude change in pain, whereas Farrar et al.[41] estimated a 20-mm change was needed to discriminate a crude change in pain. Most recently, Giraudeau et al.[52] also reported that 30 mm reflected a crude change in pain.

Idiopathic Facial Paralysis/Bell's Palsy

Incidence

Bell's palsy is a common clinical condition in which the facial nerve is unilaterally affected. It affects 20 of 100,000 people each year. Although any age group can be affected, it is most common in persons between the ages of 15 and 45 years.[64]

Etiology and Pathogenesis

The cause of Bell's palsy is uncertain; however, evidence is increasing that indicates that the primary cause of Bell's palsy is a latent herpes virus (herpes simplex type 1/herpes zoster) that has been reactivated.[19,121] Days before Bell's palsy onset, the client may recall experiencing severe pain in the area of the mastoid or a sensation of fullness in the ear. Pain suggests that this disorder is a product of an inflammatory response. Because the facial nerve lies in the auditory canal, any agent that causes inflammation and swelling creates a compression that initially causes demyelination. However, if the inflammatory response is more fulminating, ischemia will cause an axonal degeneration.

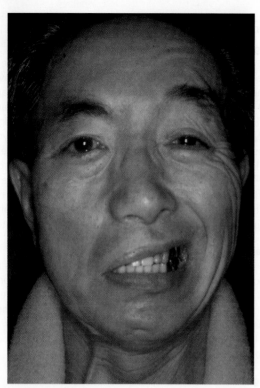

FIG. 25.10 Patient with left facial paralysis. (From Takushima A, Harii K, Hiortaka A, et al.: Fifteen-year survey of one-stage latissimus dorsi muscle transfer for treatment of longstanding facial paralysis. J. Plast Reconstr Aesthet Surg 66(1):29–36, 2013.)

In addition, centrally located structures, such as acoustic neuromas (tumor), can produce unilateral paralysis in the face by impinging on the facial nerve as it emerges from the brainstem; however, these tend to produce a slowly progressive paralysis.

Risk Factors

People with diabetes mellitus and pregnant women[19] have an increased incidence of Bell's palsy.

Clinical Manifestations

A unilateral facial paralysis develops rapidly, often overnight. Paralysis of the muscles of facial expression on one side creates an asymmetric facial appearance (Fig. 25.10). The corner of the mouth droops, the nasolabial fold is flattened, and the palpebral fissure is widened because the eyelid does not close. In addition to the motor fibers providing innervation for facial musculature, the facial nerve also innervates the stapedius muscle of the middle ear and the sensory and autonomic fibers, which innervate for taste and lacrimation and salivation, respectively. Therefore involvement of these fibers may produce additional signs and symptoms to those of facial paralysis. If the lesion is proximal to where the fibers of the chorda tympani enter the facial nerve, the client will experience loss of taste on the affected side. In a similar fashion, if the autonomic fibers are involved, the client will experience dry eye (lack of tearing) and will produce less but thicker saliva. Some clients report that sounds are louder than normal because the stapes bone of the middle ear is less able to accommodate sound when the stapedius muscle's innervation is lost.

Medical Management

Diagnosis

Ask the client to wrinkle the forehead, close the eyes tightly, smile, and whistle while you observe for facial asymmetry. In addition to the clinical presentation and history, electrodiagnostic tests can be used to demonstrate whether the lesion is one of demyelination or axonal degeneration. However, EMG as a diagnostic tool is only helpful after the nerve has degenerated; therefore testing is most accurate after 1 week. Tests of facial nerve excitability will also indicate whether the paralysis is complete.

The LMN involvement of the facial nerve can be differentiated from an upper motor neuron (UMN) involvement of this nerve because with UMN involvement the client can close the eye and wrinkle the forehead but cannot smile voluntarily. With LMN involvement, the client is unable to close the eye, wrinkle the forehead, or smile voluntarily.

Treatment

Because the outcome (demyelination or degeneration) is unknown initially, prophylactic administration of high-dose corticosteroids for 5 days, followed by a tapered dose for 5 days, has been advocated. For more severe involvement, this treatment is reported to help prevent permanent damage. Treatment should begin as soon as possible and no later than 10 days after onset of signs of paralysis. The association that has been discovered between herpes simplex virus and Bell's palsy suggests that treatment with antiviral medications, such as acyclovir or acyclovir paired with corticosteroids, may aid in recovery.[62] Patients who received a combined treatment of acyclovir (antiviral) with prednisolone (corticosteroid) had a recovery rate of 95.7% (better than corticosteroids alone, 89%). Treated within 3 days on onset of paralysis, a 100% recovery has been reported; the rate of recovery drops to 86% when treatment was delayed until day 4. Benefits of antiviral medications or nerve root decompression have not been established definitely.[56,63] Yet controversies exist related to the medical management of Bell's palsy. One systematic review reports that available evidence does not show significant effects of corticosteroids,[131] whereas a meta-analysis found that corticosteroids provided both clinically and statistically significant recovery of motor function in facial nerve–innervated musculature.[125] Studies of Bell's palsy in children have indicated that there is no supporting evidence for the use of steroids or antiviral medications in children.[132]

To protect the cornea, the client should cover the eye with a patch or glasses and use artificial tears. Other palliative treatments, such as gentle massage and gentle heat, may also be used.[1]

Prognosis

Ninety-four percent of individuals with incomplete involvement make a full recovery, generally within 3 weeks. For complete involvement, 75% recover normal motor function, although the time course of recovery is longer.[64] Factors associated with a poorer outcome include age greater than 60 years, presence of systemic comorbidities such as diabetes mellitus and hypertension, and symptoms indicating a lesion with autonomic involvement.[16] Plastic surgery, using fascial slings to replace active muscle contraction, can help restore facial function when recovery does not occur. Another complication that can occur during recovery is a phenomenon called *motor synkinesis* (crocodile tears), which occurs when motor fibers of the facial nerve cross-innervate the autonomic branch of the greater superficial petrosal nerve. When muscles of the face contract, tears appear. This has been noted up to 1 year after the start of treatment.[146]

25.3 Special Implications for the PTA: Bell's Palsy Because experiments using animals have indicated that electrical stimulation suppresses neuronal sprouting, some scientists have proposed that electrical stimulation should not be used. To promote enhanced motor control of fascial musculature and recovery of function, a twice-daily exercise program emphasizing facial movement has been proposed. Progress can be assessed using the facial grading scale, paresis index, and question score.[16]

Tardy Ulnar Palsy/Retroepicondylar Palsy

Anatomy

The ulnar nerve arises from the lower trunk of the brachial plexus and carries fibers from C8 and T1 nerve roots. At the elbow, it passes behind the medial epicondyle and then passes between the two heads of the flexor carpi ulnaris (FCU) through the forearm to the wrist (Fig. 25.11). The distal portion of the nerve enters the palm by crossing the flexor retinaculum and divides into a superficial and deep branch in the hand.

Etiology

Because of its anatomic location, ulnar nerve palsy is a common complication of fractures in the region of the elbow. A late or tardy ulnar palsy may occur years after a fracture and is associated with callus formation or a valgus deformity of the elbow. These produce a gradual stretching of the nerve in the ulnar groove of the medial epicondyle.

Risk Factors

A similar type of tardy ulnar palsy occurs with repeated trauma for relatively long periods of time in clients with a shallow ulnar groove at the elbow. Ulnar neuropathy from entrapment at the elbow is the second most frequent upper extremity neuropathy (after carpal tunnel).

Pathogenesis

The mechanism of injury compressing the ulnar nerve has been attributed to recurrent microtrauma associated with fracture and fibrous bands or recurrent cubital subluxations, as well as entrapment at the entrance or exit of the cubital tunnel.[91] Elbow flexion aggravates symptoms. Compression will initially cause a neurapraxia with demyelination of the nerve; if the pressure goes unrelieved, this will progress to an axonotmesis, with denervation occurring below the level of the elbow.

Clinical Manifestations

Expect a clawhand deformity with metacarpophalangeal (MCP) extension and interphalangeal (IP) flexion of the ring and little fingers because of the unopposed action of the extensor muscle group and paralysis of the third and fourth lumbricals that normally flex the MCPs and extend the IPs (Fig. 25.12). Flattening of the hypothenar eminence along with abduction of the little finger coincides with weakness of the palmaris brevis and

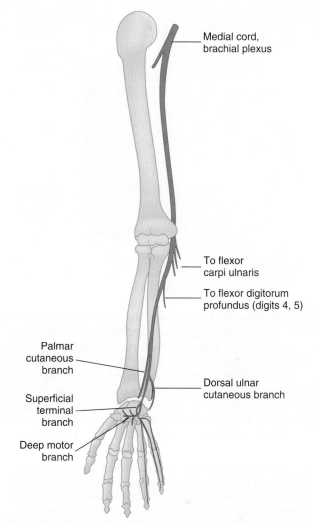

FIG. 25.11 Distribution of the ulnar nerve. A tardy ulnar palsy impinges the ulnar nerve as it passes behind the medial epicondyle of the humerus. (Redrawn from Stewart JD: Focal peripheral neuropathies, ed 4, West Vancouver, Canada, JBJ Publishing, 2010.)

abductor digiti minimi. Marked atrophy of the interossei on the dorsal surface of the hand with guttering between the extensor tendons indicates the presence of denervation. Abduction and adduction movements of the fingers are impaired. Paralysis of the FCU produces a radial deviation of the hand when wrist flexion is attempted. Sensory loss is variable, but impaired sensation may be expected involving the little finger and the ulnar aspect of the ring finger and along the ulnar aspect of the palm of the hand to the wrist. Occasionally, sensory symptoms extend proximally to the wrist (see Fig. 25.12).

Medical Management

Diagnosis

Percussion of or bending the elbow can replicate sysmptoms.[91] NCV studies are helpful only when sufficient nerve damage has occurred to produce definite strength or sensory changes in the hand. NCVs are slowed through the involved region but are relatively normal above and below the epicondyle. EMG reports slowing of sensory or motor NCV across

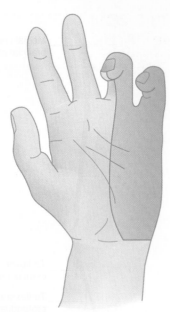

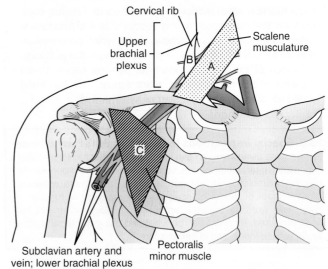

FIG. 25.13 Schematic relationship of structures in development of thoracic outlet syndrome. Compression of the neurovascular bundle can occur with (A) hypertrophy of scalene musculature impinging on structures lying between middle and anterior scalene; (B) the presence of cervical rib or fibrous bands between the cervical and first rib; or (C) compression by pectoralis minor during hyperabduction. (From Rakel RE: Textbook of medicine, ed 7, Philadelphia, 2007, Saunders.)

FIG. 25.12 Clawing of the ring and little fingers (hyperextension of the metacarpophalangeal joint and flexion of the interphalangeal joints) from unopposed action of extensor musculature combined with paralysis of the intrinsic muscles of the hand occurs when there is involvement of the ulnar nerve. Shaded area represents ulnar nerve sensory distribution in the hand. (Redrawn from Ellis H, Mahadevan V: Clinical anatomy: applied anatomy for students and junior doctors, ed 13, Chichester, West Sussex, UK, Wiley-Blackwell, 2013.)

the elbow, prolonged conduction (termed a *latency*) to the FCU, along with changes in amplitude, duration, or shape of the sensory potential across the elbow. Sensory fibers were affected first. Detection of an abnormal latency requires accurate measurement of ulnar nerve segment length.[105]

Treatment
Mild entrapments are managed conservatively; moderate and severe compression require surgery. To relieve the compression, either decompression, the preferred method (medial epicondylectomy), or transposition of the ulnar nerve to the anterior aspect of the elbow is performed.[13,148] Symptomatically, the clawhand deformity should be treated with a splint that blocks MCP hyperextension (lumbrical bar) and allows the extensor digitorum to extend the IP joints.

Prognosis
Results of surgery are normally good when the individual has not had a chronic tardy ulnar involvement. Decompression surgery should have complete restoration of function quickly, but recovery after transposition surgery may take up to 6 months. Surgery to treat chronic involvement (more than 3 months) may have a less certain restoration of function.[148] After nerve transposition, most NCVs at follow-up are improved. However, the magnitude of change in the motor conduction velocity does not correlate well with clinical improvement. One factor that has been identified to effect outcome is body mass index; increased body weight is related slightly to patient's perception of poorer improvement.[109]

Thoracic Outlet Syndrome
Because clients diagnosed with TOS have vague symptoms or symptoms that are difficult to interpret, TOS remains a controversial diagnosis. Because this disorder is complex and poorly defined, many clients have been labeled neurotic.

Definition
TOS is an entrapment syndrome caused by pressure from structures in the thoracic outlet on fibers of the brachial plexus at some point between the interscalene triangle and the inferior border of the axilla. In addition, vascular symptoms can occur because of pressure on the subclavian artery (Fig. 25.13).

Etiology
The anatomy of the region of the thoracic outlet is extremely complex. Spinal nerve roots of the brachial plexus interact with surrounding bony ribs, muscles, and tendons (subclavius, anterior and middle scalene, and pectoralis minor) and the vascular supply (subclavian artery and vein) to the region. In addition to neurologic structures becoming entrapped, arterial and venous structures also may be affected individually or in combination. Thus multiple specialists may be involved in a person's care. Practically, TOS can be divided into three groups: neurogenic (compression of brachial plexus), vascular (compression of subclavian artery and/or vein), and disputed (nonspecific TOS with chronic pain and symptoms of brachial plexus involvement).[12,67]

Risk Factors
Postural changes associated with growth and development, trauma to the shoulder girdle, and body composition have all been identified as contributing to the development of TOS. The human upright posture has contributed to the development of TOS because gravity pulls on the shoulder girdle creating traction on the structures. Additionally, congenital factors that

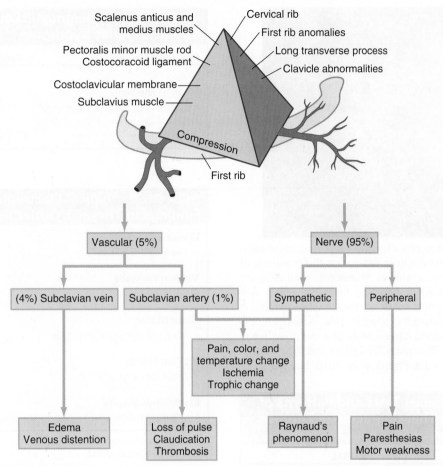

FIG. 25.14 Relationship of thoracic outlet abnormalities and impairments. (From Marx RS, Hockberger RS, Walls RM: Rosen's emergency medicine: concepts and clinical practice, ed 8, Philadelphia, 2014, Saunders.)

affect the bony structures, such as a cervical rib or fascial bands, also compress the neurovascular bundle.

Pathogenesis

Chronic compression of nerve roots or proximal plexus and arteries between the clavicle and first rib or impinging musculature results in edema and ischemia in the nerves (see Fig. 25.13). This compression initially creates a neurapraxia in which the axons are preserved, but segmental demyelination occurs. After loss of myelin, the axons are more vulnerable to unrelieved compression. The neurapraxia can progress to an axonotmesis in which axon continuity is lost and wallerian degeneration occurs.

Clinical Manifestations

Signs and symptoms reflect the structures that have been compressed. When the nerves are compressed, most people report paresthesias and pain in the arm; most often these are nocturnal. Other symptoms may include pain, tingling, and paresis. If the upper nerve plexus is involved (C5 to C7), pain is reported in the neck; this may radiate into the face (sometimes with ear pain) and anterior chest as well as over the scapulae. Symptoms may also extend over the lateral aspect of the forearm into the hand. If the lower plexus is compromised (C7 to T1), pain and numbness occur in the posterior neck and shoulder, medial arm and forearm, and radiate into the ulnarly innervated digits

of the hand. Weakness is usual in the muscles corresponding to nerve root innervation, and atrophy occurs in severe cases. Vascular symptoms may include coldness, edema in the hand or arm, Raynaud's phenomenon (cyanosis), fatigue in hand and arm, and superficial vein distention in the hand (Fig. 25.14).

The clinical presentation usually relates to posture and activities that aggravate symptoms. Overhead and lifting activities, along with movements of the head, produce symptoms in the upper plexus.

Medical Management

Diagnosis

Provocative tests are used to elicit symptoms of TOS, but these tests have a high false-positive response. Maneuvers are performed bilaterally, and the pulse is monitored to note a change in its quality. Based on the belief that the anterior scalene compresses the neurovascular bundle, the individual is positioned to elicit the symptoms. However, mere obliteration of the peripheral pulse does not necessarily mean that TOS exists as an entrapment problem; sensory symptoms must be reproduced. For persons with a vascular component, blood pressure may differ from side to side. Although there is no universally accepted reliable diagnostic test for TOS, *Adson's maneuver* (Fig. 25.15) appears among the most effective. Several other maneuvers with a positional component

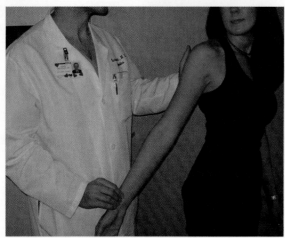

FIG. 25.15 Adson's test is one of many diagnostic tests used to examine the upper extremity to determine the presence of thoracic outlet syndrome: arterial or neurologic. Hold patient's arm in slight abduction while palpating the radial pulse. Ask the patient to inhale and hold his or her breath while extending the neck and rotating toward the affected side. Adson's test is positive if the patient reports paresthesias or if the pulse fades away. (From Miller MD, Thompson SR: DeLee and Drez's orthopaedic sports medicine, ed 3, Philadelphia, 2010, Saunders.)

TABLE 25.6 **Special Tests and Patterns of Positive Findings That Characterize Thoracic Outlet Syndrome[a]**

| Vascular Component | NEURAL | |
	Upper Plexus	Lower Plexus
3-minute elevated test	Point tenderness over C5-C6	Pressure above clavicle elicits pain
Adson's sign	Pressure over lateral neck elicits pain or numbness	Ulnar nerve tenderness when palpated under axilla or along inner arm
Swelling (hand, arm)		
Discoloration of hand	Pain with head turn or tilted to opposite side	
Costoclavicular test		Tinel's test for ulnar nerve in axilla
Hyperabduction test	Weak biceps	Hypoesthesia in ulnar nerve distribution
Upper extremity claudication	Weak triceps	
Differences in blood pressure from side to side	Weak wrist	Serratus anterior weakness
	Hypoesthesia in radial nerve distribution	Weak handgrip
Skin temperature changes	3-minute abduction stress test	
Cold intolerance		

[a]With the use of special tests, pattern of position objective findings may help characterize thoracic outlet syndrome.
From Goodman CC, Synder TEK: Differential diagnosis for physical therapists: screening for referral, ed 5, St. Louis, 2013.

of the head, shoulder, or arm have been found to compress vascular or neural structures and thus evoke symptoms. These tests include the Allen's, Wright's, Halsted's, costoclavicular, Roos/elevated arm stress test, and provocative elevation tests (Table 25.6).[95] The sensitivity and specificity of Adson's test improve when used in combination with the hyperabduction test (symptom replication), the Wright's test (symptom replication), or the Roos test (Table 25.7).[50]

Radiographic Tests
Radiographic procedures are used to identify bony abnormalities. Presence of a cervical rib may indicate that the nerve has

TABLE 25.7 **Diagnostic Utility of Tests for Thoracic Outlet Syndrome**

Provocation Test	Sensitivity	Specificity
Adson's	0.79	0.76
HA, pulse abolition	0.84	0.4
Adson's + HAs (symptom replication)	0.72	0.88
Adson's + Wright's	0.54	0.94
Adson's + Roos	0.72	0.82

HA, Hyperabduction.

BOX 25.2 **Typical Electrophysiologic Findings in Thoracic Outlet Syndrome**

Upper Sensory
- Decreased amplitude

Median Sensory
- Normal

Ulnar Motor
- Normal or decreased amplitude

Median Motor
- Decreased amplitude

Electromyography
- +Fibrillation potentials: first dorsal interosseous

Adapted from Huang JH, Zager EL: Thoracic outlet syndrome, Neurosurgery 55:897–903, 2004.

been compressed; however, presence of the rib alone does not necessarily replicate symptoms. Plane films are used to distinguish between a C7 to T1 diskogenic lesion and TOS.

Electrophysiologic Studies
Because symptoms of TOS are related to neural compression, electrophysiologic studies are valuable in documenting the presence of neuropathy. NCV allows the examiner to pinpoint the lesion, either because of a change in amplitude or a slowing in conduction velocity (Box 25.2). Other, more refined electrophysiologic techniques, including somatosensory evoked potentials and F waves, are used to confirm a diagnosis of nerve root entrapment.

Differential Diagnosis
TOS must be distinguished from other disorders with similar symptoms. These include cervical radiculopathy, reflex sympathetic dystrophy (RSD), tumors of the apex of the lung, and ulnar nerve compression at either elbow or wrist. The sensory pattern of TOS distinguishes it from an ulnar neuropathy such as tardy ulnar palsy. Because the nerve roots are affected, the sensory changes extend above the hand and wrist into the forearm in TOS and follow a dermatomal pattern. Myofascial pain patterns may also mimic TOS symptoms.

Treatment
Management is divided into conservative and surgical approaches. The initial treatment of the person with TOS is conservative when symptoms are mild to moderate in se-

---

BOX 25.3 Surgical Procedures and Approaches for Thoracic Outlet Syndrome

Procedures

- Scalenotomy
- Scalenectomy
- Clavicle resection
- Pectoralis minor release
- First rib resection
- Cervical rib resection

Approaches

- Axillary
- Supraclavicular
- Combined axillary and supraclavicular
- Posterior
- Subclavicular
- Transclavicular

25.4 Special Implications for the PTA: Thoracic Outlet Syndrome One of the reasons TOS has been difficult to diagnose relates to the client's subjective report. Frequently, signs and symptoms do not correspond to a single lesion, but to multifocal lesions, either of vascular and/or neurogenic origin. For clients who do not respond to treatment, some believe that compression at a proximal or distal source might increase the vulnerability of nerves, making them more susceptible to compression at another site.

---

verity. Postural and breathing exercises and gentle stretching are the cornerstones of the initial conservative program. This is followed by strengthening exercises for shoulder girdle musculature, especially the trapezius, levator scapulae, and rhomboids. Initially, overhead exercises should be avoided because they tend to evoke symptoms. PTAs are cautioned against forceful stretching to mobilize the first rib.[88,166]

Surgical management of TOS is reserved for cases that are refractory to postural and exercise correction and those with vascular compromise.[20] Once the decision for surgical intervention has been made, the physician must select a procedure and the anatomic approach. There are at least six different surgical procedures and six different anatomic approaches (Box 25.3). In scalenotomy, the muscle is detached from the first rib; unfortunately, with this approach a high percentage of people experience recurring symptoms. Scalenectomy, removal of the scalene muscle, is advocated for people who have had recurrence of their symptoms. Clavicle resection is indicated primarily when the clavicle is damaged. When scalenectomy with or without first rib resection is the surgical approach used, its 5-year success rate is about 70%.[133]

Prognosis

After surgery, 70% of cases have a good or excellent response using a supraclavicular or transaxillary resection of the first rib. Improvement in pain symptoms ranges from 70% to 80%, some patients require occasional analgesics, and 10% note no improvement. In individuals with signs and symptoms and electrophysiologic changes consistent with classic TOS, no improvement in strength is noted when atrophy was present before surgery.[20] Complications during surgery include pneumothorax, nerve compression, and transient winging of the scapula because the upper digitations of the serratus are detached.

A 4-year follow-up reported no significant difference in return to work or symptom severity when the first rib was resected compared with a conservative, nonoperative approach.[85] Factors that are associated with long-term disability include preoperative depression, single status, and less than high school education.[6]

Saturday Night Palsy/Sleep Palsy
Definition and Etiology

Saturday night palsy is associated with radial nerve compression in the arm. It results from direct pressure against a firm object and typically follows deep sleep on the arm with compression of the radial nerve at the spiral groove of the humerus in a person who is sleeping after becoming intoxicated. Sleep palsy has also been associated with lipoma compressing the radial nerve.[43] If the radial nerve is compressed in the axilla, the damage is often referred to as a crutch palsy.

Pathogenesis

Compression of the nerve causes segmental demyelination.

Clinical Manifestations

Symptoms of radial nerve paralysis depend on the level of the lesion. The more proximal the involvement, the more extensive is the paralysis. When involvement occurs in the axilla, weakness occurs in elbow extension (triceps), elbow flexion (brachioradialis), and supination (supinator). If the nerve is damaged in the upper arm the triceps is spared. In addition, in both instances there will be paralysis of wrist extensors and the extensors of the fingers and thumb, diminishing grip strength. Sensory loss with radial nerve involvement is variable. If present, it is typically confined to the dorsum of the hand but may extend to the dorsum of the forearm.

Medical Management
Diagnosis

Diagnosis is by history, clinical examination, and electrophysiologic examination. This type of paralysis is usually classified as a neurapraxia or conduction block, signifying demyelination. There is slowing of nerve conduction in both motor and sensory fibers across the lesion site.

Treatment

Medical management is aimed at asymptomatic management. A cock-up splint is used to maintain the wrist in an extended position until return of function.

Prognosis

If a neurapraxia is reported, normal conduction can be anticipated within a few months because the paralysis is related to a focal demyelination.[58]

Morton's Neuroma

Morton's neuroma is a common entrapment neuropathy in the forefoot, also called *interdigital perineural fibroma*, and most often involving the third toe interspace.

Definition and Etiology

No incidence or prevalence for Morton's neuroma has been published in any study. However, the average age of individuals diagnosed with Morton's neuroma is reported between 45 and 60 years, with women affected 5:1 more than men. Bilateral involvement is uncommon.[18]

Pathogenesis

Three common digital nerves, two arising from the medial plantar nerve and third from the lateral plantar nerve, pass between divisions of the plantar aponeurosis where each bifurcates into two interdigital nerves. The first common digital nerve supplies adjacent sides of the great and second toe, those of the second common digital nerve supply adjacent sides of the second and third toes, and the sides of the third and fourth toes are supplied by the third common digital nerve (Fig. 25.16). Mechanical irritation resulting from intrinsic factors, such as diminished intermetatarsal head distance[89] and poor foot mechanics (excessive pronation during gait) that pulls the nerve more medially than normal and taut as the toes extend during terminal stance. Irritation also results from extrinsic factors, such as high heels in which the weight is transferred onto the forefoot, maintaining the nerve in a taut condition; narrow toe box on shoe that creates a greater compression in the area; and thin-soled shoes where ground forces interact with the deep transverse metatarsal ligament, causing compression in this confined space, have been implicated as contributing to this condition. Additional inflammatory conditions, such as arthritis, and activities that involve application of repetitive forces to the plantar nerves, such as jogging on a hard surface, produce shear forces that can irritate the nerve.

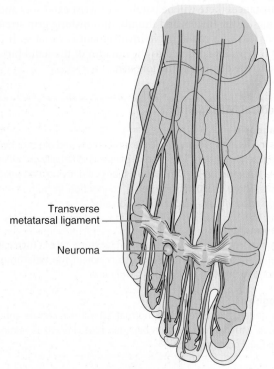

Transverse
metatarsal ligament —

Neuroma —

FIG. 25.16 Morton's neuroma involves the common digital nerve. The most frequent location is between third and fourth metatarsals. (From Frontera WR, Silver JK, Rizzo TD: *Essentials of physical medicine and rehabilitation*, ed 3, Philadelphia, 2015, Saunders.)

Entrapment produces some or all of the following histopathology: thickening of the endoneurium, hyalinization of endoneurial vessels, thickened perineurium, and demyelination of nerve fibers.[18,135]

Clinical Manifestations

Symptoms include burning, tingling, or sharp lancinating pain in one of the interspaces of the forefoot that occurs while walking. Pain may radiate into adjacent toes or proximally into the foot. Individuals may state that they must stop, remove their shoe, and massage their foot to relieve the symptoms. At its worst, the person may be apprehensive about stepping with the involved foot. Symptoms occur paroxysmally over many years.

Medical Management

Diagnosis

Typically, history and clinical examination have been used to diagnose this disorder. Two tests that provoke symptoms include plantar palpation of the involved space at the metatarsal heads as mediolateral compression is applied to the metatarsal heads (Mulder's sign) and dorsiflexion of the involved toe producing symptoms and plantarflexion of the toe relieving them (Lasègue's sign).[45] The reported positive predictive values of these clinical tests vary widely. Recently sonography and MRI have been used to assess the presence of Morton's neuroma. Whereas the sensitivity for predicting the presence of Morton's neuroma is reported at 0.79 and 0.86, respectively, the specificity of both sonography and MRI is 1.0[143] and has been used to diagnose Morton's neuromas.[124,155]

Differential diagnoses considered would include metatarsal stress fractures, metatarsalgia, and metatarsal phalangeal derangement.

Treatment

Conservative, nonoperative management is directed at pressure relief and involves use of a soft orthosis (insoles) or metatarsal pad. These may provide symptom relief as long as the shoes the person is wearing have a wider toe box and a lower heel. If symptoms continue, injection of a local anesthetic or corticosteroid from the dorsal direction may be helpful. Finally, surgical treatment involves either neural decompression by releasing the intermetatarsal ligament or neurectomy, proximal to the location of the neuroma to allow retraction of the plantar nerve away from the weight-bearing surface.

Prognosis

A systematic review of these interventions reports that for studies in which orthoses have been used, 45% to 50% of the participants reported pain relief of more than 50% up to 1 year postintervention. For various surgical approaches, pain relief of more than 50% occurred in 65% to 100% of patients up to 3 years postsurgery.[157]

Neurotmesis
Definition

A neurotmesis occurs after total loss of axon and connective tissue continuity; the nerve is severed.

Etiology

Neurotmesis occurs after a gunshot wound, stab wound, or avulsion injury.

Pathogenesis

When the axon is lacerated, *wallerian degeneration* occurs distally and proximally the cell body also responds to the trauma. It swells and undergoes chromatolysis. The ribosomes that normally make protein for the cell disperse throughout the cytoplasm. *Chromatolysis* reflects a change in the metabolic priority of the cell as it switches from daily needs to a repair mode. Distally the axon begins to degenerate and myelin fragments within 12 hours of the lesion (see Fig. 25.3C). This material is removed by macrophages responding to the inflammatory process.

As long as the cell body remains viable, a regenerative process begins with sprouting of a growth cone as soon as new cytoplasm is synthesized and transported down the axon from the cell body (see Fig. 25.3D). As the growth cone grows, it releases proteases that dissolve material and permit the axon to enter the tissue more easily. Filopodia, which are fingerlike projections extending from the growth cone, sample the environment searching for chemical and tactile cues to guide the regenerating axon; however, because the tactile cues provided by the endoneurium are absent, many times these fibers become misguided and form a neuroma. The standard used to anticipate return of function is based on a growth rate of 1 mm a day or 1 inch a month. In reality, this is an average reflecting the delays that occur, whereas the growth cone crosses the repair site and makes connection with sensory end organs or motor endplate. Growth occurs faster nearer the lesion site (3 mm/day) and slower as the length of the axon increases (1 mm/day).[114]

Clinical Manifestations

The degree of involvement relates to the nerve involved and its level of involvement. In any case, an immediate flaccid paralysis occurs in muscles distal to the lesion. Rapid atrophy ensues because of loss of the trophic influences of the nerve that innervated the muscle fibers. Sensory function is also lost below the level of the lesion.

Medical Management

Diagnosis

History and clinical examination are used to diagnose neurotmesis. In addition, electrophysiologic studies may be performed after a week. EMG will demonstrate the presence of fibrillation potentials and positive sharp waves, indicating denervation of muscle fiber. EMG can be used to determine whether the lesion is complete or partial.

Treatment

Surgical management is needed to suture the connective tissue bundles together to guide the regenerating growth cone. Various microsurgical techniques (cable and interfascicular grafts) are used to try and direct the axon into the appropriate fascicle by restoring connective tissue continuity. After complete axonal transection, the neuron undergoes a number of degenerative processes, followed by attempts at regeneration. A distal growth cone seeks out connections with the degenerated distal fiber. The current surgical standard is epineurial repair with nylon suture. To span gaps that primary repair cannot bridge without excessive tension, nerve-cable

interfascicular autografts are used. Unfortunately, results of nerve repair have been no better than fair, with only 50% of patients regaining useful function. There is much ongoing research regarding pharmacologic agents, immune system modulators, enhancing factors, and entubulation chambers. Clinically applicable developments from these investigations will continue to improve the results of treatment of nerve injuries.[87] Ideally, a primary repair will be performed; operative delays lead to shrinkage and fibrosis of the distal connective tissue support structures.[65]

Other treatments are symptomatic. For the PTA, this means splinting to support structures. Use of electrical stimulation to maintain muscle bulk is controversial; recent studies have shown that the chemical signal guiding the nerve (neural cell adhesion molecule) disappears when denervated muscle receives electrical stimulation.[134] However, muscle bulk is maintained for up to 4 weeks. Because denervated skin does not wrinkle after it has been soaked in water, this has been used to evaluate denervation patterns.[122]

Prognosis

Recovery after neurotmesis depends on whether the nerve was repaired and the length of nerve that must be regenerated. Following transection, muscles atrophy rapidly, and after 2 years, they have undergone irreversible changes and have become fibrotic. If reinnervation occurs after 1 year, function is poor; with a delay of 18 to 24 months there is no hope for return of function.

METABOLIC NEUROPATHIES

Diabetic Neuropathy

Definition

A consensus conference has agreed that a detailed definition of *diabetic neuropathy* (DN) is "a descriptive term meaning a demonstrable disorder, either clinically evident or subclinical, that occurs in the setting of diabetes mellitus without other causes for peripheral neuropathy."[3,89] DN is a common complication associated with diabetes mellitus composed of a heterogeneous group of progressive syndromes with diverse clinical manifestations. Neuropathies may be focal or diffuse and involve the autonomic or somatic PNS.[11,12,164] Typically, the involvement occurs in a distally, symmetric pattern, termed *diabetic polyneuropathy*, although single, focal nerve involvement may be seen.

Incidence

In the United States diabetes mellitus affects more than 20 million people, and this number is expected to increase by 5% every year. The prevalence of DN is greater (54%) in type 1 diabetes (insulin-dependent diabetes mellitus) than the prevalence of DN in type 2 diabetes (non–insulin-dependent diabetes mellitus), which is 30%. The most reliable estimates from clinical studies report that DN, although present in individuals with diabetes lasting longer than 25 years, is present in 7% of people within 1 year of diagnosis with diabetes.[145]

Etiology

DN is probably caused by the chronic metabolic disturbances that affect nerve cells and Schwann cells in diabetes. For years, hyperglycemia was considered the sole cause of these secondary complications of diabetes. Although consequences of hyperglycemia include elevated levels of sorbitol and fructose, which coincides with deficiencies of sodium-potassium and adenosine triphosphate (ATP) that alter the function of peripheral nerves, chronic hyperglycemia leads to abnormalities in microcirculation, creating endothelial capillary changes and local ischemia that affect the nerve. Excess sorbitol also damages Schwann cells. Most recently, researchers have suggested that alterations in insulin levels alter its regulatory roles in gene-regulation of neurotrophic factors, cell–cell adhesion molecules, and modification of proteins.[145]

Risk Factors

Although hyperglycemia is not directly attributed to damaging nerve fibers causing DN, it is a contributing factor. Conversely, some people develop neuropathies when glycemic control is good. A clear relationship does exist between duration of diabetes and development of DN. After the onset of neuropathy, control of hyperglycemia is known to enhance the possibility of regeneration of fibers. Although studies have confirmed a genetic predisposition to diabetes, they have not confirmed such a predisposition to development of DN nor has a familial tendency been reported. Up to 50% of all people with diabetes never develop symptoms of neuropathy.

Pathogenesis

Many hypotheses exist for the pathogenesis of this disorder. The metabolic effect of hyperglycemia exposes nerves and their associated Schwann cells to glucose. The most prominent change in DN is loss of both myelinated and unmyelinated axons. Nerves are affected distally more than proximally. Subtle changes have been reported at the nodes of Ranvier in nerves of people with DN. This is associated with slowing of the NCV.[163]

A number of studies suggest that vascular changes affect peripheral nerves in diabetes. Evidence demonstrates endoneurial microvascular thickening. In the sural nerve, this has resulted in increased numbers of closed capillaries, which are believed to cause multifocal regions of ischemia and hypoxia in the nerve, resulting in an axonal degeneration.

Another explanation for the development of DN proposes that the concentration of nerve growth factor (NGF), which has a structure that is molecularly and physiologically similar to insulin, is reduced. Because NGF acts as a trophic factor, its reduction also reduces nutrition to the nerve.

Clinical Manifestations

DN has been classified in a number of ways: presumed etiology, pathologic features, anatomic location, and a mixture of these. The most recent classification reflects the disturbances that occur in DN (Box 25.4).

Rapidly reversible neuropathy

Hyperglycemic neuropathy. Hyperglycemic neuropathy occurs in individuals with poorly controlled diabetes, and in those who have been newly diagnosed, rapidly reversible nerve conduction abnormalities have been reported. These abnormalities are accompanied by distally symmetric sensory changes such as burning, paresthesias, and tenderness in the feet and legs. Symptoms disappear when the individual's blood sugar is controlled, although abnormalities in nerve conduction may persist.[12]

> **BOX 25.4**   **Classification of Diabetic Neuropathy**
>
> **Rapidly Reversible**
> - Hyperglycemic neuropathy
>
> **Generalized Symmetric Polyneuropathies**
> - Acute sensory
> - Chronic sensorimotor
> - Autonomic
>
> **Focal Neuropathies**
> - Cranial
> - Focal limb

Adapted from Boulton AJ, Vinik AI, Arezzo JC, et al.: Diabetic neuropathies: a statement by the American Diabetes Association, Diabetes Care 28:956–962, 2005.

Generalized symmetric polyneuropathies

Acute sensory neuropathy. Hallmarks of acute sensory neuropathy, are the rapid onset of severe burning pain, deep aching pain, a sudden sharp "electric shock–like" sensation, and hypersensitivity of the feet that is often worse at night. Signs of this painful diabetic polyneuropathy (DPN) are relatively normal: normal motor examinations in which the tendon reflexes are normal or reduced at the ankle. The patient may have no or only mild symmetric sensory loss, with allodynia. Testing procedures to confirm allodynia should apply the following concepts. Apply a phasic stimulus (rub) to various parts of the body and ask the person whether burning occurs in a nearby region; a cotton ball or Semmes–Weinstein monofilament is not applied long enough for the slow summation required for allodynia. Place a towel on the patient's body and wait for a period of time before asking whether the cover creates pain; *do not* use a sharp–dull to test for allodynia because it is pain from nonpainful stimuli. Nociceptive stimuli are perceived normally in acute sensory neuropathy. Electrophysiologic studies (NCVs) may be normal or show minor changes. If the person can achieve and maintain stable blood glucose, recovery can occur within 1 year, even with severe symptoms.[12]

Chronic sensorimotor neuropathy. Chronic sensorimotor neuropathy, or DPN, is the most common type of DN and up to 50% of patients may develop this condition. Typically, its onset is insidious, but occasionally signs and symptoms appear acutely. DPN's clinical features include sensory loss, occasionally with selective fiber type involvement. Small fiber involvement leads to burning pain, and paresthesias, such as those described for acute sensory neuropathy, and are more profound at night in the feet and lower legs (stocking pattern). Large fiber involvement results in painless paresthesia with impaired vibration, proprioception, touch, and pressure along with loss of ankle DTRs. Clients may report that they feel as if they were walking on cotton or clouds. In DPN, motor weakness is mild (presence of hammer toes and/or pes cavus) with wasting of small muscles in the feet and hands in more advanced cases. The presence of pronounced motor involvement implies that this is not DPN. DPN may be accompanied by clinical or subclinical autonomic involvement that can include cardiovascular and sympathetic disturbances resulting in sweating, orthostatic hypotension, and resting tachycardia (<100 beats/minute at rest).[12]

BOX 25.5 Manifestations of Autonomic Diabetic Neuropathy

Cardiovascular
- Tachycardia
- Exercise intolerance
- Orthostatic hypotension
- Dizziness

Gastrointestinal
- Esophageal motility dysfunction
- Diarrhea
- Constipation

Genitourinary
- Neurogenic bladder
- Bladder urgency, incontinence
- Erectile dysfunction

Other
- Sweating, heat intolerance
- Dry skin
- Pupillary dysfunction, blurred vision

Adapted from Boulton AJ, Malik RA, Arezzo JC, et al.: Diabetic somatic neuropathies, Diabetes Care 27:1458–1486, 2004.

Autonomic neuropathy. Sympathetic and parasympathetic involvement may occur in both type 1 and type 2 diabetes; however, in type 2 diabetes, parasympathetic functions are more affected. After 10 to 15 years, 30% of patients have subclinical manifestations of autonomic involvement. Major manifestations associated with autonomic involvement are shown in Box 25.5.[126]

Focal neuropathies

Mononeuropathies. Mononeuropathies in the limbs or cranial nerves may occur in diabetes less often than the generalized, symmetric patterns. The median, ulnar, and peroneal nerves are most commonly affected in limb focal neuropathies. The somatic division of the oculomotor nerve is most commonly involved.

Medical Management

Diagnosis

The diagnosis is based on the history, clinical examination, electrodiagnostic studies, quantitative sensory evaluation, and autonomic function testing. Diagnosis of DN should not be based on a single symptom, sign, or test; a minimum of two abnormalities (signs and symptoms from NCV, sensory, or autonomic tests) has been recommended.[3] Tools required for the sensory examination include a 128-Hz tuning fork to assess vibration and a 1-g monofilament for touch. Autonomic functions can initially be assessed by blood pressure and heart rate response at rest, in standing and with exercise. Because diabetes is a common disorder and because neuropathies may be related to other causes, mere association of neuropathic signs and symptoms in a person with diabetes is not sufficient to diagnose DN. Other causes must be excluded.[60]

Sensory, motor, and F responses are important to assess nerve function at baseline and intermittently at follow-up visits. The most common electrical change is a reduced amplitude in the sensory action potential (SNAP), which suggests axonal degeneration. A recent report found that a high percentage of newly diagnosed patients with type 2 diabetes have reduced SNAP in upper extremity nerves.[129] Slowing of sensory and/or motor NCV suggests a demyelinating neuropathy, and pronounced slowing suggests that an alternative diagnosis should be explored.[8] Sensory fibers are generally affected first before motor fibers.

Treatment

Management is divided into general and specific measures. General measures include control of hyperglycemia,[162] and specific measures address the symptomatic management of the disorders. Because there is evidence that further complications can be reduced by maintaining control of the diabetes, this is one specific area addressed by health care professionals. In addition, specific drug therapies are being evaluated. Currently, studies on medications and biochemical factors, such as gangliosides and NGFs, are being conducted and some show promise. Tricyclic antidepressants are used alone or in combination with fluphenazine to treat painful neuropathies, and gabapentin or carbamazepine is efficacious in managing pain in focal neuropathies.[162] Although topical capsaicin has been recommended for allodynia, a systematic review concluded that it had moderate to poor efficacy in the management of chronic pain.[102] Angiotensin-converting enzyme inhibitors act on the vascular dysfunction and prevent the development and progression of DN.[99] In a systematic analysis of seven qualifying studies, researchers found vitamin B_{12} (either as B_{12} complex or methylcobalamin, one of two coenzyme forms of B_{12}) had beneficial effects on pain and paresthesia more than electrophysiologic changes. Methylcobalamin improved autonomic symptoms in three studies.[150]

If the person has a painful DN, an algorithm has been developed that begins with physical modalities to manage pain. This is combined with simple analgesics. Further management may include a trial of topical or benign drugs.[163] A common complication of DN is the development of neuropathic foot ulcers. When great toe and ankle joint mobility is limited greater forefoot pressures occur during gait, which may place patients with diabetes (type 1 or 2) at risk for development of metatarsal ulceration.[175] In type 2 diabetes, early detection of DN along with prophylactic foot care regimens has led to fewer foot ulcerations and amputations.[141] Institution of foot care procedures is essential. With the development of a foot drop gait, orthotic devices should be considered for the person's safety. The type of orthosis and shoe construction prescribed should be carefully considered based on the sensory picture and the person's ability to demonstrate appropriate foot care.

Prognosis

DN is a slowly progressive disorder. Because it is a metabolic disorder, other systems are often affected. Estimates are that more than 50% of nontraumatic amputations in the United States are performed in diabetic clients. The presence of autonomic involvement is associated with an increased mortality risk.

Alcoholic Neuropathy

Peripheral neuropathies, typically with distally symmetric involvement, appear in alcoholics after years of chronic alcohol abuse.

Etiology and Risk Factors

Although the exact pathogenesis of alcoholic neuropathy remains unclear,[165] lesions affecting the peripheral nerves have been attributed to both the direct toxic effects of alcohol on nerve and nutritional deficiencies in thiamine and other B vitamins from poor dietary habits. However, there is evidence that neither age nor nutritional status play a part in development of alcoholic neuropathies. Rather, alcohol-related neuropathies appear to be caused by the total lifetime accumulation of ethanol.[38] Patients exhibiting alcoholic neuropathy were divided into those with and without a coexisting thiamine deficiency. Researchers reported that patients without thiamine deficiency tended to have a more slowly progressive disorder in which sensory symptoms were dominant, primarily pain or a burning sensation. Along with these symptoms, the nerve biopsy demonstrated greater small fiber axonal loss. Those with alcoholic neuropathy with thiamine deficiency had large fiber involvement with segmental demyelination, and an acutely progressive motor dominant pattern along with loss of superficial and deep sensation was noted. These findings further support the view that alcohol directly affects nerve fibers.[81]

Pathogenesis

The exact pathogenesis of alcoholic neuropathy remains unclear. Segmental demyelination and axonal degeneration have been described in persons with alcoholic polyneuropathy; these differences may relate to the presence of vitamin deficiencies, as noted previously. Changes occur distally at first and become more marked and proximal.[53]

Clinical Manifestations

Mild forms of alcoholic neuropathy exhibit minor loss of muscle bulk, diminished ankle reflexes, impaired sensation in the feet, and aching in the calves. Distal sensory changes include pain, paresthesia, and numbness in a symmetric stocking-glove pattern. In addition, vibratory perception is impaired. It begins insidiously and progresses slowly; occasionally the onset may occur acutely. In the most advanced cases, symptoms involve all four extremities. Weakness and atrophy of distal musculature should be anticipated, with lower extremity involvement greater than upper extremity. Bilateral foot drop is observed during gait, and a wrist drop contributes to a diminished grip strength because of the client's inability to extend the wrist. Both of these features are often combined with varying amounts of peripheral weakness in other muscles.

Medical Management

Diagnosis and Treatment

The diagnosis is made by history, clinical examination, and electrodiagnostic testing showing loss of action potential amplitude (sensory and motor). Although diet is no longer implicated as a contributing factor in the development of alcoholic neuropathies, diet to improve nutritional status, along with vitamin supplements and abstinence from alcohol, is the treatment of choice to slow progression. All other treatment is symptomatic. Orthotic devices, such as ankle-foot orthoses and cock-up splints, are used to manage weakness and improve function. Medications for sensory changes include carbamazepine, salicylates, and amitriptyline.

Prognosis

If the client totally abstains from alcohol, mild improvement can be expected, but recovery is slow (months to years) and incomplete when axonal degeneration has occurred.[116] Therefore, to anticipate the outcome, review the client's electrophysiologic studies to determine whether demyelination or degeneration is present.

Compression neuropathies, such as Saturday night palsy or peroneal nerve compression, may result from a bout of chronic alcohol intoxication in which prolonged pressure compromises nerve function. Excessive alcohol intake may also produce rhabdomyolysis, which produces proximal muscle weakness, swelling, and pigmented urine. Rhabdomyolysis (destruction of skeletal muscle tissue that results in muscle cell contents being released into bloodstream) occurs as product of renal failure after drinking.

Chronic Renal Failure
Clinical Manifestations

Neurologic. Alteration of CNS and PNS function often occurs with chronic renal failure associated with uremia. CNS involvement (uremic encephalopathy) is manifested by recent memory loss, inability to concentrate, perceptual errors, and decreased alertness. Uremic toxins contribute to atrophy and demyelination of both sensory and motor nerves of the PNS. The lower extremities are much more commonly affected than the upper extremities; neurologic changes are typically symmetric and can also be manifested as peripheral neuropathy or restless leg syndrome, which is more pronounced at rest.

Anemia

CNS symptoms can develop in cases of severe pernicious anemia, whereas neuropathy is observed in early cases of B_{12} deficiency, allowing for early identification. The findings typically consist of a symmetric sensory neuropathy that begins in the feet and lower legs, although it rarely may involve the upper extremities, especially fine motor coordination of the hands. This upper extremity neuropathy may clinically manifest as problems with deteriorating handwriting. Affected individuals may also describe moderate pain or paresthesias of the extremities, especially the feet. The person may interpret the neuropathy as difficulty with locomotion when in fact they are experiencing the loss of proprioception. The affected individual may need to hold on to the wall, countertops, or furniture at home as a result of difficulties maintaining balance. There may be an associated positive Romberg sign. Loss of motor function is a late manifestation of B_{12} deficiency. Although a symmetric neuropathy is the usual pattern, B_{12} deficiency occasionally presents as a unilateral neuropathy and/or bilateral but asymmetric neuropathy. Rarely, subacute degeneration of the spinal cord caused by

TABLE 25.8   Guillain–Barré Syndrome and Its Variants

Abbreviation	Name	Clinical Characteristics
AIDP	Acute inflammatory demyelinating polyneuropathy	Primary demyelination: progressive paralysis, areflexia
AMAN	Acute motor axonal neuropathy	Axonal variant, more severe: frequent respiratory involvement/ventilator dependence and significant residual impairments
ASAN	Acute sensory ascending neuropathy	Sensory changes more prominent than weakness
AMSAN	Acute motor and sensory axonal neuropathy	
	Acute autonomic neuropathy	Manifested by postural hypotension, impaired sweating, lacrimation, bowel and bladder function
	Miller Fisher syndrome	Ophthalmoplegia, ataxia, areflexia with significant weakness
CIDP	Chronic inflammatory demyelinating polyneuropathy	Slower onset, relapses and remissions or progressive course over year

vitamin B$_{12}$ deficiency can occur in pernicious anemia, characterized by pyramidal and posterior column deficits. CNS manifestations may include headache, drowsiness, dizziness, fainting, slow thought processes, decreased attention span, apathy, depression, and irritability.

INFECTIONS/INFLAMMATIONS

Guillain–Barré Syndrome

Overview and Definition

Guillain–Barré syndrome (GBS) was originally described by and named for the French neurologists who published case reports describing a syndrome of flaccid paralysis, areflexia, and albuminocytologic dissociation. More recently, the syndrome has been viewed as having distinct subtypes with varying distributions worldwide. Since the virtual elimination of poliomyelitis, GBS is the most common cause of rapidly evolving motor paresis and paralysis and sensory deficits. Individuals affected with GBS typically reach maximal weakness within 2 to 3 weeks but spend weeks to months recovering. The most common form of GBS is also known as acute inflammatory demyelinating polyradiculoneuropathy.

Incidence

Annual incidence varies from 1 to 2 cases per 100,000 people. Although GBS occurs at all ages, peaks in frequency can be seen in young adults and in the fifth through the eighth decades. Occurrence is slightly greater for men than women and for whites more than blacks. Some researchers have noted a seasonal relationship associated with infections.

Etiology and Risk Factors

Evidence supports the view that GBS is an immune-mediated disorder. Bacterial (*Campylobacter jejuni*) and viral (*Haemophilus influenza*, Epstein–Barr virus, and cytomegalovirus [CMV]) infections, surgery, and vaccinations have been associated with the development of GBS. Of the two-thirds of persons reporting an acute infection within 2 months preceding onset of GBS, 90% had illnesses (e.g., respiratory or gastrointestinal) during the preceding 30 days.[118]

Pathogenesis

Lesions occur throughout the PNS from the spinal nerve roots to the distal termination of both motor and sensory fibers. Originally, GBS was classified as a single entity characterized by PNS demyelination. Now, however, it is defined as

several heterogeneous forms (Table 25.8). *C. jejuni* is associated more commonly with the axonal form, whereas greater sensory involvement is seen following CMV.[68] The axonal pattern of involvement can involve motor fibers only or in the more severely involved form, motor and sensory fiber degeneration. Finally, Miller Fisher syndrome is characterized by an acute onset of extraocular muscle paralysis with sluggish pupillary light reflexes, a peripheral sensory ataxia, and loss of DTRs with relative sparing of strength in the extremities and trunk. Facial weakness and sensory loss in the limbs may also occur.

Molecular mimicry, an autoimmune theory, is the primary theory for the cause of GBS because evidence exists for antibody-mediated demyelination. Myelin of the Schwann cell is the primary target of attack. Researchers theorize that circulating antibodies to gangliosides penetrate and bind to an antigen on the surface of the myelin and activate either complement or an antibody-dependent macrophage.[69] The earliest pathologic changes in the PNS take the form of a generalized inflammatory response. Lymphocytes (T cells) and macrophages are the inflammatory cells present. Demyelination, initiated at the node of Ranvier, occurs because macrophages, responding to inflammatory signals, strip myelin from the nerves. After the initial demyelination, the body initiates a repair process. Schwann cells divide and remyelinate nerves, resulting in shorter internodal distances than were present initially.

In addition to the demyelination, there is another process that has longer lasting effects. Although there is an axonal subtype, axonal degeneration to some degree occurs in most cases of demyelinating GBS. In the latter, many believe that the axons are damaged during the inflammatory process, according to what has been called a "bystander effect." Products that are liberated by the macrophages as they strip myelin (e.g., free oxygen radicals and proteases) also damage axons.

Axonal patterns of involvement display a diminished or absent inflammatory response seen in demyelination. Researchers have reported the presence of macrophages that invade periaxonal spaces, causing the axon to degenerate within the ventral roots. Recovery for this wallerian-like degeneration would require an extremely long period. For those individuals with acute motor axonal neuropathy, another mechanism may promote rapid recovery for what appears to be axonal involvement. Binding of antibodies to the nodes of Ranvier may cause blocking of nerve conduction by altering sodium channel conductance, which has been established in rabbits. Although the autoimmune theory is the main one advanced for this disorder, it may not be the only reason for the development of GBS. Cases of GBS have been reported in immunosuppressed individuals after renal transplant.

Clinical Manifestations

Various subtypes of GBS exist; however, the "classic" picture is an acute form in which the time from onset to peak impairment is 4 weeks or less. A recurrent form of GBS is reported in up to 10% of cases. Acute relapses may occur in GBS, and this characteristic may make it difficult to differentiate the acute from the chronic form, called *chronic inflammatory demyelinating polyradiculoneuropathy* (CIDP). Most cases of CIDP progress over a period of months instead of weeks.

In GBS, symptoms are characterized by a rapidly ascending symmetric motor weakness and distal sensory impairments. The first neurologic symptom is often paresthesia in the toes. This is followed within hours or days by weakness distally in the legs. Weakness spreads to involve arms, trunk, and facial muscles. Flaccid paralysis is accompanied by absence of DTRs. Occasionally, sensory and motor symptoms begin in the hands and arms instead of the feet and legs. Palatal and facial muscles become involved in about half of all cases; even the muscles of mastication may be affected, but nerves to extraocular muscles typically are not involved. Up to 30% of all cases require mechanical ventilation.

Because the preganglionic fibers of the ANS are myelinated, they, too, may be subject to demyelination. If this occurs, tachycardia, abnormalities in cardiac rhythm, blood pressure changes, and vasomotor symptoms occur.

In 50% of the cases, progression of symptoms generally ceases within 2 weeks and in 90% of the cases, progression ends by 4 weeks. After the progression stops, an event known as nadir, a static phase begins, lasting 2 to 4 weeks before recovery occurs in a proximal to distal progression. This recovery may take months or even years.

Medical Management

Diagnosis

Careful clinical and neurophysiologic examinations and laboratory tests are needed to diagnosis GBS. Criteria have been developed by the National Institute of Neurologic and Communicative Disorders and Stroke (Box 25.6); however, these criteria omit the variants that have been identified.[15]

After symptoms have existed for 1 week, a lumbar puncture can be performed to withdraw cerebrospinal fluid (CSF). Albumin (a protein) is elevated in the CSF with 10 or fewer mononuclear leukocytes present. Electrophysiologic tests will reveal slowed NCVs the entire length of the nerve when demyelination is present, as well as fibrillation potentials when axonal degeneration occurs. When both axonal involvement and demyelination occur, the amplitude of the evoked (NCV) potential will be reduced and the velocity is slowed, respectively.

These abnormalities may not be apparent during the first few weeks of the illness. In addition, to determine the ex-

---

BOX 25.6   Criteria for Diagnosis of Guillain–Barré Syndrome

Symptoms Required for Diagnosis
- Progressive weakness in more than one extremity
- Loss of deep tendon reflexes

Symptoms Supportive of Diagnosis (in Order of Importance)
- Weakness developing rapidly that ceases to progress by 4 weeks
- Symmetric weakness
- Mild sensory symptoms and signs
- Facial weakness common and symmetric; oral-bulbar musculature may also be involved
- Recovery usually begins 2 to 4 weeks after GBS ceases to progress
- Tachycardia, cardiac arrhythmias, and labile blood pressure may occur
- Absence of fever

CSF Features
- CSF protein levels increased after 1 week; continue to increase on serial examinations
- CSF contains 10 or fewer mononuclear leukocytes/mm³

Electrodiagnostic Features
- Nerve conduction velocity slowed

CSF, Cerebrospinal fluid; *GBS,* Guillain–Barré syndrome.
Adapted from Hund EF, Borel CO, Cornblath DR, et al.: Intensive management and treatment of severe Guillain-Barré syndrome, Crit Care Med 21:435, 1993.

---

tent of demyelination of the more proximal nerve roots, an F wave electrophysiologic test may be performed; it is often prolonged or absent. As recovery occurs, slowed NCVs persist, even though the person has made a full clinical recovery. Although electrophysiologic studies are used for diagnosis, the distal compound motor action potential (CMAP) is a predictor of prognosis. If the CMAP amplitude is less than 20% of normal limits at 3 to 5 weeks, it predicts a prolonged or poor outcome.[123]

Differential Diagnosis

Hysteria is the most common misdiagnosis. Because of the speed of onset, a stroke involving the brainstem will also be considered. Less common causes of acute neuropathies must also be considered, including tick paralysis, West Nile virus, and metabolic disorders such as porphyria.

Treatment

Because GBS is believed to be an autoimmune disease, treatment has been aimed at controlling the response. In two major trials, plasmapheresis, a technique (also called plasma exchange [PE]) that removes plasma from circulation and filters it to remove or dilute circulating antibodies, has been shown to significantly improve the impairments in GBS. Typically, the client will have four to six exchanges of 500 mL per treatment over a week. Time on a respirator and time to independent ambulation (53 days) were both shorter than in the control group (85 days). Plasmapheresis is instituted when respiratory function drops precipitously (to 1.0 to 1.5 L), and the person is placed on a respirator.

High-dose intravenous (IV) administration of immunoglobulin (Ig; a protein the immune system normally uses to attack foreign organisms) has been found safe and effective in the treatment of GBS.[160] The therapeutic dose is 0.4 g/kg per day for 5 days.[70] Practice parameter recommendations made after a review of PE and IV Ig studies are that PE should be administered in nonambulatory adults seeking treatment within 4 weeks of GBS onset or ambulatory adults within 2 weeks of onset. IV Ig was recommended in nonambulatory adults within 2 weeks of onset. Outcomes for either approach were equivalent. For children with severe GBS, either treatment approach is an option.[70]

Prognosis

The primary methods of managing GBS have helped to improve mortality rates, which can exceed 5%. Factors that predict a poor outcome include onset at an older age, a protracted time before recovery begins, and the need for artificial respiration. An important objective evaluation finding that predicts a poor outcome is significantly reduced evoked motor potential amplitude, which correlates with the presence of axonal degeneration. Although most persons recover, up to 20% can have remaining neurologic deficits. After 1 year, 67% of clients have complete recovery, but 20% remain with significant disability.[42] Even after 2 years, 8% have not recovered.

25.5 Special Implications for the PTA: Guillain–Barré Syndrome

Physical therapy is initiated at an early stage in this condition to maintain joint ROM within the client's pain tolerance and to monitor muscle strength until active exercises can be initiated. During the ascending phase when the person is losing function and becoming weaker, he or she can become easily fatigued and overwhelmed. Focus is toward prevention of complications associated with immobilization.

Meticulous skin care is required by all staff members to prevent skin breakdown and contractures. A strict turning schedule is usually established by the nursing staff and should be followed by all other health care staff as well. After each position change, inspect the skin (especially the sacrum, heels, ankles, shoulders, and greater trochanter). Massage to pressure points stimulates circulation; family or other caregivers can be instructed to perform this on a regular basis. High-top gym shoes can help prevent plantar flexion contractures while the patient is confined to bed.

Care in the intensive care unit (ICU) requires observation of arterial blood gas measurements. Because the disease results in primary hypoventilation with hypoxemia and hypercapnia, watch for a Po_2 less than 70 mm Hg, which signals respiratory failure. Report any signs of rising Pco_2 (e.g., confusion, tachypnea). Pulse oximetry may be used to monitor peripheral oxygen saturation. Auscultate breath sounds, turn and position the person, and encourage coughing and deep breathing to maintain clear airways and prevent atelectasis. The PTA must also follow universal precautions to help prevent any respiratory infection for the client. Respiratory support is needed at the first sign of dyspnea (in adults, vital capacity less than 800 mL; in children, less than 12 mL/kg of body weight) or decreasing Po_2.

Ventilation is instituted when pulmonary function is compromised by loss of respiratory skeletal muscle control. Coughing and clearing of tracheal secretions becomes difficult. In addition, weakness of laryngeal and pharyngeal muscles makes swallowing difficult and increases the risk of aspiration. Early tracheostomy is indicated in people with clinical and EMG evidence of axonal involvement together with respiratory failure.

Clinical indications for weaning from the ventilator include improved forced vital capacity and improved inspiratory force concomitant with improved muscle stretch. Finally, the chest should be clear of atelectasis. Communication using a communication board or other method is needed during ventilatory support.

Exercise and Guillain–Barré Syndrome

When the person's condition stabilizes, a therapeutic pool or Hubbard tank can be used to initiate movement in a controlled environment. A major precaution during the early treatment phase is to provide gentle stretching and active or active-assistive exercise at a level consistent with the person's muscle strength. Overstretching and overuse of painful muscles may result in a prolonged recovery period or a lack of recovery. During the descending phase, when the paralysis slowly recedes and physical function returns, neuromuscular facilitation techniques (such as proprioceptive neuromuscular facilitation) may be integrated into the active and resistive exercises.

Deep muscular discomfort or pain in the proximal muscles may be reported by clients. Paresis or paralysis requires positioning and appropriate splinting, which can help alleviate muscle and joint pain. Bed cages may reduce dysesthesias that are present in the feet. Palliative modalities, such as hot packs and gentle massage, may also bring relief of musculoskeletal pain.

Foster and Mulroy reported that the average length of stay (LOS) for individuals in a rehabilitation facility was 63 days. Longer LOS correlated with presence of muscle belly tenderness, extreme lower limb weakness as measured by manual muscle test, and functional independence measure scores at admission. Although the presence of axonal involvement was not significantly related to LOS, it does affect severity of involvement and the need for ventilator and orthosis, which tended to require longer stays.[48] The length of time to maximum impairment (respiratory compromise and motor involvement) has not been found to correlate with outcome. Generally, the shorter the time it takes for recovery to begin after maximum impairment has been reached, the less likely it is that long-term disability will occur.[110]

Discharge Planning

Patients usually participate in outpatient rehabilitation following discharge from the hospital. When the person is discharged from therapy, recovery may not be complete. Impaired function may require the continued use of assistive devices and possibly even mobility equipment such as a wheelchair or scooter. The home may require modifications, which should be evaluated and planned for before discharge.

Postpolio Syndrome/Postpolio Muscular Atrophy
Overview

Poliomyelitis (polio) virus infection was virtually eradicated in the United States with the advent of the Salk vaccine in the 1950s and the Sabin vaccine in the 1960s. Clinically, the disease was characterized as one of three patterns: (1) an asymptomatic or (2) nonparalytic infection that produced gastrointestinal, flulike symptoms and muscular pain or (3) a paralytic infection that also began with flulike symptoms. The paralytic form generally developed within a week after the onset of the symptoms. The virus invaded and damaged motor cell bodies. The extent of the asymmetric paresis and paralysis that ensued depended on the degree of anterior horn cell involvement. When cell bodies were killed, motor axons underwent wallerian degeneration and muscles rapidly atrophied. Of those persons developing acute paralysis, equal numbers (30%) recovered, had mild residual paralysis, or were left with moderate to severe paralysis. Ten percent died from respiratory involvement. Recovery was attributed to the recovery of some anterior horn cells, as well as collateral sprouting from intact peripheral nerves and to hypertrophy of spared muscle fibers.[30]

Polio was a unique neuropathy that created only focal and asymmetric motor impairments, rather than the typical distal, symmetric motor and sensory losses associated with other neuropathies. For decades it was considered a static disease; after the initial episode there was no further progression of the disease. The last major epidemics of polio occurred in the early 1950s; thus most of the people who had paralytic polio are at least 50 years old today. Most people had significant recovery of function and went on to live very productive lives.

Definition

Postpolio syndrome (PPS), or postpolio muscular atrophy, refers to new neuromuscular symptoms that occur decades (average postpolio interval is 25 years) after recovery from the acute paralytic episode.[119]

Incidence and Risk Factors

It is estimated that there are 1.63 million polio survivors in the United States and that one-fourth to one-half of them will develop PPS.[59] A previous diagnosis of polio is essential for this diagnosis. Also, the degree of initial motor involvement as measured by weakness in the acute stage is a factor in the development of PPS. These combine with long-term overuse of muscle that places increased demands on joints, ligaments, and muscle.

Etiology

PPS appears to be related to the initial disorder of the motor neuron cell body affected by the poliovirus. Much of the recovery of muscle strength that occurred after the axonal degeneration can be attributed to reinnervation of denervated muscle fibers by collateral spouts from other nearby surviving axons. That is, surviving axons increased the size of their innervation ratio. For example, instead of one axon innervating 3000 muscle fibers in the quadriceps, one axon innervated 5000 fibers. Studies confirm that denervation progresses in patients with prior poliomyelitis in both clinically affected and unaffected muscles, and indicate that this progression is more rapid than that occurring in normal aging. Overall, there was a 13.4% reduction in motor-unit number and an 18.4% diminution in M-wave amplitude ($p < 0.001$). The rate of motor-unit loss was twice that occurring in healthy subjects older than age 60 years.[103]

Pathogenesis

Muscle biopsy and EMG both indicate ongoing muscle denervation. PPS seems to be an evolution of the original motor neuron dysfunction that began after the poliovirus affected the alpha motor neuron. PPS is manifested when the compensated reinnervation that occurred cannot maintain that muscle fiber innervation. The nervous system is pruning back axonal sprouts in this enlarged motor unit that it no longer has the metabolic ability to support; thus new denervation results. Symptoms are related to an attrition of

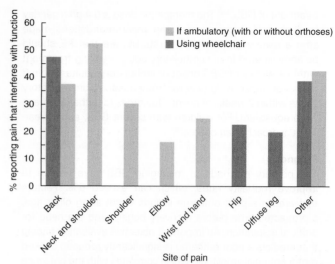

FIG. 25.17 Location of pain reported in ambulatory and wheelchair-bound persons diagnosed with postpolio syndrome. (Data from Department of Physical Therapy, Institute for Rehabilitation and Research, Houston, TX: An instructional course on physical therapy management of postpoliomyelitis: new challenges. Presented at the 65th American Physical Therapy Association Annual Conference, Chicago, June 1986.)

oversprouting motor neurons that can no longer support these axonal sprouts.[22]

Clinical Manifestations

Symptoms vary, but generally muscle strength declines in all people, with periods of stability for 3 to 10 years in muscles that had previously been affected by polio and had fully or partially recovered. Administration of an index of postpolio sequelae has shown that pain, atrophy, and bulbar (respiratory and swallowing) problems are the three most prominent sequelae from poliomyelitis.[73] Affected persons have also reported myalgias, joint pain, increased muscle atrophy, and new weakness, as well as excessive fatigue with minimal activity, vasomotor abnormalities, and diminishing endurance. These all combine to contribute to a loss of function. Researchers report that the rate of strength deterioration is faster than would occur in normal aging. Deterioration in the lower extremity predisposes individuals to overuse of upper extremity musculature to compensate.[79]

Typically, symptoms are related to the individual's activities of daily living: crutch walking, wheelchair propulsion (Fig. 25.17). Pain is commonly located in the low back and joints of the upper extremity in women; it is worse at night and increases with physical activity and changes in climate.

Medical Management

Diagnosis

PPS is a clinical diagnosis requiring the exclusion of other medical, neurologic, orthopedic, or psychiatric disorders that could explain the new symptoms. Routine EMG can be used to confirm any new denervation, as can muscle biopsies. Single-fiber EMG and spinal fluid studies are rarely needed to establish a diagnosis.[22]

Treatment

Medical management is aimed at symptomatic treatment and modification of lifestyle. Surgery for residual calcaneovalgus deformities at the ankle include triple arthrodesis.[40] Perimalleolar tendon transfers have been performed to compensate for triceps surae insufficiency.[31]

Prognosis

PPS is a slowly progressive disorder with stable periods that last 3 to 10 years. A decline in functional status is reported to correlate with a poorer quality of life in individuals affected by PPS.[80]

25.6 Special Implications for the PTA: Postpolio Syndrome
Of importance to PTAs is the ongoing question of the use of exercise in the management of this disorder. Partially denervated muscle does not have the physiologic capacity to respond to a conventional strengthening program. Instead, programs aimed at nonexhaustive exercise and general body conditioning are preferable.[57] The client should never exercise to the point of fatigue, and vital signs are monitored before and after exercise to assess the client's response to even mild activity. Caution the client to stop if pain persists or weakness increases. Because individuals with PPS have decreased peak workloads and decreased oxygen uptake, functional exercises of submaximal intensity are stressed with the goal of maintaining and improving endurance and functional capacity. For those with relatively good strength, a program to improve aerobic fitness is appropriate; for those with weaker leg musculature, a generalized fitness program should be aimed at endurance and improving work capacity.[172] Additionally, clients with PPS may also benefit from lifestyle modifications, including energy conservation techniques. Late-onset weakness, pain, and fatigue have been reported in individuals who had not developed the paralytic form of the disease.[59]

Posturally induced mechanical strain and overuse have led to degenerative changes and pain, as well as unstable joints. For these deformities to be reversed, the PTA should explore the use of orthoses, especially for gait. Many clients who have developed PPS are former brace users and may have an aversion to orthoses, but the braces they formerly used were not the cosmetic lightweight braces that can be fabricated today.

Herpes Zoster/Postherpetic Neuralgia

Varicella-zoster virus is a common herpes virus that affects the nervous system. It is the virus that causes chickenpox in children. After recovery from that childhood disease, the virus is not eliminated from the body; it lies dormant within sensory ganglia of cranial and spinal nerves and can become activated later in life to cause herpes zoster (HZ), or shingles.

Incidence

Annually, approximately 1% of the adult population older than age 80 years develops HZ each year[128] and of those, about 20% develop postherpetic neuralgia. Immunocompromised individuals are also at risk.

Pathogenesis

HZ primarily affects the sensory ganglia of the spinal cord or cranial nerves. When reactivated, the virus causes a generalized inflammatory response beginning in the sensory ganglion and spreading along spinal and peripheral nerves to produce demyelination and degeneration.

Clinical Manifestations

The inflammation produces pain and tingling in the involved dermatome with a rash followed by development of vesicles (blisters) that burst and encrust in the same dermatome. The skin lesions last up to 1 month and disappear as the effects of the virus resolve. Thoracic and trigeminal dermatomes are involved most often. Occasionally, the inflammation may affect motor neurons and produce LMN signs and symptoms. The pain resolves over time, but in individuals that develop postherpetic neuralgia, it may linger for weeks or months. Postherpetic pain is possibly related to hyperirritable primary afferent nociceptors that provide input to an already synthesized CNS.[120] The type of pain has been described as a constant aching or burning or a cutting or stabbing pain.

Medical Management

Diagnosis and Treatment

The diagnosis is made by clinical presentation. The disorder is treated symptomatically unless there is widespread involvement. Oral antiviral medications, such as acyclovir, are used to control the response and accelerate the resolution of the pain, hypoesthesia, burning, and itching associated with the neuralgia. Although analgesic drugs may be prescribed to relieve pain, a randomized controlled trial using topical lidocaine patches, gabapentin, and controlled-release oxycodone shows better pain relief. Nortriptyline, a tricyclic antidepressant, also provides analgesia and may be tolerated better than other medications.[74]

Prognosis

For immunosuppressed clients, there is a greater risk of developing postherpetic neuralgia and painful dysesthesias as a complication of HZ. Postherpetic pain is very resistant to treatment. Signs of the disorder in immunocompetent persons resolve within a month, but the area that was affected may be partly insensitive. Up to 20% of people who experience HZ will experience a second attack.

Trigeminal Neuralgia/Tic Douloureux

Trigeminal neuralgia (TN), or tic douloureux, is a disorder of the trigeminal (fifth cranial) nerve in which there are intense paroxysms of lancinating pain within the nerve's distribution.

Incidence

TN is not a common disorder (5 cases per 100,000). It typically occurs in women between the ages of 50 and 70 years.

Etiology

TN arises from many causes: herpes zoster, multiple sclerosis, vascular lesions, or tumors that can affect the nerve to produce the painful sensations. Many times it will be referred to as idiopathic because the cause remains undetermined. Physical triggers can elicit paroxysms of pain.

Pathogenesis

Researchers hypothesize that the pain is caused by ectopic activity generated at the site of involvement. Demyelinated fibers become hyperexcitable. Light mechanical stimulation recruits nearby pain fibers causing them to discharge and create the sensation of intense pain.

Clinical Manifestations

The pain associated with TN has a sudden onset and has been described as sharp, knifelike, lancinating, and "like a lightning bolt inside my head that lasts for seconds to minutes." The sensation is typically restricted to the maxillary (V2) division of the nerve, but it may involve the maxillary and mandibular divisions together. Less likely is involvement of the ophthalmic (V1) division.

The painful sensation often occurs in clusters. Any mechanical stimulation, chewing, smiling, or even a breeze can trigger an attack. Clients avoid stimulating the trigger zone. Remissions occur between attacks, but these remission periods shorten and attacks become more frequent over the course of the disorder. In about 10% of the cases the pain occurs bilaterally.

Medical Management

Diagnosis

Subjective reports of pain in the typical pattern are the basis for the diagnosis. No impairment or loss of sensation or motor control is obvious on evaluation. The person can identify the trigger site. Skull radiographs, CT scans, and MRI are used to rule out tumors and vascular causes.

Treatment

The preferred treatment of TN is oral carbamazepine (Tegretol, an anticonvulsant). Pain can be controlled with appropriate dosage in about 75% of clients with TN. Side effects of this medication include blurred vision, dizziness, and drowsiness, as well as hematologic changes (anemia) and altered liver function. In addition, because carbamazepine has teratogenic effects, it should not be used in the first trimester of pregnancy and should not be used by nursing mothers.[51] Other medications, such as phenytoin (Dilantin), are less effective but should be tried in those who cannot tolerate carbamazepine. Promising new medications to manage TN include pimozide, tizanidine hydroxychloride, and topical capsaicin.[28]

In persons whose pain is refractory to medications, neurosurgical procedures are advised. Radiofrequency rhizotomy is preferred over trigeminal nerve section or alcohol ablation. Microvascular surgery has also been used when small blood vessels have been found to constrict the trigeminal nerve near its root. This procedure provides immediate pain relief; however, it is a major and difficult surgery.

Prognosis

The efficacy of evaluating treatments for TN is complicated by the fact that the disorder may remit spontaneously. Remissions that occur soon after onset of TN may last for years. For those who do not remit, TN can be managed medically in most cases. The Trigeminal Neuralgia Association provides information and support for persons with this diagnosis.

Human Immunodeficiency Virus Advanced Disease (Acquired Immunodeficiency Syndrome)

Peripheral neuropathy, disease- or drug-induced myopathy, and musculoskeletal pain syndromes occur most often in advanced stages of human immunodeficiency virus (HIV) disease but can occur at any stage of HIV infection and may be the presenting manifestation. During the early phases of HIV when the immune system has altered responsiveness, GBS tends to develop. When immunoincompetence is severe, distal symmetric peripheral neuropathies occur; however, other parts of the body may be affected such as the face or trunk. The polyneuropathies are predominantly sensory. Painful dysesthesias characterized by burning, tingling, contact sensitivity, and proprioceptive losses begin in the soles and ascend. Upper extremity involvement rarely occurs.[36] In severe cases, secondary motor deficits occur. In the individual with HIV and newly acquired neuropathy with a strong major motor component, vasculitis may be the underlying etiology. Involvement of the upper extremities can occur, but this is less common and usually later in the disease progression.

Vasculitis

Vasculitis can occur as a primary inflammation and necrosis of blood vessel walls (polyarteritis nodosa) or as a secondary process associated with autoimmune responses (rheumatoid vasculitis or systemic lupus erythematosus vasculitis), infections (hepatitis C with vasculitis), toxins, or drug exposure. Vasculitis can involve blood vessels of any size, type, or location and can affect any organ system, including blood vessels that supply the PNS, as well as the CNS. However, because the watershed zones between major vascular supplies exist in the PNS, peripheral nerves are apt to sustain ischemia.[108] Vasculitis may range from acute to chronic. Distribution of lesions may be irregular and segmental rather than continuous.

Pathology

Immune (antibody–antigen) complexes to each disorder are deposited in the blood vessels resulting in varying symptoms, depending on the organs affected. In the case of vasculitic neuropathy, the formation of antibody–antigen complexes activates the complement cascade with generation of C3a and C5a (chemotactic agents that recruit polymorphonuclear leukocytes to the vessel walls). Phagocytosis of the immune complexes takes place, and release of free radicals and proteolytic enzymes disrupt cell membranes and damage blood vessel walls. The complement cascade generates the formation of a complement membrane attack complex that also contributes to endothelial damage. The resulting damage to endothelial cells results in thickening of the vessel wall, occlusion, and ischemia to the affected nerves with axonal degeneration and the resultant neuropathy. Classification is usually according to the size of the predominant vessels involved. In either case, the resulting ischemia may affect peripheral nerves.

Symptomatic presentation of vasculitic neuropathy. Symptoms of a vascular neuropathy reflect the distribution of the peripheral nerve involved. Onset is generally acute, and individuals complain of burning pain in the nerve's distribution. In addition, motor weakness can be anticipated. Although a single nerve may be involved (mononeuritis), overlapping asymmetric polyneuropathies are relatively common.[55]

Peripheral neuropathy is a well-known and frequently early manifestation of many vasculitis syndromes. The pattern of neuropathic involvement depends on the extent and temporal progression of the vasculitic process that produces ischemia. A severe, burning dysesthetic pain in the involved area is present in 70% to 80% of all cases. Other symptoms may include paresthesias and sensory deficit; severe proximal muscle weakness and muscular atrophy can occur secondary to the neuropathy. In the early phase, one nerve is affected and causes symptoms in one extremity (mononeuritis multiplex) but can involve other

TABLE 25.9   Paraneoplastic Antibodies, Associated Carcinoma, and Symptoms that Develop

Antibody	Associated Carcinoma	Paraneoplastic Syndrome	Antibody Reactions with Region Involved	Signs and Symptoms
Anti-Hu	SCLC; oat cell	Paraneoplastic sensory/ sensorimotor neuropathy	Antibody affects neuronal nuclei in PNS and produces peripheral neuropathies (acute, subacute, or chronic)	Sensory neuropathy Encephalomyeloneuropathy
	SCLC	Paraneoplastic encephalo-myeloneuritis	Multifocal disorder; antibody affects all neuronal nuclei in PNS and CNS and produces both peripheral neuropathies and cerebellar, brainstem, cerebral, and spinal signs ANS involvement may occur	Sensory neuropathy plus: Cerebellar ataxia, dysarthria, nystagmus Vertigo Confusion Areflexia
	SCLC Lymphomas	Subacute motor neuropathy	Loss of anterior horn cells in spinal cord	Impaired motor function; sensation is spared
Anti-Yo	SCLC	LEMS	Antibodies directed against voltage-gated calcium channels that regulate ACh release in neuromuscular junction	Proximal muscle weakness
Anti-Tr	Ovarian, breast, uterine	Pancerebellar syndrome, dysarthria and nystagmus	Purkinje cell cytoplasm and deep cerebellar neurons: subacute (weeks to months) cerebellar symptoms (limb and truncal ataxia, dysarthria, nystagmus)	Cerebellar ataxia
Anti-Ri	Hodgkin's lymphoma	Slowing developing cerebellar syndrome	Purkinje cell cytoplasm	Cerebellar ataxia
Antiamphiphysin	Breast, small cell lung	Opsoclonus-myoclonus	CNS nuclei: Opsoclonus (involuntary conjugate multidirectional saccades)	Opsoclonus
Anti-VGC	Breast	Stiff person syndrome		
Anti-Ta	SCLC Testicular	LEMS Limbic encephalitis	Limbic and brainstem neuronal nuclei	Proximal weakness

ACh, Acetylcholine; *ANS,* autonomic nervous system; *CNS,* central nervous system; *LEMS,* Lambert–Eaton myasthenic syndrome; *PNS,* peripheral nervous system; *SCLC,* small cell lung carcinoma.

nerves as the disorder progresses. The PTA should watch for anyone with neuropathy who exhibits constitutional symptoms such as fever, arthralgia, or skin involvement. This may herald a possible vasculitis syndrome and requires medical referral for accurate diagnosis. Early recognition of vasculitis can help prevent a poor outcome. Untreated or with a poor outcome to intervention, CNS involvement (e.g., encephalopathy, ischemic and hemorrhagic stroke, cranial nerve palsy) can occur late in the course of vasculitis.

When corticosteroids (e.g., prednisone alone or sometimes in combination with other medications) are used (such as in the case of vasculitic neuropathy), the PTA must be aware of the need for osteoporosis prevention and attend to the other potential side effects from the chronic use of these medications. Alternative methods of pain control may be offered in a rehabilitation setting such as biofeedback, TENS, and physiologic modulation (e.g., using handheld temperature sensor to control ANS function).

CANCER INDUCED

Paraneoplastic Neuropathies

A little more than 50 years ago the symptoms of two individuals were reported whose autopsy revealed bronchial carcinoma. Both had developed a sensory neuropathy. Although subsequent reports of similar sensory neuropathies associated with other carcinomas have been reported, paraneoplastic syndromes can affect any portion of the nervous system (Table 25.9).

Etiology

In most individuals diagnosed with paraneoplastic neuropathy, the development of symptoms occurs subacutely or chronically over weeks to months and precedes the discovery of the tumor from months to years. The clinical features and electrophysiologic abnormalities indicate that the cell body is the primary site of involvement. Large-diameter neurons are preferentially affected.

Incidence

Numbers vary depending on how the disorder is defined, but estimates range from 10% to 50% of individuals with cancer will develop a paraneoplastic syndrome at some time during the course of their disease. Using a restrictive definition, paraneoplastic syndromes are rare.

Pathogenesis

The current theory is that an autoimmune response, initially directed against the cancer's antigen, subsequently attacks membrane receptors on or receptors within (antinuclear) neurons.

Clinical Manifestations

The most common symptoms are numbness and paresthesias, initially asymmetric, but progressing to involvement of all extremities. Burning and aching or lancinating pain is common. Although individuals exhibit symptoms of areflexia, weakness is not common, and when it occurs it generally is related to an inability to sustain the contraction secondary to impaired proprioceptive feedback. Many individuals with paraneoplastic neuropathy develop additional symptoms demonstrating a progressive involvement of central neural structures. This includes dysarthria, cerebellar ataxia (limb and truncal), ocular nystagmus, memory loss, and ANS involvement. When these central structures are involved, the diagnosis is termed *paraneoplastic encephalomyeloneuritis.*[23]

Medical Management

Diagnosis

The differential diagnosis of paraneoplastic neuropathy is extensive and includes many disorders identified in this chapter that affect sensory nerve fibers or neurons. In addition to electrophysiology findings of severely reduced amplitude or absence of sensory nerve potentials, with normal to slightly slowed sensory NCVs, nerve biopsies show non-specific axonal degeneration and a reduction in myelinated fibers. Lumbar puncture and serum assays for antibodies may be included in the diagnostic workup. High serum titers for antibodies are suggestive of an occult tumor, but the sensitivity and specificity of these tests yields false positives and negatives. CT and MRI scanning are used to locate the tumor.[34]

Treatment

Typical treatments for autoimmune disorders, such as immunosuppression using prednisone, cyclophosphamide, IV Ig, or plasmapheresis, generally do not work with antinuclear antibodies because receptors are located within the nucleus of the neuron.

Prognosis

The course is fairly stereotypical. Individuals deteriorate over weeks or months and then stabilize at a level of severe disability; for example, sensory polyneuropathies progress proximally, then ataxias develop and become progressively greater. Neurologic improvement is rare.

TOXINS

In addition to toxic substances in the environment, some medications prescribed to treat medical conditions can be toxic to the PNS (Table 25.10).[4]

Lead Neuropathy

Definition

Toxic substances, such as lead, affect peripheral myelin or axons.

Etiology and Risk Factors

Although lead has been virtually eliminated in urban environments, it may exist in third-world countries or in some industries such as ceramics. The leading cause of lead neuropathy is the ingestion of lead from paint by children who live in old homes predating 1925. However, lead exposure may also occur after inhaling fumes from car batteries, and after drinking contaminated water or moonshine whiskey. Lead neuropathies also occur in workers in industries that use materials containing lead or who live near lead smelters. Most recently, the Consumer Product Safety Commission has identified inexpensive plastic miniblinds as a source of lead exposure. As the blind is exposed to sunlight, the plastic disintegrates and sheds dust that is high in lead.

Pathogenesis

Both the CNS and PNS can be affected. In the PNS, lead exposure initially causes segmental demyelination, but with prolonged exposure damage to axon cell bodies causes axonal degeneration.[51]

TABLE 25.10 Medications Toxic to Peripheral Nerves

Medication	Use
Doxorubicin (Adriamycin)	Cancer
Amiodarone	Irregular heartbeat
Chloramphenicol	Antibiotic
Cisplatin	Cancer
Dapsone	Skin diseases
Phenytoin (Dilantin)	Seizures and pain
Disulfiram (Antabuse)	Alcoholism
Ethionamide	Tuberculosis
Metronidazole (Flagyl)	*Trichomonas* infection
Gold	Rheumatoid arthritis
Isoniazid	Tuberculosis
Lithium	Manic depression and headache prevention
Nitrofurantoin (Furadantin)	Urinary tract infection
Nitrous oxide	Anesthetic
Penicillamine	Rheumatoid arthritis
Suramin	Cancer
Paclitaxel (Taxol)	Cancer
Vincristine	Cancer

Adapted from Asbury AK: Disorders of peripheral nerve. In Asbury AK, McKhann GM, McDonald WI, editors: *Disease of the nervous system: clinical neurobiology*, Philadelphia, 1986, Saunders, pp 326–327.

Clinical Manifestations

Unlike most neuropathies, lead neuropathies primarily affect neurons innervating muscles in the upper extremity. After months of exposure, persons with a lead peripheral neuropathy will develop wrist drop.

Medical Management

Diagnosis, Treatment, and Prognosis

Diagnosis is based on the history, clinical examination, and motor NCVs, which will be slowed. If axonal degeneration has occurred, EMG will reveal fibrillation potentials, demonstrating loss of axonal innervation. Other tests to check for concentration of lead in the body are urine evaluation and radiographs to reveal a lead line at the metaphysis in the iliac creases, long bones, and tips of the scapula.

Treatment consists of the removal of the source of the lead toxin along with the introduction of the chelating agent, edetate calcium disodium, administered twice daily, to rid the body of lead. Symptomatic management consists of cock-up splints for the wrist drop. Recovery depends on the length of exposure and removal of the toxin.

Pesticides and Organophosphates

Etiology

Insecticides are used extensively worldwide in industry and agriculture. Some compounds have contaminated cooking oils, and outbreaks of organophosphate poisoning have been reported after ingestion. Parathion has been responsible for more accidental poisonings and deaths than any other organophosphate.

Pathogenesis and Clinical Manifestations

All organophosphate compounds inhibit cholinesterase activity, thus creating an acute cholinergic crisis. Acutely, organophosphate toxins affect systemic functions throughout the body; they are also capable of producing a less acute, more chronic neuropathy. Nausea and vomiting, diarrhea, muscle fasciculations, weakness, and paralysis, including sudden paralysis of the respiratory musculature, can occur after overstimulation at the neuromuscular junction. Death can result from vasomotor collapse that coincides with respiratory paralysis. Symptoms of peripheral nerve involvement appear within 1 to 4 days and because they arise quickly, may resemble GBS. A chronic peripheral neuropathy may persist for months or years, or a delayed neuropathy may have its onset weeks after exposure.[136]

Medical Management

Diagnosis
Overexposure to organophosphates will reduce cholinesterase activity of erythrocytes to less than 25% of normal. History and clinical evaluation may be accompanied by electrophysiologic studies to indicate the severity of the neuropathy (e.g., segmental demyelination or axonal degeneration or both).

Treatment
Insecticides should be washed from the skin and hair; if toxins have been ingested, emesis or lavage should be performed. Acutely, atropine is given in doses every 10 minutes until the pupils are dilated, the skin flushed and dry, and the pulse rate rises. Neuromuscular paralysis can be reversed by injection of pralidoxime, a cholinesterase reactivator. Endotracheal intubation and ventilation may be required in the presence of respiratory paralysis. Strictly neuropathic management is aimed at symptomatic management.

Prognosis
Recovery is based on removal from the toxin and the degree of involvement. If only segmental demyelination occurs, recovery will occur in weeks to months, but if axonal degeneration is present, recovery will take months to years.

MOTOR ENDPLATE DISORDERS

Myasthenia Gravis

Overview and Definition
Myasthenia gravis (MG) is the most common of the disorders of neuromuscular transmission. It is characterized by fluctuating weakness and fatigability of skeletal muscles.

Incidence
The incidence of MG is estimated at one in 200,000. Estimates from the National Myasthenia Gravis Foundation are that there are more than 100,000 clients with MG and an additional 25,000 undiagnosed cases. It can affect people in any age group, but peak incidences occur in women in their twenties and thirties and in men between 60 and 80 years old. Overall, the ratio of women affected compared with men is 3 : 2.

Etiology
MG is an autoimmune disorder whose action takes place at the site of the neuromuscular junction and motor endplate.

Risk Factors
Disorders associated with an increased incidence of MG are thymic disorders such as hyperthyroidism, thymic tumor, or thyrotoxicosis. There is an association with diabetes and immune disorders such as rheumatoid arthritis or lupus. Exacerbations may occur before the menstrual period or shortly after pregnancy. Chronic infections of any kind can exacerbate MG. Five to seven percent appear to have a familial association.

Pathogenesis
In MG, the fundamental defect is at the neuromuscular junction. Receptors at the motor endplate normally receive acetylcholine (ACh) from the motor nerve terminal. An action potential occurs that leads to a muscle contraction. In MG the number of ACh receptors are decreased and those that remain are flattened, which results in decreased efficiency of neuromuscular transmission. The neuromuscular junction can normally transmit at high frequencies so that the muscle does not fatigue. Without ACh, the nerve impulses fail to pass across the neuromuscular junction to stimulate muscle contraction. The neuromuscular abnormalities in MG are brought about by an autoimmune response mediated by specific anti-ACh receptor antibodies. The antibodies may block the site that normally binds ACh, or the antibodies may damage the postsynaptic muscle membrane. There may be endocytosis (pinching off of regions of the cell's membrane) of the receptor site.

Although the cause of the autoimmune response in MG is not well understood, the thymus appears to play a role in the disease; 75% of persons with MG have abnormalities of the thymus (e.g., thymic hyperplasia or thymoma). Cells within the thymus bear ACh receptors on their surface, and may serve as a source of autoantigen to trigger the autoimmune reaction within the thymus gland when an immunologic abnormality causes a breakdown an autoimmune attack on ACh receptors.[33]

Clinical Manifestations
Although MG encompasses a spectrum of mild to severe, its cardinal features are skeletal muscle weakness and fatigability. Repetition of activity causes fatigue, whereas rest restores activity. Other than weakness, neurologic findings are normal. A system of four major categories is used to classify MG: ocular, mild generalized, acute fulminating, or late severe.

The distribution of muscle weakness has a dichotomous pattern affecting only the ocular muscles, or a more variable, generalized pattern occurs. In approximately 85% of persons with MG, the weakness is generalized and affects the limb musculature. This fluctuating weakness is often more noticeable in proximal muscles.

Cranial muscles, particularly the eyelids and the muscles controlling eye movements, are the first to show weakness. Diplopia (double vision) and ptosis (drooping eyelids) are common early signs causing the person to tilt the head back to see (Fig. 25.18). Weak neck muscles may cause head bobbing in this position.

Chewing of meat produces fatigue, and the facial expression is one that seems to be snarling because the lips do not close. Speech tends to be nasal. Difficulty in swallowing may occur as a result of palatal, pharyngeal, and tongue weakness. Nasal regurgitation or aspiration of food is common.

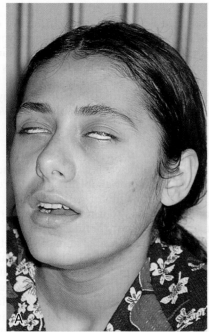

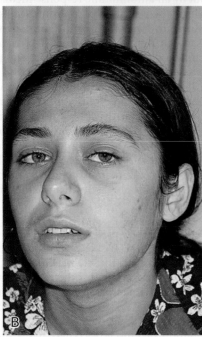

FIG. 25.18 (A) Facial weakness with myasthenia gravis is easily identified when the patient is asked to perform repeated facial movement. Note inability to fully open eyelids and the open jaw. (B) Edrophonium (Tensilon) test can be used to confirm the diagnosis. Edrophonium chloride is a short-acting anticholinesterase that is injected intravenously. In myasthenia gravis, the facial weakness is rapidly relieved by this test. Similar responses occur elsewhere in the body. (From Goldman L, Ausiello D: Cecil textbook of medicine, ed 22, Philadelphia, 2004, Saunders.)

Medical Management

Diagnosis

History and clinical observation of symptoms of weakness with continued use and improvement with rest are important in diagnosing MG. Several conditions that cause weakness of cranial, or somatic, muscles must also be considered. These include drug-induced myasthenia, hyperthyroidism, botulism, intracranial mass lesions, and progressive disorders of the eye. Lambert–Eaton syndrome is a presynaptic disorder of the neuromuscular junction that can cause symptoms similar to those of MG. Lambert–Eaton syndrome is an autoimmune disorder associated with neoplasm, most commonly small cell (oat cell) carcinoma of the lung, which is believed to trigger the autoimmune response.

The three methods used to diagnose MG are (1) immunologic, (2) pharmacologic, and (3) electrophysiologic testing.[104] Immunologic testing detects anti-ACh receptor antibodies in the serum. The presence of anti-ACh receptor antibodies is virtually diagnostic of MG, but a negative test does not exclude diagnosis of the disease. There is no correlation between the amount of anti-ACh receptor antibodies and the severity of the disease. However, in a person with MG a treatment-induced fall in the antibody level often correlates with clinical improvement.

The drug edrophonium (Tensilon) is used to demonstrate improvement in the myasthenic muscles by inhibiting acetylcholinesterase (AChE), an enzyme required for ACh uptake. Muscle strength and endurance are measured before and after administration of the drug. This test confirms that ACh uptake is part of the pathologic status; however, a control test of saline should also be used for comparison.

Electrophysiologic testing of myasthenic disorders demonstrates a normal EMG at rest. Specialized testing must be performed using repetitive stimulation to demonstrate a rapid decrement in the motor action potential's amplitude. Absence of sensory deficits and retention of tendon reflexes throughout the course of the disease also tend to confirm the diagnosis of MG. Because respiratory impairment is a serious complication of MG, measurements of ventilatory function should be performed.[156]

Treatment

AChE inhibitor medication provides for improvement of weakness but does not treat the underlying disease. Administration of this medication is tailored to the individual's requirements throughout the day. For example, a person with difficulty chewing and swallowing would take the medication before meals. Side effects of AChE inhibitors include gastrointestinal effects such as nausea and vomiting, abdominal cramping, and increased bronchial and oral secretions.

Surgical removal of the thymus is successful in 85% of persons with MG. Up to 35% of those undergoing thymectomy achieve a drug-free remission, although this may take years.

Immunosuppression using drugs, such as corticosteroids (prednisone) and azathioprine, are effective in nearly all persons with MG. Initially, high daily doses are begun and then followed by alternate-day high doses that are tapered slowly over a period of months. Unfortunately, adverse side effects are associated with high-dose steroids. These include cushingoid appearance, weight gains, hypertension, and osteoporosis.

Plasmapheresis is performed to remove substances that affect ACh receptors. However, plasmapheresis produces only short-term reduction in anti-AChE antibodies and is not effective for long-term symptom control.

Prognosis

The course of MG is variable, typified by remissions and exacerbations, especially within the first year after onset. Symptoms often fluctuate in intensity during the day. This daily variability is superimposed on longer term spontaneous relapses that may last for weeks. Remissions are rarely complete or permanent. This disorder follows a slowly progressive course. Onset of other systemic disorders and infections may precipitate an exacerbation of the disease and are the most common cause of a crisis. A myasthenic crisis is a medical emergency requiring attention to life-endangering weakening of the respiratory muscles. A myasthenic crisis requires ventilatory assistance. Treatment of a crisis occurs in the ICU because the client requires careful, immediate control of medications for survival.[174]

When MG begins in children, it is important to establish the form it takes. Because AChE antibodies cross the placenta, 10% of newborns of mothers with MG develop a myasthenic reaction. Newborns with neonatal MG have a weak suck and cry and are hypotonic. Fortunately, this resolves in a few weeks.

25.7 Special Implications for the PTA: Myasthenia Gravis

Physical and occupational therapy may be indicated as supportive care to assist the client with MG. In the acute care setting, the PT and PTA must establish an accurate neurologic and respiratory baseline. Tidal volume, vital capacity, and inspiratory force should be monitored regularly during treatment. Deep breathing and coughing should be encouraged. When eating, the person should be instructed to sit upright and to swallow when the chin is tipped slightly downward toward the chest and never with the neck extended because of the risk of aspiration. Finally, the client should never speak with food in the mouth.

The PTA must also be alert to signs of an impending myasthenic crisis (increasing muscle weakness; respiratory distress; or difficulty while talking, chewing, or swallowing). Make sure the client recognizes the side effects and signs of toxicity of AChE inhibitor medications. For those receiving a prolonged course of corticosteroids, report adverse side effects to the physician.

Plan therapy and teach the client to plan activities to coincide with periods of maximum energy. The home should be arranged to help prevent unnecessary energy expenditure. Frequent rest periods help conserve energy and give muscles a chance to regain strength. The person with MG should avoid strenuous exercise, stress, and excessive exposure to the sun or cold weather. All of these can exacerbate signs and symptoms.

Researchers report that a strength training program eliciting maximal isometric contractions could be instituted in clients with mild-to-moderate MG. As long as participants were monitored for fatigue during periods of exercise, improvements were noted in all muscles.[92] After 3 months, participants' knee extensor muscles showed the most significant strength gains without adverse reactions. Recently a cooling vest was worn to decrease core body temperature to determine whether pulmonary function and subjective perceptions of strength and fatigue would improve. All measures were improved in the majority of participants.[106]

Because individuals diagnosed as having MG are placed on long-term corticosteroid medication, the treatment may induce a secondary condition: osteoporosis. These individuals should be encouraged to undergo dual energy x-ray absorptiometry (previously DEXA, now DXA) scan and to receive calcium supplements to counteract osteoporosis.[90]

The Myasthenia Gravis Foundation (www.myasthenia.org) publishes educational materials that can be helpful to the client and family.

BOTULISM

Definition and Incidence

Botulism is a rare, often fatal condition (20% mortality) caused by ingestion of a potent neurotoxin produced by *Clostridium botulinum*, which is found in improperly preserved or canned foods, as well as in contaminated wounds. The Centers for Disease Control and Prevention recognizes four categories of botulism: (1) foodborne, (2) wound, (3) infant, and (4) unclassified.[29] Approximately 10 adult cases and 100 cases of infant botulism are reported each year in the United States.

Etiology and Pathogenesis

The anaerobic bacillus releases a protein neurotoxin that is heat labile; it is destroyed by boiling food for 10 minutes. Therefore inadequate food preparation allows the neurotoxin to be ingested.

Infant botulism affects babies aged from 3 weeks to 9 months; the most common source of infant botulism arises from the ingestion of honey, which is why children of less than 1 year are not allowed to have honey.

Botulism is not always ingested orally. Some cases occur after wounds are contaminated with soil, in chronic drug abusers, after cesarean delivery, and may even occur when antibiotics are administered to prevent wound infection.

When the neurotoxin is ingested, digestive acids and proteolytic enzymes cannot destroy the molecules of the toxin and it is absorbed into the blood from the small intestine. Minute amounts of circulating toxin reach the cholinergic nerve endings at the motor endplate and bind to gangliosides of the presynaptic nerve terminals. Flaccid paralysis is caused by inhibition of ACh released from cholinergic terminals at the motor endplate. Inhibition of ACh release causes a symmetric paralysis with normal sensory and mental status.

Clinical Manifestations

Onset of symptoms develops 12 to 36 hours after ingestion of food containing the toxin. Signs and symptoms include malaise, weakness, blurred and double vision (diplopia), dry mouth, and nausea and vomiting. Progression is variable, but respiratory failure can occur in 6 to 8 hours. People may also report difficulty swallowing (dysphagia), dysarthria (slurred speech), and photophobia. Because the motor endplate is involved, there are no sensory changes. Motor weakness of the face and neck muscles progresses to involve the diaphragm, accessory muscles of respiration, and muscles controlling the extremities. Secondary effects from the flaccid paralysis, such as severe muscle wasting, pressure sores, and aspiration pneumonia, occur.

Medical Management

Diagnosis, Treatment, and Prognosis

A history suggesting a food source and toxin identification made by serum or stool analysis aids in the diagnosis. EMG testing demonstrates a decreasing amplitude and facilitation of muscle action potential after tetanic stimulation. Differential diagnosis includes disorders that also display a rapidly evolving flaccid paralysis, such as GBS, MG, and tick paralysis.

Immediate treatment is directed toward neutralizing the toxin using injectable trivalent ABE serum, which is an antitoxin. Antitoxin prevents further binding of free botulism toxin to the presynaptic endings. If paralysis occurs because of wound botulism, care should include debridement and antibiotics.

Removal of unabsorbed toxin from the gastrointestinal tract is accomplished by gastric lavage and induced emesis. Finally, supportive measures should be instituted in the hospital; intubation and mechanical ventilation are needed when the individual's vital capacity is compromised.

If untreated, this disorder can be fatal within 24 hours of ingestion. Respiratory failure leads to death. In mild to moderate cases, a gradual recovery of muscle strength can take as long as 12 months after onset. After hospitalization, graded rehabilitation is instituted to treat muscle wasting, deconditioning, and orthostatic hypotension.

ABNORMAL RESPONSE IN PERIPHERAL NERVES

Complex Regional Pain Syndrome/Reflex Sympathetic Dystrophy/Causalgia

RSD is a syndrome, first described in 1864, that changes over time and varies by etiology. Now, the preferred terminology for the syndrome that develops after trauma is complex regional pain syndrome, type I (CRPS I). Early on, pain is greater than expected for the degree of tissue trauma that has been sustained. The pain spreads from localized to a regional distribution, characterized by a burning sensation that occurs spontaneously and at an intensity that does not correspond with the stimulus that elicited it. If the trauma that was sustained involves a major nerve and the clinical syndrome develops, it is causalgia, or CRPS type II (CRPS II).[98]

Incidence

CRPS I may occur after 5% of all injuries. Because the diagnosis is often delayed, some very mild cases may resolve and others may progress to become a chronic, debilitating disorder. Although the average age of an individual with CRPS is in the mid-thirties, it has been reported in all age groups, including children as young as 3 years.

Etiology

RSD has its origin in a variety of conditions: it can follow surgery, such as arthroscopy; it can occur after a UMN lesion arising from traumatic brain injury, cerebrovascular accidents (creating a shoulder–hand syndrome), or destructive lesions of the CNS; or it can occur after LMN disorders from peripheral nerve injuries, neuropathies, and entrapments. CRPS I occurs without an overt nerve injury, and CRPS II is associated with peripheral nerve trauma.

Pathology

An injury at one somatic level initiates sympathetic efferent activity that affects many segmental levels. CRPS is thought to represent a reflex neurogenic inflammation. Facilitation of the sympathetic nervous system (SNS) and its neurotransmitters, catecholamines, activates primary afferent nociceptors to create the sensation of pain. Thermal dysfunctions are related to either the inhibition of SNS vasoconstriction or facilitation of the SNS causing excessive vasoconstriction (Fig. 25.19). Clinical studies have shown abnormal SNS reflexes that indicate CNS dysfunction exists as well.[170]

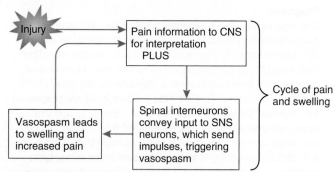

FIG. 25.19 Exaggerated pain associated with sympathetic response over activity occurs after minor trauma. Normally, the response of the sympathetic nervous system after injury causes cutaneous blood vessels to contract. This response shuts down appropriately within minutes to hours. In complex regional pain syndrome, the sympathetic nervous system functions abnormally and causes vasospasm, which creates cycles of swelling and pain. Initially, vasodilation occurs that increases skin temperature. Later in the course of the disorder, symptoms consist of cyanosis and coldness in the involved extremity.

Clinical Manifestations

CRPS has overlapping but identifiable clinical stages (Table 25.11). Although sensory impairments are often most the hallmark of CRPS, movement disorders also occur. Motor symptoms may precede the appearance of other impairments by weeks or months or may appear on the contralateral extremity in a mirror fashion, but most often they occur concomitantly with autonomic changes and pain.

The primary clinical features of CRPS I are pain, ANS dysfunction, edema, movement disorders including inability to initiate movement, weakness, tremor, muscle spasms, dystrophy, and atrophy.[61] The pain that occurs is disproportionate to the pain that would be expected. Even tactile stimulation may be perceived as pain (allodynia).[78] All contribute to functional impairments. Despite the fact that three stages of CRPS were originally identified and are still referred to, the course of this disorder is more unpredictable than the stages imply.[78] Individuals typically remain in a specific stage for 6 to 8 months; however, some may progress rapidly to and through the next stage. As the condition progresses, symptoms may spread proximally and even spread to affect other extremities. In a few cases, the entire body may become involved.[98]

Three abnormal vasomotor patterns have been identified; these relate to the temperature and color of the extremity and the acuity of CRPS. Other vasomotor changes include changes in the nails in which they become thick, brittle, and ridged.

Medical Management

Diagnosis

Diagnosis of CRPS is based primarily on the clinical examination and history. A combination of diagnostic tests aimed at assessing secondary changes (radiographic examinations, thermographic studies, and laser Doppler flowmetry) may aid in establishing a diagnosis. Because of the evolutionary nature of CRPS, a correct diagnosis may be delayed, especially in children.[35]

TABLE 25.11 CRPS: Progressive Clinical Stages

Stage		Classic Signs and Symptoms
Stage I: Acute inflammation: denervation and sympathetic hypoactivity	Begins up to 10 days following injury; lasts 3-6 months	**Pain:** more severe than expected; burning or aching character; increased by dependent position, physical contact or emotional disturbances **Hyperalgesia** (lower pain threshold, increased sensitivity), **allodynia** (all stimuli are perceived as pain), and **hyperpathia** (threshold to pain is increased, once exceeded, sensation intensity increased more rapidly and greater than expected) **Edema:** soft and localized **Vasomotor/thermal changes:** affected limb is warmer **Skin:** hyperthermia and dry Increased hair and nail growth
Stage II: Dystrophic: paradoxical sympathetic hyperactivity	Occurs 3-6 months after onset of pain, lasts about 6 months	**Pain:** worsens: constant, burning and aching **Allodynia, hyperalgesia,** and **hyperpathia** almost always present **Edema:** becomes hard causing joint stiffness **Vasomotor/thermal changes:** neither warm, nor cold **Skin:** thin, glossy, cool (vasoconstriction) and sweaty Thin, ridged nails X-rays reveal **osteoporosis,** cystic and subchondral bone erosion
Stage III: Atrophic	Begins about 6-12 months after onset; may last for years, or may resolve and recur	**Pain:** spreads proximally, occasionally to entire skin surface or plateaus **Edema:** continues to harden **Vasomotor/thermal changes:** SNS regulation is decreased on affected extremity, affected limb is cooler **Skin:** is thin, shiny, cyanotic and dry Fingertips and toes on involved extremity are atrophic Fascia is thickened; contractures may occur X-ray demonstrate bony **demineralization and ankylosis**

SNS, Sympathetic nervous system.

Treatment

Treatment for CRPS tends to be multifactorial and prolonged. Successful treatment depends on early diagnosis, treatment of the underlying cause, and aggressive and sustained physical therapy.[66] Although stellate ganglion blocks or sympathectomy are used to alleviate pain and early symptoms, this approach is based on weak evidence.[97] All of the following treatments have limited evidence for their effectiveness.[47] Acupuncture, corticosteroids, and NSAIDs have been used early in stage I. They provide pain relief in up to 20%. Amitriptyline has been used to facilitate sleep and relieve depression. Calcium channel blockers help to improve peripheral circulation through their effect on the SNS.

Long-term intrathecal baclofen is used to control symptoms of motor dystonia. Its use is supported by the fact that γ-aminobutyric acid (GABA)-ergic inhibition is involved in motor function.

Although external TENS units have been minimally effective, implanted dorsal column stimulation has been shown to decrease pain intensity and perception of pain in randomized trials. Health-related quality of life improved only in individuals receiving spinal cord stimulation. It works best for intractable pain in one extremity.[98]

Prognosis

CRPS is a complex syndrome with varying severity and disability. In many cases, the pain continues for years, or less frequently, it may remit, then recur after another injury. In some cases, malingering for secondary gain has been documented.[177] Outcome measures for CRPS I typically concentrate on impairments, leaving measurement of disability, which is the most relevant to function, with few assessments.[136] Physical therapy is indicated, particularly as part of a program of pain control. Although the goal is to maintain function so that the individual can perform normal activities, a vigorous approach is not indicated. Current research is aimed at understanding physiologic processes and finding the most effective interventions.

25.8 Special Implications for the PTA: Complex Regional Pain Syndrome Goals for physical therapy include educating the client and encouraging normal use of the involved extremity while minimizing pain. Although modalities are used to provide pain relief, the greatest success occurs when they are administered during earlier stages of CRPS. External TENS units are reported to be minimally effective.[35] Recently, when TENS was applied contralateral to the lesion, high-frequency stimulation decreased mechanical allodynia and low-frequency stimulation decreased thermal allodynia in Sprague–Dawley rats.[147] When the lower extremity is involved, pool exercises are helpful for improving mobility when weight bearing on land is problematic.

REFERENCES/SUGGESTED READINGS

To enhance this text and add value for the reader, references and suggested readings are included on the companion Evolve site that accompanies this textbook. The reader can view the source and access it online whenever possible.

INDEX

Page numbers followed by *f* indicate figures; *t*, tables; *b*, boxes; and *e*, online only.

774